Diagnosis for
PHYSICAL
THERAPISTS

A Symptom-Based Approach

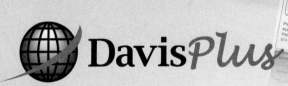

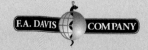

Diagnosis for PHYSICAL THERAPISTS

A Symptom-Based Approach

Todd E. Davenport, PT, DPT, OCS
Assistant Professor
University of the Pacific
Department of Physical Therapy
Thomas J. Long School of Pharmacy and
    Health Sciences
Stockton, California

Kornelia Kulig, PT, PhD, FAPTA
Associate Professor of Clinical Physical
    Therapy
University of Southern California
Division of Biokinesiology and Physical
    Therapy
Los Angeles, California

Chris A. Sebelski, PT, DPT, OCS, CSCS
Assistant Professor
Saint Louis University
Department of Physical Therapy & Athletic
    Training
Doisy College of Health Sciences
Saint Louis, Missouri

James Gordon, PT, EdD, FAPTA
Associate Dean and Chair
University of Southern California
Division of Biokinesiology and Physical
    Therapy
Los Angeles, California

Hugh G. Watts, MD
Adjunct Associate Professor
University of Southern California
Division of Biokinesiology and Physical
    Therapy
Los Angeles, California

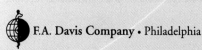

F.A. Davis Company • Philadelphia

F. A. Davis Company
1915 Arch Street
Philadelphia, PA 19103
www.fadavis.com

Printed in the United States of America

Last digit indicates print number: 10 9 8 7 6 5 4 3 2 1

Editor-in-Chief: Margaret M. Biblis
Manager of Content Development: George W. Lang
Developmental Editor: Peg Waltner
Art and Design Manager: Carolyn O'Brien

As new scientific information becomes available through basic and clinical research, recommended treatments and drug therapies undergo changes. The author(s) and publisher have done everything possible to make this book accurate, up to date, and in accord with accepted standards at the time of publication. The author(s), editors, and publisher are not responsible for errors or omissions or for consequences from application of the book, and make no warranty, expressed or implied, in regard to the contents of the book. Any practice described in this book should be applied by the reader in accordance with professional standards of care used in regard to the unique circumstances that may apply in each situation. The reader is advised always to check product information (package inserts) for changes and new information regarding dose and contraindications before administering any drug. Caution is especially urged when using new or infrequently ordered drugs.

Library of Congress Cataloging-in-Publication Data

Diagnosis for physical therapists : a symptom-based approach / Todd E. Davenport ... [et al.].
  p. ; cm.
Includes bibliographical references and index.
ISBN 978-0-8036-1528-1 — ISBN 0-8036-1528-0
I. Davenport, Todd E.
[DNLM: 1. Diagnostic Techniques and Procedures. 2. Physical Therapy Modalities. 3. Signs and Symptoms. WB 141]

616.07'5—dc23   2012002507

Direct access to physical therapy is a central tenet of the American Physical Therapy Association's *Vision 2020* statement. *Vision 2020* anticipates physical therapists being "recognized by consumers and other health care professionals as the practitioners of choice to whom consumers have direct access for the diagnosis of, interventions for, and prevention of impairments, functional limitations, and disabilities related to movement, function, and health."[1] One clear assumption of *Vision 2020* – with its emphasis on consumer direct access – is that physical therapists must function autonomously to determine whether physical therapy is appropriate for their patients. This function involves being able to decide whether to begin physical therapy, refer their patient to another health care provider for additional consultation or management, or both. If the decision to refer to another health care provider is made, then the appropriate disposition and urgency must be established.

Determining the appropriateness of physical therapy for patients assumes physical therapists must engage in a process of diagnostic reasoning as part of their overall evaluation. Diagnostic reasoning allows physical therapists to develop a well-reasoned plan for addressing the patient's concerns, adequately communicate with other members of the health care team using the universal language of the health care system, and appropriately educate patients. In order to adequately determine the appropriateness of physical therapy for patients, this diagnostic process must lead to a decision regarding the probable pathological or pathophysiological source of the patient's problem. It must be emphasized that *Vision 2020*, with its emphasis on direct access, presupposes that the physical therapist will be able to reach that decision without provision of a diagnostic label beforehand by a physician or other health care professional. However, to date, no resource exists to support daily efforts of physical therapists to engage in diagnostic reasoning and student physical therapists to learn diagnostic reasoning.

The purpose of this book is to present a framework and body of content necessary to support the acquisition and maintenance of diagnostic reasoning skills for physical therapists. Special emphasis in this book is placed on diagnostic reasoning at the level of pathology. This book proposes a detailed approach for diagnosis at the level of pathology, based on the notion that physical therapists must begin with the patient's symptoms and signs as the starting point for reasoning. The book's format supports the needs of both clinicians who must make rapid decisions in the context of a busy clinic environment, as well as students who are in the initial stages of learning and refining their diagnostic reasoning skills.

For established clinicians:

- The diagnostic reasoning framework presented in the book encourages a systematic yet flexible approach to diagnostic reasoning
- Organization of the book into Adult Pain, Adult Non-Pain, and Children sections ensure usefulness of the book across areas of practice and the lifespan
- Symptoms of special diagnostic concern are presented at the beginning of each chapter, so this important information is available at a glance
- Chapter previews organize possible conditions by a pathologic category and the likelihood of causing the symptom of chief concern
- Conditions are divided among remote and local pathologies that may manifest as the symptom of chief concern
- Succinct descriptions of each condition include details regarding their clinical presentation, contributing pathology/pathophysiology, confirmatory tests, and potential treatments

For physical therapy students and instructors:

- A series of foundational chapters provide the basic rationale for diagnosis by physical therapists

- The framework for diagnostic reasoning presented in this book will integrate seamlessly with existing coursework in pathology/pathophysiology and clinical management
- Chapters are presented in a similar format that enunciates each step of the diagnostic reasoning process
- Pathologic categories are presented using a mnemonic 'TIM VaDeTuCoNe' in order to assist recall of categories of pathology that may contribute to the patient's symptom of chief concern
- Case chapters demonstrate the stepwise application of the diagnostic reasoning process presented in this book

Despite the overwhelming need for more systematic approaches to diagnosis by physical therapists, there remains a level of controversy surrounding the topic of diagnosis by physical therapists, particularly as it relates to pathology.

Many physical therapists have developed excellent diagnostic skills, but these skills were hard-earned through independent study, on-the-job training, and trial and error. In order to reach the goal of direct access as described in *Vision 2020*, the physical therapy profession must continue to develop systematic, evidence-based approaches for diagnosis that are taught in entry-level curricula and refined in post-graduate educational programs, so that all physical therapists demonstrate a certain level of skill in diagnosis. This book represents a first attempt to describe and formalize diagnostic reasoning by physical therapists at the level of pathology. Much like the collective understanding that it represents and to which it contributes, the material presented in this book remains an exciting and dynamic work in progress.

Reference

1. www.apta.org/vision2020. Accessed 13 April 2012.

Contributors

Ragen L. Agler, PT, DPT, ATC
Physical Therapy Faculty
USC Lung Transplant Program
Los Angeles, California

Michael A. Andersen, PT, DPT, OCS
Adjunct Instructor of Clinical Physical
Therapy
University of Southern California
Division of Biokinesiology and Physical
Therapy
Los Angeles, California

Lucinda L. Baker, PT, PhD
Associate Professor
University of Southern California
Division of Biokinesiology and Physical
Therapy
Los Angeles, California

Kyle F. Baldwin, PT, DPT
Adjunct Assistant Professor of Clinical
Physical Therapy
University of Southern California
Division of Biokinesiology and Physical
Therapy
Los Angeles, California

Robin I. Burks, PT, DPT, CHT*
Former Instructor of Clinical Physical Therapy
University of Southern California
Division of Biokinesiology and Physical
Therapy
Los Angeles, California

Julia L. Burlette, PT, DPT, OCS
Assistant Professor of Clinical Physical Therapy
University of Southern California
Division of Biokinesiology and Physical Therapy
Los Angeles, California

Jason R. Cozby, PT, DPT, OCS
Adjunct Instructor of Clinical Physical Therapy
University of Southern California
Division of Biokinesiology and Physical
Therapy
Los Angeles, California

Bernadette M. Currier, PT, DPT, MS, NCS
Adjunct Instructor of Clinical Physical
Therapy
University of Southern California
Division of Biokinesiology and Physical
Therapy
Los Angeles, California

Todd E. Davenport, PT, DPT, OCS
Assistant Professor
University of the Pacific
Department of Physical Therapy
Thomas J. Long School of Pharmacy and
Health Sciences
Stockton, California

Sharon K. DeMuth, PT, DPT, MS
Adjunct Assistant Professor of Clinical
Physical Therapy
University of Southern California
Division of Biokinesiology and Physical
Therapy
Los Angeles, California

Jesus F. Dominguez, PT, PhD
Assistant Professor of Clinical Physical
Therapy
University of Southern California
Division of Biokinesiology and Physical
Therapy
Los Angeles, California

Kathy Doubleday, PT, DPT, OCS
Physical Therapy Affiliate
Pacifica Spine
Ojai, California

Elizabeth L. Ege, PT, DPT
Adjunct Instructor of Clinical Physical
Therapy
University of Southern California
Division of Biokinesiology and Physical
Therapy
Los Angeles, California

*Deceased.

Daniel Farwell, PT, DPT
Adjunct Assistant Professor of Clinical
  Physical Therapy
University of Southern California
Division of Biokinesiology and Physical
  Therapy
Los Angeles, California

Beth E. Fisher, PT, PhD
Associate Professor of Clinical Physical
  Therapy
University of Southern California
Division of Biokinesiology and Physical
  Therapy
Los Angeles, California

James Gordon, PT, EdD, FAPTA
Associate Dean and Chair
University of Southern California
Division of Biokinesiology and Physical
  Therapy
Los Angeles, California

Rose Hamm, PT, DPT, CWS, FACCWS
Assistant Professor of Clinical Physical
  Therapy
University of Southern California
Division of Biokinesiology and Physical
  Therapy
Los Angeles, California

Julie Hershberg, PT, DPT, NCS
Instructor of Clinical Therapy
University of Southern California
Division of Biokinesiology and Physical
  Therapy
Los Angeles, California

Larry Ho, PT, DPT, OCS
Adjunct Assistant Professor of Clinical
  Physical Therapy
University of Southern California
Division of Biokinesiology and Physical
  Therapy
Los Angeles, California

Sally Ho, PT, DPT, OCS
Adjunct Assistant Professor of Clinical
  Physical Therapy
University of Southern California
Division of Biokinesiology and Physical
  Therapy
Los Angeles, California

Robbin Howard, PT, DPT, NCS
Assistant Professor of Clinical Physical Therapy
University of Southern California
Division of Biokinesiology and Physical
  Therapy
Los Angeles, California

John M. Itamura, MD
Associate Professor of Clinical Orthopaedic
  Surgery
USC University Hospital
Los Angeles, California

Stephanie A. Jones, PT, DPT, OCS, NCS
Clinical Assistant Professor
MGH Institute of Health Professions
School of Health and Rehabilitation Sciences
Department of Physical Therapy
Boston, Massachusetts

Rob Landel, PT, DPT, OCS, CSCS, FAPTA
Professor of Clinical Physical Therapy
University of Southern California
Division of Biokinesiology and Physical
  Therapy
Los Angeles, California

Covey J. Lazouras, PT, DPT, NCS
Adjunct Instructor of Clinical Physical
  Therapy
University of Southern California
Division of Biokinesiology and Physical
  Therapy
Los Angeles, California

Della Lee, PT, DPT, OCS, ATC
Adjunct Instructor of Clinical Physical Therapy
University of Southern California
Division of Biokinesiology and Physical
  Therapy
Los Angeles, California

Kim Levenhagen, PT, DPT, WCC
Instructor of Physical Therapy
Saint Louis University
Department of Physical Therapy & Athletic
  Training
Doisy College of Health Sciences
Saint Louis, Missouri

J. Raul Lona, DPT, OCS, ATC
Managing Partner & Co-owner
Wilshire Linden Physical Therapy
Beverly Hills, California

**Munesha Ramsinghani Lona,
PT, DPT, PCS**
Pediatric Physical Therapist
California Children's Services
Reseda, California

Jennifer Lundberg, PT, DPT
Instructor of Clinical Physical Therapy
University of Southern California
Division of Biokinesiology and Physical
 Therapy
Los Angeles, California

Bach T. Ly, PT, DPT
Clinical Instructor of Physical Therapy
University of Southern California
Division of Biokinesiology and Physical
 Therapy
Los Angeles, California

Jill S. Masutomi, PT, DPT, PCS
Instructor of Clinical Physical Therapy
University of Southern California
Division of Biokinesiology and Physical
 Therapy
Los Angeles, California

Yogi Matharu, PT, DPT, OCS
Director of Physical Therapy Clinical Services
University of Southern California
Division of Biokinesiology and Physical
 Therapy
Los Angeles, California

Didi Matthews, PT, DPT, NCS
Adjunct Assistant Professor of Clinical
 Physical Therapy
University of Southern California
Division of Biokinesiology and Physical
 Therapy
Los Angeles, California

Wendi W. McKenna, PT, DPT, PCS
Clinical Instructor of Physical Therapy
University of Southern California
Division of Biokinesiology and Physical
 Therapy
Los Angeles, California

Lisa Meyer, PT, DPT, OCS
Adjunct Instructor of Clinical Physical Therapy
University of Southern California
Division of Biokinesiology and Physical
 Therapy
Los Angeles, California

Phibun Ny, PT, DPT
Clinical Instructor of Physical Therapy
University of Southern California
Division of Biokinesiology and Physical
 Therapy
Los Angeles, California

**Michael O'Donnell, PT, DPT, OCS,
FAAOMPT**
Assistant Professor of Clinical Physical
 Therapy
University of Southern California
Division of Biokinesiology and Physical
 Therapy
Los Angeles, California

Shelly Olivadoti-Santoro, PT, DPT
Clinical Instructor of Physical Therapy
University of Southern California
Division of Biokinesiology and Physical
 Therapy
Los Angeles, California

Marisa Perdomo, PT, DPT
Assistant Professor of Clinical Physical
 Therapy
University of Southern California
Division of Biokinesiology and Physical
 Therapy
Los Angeles, California

Amy B. Pomrantz, PT, DPT, OCS, ATC
Assistant Professor of Clinical Physical
 Therapy
University of Southern California
Division of Biokinesiology and Physical
 Therapy
Los Angeles, California

Elizabeth M. Poppert, PT, DPT, MS, OCS
Adjunct Instructor of Clinical Physical
 Therapy
University of Southern California
Division of Biokinesiology and Physical
 Therapy
Los Angeles, California

Michelle G. Prettyman, PT, DPT, MS
Assistant Professor
University of Maryland School of Medicine
Department of Physical Therapy and
 Rehabilitation Science
Baltimore, Maryland

Stephen F. Reischl, PT, DPT, OCS
Adjunct Associate Professor
University of Southern California
Division of Biokinesiology and Physical
Therapy
Los Angeles, California

Jeffrey S. Rodrigues, PT, DPT, CCS
Instructor of Clinical Physical Therapy
University of Southern California
Division of Biokinesiology and Physical
Therapy
Los Angeles, California

Cassandra Sanders-Holly, PT, DPT, PCS
Clinical Instructor of Physical Therapy
University of Southern California
Division of Biokinesiology and Physical
Therapy
Los Angeles, California

Alison R. Scheid, PT, DPT, OCS, NCS
Staff, Financial District Clinic
San Francisco Sport and Spine Physical Therapy
San Francisco, California

Stephen Schnall, MD
Specialist, Orthopaedic Surgery — Hand
USC Center for Spinal Surgery
Los Angeles, California

Chris A. Sebelski, PT, DPT, OCS, CSCS
Assistant Professor
Saint Louis University
Department of Physical Therapy & Athletic
Training
Doisy College of Health Sciences
Saint Louis, Missouri

Cheri Kay Sessions, PT, DPT, ATC
Clinical Instructor of Physical Therapy
University of Southern California
Division of Biokinesiology and Physical
Therapy
Los Angeles, California

Robert C. Sieh, PT, DPT
Pediatric Physical Therapist
Mercy Riverside Rehabilitation
Des Moines, Iowa

Michael S. Simpson, PT, DPT
Assistant Professor of Clinical Physical Therapy
University of Southern California
Division of Biokinesiology and Physical
Therapy
Los Angeles, California

Christy L. Skura, PT, DPT, PCS
Physical Therapist
Therapy West Inc. and Play Studio
Los Angeles, California

Claire Smith, PT, DPT, NCS
Adjunct Instructor of Clinical Physical
Therapy
University of Southern California
Division of Biokinesiology and Physical
Therapy
Los Angeles, California

Josiane Stickles, PT, DPT
Clinical Instructor of Physical Therapy
University of Southern California
Division of Biokinesiology and Physical
Therapy
Los Angeles, California

Katherine J. Sullivan, PT, PhD, FAHA
Associate Professor of Clinical Physical
Therapy
University of Southern California
Division of Biokinesiology and Physical
Therapy
Los Angeles, California

Shirley Wachi-See, PT, DPT, OCS
Clinical Instructor of Physical Therapy
University of Southern California
Division of Biokinesiology and Physical
Therapy
Los Angeles, California

Hugh G. Watts, MD
Adjunct Associate Professor
University of Southern California
Division of Biokinesiology and Physical
Therapy
Los Angeles, California

Katherine M. Weimer, PT, DPT, NCS
Adjunct Instructor of Clinical Physical
Therapy
University of Southern California
Division of Biokinesiology and Physical
Therapy
Los Angeles, California

Ronald P. Andrews, PT, PhD
Associate Professor
University of New Mexico
School of Medicine
Department of Orthopaedics/Physical
    Therapy Program
Albuquerque, New Mexico

Theresa Geraldine Bernsen, PT, MA
Assistant Professor
Saint Louis University
Doisy College of Health Sciences
Department of Physical Therapy
Saint Louis, Missouri

Mark W. Cornwall, PT, PhD, CPed
Chair
Northern Arizona University
Department of Physical Therapy
Flagstaff, Arizona

Janet P. Dolot, PT, DPT
Assistant Professor of Clinical Physical
    Therapy
New York Medical College
School of Health Sciences and Practice
Doctor of Physical Therapy Program
Valhalla, New York

Jacqueline S. Drouin, PT, PhD
Associate Professor
Oakland University
School of Health Sciences
Physical Therapy Program
Rochester, Michigan

Lisa L. Dutton, PT, PhD
Associate Professor
St. Catherine University
Henrietta Schmoll School of Health
Doctor of Physical Therapy Program
Minneapolis, Minnesota

Staffan Elgelid, PT, PhD, MT, CFP
Former Assistant Professor
Arkansas State University
Department of Physical Therapy
Jonesboro, Arkansas

Donald L. Gabard, PT, PhD
Professor
Chapman University
Department of Physical Therapy
Orange, California

Judith Gale, PT, DPT, MPH, OCS
Associate Professor
Creighton University
School of Pharmacy and Health Professions
Department of Physical Therapy
Omaha, Nebraska

Charles J. Gulas, PT, PhD, GCS
Dean, Associate Professor
Maryville University
School of Health Professions
Saint Louis, Missouri

Kevin Helgeson, PT, DHSc, SCS
Faculty
Rocky Mountain University of Health
    Professions
Doctor of Physical Therapy Program
Provo, Utah

Eric Johnson, PT, DSc
Professor
Loma Linda University
School of Allied Health Professions
Department of Physical Therapy
Loma Linda, California

David Krause, PT, MBA, DSc, OCS
Faculty
Mayo School of Health Sciences
College of Medicine
Physical Therapy Doctoral Program
Rochester, Minnesota

David A. Lake, PT, PhD
Interim Department Head / Professor
Armstrong Atlantic State University
College of Health Professions
Department of Physical Therapy
Savannah, Georgia

James J. Laskin, PT, PhD
Executive Director, Associate Professor
The University of Montana
The College of Health Professions and
    Biomedical Sciences
School of Physical Therapy & Rehabilitation
    Science
Missoula, Montana

Everett B. Lohman, III, PT, DSc, OCS
Professor and Assistant Dean of Graduate
    Academic Affairs
Loma Linda University
School of Allied Health Professions
Department of Physical Therapy
Loma Linda, California

Venita Lovelace-Chandler, PT, PhD, PCS
Professor and Associate Director
Texas Woman's University
School of Physical Therapy
Dallas, Texas

John D. Lowman, PT, PhD, CCS
Assistant Professor
University of Alabama at Birmingham
School of Health Professions
Department of Physical Therapy
Birmingham, Alabama

Susanne M. Morton, PT, PhD
Assistant Professor
University of Iowa
Graduate Program in Physical Therapy &
    Rehabilitation Science
Iowa City, Iowa

Rose Marie Ortega, PT, DPT
Former Professor and Academic Coordinator
    of Clinical Education
Stony Brook University
Physical Therapy Program
Stony Brook, New York

Jaime C. Paz, PT, MS
Part Time Faculty
Simmons College
School of Nursing and Health Sciences
Department of Physical Therapy
Boston, Massachusetts

Andrew Priest, MPT, EdD
Chair and Associate Professor
Clarke College
Physical Therapy Department
Dubuque, Iowa

Pamela D. Ritzline, PT, EdD
Associate Professor
Director of Graduate Programs
The University of Tennessee Health Science
    Center
College of Allied Health Sciences
Department of Physical Therapy
Memphis, Tennessee

Joellen Roller, PT, DPT, EdD
Chair, Division of Human Performance
    Sciences
Chair, Department of Physical Therapy
University of Mary
Bismarck, North Dakota

Summer San Lucas, PT, DPT
Contract Instructor
Loma Linda University
School of Allied Health Professions
Department of Physical Therapy
Loma Linda, California

David Scalzitti, PT, PhD, OCS
Associate Director - Research Department
American Physical Therapy Association
Alexandria, Virginia

Frank B. Underwood, PT, PhD, ECS
Professor
University of Evansville
College of Education and Health Sciences
Department of Physical Therapy
Evansville, Indiana

Shelly D. Weise, PT, EdD
Associate Professor
Angelo State University
Department of Physical Therapy
San Angelo, Texas

Shiren Assaly, PT, DPT
Physical Therapist
Physical Rehabilitation Network
Sunnyvale, California

Emily Bannister, PT, DPT
Physical Therapist
Santa Clara Valley Medical Center
San Jose, California

Sara J. Belluomini, PT, DPT
Physical Therapist
Central Valley Physical Therapy
Stockton, California

Jill Dietmeyer, PT, DPT, LMT
Physical Therapist
REHAB at Nu'uanu
Honolulu, Hawaii

Kristina M. Gibson, PT, DPT
Physical Therapist
Andersen Physical Therapy
Modesto, California

Kristen M. Judson, PT, DPT
Physical Therapist
Sutter Medical Foundation
Fairfield, California

Rachel Gail Lee, PT, DPT
Physical Therapist
Southland Physical Therapy
Irvine, California

Zachary J. Mertz, PT, DPT
Physical Therapist
Lodi Physical Therapy
Lodi, California

Sheila H. Mistry, PT, DPT
Acute/ICU Physical Therapist
VA Palo Alto Health Care System
Palo Alto, California

Jennifer L. Myers, PT, DPT
Physical Therapist
ProActive Orthopedic and Sports Physical
    Therapy, LLC
Vancouver, Washington

Nella Tay, PT, DPT
Physical Therapist
Marin General Hospital
Greenbrae, California

Bryan Van Vliet, PT, DPT
Physical Therapist
Tower Physical Therapy
Turlock, California

Acknowledgments and Dedication

This book owes its very existence to the passion, dedication, and support of a host of people:

The dedicated and expert physical therapists who strive to provide efficient and high quality healthcare for their patients every day, as well as the talented students who are training to become physical therapists. Without them, this book would not be necessary.

The many leaders and luminaries in the physical therapy profession who have advocated for the professional responsibility of physical therapists to determine the appropriateness of physical therapy for their patients. Without them, this book would not be relevant.

The individuals who contributed to this textbook, including its authors, editors, illustrators, and publishers. All their contributions are the result of their knowledge and hard work; they have indelibly shaped our collective understanding of diagnostic reasoning by physical therapists. Without them, this book would not be possible.

Our families, close friends, and colleagues, whose encouragement sustained the process of creating this book. Each page of this book is infused with their influences, ranging from the ideas that stemmed from countless hours of conversation to the inspiration of knowing that they may someday benefit from the application of this book's content by a physical therapist. Without them, this book would not be meaningful.

We offer this book in memory of Robin I. Burks, PT, DPT, CHT, our friend and colleague, whose life was cut short by a brain tumor during the creation of this book. His family, friends, colleagues, students, and patients miss his caring and gentle manner, his sense of humor, and the simple personal wisdom that complemented his expansive professional knowledge. As Dr. Burks encouraged the Doctor of Physical Therapy students at the University of Southern California in his 2008 White Coat Ceremony address, we similarly urge you to "…put on your coat, roll up your sleeves, and make the world a better place."

Contents in Brief

Contents

CHAPTER **1**

Why Should Physical Therapists Know About Diagnosis?

■ *James Gordon, PT, EdD, FAPTA* ■ *Hugh G. Watts, MD*

IN THIS CHAPTER:
- Development of professional responsibility and education in physical therapy
- Role of diagnosis in the professional vision for the future of physical therapy
- Definition of diagnosis
- Conceptualization of diagnosis by physical therapists

Introduction

The close of physical therapy's first 100 years marks a new direction in its history as a young profession—establishing the autonomy necessary to ensure patients can benefit from safe, efficient, and universal direct access to physical therapy. Direct access to physical therapy is a central tenet of the American Physical Therapy Association's *Vision 2020* statement, which looks forward to physical therapists being "recognized by consumers and other health care professionals as the practitioners of choice to whom consumers have direct access for the diagnosis of, interventions for, and prevention of impairments, functional limitations, and disabilities related to movement, function, and health."[1] One clear assumption of *Vision 2020*, with its emphasis on direct access, is that physical therapists must be able to engage in the **diagnostic process** as part of their overall evaluation, in order to develop a well-reasoned intervention plan for addressing the patient's problems. This process must lead to a decision regarding the probable pathological or pathophysiological cause of the patient's problem, followed by a determination of whether physical therapy intervention is the most appropriate to address the underlying pathology of the patient's condition. Again, it must be emphasized that *Vision 2020*, with its emphasis on direct access, presupposes that the physical therapist will be able to reach that decision without provision of a diagnosis beforehand by a physician or other health care professional.

The development of diagnostic skills by physical therapists is a critical step to establishing the autonomy necessary for universal direct access to physical therapy. Since the introduction of a groundbreaking textbook on medical screening in 1990,[2] physical therapists have made considerable progress toward the development of systematic approaches to the consideration of pathology. Despite these advances, however, the profession lacks a strong tradition of diagnosis.[3] Many experienced physical therapists have developed excellent diagnostic skills, but they have succeeded the hard way—by independent study, on-the-job training, and trial and error. To reach the goal of direct access, the physical therapy profession must continue to develop systematic, evidence-based approaches for diagnosis that are taught in entry-level curricula, so that all physical therapists can be presumed to have adequate skill in diagnosis.

This textbook adds to the effort to develop physical therapists' diagnostic skills for recognizing pathologies in a significant and unique way. The purpose of this book is to present a framework for physical therapists to become more skilled diagnosticians of pathology and provide a ready resource to support the work of physical therapists in direct access environments. It proposes a detailed symptom-based approach for diagnosis based on the notion that, in starting the process of diagnostic investigation, the physical therapist must begin with the patient's symptoms and signs. Much like the collective understanding that it represents and to which it contributes, the material presented in this textbook remains a work in progress.

Five Critical Issues Frame the Topic of Diagnosis by Physical Therapists

Despite the overwhelming recognition of the need for more systematic approaches to diagnosis by physical therapists—especially approaches that can be taught to physical therapists during entry-level educational programs—considerable controversy surrounds the topic of diagnosis by physical therapists, particularly as it relates to pathology.

The rest of this chapter is devoted to discussing a conceptual perspective about diagnosis by physical therapists. In understanding the physical therapist's role as a diagnostician, we must agree to acknowledge two items. First, physical therapists fill similar professional roles, despite often substantial differences in practice area and physical proximity to referring physicians. With this in mind, we will develop a unifying philosophy regarding the role of diagnostic reasoning in physical therapy.

Second, ongoing changes in the health care environment shape the needs of patients and clients and, as a result, the requisites of physical therapy as a profession. Therefore, our discussion is a snapshot in time of current thinking on this topic that continues to evolve.

In addressing the current controversy regarding diagnosis by physical therapists, we believe five critical issues must be discussed:

1. *What is a diagnosis?* We assert that forming a diagnosis is a clinical reasoning process related to the patient's underlying pathology that concludes with a clinical label. The fundamental relevance of the diagnostic label in mainstream health care is as an identifier of the underlying pathology that is the cause of the patient's condition. Physical therapists also use diagnostic reasoning to determine working hypotheses regarding the physical impairments that may either result from, or contribute to, their patients' presenting pathology.

2. *Should physical therapists diagnose pathology?* We propose that physical therapists are profoundly involved in the diagnostic investigation of the patient's pathology and that they make critical decisions based on their conclusions about the nature, location, and severity of the pathology. Even when making the most basic determination of whether a patient's or client's condition is amenable to physical therapy, the physical therapist makes a diagnostic decision.

3. *Should physical therapists adopt a different definition for diagnosis than other health professionals?* We contend that it is a mistake to have a separate "physical therapy diagnosis," because the diagnostic label belongs to the patient or client and not a specific profession. We also propose that physical therapists' use of diagnostic reasoning to determine the underlying mechanical etiology for the presenting pathology is similar to the process by which many other health care providers use their unique expertise to elaborate on the diagnostic label in order to determine a prognosis and appropriate interventions for a patient or client.

4. *Should physical therapists be expected to diagnose given the current legal environment?* We propose that physical therapists have an ethical responsibility to use their skills to ensure

that patients receive the best possible care and that this responsibility need not conflict with legal restrictions.

5. *What information should physical therapists use to make decisions about treatment and prognosis?* We suggest that detailed investigations of the causes of movement dysfunction, and classification systems based on clinical decision rules, are important evaluative processes conducted by physical therapists that characterize the search for an underlying etiology. These approaches will be strengthened by an association with the diagnosis of pathology made by physical therapists, because they cannot be considered conclusive without considering pathology.

Each of these critical issues is discussed in greater detail throughout the remainder of this chapter.

Critical Issue 1: What is a Diagnosis?

As it is ordinarily understood in health care, **diagnosis** is defined as the process and product of a clinical investigation related to the pathology underlying a patient's or client's symptoms and signs. The process of diagnosis involves a combination of inductive and deductive reasoning. The product of the clinical reasoning process of diagnosis is a label, which serves as shorthand communication between providers. This label is called a *diagnosis*. We put forward that the term *diagnosis* should be used by physical therapists in the same manner as the rest of the health care system. To be certain, all health care practitioners are constrained by their training, resources, practice-related legislation, and current knowledge. Therefore, there are many instances throughout the health care system in which the precise cause of the condition cannot be determined due to a lack of knowledge. In these cases, the diagnostic label will necessarily be descriptive. Nevertheless, even in these cases, the presumption is that the label would identify the pathology if more information were available.

Because the result of diagnostic reasoning is a label that may lack pathological specificity, Sackett and colleagues[4] proposed that we might think of diagnostic labeling as an attempt to identify the target disorder, rather than consider it as a well-characterized, specific label of pathology or pathophysiology. Sackett defined the **target disorder** as:

> *The anatomical, biochemical, physiologic, or psychological derangement whose etiology (if known), maladaptive mechanisms, presentation, prognosis, and management we read about in medical texts. Although this element is usually called the disease, the usefulness of this ambiguous term is hampered by the inability of both patients and health scientists to agree on its application to specific situations. Accordingly, we shall call this element of patient's sickness the target disorder when it becomes the objective of the diagnostic process.[4]*

In this passage, Sackett and his colleagues[4] are expressing what is generally accepted about diagnostic labels: the diagnostic label frequently fails to precisely identify the disease or pathology. Nevertheless, a clinician's application of a diagnostic label represents the best attempt at a shorthand categorization of the patient's or client's condition with a link to the underlying cause of the patient's signs and symptoms.

Physical therapists must make a decision regarding the nature of the pathology and its severity in order to determine whether physical therapy is appropriate to address the patient's condition. In Chapter 2, Dr. Rob Landel discusses how physical therapists make decisions based on diagnostic information. For this discussion, deciding that the pathology causing a patient's pain is *not* cancer or *not* myocardial infarction or *not* an infection in the kidney requires the physical therapist to undertake a diagnostic process in which the nature of the pathology is investigated, and these pathologies are ruled as less likely causes of the patient's symptoms. Although the physical therapist does not always make the definitive determination of the diagnostic label that will go in the patient's medical record, this does not mean that the therapist is not actively engaged in diagnosing pathology. Therefore, we propose that two intermediate stages of labeling are important for physical therapists:

- Physical therapists may form a **diagnostic impression**, which is a working diagnosis requiring further verification. In documentation, the therapist may use the term *impression* to put forward a possible diagnostic label, or he or she may state that a patient's signs and symptoms "are consistent with" a certain diagnostic label.

- An even more preliminary stage between the diagnostic process and a label is the **diagnostic decision**. This is the situation in which the physical therapist does not definitively label the condition, but makes a decision based on a presumptive label. For example, when a physical therapist decides on a referral disposition, such as to send a patient back to the referring physician instead of activating the emergency medical system, the therapist has made a diagnostic decision. This decision is based on conclusions that the therapist has drawn about the pathology and its severity.

Despite the less specific nature of diagnostic labeling implied by *diagnostic impression* and *diagnostic decision*, a systematic and rigorous diagnostic clinical reasoning process should inform physical therapists' diagnostic impressions and diagnostic decisions. Dr. Todd Davenport discusses the theory and application of cognitive science related to diagnostic judgments and decision making in Chapter 3. In Chapter 4, Dr. Hugh Watts describes a process for arriving at a diagnostic label, diagnostic impression, or diagnostic decision that describes the target disorder. Subsequently, Dr. Watts provides a case example to demonstrate the specific process for diagnosis around which this book is arranged.

Critical Issue 2: Should Physical Therapists Diagnose Pathology?

Physical therapists are often essential participants in the process of identifying the pathology that is causing a patient's condition. In many instances, physical therapists further specify the nature of the pathology or its precise anatomical location when the diagnosis is within the physical therapist's scope of practice. In some cases, this means refining or correcting an initial diagnosis by bringing new information to the attention of the referring practitioner.

In a recent multicenter retrospective study involving referral diagnoses provided by physicians for patients presenting to outpatient orthopedic physical therapy clinics, Davenport and colleagues[5] found that less than a third of referrals to physical therapy practices were specific as to the nature of the pathology and anatomical location. Many referral diagnoses were not much more than a restatement of the patients' symptoms. This suggests that at least some portion of physical therapists' time in the initial evaluative process is spent on two functions: (1) deciding whether the patient presents with pathology that is amenable to physical therapy interventions and (2) how the nature and acuity of the pathology will shape the intervention plan. This makes the diagnosis of pathology by physical therapists an important professional function.[6]

First and foremost, it is the physical therapist's responsibility to determine whether the patient's condition is appropriate for physical therapy intervention. During the course of assessing and reassessing the patient, information is often uncovered that may necessitate modification of the original diagnosis. In this case, it is the legal and professional responsibility of the physical therapist to bring this information to the attention of the referring practitioner. The direct access environment places special importance on this function, because physical therapists are charged with making the initial observations that suggest the nature of the underlying pathology. This information is used to refer the patient to a physician or other health care provider if further investigation or treatment is warranted, or if the treatment of the specific pathology is outside the scope of physical therapy.

Critical Issue 3: Should Physical Therapists Adopt a Different Definition for Diagnosis Than Other Health Professionals Use?

Physical therapists should use the common definition of diagnosis as a clinical reasoning process and its resultant label for a variety of reasons. Perhaps most importantly, a common terminology is essential for physicians to understand which diagnoses are appropriate for referral to a physical therapist. As a practical matter, the reimbursement systems as well as most large outcome databases are inextricably linked to diagnoses. Finally, the database of clinical research evidence that physical therapists both use and contribute to is primarily organized around the mainstream pathology-based diagnostic system.

Adoption of a differing definition for diagnosis may expose physical therapists and the physical therapy profession to a communication disconnection from the mainstream health care community. One example of such ambiguity arises in the term **physical therapy diagnosis**, which is often used in contradistinction to the term **medical diagnosis**. This seems acceptable if these terms refer to the *processes* of diagnosis in which physical therapists and physicians engage, respectively, although it would be more precise, then, to refer to a physical therapist's diagnosis and a physician's diagnosis. However, more often these two terms appear to be used to distinguish the diagnostic labels that are assigned by physical therapists and physicians. With this definition, *physical therapy diagnosis* implies that when a physical therapist engages in diagnosis, a different type of label results than when a physician engages in diagnosis. We assert that there should not be a *physical therapy diagnosis* that is separate and distinct from the *medical diagnosis*. In the mainstream health care community, there is simply *the diagnosis* and it belongs to the patient—not to a specific health care discipline.

At best, introducing a separate category of diagnostic label for physical therapists invites confusion; at worst, this separate category will invite derision and isolation from colleagues in the health care community. The nursing profession's attempts to establish *nursing diagnoses* were unsuccessful. If the physical therapy profession adopts a complementary and alternative diagnostic language, it risks being viewed as providers of complementary and alternative treatments. Indeed, a private diagnostic system in the physical therapy profession will not help it to foster optimal communication using a common language.

It might seem politically advantageous to avoid conflict with physicians by using the term **medical screening** in place of diagnosis of pathology; however, this also leads to confusion by redefining a word that has a common and consistent usage in medicine. When a

physical therapist engages in the screening process, the patient is asked a series of general questions, often referred to as the *systems review*.[7] The goal of this part of the history taking is not to define a diagnosis, but to make sure that the patient has not neglected to mention an issue that may have an impact on the patient's overall well-being. By contrast, the diagnostic interview uses *directed* questions and *focused* physical examination tests to answer the specific question "What is the disease process that is causing my patient's symptoms?" Indeed, physical therapists should be prepared to engage in both diagnosis and medical screening, because they serve different and important functions in practice.

Critical Issue 4: Should Physical Therapists be Expected to Diagnose Given the Current Legal Environment?

Certainly, several legal and economic barriers impede diagnosis by physical therapists who practice in many areas. These include state practice act restrictions on diagnostic labeling and ordering of diagnostic tests, as well as the lack of reimbursement by third-party payers for services related to diagnosis performed by physical therapists. Any meaningful discussion of the complexity of the laws, regulations, and payment related to physical therapist practice is beyond the scope of this textbook. Nevertheless, we reiterate our assertion that the physical therapist has a professional and ethical responsibility, *regardless of how the state practice act may read*, to use his or her professional judgment to make the most accurate determination of the underlying pathology, to inform the physician of findings that may conflict with the physician's diagnosis, or to suggest tests that might clarify the diagnosis. Indeed, in the modern health care system, such a collaborative approach to diagnosis has become more the rule than the exception; physicians and health care professionals of different specialties all provide input to the diagnostic decision-making process.

To summarize, physical therapists use diagnostic skills to first differentiate whether a patient's presenting pathology appears amenable to physical therapy intervention. In turn, this information is used to determine whether the patient should receive physical therapy treatment, be referred to another health care provider for additional testing or treatment, or both. Also, physical therapists should determine the appropriate disposition and speed of referral based on their estimate of the nature and acuity of the underlying pathology.

Implicit in these decisions is a specific consideration by physical therapists of how each form of pathology presents and contributes to the patient's symptoms or disablement. As we discussed previously, the specificity of the diagnostic label that the physical therapist provides reflects the training of physical therapists, constraints on ordering tests, and the perceived acuity of the patient's condition. Physical therapists also use information regarding the nature of pathology in making treatment decisions when that pathology has been determined to respond to physical therapy interventions (i.e., tendinitis versus tendinosis). If the diagnosis of pathology is excluded from physical therapist practice out of concern about inappropriate consideration of the systemic disorders beyond the scope of physical therapy, this also would preclude the ability to diagnose musculoskeletal and neuromuscular pathologies to the extent that physical therapy treatment decisions can be made.

Critical Issue 5: What Information Should Physical Therapists Use to Make Decisions About Treatment and Prognosis?

Since the publication of several papers in the 1980s advocating for more detailed evaluative processes by physical therapists, several different systems have developed. Some have suggested that physical therapists should classify problems according to the constellations of impairments.[3] Others have developed systems that are intended to identify the relationships between impairments and functional limitations, using disablement models.[8] Still others have argued for classification systems based on clinical decision rules that identify the intervention of choice.[9–11] In principle, none of these approaches is mutually exclusive. In fact, it appears that different approaches are considered more useful for different patients

and different practice patterns within the physical therapy profession. It is critical for physical therapists to elaborate on the referral diagnosis with information that further refines the description of patients' disablement, or to further classify the patient within an accepted schema to define the appropriate treatment. Indeed, the first assumption in any of these approaches is that physical therapy is appropriate for the patient. Therefore, diagnosis of pathology by physical therapists should play a prominent role in physical therapist practice, similar to the search for an underlying etiology that is represented by the classification of patient clinical presentation according to disablement models, impairment clusters, and clinical decision rules that predict response to treatment.

We propose that, in the long run, linking classification-driven evaluative systems with pathology-based diagnosis will strengthen the physical therapy profession by establishing relationships between our unique professional reasoning and knowledge and the established diagnostic language of health care.

Conclusion

The physical therapy profession has set as one of its highest priorities the achievement of direct access. Refining the ability of all physical therapists to carry out the process of diagnosis of pathology is a necessary prerequisite for direct access and, thus, is the focus of this textbook. We do not believe that accomplishment of this objective will result from downplaying the importance of diagnostic skills. Indeed, the major argument of organized opposition to direct access is that physical therapists are inadequately trained to recognize serious diseases. Over the long term, the physical therapy profession will achieve direct access by continuing to demonstrate that physical therapists are well trained to systematically investigate the disease processes that cause physical disablement with sufficient specificity to assist in the achievement of an accurate diagnosis within the context of the health care team.

References

1. American Physical Therapy Association. *Vision 2020.* http://www.apta.org/vision2020. Accessed June 20, 2009.

2. Goodman C, Snyder T. *Differential Diagnosis in Physical Therapy*. Philadelphia: WB Saunders; 1990.

3. Sahrmann S. Are physical therapists fulfilling their responsibilities as diagnosticians? *J Orthop Sports Phys Ther*. 2005;35(9):556–558.

4. Sackett DL, Straus SE, Richardson WS, Rosenberg W, Haynes RB. *Evidence-Based Medicine: How to Practice and Teach EBM*. 2nd ed. New York, NY: Churchill Livingstone; 2000.

5. Davenport TE, Watts HG, Kulig K, Resnik C. Current status and correlates of physicians' referral diagnoses for physical therapy. *J Orthop Sports Phys Ther*. 2005;35(9):572–579.

6. Davenport TE, Kulig K, Resnik C. Diagnosing pathology to decide the appropriateness of physical therapy: what's our role? *J Orthop Sports Phys Ther*. 2006;36(1):1–2.

7. American Physical Therapy Association. Guide to physical therapist practice, second edition. *Phys Ther*. 2001;81(1):9–746.

8. Sullivan KJ. Role of the physical therapist in neurologic differential diagnosis: a reality in neurologic physical therapist practice. *J Neurol Phys Ther*. 2007;31(4): 236–237.

9. Fritz JM, Cleland JA, Childs JD. Subgrouping patients with low back pain: evolution of a classification approach to physical therapy. *J Orthop Sports Phys Ther*. 2007;37(6):290–302.

10. Childs JD, Fritz JM, Piva SR, Whitman JM. Proposal of a classification system for patients with neck pain. *J Orthop Sports Phys Ther*. 2004;34(11):686–696; discussion 697–700.

11. Delitto A, Erhard RE, Bowling RW. A treatment-based classification approach to low back syndrome: identifying and staging patients for conservative treatment. *Phys Ther*. 1995;75(6):470–485; discussion 485–489.

CHAPTER 2

Beyond the Diagnosis: The Search for Underlying Etiology

■ *Rob Landel, PT, DPT, OCS, CSCS, FAPTA*

IN THIS CHAPTER:
- How physical therapists use and elaborate on diagnostic labels
- A process physical therapists use to search for underlying etiology

Introduction

In the previous chapter, a process for symptom-based diagnosis was described. The outcome of that process is the diagnostic label, which is the pathology or the pathological process that is the root cause of the patient's or client's chief concern.[1-3] Once a diagnosis has been established, the clinician's evaluation must continue until the etiology of the pathology is uncovered. The focus of this investigation is specific to the discipline of the searcher. Once a diagnosis of myocardial infarction is

reached, for example, the cardiac surgeon looks for the offending coronary artery, the internist measures cholesterol and blood pressure, the dietician looks at eating habits, and the physical therapist examines exercise patterns. Each health care provider goes beyond the diagnosis in search of the underlying etiology, in order to provide the optimal management plan.

The process of searching for an underlying etiology by a physician may be more familiar to some than the search for an underlying etiology by a physical therapist. This chapter provides an overview of the ways physical therapists use diagnostic labels in making treatment and prognosis decisions, as well as how physical therapists search for the underlying etiology of a pathology.

Many health care providers wish to identify the tissue or pathology responsible for a patient's symptoms, and they strive to understand the root cause of the chief concern. Physical therapists use and elaborate on the diagnostic label for purposes of treatment. Perhaps the most intuitive manner in which the physical therapist can elaborate on the diagnostic label is to revise it with their diagnostic label, impression, or decision as described in the previous chapter. For example, a patient referred to a physical therapist with a diagnosis of *Back Pain* may be referred back to the physician after a physical therapy evaluation with the diagnostic impression of *Kidney Stone vs. Urinary Tract Infection*. In this example, the physical therapist is elaborating on the initial diagnostic label by advocating additional testing that may result in the label's revision. Physical therapists, like other health care providers, also use and elaborate on the diagnostic label to create a plan for intervention and prognosis. This involves a search for the underlying etiology of the pathology denoted by the diagnostic label. Diagnostic reasoning at the level of pathology is a similar process for both physicians and physical therapists and also for other health care providers in allopathic settings. The search for the underlying etiology, however, is specific to the discipline, and therefore physical therapists' unique professional focus and expertise characterize their search.

Physical Therapists Use the Diagnostic Label

Given a particular patient problem, the first goal of the physical therapist's evaluation is to determine if managing the causative pathology is within the scope of physical therapy. This critical first step ensures the safety of the patient, integrates the physical therapist into the health care system on a collegial basis, and results in an appropriate plan of care. This first decision-making process leads to three possible outcomes:

- Physical therapy is not indicated,
- Physical therapy is indicated but a consultation to another health care provider is required, or
- Physical therapy can proceed independent of additional consultation.

If physical therapy is not indicated, then the physical therapist must decide how urgently the referral should be made. The physical therapy episode of care ends when it becomes apparent that referral to another health care provider for additional evaluation and treatment will be more beneficial to the patient than either beginning or continuing physical therapy. This may be immediately apparent, for example, in the patient referred for shoulder pain who presents with shortness of breath, bilateral extremity edema, general pallor, and tachycardia. At the other end of the spectrum, it may not be until the patient has had several treatment sessions but has failed to meet expected goals for improvement that physical therapy is halted and referral to another health care provider is made. Either way the diagnostic process should still be completed beyond the simple identification of the presence of *Red Flags*. For example, a 67-year-old male patient's report of left shoulder pain

might well be referred to physical therapy with a referral diagnosis of *Shoulder Pain*. Upon questioning, however, it becomes apparent that the pain is aggravated by activities such as walking or ascending stairs. A review of his medical history reveals he is a smoker, has high blood pressure and hypercholesteremia, is sedentary, and had parents who died young of a stroke and a heart attack, respectively. Another patient is referred for a diagnosis of *Balance Retraining* who in her history relates no imbalance but does have short-duration dizzy spells that occur only when she rolls over in bed onto her left side. Whereas the first patient requires an urgent referral to a cardiologist to investigate his angina, the second patient can be treated effectively for benign paroxysmal positional vertigo by the physical therapist in one or two visits and a physician consult is not needed.

In cases where caution is indicated as the examination proceeds, the physical therapist must decide if the examination (and subsequent intervention) can proceed without the need for further consultation with other health care providers. If so, in a patient with ankle pain who does not meet the criteria necessitating radiographs,[4,5] for example, or a patient with transient dizziness whose clinical examination reveals benign positional paroxysmal vertigo,[6–9] the diagnostic process continues until the underlying cause is found. Clearly, if the physical therapist's evaluation does not reveal a specific pathology, then a consultation request made to a provider in the area of practice most likely to uncover the diagnosis is warranted. It is likely that most cases will require this type of referral. The physical therapist should proceed with the diagnostic process as far as is safely possible in order to provide the consultant with as much information as possible.

Even if physical therapy is deemed the appropriate management strategy for the patient's disablement, it remains essential to identify the presence of a medical condition that will affect the outcome of any physical therapy intervention. Medical comorbidities must be taken into consideration when designing a physical therapy intervention. For example, the presence of osteoporosis may affect the nature of any intervention provided to a patient with a history of thoracic spine pain, since the patient's symptoms may be related to compression fractures. Because confirmation and grading of osteoporosis requires access to imaging modalities outside the scope of practice for physical therapists to order, referral to a physician for additional testing if a high index of clinical suspicion is present would be prudent, even though osteoporosis itself is not a life-threatening condition and would warrant a nonemergent referral.

Establishment of a *tissue-specific diagnosis* is important when the physical therapy intervention itself can directly influence the course of the pathology. An example of this is the presence of aseptic inflammation. Physical therapy includes anti-inflammatory interventions that can directly treat the inflammation: ice, iontophoresis, and phonophoresis. Iontophoresis, in particular, needs precise placement in order to be effective, so knowledge of the precise location of pathology is required. Shoulder impingement, for example, is a common diagnosis in patients referred for physical therapy, yet the diagnosis is not specific enough to direct the application of iontophoresis. Further investigation must be done to identify the exact location of the pathology (differentiating between the supraspinatus or infraspinatus tendon, for example).

Another specific tissue pathology directly amenable to physical therapy intervention is tendinopathy. Tendinopathy may present either as tendinitis or tendinosis, but the underlying pathologies are different and the interventions differ accordingly. Tendinitis implies an inflammatory process, and appropriate anti-inflammatory measures should improve the condition. Tendinosis, however, is an alteration in the structure of the tendon and requires rest followed by progressive reloading of the tendon through exercise.[10] Providing an inappropriate treatment due to misdiagnosis will at best fail to improve the patient's condition (eg, using ice on a tendinopathy) and at worst exacerbate it (eg, exercising an inflamed tendon).

Physical Therapists Elaborate on the Diagnostic Label

Physical therapists, like all other members of the health care team, interpret the diagnostic label to determine the most appropriate intervention and prognosis. Physicians can often treat the pathology directly, whereas physical therapists can do so only in some cases (e.g., treating inflammation as noted above). Most interventions that a physical therapist can employ do not directly address the pathological tissue. For example, physical therapy interventions cannot *directly* address an intervertebral disk defect, heal a torn meniscus, or repair a sprained ankle. Rather, the role of the physical therapist is to provide an optimal healing environment for the tissue that is injured, reduce abnormal mechanical stresses placed on the injured tissue, and restore optimal movement once the tissue is healed. Ameliorating the contributing or associated physical impairments can achieve these goals. Therefore, even if the pathology is known, the physical therapist must go beyond the diagnostic label and identify how it relates to the patient's impairments, activity levels, participation, and health. In addition, the physical therapist must determine which impairments are causing the activity and participation restrictions, and how they are doing so. Accomplishing this provides the best chance at intervening with respect to the most relevant impairments.

Physical therapists' professional emphasis on movement creates a unique and specialized goal in the search for underlying etiology, in that physical therapists typically infer cause-and-effect relationships between tissue pathology and a client's movement patterns based on skilled assessment. One of the major factors a physical therapist must determine is whether the abnormal movement *resulted from* the tissue pathology, or whether abnormal movement *caused* the tissue pathology. For example, a patient with a chief concern of knee pain without a history of traumatic onset may receive a tissue-specific diagnosis from the physician that is related to the root cause, such as a sprained medial collateral ligament of the knee. One could argue that, upon having identified the pathology and arrived at the diagnosis of the sprained ligament, the differential diagnostic process is completed. In this case, however, the sprained ligament is not the result of a single traumatic event, but due to overuse. Confronted with this situation, the physical therapist must now identify whether any abnormal movement patterns led to the overuse and overstress of the sprained ligament, and then implement an intervention strategy that will alleviate stress on the ligament. Suppose movement analysis of the patient revealed a knee valgus thrust during each weight acceptance phase of running, which would repeatedly stress the medial collateral ligament. Knowing that the hip abductor muscles should control this aberrant movement, their strength is tested and they are found to be weak. The result of this search for the underlying etiology of medial knee pain is a hip strengthening program. This case illustrates the direction of investigation specific to physical therapy that extends beyond the pathology identified by the medical practitioner.

Physical therapists often attempt to isolate the patient's or client's movement dysfunction to the narrowest practical level in order to provide treatment. Often, this involves a hierarchical organization of the movement-related disablement using enablement/disablement models. Physical therapists commonly consider the interrelationships among physical impairments, activity limitations, and participation limitations.[1,3,11–13] Physical therapists identify and manage movement dysfunctions as their unique elaboration on the diagnostic label, and this allows for the enhancement of physical and functional abilities through focused intervention. They restore, maintain, and promote not only optimal physical function, but also optimal wellness and fitness and optimal quality of life as it relates to movement and health. Finally, they prevent the onset and progression of symptoms due to impairments, functional limitations, and disabilities that may result from diseases, disorders, conditions, or injuries. Thus, the physical therapist must identify abnormal movement when it exists in a patient and restore optimal movement.[1]

The Diagnostic Label Alone is Insufficient to Guide Physical Therapists

A basic precept of patient management is that it is important to determine the anatomical or pathological source of symptoms and to determine the stage of healing, so that appropriate treatment is directed to the appropriate tissue at the appropriate time. In medicine, when a specific cause or source of the problem is known and amenable to treatment, treatment of the cause or source is usually considered more effective than treating individual signs and symptoms. Likewise, in physical therapy, identifying specific patterns of movement dysfunction (for example, aberrant movement patterns[14]) may be a more effective basis for determining interventions than managing individual impairments as isolated phenomena. This concept has become known as *essentialism*.[15]

The essentialist approach to diagnostic classification states that an etiologic mechanism exists for every disease, whether or not that mechanism has been discovered. This approach arose from the discovery of microorganisms as a causative agent for disease. The fact that a specific microorganism could be the cause of a specific disease suggested that each and every disease must also have a singular cause. Furthermore, regardless of our current limitations in knowledge, it appears to be only a matter of time before science identifies and explains the diagnosis for every malady. Essentialism is the driving force behind science's relentless pursuit to identify the origins for all manner of disease causes. After the narrowest possible level of cause has been identified, an essentialist approach to treatment is to eliminate or modify the cause.[15]

Important limitations exist in the essentialist approach to diagnosis in consistently guiding physical therapists' interventions and prognoses. As mentioned earlier, the outcome of the differential diagnostic process, the diagnostic label, should provide clues as to the proper intervention and prognosis. In other words, the diagnosis is just one driver of the choice of intervention. Unfortunately, the referral diagnosis provided to physical therapists by a physician is tissue specific less than one-third of the time.[16] Over two-thirds of referrals to outpatient physical therapy clinics have as a "diagnosis" terms like *Shoulder Pain, Low Back Pain, Knee Pain*, and so on. Even a casual look reveals that these are not diagnoses at all, but are simply restatements of a patient's or client's symptoms. They are not specific regarding the pathology or tissue involved and provide no indication of the appropriate intervention. Therefore, the ability for physical therapists to establish a diagnosis and search for underlying etiology even in the case of vague referral diagnoses becomes critical to making treatment and prognosis decisions.

A Process Guides Physical Therapists' Search for an Underlying Etiology

So how do we proceed after a diagnosis is established? The foregoing situation reveals a significant shortcoming of the essentialist approach. With the patient sitting in our clinic we do not have time for science to "catch up" and deliver us a clear treatment plan for each individual. We must act as best we can with the information currently available to develop a plan of care. In contrast to essentialism, the *nominalist* approach to diagnostic classification uses groupings of signs and symptoms as the basis for establishing and labeling a disease.[15] A classic example of nominalism is the management of a patient with the chief concern of low back pain. The literature has established that lumbar pathoanatomy correlates poorly with symptoms,[17–21] leading to findings that 85% of the time the exact cause of low back pain remains undiagnosed.[22] Of course, this does not mean low back pain cannot be treated effectively. The impairments relative to the chief concern such as pain, or activity limitations such as the inability to stand, sit, or walk, or participation limitations such as the inability to work can still be identified and guide formation of a plan of care. If specific impairments can be identified that are directly related to the chief concern, and these impairments are addressed through an appropriate intervention plan, then the patient stands the best chance of realizing a positive change in their chief concern.

Impairment-based classification systems have developed because of the physical therapist's emphasis on intervening at the level of physical impairments. Because the classification of disablement according to enablement/disablement models and physical impairments takes on the characteristic of a nominalist diagnostic system, some authors have gone so far as to label them forms of physical therapy diagnosis.[23–25] Although relatively recently introduced into physical therapy practice, there is some support for the value of a specific movement classification to help guide physical therapy intervention.[2,15,26–30] Impairment-based classification systems are problematic, however, when they fail to account for pathoanatomical and psychosocial factors and the stage of the disorder.[31] In addition, although movement and motor control impairments certainly manifest themselves in common ways for particular diagnoses, there is no certainty of cause and effect without the relevance provided by the context of movement. For example, directing intervention at the movement impairments resulting from neuropathic or inflammatory pain would be ineffective compared to treating the cause of the pain directly. Similarly, psychological processes such as depression, stress, and anxiety can produce impairments that affect movement. Identifying and treating impairments alone irrespective of other contributing factors will result in physicians and physical therapists alike missing a significant aspect of the patient's disorder and thereby rendering care that results in poor outcomes.[31]

The health care community accepts nominalist diagnoses on the basis of consensus. There is much research, debate, and revision that occurs prior to reaching a strong enough consensus that nominalist diagnoses should become a part of the general standard of care. Along these lines, more research is necessary to determine the validity and reliability of and the clinical outcomes related to the proposed nominalist approaches that involve classification according to impairment clusters before they can be universally accepted. Indeed, the search appears to continue for a nominalist classification system for movement in health and disease. In the meantime, considering the patient as a whole—including hypothetical cause-and-effect relationships among pathology, psychology, sociology, symptoms, and movement dysfunction—will remain the physical therapist's challenge.

Physical therapists' search for underlying causes requires impairments to be identified and linked to function. Since the goal of physical therapy care is restoring function and reducing disability, and interventions may be directed toward ameliorating impairments, it is imperative for the impairments being treated to be linked to the patient's functional losses and disabilities using a systematic approach. This approach involves three steps:

1. Careful identification of the functional chief concern,
2. Completion of a task and movement analysis, and
3. Testing of hypothetical relationships between physical impairments and functional limitations during physical examination.

This specialized approach is dynamic and continues throughout an episode of care.

Physical Therapists Identify the Functional Chief Concern

The first step to linking function and impairments is to ask what impairments could be the cause of a given set of activity limitations or, conversely, to ask *"What activity limitations could ensue for a given set of impairments?"* In most orthopedic settings, the patient's chief concern corresponds to an impairment. For example, a patient with a torn meniscus may report having pain. Given this impairment, the physical therapist must ask not only what pathology could be the source of the pain, but also what activity and participation limitations arise as a result of that pain. The key question for the patient is "What does this pain prevent you from doing?" Possible answers may be an inability to squat, rise from a chair, or negotiate stairs. In the neurological setting, the patient's presenting concern commonly and conveniently identifies the functional limitation, such as "I can't walk" or "I can't get up from a chair."

Physical Therapists Perform Task and Movement Analyses

Once the activity limitation has been identified, the second step in linking impairment to function is to perform a task analysis, that is, *to compare how the patient does the activity and how someone in good health would optimally do it.*[32] For example, when a patient states she cannot rise from a chair, one can ask how a healthy individual would accomplish this task. The healthy individual possesses the resources necessary for successful task completion: a prerequisite amount of joint motion, strength, motor control, proprioception, and so on. These resources are readily available to the person who is able to rise from the chair without difficulty. We can observe the patient's performance of the task, compare it to the optimal performance, and hypothesize what resources are lacking to interfere with task accomplishment. This lack of resources is synonymous with impairments.

Physical Therapists Create and Test Hypothetical Relationships

The third step to linking impairment and function is *testing the hypotheses via the physical examination.* To thoroughly test the hypotheses, appropriate tests and measures must be chosen. Thus, for a patient having difficulty rising from a chair, we would ensure there is enough hip flexion mobility,[33] ensure there is sufficient hip extensor strength,[34] and so on. Any impairments found would very likely underlie the functional limitation; amelioration of these specific impairments would stand an excellent chance of decreasing the functional limitation.

A very important by-product of this approach is that the choice of tests and measures used in the physical examination is dictated by the predictions made during the task analysis. For example, if strength is required to perform the task optimally, then the clinician has no choice but to measure strength to determine if weakness prevents optimal performance. The clinician can choose *how* to determine if the impairment is present, for example, testing strength using manual muscle testing, hand-held dynamometry, or isokinetic dynamometry, but not *whether* it will be tested.

Several advantages emerge from this process. First, the resulting physical examination is focused and efficient, because unnecessary tests are avoided. Second, the findings have meaning, because they relate to the patient's concerns. Third, since the impairments stand a reasonable chance of being linked to activity and participation limitations, intervening in those impairments will have the highest likelihood of producing positive results in the activity and participation limitations.

The Search for an Underlying Etiology is Dynamic and Ongoing

As noted previously, there are times when a hypothesis is made about the pathology that causes a patient's or client's disablement. Based on this hypothesis, an intervention plan is designed, complete with objectively measurable goals that have a time frame for success. At the conclusion of this time frame, remeasurement is completed to determine whether the patient or client has met the treatment goals. If the goals have been met, then not only was the intervention a success, but it is also possible that the initial diagnostic hypothesis was correct. For example, in the case of a patient with unilateral low back pain of nontraumatic onset, aggravated by extension and ipsilateral lateral flexion, one might surmise based on the history and physical examination that the symptoms are due to a facet joint impingement. Following this biomechanically based hypothesis, a decision might be made to initiate interventions that decompress the offending facet joint. If the patient improves, this might provide indirect evidence supporting the initial treatment hypothesis. This type of thinking is often used as a form of content validity for clinical reasoning; however, it neglects the possibility that many other structures could have been positively affected as the facet joint was decompressed (eg, the surrounding musculature could have been stretched). It would be better to know the exact underlying pathology, of course, using tests and measures that have criterion-related validity (in this example, a diagnostic facet joint block), but this is not always feasible, practical, or possible. As noted previously, a gold standard diagnostic criterion may not exist. Alternatively, the patient may fail to improve within the specified time frame or even worsen, which may be interpreted as evidence against the initial hypothetical underlying etiology. *Thus, the search for underlying etiology considers not only information gathered from the history and examination, but also the response to treatment.*

Determining whether the response to treatment was appropriate implies that progress is compared to an expected outcome. If the expected goals have been met, the outcome is clear and the patient is discharged. When the goals have not been met, however, the therapist must assess each step taken during the episode of care to determine the cause for lack of progress. The first step to review is the implementation of the intervention. If not done well, treatment is repeated with improved implementation and the problem is reassessed. If the treatment was implemented properly but the goals were still not met, the choice of treatment is reassessed. For example, when mobilizing a joint to gain range of motion fails to yield positive results, perhaps stretching the muscles will. If the choice of interventions was appropriate but the goals were still not met, then perhaps the overall strategy was incorrect and needs to be rethought. In this case, perhaps the problem was not lack of range of motion, but lack of strength.

Conclusion

Determining a tissue-specific diagnosis initially drives decisions regarding intervention and prognosis. Arriving at a diagnosis, however, is not always the end of the process for determining the best possible intervention and prognosis in physical therapy. In some cases, it is impossible to arrive at a diagnosis for lack of adequate differentiating tests or current medical understanding. In some cases, although the offending tissue is identified, the interventions available to the physical therapist do not allow direct treatment of the tissue itself.

In all cases, the physical therapist must proceed beyond the diagnosis and determine the presence of movement abnormalities. Furthermore, the therapist must determine whether identified movement abnormalities are the cause or result of the pathology. The physical therapist must create hypothetical links between function and individual physical impairments, and then test the hypotheses. This requires a clear understanding of the patient's or client's functional chief concern, a thorough task and movement analysis, and testing hypothesized movement deficits during the physical examination. Finally, the patient's or client's response to treatment—or lack thereof—serves to verify or disconfirm the diagnosis.

References

1. American Physical Therapy Association. Guide to physical therapist practice, second edition. *Phys Ther.* 2001;81(1):9–746.

2. Guccione AA. Physical therapy diagnosis and the relationship between impairments and function. *Phys Ther.* 1991;71:499–504.

3. Nagi S. Disability concepts revisited: implications for prevention. In: Pope A, Tarlov A, eds. *Disability in America: Toward a National Agenda for Prevention.* Washington, DC: Institute of Medicine, National Academy Press; 1991.

4. Stiell IG, Greenberg GH, McKnight RD, Nair RC, McDowell I, Worthington JR. A study to develop clinical decision rules for the use of radiography in acute ankle injuries. *Ann Emerg Med.* 1992;21(4):384–390.

5. Bachmann LM, Kolb E, Koller MT, Steurer J, ter Riet G. Accuracy of Ottawa ankle rules to exclude fractures of the ankle and mid-foot: systematic review. *BMJ.* 2003;326:417.

6. Korres SG, Balatsouras DG. Diagnostic, pathophysiologic, and therapeutic aspects of benign paroxysmal positional vertigo. *Otolaryngol Head Neck Surg.* 2004;131(4):438–444.

7. Hilton M, Pinder D. The Epley (canalith repositioning) manoeuvre for benign paroxysmal positional vertigo [update of Cochrane Database Syst Rev. 2002;(1): CD003162; PMID: 11869655]. *Cochrane Database Syst Rev.* 2004(2):CD003162.

8. Parnes LS, Agrawal SK, Atlas J. Diagnosis and management of benign paroxysmal positional vertigo (BPPV). *CMAJ.* 30 2003;169(7):681–693.

9. Tusa RJ. Benign paroxysmal positional vertigo. *Curr Neurol Neurosci Rep.* 2001;1(5):478–485.

10. Davenport TE, Kulig K, Matharu Y, Blanco CE. The EdUReP model for nonsurgical management of tendinopathy. *Phys Ther.* 2005;85(10):1093–1103.

11. Gray DB, Hendershot GE. The ICIDH-2: developments for a new era of outcomes research. *Arch Phys Med Rehabil.* 2000;81(suppl 2):S10–S14.

12. Stucki G, Ewert T. How to assess the impact of arthritis on the individual patient: the WHO ICF. *Ann Rheum Dis.* 2005;64:664–668.

13. Stucki G, Ewert T, Cieza A. Value and application of the ICF in rehabilitation medicine. *Disabil Rehabil.* 2002;24(17):932–938.

14. Sahrman SA. *Diagnosis and Treatment of Movement Impairment Syndromes.* St. Louis, MO: Mosby; 2002.

15. Zimny NJ. Diagnostic classification and orthopaedic physical therapy practice: what we can learn from medicine . . . including commentary by O'Sullivan P, Moffat M, and Delitto A with author response. *J Orthop Sports Phys Ther.* 2004;34(3):105–115.

16. Davenport TE, Watts HG, Kulig K, Resnik C. Current status and correlates of physicians' referral diagnoses for physical therapy. *J Orthop Sports Phys Ther.* 2005; 35(9):572–579.

17. Borenstein DG, O'Mara JW Jr, Boden SD, et al. The value of magnetic resonance imaging of the lumbar spine to predict low-back pain in asymptomatic subjects: a seven-year follow-up study. *J Bone Joint Surg Am.* 2001;83–A(9):1306–1311.

18. Carragee EJ, Paragioudakis SJ, Khurana S. 2000 Volvo Award winner in clinical studies: lumbar high-intensity zone and discography in subjects without low back problems. *Spine.* 2000;25(23):2987–2992.

19. Stadnik TW, Lee RR, Coen HL, Neirynck EC, Buisseret TS, Osteaux MJ. Annular tears and disk herniation: prevalence and contrast enhancement on MR images in the absence of low back pain or sciatica. *Radiology.* 1998;206(1):49–55.

20. Savage RA, Whitehouse GH, Roberts N. The relationship between the magnetic resonance imaging appearance of the lumbar spine and low back pain, age and occupation in males. *Eur Spine J.* 1997;6(2):106–114.

21. Jensen MC, Brant ZMN, Obuchowski N, Modic MT, Malkasian D, Ross JS. Magnetic resonance imaging of the lumbar spine in people without back pain [see comments]. *N Engl J Med.* 1994;331(2):69–73.

22. Dillingham T. Evaluation and management of low back pain: an overview. *State of the Art Rev.* 1995;9: 559–574.

23. Zimny NJ, Goodman CC, Orest M, Delitto A, Snyder-Mackler L. Physical therapy diagnosis . . . "The diagnostic process: examples in orthopedic physical therapy" (March 1995). *Phys Ther.* 1995;75(7):635–638.

24. Guccione AA. Physical therapy diagnosis and the relationship between impairments and function . . . including commentary by Jette AM with author response. *Phys Ther.* 1991;71(7):499–504.

25. Rose SJ. Physical therapy diagnosis: role and function. *Phys Ther.* 1989;69(7):535–537.

26. Delitto A, Erhard RE, Bowling RW. A treatment-based classification approach to low back syndrome: identifying and staging patients for conservative treatment. *Phys Ther.* 1995;75(6):470–485.

27. Jull G, Bogduk N, Marsland A. The accuracy of manual diagnosis for cervical zygapophysial joint pain syndromes. *Med J Australia.* 1988;148(5):233–236.

28. Fritz JM, Delitto A, Erhard RE. Comparison of class based physical therapy with therapy based on CPGs for patients with acute LBP. *Spine.* 2003;28:1363–1372.

29. Delitto A, Cibulka MT, Erhard RE, Bowling RW, Tenhula JA. Evidence for use of an extension-mobilization category in acute low back syndrome: a prescriptive validation pilot study. *Phys Ther.* 1993;73(4):216–228.

30. Erhard RE, Delitto A, Cibulka MT. Relative effectiveness of an extension program and a combined program of manipulation and flexion and extension exercises in patients with acute low back syndrome. *Phys Ther.* 1994;74(12):1093–1100.

31. O'Sullivan PB. Invited commentary: diagnostic classification and orthopedic physical therapy practice: what we can learn from medicine. *J Orthop Sports Phys Ther.* 2004;34:110–111.

32. Fisher B, Yakura J. Movement analysis: a different perspective. *Orthop Phys Ther Clin N Am.* 1993;2:1–14.

33. Riley PO, Krebs DE, Popat RA. Biomechanical analysis of failed sit-to-stand. *IEEE Trans Rehabil Eng.* 1997; 5(4):353–359.

34. Schultz AB, Alexander NB, Ashton-Miller JA. Biomechanical analyses of rising from a chair. *J Biomech.* 1992;25(12):1383–1391.

CHAPTER 3

Diagnostic Reasoning

Todd E. Davenport, PT, DPT, OCS

IN THIS CHAPTER:

- The difference between diagnosis and medical screening
- Cognitive models of diagnostic reasoning

Introduction

In the previous chapter, the case was made for why physical therapists need to know about diagnosis. The idea emphasized in that chapter was that physical therapists have the ethical obligation to engage in a systematic process of diagnosing a disorder by differentiating between the many diseases that may cause the symptom. Diagnostic reasoning is one component of clinical reasoning by expert physical therapists. According to Edwards and colleagues, diagnostic reasoning includes the "... formation of a diagnosis related to physical disability and impairment with consideration of associated pain mechanisms, tissue pathology. . . ."[1 (p322)] Indeed, determining the cause of a patient's symptoms is the initial stage of deciding how to treat a patient. As previous chapters have pointed out, the term *diagnosis* has dual meanings. It refers to the *clinical reasoning process* of determining the sources of a patient's symptoms. This term is also used to describe the outcome of the clinical reasoning process, which is a *label* that serves as shorthand communication among different health care providers. When the diagnostic label is coded, it can then be used to inform the processes of disease tracking and insurance reimbursement. The purpose of this chapter is to discuss a clinical reasoning process aimed at determining the pathology responsible for a patient's symptom(s), using the presenting symptom as the starting point.

Both Diagnosis and Medical Screening Have Roles in Physical Therapy

Systems-based processes for medical screening have been proposed for use by physical therapists in order to move from diagnostic uncertainty to a sufficient level of certainty to determine if the patient/client requires referral to another health care provider. However, *medical screening* is different than *diagnosis*. As part of any effective assessment by a physical therapist, the patient is asked a series of questions, commonly called the *review of systems*. The goal of the medical screening portion of the subjective examination is not to determine the pathology or pathophysiology underlying a patient/client's clinical presentation, but to ensure that nothing that may impact the patient's well-being has been overlooked. The organization of the review of systems is based on anatomical structures or physiological systems.[2] Typically, these questions are integrated into a thorough questionnaire format that is designed to cover all areas and systems.

The clinical data acquired from the review of systems or medical screening is then typically examined by the physical therapist for the presence of *Red Flags*. In 1994, the U.S. Agency for Health Care Policy and Research[3] released a brochure describing symptoms and signs that may indicate the presence of serious pathology in patients with low back pain, which have become known as *Red Flags*. Red Flags are commonly interpreted to signal an automatic need for patient/client referral to another health care provider.[4,5] However, emerging literature indicates a lack of diagnostic accuracy for individual Red Flags.[6] Indeed, the diagnostic relevance of individual or clusters of Red Flags must be interpreted for a given patient situation; a symptom or sign considered a Red Flag for one patient/client may not necessarily be a Red Flag for another. For example, a patient who received gastric bypass and a patient with malignant cancer may both demonstrate significant weight change; however, the etiology of weight change is far less insidious in the patient who received a gastric bypass than in the one with metastatic cancer. Also, a history of smoking may not be considered a Red Flag by itself, but it takes on significant diagnostic relevance in a patient with shoulder pain and upper extremity paresthesias due to the elevated risk for a Pancoast tumor.

Some authors advocate screening for multiple Red Flags in order to screen for certain forms of pathology.[7] Scientific determination of symptoms and signs that have the highest likelihood of indicating a disease is important. However, organizing this information around the details of a specific patient's case may be more clinically meaningful than synthesizing a collection of unrelated facts, as we discuss in a later section of this chapter. Organizing the search for underlying pathology around a process rather than fragments of information enhances the search's consistency and speed, because the clinician can recognize features of the case that point to a diagnosis rather than needing to remember all of the Red Flags in a cluster. In addition, the patient/client does not always present with signs and symptoms that fit dysfunction in a well-defined physiological system. Memorization of Red Flag clusters would impair perception of the necessary cues to integrate diagnostic information from across body systems.

These issues reinforce the importance of establishing a diagnostic process that is flexible enough to allow physical therapists to consider how pathology may cause an individual patient's symptoms and signs given the patient's unique situation.

Diagnosis is a Unique Combination of Reasoning Patterns

The goal of the diagnostic process is to move from uncertainty to a sufficient level of certainty regarding the cause of a patient's presenting symptoms or signs for referral and treatment decisions to be made. It is this certainty that allows for labeling of the pathology hypothesized to be responsible for the patient's clinical presentation. To achieve this goal, physical therapists must answer a fundamental question: "What disease is causing the patient's symptoms?" A formal process for finding the answer to this question is necessary, because the rate of errors in medical decision making has been shown to decrease with implementation of formal processes.

Several characteristics are important in a well-designed diagnostic process. The process should allow consideration of all the important clinical data without missing any data that might be salient to the patient's case. At the same time, the process must be efficient and flexible to allow consistent application throughout the day and for different clinical presentations and clinicians at various levels of knowledge and skill. Efficiency and flexibility in a diagnostic process relates to the ability of clinicians to integrate several patterns of diagnostic thinking within the process. Each of these patterns is discussed in the following sections.

Backward Reasoning Involves Creation and Testing of Clinical Hypotheses

Backward reasoning involves the creation of hypotheses to be tested. The process of testing hypotheses has been referred to as the **hypothetico-deductive model**. Pure use of this form of diagnostic reasoning would suggest that a clinician should collect all the possible data by taking an absolutely complete history from the patient. This would be followed by an exhaustive physical examination and collation of an exhaustive set of tests. At that point, all data would be sorted by the probabilities of a specific disease being found in a patient or client based on relevant demographic characteristics and clinical test results until the most likely diagnosis is reached. Although backward reasoning is a pattern that aims to carefully consider much information, this pattern is also characterized by a slower processing time and a higher potential for distractions that affect decision accuracy.[8]

The exhaustive nature of pure backward reasoning models makes them too time consuming for consistent use in the clinic, although their use has merit in computer models. One example of backward reasoning computer modeling is the use of **expert systems** or **decision support systems**. A decision support system is a computer system that is intended to simulate the knowledge and expertise of a human expert. The system is composed of a large computer database containing information related to the diagnosis and treatment of disease. The database can be searched using an inference engine, and the computer is programmed with software that provides a set of rules for basic deductions. After the patient's presenting symptoms and signs have been entered into the search engine, the computer yields a likely diagnosis and treatment options. Of course, there are many advantages to this type of system, which are beyond the scope of this chapter to discuss in detail.[9,10] However, computerized decision support systems have yet to be widely implemented into health care, emphasizing the need for clinicians to continue to develop hypothetico-deductive reasoning skills.

Forward Reasoning Involves the Attempt to Recognize Patterns in Clinical Presentation

Forward reasoning (or forward-inductive reasoning) is the attempt to recognize patterns in clinical presentation that may indicate pathology. This approach also is called **pattern recognition**. In this manner, hypothesis generation is triggered by the patient's presentation.[11] Certain features of the patient's clinical presentation commonly facilitate hypothesis formation. These features include clinicians' judgments about how representative the patient's clinical picture is with respect to the perceived frequency, variability, causation, and prototype of a disease.[12]

Clinicians may make rapid judgments about the perceived *frequency* of a disease based on specific variables that are identified. For example, you might consider a genetic basis to be more likely in children with motor delay and a family history of a heritable genetic disease than in children with motor delay and no family history.

Judgments regarding disease *variability* occur when a clinician makes inferences about the entire population with a disease based on a small subset. In this manner, you might infer that the entire population of patients with diffuse leg pain has peripheral vascular disease based on your experience with a few individuals with peripheral vascular disease.

Clinicians may rapidly consider *causation* in determining whether a patient has a disease. In this scenario, you might consider the probability of brain trauma to be most prominent in a patient with loss of consciousness following a motor vehicle accident.

In making judgments about a *prototype* to determine if Mrs. Juarez has a certain disease, you would compare Mrs. Juarez's presentation to what you saw last week in Mrs. Smith. If Mrs. Juarez and Mrs. Smith have the same symptoms and signs, they must have the same pathology.

The pure use of forward reasoning has both advantages and disadvantages. One advantage of forward reasoning is that decisions can be made faster than with backward reasoning.[8] Problems with the use of forward reasoning alone relate to the fact that forward reasoning is subject to errors,[13,14] especially by novice clinicians.[12] These errors would be addressed if a clinician has seen at least a representative sample of all pathologies, which is impractical and impossible. The need for experience with different patient presentations to engage in a forward reasoning process is supported by studies that suggest expert clinicians demonstrate behaviors consistent with forward reasoning processes more frequently than beginners,[15–17] and also demonstrate better recognition memory for salient and nonsalient clinical information than beginners.[18] However, our experience indicates that variations among patients can make it more difficult to recognize underlying similarities. This trend is particularly true for novice clinicians, although expert clinicians may be subject to **cue interference**, in which conflicting pieces of information are present in a patient's case. Perhaps for this reason, interfering pieces of information may cause even clinical experts to participate in a more backward reasoning pattern.[19]

Experts Create "Small Worlds" of Information to Use in Diagnostic Reasoning

Most recently, the **small worlds hypothesis** was created to model diagnostic reasoning by experts.[20] This hypothesis suggests that clinicians use both forward and backward reasoning through "chunking" clinical information into manageable pieces that are used to establish diagnostic certainty. Our experience indicates the experienced clinician sorts through a series of diagnostic *possibilities* by choosing those with the highest *probabilities* given the patient's gender, age, locale of habitation, and occupation. The questions then asked during the subjective examination are specifically directed to eliminate as many causes as possible. Questions are chosen to be *most differentiating*; that is, the answer to the question should eliminate as many inappropriate diseases as possible. At that point, a quick mental sorting provides a more limited array of possibilities that must be differentiated by selecting a narrow, yet specific set of physical examination tests.

If final selection of a single diagnosis cannot be made, referral for appropriate laboratory or imaging tests may be required. In the case of most physical therapists, this latter step will require referral to a physician. However, narrowing down the group of likely causes and pathologies will help the physical therapist to decide the urgency and direction of the referral.

Preferred Diagnostic Reasoning Processes Depend on the Clinician and the Case

Experienced clinicians tend to employ more inductive reasoning than less experienced clinicians to achieve diagnostic certainty, bringing up an important relationship between expertise and diagnostic reasoning processes. The interaction between knowledge and process can be summarized in the following example from Norman and Eva,[21] involving three individuals who encounter a white dog on the street:

> The first ... says, "It looks like Lassie. It's a dog." The second ... says, "Well, it has 4 legs, floppy ears and it weighs about 20 kg. It barked a minute ago. It's furry. It must be a dog." His brother ... who recently arrived from the Aleutians and has only encountered husky dogs, says, "It might be a dog because it has 4 legs, a tail and floppy ears. On the other hand, it could be a baby polar bear, because it's white. And I thought I heard it growl a minute ago, so maybe it's a wolf."

The first individual used a pattern recognition approach to quickly arrive at the answer, while the other two individuals appeared to actively consider competing hypotheses in a more hypothetico-deductive manner. The latter two individuals differed in their experience with similar animals, and the number of competing hypotheses increases in parallel with inexperience.[22] Therefore, these less experienced individuals would need to adopt a more hypothetico-deductive approach to determining the appropriate label for the animal, by collecting additional data to assist in distinguishing among the different possibilities.

This trend toward more forward reasoning patterns by clinical experts is supported by various scientific studies. For example, in one study expert dentists ordered fewer diagnostic examinations than beginners, and tended to make decisions based on prior patient experiences rather than didactic coursework.[16] In addition, analyses of self-reported thought processes indicate that forward reasoning is used more frequently by more experienced medical residents in the critical care setting than novices.[17] To say that the use of forward and backward reasoning is mutually exclusive, however, may be an oversimplification; experts and novices alike may use both patterns of reasoning, but simply may display a predilection toward one over the other.[23,24] It seems necessary then, for a symptom-based diagnostic process to be flexible enough for clinicians to preferentially use the pattern of reasoning that best fits the situation and the clinician's level of experience.

Characteristics of the case also influence the type of reasoning processes selected. Findings from one study established that straightforward cases were better processed by medical residents than ambiguous ones, although the memory for facts that characterized the cases was higher in the ambiguous case than the simple case.[25] In another study, the time spent on the diagnosis, the memory for case findings, and the number of inferences from case findings were found to be significantly elevated in a problematic case compared to a case that was seen as simple.[26] Medical specialists also processed cases in their specialties faster and more accurately than cases outside their expertise, although recall for findings within the cases and pathophysiological explanations were not significantly different.[27] These findings indicate the importance of case complexity or ambiguity to the pattern of clinical reasoning employed, in which cases that are perceived as complex are characterized by a more careful backward approach, and cases that are perceived as simpler are characterized by a faster forward approach. Although the rate of recall for findings between ambiguous and simple cases may differ with clinical expertise, the goal of the diagnostic process remains to identify underlying pathophysiological explanations for patients' symptoms and signs regardless of case complexity.

Conclusion

Diagnostic reasoning involves a combination of pattern recognition and hypothetico-deductive reasoning. The type of reasoning that is involved with diagnosis depends on the expertise of the clinician. This highlights the need for a diagnostic process for physical therapists that is flexible yet thorough to accommodate for all levels of experience. Subsequent chapters in this book are organized around a process for symptom-based diagnosis, which is described in the next chapter. This approach supports the need for thoroughness and efficiency, as well as the flexibility needed for the various patient/client presentations and types of clinical thinking displayed by clinicians at all levels of experience.

References

1. Edwards I, Jones M, Carr J, Braunack-Mayer A, Jensen GM. Clinical reasoning strategies in physical therapy. *Phys Ther.* 2004;84(4):312–330; discussion 331–335.

2. Guide to Physical Therapist Practice. Second Edition. American Physical Therapy Association. *Phys Ther.* 2001;81(1):9–746.

3. *Clinical Practice Guideline, Acute Low Back Problems in Adults.* Silver Spring, MD: Agency for Health Care Policy and Research Publications Clearinghouse; 1994.

4. Boissonnault WG. *Examination in Physical Therapy Practice: Screening for Medical Disease.* New York, NY: Churchill-Livingstone; 1995.

5. Sizer PS, Jr., Brismee JM, Cook C. Medical screening for red flags in the diagnosis and management of musculoskeletal spine pain. *Pain Pract.* 2007;7(1):53–71.

6. Leerar PJ, Boissonnault W, Domholdt E, Roddey T. Documentation of red flags by physical therapists for patients with low back pain. *J Man Manip Ther.* 2007;15(1):42–49.

7. Henschke N, Maher CG, Refshauge KM. A systematic review identifies five "red flags" to screen for vertebral fracture in patients with low back pain. *J Clin Epidemiol.* 2008;61(2):110–118.

8. De Neys W. Automatic-heuristic and executive-analytic processing during reasoning: chronometric and dual-task considerations. *Q J Exp Psychol (Colchester).* 2006;59(6):1070–1100.

9. Lobach DF, Hammond WE. Computerized decision support based on a clinical practice guideline improves compliance with care standards. *Am J Med.* 1997;102(1):89–98.

10. Sucher JF, Moore FA, Todd SR, Sailors RM, McKinley BA. Computerized clinical decision support: a technology to implement and validate evidence based guidelines. *J Trauma.* 2008;64(2):520–537.

11. Crowley RS, Naus GJ, Friedman CP. Development of visual diagnostic expertise in pathology. *Proc AMIA Symp.* 2001:125–129.

12. Payne VL, Crowley R. Assessing the use of cognitive heuristic representativeness in clinical reasoning. *AMIA Annu Symp Proc.* 2008:571–575.

13. Dawson NV. Physician judgment in clinical settings: methodological influences and cognitive performance. *Clin Chem.* 1993;39(7):1468–1478; discussion 1478–1480.

14. Elstein AS. Heuristics and biases: selected errors in clinical reasoning. *Acad Med.* 1999;74(7):791–794.

15. Noll E, Key A, Jensen G. Clinical reasoning of an experienced physiotherapist: insight into clinician decision-making regarding low back pain. *Physiother Res Int.* 2001;6(1):40–51.

16. Crespo KE, Torres JE, Recio ME. Reasoning process characteristics in the diagnostic skills of beginner, competent, and expert dentists. *J Dent Educ.* 2004;68(12):1235–1244.

17. Young JS, Smith RL, Guerlain S, Nolley B. How residents think and make medical decisions: implications for education and patient safety. *Am Surg.* 2007; 73(6):548–553; discussion 553–554.

18. Norman GR, Brooks LR, Allen SW. Recall by expert medical practitioners and novices as a record of processing attention. *J Exp Psychol Learn Mem Cogn.* 1989;15(6):1166–1174.

19. Patel VL, Groen GJ, Arocha JF. Medical expertise as a function of task difficulty. *Mem Cognit.* 1990; 18(4):394–406.

20. Kushniruk AW, Patel VL, Marley AA. Small worlds and medical expertise: implications for medical cognition and knowledge engineering. *Int J Med Inform.* 1998;49(3):255–271.

21. Norman GR, Eva KW. Doggie diagnosis, diagnostic success and diagnostic reasoning strategies: an alternative view. *Med Educ.* 2003;37(8):676–677.

22. Joseph GM, Patel VL. Domain knowledge and hypothesis generation in diagnostic reasoning. *Med Decis Making.* 1990;10(1):31–46.

23. Ferreira MB, Garcia-Marques L, Sherman SJ, Sherman JW. Automatic and controlled components of judgment and decision making. *J Pers Soc Psychol.* 2006; 91(5):797–813.

24. May S, Greasley A, Reeve S, Withers S. Expert therapists use specific clinical reasoning processes in the assessment and management of patients with shoulder pain: a qualitative study. *Aust J Physiother.* 2008;54(4): 261–266.

25. Mamede S, Schmidt HG, Rikers R. Diagnostic errors and reflective practice in medicine. *J Eval Clin Pract.* 2007;13(1):138–145.

26. Mamede S, Schmidt HG, Rikers RM, Penaforte JC, Coelho-Filho JM. Breaking down automaticity: case ambiguity and the shift to reflective approaches in clinical reasoning. *Med Educ.* 2007;41(12):1185–1192.

27. Rikers RM, Schmidt HG, Boshuizen HP, Linssen GC, Wesseling G, Paas FG. The robustness of medical expertise: clinical case processing by medical experts and subexperts. *Am J Psychol.* 2002;115(4):609–629.

CHAPTER 4

How to Use This Book

■ *Hugh G. Watts, MD*

IN THIS CHAPTER:

■ A detailed description of the process for symptom-based diagnosis that is used throughout this book

Introduction

In the first chapter, two definitions of the term *diagnosis* were given. The term can refer to (1) the *process* of deciding the cause of an illness as well as to (2) the result of that process, which is a *label* that indicates the putative cause of the problem. The focus of this book is the first definition, that is, the systematic technique of making a diagnosis. This chapter provides a method by which a diagnosis can be made and is the method that is used throughout this book.

Principle of "Economy of Diagnoses"

If a patient has left shoulder pain and a cough, has reported paresthesias in the left hand, and on examination demonstrates a constricted pupil in the left eye, what is the likely cause?

One could explain the shoulder pain as due to a rotator cuff tear, the cough due to a common cold, the hand paresthesias due to carpal tunnel syndrome, and the pupillary constriction to a congenital abnormality. Although it is possible that the problems could have been caused by four different diagnoses, health care thinking, and science in general, prefers the simplest hypothesis that can reasonably explain the multiple phenomena—in this case a Pancoast tumor of the upper lung invading into the region of the brachial plexus and the sympathetic ganglia, resulting in Horner's syndrome.

William of Occam, a 14th-century philosopher-theologian,[1] is credited with enunciating the principle that when having to choose among competing hypotheses, one should favor the simplest one. Or stated differently, when multiple explanations are available for a phenomenon, the simplest version is preferred. This concept is commonly known as "Occam's razor" (where *razor* refers to a tool in a logical argument used to cut absurdities from philosophical discourse).

The concept of parsimony of diagnosis has not gone unchallenged. Saint's triad, by Hilliard and Weinberger, emphasizes the importance of considering the possibility of multiple separate diagnoses in a patient *whenever his or her history and the results of the physical examination are atypical of any single condition*.[2] Although in the medical care of children, the probability of several disease processes occurring simultaneously is less likely, be aware that, as the patient ages, there is an increasing likelihood of disease developing in multiple organ systems.

Was Occam wrong? No. Occam did not state that the simpler explanation is always right or that the more complex explanation is always wrong. He emphasized that one should *start from the simplest possible explanation* and only make it more complex when absolutely necessary. This principle—the *economy of diagnoses*—has been a cornerstone of differential diagnosis and is still the best approach to making a differential diagnosis.

The process of making a diagnosis outlined in this chapter is modulated by the need for efficiency by the physical therapist. A physical therapist cannot spend several hours with each patient. It is important to develop a clinically viable process that gets to the diagnosis as efficiently as possible.

The Diagnostic Process

Barriers to Communication

In order for a physical therapist to make a reasonable diagnosis, information must flow freely between the patient and the therapist. Barriers to communication are those situations that may interfere with this proper flow of information.

Why then does our discussion of the diagnostic process begin by listing barriers to communication? Any information that is gathered is always filtered. Hence, the physical therapist should be aware of the presence of possible biases so that the information that is collected can be as free of distortions as possible.

In trying to make a diagnosis, obtaining accurate information is paramount. Anything that interferes with the proper flow of information needs to be identified and dealt with. Barriers to communication warn the therapist to recognize possible interactions between the therapist and the patient that may lead the therapist astray when trying to make a diagnosis. An obvious example would be a patient who does not speak the same language as the therapist. Even among patients who think they are speaking the same language, slang and other alternative word usages can impair communication. Wide cultural differences between the patient and the local community, wide generational gaps, or gender-sensitive issues may also impede the flow of information.

Another barrier to communication is the *informal referral*. Physical therapists are frequently subject to direct informal referrals. These are the people, often fellow workers or relatives, who casually ask about a medical problem concerning them or a friend or relative. A coworker might come to you in a hallway and say, "I fell this weekend and now my knee is swollen. Would you take a look and tell me if I need to see a physician?" In this informal situation, the questions you ask of "the patient" and the physical examination might not be as complete as in a formal situation. There will be no record of the visit, nor will a follow-up visit be arranged. This potentially dangerous situation is compounded by the personal relationship, because we are unlikely to think of some of the very serious diseases that might be involved, or that this friend or relative is subject to socially stigmatized activity that might be the basis of a sexually transmitted disease.

The Starting Point: Identify the Patient's Chief Concern

The process of making a diagnosis starts with the patient's presenting concern or symptom. Classically, the subject of differential diagnosis has been taught to physical therapy students using a body system approach. Here the term system refers to the anatomical or physiological system of the body involved in the disease such as the cardiac or neurological system. Early on, physical therapists learn about the pain that can result from cardiac disease or the particular limp that might result from a neurological disease. Patients, however, do not arrive at the clinic or office announcing that they have a cardiac or a neurological problem. Instead, a patient presents, for example, with shoulder pain. That shoulder pain could be caused by cardiac disease or gallbladder inflammation irritating the underside of the diaphragm or cervical disk disease or a rotator cuff tear. Another patient might be concerned about a feeling of generalized weakness that could be secondary to a metabolic disorder, a neurological disease, or psychological depression. Hence, the method taught here begins with a patient who presents with a symptom, the cause of which may originate in any of a number of different body systems.

Is a system approach the wrong way to initially teach students differential diagnosis? We believe not. The student first needs a grounding of information to work with. Ultimately, however, the student needs a method for integrating this knowledge learned from the *system* texts into a useful clinical tool.

Symptoms Versus Signs

We have based this text on the symptoms that a patient brings to our attention. Some of the chapter titles suggest signs rather than symptoms. Is there a significant difference between terms symptom and sign? By some definitions[2] a symptom is "a subjective indication of a disease or change in condition as perceived by the patient," whereas a sign is "an objective finding perceived by the examiner."[2,3] Other definitions,[4,5] however, do not make as clear a differentiation. Instead, they define a symptom as "a characteristic sign or indication of a disorder or disease." In practice also, the distinction is not always clear. If a patient limps in to your clinic and says, "I limp," is that a sign or a symptom or both? If the mother of a child says, "My child limps," is the limp the mother has observed a sign or a symptom? We feel that this is not a productive debate and, therefore, use the term *chief concern* as including both signs and symptoms.

Special Concerns

In this book, the term *special concerns* denotes situations in which the therapist needs to be especially wary. It does *not* mean that the therapist should stop thinking through the diagnostic possibilities and immediately refer the patient elsewhere.

We are all aware that some cardiac pathology may be felt by the patient as pain in the medial aspect of the upper arm on the left. Understandably, most therapists would be alarmed if a patient stated that the upper medial arm hurt, especially if the pain was worsened by exertion. However, therapists are less likely to be aware that gallbladder inflammation irritating the underside of the diaphragm may give right-sided shoulder pain, or that hip disease can be felt as pain in the anteromedial aspect of the knee. Although the consequences of missing these connections are less grave than with the cardiac disease, these cautions need to be heeded.

Some *special concerns* need to be individualized to the presenting symptom. The information that a 45-year-old male smokes three packs of cigarettes a day would certainly represent a cause for caution if he were presenting with shoulder pain because of the possibility of a malignant lung tumor as the cause, but not necessarily if he was concerned with foot pain that appears to be secondary to plantar fasciitis.

Some situations that require special attention are patients who arrive with:

- A nonspecific diagnosis from a referring physician. A patient referred with a diagnosis of *Shoulder Pain, Low Back Pain,* or *Neck Pain* should be seen as one who arrived with no diagnosis. Pain is a symptom, not a pathology. The fact that a patient's symptom is translated into Latin (eg, *cervicalgia* for "neck pain") does not change the situation that this is a patient who arrived without a diagnosis.

- Changes in symptoms since the last visit or since the patient last saw the referring physician.

- Unusual pain patterns.

- Night pain that is felt as a deep ache and not affected by positional change. However, note that the isolation and silence of darkness often makes patients feel worse at nighttime.

- Unrelenting pain.

- Migratory pains.

- Nonanatomical distribution of pains.

- Acute changes:
  - with increased body temperature
  - sudden weakness
  - sudden inability to bear weight.

- Signs of ischemia, for example:
  - decreased pulses in the extremities
  - smooth, shiny skin
  - loss of hair over extremities.

- Sensory changes:
  - paresthesias
  - sensory loss
  - pain that radiates.

- Recent unintended weight loss.

- Genitourinary problems, especially urinary retention.

- Rapid onset of limited coordination, impaired special senses, or other neurological signs.

When such conditions are noted, this does not mean that the patient needs immediate referral back to the physician, because the conditions may well be part of the disease for which the patient was referred to the physical therapist to begin with. For example, a patient might be referred for a program to regain range of motion of the hip following a hemorrhage in the psoas muscle resulting from anticoagulant therapy for her atrial fibrillation (Box 4-1).

TIM VaDeTuCoNe: A Database of Possible Causes

When using our method of making a diagnosis, one cannot overemphasize the importance of making a list, mentally or written, of all possible causes. This is the database from which the diagnosis is determined and forms the basis for future decisions concerning intervention. This list is a starting point and needs to be sorted by the discriminating questions asked during the history taking followed by the re-sorting done with the help of the appropriately discriminating physical findings.

Such a list of possible causes of a symptom can be very long, making it difficult to remember them all. Lists of diagnoses, subdivided by anatomical/physiological system, such as those given in the American Physical Therapy Association's *Guide to Physical Therapy Practice*,[6] are not as useful to a physical therapist whose starting point is the patient's presenting symptom. Just listing diseases as they come to mind, however, also is not an efficient approach.

The physical therapist needs to organize the disease processes in some way to facilitate the use of the method. One convenient approach is to use a mnemonic. A *mnemonic* is an aid to memory (from the Greek *mnemos*, meaning "memory"). We have developed a mnemonic that we have found helpful in teaching the method of differential diagnosis to physical therapists: TIM VaDeTuCoNe (Box 4-2).

Who is TIM VaDeTuCoNe? TIM VaDeTuCoNe is an artificial construct. It was designed to allow the physical therapist to list the potential diseases in an organized fashion. The order chosen for those items was one that would be relevant to a physical therapist. Why are some letters in uppercase and some in lowercase?—Simply to provide enough vowels to make the word easier to sound out and to remember. To someone new to this mnemonic, it may seem clumsy and no more convenient than other mnemonics or than not using a mnemonic at all. However, we have used this very effectively with both entry-level doctoral students and post-professional DPT students with many years of clinical expertise. They have found it easy to remember and that it guides them in making a list of possible diagnoses so that uncommon problems are not overlooked. Many students refer to it as the "TIM list."

In this book, each chapter that describes possible causes of a symptom will begin with a Chapter Preview (see Chapter 7). The previews are sorted using TIM VaDeTuCoNe, and also by the estimates of the condition's prevalence in society.

BOX 4-1 **Getting Started with the Diagnostic Process**

- Barriers to communication are potential problems with any patient who arrives with any symptom; hence, we have not listed them in each of the following chapters.

- Special concerns may differ from one presenting symptom to another. As a consequence, we have listed them at the top of every diagnostic list in the following chapters.

BOX 4-2 **TIM VaDeTuCoNe—An Artificial Construct**

Trauma

Inflammation

Metabolic

Vascular

Degenerative

Tumor

Congenital

Neurogenic/Psychogenic

Into which category does a particular disease fit? That can be a problem. There may be more than one process going on. Infection in a bone may cause ischemia of the bone tissue, which in turn will cause inflammation in the surrounding viable bone. However, for simplicity, we have arbitrarily chosen the primary process as the one for categorizing.

Sometimes it is difficult to choose between categories. For example should an arteriovenous (AV) malformation be considered a "vascular disease" or a "tumor" or perhaps a "congenital malformation"? All could fit. In this situation, we have found that most physical therapists think of an AV malformation as a vascular problem, hence we have put it into that category. By that same thinking we have made several arbitrary decisions for consistency across the many chapters of the book.

The choices we have made do not reflect our concept of the pathophysiology. For example, consider a prolapsed intervertebral disk. Should it go under the "Trauma" or "Degeneration" category? That might depend on whether the prolapse occurred in a 15-year-old as a result of a motor vehicle accident or in a 45-year-old after lifting a heavy load. We also recognize that ultimately, the prolapsed disk will irritate the nerve root through local inflammation. So should the disease be listed under "Inflammation"? We have made an arbitrary decision to categorize all nerve compression under Trauma.

Do "Neurogenic" and "Psychogenic" really belong together? We still needed a category to place items such as schizophrenia, anxiety, malingering, or, for example, dystonia musculorum as a cause of torticollis. Ultimately, all disease processes that occur in the brain (whether neurogenic or psychogenic) have a common pathway of electrical impulses traveling between cells, so the separation into a duality is artificial. Hence, we feel that these terms can be grouped together.

We have studiously avoided a "Miscellaneous" category. If such a category were used, it could contain so many diagnoses that were difficult to remember that the process would be counterproductive.

Let's take a look now at what the individual categories of TIM VaDeTuCoNe include.

Trauma (T)

The Trauma category may include:

- Rupture of a tendon or muscle.
- Strain: a tear of muscle tissue.
- Sprain: a tear of joint ligaments.
- Fracture:
  - Cortical or metaphyseal
  - Stress
  - Avulsion: piece of bone to which muscle is attached is pulled off but the muscle is intact
  - Osteochondral
  - Physeal.
- Dislocation.
- Mechanical includes the obvious causes above but we have also included nerve entrapment and nerve instability.

Inflammation (I)

The inflammation category has been divided into "Aseptic" and "Septic." The Aseptic subcategory has been put first, because, again, this is a category of illness that may be more likely to be overlooked. Aseptic processes are those that are not directly involved with microorganisms, whereas septic conditions are caused by microorganisms such as bacteria. Although some aseptic conditions are the result of the body responding to the antigens on the microorganism (eg, Lyme disease), the condition might not be considered a septic process. However, most physical therapists would put it under Septic, so that is where we have placed it.

This category *may* include:

- **Aseptic** (ie, noninfectious):
  - Autoimmune diseases such as rheumatoid arthritis, and associated rheumatoid diseases such as lupus and scleroderma, arthritis associated with inflammatory bowel disease, or psoriasis.
  - Reactive arthritis (Reiter's, hepatitis B, allergic). Some would include all of the associated rheumatoid diseases mentioned above under reactive arthritis.
  - Postsurgical capsulitis tendinitis when tendon inflammation is truly present. Some pathologies are sometimes called tendinitis but are not associated with an inflammatory response. These are now

more commonly termed tendinoses, or tendinopathies, such as rotator cuff, and are listed under the "Degenerative" column.

- **Septic** (ie, infectious):
  - *Acute:* bacterial (eg, *Staphylococcus*), fungal, or parasitic.
  - *Chronic:* bacterial (eg, *tuberculosis*), viral, fungal, or parasitic.

Metabolic (M)

The Metabolic category may include:

- Diabetes, gout, hyperparathyroidism, endocrine disorders, and issues related to pregnancy.
- Toxic (eg, lead poisoning).
- Envenomation (eg, black widow spider bites).
- Ethanol-induced polyneuropathy.
- Chronic drug use—either illegal drugs or overuse of legal drugs—a problem that is easily overlooked.
- Pulmonary insufficiency caused, for example, by asbestos inhalation.

Vascular (Va)

The Vascular category may include:

- Cardiac.
- Arterial: "too little" (eg, ischemia, acute [infarction], chronic insufficiency, avascular necrosis) or "too much" (eg, bleeding or hematoma).
- Venous (eg, thrombosis).
- Lymphatic (eg, lymphedema).

Degenerative (De)

The Degenerative category may include:

- *Tendinoses:* As outlined above, some pathologies that are sometimes called tendinitis but are not associated with an inflammatory response are now more commonly termed tendinoses, or tendinopathies, such as a rotator cuff tear.
- *Arthroses:* Similar to conditions of the tendon, joint pathologies formerly known as osteoarthritis are now more commonly known as osteoarthrosis and are considered degenerative.

Tumor (Tu)

The Tumor category may include:

- *Malignant Primary:* A malignant primary tumor is one at its site of origin, for example,

an osteosarcoma in the femur or a bronchogenic carcinoma in the lung.

- *Malignant Metastatic:* This type of tumor is the result of spread of the primary tumor away from the organ of origin to a new and distant site. In the past, the term *secondary tumor* was used synonymously with *metastatic tumor*. Now the term secondary tumor refers to a new tumor, of a different tissue origin than the first, caused by the effects of the treatment of the first tumor. An example would be an osteosarcoma of the ileum resulting from radiation treatment to a Ewing's sarcoma in the pelvis several decades earlier.
- *Benign:* Benign tumors are ones that characteristically do not metastasize and usually are not a threat to life but can be locally aggressive and destructive (ie, pigmented villonodular synovitis).

Congenital (Co)

The Congenital category may include:

- Congenital anomalies.
- Developmental conditions, such as developmental dislocation of the hip.
- Hereditary diseases.

Neurogenic/Psychogenic (Ne)

The Neurogenic/Psychogenic category may include:

- Psychological diseases such as neuroses and psychoses and malingering conditions such as amyotrophic lateral sclerosis or spinal muscular atrophy.

Note that spinal cord injuries have been placed under the Trauma category.

Does this system work for nonpain symptoms such as weakness, tripping, palpitations, and joint contractures? We have found that it does. However, the differentiation into *remote* versus *local* sources of the problem is not relevant to these diagnoses, so it has been omitted.

Remote Versus Local Source of Pain

We all have a tendency to look for causes of pain that are found locally in the region where the patient complains of the symptom.

A moment's reflection shows that such an approach is inappropriately limited. The source of such a pain could be *remote* instead of *local*. By **local** pain we mean pain caused by a pathologic process in the immediate region of the symptom, eg, muscle tissue rupture. By **remote pain** we mean the pain that is caused at some other point than where the patient feels the symptom, for example, pain felt in the foot as a result of a tumor at the fibular head pressing on the peroneal nerve or referred pain felt in the anteromedial aspect of the knee due to a pathologic process in the ipsilateral hip. Because physical therapists are more likely to overlook remote causes of pain, we give emphasis to these remote sources of pain. For this same reason, in the diagnostic lists in the individual chapters of this book, the remote possibilities are always given first so they will be less likely to be overlooked.

When dealing with pain in the knee the difference between *Remote* and *Local* causes is reasonably clear. However, the closer the pain is to the trunk, the more difficult this differentiation becomes. For example, when considering neck pain-is a disk impingement on the nerve roots at the neck *Remote* or *Local*? Is mid-lumbar back pain that is the result of pancreatitis *Remote* or *Local*? To answer these questions, ponder how most physical therapists think about the particular clinical problem. In the neck, most physical therapists would certainly think of cervical disk disease as a source of pain in the neck, hence we have included this under *Local*. However, with mid-lumbar pain, many physical therapists would not think about pathology in an abdominal organ (eg, pancreatitis) or great vessel pathology (eg, an aortic aneurysm) as being a source of the pain so could benefit from being reminded about the other possible sources of the pain. Thus they are listed under *Remote*.

Some readers may be unsure whether we consider systemic diseases, such as gout or rheumatoid arthritis, *Remote* or *Local*. We consider them as *Local*, in that the pathology, ie, the swollen, hot joint is local.

Is *Remote pain* the same as *Referred pain*? **Referred pain**, as it is usually understood, comes from confusion on the part of the brain at deciphering the source of pain. When dealing with body organs that have no surface component, the brain has difficulty deciding where the pain originates. It will assign the source to the region on the surface that shares the same innervation as the structure deep inside. Hence pain from the heart may be misinterpreted as coming from the medial aspect of the upper arm or axillary region. Pain in the hip may be misinterpreted as coming from the anteromedial aspect of the knee that shares the same innervation by the obturator nerve. However, the pain experienced in the hand secondary to a thoracic outlet compression of the nerves is not *referred* pain. The brain is not confused as it is when a patient feels pain in the axilla after injury to the heart muscle. Thus we have two separate ways in which a pathologic process that takes place in one location is felt in another. We have combined these two and use the term *Remote Pain*.

What Follows the Making of a TIM VaDeTuCoNe List?

A diagnosis begins by gathering a complete list of potential diagnoses that could result in the patient's symptoms. These are then sorted by the likelihood of occurrence given the patient's demographics. Directed questions are then asked to eliminate as many inappropriate diagnoses as possible. Specific physical examination tests are selected to sort the remaining diagnoses to eliminate inappropriate ones.

We have provided Case Demonstration chapters throughout this textbook to show the application of the diagnostic process to example patient cases. These chapters are structured around the steps of the diagnostic process presented in Box 4-3, which are discussed in more detail next:

1. Identify the patient's chief concern.
2. List *barriers to communication*.
3. List *special concerns*.
4. Draw a timeline and sketch the anatomy if needed. It is often useful to sketch a horizontal line, to an approximate scale, representing the time over which the patient's various symptoms and signs appeared, marking significant events (Fig. 4-1). Drawing the anatomy can be especially useful for remembering the location of the

BOX 4-3 **Steps of the Diagnostic Process**	
Step 1 Identify the patient's chief concern.	**Step 8** Re-sort the diagnostic hypothesis list based on the patient's responses to specific questioning.
Step 2 Identify *barriers to communication.*	
Step 3 Identify *special concerns.*	**Step 9** Perform tests to differentiate among the remaining diagnostic hypotheses.
Step 4 Create a symptom timeline and sketch the anatomy (if needed).	
Step 5 Create a diagnostic hypothesis list considering all possible forms of *remote* and *local* pathology that could cause the patient's chief concern.	**Step 10** Re-sort the diagnostic hypothesis list based on the patient's responses to specific tests.
	Step 11 Decide on a diagnostic impression.
Step 6 Sort the diagnostic hypothesis list by epidemiology and specific case characteristics.	**Step 12** Determine the appropriate patient disposition.
Step 7 Ask specific questions to rule specific conditions or pathological categories less likely.	

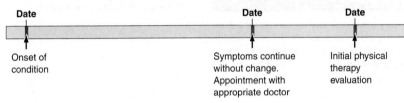

Date

Date

Date

↑ Onset of condition

↑ Symptoms continue without change. Appointment with appropriate doctor

↑ Initial physical therapy evaluation

FIGURE 4-1 Sample timeline.

internal organs in regard to remote causes of pain. This can be particularly useful if the reader's knowledge of visceral anatomy is not strong.

5. List possible *remote* and *local* diagnoses. These are listed first since these are more readily overlooked:
   - List the anatomic regions possibly involved: thorax, abdomen, pelvis, etc.
   - Within each anatomic region, list the possible organs that could cause the symptom: abdomen, pancreas, gallbladder, liver, spleen, great vessels, etc.

For each of the organs, one could make a TIM list of possible diagnoses, but that would be excessively tedious. If a reader's knowledge of visceral anatomy is not strong, however, then he or she should consider this step.

6. Sort all of the potential causes into clusters based on the patient's demographics:
   - Reasonably likely
   - Possible
   - Unlikely.

7. Take a history. Ask the *most discriminating* relevant questions to rule out as many options as possible with the fewest questions. Ask yourself, "Does this question asked exclude or minimize the likelihood of one or more of the diagnoses on the TIM list?" If not, change or eliminate the question.

8. Based on the answers to the questions, re-sort the potential causes into clusters as you did in step 6:
   - Reasonably likely
   - Possible
   - Unlikely.

9. Conduct a physical examination. Look for the *most discriminating* physical findings to rule out as many options as possible with the fewest tests. Again, ask yourself, "Does this physical test that I'm doing exclude or minimize the likelihood of one or more of the diagnoses on the TIM list?"

10. Once again, re-sort the potential causes into clusters:
    - Reasonably likely
    - Possible
    - Unlikely.

11. Select the most probable diagnosis (the *diagnostic impression*) for further evaluation to establish a treatment plan. Remember the principle of economy of diagnoses (Occam's razor).

12. Determine the appropriate patient disposition.

Conclusion

This chapter described the process for making a diagnosis. The process begins with identification of the patient's chief concern, communication barriers, and features of the case that raise special concerns. It continues with the formation of a diagnostic hypothesis list—a database—consisting of all possible local and remote causes of the symptoms and signs. The database is then sorted by probability on the basis of epidemiology, specific questions, and specific physical examination findings. Now turn to the next chapter for an example of how one might go through the process.

References

1. Drachman D. Occam's razor, geriatric syndromes, and the dizzy patient. *Ann Intern Med.* 2000;132:403–404.
2. *Mosby's Medical, Nursing, and Allied Health Dictionary.* 4th ed. St. Louis, MO: Mosby; 1994.
3. *Merriam-Webster's Collegiate Dictionary.* 11th ed. Springfield, MA: Merriam-Webster; 2003.
4. *Stedman's Medical Dictionary.* 27th ed. Philadelphia, PA: Lippincott Williams & Wilkins; 2004.
5. *Oxford English Dictionary.* 2nd ed. New York: Oxford University Press; 1989.
6. *Guide to Physical Therapist Practice.* 2nd ed. Alexandria, VA: American Physical Therapy Association; 2003.

CHAPTER 5

Case Demonstration: Shoulder

■ *Hugh G. Watts, MD*
Acknowledgment: Susan Layfield, PT, DPT, OCS

NOTE: This case demonstration was developed using the diagnostic process described in Chapter 4 and is designed to demonstrate that process. As Chapter 4 discussed, the diagnostic process begins with identification of the patient's chief concern. Communication barriers are then identified in order to establish features of the case that may influence the ability to gather information during the diagnostic process. Features of the case that raise special concerns are then established, in order to prioritize the additional information gathering required.

The process continues with the formation of a diagnostic hypothesis list consisting of all possible local and remote causes of the symptom. The hypothesis list is then sorted by probability on the basis of epidemiology, specific questions, and specific physical examination findings. The reader is encouraged to use this diagnostic process in order to ensure that thorough diagnostic clinical reasoning has been applied to all patient encounters. A brief list of the steps in the diagnostic process is given next. If more elaboration is required on the information presented in this chapter, please consult Chapters 1 through 4.

THE DIAGNOSTIC PROCESS

Step 1 Identify the patient's chief concern.
Step 2 Identify *barriers to communication*.
Step 3 Identify *special concerns*.
Step 4 Create a symptom timeline and sketch the anatomy (if needed).
Step 5 Create a diagnostic hypothesis list considering all possible forms of *remote* and *local* pathology that could cause the patient's chief concern.
Step 6 Sort the diagnostic hypothesis list by epidemiology and specific case characteristics.
Step 7 Ask specific questions to rule specific conditions or pathological categories less likely.

Step 8 Re-sort the diagnostic hypothesis list based on the patient's responses to specific questioning.
Step 9 Perform tests to differentiate among the remaining diagnostic hypotheses.
Step 10 Re-sort the diagnostic hypothesis list based on the patient's responses to specific tests.
Step 11 Decide on a diagnostic impression.
Step 12 Determine the appropriate patient disposition.

Case Description

Charles T. is a 58-year-old male with a referral to physical therapy by an orthopedic surgeon with the diagnosis of *Left Rotator Cuff Tendinitis*. His chief concern is an intermittent sharp left anterior shoulder pain, the onset of which was 2 weeks ago. He seems concerned because he cannot recall a mechanism of injury nor does he comment on any swelling in his shoulder or arm. The pain is aggravated by initial exposure to a cold draft, for example, when taking out the trash, and when square dancing with his wife during the first two to three twirls with his left arm lifted up and outstretched. Over the past 2 weeks, he believes his symptoms have not changed in frequency or intensity. He denies any associated pain or symptoms in his midback or upper extremity.

Mr. T is an accountant. His recreation includes square dancing two to three times a week. On the verbal confirmation of his intake form, Mr. T does not report any recent health issues or significant medical or surgical history. Recently, he has been attempting to stay on a diet that his wife initiated for him. His weight loss is inconsistent per his report. He believes he has lost 5 lbs in the past 4 weeks. Mr. T has a smoking history of 20 years and quit 10 years ago. In his family history, his father died of a heart attack at age 70 and his mother is 80 years old and healthy.

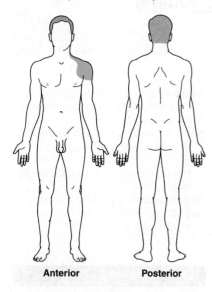

Anterior   **Posterior**

Teaching Comments: Clinicians need to view the anatomical representation of the region where the pain is located with care. Reliance on the accuracy of the patient's interpretation of the location of pain should not supersede the clinical reasoning process nor prohibit the therapist from examining the patient for other sources of pain. Instead it should serve as a potential starting point.

STEP #1: Identify the patient's chief concern.

- Intermittent sharp left shoulder pain that interferes with recreational activities

STEP #2: Identify *barriers to communication*.
- None

STEP #3: Identify *special concerns*.
Several special concerns were identified during the initial intake and questioning that raised concern regarding potential underlying etiologies of the patient's chief concern. These include:

- Age of the patient
- History of smoking
- Obesity
- Sedentary profession.

Teaching Comments: One body of literature that is helpful is the data collected for the Framingham Heart Study. The Framingham study is a long-term project that originally began in 1948 and has since been expanded to a third generation with the objective of identifying common factors or characteristics that contribute to cardiovascular disease (CVD) by following its development over a long period of time in a large group of participants who had not yet developed overt symptoms of CVD or experience a heart attack or stroke.

STEP #4: Create a symptom timeline and sketch the anatomy (if needed).

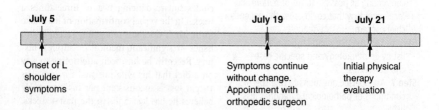

July 5	July 19	July 21
Onset of L shoulder symptoms	Symptoms continue without change. Appointment with orthopedic surgeon	Initial physical therapy evaluation

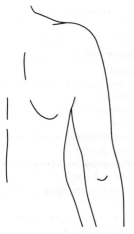

Example of PT's sketch

Teaching Comments: In the case of Mr. T, this step may seem irrelevant because his timeline is simple. However, it does illustrate the lack of change during the 2-week period of aggravation. It also allows you to appreciate the temporal features of competing diagnoses. The length of his symptoms illustrates that it is unlikely that any acute perforations or ruptures are the cause of his pain. This temporal feature combined with the intensity of his symptoms (he continues to work, perform household chores, and participate in square dancing) furthers the unlikelihood that he has experienced any acute perforations or rupture as the cause of his pain.

Teaching Comments: Clinicians need to remind themselves of the proximity of various organs to the region of the symptoms their patients are reporting. Perhaps even more important is the review of the neurotube development of various organs, which is the theory behind referred pain.

STEP #5: Create a diagnostic hypothesis list considering all possible forms of *remote* and *local* pathology that could cause the patient's chief concern.

Teaching Comments: As recommended in Chapter 4, it may be helpful for the clinician to break this step down even further to reduce the risk of "missed" potential hypotheses.

STEP #6: Sort the diagnostic hypothesis list by epidemiology and specific case characteristics.

Teaching Comments: Conditions that are shown with a strikethrough are those that are determined to be less likely based on the reasons that follow the hypothesis. It is understood that some may return to the list following questioning.

Remote

T   Trauma

   Cervical spine disk herniation
   Internal organ injuries:

   • Diaphragm
   • Liver
   • Lung
   • Spleen

Remote

T   Trauma

   Cervical spine disk herniation
   ~~Internal organ injuries~~ (very unlikely due to lack of trauma to the trunk)

   • ~~Diaphragm~~
   • ~~Liver~~
   • ~~Lung~~
   • ~~Spleen~~

Post–laparoscopic procedure	~~Post–laparoscopic procedure~~ (no surgical history)
Thoracic outlet syndrome	Thoracic outlet syndrome

I   Inflammation

I   Inflammation

Aseptic

Aseptic

Acute cholecystitis	~~Acute cholecystitis~~ (presentation, no scapular pain)
Costochondritis	~~Costochondritis~~ (presentation, no scapular pain)
Gaseous distention of the stomach	~~Gaseous distention of the stomach~~ (presentation)
Inflammatory bowel disease	~~Inflammatory bowel disease~~ (absent medical history)

Rheumatoid arthritis–like diseases of the cervical spine:
- Inflammatory muscle disease
- Psoriatic arthritis
- Scleroderma
- Systemic lupus erythematosus

Rheumatoid arthritis–like diseases of the cervical spine:
- Inflammatory muscle disease
- Psoriatic arthritis
- ~~Scleroderma~~ (presentation, patient sex)
- ~~Systemic lupus erythematosus~~ (presentation, patient sex)

Septic

Septic

Acute viral/idiopathic pericarditis	~~Acute viral/idiopathic pericarditis~~ (presentation, time course)
Cat-scratch disease	~~Cat-scratch disease~~ (presentation)
Cervical epidural abscess	Cervical epidural abscess
Cervical lymphadenitis	~~Cervical lymphadenitis~~ (presentation)
Gastric ulcer	~~Gastric ulcer~~ (presentation)
Hepatitis	~~Hepatitis~~ (presentation)
Perihepatitis	~~Perihepatitis~~ (presentation)
Pleuritis	~~Pleuritis~~ (presentation)
Pneumonia	~~Pneumonia~~ (presentation)
Subphrenic abscess	~~Subphrenic abscess~~ (presentation)

M   Metabolic

M   Metabolic

Osteomalacia	Osteomalacia

Va   Vascular

Va   Vascular

Aneurysm	Aneurysm
Coronary artery insufficiency	Coronary artery insufficiency
Myocardial infarction	~~Myocardial infarction~~ (presentation, time course)
Pulmonary embolism	~~Pulmonary embolism~~ (presentation, time course)
Sickle cell pain crisis	~~Sickle cell pain crisis~~ (presentation, time course)

De   Degenerative

De   Degenerative

Osteoarthritis of the cervical spine	Osteoarthritis of the cervical spine

Tu   Tumor

Tu   Tumor

Malignant Primary, such as:
- Breast tumor
- Pancoast tumor

Malignant Primary, such as:
- Breast tumor
- Pancoast tumor

Malignant Metastatic:
Not applicable
Benign:
Not applicable

Co Congenital

Not applicable

Ne Neurogenic/Psychogenic

Not applicable

Malignant Metastatic:
Not applicable
Benign:
Not applicable

Co Congenital

Not applicable

Ne Neurogenic/Psychogenic

Not applicable

Teaching Comments: "Not applicable" means that the author of that chapter or case was unable to locate a reasonable diagnosis to place under that diagnostic category. The user of the textbook may be able to discover a diagnosis that would be appropriate or may choose a different category for a previously mentioned diagnoses. Each of these discrepancies would be considered acceptable. The algorithmic steps are designed to enhance the clinical reasoning, not stifle it.

Local

T   Trauma

Dislocation such as acromioclavicular, glenohumeral, or sternoclavicular joints
Fractures
Glenohumeral joint sprain/subluxation
Glenoid labrum tear
Muscle strain, such as pectoralis major, rotator cuff, upper trapezius, levator scapulae
Subacromial impingement syndrome

I   Inflammation

Aseptic
Adhesive capsulitis
Biceps tendinitis
Bursitis
Complex regional pain syndrome

Fibromyalgia

Myofascial pain syndrome

Neuralgic amyotrophy
Polymyalgia rheumatica

Local

T   Trauma

~~Dislocation such as acromioclavicular, glenohumeral, or sternoclavicular joints~~ (presentation)
~~Fractures~~ (presentation)
Glenohumeral joint sprain/subluxation
Glenoid labrum tear
Muscle strain, such as pectoralis major, rotator cuff, upper trapezius, levator scapulae
Subacromial impingement syndrome

I   Inflammation

Aseptic
~~Adhesive capsulitis~~ (presentation)
Biceps tendinitis
Bursitis
~~Complex regional pain syndrome~~ (presentation)
~~Fibromyalgia~~ (patient sex, age, presentation)
~~Myofascial pain syndrome~~ (presentation, time course)
~~Neuralgic amyotrophy~~ (initial presentation)
~~Polymyalgia rheumatica~~ (initial presentation with activity)

Reiter's syndrome

Reiter's syndrome (presentation, time course)

Rheumatoid arthritis

Rheumatoid arthritis (patient age, presentation, medical history)

Rheumatoid arthritis–like diseases of shoulder:
- Inflammatory muscle disease

- Psoriatic arthritis

- Scleroderma

- Systemic lupus erythematosus

Rheumatoid arthritis–like diseases of shoulder:
- Inflammatory muscle disease (patient sex, age, presentation)

- Psoriatic arthritis (patient sex, age, presentation)

- Scleroderma (patient sex, age, presentation)

- Systemic lupus erythematosus (patient sex, age, presentation)

Rotator cuff tendinitis

Rotator cuff tendinitis

Septic
Osteomyelitis

Septic arthritis
Skeletal tuberculosis

Septic
Osteomyelitis (presentation, medical history)

Septic arthritis (presentation)
Skeletal tuberculosis (presentation, medical history)

M Metabolic

Amyloid arthropathy
Gout
Hereditary neuralgic amyotrophy

Heterotopic ossification
Pseudogout

M Metabolic

Amyloid arthropathy (presentation)
Gout
Hereditary neuralgic amyotrophy (presentation, medical history)
Heterotopic ossification (medical history)
Pseudogout (patient sex)

Va Vascular

Aneurysm
Avascular necrosis of the humeral head
Compartment syndrome
Deep venous thrombosis, upper extremity
Quadrilateral space syndrome

Va Vascular

Aneurysm
Avascular necrosis of the humeral head
Compartment syndrome
Deep venous thrombosis, upper extremity
Quadrilateral space syndrome (patient age, presentation)

De Degenerative

Biceps tendinopathy
Osteoarthritis/osteoarthrosis
Rotator cuff tear/tendinopathy

De Degenerative

Biceps tendinopathy
Osteoarthritis/osteoarthrosis
Rotator cuff tear/tendinopathy

Tu Tumor

Malignant Primary, such as:
- Chondrosarcoma
- Lymphoma
- Osteosarcoma
- Synovial sarcoma
Malignant Metastatic, such as:
- Metastases, including from primary breast, kidney, lung, prostate, and thyroid disease

Tu Tumor

Malignant Primary, such as:
- Chondrosarcoma
- Lymphoma
- Osteosarcoma
- Synovial sarcoma
Malignant Metastatic, such as:
- Metastases, including from primary breast, kidney, lung, prostate, and thyroid disease

Benign, such as:
- Enchondroma
- Lipoma
- Osteoblastoma
- Osteochondroma
- Osteoid osteoma
- Unicameral bone cyst

Co Congenital

Not applicable

Ne Neurogenic/Psychogenic

Erb's palsy
Neuropathic arthropathy

Benign, such as:
- ~~Enchondroma~~ (patient age, presentation)
- ~~Lipoma~~ (patient age, presentation)
- Osteoblastoma
- ~~Osteochondroma~~ (patient age, presentation)
- Osteoid osteoma
- Unicameral bone cyst

Co Congenital

Not applicable

Ne Neurogenic/Psychogenic

~~Erb's palsy~~ (patient age, presentation)
~~Neuropathic arthropathy~~ (patient age, presentation, family history)

STEP #7: Ask specific questions to rule specific conditions or pathological categories less likely.

> **Teaching Comments:** The therapist should strive to ask the most discriminating relevant questions to rule less likely as many options as possible with the least number of questions to the patient. The phrase "makes less likely" is used rather than "rules out" because there are enough exceptions to the usual behavior of diseases that the less concrete term is less liable to lead one astray.

- **Do you have neck pain?** *Answer: No.*
- **Does your shoulder hurt if you move your neck?** *Answer: No.* Makes less likely cervical spine disk herniation, levator scapula and upper trapezius strain, rheumatoid arthritis–like disease of the cervical spine, and osteoarthritis/osteoarthrosis of the cervical spine.
- **Do you have any restriction in your range of shoulder motion?** *Answer: No.* Makes less likely avascular necrosis of humeral head, tendinitis, osteomyelitis of shoulder, osteoarthritis/osteoarthrosis of the shoulder complex joints, and unicameral bone cyst.
- **Is the pain constantly present?** *Answer: No.* Makes less likely avascular necrosis/osteonecrosis of humeral head and unicameral bone cyst.

- **Do you have stiffness or pain in other joints of your body?** *Answer: No.* Makes less likely gout of the shoulder, osteomalacia, and pathologies of the cervical spine.
- **Has there been any swelling, redness, or warmth in area?** *Answer: No.* Makes less likely deep venous thrombosis such as the subclavian, gout within the shoulder, septic arthritis of glenohumeral joint, osteoid osteoma, and unicameral bone cyst.

> **Teaching Comments:** The user should note that the majority of questions were asked specifically to rule less likely a number of the diagnoses or diagnostic categories that were remaining on the potential list for Mr. T's chief concern. This is an efficient method of questioning—not only questioning the patient for the answer but asking questions specifically toward a particular diagnoses or diagnostic category.

STEP #8: Re-sort the diagnostic hypothesis list based on the patient's responses to specific questioning.

Remote

T Trauma

~~Cervical spine disk herniation~~ (absent neck pain, shoulder pain with neck movement)
Thoracic outlet syndrome

I   Inflammation

Aseptic

~~Rheumatoid arthritis–like diseases of the cervical spine:~~
- ~~Inflammatory muscle disease~~ (absent neck pain, shoulder pain with neck movement)
- ~~Psoriatic arthritis~~ (absent neck pain, shoulder pain with neck movement)

Septic
Not applicable

M   Metabolic

~~Osteomalacia~~ (no pain in other joints)

Va   Vascular

Aneurysm
Coronary artery insufficiency

De   Degenerative

~~Osteoarthritis of the cervical spine~~ (absent neck pain, shoulder pain with neck movement)

Tu   Tumor

Malignant Primary, such as:
- Breast tumor
- Pancoast tumor

Malignant Metastatic:
Not applicable
Benign:
Not applicable

Co   Congenital

Not applicable

Ne   Neurogenic/Psychogenic

Not applicable

Local

T   Trauma

Glenohumeral joint sprain/subluxation
Glenoid labrum tear
~~Muscle strain, such as pectoralis major, rotator cuff, upper trapezius, levator scapulae~~ (absent neck pain, shoulder pain with neck movement)
Subacromial impingement syndrome

I   Inflammation

Aseptic

~~Biceps tendinitis~~ (no restriction in shoulder range of motion)
Bursitis

~~Rotator cuff tendinitis~~ (no restriction in shoulder range of motion)

Septic
Not applicable

M   Metabolic

~~Gout~~ (no stiffness/pain in other joints, no swelling/redness/warmth)

Va   Vascular

Aneurysm
~~Avascular necrosis of the humeral head~~ (no restriction in shoulder range of motion, no constant pain)
Compartment syndrome
Deep venous thrombosis, upper extremity

De   Degenerative

Biceps tendinopathy
~~Osteoarthritis/osteoarthrosis~~ (no restriction in shoulder range of motion)
Rotator cuff tear/tendinopathy

Tu   Tumor

Malignant Primary, such as:
- Chondrosarcoma
- Lymphoma
- Osteosarcoma
- Synovial sarcoma

Malignant Metastatic, such as:
- Metastases, including from primary breast, kidney, lung, prostate, and thyroid disease

Benign, such as:
- Osteoblastoma
- ~~Osteoid osteoma~~ (no swelling/redness/warmth)
- ~~Unicameral bone cyst~~ (no restriction in shoulder range of motion, no constant pain, no swelling/redness/warmth)

Co   Congenital

Not applicable

Ne   Neurogenic/Psychogenic

Not applicable

STEP #9: Perform tests to differentiate among the remaining diagnostic hypotheses.

Teaching Comments: Clinicians should look for the most discriminating physical findings to rule out as many options as possible with the fewest tests.

- **Shoulder active range of motion.** Full and pain free. Makes less likely biceps and rotator cuff tendinopathy, chondrosarcoma, bursitis, and osteoblastoma.
- **Palpate for mass; listen for bruit over region including auscultation over lungs.** Negative. Makes less likely breast tumor.

Teaching Comments: Breast cancer in males exhibits similar signs as in females with a lump or swelling in the breast tissue, skin dimpling, nipple retraction or discharge from the nipple, and/or redness of the nipple/breast skin.

STEP #10: Re-sort the diagnostic hypothesis list based on the patient's responses to specific tests.

Remote

T   Trauma

~~Thoracic outlet syndrome~~ (pain-free shoulder range of motion)

I   Inflammation

Aseptic
Not applicable

Septic
Not applicable

M   Metabolic
Not applicable

Va   Vascular

~~Aneurysm~~ (no bruits on auscultation)
Coronary artery insufficiency

De   Degenerative
Not applicable

Tu   Tumor

Malignant Primary, such as:
- ~~Breast tumor~~ (negative palpation)
- Pancoast tumor

Malignant Metastatic:
Not applicable

Benign:
Not applicable

Co   Congenital
Not applicable

Ne   Neurogenic/Psychogenic
Not applicable

Local

T   Trauma

~~Glenohumeral joint sprain/subluxation~~ (pain-free shoulder range of motion)
~~Glenoid labrum tear~~ (pain-free shoulder range of motion)
~~Subacromial impingement syndrome~~ (pain-free shoulder range of motion)

I   Inflammation

Aseptic
~~Bursitis~~ (pain-free shoulder range of motion)

Septic
Not applicable

M   Metabolic
Not applicable

Va   Vascular

~~Aneurysm~~ (auscultation negative for bruits)
Compartment syndrome
Deep venous thrombosis, upper extremity

De   Degenerative

~~Biceps tendinopathy~~ (pain-free shoulder range of motion)
~~Rotator cuff tear/tendinopathy~~ (pain-free shoulder range of motion)

Tu   Tumor

Malignant Primary, such as:
- ~~Chondrosarcoma~~ (pain-free shoulder range of motion)
- Lymphoma
- Osteosarcoma
- Synovial sarcoma

Malignant Metastatic, such as:
- Metastases, including from primary breast, kidney, lung, prostate, and thyroid disease

Benign, such as:
- ~~Osteoblastoma~~ (pain-free shoulder range of motion)

Co	**Congenital**

Not applicable

Ne	**Neurogenic/Psychogenic**

Not applicable

STEP #11: Decide on a diagnostic impression.

- Remaining conditions include coronary artery insufficiency, Pancoast tumor, compartment syndrome, upper extremity deep venous thrombosis, as well as local malignant primary and metastatic tumors.

STEP #12: Determine the appropriate patient disposition.

- Refer the patient to a physician for additional testing and treatment, because none of the remaining health conditions is amenable to physical therapy independently.

- Clear communication with the referral source and potentially the patient's family physician should be the immediate next step.

Case Outcome

At this point, Mr. T.'s treating physical therapist was unsure as to a specific diagnosis, but was certain that his symptoms warranted further medical evaluation. Mr. T. was referred to his family physician after first telephoning him. Mr. T. later called to report that his physician wasted no time in performing cardiac function tests and cardiac bypass surgery was performed successfully within a week. Note that this patient had gone to the physical therapist and had filled in a "screening form" where the patient's answers were interpreted as indicating that his symptom was due to a process that could be construed as appropriate for treatment by a physical therapist.

CHAPTER **6**

Diagnostic Considerations of Pain

■ *Todd E. Davenport, PT, DPT, OCS* ■ *Lucinda L. Baker, PT, PhD*

IN THIS CHAPTER:
- Anatomy and physiology of pain
- Pain perception and clinical presentation

OUTLINE

Introduction

Disability and distress related to pain are among the most common reasons that lead people to seek rehabilitation. Pain is a somatosensory modality—along with thermoreception, touch, and proprioception—that is defined as the unpleasant sensory experience associated with actual or potential tissue damage.[1] Pain serves sensory, emotional, and cognitive functions.[2,3] Pain's *sensory-discriminative function* allows for self-preservation. When a hand is placed on a hot stove, the sensory-discriminative function of pain compels the withdrawing of the hand and inspecting for tissue damage. Tissue damage results when the sensory-discriminative function of pain is impaired. One example of this phenomenon is the skin ulceration often seen on the plantar surfaces of the feet in people with diabetic polyneuropathy. The *affective function* of pain provides emotional unpleasantness to pain sensations. This causes people to avoid additional pain and the tissue damage that pain represents. The *cognitive-evaluative function* serves to encourage learning and foster behavioral adaptation. Disorder involving the affective and cognitive-evaluative functions of pain may result in maladaptive behavioral responses to pain, such as a disabling avoidance of work, family, and recreational activities.

The same basic anatomical and physiological processes that generate and conduct pain sensations are found in all people. However, there are vast differences in how people respond to pain sensations. This causes a great variation in how people will demonstrate pain in the clinic. Individual differences in how pain sensation is processed often make it difficult to interpret for both patients and clinicians in the diagnostic process. This chapter discusses pain as it relates to the diagnostic process. The chapter first describes the processes that all people have in common, and then describes anatomical and physiological reasons for individual differences in pain perception.

All People Share Common Nociceptive Processes

The association between pain and actual tissue damage suggests that all people share common anatomy and physiology that mediate pain perception. *Nociception* occurs when pain is perceived through the activation of peripheral pain receptors due to tissue damage.

Nociceptors Respond to Various Forms of Tissue Injury

Pain receptors are free nerve endings called *nociceptors*. Nociceptors are broadly categorized by their location. Nociceptors located throughout the skin and musculoskeletal structures are called *somatic nociceptors*. Somatic nociceptors are primarily classified by their *adequate stimuli*—stimuli to which they respond. *Mechanical nociceptors* are activated by intense pressure.[4] *Thermal nociceptors* respond to temperatures less than 5°C and greater than 45°C. Mechanical and thermal nociceptors transmit action potentials along Aδ axons when activated. The Aδ axons are thinly myelinated and conduct at velocities of 5 to 30 m/s.[4] *Polymodal nociceptors* are activated by mechanical, thermal, and chemical stimuli, sending action potentials along C fibers to the spinal cord when activated.[4] The C fibers are small, unmyelinated axons that conduct at velocities less than 1 m/s.

Visceral nociceptors transmit information about distention, ischemia, and chemical irritation of the deep organs along C fibers.[5] Visceral nociceptors are further classified by their activation thresholds into low, high, and silent nociceptors.[6] Low-threshold nociceptors

are most likely to transmit information at low levels of an adequate stimulus, whereas silent nociceptors are characterized by such high activation thresholds that they must be sensitized by inflammatory chemicals to facilitate their function (Box 6-1).[7]

Nociceptors Transmit Pain Signals Along Organized Neural Pathways

Axons transmitting nociceptive information from the periphery project onto the dorsal horn of the spinal cord. Six subdivisions of dorsal root ganglion receive input from axons transmitting information about one nociceptive modality each.[8] The Aδ axons of mechanical and thermal nociceptors make unisynaptic connections with neurons that transmit pain signals to the central nervous system, referred to as projection neurons. In addition, Aδ axons synapse with wide dynamic range neurons that integrate pain signals from multiple regions of the body. The C axons of polymodal nociceptors make multisynaptic connections with projection neurons by way of interneurons in the substantia gelatinosa of the spinal cord. The functional relevance of these local neural circuits is discussed in a later section.

BOX 6-1 A "Toxic Soup" Sensitizes Nociceptors

Among their many functions, inflammatory substances released during tissue injury sensitize nociceptors, enhancing the *primary hyperalgesia* that results from mechanical stimulation of nociceptors.[2] Histamine, the first chemical released in the inflammatory process through mast cell degranulation, activates polymodal nociceptors. Bradykinins are potent pain-producing substances that result from conversion of a plasma protein in the blood clotting cascade. Prostaglandins and leukotrienes are derivatives of arachidonic acid formed after damage to the cell membranes that sensitize nociceptors. The neuropeptide substance P is released from activated nociceptors, leading to additional nociceptor sensitization. Other inflammatory chemicals increase nociception by promoting tissue damage adjacent to the initial area of injury, including cytokines and oxygen free radicals. These substances serve to sensitize surrounding nociceptors, producing a *secondary hyperalgesia*.

Projection neurons transmit action potentials along five organized tracts within the ventral and lateral regions of the spinal cord.[4,9] Their axons are called the anterolateral system of the spinal cord because of their location. Axons of the anterolateral system cross sides within one to two spinal levels rostral to the input level before ascending to target nuclei in the brainstem, hypothalamus, and thalamus. The spinothalamic tract is the most prominent in the anterolateral system, transmitting nociceptive signals to cortical processing centers by way of thalamic interneurons. The spinohypothalamic tract transmits nociceptive signals to supraspinal autonomic centers that mediate neuroendocrine and cardiovascular control. Many spinohypothalamic axons do not cross sides.

The spinoreticular tract projects onto the reticular formation and thalamus for control of consciousness and relay to cortical centers, respectively. Neurons composing the spinomesencephalic tract project onto the periaqueductal gray matter in the midbrain that inhibits the transmission of pain signals from the periphery. In addition, neurons from the spinomesencephalic tract project onto the insula, which may also mediate the autonomic control of pain perception. The cervicothalamic tract originates in the lateral cervical nucleus and ascends along the dorsal column–medial lemniscal pathway. This tract may be significant for people with neck pain.

The Perception of Pain Severity Depends on Anatomical, Physiological, and Cognitive Factors

One would think that the most severe injuries would cause the most incapacitating pain. However, some people may report incapacitating pain levels due to an undetectable tissue injury. There are also numerous stories of people reacting meaningfully to their environment despite sustaining severe injuries in combat. Clearly, the perception of pain severity is modulated by a variety of anatomical, physiological, and cognitive processes. This challenges attempts at reproducible and meaningful measurement of pain severity (Box 6-2).

BOX 6-2 Pitfalls of Measuring Pain Severity

Change in pain severity is commonly considered useful to estimate treatment efficacy. Unfortunately, health care providers are poor at estimating patients' levels of pain.[49] Accurate estimation of pain severity is crucial—overestimation may lead to overtreatment and vice versa. The visual/verbal analog scale (V/VAS), in which the patient rates pain on a scale from 0 (lowest) to 10 (greatest), is widely used because of its intuitive appeal and convenience. However, V/VAS ratings do not predict the need for analgesic medication,[50] and the magnitude of clinically meaningful change for V/VAS ratings has yet to be determined. Measurements of pain-related function, anxiety level, or disability beliefs may serve as more effective indicators of treatment efficacy.

Melzack and Wall[10] first described the *gate control hypothesis* to explain how the anatomy and physiology of the central nervous system control the transmission of information about pain all along the neuraxis. This theory has been greatly elaborated since it was first proposed. The mechanisms responsible for the gate include the morphology of axons carrying somatosensory information, the structure of local neural circuits, and the nature of interconnections between local neural circuits and supraspinal centers. Interactions among different regions of the central nervous system are also responsible for creating thoughts, feelings, learning, and behaviors related to pain. These cognitive processes may also modulate the severity of a person's pain sensations.

A "Gate" Controls the Transmission of Pain Signals at the Spinal Cord and Elsewhere

Neural networks that transmit sensory information about light cutaneous pressure from the periphery compete with the transmission of pain signals within the spinal cord. Touch receptors transmit along large-diameter Aβ axons to the dorsal horn of the spinal cord.[4,9] This arrangement allows integration of touch, temperature, and pain signals before transmission to the thalamus. The larger diameter and thicker myelination of the Aβ axons also provide faster conduction speeds than the Aδ and C axons that carry pain signals. Because light-touch sensation signals reach the wide dynamic range neuron faster than pain signals, light-touch sensation is perceived first.

Interaction among Aβ, C, and inhibitory interneurons also modulates the transmission of pain signals at the level of the spinal cord (Fig. 6-1A). In addition to their synaptic connection to a wide dynamic range neuron, Aβ axons also make an excitatory synapse onto inhibitory interneurons that project onto the wide dynamic range neuron. Normally, the inhibitory interneuron prevents the activation of the wide dynamic range neuron. Consequently, the inhibitory interneuron normally inhibits the perception of pain. Touch input increases the level of inhibition of the wide dynamic range neuron and decreases the perception of pain (Fig. 6-1B). The C axon makes an inhibitory synapse with the inhibitory interneuron. When C axonal input is greatest,

the inhibitory interneuron is itself inhibited, causing an increase in activation of the wide dynamic range neuron and perception of pain (Fig. 6-1C). When both the Aβ and C axons provide input, pain signal transmission by the wide dynamic range neuron is modulated (Fig. 6-1D).

Input from the Cerebral Cortex and Midbrain Also Plays a Role in the Gate's Function

Descending inputs to the dorsal horn of the spinal cord from the midbrain and cerebral cortex modulate pain perception by way of two interrelated neurotransmitter systems: serotonin and enkephalin. Neurons in the periaqueductal gray matter of the midbrain synapse onto serotonergic projection neurons in the raphe nuclei of the medulla. These serotonergic projection neurons descend to the dorsal horn of the spinal cord, reducing pain perception by two mechanisms (Fig. 6-1E).[9]

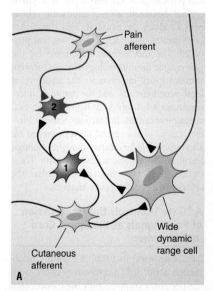
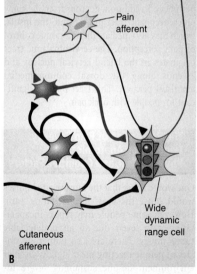

A   **B**

FIGURE 6-1 (A) Somatosensory afferents also synapse with two different types of neurons—one excitatory synapse with an excitatory interneuron (1) and one excitatory synapse with the wide dynamic range cell. The excitatory interneuron makes an excitatory synapse with the inhibitory interneuron and the wide dynamic range cell. Nociceptive afferent makes two synapses—one inhibitory synapse with an inhibitory interneuron (2) and one excitatory synapse directly with the wide dynamic range cell. The inhibitory interneuron synapses with the wide dynamic range cell. (B) When somatosensory input is greatest, touch signals are propagated in two ways. The cutaneous afferent excites the wide dynamic range cell directly and indirectly through activating the excitatory interneuron.

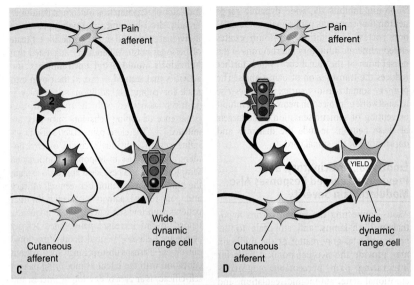

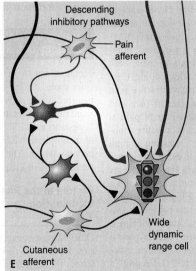

FIGURE 6-1—cont'd (C) When nociceptive input is greatest, pain signals are propagated in two ways. The pain afferent excites the wide dynamic range cell directly and indirectly by inhibiting the inhibitory interneuron. (D) When somatosensory and nociceptive input are present, input from the somatosensory afferent mitigates the transmission of pain signals by activating the inhibitory interneuron. (E) Descending inhibitory input from serotonergic projection neurons in the raphe nucleus of the medulla reduces the transmission of nociceptive signals directly by inhibiting the wide dynamic range cell and indirectly by exciting the inhibitory interneuron.

Serotonin inhibits the wide dynamic range neuron that transmits pain signals to the cerebral cortex. In addition, serotonin excites enkephalinergic inhibitory interneurons in the dorsal horn of the spinal cord, which further reduces the transmission of pain signals. The primary somatosensory cortex also gives rise to a network of projection neurons that inhibit perception of somatic sensation.[9] The targets of these neurons include the thalamus and dorsal horn of the spinal cord.

Emotional, Anticipatory, and Previously Learned Responses Also Modulate Pain Severity

Axons connecting the frontal cortex, hypothalamus, thalamus, and amygdala to the periaqueductal gray matter of the midbrain may provide the neuroanatomical basis for integrating pain perception, cognitive-emotional state, autonomic regulation, and motor activity.[11] This neural circuit appears at least partially responsible for the unique psychological features of people that powerfully influence how pain is perceived. Emotional and cognitive aspects of pain both positively and negatively affect coping. Cognitive factors that negatively influence pain coping include increased fear of pain and catastrophizing about pain. **Fear of pain** is defined as "a highly specific negative emotional reaction to pain involving a high degree of mobilization for escape/avoidance behavior,"[12] which relates to excessive anxiety about pain. Otherwise healthy people with a high fear of pain report a higher severity of experimentally induced acute pain than people with a low fear of pain. **Catastrophizing** is defined as "an exaggerated negative mental act brought to bear during an actual or anticipated painful experience,"[13] reflecting "a tendency to focus on pain and negatively evaluate one's own ability to cope with pain."[14] Although fear of pain and catastrophizing are related, catastrophizing behavior more strongly predicts the self-reported severity of experimentally induced acute pain than fear of pain itself.[15]

The importance of metacognitive processes on pain perception has led some authors to hypothesize that self-efficacy is an important indicator of rehabilitation outcomes. Bandura[16] broadly describes efficacy expectations as an individual's task- and situation-specific estimate of personal mastery. Bandura[16] suggested that individuals would avoid environments and activities that seemed to exceed their own estimate for coping. In addition, self-efficacy is positively associated with the magnitude and persistence of coping behaviors once they are initiated.[17-19] Therefore, pain-related self-efficacy influences an individual's choice of environment and activities in response to anticipated symptom coping. These ideas appear to explain the significant association between self-efficacy and pain-related activity avoidance, in that patients with low self-efficacy more frequently tended toward increased pain-related activity avoidance beliefs[12,20-22] and poorer functional outcomes.[23] Perhaps unsurprisingly then, patient education with the intent of modifying patient self-efficacy is an area of developing interest and research in physical therapy.[24]

Timing of Pain Suggests the Etiology of Underlying Pathology

Temporal aspects of pain provide important clues about affected tissues and the nature of pain-producing pathology. Short-term pain is more often the result of an active pathology. Long-term pain is more likely to be the result of neuroplastic changes within the central nervous system. The nature of these changes are discussed in a later section of this chapter.

Factors in the History and Physical Examination Can Implicate Affected Tissues

Differentiation among pain-producing pathologies depends on their dissimilar patterns of factors that aggravate, alleviate, and associate with the perception of pain. *Aggravating factors* are those activities of daily living, exercise, work, or recreation; active, passive, or resisted movements; or palpation that worsen pain. Conversely, *alleviating factors* relieve pain. *Associated factors* include a wide variety of constitutional, dermatological, mental, and neurological signs and symptoms that may appear simultaneously with pain. To be certain, clinicians should also be alert for aggravating, alleviating, and associated factors that indicate an immediate need to refer for additional medical treatment. These are listed at the beginning of each chapter discussing pain in each body region.

Three sources of lower extremity pain—lumbar herniated intervertebral disk, lumbar spinal stenosis, and peripheral vascular disease—may be distinguished on the basis of different movements that aggravate or alleviate pain. People with a displaced lumbar disk classically report pain that worsens during positions of lumbar flexion that include bending, kneeling, sitting, and squatting. Conversely, symptoms associated with herniated lumbar disk are most likely alleviated in positions of extension, such as standing. People with lumbar spinal stenosis classically report pain that worsens with the positions of lumbar extension, and pain relief during positions of flexion.[25] People with peripheral vascular disease of the lower extremities also report pain during standing and walking—which involves lumbar extension—and relief with sitting—which involves lumbar flexion.

The stoop test,[26] in which an individual assumes a squat position, places the lumbar spine in a position of relative flexion. Reproduction of symptoms with the stoop test may rule out lumbar spinal stenosis and confirm the presence of a lumbar herniated disk. Alleviation of symptoms with this test may rule out the herniated lumbar disk as a likely cause of symptoms and confirm the presence of either lumbar spinal stenosis or peripheral vascular disease. The bicycle test,[27] in which an individual performs aerobic exercise on a bicycle, maintains the spine in a relatively flexed position while challenging the cardiovascular system. Reproduction of symptoms with the bicycle test implicates peripheral vascular disease as a cause of the individual's lower extremity pain. The effectiveness of all history and physical examination tests may be represented by their statistical properties (Box 6-3).

Descriptions of Pain May Relate to Either Injured Tissues or Emotional Features

Words selected to describe the internal and deeply personal phenomenon of pain may provide useful information regarding its underlying pathology. An anecdotal relationship between

> **BOX 6-3 How "Good" Are History and Physical Examination Findings?**
>
> Various statistical properties are used to represent the effectiveness of questions and tests for purposes of diagnosis.[51] Sensitivity is the proportion of people who give a positive result for the disorder a test is intended to reveal. Specificity is the probability that a test will not give a positive result for people in whom the target disorder is absent. Positive predictive value is the ratio of people with the disease that test positive to the entire population of people with the disorder regardless of test result. Negative predictive value is the ratio of people without the disease that test negative to the entire population of people without the disorder regardless of test result. Use of several questions and tests in clusters is common to help compensate for the low sensitivity, specificity, and predictive values of many questions and physical examination tests.

an individual's description and corresponding pain-generating structure is known to exist, such as cardiac ("crushing"), neuropathic ("shooting and stinging"), muscular ("sharp"), vascular ("cramping"), and visceral ("dull and diffuse"). Although the relationship between description and pathology can vary, it provides one shorthand approach to ruling out pathology in the differential diagnostic process.

Words such as "punishing," "sickening," and "excruciating" suggest that an individual attributes a strong emotional meaning to pain. The McGill Pain Questionnaire[28,29] is a psychometric test that measures the frequency of emotionally charged terms that individuals use to describe their perception of pain, reflecting the state of individuals' emotional reasoning about their pain experience. An increased frequency of affective descriptions of pain may relate to symptoms of depression and anxiety. In turn, depression and anxiety may lead to difficulty soliciting necessary information during the history and lead to poor treatment outcomes.

Locations of Pain and Its Underlying Cause May Differ

"Where does it hurt?" is one of the first questions a clinician often asks a patient who presents with pain. The answer may be misleading. Pathology that is remote or local to the painful area may be responsible for the patient's symptoms. *Local pain* is perceived at the location of tissue damage (Fig. 6-2A). *Remote pain* is perceived at a distance from the location of the responsible pathology.[30] Pathology causing remote pain is often confused with pathology causing local pain, making it important to consider remote causes of pain first in the diagnostic process.

Remote pain may be neuropathic or referred. *Neuropathic pain* occurs with damage to the nociceptive system itself. Examples of neuropathic pain syndromes include diabetic polyneuropathy, post-herpetic neuralgia, and traumatic nerve injury (formerly referred to as complex regional pain syndrome type II). *Radicular pain* is a type of neuropathic pain that occurs when mechanical impingement of a spinal nerve root causes the sensation of pain in a *dermatome*, or peripheral distribution of a spinal nerve root (Fig. 6-2B). One example of radicular pain is medial forearm pain due to C7–T1 herniated nucleus pulposus with impingement of the C8 nerve root. Radicular

pain is a specific type of *neuropathic pain*, which originates from a lesion of the nervous system. *Projected pain* is another type of neuropathic pain that occurs when injury to a peripheral nerve occurs along its course (Fig. 6-2C). One example of projected pain is medial forearm pain due to an ulnar nerve entrapment at the cubital tunnel. *Referred pain* is perceived at a distance from the site of pathology, though not secondary to irritation of a spinal or peripheral nerve. Pain may be referred from one somatic structure to another, a visceral structure to a somatic structure, or one visceral structure to another (Fig. 6-2D).[31] Pain referred from one somatic structure to another often follows predictable, irregular soft tissue patterns called *sclerotomes*.[32] Pain referred from a visceral structure to a somatic structure may also follow a dermatomal distribution.[33]

Misinterpretation by the Central Nervous System Causes Referred Pain

While direct activation of the nociceptive pathway causes local pain, referred pain results

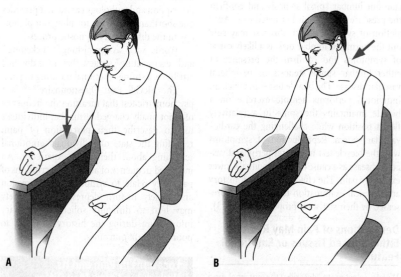

A   **B**

FIGURE 6-2 Possible causes of medial elbow pain (red ellipse) include (A) local pain secondary to medial epicondylosis; (B) radicular pain secondary to C7–T1 herniated nucleus pulposus (*arrow*);

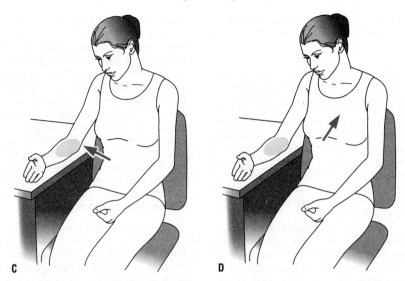

FIGURE 6-2—cont'd (C) projected pain due to cubital tunnel syndrome (*arrow*); and (D) referred pain secondary to myocardial infarction (*arrow*).

from a misinterpretation of the origin of pain signals by the central nervous system. As sensory information is passed rostrally along the neuraxis, sensory information from somatic and visceral structures converges. Convergence of afferent inputs in spinal and supraspinal centers, such as the thalamus and cerebral cortex, results in the loss of region specificity in processing of pain signals. Convergent processing of several body regions leads to the perception of poorly localized pain that exists beyond the area of tissue injury. In addition, excitability of the dorsal horn neurons leads to an expansion of their receptive fields, also leading to an overlap in processing of nociceptive inputs from various somatic and visceral structures.[34,35] Parallel processing of information carried by a segmental innervation shared by somatic and visceral structures also causes referral from a visceral structure to a somatic structure. For example, sensory innervation of the heart, shoulder, and jaw overlap.[33] Because experience with shoulder and jaw pain from local pathology is more common than pain originating from heart pathology, pain associated with heart pathology is often erroneously attributed to the jaw and shoulder.

Long-Term Pain Causes Cyclic Anatomical, Physiological, and Cognitive-Behavioral Changes

Long-term pain is a prevalent and disabling chronic health issue. **Chronic pain** is defined as persisting beyond 3 months, which has been established as a reasonable average tissue healing time. In addition, chronic pain has no biological value because it provides no useful sensory-discrimination information.[1] Chronic pain is a negative result of learning, characterized by structure-function maladaptations throughout the nervous system due to psychosocial pain behavior reinforcement and psychological predisposition. Although *chronic pain* is an accepted term in the neurophysiology literature, *persistent pain* may be a more acceptable term for use in the clinic because of the negative connotation of chronic pain. Persistent pain has also been adopted by some authors. In general, authors may also differentiate between chronic pain due to malignant disease and chronic pain not caused by malignant disease.

Prolonged Activation of Nociceptive Pathways Causes Maladaptations Throughout the Nervous System

Nociceptive pathways constantly adapt to optimally transmit and respond to information about noxious stimuli. Prolonged activation of nociceptive pathways results in a whole host of structural and functional maladaptations at various levels of the central nervous system. These maladaptations may lead to the perception of chronic pain.

Receptors located on neuronal cell membranes provide the cellular basis for learning and memory at all levels of the central nervous system, called *long-term potentiation*. Certain neuronal membrane receptors, called *ion channels*, respond to binding of specific substances by permitting an influx of ions from the extracellular space.[36] This causes a change in voltage across the neuronal cell membrane.[37] If enough ion channels respond simultaneously to depolarize the cell membrane at the soma, a critical voltage threshold is reached that allows generation of an action potential.[38]

In the dorsal horn of the spinal cord, wide dynamic range neurons accepting input from nociceptive axons have three classes of membrane receptors[39]:

- *Ligand-gated ion channels* that open in response to binding of a neurotransmitter, neuropeptide, or other molecules. These are common at the soma, providing for the small changes in membrane voltage that may culminate in an action potential. Ligand-gated ion channels on wide dynamic range nociceptive neurons are responsive to substance P, calcitonin gene-related peptide, and other molecules.
- *Voltage-gated ion channels* that open in response to changes in voltage across the cell membrane. These are common along the axon, allowing for propagation of an action potential to the axon terminal.[38]
- *Ligand- and voltage-gated ion channels* that open in response to binding of a neurotransmitter, neuropeptide, or other molecule in the presence of a sufficient membrane voltage. These are also commonly located on the soma. A crucial ligand- and voltage-gated ion channel to long-term potentiation is the NMDA receptor. NMDA receptors allow the influx of calcium ions across the neuronal membrane. NMDA receptors are responsive to binding of the neurotransmitter glutamate (the ligand gate), although the ion channel associated with it has a "cap" of magnesium ions that must be removed by a sufficiently high membrane potential (the voltage gate) to allow the influx of calcium ions.

Long-term potentiation in nociceptive wide dynamic range neurons depends on NMDA receptor activity.[40] Substance P[41] and calcitonin gene-related peptide bind to ligand-gated ion channels on wide dynamic range nociceptive neurons, causing a change in membrane potential that removes the "cap" of magnesium ions from the NMDA receptor. If glutamate also binds to the NMDA receptor at this time, the calcium ion channel associated with the NMDA receptor opens. The resulting influx of calcium ions initiates a cascade of intracellular processes that causes structural changes to the wide dynamic range neuron to facilitate its transmission of pain signals. Long-term potentiation of nociceptive pathways is also referred to as *central sensitization* or *wind-up*.

Neuroanatomical changes eventually result from maladaptive learning by the central nervous system. Hypothesized changes in the spinal dorsal root ganglion include disinhibition of spinal cord neurons,[42] axonal sprouting by local spinal interneurons outside their normal distribution,[16,43] and formation of noradrenergic axons where they did not previously exist.[44] Neuroanatomical changes are also present in supraspinal structures. Changes in cerebral cortex activation also contribute to persistent pain, paralleling cognitive and behavior changes. People with persistent lower back pain demonstrate a larger representation of the lower back in the primary sensory cortex than healthy people.[17] In addition, experimental induction of prolonged cutaneous and muscle pain reduces primary motor cortex excitability.[18–21]

The Sympathetic Nervous System Can Contribute to the Perception of Pain

Abundant research and clinical evidence suggest that the sympathetic autonomic nervous system can contribute to chronic pain disorders involving neuropathic pain. Complex regional pain syndrome (CRPS) refers to a group of chronic neuropathic pain disorders. CRPS is divided into two types based on etiology[22]:

- CRPS I refers to chronic neuropathic pain without identifiable nerve trauma (formerly known as reflex sympathetic dystrophy).
- CRPS II refers to chronic neuropathic pain that corresponds with previous nerve trauma (formerly known as causalgia).

CRPS I and II share a common pathological progression, which has been divided into three hypothetical stages[23]:

- *Acute/warm phase*—The first phase of CRPS occurs immediately after the precipitating event, if one is present. The affected limb is warm and swollen. There may be increased hair and nail growth, spontaneous burning pain, and pain with normal non-noxious sensory stimulation (allodynia).
- *Instability/dystrophic phase*—This second phase of CRPS typically begins 3 months after the precipitating event, and is characterized by pain in a more extended area, limitation of movement, joint stiffness. Osteoporosis and muscle wasting are typically evident in the second stage of CRPS.
- *Atrophic phase*—This third phase of CRPS generally presents 6 months after the initiation of symptoms. In this stage, pain may actually decrease, although the skin over the affected area becomes cool, cyanotic, smooth, and glossy.

Surgical ablation of the sympathetic chain has long been known to partially or completely resolve CRPS in some patients, even though the sympathetic autonomic nervous system does not directly participate in nociception. This suggests that the nociceptive afferent and autonomic nervous systems may become coupled outside the spinal cord, where nociceptors become abnormally sensitized to sympathetic autonomic signaling. Coupling of nociceptive and sympathetic autonomic nervous systems may be direct or indirect.[45] Direct coupling occurs after complete or partial nerve injury, when nociceptors become sensitized to autonomic signal molecules called *catecholamines*. Catecholamines may also cause indirect coupling by triggering the formation of prostaglandins during tissue inflammation that, in turn, sensitize nociceptors.

Psychological and Social Factors Perpetuate Pain Through Behavior Reinforcement

Continual activation of nociceptive pathways may cause cyclic disorders in thoughts, beliefs, emotions, and consequent interaction with the environment. Fear and avoidance of pain after tissue injury initially serve an adaptive role by allowing damaged tissues to heal. In some people, initial pain avoidance behavior causes a maladaptive anxiety involving movements and activities that may cause pain. Increased fear and anxiety regarding pain result in the formation of *fear avoidance beliefs*. Correspondingly, fear avoidance beliefs cause initially adaptive pain avoidance behaviors—intended to avoid pain—to become maladaptive *fear avoidance behaviors*—intended to avoid anxiety related to movements and activities that cause pain. Fear avoidance beliefs and behaviors are maintained and amplified through social and environmental reinforcements, such as rest, medication, attention, or compensation.[2] Eventually, fear avoidance beliefs and behaviors may be more disabling than pain severity itself.[46] Fear avoidance beliefs and behaviors may become magnified by a spiraling cycle of decline, in which progressive disuse and deconditioning contribute to additional fear avoidance.

Cognitive factors that influence the perception of acute pain severity also play important roles in the perception of chronic pain. Catastrophizing is associated with limited confidence in one's own ability to cope with symptoms, leading to the perception of pain as inescapable and unpredictable. This perception of pain reinforces fear avoidance beliefs and contributes to learned helplessness. *Learned helplessness* relates to an individual's belief that negative outcomes due to pain are inevitable.[15,47] Helplessness interferes with learning of new coping strategies. Learned helplessness eventually leads to *hopelessness*, when all efforts to improve pain are perceived as futile.[15] Helplessness and hopelessness result in cessation of an individual's efforts to self-manage symptoms. Both helplessness and hopelessness are reversible processes.[48] Interdisciplinary treatment involving medical, rehabilitation, and mental health professionals may be effective to reduce functional limitation and disability in people with persistent pain.

Conclusion

Pain is among the most common reasons that individuals seek physical therapy. A common set of stimulus-specific anatomical structures and physiological processes are present in almost all people, and a growing body of clinical and scientific evidence also indicates there are substantial differences in how patients respond to pain. Thus, a careful approach to the diagnosis of pain's underlying causation requires a thorough understanding of pain's anatomy, physiology, and psychology.

References

1. Anonymous. Pain terms: a list with definitions and notes on usage. Recommended by the IASP Subcommittee on Taxonomy. *Pain.* 1979;6(3):249.
2. Fields H. *Pain.* New York, NY: McGraw-Hill; 1987.
3. Melzack R, Casey K. Sensory, motivational, and central control determinants of pain. In: Kenshalo D, ed. *The Skin Senses.* Springfield, IL: Charles C. Thomas; 1968:423–439.
4. Basbaum A, Jessell T. The perception of pain. In: Kandel E, Schwartz J, Jessell T, eds. *Principles of Neural Science.* 4th ed. New York, NY: McGraw-Hill; 2000:472–490.
5. Ness T, Gebhart G. Visceral pain: a review of experimental studies. *Pain.* 1990;41(2):167–234.
6. Sengupta J, Gebhart G. Characterization of mechanosensitive pelvic nerve afferent fibers innervating the colon of the rat. *J Neurophysiol.* 1994;71(6):2046–2060.
7. McMahon S, Koltzenburg M. Silent afferents and visceral pain. Pharmacological approaches to the treatment of chronic pain: new concepts and critical issues. In: *Progress in Pain Research and Management.* Vol 1. Seattle, WA: IASP Press; 1994:11–30.
8. Raja S, Campbell J, Meyer R. Evidence for different mechanisms of primary and secondary hyperalgesia following heat injury to the glabrous skin. *Brain.* 1984;107(pt 4):1179–1188.
9. Martin J. *Neuroanatomy: Text and Atlas.* 3rd ed. New York, NY: McGraw-Hill; 2003.
10. Melzack R, Wall P. Pain mechanisms: a new theory. *Science.* 1965;150(699):971–979.
11. Bandler R, Shipley MT. Columnar organization in the midbrain periaqueductal gray: modules for emotional expression? *Trends Neurosci.* 1994;17(9):379–389.
12. McNeil D, Au A, Zvolensky M, McKee D, Klineberg I, Ho C. Fear of pain in orofacial pain patients. *Pain.* 2001;89(2–3):245–252.
13. Sullivan M, Thorn B, Haythornthwaite J, et al. Theoretical perspectives on the relation between catastrophizing and pain. *Clin J Pain.* 2001;17(1):52–64.
14. Keefe F, Rumble M, Scipio C, Giordano L, Perri L. Psychological aspects of persistent pain: current state of the science. *J Pain.* 2004;5(4):195–211.
15. Sullivan M, Thorn B, Rodgers W, Ward L. Path model of psychological antecedents to pain experience: experimental and clinical findings. *Clin J Pain.* 2004;20(3): 164–173.
16. Bandura A. Self-efficacy: toward a unifying theory of behavioral change. *Psychol Rev.* 1977;84(2):191–215.
17. Bandura A, Adams NE, Beyer J. Cognitive processes mediating behavioral change. *J Pers Soc Psychol.* 1977;35(3):125–139.
18. Bandura A, Cervone D. Self-evaluative and self-efficacy mechanisms governing the motivational aspects of goal systems. *J Pers Soc Psychol.* 1983;45:1017–1028.
19. Bandura A, Cervone D. Differential engagement of self-reactive influences in cognitive motivation. *Organ Behav Hum Decis Process.* 1986;38:92–113.
20. Le Pera D, Graven-Nielsen T, Valeriani M, et al. Inhibition of motor system excitability at cortical and spinal level by tonic muscle pain. *Clin Neurophysiol.* 2001;112(9):1633–1641.
21. Valeriani M, Restuccia D, Di Lazzaro V, et al. Inhibition of biceps brachii muscle motor area by painful heat stimulation of the skin. *Exp Brain Res.* 2001;139(2):168–172.
22. Merskey H, Bogduk N. *Classification of Chronic Pain: Descriptions of Chronic Pain Syndromes and Definitions of Pain Terms.* Seattle, WA: IASP Press; 1994.
23. Bonica JJ. Causalgia and other reflex sympathetic dystrophies. In: Bonica JJ, ed. *Management of Pain.* 2nd ed. Philadelphia, PA: Lea & Febiger; 1990: 220–243.
24. Rundell SD, Davenport TE. Patient education based on principles of cognitive behavioral therapy for a patient with persistent low back pain: a case report. *J Orthop Sports Phys Ther.* 2010;40(8):494–501.
25. Katz J, Dalgas M, Stucki G, et al. Degenerative lumbar spinal stenosis. Diagnostic value of the history and physical examination. *Arthritis Rheum.* 1995;38(9):1236–1241.
26. Dyck P. The stoop-test in lumbar entrapment radiculopathy. *Spine.* 1979;4(1):89–92.
27. Dyck P, Doyle J, Jr. "Bicycle test" of van Gelderen in diagnosis of intermittent cauda equina compression syndrome. Case report. *J Neurosurg.* 1977;46(5): 667–670.
28. Melzack R. The short-form McGill Pain Questionnaire. *Pain.* 1987;30(2):191–197.
29. Melzack R. The McGill Pain Questionnaire: major properties and scoring methods. *Pain.* 1975;1(3):277–299.
30. Arendt-Nielsen L, Svensson P. Referred muscle pain: basic and clinical findings. *Clin J Pain.* 2001;17(1):11–19.

31. Al-Chaer E, Traub R. Biological basis of visceral pain: recent developments. *Pain.* 2002;96(3):221–225.

32. Inman V, Saunders J. Referred pain from skeletal structures. *J Nerv Ment Dis.* 1944;99:660–667.

33. Foreman RD. Mechanisms of cardiac pain. *Annu Rev Physiol.* 1999;61:143–167.

34. Hoheisel U, Mense S. Response behaviour of cat dorsal horn neurones receiving input from skeletal muscle and other deep somatic tissues. *J Physiol.* 1990;426: 265–280.

35. Hoheisel U, Mense S, Simons D, Yu X. Appearance of new receptive fields in rat dorsal horn neurons following noxious stimulation of skeletal muscle: a model for referral of muscle pain? *Neurosci Lett.* 1993;153(1):9–12.

36. Siegelbaum S, Koester J. Ion channels. In: Kandel E, Schwartz J, Jessell T, eds. *Principles of Neural Science.* 4th ed. New York, NY: McGraw-Hill; 2000:105–123.

37. Koester J, Siegelbaum S. Membrane potential. In: Kandel E, Schwartz J, Jessell T, eds. *Principles of Neural Science.* 4th ed. New York, NY: McGraw-Hill; 2000:125–139.

38. Koester J, Siegelbaum S. Propagated signaling: the action potential. In: Kandel E, Schwartz J, Jessell T, eds. *Principles of Neural Science.* 4th ed. New York, NY: McGraw-Hill; 2000:150–170.

39. Berne R, Levy M, Koeppen B, Stanton B. *Physiology.* 4th ed. St. Louis, MO: Mosby; 1998.

40. Woolf C, Thompson S. The induction and maintenance of central sensitization is dependent on N-methyl-D-aspartic acid receptor activation; implications for the treatment of post-injury pain hypersensitivity states. *Pain.* 1991;44(3):293–299.

41. Khasabov S, Rogers S, Ghilardi J, Peters C, Mantyh P, Simone D. Spinal neurons that possess the substance P receptor are required for the development of central sensitization. *J Neurosci.* 15, 2002;22(20):9086–9098.

42. Woolf CJ, Mannion RJ. Neuropathic pain: aetiology, symptoms, mechanisms, and management. *Lancet.* 1999;353(9168):1959–1964.

43. Woolf CJ, Shortland P, Coggeshall RE. Peripheral nerve injury triggers central sprouting of myelinated afferents. *Nature.* 2, 1992;355(6355):75–78.

44. McLachlan EM, Janig W, Devor M, Michaelis M. Peripheral nerve injury triggers noradrenergic sprouting within dorsal root ganglia. *Nature.* 1993;363(6429):543–546.

45. Baron R, Levine J, Fields H. Causalgia and reflex sympathetic dystrophy: does the sympathetic nervous system contribute to the generation of pain? *Muscle Nerve.* 1999;22(6):678–695.

46. Waddell G, Newton M, Henderson I, Somerville D, Main CJ. A Fear-Avoidance Beliefs Questionnaire (FABQ) and the role of fear-avoidance beliefs in chronic low back pain and disability. *Pain.* 1993;52(2):157–168.

47. Seligman M. Chronic fear produced by unpredictable electric shock. *J Comp Physiol Psychol.* 1968;66(2):402–411.

48. Seligman M, Maier S, Geer J. Alleviation of learned helplessness in the dog. *J Abnorm Psychol.* 1968;73(3):256–262.

49. Luger T, Lederer W, Gassner M, Lockinger A, Ulmer H, Lorenz I. Acute pain is underassessed in out-of-hospital emergencies. *Acad Emerg Med.* 2003;10(6):627–632.

50. Blumstein H, Moore D. Visual analog pain scores do not define desire for analgesia in patients with acute pain. *Acad Emerg Med.* 2003;10(3):211–214.

51. Sackett D. *Evidence-Based Medicine: How to Practice and Teach EBM.* 2nd ed. New York, NY: Churchill Livingstone; 2000.

CHAPTER 7

Headaches

■ *Michael O'Donnell, PT, DPT, OCS, FAAOMPT*

Description of the Symptom

This chapter describes pathology that may lead to headaches. **Local causes** are defined as pathology occurring within the cranial vault, as well as the temporomandibular joint (Fig. 7-1). **Remote causes** are defined as occurring outside this region. Each symptom description in this chapter is followed by a brief summary of clinical presentation.

Special Concerns
Headache with:

- Awakening from sleep
- History of head trauma inside of 2 weeks
- Neurological symptoms, such as dizziness, paresthesias, or weakness
- New onset after age 50
- New onset of headache in patient with risk factors for cancer or HIV infection
- Progressing intensity or frequency
- Signs of illness, such as fever, nuchal rigidity, or rash
- Signs of papilledema
- Sudden onset of headache
- Worsening with exertion or Valsalva maneuver

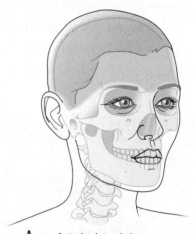
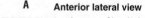

A Anterior lateral view

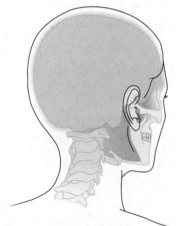

B Posterior lateral view

FIGURE 7-1 Local causes of headache include cranium, contents of the cranial vault, articular and periarticular structures of the temporomandibular joint, and nasal sinuses. (A) Anterior lateral view; (B) posterior lateral view.

CHAPTER PREVIEW: Conditions That May Lead to Headache

T Trauma

REMOTE	LOCAL
COMMON	
Cervicogenic headache 57	Post-traumatic headache 67
UNCOMMON	
Not applicable	Temporomandibular dysfunction 71
RARE	
Not applicable	Not applicable

I Inflammation

REMOTE	LOCAL
COMMON	
Not applicable	**Aseptic** Not applicable **Septic** Fever-induced headache 63 Meningitis 66 Sinusitis 68
UNCOMMON	
Not applicable	**Aseptic** Encephalitis 62 Temporal arteritis 70 **Septic** Not applicable
RARE	
Not applicable	Not applicable

M Metabolic

REMOTE	LOCAL
COMMON	
Not applicable	Hypoglycemia 63 Medication overuse headache 65
UNCOMMON	
Not applicable	Not applicable
RARE	
Not applicable	Benign exertional headache 60 Benign sexual headache 61 Hypoxia 64

(continued)

Va Vascular

REMOTE	LOCAL
COMMON	
Not applicable	Not applicable
UNCOMMON	
Not applicable	Arterial dissection (carotid and vertebral) 60
	Carotid artery dissection 60
	Idiopathic intracranial hypertension
	(pseudotumor cerebri) 64
	Idiopathic intracranial hypotension 65
	Stroke or transient ischemic attack 68
	Subdural hematoma 69
RARE	
Not applicable	Arterial dissection (carotid and vertebral) 60
	Subarachnoid hemorrhage 69
	Vertebral artery dissection 60

De Degenerative

REMOTE	LOCAL
COMMON	
Not applicable	Not applicable
UNCOMMON	
Not applicable	Not applicable
RARE	
Not applicable	Not applicable

Tu Tumor

REMOTE	LOCAL
COMMON	
Not applicable	Not applicable
UNCOMMON	
Not applicable	Not applicable
RARE	
Not applicable	Tumors (brain) 72
	Tumors leading to headaches:
	• Acoustic neuroma 72
	• Central nervous system 72
	• Leptomeningeal metastasis 72
	• Meningeal tumors 72
	• Primary brain tumors 72
	• Skull base tumors 72

Co Congenital

REMOTE	LOCAL
COMMON	
Not applicable	Not applicable
UNCOMMON	
Not applicable	Not applicable
RARE	
Not applicable	Not applicable

Ne Neurogenic/Psychogenic

REMOTE	LOCAL
COMMON	
Not applicable	Migraine 66
	Tension-type headache 71
UNCOMMON	
Not applicable	Not applicable
RARE	
Not applicable	Cluster headaches 61

Note: These are estimates of relative incidence because few data are available for the less common conditions.

Overview of Headache

The International Headache Society (IHS) recognizes 14 broad categories and 300 different types of headaches.[1,2] Headaches are divided among primary and secondary headaches. Primary headaches are unrelated to a specific causative pathology (eg, migraine), whereas secondary headaches occur due to an underlying pathological process (eg, brain tumor). Each headache is characterized by a hallmark frequency, duration, and time course, which may be helpful to distinguish among the different types of headaches (Table 7-1). While it is true that headaches could be the harbinger of grave pathological conditions, only 2% of all headache complaints are caused by serious disease or pathological conditions.[3] Most pathology that necessitates a patient's or client's referral to a physician for consultation can be ruled less likely with a history and a clinical examination, whereas tests such as neuroimaging and electroencephalograms rarely contribute to the diagnosis of headache.

Description of Conditions That May Lead to Headache

Remote

■ Cervicogenic Headache

Chief Clinical Characteristics

This presentation typically is characterized by unilateral head pain associated with neck movement; sustained or awkward cervical posture; restricted cervical range of motion; and ipsilateral neck, shoulder, or arm pain.[4] This condition is characterized by moderate to severe episodic pain that originates in the neck or suboccipital region and spreads to the head. Pain attacks last from 3 weeks to 3 months, and may vary in frequency from occurring every 2 days to 2 months. People with cervicogenic headache describe symptoms that do not change sides during an attack,[5] and may also present with nausea, dizziness, and phonophobia or photophobia that is unresolved with migraine medications.

TABLE 7-1 ■ Diagnosis of Headache Based on Features of the Symptom Timeline

RELATIVE DURATION OF SYMPTOMS

	Hours	Days	Weeks	Months	Constant
Frequency of Symptoms					
Hourly	• Cluster headaches				
Daily	• Chronic migraine • Cluster headaches • Hypoxia	• Cervicogenic headache • Chronic migraine • Hypoxia • Idiopathic intracranial hypotension (lumbar puncture)	• Acute post-traumatic headache • Cervicogenic headache • Hypoxia • Idiopathic intracranial hypotension (lumbar puncture) • Idiopathic intracranial hypotension (fistula)	• Cervicogenic headache • Chronic post-traumatic headache • Idiopathic intracranial hypotension (fistula)	• Medication overuse headache
Weekly	• Chronic migraine • Cluster headaches	• Cervicogenic headache • Chronic migraine	• Cervicogenic headache	• Cervicogenic headache • Migraine	
Monthly	• Chronic migraine	• Chronic migraine			
Yearly	• Chronic migraine	• Chronic migraine			
Constant					• Temporal arteritis
Variable	• Benign exertional headache • Benign sexual headache • Hypoglycemia • Subarachnoid hemorrhage • Tension-type headache	• Arterial dissection (carotid) • Benign exertional headache • Benign sexual headache • Meningitis • Sinusitis • Stroke or transient ischemic attack	• Arterial dissection (carotid) • Arterial dissection (vertebral) • Benign sexual headache • Encephalitis • Intracranial hypotension (lumbar puncture)	• Arterial dissection (vertebral) • Encephalitis • Intracranial hypotension (fistula) • Meningitis • Sinusitis • Stroke or transient ischemic attack	• Fever-induced headache

TABLE 7-1 ■ Diagnosis of Headache Based on Features of the Symptom Timeline—cont'd

RELATIVE DURATION OF SYMPTOMS

	Hours	Days	Weeks	Months	Constant
Variable					
		• Subarachnoid hemorrhage • Subdural hematoma • Temporo-mandibular dysfunction • Tension-type headache	• Intracranial hypotension (fistula) • Meningitis • Sinusitis • Stroke or transient ischemic attack • Subarachnoid hemorrhage • Subdural hematoma • Temporo-mandibular dysfunction • Tension-type headache	• Subdural hematoma • Temporo-mandibular dysfunction • Tension-type headache • Tumor	

Background Information

Initial management includes amelioration of cervical spine musculoskeletal impairments. Nerve blockade may be effective in recalcitrant cases. A favorable response to this intervention also is pathognomic.[6] Typical management of cervicogenic headache involves rehabilitative interventions.

Clinical Features of Cervicogenic Headache

Pain Character	Dull, nonthrobbing, and nonlancinating. Intensity can be moderate to severe.
Location	Side locked unilaterally. Localized to upper cervical or occipital region. Pain may radiate to frontal or orbital region, vertex, temples, or ears.
Precipitants	Trauma, sustained neck postures, mechanical faults such as painful restricted cervical mobility, crepitations[6] with movement, unilateral feeling of tension, pain aggravated by head movements, pressure on ipsilateral trigger points.
Onset	Acute (trauma) or prolonged insidious onsets (degenerative joint disease of upper cervical vertebrae).
Duration	3 weeks to 3 months.
Frequency	Every 2 days to every 2 months.
Time Course	May be present when awakening and worsen as day goes on; activity dependent.
Associated Symptoms/ Signs	Phonophobia, dizziness, ipsilateral eyelid edema, ipsilateral blurred vision.

Local

■ Arterial Dissection (Carotid and Vertebral)

Chief Clinical Characteristics

This presentation often involves steady pain in a pattern that loosely follows the distribution of the affected artery, associated with Horner's syndrome, ipsilateral tongue weakness, diplopia, syncope, tinnitus, amaurosis fugax, or dysgeusia.

Background Information

Dissections are typically seen in people ages 30 to 39 as compared to cerebral ischemia. The most common symptoms of internal carotid artery dissection (ICAD) are headache and/or cervical pain.[7] Zetterling reports the characteristic pain to have a sudden onset,[7] whereas Biousse reports that 85% of patients with ICAD have a gradual onset of pain.[8] The headache pain is severe and is located in the ipsilateral periorbital, periauricular, or upper cervical region. Dodick states that components of the clinical presentation greatly assist in making the diagnosis. He states that the onset of pain is frequently temporally related to cervical manipulation, sustained exertion, or trauma. Horner's syndrome accompanies the headache and there may be ipsilateral tongue weakness.[3] Vertebral artery dissection is less common than ICAD and may go unrecognized until an ischemic event occurs.[3] Pain is localized to the occiput or posterior neck bilaterally or the frontal region unilaterally. Vertebral artery dissection (VAD) can produce brainstem or cerebellar ischemia. This can result in Wallenberg's syndrome. A young person with occipital or posterior neck pain presenting with Wallenberg's syndrome is highly likely to have a VAD.[8] Individuals suspected of this condition require emergent medical attention.

Clinical Features of Headache Secondary to Arterial Dissection

Pain Character	Severity ranges from mild to excruciating.
	Carotid artery—constant, steady ache.
	Vertebral artery—steady pressure or throbbing.
Location	Carotid artery—neck pain or headache that radiates to eye, ear, or face.
	Vertebral artery—bilateral occipital, unilateral frontal.
Precipitants	Sustained exertion, trauma, or cervical manipulation.
Onset	85% of cases of headache are characterized by gradual onset. On occasion, onset can be sudden with "thunderclap" qualities.
Duration	Carotid artery-related headaches resolve within 1 week. Vertebral artery-related headaches may last 5 weeks.
Frequency	Related to the precipitating incident.
Time Course	Headache may appear 1 hour to 90 days prior to dissection.
Associated Symptoms/ Signs	Horner's syndrome, hypoglossal nerve palsy (ipsilateral tongue weakness), diplopia, syncope, tinnitus, amaurosis fugax, dysgeusia.

■ Benign Exertional Headache

Chief Clinical Characteristics

This presentation involves head pain that is associated with exertion or a Valsalva-type maneuver.

Background Information

When the headache occurs with a sudden onset, it is thought to be due to acute venous distention.[9] In cases with a more gradual onset, it has been shown to be due to arterial spasm.[10] Despite having a vascular nature, Sjaastad and others have demonstrated there is no convincing association between this condition and migraines.[4,10] Sentinel headache associated with subarachnoid hemorrhage or subdural hematoma must be ruled less likely in individuals suspected of benign exertional headache. A combination of avoidance or modification of aggravating activities and nonsteroidal anti-inflammatory or beta-blocker medications is typically considered in order to manage exertional headaches.

Clinical Features of Benign Exertional Headache

Pain Character	Throbbing or pulsatile.
Location	Bilateral.
Precipitants	Physical exertion, particularly in hot weather, high humidity, or high altitudes.
Onset	Rapid.
Duration	5 minutes to 24 hours.
Frequency	Related to precipitating activity.
Time Course	Begins quickly following activity.
Associated Symptoms/ Signs	May be characterized by migraine-like symptoms in those who are susceptible to migraines.

■ Benign Sexual Headache

Chief Clinical Characteristics

This presentation may include variable head and facial symptoms related to sexual activity. Three different subtypes of headache related to sexual activity have been identified. The first, regarded as the dull type, comes on as the sexual excitement increases.

Background Information

Sentinel headache associated with subarachnoid hemorrhage or subdural hematoma must be ruled less likely in individuals suspected of benign sexual headache. A combination of avoidance or modification of aggravating activities and nonsteroidal anti-inflammatory or beta-blocker medications is typically considered in order to manage exertional headaches.

Clinical Features of Benign Sexual Headache

Pain Character	Dull, throbbing, or explosive.
Location	Bilateral occipital, temporal, or facial.
Precipitants	Sexual activity or posturally related.
Onset	Depending on type, may be gradual onset, which increases as sexual excitement increases, or may have sudden onset in the case of orgasmic headaches.
Duration	May last up to 48 hours following sexual activity.
Frequency	Related to precipitating activity.
Time Course	Preorgasmic type—occurs with sexual activity and intensifies with sexual excitement. Orgasmic type—very sudden onset occurs with orgasm.
Associated Symptoms/ Signs	Neck and jaw pain.

■ Cluster Headaches

Chief Clinical Characteristics

This presentation can include an excruciating unilateral headache in the trigeminal distribution, lasting a short period of time but occurring relatively frequently, and associated with ipsilateral facial autonomic signs (Fig. 7-2A). This condition generally comes in bouts of several headaches of short duration that occur several times a day over a period of several weeks. It is rare and occurs more commonly in males than females.[11,12] The pain associated with cluster headaches is very severe and is often described as "boring, stabbing, or a hot poker in the eye."[13] This condition is localized to the orbital and temporal region. Attacks of pain are accompanied by one or more autonomic features ipsilateral to the pain. These signs include ptosis, miosis, lacrimation, nasal congestion, and rhinorrhea or conjunctiva injection. Each attack may last anywhere from 15 minutes to 3 hours and the attacks come in clusters of one per day to as many as eight per day. Cluster periods can last from 7 days to 1 year. In the episodic state there are periods of remission that last from 6 to 12 months.

Background Information

This condition is triggered by alcohol consumption, although it does not appear to precipitate headaches during periods of remission.[12] Other vasodilators have also been shown to induce attacks, such as nitroglycerin tablets and histamine.[14] Altitude hypoxemia and sleep apnea–induced hypoxemia also have been documented to induce cluster headaches during cluster periods.[15] A seasonal

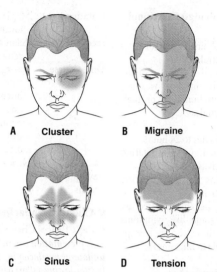

A   Cluster   **B**   Migraine

C   Sinus   **D**   Tension

FIGURE 7-2   Locations for common types of headaches: (A) cluster; (B) migraine; (C) sinus; (D) tension.

preponderance of cluster attacks occurs in the spring or fall. There is also a clock-like regularity with the onset of individual attacks.[12] The pathophysiology of cluster headaches remains unclear, but the trigeminovascular system, hypothalamus, and autonomic nervous system appear to be important components. Lifestyle modification to reduce risk factors, abortive medication, and prophylactic medication may be considered in the management of cluster headaches.

Clinical Features of Cluster Headaches

Pain Character	Excruciating intensity, boring or tearing, described as "hot poker" or "eye being pushed out."
Location	Almost always unilateral in a trigeminal distribution, typically orbital, retro-orbital, temporal, supra-orbital, and infraorbital.
Precipitants	Smoking, ethanol consumption, other vasodilators such as nitroglycerin tablets, histamine, altitude hypoxemia, sleep apnea.
Onset	Rapid onset reaching its peak in 10 to 15 minutes.
Duration	15 minutes to 3 hours.
Frequency	Range from one per week to eight or more per day.
Time Course	One to 4 months separated by remission that can last 6 to 24 months. Chronic cluster headaches continue for 1 year without remission.
Associated Symptoms/ Signs	Parasympathetic overactivity causes lacrimation, nasal stuffiness, runny nose, forehead and facial sweating. Partial sympathetic paralysis causes ptosis, miosis (Horner's syndrome).

■ Encephalitis

Chief Clinical Characteristics

This presentation often involves an abrupt onset of severe bifrontal headache associated with fever, confusion, altered level of consciousness, focal neurological deficits, and seizures.

Background Information

Several viral sources can lead to encephalitis (eg, arbovirus, mumps, herpes simplex and herpes zoster, Epstein-Barr, measles, and chickenpox), but the specific virus often cannot be identified.[16] Sudden and severe headaches may occur early and may be the only manifestation of encephalitis.[3] Magnetic resonance imaging is the imaging procedure of choice to confirm the diagnosis.[3] Individuals suspected of this condition require emergent medical attention.

Clinical Features of Headache Secondary to Encephalitis

Pain Character	Abrupt and severe.
Location	Bifrontal.
Precipitants	Viral or bacterial infection, such as herpes simplex, *Coxiella burnetii*, and *Listeria monocytogenes*.
Onset	Rapid.
Duration	Several days to 4 to 5 months in some chronic forms.
Frequency	Incidental to underlying disease.
Time Course	Headache occurs with encephalitis. Resolves within 3 months after infection is treated effectively with antibiotics or spontaneously ends.
Associated Symptoms/ Signs	Fever, confusion, altered level of consciousness, focal neurological deficits, seizures.

■ Fever-Induced Headache

Chief Clinical Characteristics
This presentation may be characterized by a bilaterally distributed diffuse headache that is associated with fever, nausea, vomiting, malaise, chills, photophobia, skin rash, and myalgias.

Background Information
Noncephalic causes may be viral in nature such as influenza or adenovirus. Bacterial causes include Rocky Mountain spotted fever and *Rickettsia*. The cause of headache in these acute cases is unclear but may be related to the interaction of inflammatory mechanisms with pain transmission. Some infective agents have a predilection for the central nervous system. They may invade the brainstem nuclei where the release of toxins activates headache mechanisms. In more chronic situations, headache may be caused by delayed septicemia. Viral illnesses such as herpes simplex or Epstein-Barr

appear to be related to more chronic presentations in which headache occurs after fever subsides. In these cases the headache may be caused by meningeal involvement. Management of fever-induced headaches involves treatment of the underlying bacterial infection or supportive intervention for viral causes.

Clinical Features of Fever-Induced Headache

Pain Character	Variable intensity.
Location	Bilateral and diffuse; occipital, frontal, or retro-orbital.
Precipitants	Viral or bacterial infection.
Onset	May occur concurrently with or following onset of fever.
Duration	Related to acute phase of illness. Resolves in less than 1 month after successful treatment or spontaneous remission of infection.
Frequency	Occurs with frequency of underlying disease.
Time Course	Variable.
Associated Symptoms/ Signs	Fever, nausea, vomiting, malaise, chills, photophobia, skin rash, myalgia.

■ Hypoglycemia

Chief Clinical Characteristics
This presentation includes a pressing or pounding bifrontal headache occurring within 16 hours after fasting or 30 minutes of ingesting food. Headaches due to hypoglycemia are more common in individuals with diabetes mellitus and those who skip meals. Headaches due to this condition also may be associated with nausea, light-headedness, confusion, and lethargy.

Background Information
Headaches associated with fasting may result from metabolic changes such as hypoglycemia or the accumulation of certain metabolites.[17] In those individuals who suffer from more chronic types of headache such as migraine or tension-type headaches, hypoglycemia may be a precipitating factor.[18] A small percentage of individuals have the onset of headache within 30 minutes of breaking their fast. This could be due to postprandial hypoglycemia. Management of headaches secondary

to hypoglycemia includes lifestyle and dietary modifications. Individuals with diabetes mellitus who are suspected of having hypoglycemia may require consultation regarding their current regimen of insulin therapy.

Clinical Features of Headache Secondary to Hypoglycemia

Pain Character	Pressing or pounding.
Location	Bitemporal or bifrontal.
Precipitants	Diabetes mellitus, fasting, or skipping meals.
Onset	Within 16 hours after fasting.
Duration	15 to 30 minutes following the ingestion of food.
Frequency	Incidental to individual's diet and activity level.
Time Course	Resolves within 15 to 30 minutes of nutrition intake.
Associated Symptoms/ Signs	Nausea, light-headedness, confusion, lethargy.

■ Hypoxia

Chief Clinical Characteristics

This presentation involves a pounding frontal headache within 24 hours of ascent to a high altitude, which may be associated with nausea, vomiting, vertigo, palpitations, and impaired vision.

Background Information

Situations that can produce hypoxia may be environmental with reduced ambient oxygen, such as high altitude or normal altitude with low O_2 conditions. This condition also may occur in disease conditions such as pulmonary disease or disorders of oxygen delivery such as anemia, cardiac failure, or carbon monoxide poisoning. The etiology of headaches associated with this condition is unclear, although the increase in cerebral blood flow associated with hypoxia may be the underlying cause. The increase in cerebral blood flow is caused by vasodilation, which can produce pain by stretching of the vessel exciting trigeminal sensory afferents, which in turn innervate the large pain-producing cranial vessels.[18] Headaches secondary to hypoxia are managed with supplemental oxygen. In particular, individuals with cardiopulmonary disease or other disorders of oxygen transport who are

suspected of headaches due to hypoxia should be referred for evaluation.

Clinical Features of Headache Secondary to Hypoxia

Pain Character	Pounding.
Location	Frontal; 25% are unilateral.
Precipitants	Pulmonary disease and other disorders of oxygen delivery (eg, anemia, carbon monoxide intoxication), sudden ascent to high altitude (10,000 ft), or exertion at high altitude.
Onset	Within 24 hours of hypoxic incident.
Duration	Up to 48 hours.
Frequency	Incidental to individual's diet and activity level.
Time Course	Occurs within 24 hours of being exposed to hypoxic state and resolves within 48 hours of returning to normal atmospheric conditions.
Associated Symptoms/ Signs	Nausea, vomiting, vertigo, palpitations, impaired vision.

■ Idiopathic Intracranial Hypertension (Pseudotumor Cerebri)

Chief Clinical Characteristics

This presentation can include a gradual onset of throbbing, pressing headache that involves the entire cranium.

Background Information

This condition exists when an increase in intracranial pressure occurs that is caused by hydrocephalus or intracranial mass. Along with headaches the condition is characterized by papilledema, but there are no abnormalities in the composition of the cerebrospinal fluid and there are no localizing neurological signs. The exact cause is unknown but several hypotheses have been suggested. The most commonly accepted hypotheses are an increase in the brain water content, increased resistance to cerebrospinal fluid outflow, or a hypothalamic-pituitary disturbance. Management of this health condition may range from medications to lower intracranial pressure to emergency surgical intervention in patients with deteriorating visual field impairments.[19]

Clinical Features of Headache Secondary to Idiopathic Intracranial Hypertension (Pseudotumor Cerebri)

Pain Character	Throbbing or pressing.
Location	Can be the entire cranium or may be unilateral.
Precipitants	Obstruction of the cerebrospinal fluid flow at any of several sites.
Onset	Acute or gradual.
Duration	Typically 1 week (in the case of lumbar puncture), or may be several weeks or months (in the case of fistula).
Frequency	Daily.
Time Course	Prolonged. The condition is not always self-limiting.
Associated Symptoms/ Signs	Papilledema, visual field defects, loss of visual acuity, nausea, and to a lesser degree vomiting. Occasionally hearing difficulties and tinnitus.

■ Idiopathic Intracranial Hypotension

Chief Clinical Characteristics
This presentation typically involves a deep, aching headache that occurs rapidly after assuming an upright posture. This condition most commonly is caused by a lumbar puncture. In the case of post–lumbar puncture headache, onset is within 7 days and resolves within 14 days. Headaches are worse when standing and decrease when lying down. Those that do not resolve within 14 days may be due to a persistent fistula.

Background Information
In either case the underlying problem is a leak of cerebrospinal fluid. Major trauma, neurosurgery, or erosive lesions also may cause cerebrospinal fluid leaks. With a decrease of cerebrospinal fluid, there is a decrease in pressure and volume that causes cerebral veins to dilate. The brain then loses its cerebrospinal fluid cushion. Management may include options ranging from bed rest, epidural blood patching, percutaneous fibrin sealant placement, and surgical leak repair.[20]

Clinical Features of Headache Secondary to Idiopathic Intracranial Hypotension

Pain Character	Aching, dull, deep, constricting, or throbbing.
Location	Bilateral, frontal, occipital, or generalized.
Precipitants	Lumbar puncture or development of fistula in which upright position produces headache rapidly.
Onset	Rapid—within 20 seconds of assuming upright posture.
Duration	Typically 1 week (in the case of lumbar puncture), or may be several weeks or months (in the case of fistula).
Frequency	Incidental.
Time Course	Initially headache occurs rapidly when assuming upright position. In the case of lumbar puncture headache comes on more gradually over the course of 1 week.
Associated Symptoms/ Signs	Dizziness, nausea, vomiting. Occasionally hearing difficulties and tinnitus.

■ Medication Overuse Headache

Chief Clinical Characteristics
This presentation may involve progressively worsening daily headaches present greater than 15 days per month in the presence of regular overuse of a medication for greater than 3 months.[21] Headaches due to medication overuse resolve or revert to their previous pattern within 2 months of ceasing the overused medication. Headache intensity may be widely variable from day to day.

Background Information
Inappropriate use of headache medications—such as ergotamine, triptans, opioids, and simple or combination analgesics—may contribute to the development of chronic daily headaches.[22] This condition also is known as analgesic rebound headache, chronic daily headache, chronic migraine, medication-induced migraine, or transformed migraine.

In addition, cardiovascular drugs (eg, calcium channel blockers, antiarrhythmics, phosphodiesterase inhibitors, alpha-1 agonists and antagonists, beta-adrenergic antagonists, angiotensin converting enzyme inhibitors, angiotensin II receptor antagonists, and organic nitrates), anti-infective agents (eg, various antibacterial, antifungal, and antiretroviral drugs), immunomodulatory drugs, anti-inflammatory drugs, antihistamines, medications used to treat asthma, and tricyclic antidepressants are most commonly implicated in promoting headaches.[23–25] A retrospective diagnosis is made when the offending agent is withdrawn and the headache pattern ceases to be daily. Although discontinued use of these medications can relieve the undesirable symptoms, discontinuation should occur with appropriate medical consultation including appropriate substitution as needed.

Clinical Features of Headache Secondary to Medication Overuse

Pain Character	Dull.
Location	Variable.
Precipitants	Ingestion of antipyretic or anti-inflammatory analgesics, triptans, ergotamine, or opioids.
Onset	Weeks or months after initiating use of offending medications.
Duration	Constant.
Frequency	Daily.
Time Course	Typically begins after a 3-month or more period of taking offending medications. Resolves within a few days after discontinuing the medication.
Associated Symptoms/ Signs	Typically absent of migraine-like symptoms.

■ Meningitis

Chief Clinical Characteristics

This presentation can involve a rapid onset of progressive frontal or generalized headache that is associated with fever, cough, skin rash, lethargy, altered level of consciousness, nuchal rigidity, or photophobia. Headache secondary to meningitis may last several days to 3 months. Symptoms may radiate to the cervical region and into the upper thoracic region and even the extremities.[16]

Background Information

The headache associated with this condition may be caused by meningeal irritation with direct stimulation of the sensory terminal in the meninges.[16] It may also be due to increased intracranial pressure caused by an accumulation of exudates, which obstructs the circulation of cerebrospinal fluid.[3] In addition, this headache may be caused by a distant infection.[26] To properly identify the infective organism for the most appropriate treatment, a lumbar puncture must be performed.[16] Identification of the infective organism guides management of this health condition.

Clinical Features of Headache Secondary to Meningitis

Pain Character	Moderate or severe.
Location	Frontal or generalized.
Precipitants	Viral or bacterial infection.
Onset	Rapid.
Duration	Several days to 3 months.
Frequency	Incidental to underlying disease.
Time Course	Typically has a relatively rapid onset. Resolves within 3 months after infection is treated effectively with antibiotics or spontaneously ends.
Associated Symptoms/ Signs	Fever, cough, skin rash, lethargy, altered level of consciousness, and meningism as demonstrated by nuchal rigidity and photophobia.

■ Migraine

Chief Clinical Characteristics

This presentation often includes a severe pulsating and throbbing unilateral headache that may switch sides, associated with nausea, vomiting, diarrhea, abdominal cramps, polyuria, sweating, facial pallor, photophobia, or phonophobia (see Fig. 7-2B). This condition is a chronic condition of recurring attacks of transient focal neurological symptoms, headaches, or both.[27] Not only is this process responsible for producing headaches, the condition can also interfere with the function of other body systems.[28] *Migraines are preceded by aura in 20% of cases.[29] Even in individuals who commonly experience them, auras may not accompany every headache. Auras can be visual, somatosensory, olfactory, or involve speech disturbances. The location of headache may switch sides from episode to episode.*

Background Information

The pathophysiology of this condition is very complex. Current theories postulate that a cascade of events occurs that involves vasodilation of meningeal blood vessels, irritation of perivascular sensory nerves, and stimulation of brainstem nuclei. Additionally, extrinsic factors such as hormonal fluctuations, fatigue, or anxiety may be triggers that initiate the pathophysiological cascade. This condition also has a strong familial tendency and begins at a young age, suggesting that genetic factors may predispose individuals to migraine attacks. The use of neuroimaging is not indicated in individuals with migraine symptoms and a normal neurological exam. Certain pharmaceutical agents, such as triptans and ergots, are effective in preventing migraine attacks from becoming too severe.[30] Other medications can be considered to prevent migraine attacks.

Clinical Features of Migraine

Pain Character	Very severe and is typically described as pulsating and throbbing. The headache may start out as a dull steady ache and progress to the more characteristic features.
Location	Typically unilateral (but can switch sides). Localized to temple, forehead or eye, or back of head.
Precipitants	Stress, relaxation after stress, fatigue, too little or too much sleep, skipping meals, menstruation, weather changes, high altitudes, exposure to glare or flickering lights, loud noises, physical activity, food triggers such as red wine, food additives such as MSG, nitrates or aspartate, caffeine or caffeine withdrawal.
Onset	Males—10 to 13 years. Females—menarche.
Duration	4 to 72 hours.
Frequency	At least five attacks per year, but chronic migraines may occur daily.
Time Course	Typically upon awakening in the morning and takes several hours to build to maximum intensity.
Associated Symptoms/ Signs	Nausea, vomiting, diarrhea, anorexia, abdominal cramps, polyuria, sweating, pallor of the face, photophobia, or phonophobia. Impairment of concentration, memory impairment, depression, fatigue, anxiety, irritability, and light-headedness.

■ Post-Traumatic Headache

Chief Clinical Characteristics

This presentation may be characterized by a vertex or band-like headache that develops within 7 days after head trauma or regaining consciousness following head trauma and persists for 3 months or greater.[21] Acute post-traumatic headaches may last 2 to 8 weeks after trauma, and chronic post-traumatic headaches may last up to 6 months to 4 years. Post-traumatic headache may be associated with somatic symptoms (eg, dizziness, photophobia, phonophobia, tinnitus, blurring of vision, and rapid fatigue) and psychological symptoms (eg, depression, anxiety, apathy, insomnia, decreased libido, irritability, and frequent mood swings).

Background Information

Rebound headache must be ruled out before the diagnosis of chronic post-traumatic headache is reached.[31] The severity of the head injury does not correlate to the duration or intensity of this headache. This condition occurs in 30% to 90% of people with concussion, and it was the most common symptom reported in professional football players who sustained a mild traumatic brain injury.[32] Patients suspected of post-traumatic headaches should be monitored for signs of skull fracture, subarachnoid hemorrhage, and subdural hematoma.

Post-traumatic headaches are commonly managed with rest and nonsteroidal anti-inflammatory medication.

Clinical Features of Post-Traumatic Headache

Pain Character	Mild to moderate intensity, steady ache.
Location	May be a vertex or may be band-like around the head.
Precipitants	Trauma and, if present prior to trauma, concomitant primary form of headache.
Onset	Acute form—within 2 weeks of trauma. Chronic form—begins when amnesia resolves.
Duration	Acute form—2 to 8 weeks following trauma. Chronic form—may last up to 6 months and in about 25% of cases can persist for up to 4 years.
Frequency	Daily.
Time Course	Develops within 7 days following trauma and in the chronic form headache can last 3 months or longer.
Associated Symptoms/ Signs	Somatic symptoms include dizziness, photophobia, phonophobia, tinnitus, blurring of vision, easily fatigable. Psychological symptoms include depression, anxiety, apathy, insomnia, decreased libido, irritability, frequent mood swings.

■ Sinusitis

Chief Clinical Characteristics
This presentation typically includes a strong pressure sensation associated with facial headache and upper respiratory infection (see Fig. 7-2C).

Background Information
This condition results from inflammation of the nasal membranes and the nasal sinuses. It is caused when an upper respiratory infection produces inflammation of the nasal mucous membrane. The inflammation causes an obstruction of the orifices of the nasal sinuses. Management of headache secondary to sinusitis centers on appropriate treatment of the underlying infection.

Clinical Features of Headache Secondary to Sinusitis

Pain Character	Strong pressure sensation.
Location	Frontal—frontal region, vertex, behind eyes. Maxillary—maxillary region, upper teeth forehead. Ethmoid—behind eyes, temporal region. Sphenoid—occipital region, vertex, frontal region behind eyes.
Precipitants	Viral or bacterial infection of the upper respiratory tract.
Onset	Gradual.
Duration	Days to months.
Frequency	Variable.
Time Course	Strongest after waking.
Associated Symptoms/ Signs	Purulent discharge, swelling of eyelids, and lacrimation.

■ Stroke or Transient Ischemic Attack

Chief Clinical Characteristics
This presentation may include a sudden onset of atypical hemicranial pain ipsilateral to the affected cerebral hemisphere, associated with hemiplegia, aphasia, excessive salivation, facial symmetry, and altered level of consciousness. The presentation of headache due to a cerebrovascular event is similar to migraine and tension-type headaches except for the associated neurological signs.

Background Information
Headache occurs in about one-third of cerebral infarcts and in 10% to 15% of patients with transient ischemic attacks (TIAs).[3] Headaches associated with stroke or TIA present as a new symptom or for people with chronic headache as a different presentation of headache.[33] A sentinel or premonitory headache may occur in approximately one-third of cases.[3] According to the IHS, focal

nervous system signs or symptoms should begin within 48 hours after onset of the headache.[21] The severity, quality, and duration of headache pain associated with cerebrovascular accident (CVA) or TIA is variable as is the location of the pain. Dodick[3] reports that the headache symptoms more closely resemble tension or migraine headaches than the headaches of hemorrhagic stroke. According to Jousilahti and colleagues,[34] chronic headache is an independent predictor of stroke, especially during a short follow-up. Therefore, chronic headache may be a marker of an underlying disease process that leads to acute stroke.[34] Individuals suspected of this condition require emergent medical attention.

Clinical Features of Headache Secondary to Stroke or Transient Ischemic Attack

Pain Character	Variable, resembling migraine or tension-type headache.
Location	Hemicranial, ipsilateral to ischemic hemisphere.
Precipitants	Risk factors for stroke or transient ischemic attack, including hypertension and smoking.
Onset	Abrupt.
Duration	Hours to 2 to 3 weeks.
Frequency	Related to the precipitating incident.
Time Course	Within 48 hours preceding stroke or transient ischemic attack.
Associated Symptoms/ Signs	Hemiplegia, aphasia, drooling, facial symmetry, and altered level of consciousness.

■ Subarachnoid Hemorrhage

Chief Clinical Characteristics

This presentation can involve a sudden onset of severe and abrupt hemifacial pain that is associated with a slight change in level of consciousness, blurred vision, diplopia, asymmetrical pupil response, and nuchal rigidity. Headaches due to this condition may radiate to the cervical, thoracic, and lumbar spine.

Background Information

Subarachnoid hemorrhage accounts for 3% to 9% of all strokes and is defined as the presence of blood in the subarachnoid space that surrounds the central nervous system.[35] Ruptured aneurysms and arteriovenous malformations can lead to this condition. Hypertension and diabetes mellitus are two significant risk factors,[35] and polycystic kidney disease, Ehlers-Danlos syndrome, systemic lupus erythematosus, and pregnancy are also known risk factors.[36] Polmear[37] reported that between 50% and 60% of patients with this condition described a previous history of an atypical headache days to weeks before the event. This warning sign is known as a *sentinel headache*.[37] The headache may be accompanied by signs of meningeal irritation (which produces nuchal rigidity), along with varying degrees of neurological dysfunction such as seizures, hemiparesis, and dysphasia.[36] The diagnosis is confirmed with a CT scan without contrast along with lumbar puncture.[36] Emergent medical attention is necessary for individuals suspected of this condition.

Clinical Features of Headache Secondary to Subarachnoid Hemorrhage

Pain Character	Severe.
Location	Hemifacial with possible radiation to the cervical, thoracic, or lumbar regions.
Precipitants	Physical exertion, such as exercise or sexual intercourse.
Onset	Abrupt.
Duration	Days or weeks prior to subarachnoid hemorrhage.
Frequency	Related to the precipitating incident.
Time Course	Abrupt onset occurring within seconds of hemorrhage and can continue for several hours. The headache typically resolves within 1 to 3 weeks.
Associated Symptoms/ Signs	Slight change in level of consciousness, blurred vision, diplopia, asymmetric pupil response, and nuchal rigidity.

■ Subdural Hematoma

Chief Clinical Characteristics

This presentation involves a new onset of unilateral or occipital headache associated with a decline in level of consciousness and focal neurological deficits. Secondary symptoms include autonomic signs, vomiting, somnolence, or signs of personality change.[38]

Background Information

The location of headache depends on the location of hematoma. Somewhere between 62% and 80% of patients with chronic hematomas report headaches.[33] Symptoms develop within hours to weeks after the precipitating event. This condition may be caused by severe sneezing, coughing, strain from heavy lifting, and whiplash injury.[39] It is also a rare though well-documented sequel of lumbar punctures.[40] Predisposing factors include advanced age, alcoholism, and coagulation disorders.[38] Subdural hematomas form when bridging veins rupture and blood accumulates in the space between the arachnoid and the dura. Individuals suspected of a subdural hematoma should be referred for CT scan without contrast on an emergent basis.

Clinical Features of Headache Secondary to Subdural Hematoma

Pain Character	Mild or moderate.
Location	Unilateral side ipsilateral to hematoma with the specific region depending on site of hematoma.
Precipitants	60% to 70% of time subdural hematoma is preceded by trauma such as a fall, severe coughing or sneezing, strain from heavy lifting, or whiplash.
Onset	May occur within hours to weeks after precipitating event.
Duration	Hours or weeks.
Frequency	Related to the precipitating incident.
Time Course	May be steadily progressive or may recur after pain-free interval.
Associated Symptoms/ Signs	Changes in personality or cognitive abilities, neurological signs such as weakness, sensory changes or seizures, lethargy, drowsiness, or decreased level of consciousness. Also may be accompanied by autonomic symptoms.

■ Temporal Arteritis

Chief Clinical Characteristics

This presentation includes an acute onset of severe temporal pain in an individual over 50 years of age, associated with symptoms of jaw or tongue claudication, scalp tenderness, temporal artery swelling and pulselessness, diplopia, elevated erythrocyte sedimentation rate, altered level of consciousness, fever, weight loss, malaise, and myalgias.

Background Information

This condition, also known as giant cell arteritis, is the most common form of vasculitis in adults.[41] In individuals over 50 years old, 94.8% sensitivity and 100% sensitivity was obtained if a symptom cluster consisting of jaw claudication, new-onset headache, and abnormal temporal arteries on examination was used to diagnose this condition compared with temporal arterial biopsy.[42] The clinical manifestations of this condition are caused by local and systemic inflammatory disease. Localized arterial inflammation causes endovascular damage, vessel stenosis and occlusion, ultimately leading to tissue ischemia or necrosis.[43] This process leads to the clinical manifestations of jaw claudication and visual disturbances or loss. This condition can lead to permanent blindness if left untreated. It can be treated successfully with administration of proper steroidal medication. Even though headaches and other clinical symptoms may subside within a few days of initiating this form of treatment, it should continue for 1 to 2 years due to the continued risk of blindness.

Clinical Features of Headache Secondary to Temporal Arteritis

Pain Character	Severe and throbbing.
Location	May be diffuse or localized to temporal region. Bitemporal in half of reported cases.
Precipitants	Exposure to cold.
Onset	Acute onset of new headache in a patient/client age 50 years or older.
Duration	Typically 2 to 3 months before seeking medical care.
Frequency	Related to the precipitating incident.

HEADACHES

Time Course	Tends to be worse at night.
Associated Symptoms/ Signs	Jaw or tongue claudication, temporal artery swelling and pulselessness, diplopia, elevated erythrocyte sedimentation rate, altered level of consciousness, fever, weight loss, malaise, or myalgias.

■ Temporomandibular Dysfunction

Chief Clinical Characteristics
This presentation may be characterized by headache radiating from the muscles of mastication, the periauricular region, or the temporomandibular joint associated with abnormal jaw function, asymmetric chewing, bruxism, neck pain, tinnitus, and vertigo.

Background Information
Headache pain related to this condition may be caused by pathology of the temporomandibular joint or may be an associated symptom of another form of headache. This condition is believed to be an aggravating factor in headaches and only the cause if clearly related to the clinical signs and symptoms involving the masticatory system.[44] Typical management involves a combination of rehabilitative and pharmacological interventions for headaches related to temporomandibular dysfunction.

Clinical Features of Headache Secondary to Temporomandibular Dysfunction

Pain Character	Dull ache.
Location	Muscles of mastication, periauricular region, or the temporomandibular joint. Most often headache is unilateral but may be bilateral.
Precipitants	Abnormal jaw function, asymmetrical chewing, bruxism.
Onset	Within minutes to hours of precipitating activity.
Duration	Hours or weeks.
Frequency	Incidental to precipitating incident.
Time Course	Variable, depending on underlying cause of temporomandibular dysfunction.
Associated Symptoms/ Signs	Neck pain, tinnitus, and vertigo.

■ Tension-Type Headache

Chief Clinical Characteristics
This presentation can involve a band-like distribution of nonthrobbing headache radiating from frontal region to occiput, associated with stress, anxiety, and neck tenderness (see Fig. 7-2D).

Background Information
This condition is the most common headache presentation, accounting for more than two-thirds of all headache episodes (Rasmussen) and affecting 33% to 80% of the population.[45,46] Women are affected slightly more often than men.[45] Prevalence peaks in the 30- to 39-year-old age group[45] and is found to increase in incidence with increasing educational levels.[45] It is important to differentiate between the episodic type of tension headache and the more chronic form because the management of these two variations differs.[46] This differentiation is based entirely on the frequency and duration of occurrence. This condition lacks the IHS migraine-defining features of nausea, phonophobia, or photophobia.[45] Increased muscle hardness has been demonstrated in patients who suffer from chronic tension headaches, whether or not a headache is currently present.[47] Rehabilitative interventions, non-narcotic analgesics, and triptans may be used to manage this health condition.

Clinical Features of Tension-Type Headache

Pain Character	Mild to moderate tightness, pressure, or dull ache[48] that is nonthrobbing.[49]
Location	Usually bilateral (but may be unilateral in 10% to 15% of cases), radiating from forehead to occiput. Tenderness can radiate into the posterior cervical muscles. In more involved cases the pain distribution is "cape-like," radiating along the upper trapezius muscles covering the shoulders, scapula, and interscapular areas.[50] Also may be described as "band-like."

HEADACHES

Precipitants	Stress or anxiety,[51] not eating on time, fatigue, and lack of sleep are common precipitants in those experiencing this condition.[52]
Onset	Variable.
Duration	Can last from 30 minutes to several days.
Frequency	Infrequent episodic—less than 10 times per year. Frequent episodic—at least 10 episodes occurring more than one time but less than 15 times per month. Chronic—occurring greater than 15 times per month for more than 3 months.[1]
Time Course	Variable.
Associated Symptoms/ Signs	Tenderness is the most common physical finding in patients with this condition.[53] Palpation may reveal tenderness in pericranial muscles and tension in the nuchal musculature or trapezius.[48] This condition does not worsen with exercise.[45]

■ Tumors (Brain)

Chief Clinical Characteristics

This presentation typically includes a headache of variable intensity and location that is relieved with bending forward and associated with papilledema, nausea and vomiting, focal neurological changes, and seizures.

Background Information

It is uncommon for headache to be the only clinical manifestation of a brain tumor in a patient with a normal neurological exam. Between 50% and 60% of patients with brain tumors report having headaches and many who have them do not report severe pain.[54] Tumors most likely to be detected early are those that are rapidly growing, supratentorial (such as glioblastoma), or obstructing the outflow of cerebrospinal fluid (such as an intraventricular or posterior fossa tumor), because they are more likely to produce abnormal neurological signs and symptoms.[3] Headaches from tumors are often nondescript and are not themselves pathognomic of a diagnosis of

neoplasm. Individuals suspected of headaches related to tumor should be referred for appropriate evaluation including neuroimaging.

Headache features that are most suggestive of a space-occupying lesion include[3]:

- Headache that is subacute and progressive in nature
- New onset of headache after age 40 or significant change in an existing headache pattern
- Headache associated with:
  - Nausea or vomiting not due to migraine or illness
  - Abnormal neurological signs
  - Altered level of consciousness or seizures
  - Night pain.

Tumors leading to headaches include:

- Malignant primary, such as:
  - Meningeal tumors
  - Primary brain tumors.
- Malignant metastatic, such as:
  - Central nervous system parenchymal metastasis
  - Leptomeningeal metastasis
  - Skull base metastasis.
- Benign, such as:
  - Acoustic neuroma.

Clinical Features of Headache Secondary to Tumor

Pain Character	Mild, moderate, or severe intensity.
Location	Dependent on location of tumor. Frontal or frontotemporal is most common.
Precipitants	Bending forward.
Onset	May be gradual until tumor expands to a critical volume, then may be very rapid.
Duration	Typically 2 to 3 months before seeking medical care.
Frequency	Incidental.
Time Course	Few brain tumor headaches last more than 10 weeks without other symptoms developing.
Associated Symptoms/ Signs	Papilledema, nausea, vomiting, focal neurological changes, and seizures.

References

1. Olesen J, Lipton RB. Headache classification update 2004. *Cur Opin Neurol.* 2004;17:275–282.
2. Solomon S. Diagnosis of primary headache disorders. Validity of International Headache Society criteria in clinical practice. *Neurol Clin.* 1997;15:15–26.
3. Dodick D. Headache as a symptom of ominous disease. *J Postgrad Med.* 1997;101(5):1–12.
4. Sjaastad O. Benign exertional headache. *Headache.* 2003;43:611–615.
5. D'Amico D, Leone M, Bussone G. Side locked unilaterality and pain localization in long lasting headaches: migraine, tension-type and cervicogenic headache. *Headache.* 1994;34:526–530.
6. Sjaastad O, Fredriksen TA, Pfaffenrath V. Cervicogenic headache: diagnostic criteria. The Cervicogenic Headache International Study Group. *Headache.* 1998;38:442–445.
7. Zetterling M, Carlström C, Konrad P. Internal carotid dissection. *Acta Neurol Scand.* 2000;101(1):1–7.
8. Biousse V, et al. Carotid or vertebral artery pain. In: Olesen J, Tfelt-Hansen P, Welch KMA, eds. *The Headaches.* 2nd ed. Philadelphia: Lippincott Williams & Wilkins; 2000.
9. Goadsby PJ, Lance JW. Miscellaneous headaches associated with functional or structural lesions. In: Olesen J, Tfelt-Hansen P, Welch KMA, eds. *The Headaches.* 2nd ed. Philadelphia: Lippincott Williams & Wilkins; 2000:1026.
10. McCory P. Headaches and exercise. *Sports Med.* 2000;30(3):221–229.
11. Manzoni G. Gender ratios of cluster headaches over the years. *Cephalalgia.* 1998;18:138–142.
12. Newman LC. Cluster and related headaches. *Med Clin North Am.* 2001;85(4):997–1016.
13. Mathews N. Cluster headaches. *Semin Neurol.* 1997;17(4):313–323.
14. Zakrzewska J. Cluster headaches: a review of the literature. *Br J Oral Maxillofacial Surg.* 2001;39:103–113.
15. Kudrow L, Kudrow DB. The role of chemoreceptor activity and oxyhemoglobin desaturation in cluster headaches. *Headache.* 1993;33:483–484.
16. Marinis M, et al. Headache associated with intracranial infection. In: Olesen J, Tfelt-Hansen P, Welch KMA, eds. *The Headaches.* 2nd ed. Philadelphia: Lippincott Williams & Wilkins; 2000:841–848.
17. Mosek A, Korczyn AD. Yom Kippur headache. *Neurology.* 1995;45(11):1953–1955.
18. Goadsby P. Metabolic and endocrine disorders. In: Olesen J, Tfelt-Hansen P, Welch KMA, eds. *The Headaches.* 2nd ed. Philadelphia: Lippincott Williams & Wilkins; 2000.
19. Shah VA, Kardon RH, Lee AG, Corbett JJ, Wall M. Long-term follow-up of idiopathic intracranial hypertension: the Iowa experience. *Neurology.* 2008; 70(8):634–640.
20. Schievink WI. Spontaneous spinal cerebrospinal fluid leaks and intracranial hypotension. *JAMA.* 2006;295(19):2286–2296.
21. International Headache Society. The International Classification of Headache Disorders. *Cephalalgia.* 2004;24(suppl 1):1–160.
22. Diener HC, et al. *Headaches Associated with Chronic Use of Substances.* 2nd ed. Philadelphia: Lippincott Williams & Wilkins; 2000.
23. Rosenberg H. Trismus is not trivial. *Anesthesiology.* 1987;67(4):453–455.
24. Hinkle AJ, Dorsch JA. Maternal masseter muscle rigidity and neonatal fasciculations after induction for emergency cesarean section. *Anesthesiology.* 1993;79(1):175–177.
25. Ferrari A. Headache: one of the most common and troublesome adverse reactions to drugs. *Curr Drug Saf.* 2006;1(1):43–58.
26. van de Beek D, de Gans J, Spanjaard L, et al. Clinical features and prognostic factors in adults with bacterial meningitis. *N Engl J Med.* 2004;351:1849–1859.
27. Spierings ELH. Mechanisms of migraine and actions of antimigraine medications. *Med Clin North Am.* 2001;85(4):943–958.
28. Ferrari MD. Migraine. *Lancet.* 1998;351 (9108):1043–1051.
29. Marks DR, Rapoport AM. Diagnosis of migraine. *Semin Neurol.* 1997;17(4):303–306.
30. Maizels M. Headache evaluation and treatment by primary care physicians in an emergency department in the era of triptans. *Arch Intern Med.* 2001;161:1969–1973.
31. Warner JS. Posttraumatic headache—a myth? *Arch Neurol.* 2000;57(12):1778–1780.
32. Pellman EJ, Powell JW, Viano DC, et al, Concussion in professional football: epidemiological features of games injuries and review of literature. *Neurosurgery.* 2004;34(1):81–97.
33. Jensen TS, et al. Headache associated with ischemic stroke and intracranial hematoma. In: Olesen J, Tfelt-Hansen P, Welch KMA, eds. *The Headaches.* 2nd ed. Philadelphia: Lippincott Williams & Wilkins; 2000:781–787.
34. Jousilahti P, Tuomilehto J, Rastenyte D, Vartiainen E. Headache and the risk of stroke: a prospective observational cohort study among 35,056 Finnish men and women. *Arch Intern Med.* 2003;163:1058–1062.
35. Simpson RK, Contant CF, Fischer DK, et al. Epidemiological characteristics of subarachnoid hemorrhage in an urban population. *J Clin Epidemiol.* 1991;44(7):641–648.
36. Sawin PD, Loftus CM. Diagnosis of spontaneous subarachnoid hemorrhage. *Am Fam Physician* 1997;55(1):145–156.
37. Polmear A. Sentinel headaches in aneurysmal subarachnoid hemorrhage: what is the true incidence? *Cephalalgia.* 2003;23:935–941.
38. Nolte CH, Lehmann TN. Postpartum headache resulting from bilateral chronic subdural hematoma after dural puncture. *Am J Emerg Med.* 2004;22(3):241–242.
39. Fukutake T. Roller coaster headache and subdural hematoma. *Neurology.* 2000;37:121.
40. Davies JM, Murphy A, Smith M, O'Sullivan G. Subdural haematoma after dural puncture headache treated by epidural blood patch. *Br J Anaesthsia.* 2001;86(5):720–723.
41. Lichtstein DM, Caceres LR. Heeding clues to giant cell arteritis. *J Postgrad Med.* 2004;115(5):91–99.
42. Lee AG, Brazis PW. Temporal arteritis: a clinical approach. *J Am Geriatr Soc.* 1999;47(11):1364–1370.
43. Smetana GW, et al. Does this patient have temporal arteritis. *JAMA.* 2002;287(1):92–101.
44. Grath-Radford S, et al. Oromandibular disorders. In: Olesen J, Tfelt-Hansen P, Welch KMA, eds. *The*

Headaches. 2nd ed. Philadelphia: Lippincott Williams & Wilkins; 2000.

45. Schwartz B. Epidemiology of tension-type headache. *JAMA*. 1998;279(5):381–383.

46. Walling AD. Tension-type headache: a challenge for family physicians. *Am Fam Physician*. 2002;66:728–730.

47. Ashina M. Muscle hardness in patients with chronic tension-type headache: relation to actual headache state. *Pain*. 1999;79:201–205.

48. Millea P. Tension-type headache. *Am Fam Physician*. 2002;66(5):797–804.

49. Smetana GW. The diagnostic value of historical features in primary headaches syndromes: a comprehensive review. *Arch Intern Med*. 2000;160:2729–2737.

50. Spira P. Tension headaches. *Aust Fam Physician*. 1998;27:597–600.

51. Steiner TJ. Guidelines for all doctors in the diagnosis and management of migraine and tension-type headaches. *British Association for the Study of Headache*. Published August 2004. Accessed November 12, 2004.

52. Spierings ELH. Precipitating and aggravating factors of migraine vs. tension-type headache. *Headache*. 2001;41:554–558.

53. Ashina M. The measurement of muscle hardness. *Cephalalgia*. 1998;18:106–111.

54. Forsyth PA, et al. Intracranial neoplasms. In: Olesen J, Tfelt-Hansen P, Welch KMA, eds. *The Headaches*. 2nd ed. Philadelphia: Lippincott Williams & Wilkins; 2000:849–859.

CHAPTER **8**

Temporomandibular Joint and Facial Pain

■ *Sally Ho, PT, DPT, OCS*

Description of the Symptom

This chapter describes pathology that may lead to temporomandibular joint and facial pain. Local causes of temporomandibular and facial symptoms include pathology of the temporomandibular joint, associated articular and periarticular structures (shading), and the facial bones including the sinuses, excluding the frontal bones and pharynx. Remote causes are defined as occurring outside these areas.

Special Concerns

- Fever with jaw and tooth pain
- Pain in masseter area with changes in salivation
- Progressive limitation of mandibular ROM and increasing pain
- Severe facial pain with hypersensitivity to touch
- Sudden onset of severe headache
- Stiff neck associated with fever

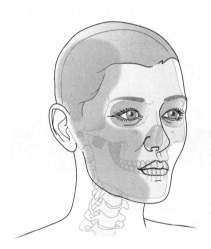

CHAPTER PREVIEW: **Conditions That May Lead to Temporomandibular Joint and Facial Pain**

T Trauma

REMOTE	LOCAL
COMMON	
Headaches: • Cervicogenic headache 81	Anteriorly displaced disk with or without reduction 86 Dental trauma: • Edentulism and denture wear 87 • Malocclusion 87 • Tooth injury 87 Dislocations: • Dislocation of the mandibular condyle into the middle cranial fossa 89 Internal derangement of the temporomandibular joint 92 Trismus 95
UNCOMMON	
Headaches: • Post-traumatic headache 82	Dislocations: • Dislocation of the mandibular condyle 89 Fractures: • Mandible 90 • Maxilla 90 • Orbit 90 • Temporal bone 91 • Zygomatic arch 91
RARE	
Not applicable	Dislocations: • Botulinum toxin–induced dislocation 89

I Inflammation

REMOTE	LOCAL
COMMON	
Aseptic Systemic lupus erythematosus 84 **Septic** Otitis media 84	**Aseptic** Adhesion of the temporomandibular joint 85 Ankylosing spondylitis 85 Capsulitis of the temporomandibular joint 86 Herpes zoster 91 Myofascial pain disorder syndrome 92 Retrodiscitis of the temporomandibular joint 94 Rheumatoid arthritis of the temporomandibular joint 94 Synovitis of the temporomandibular joint 94 Temporal arteritis 95 **Septic** Acute viral parotitis 85 Dental infection: • Tooth abscess 87 Osteomyelitis of the mandible 93

Inflammation *(continued)*

REMOTE	LOCAL
	Periodontal disease: • Alveolar osteitis 93 • Gingivitis 93 • Periodontitis 93 Sinusitis 94

UNCOMMON	
Aseptic Multiple sclerosis 82	**Aseptic** Facial nerve palsy 90
Septic Not applicable	**Septic** Not applicable

RARE	
Not applicable	Not applicable

M Metabolic

REMOTE	LOCAL
COMMON	
Chronic fatigue syndrome 80 Fibromyalgia 81	Gout of the temporomandibular joint 91 Pseudogout of the temporomandibular joint 93
UNCOMMON	
Adverse effects of medication 80	Effects of radiation/chemotherapy 90
RARE	
Not applicable	Not applicable

Va Vascular

REMOTE	LOCAL
COMMON	
Angina pectoris 80	Avascular necrosis 86
UNCOMMON	
Not applicable	Not applicable
RARE	
Not applicable	Not applicable

De Degenerative

REMOTE	LOCAL
COMMON	
Osteoarthrosis/osteoarthritis of the cervical spine 83	Ankylosis of the temporomandibular joint 86 Osteoarthrosis/osteoarthritis of the temporomandibular joint 92

(continued)

Degenerative *(continued)*

REMOTE	LOCAL
UNCOMMON	
Not applicable	Not applicable
RARE	
Not applicable	Not applicable

Tu Tumor

REMOTE	LOCAL
COMMON	
Malignant Primary, such as: • Brain tumor 84 *Malignant Metastatic:* Not applicable *Benign:* Not applicable	*Malignant Primary:* Not applicable *Malignant Metastatic:* Not applicable *Benign, such as:* • Acoustic neuroma 96 • Ganglion cyst of the temporomandibular joint 96
UNCOMMON	
Not applicable	*Malignant Primary, such as:* • External auditory canal tumor 96 • Neoplasm in the temporomandibular region 97 • Parotid gland tumor 97 *Malignant Metastatic:* Not applicable *Benign, such as:* • Osteochondroma of the mandibular condyle 97 • Parotid gland tumor 97 • Synovial cyst of the temporomandibular joint 97
RARE	
Malignant Primary, such as: • Nasopharyngeal carcinoma 84 • Oropharyngeal carcinoma 84 *Malignant Metastatic:* Not applicable *Benign:* Not applicable	*Malignant Primary:* Not applicable *Malignant Metastatic, such as:* • Metastases from adenocarcinoma of the colon 96 • Metastases from intracapsular stomach tumor 96 *Benign, such as:* • Synovial chondromatosis of the temporomandibular joint 97 • Temporal bone chondroblastoma 98

Co Congenital

REMOTE	LOCAL
COMMON	
Not applicable	Not applicable
UNCOMMON	
Not applicable	Developmental defects of the temporomandibular joint 88 Mandibular hypoplasia 92

Congenital *(continued)*

REMOTE	LOCAL
RARE	
Not applicable	Not applicable

Ne Neurogenic/Psychogenic

REMOTE	LOCAL
COMMON	
Anxiety 80	Atypical facial pain 86
Depression 81	Trigeminal neuralgia 95
Headaches:	
• Migraine 82	
• Tension-type headache 82	
UNCOMMON	
Neuralgias involving the cranial nerves:	Dislocations:
• Glossopharyngeal nerve 83	• Recurrent neurological dislocations of the temporomandibular joint 89
• Vagus nerve 83	
RARE	
Not applicable	Not applicable

Note: These are estimates of relative incidence because few data are available for the less common conditions.

Overview of Temporomandibular Joint and Facial Pain

Pain in the temporomandibular joint (TMJ) and facial area can be caused by various structures in the head, neck, and oral cavity. The proximity of these structures and their common neuron pool in the trigeminocervical nucleus (where spinal nerves C1, C2, and C3 and cranial nerves V, VII, IX, and XI converge) play a responsible role in the multifaceted symptoms of this area.[1] The condition may present with numerous associated symptoms such as headache, tinnitus, altered mandibular kinematics, TMJ noises, limited jaw opening, swallowing difficulty, toothache, dizziness, and vertigo. All of these symptoms that relate to the TMJ and facial area are defined as *temporomandibular dysfunction* (TMD).

TMJ and facial pain affects individuals of all ages. This symptom often is influenced by posture, oral habit, and stress level. Generalized poor body habit may lead to microtraumatic pathology in the TMJ and facial area, headaches, earaches, and tinnitus. Individuals

with TMD related to daily microtrauma often demonstrate a greater forward head position than individuals without TMD. The increased tension in the posterior cervical musculature caused by the forward-headed posture can set off a pathomechanical cycle of masticatory muscle imbalance, pain, disk displacement, and altered kinematics of the temporomandibular joint.[1] This cycle is exacerbated by parafunctional habits, such as bruxing, clenching, gum chewing, and fingernail biting.

Bruxing (grinding teeth) is primarily a nocturnal behavior, whereas clenching may occur during the day or at night. Both of these behaviors are involuntary. In severe cases, internal derangement and osteoarthritis may result. The microtrauma caused by daily clenching and bruxing will produce mechanical stress, which further leads to the release of free radicals. Research has suggested that the free radicals produced by mechanical stresses may cause oxidative stress, which in turns causes collapse of the lubrication system. This is considered a major initiator of internal derangement and osteoarthrosis/osteoarthritis of the temporomandibular joint.[2] After it has been determined that physical therapy is indicated, physical therapist management of TMD should address these underlying issues.

Description of Conditions That May Lead to Temporomandibular Joint and Facial Pain

Remote

■ Adverse Effects of Medication

Chief Clinical Characteristics
This presentation typically includes spasm of the masseter muscle, or trismus, associated with use of medication.

Background Information
Cardiovascular drugs (eg, calcium channel blockers, antiarrhythmics, phosphodiesterase inhibitors, alpha-1 agonists and antagonists, beta-adrenergic antagonists, angiotensin converting enzyme inhibitors, angiotensin II receptor antagonists, and organic nitrates), anti-infective agents (eg, various antibacterial, antifungal, and antiretroviral drugs), immunomodulatory drugs, anti-inflammatory drugs, antihistamines, medications used to treat asthma, and tricyclic antidepressants are most commonly implicated in promoting headaches that may involve temporomandibular joint and facial pain.[3–5] Discontinued use of these medications can relieve the undesirable symptoms, but this should occur with appropriate medical consultation including appropriate substitution as needed.

■ Angina Pectoris

Chief Clinical Characteristics
This presentation involves paroxysmal thoracic pain, often radiating to the left arm. Neck and jaw pain also may be associated with pallor, sweating, nausea, and weakness.

Background Information
This condition is most often caused by referred pain from ischemia of the myocardium and precipitated by effort or excitement. If symptoms are increased with physical exertion or cannot be reproduced with TMJ and cervical spine assessment, an emergent medical referral to assess for this condition is indicated.

■ Anxiety

Chief Clinical Characteristics
This presentation is associated with the unpleasant experience of fear in the absence of an object or activity that would justify this response. The Diagnostic and Statistical Manual of Mental Disorders,[6] text revision (DSM-IV-TR) classifies several anxiety disorders that preclude normal activities of daily living, each with its own unique symptom clusters.

Background Information
Anxiety and fear may occur either as a cause or consequence of temporomandibular and facial pain. Anxiety and fear occur as a typical response to injury, but they should be addressed when they appear to occur out of scale with symptoms, or if anxiety causes significant disablement. Patients with muscle pain related to acute TMD are more likely to have personality characteristics of anxiety.[7] Patients with chronic TMD report more stress-related impairment of daily activities than patients with acute TMD.[8] Therefore, a comprehensive team approach that combines medicine, physical therapy, psychological counseling, behavioral modification, and stress management may ensure optimal outcome of chronic pain control.[9,10]

■ Chronic Fatigue Syndrome

Chief Clinical Characteristics
This presentation is defined as a new onset of unexplained or persistent or recurrent physical or mental fatigue that substantially reduces activity level, postexertional malaise, and exclusion of other potentially explanatory medical or psychiatric conditions; also requires at least one symptom from each of the two of the following categories: autonomic manifestations, neuroendocrine manifestations, and immune manifestations.[11]

Background Information
Other possible clinical features include pain, which may serve as the chief symptom that directs patients toward physical therapists for management, and sleep dysfunction. This health condition is diagnosed on the basis of clinical examination. There is significant diagnostic overlap with major depression, fibromyalgia, and systemic lupus erythematosus. Optimal treatment includes activity modification and stress management, anaerobic

reconditioning, and medication for relief of associated symptomatology.

■ Depression

Chief Clinical Characteristics
This presentation usually involves sadness or grief in combination with loss of interest in daily activities. Major depressive disorder is one of several mood disorders categorized by the DSM-IV-TR.[6]

Background Information
Depression may occur either as a cause or consequence of TMJ and facial pain. Depressed mood may occur as a typical response to injury, but it should be addressed when it appears to occur out of scale with symptoms or if depression causes significant disablement. Patients with chronic muscular TMD demonstrate increased depression scores compared to pain-free controls and patients diagnosed with displacement of the temporomandibular articular disk.[12,13] Patients' psychological state may influence the outcome of treatment for patients with TMD. Therefore, a comprehensive team approach that combines medicine, physical therapy, psychological counseling, behavioral modification, and stress management may ensure optimal outcome of chronic pain control.[9,10]

■ Fibromyalgia

Chief Clinical Characteristics
This presentation is defined as chronic (greater than 3 months) widespread pain throughout the body, tender to 4 kg of palpation pressure at 11 out of 18 specific anatomically defined sites. Patients with this syndrome often experience associated symptoms of morning stiffness, sleep disturbance, generalized fatigue, depression, headaches, and temporomandibular pain/dysfunction.

Background Information
Reported estimates regarding the prevalence of fibromyalgia range from 0.7% to 10.5% in various countries worldwide.[14] It primarily occurs in women of childbearing age, but men and patients across the life span also can be affected. In addition to the clinical signs and symptoms, lab tests are used to confirm this diagnosis; individuals with fibromyalgia have a low serotonin level in the blood and cerebrospinal fluid, and show elevated levels of substance P in the cerebrospinal fluid. Preferred management of fibromyalgia typically occurs through a comprehensive team approach including medication, physical therapy, psychotherapy, and aerobic reconditioning.

HEADACHES

■ Cervicogenic Headache

Chief Clinical Characteristics
This presentation typically includes unilateral head pain associated with neck movement; sustained or awkward cervical posture; restricted cervical range of motion; and ipsilateral neck, shoulder, or arm pain.[15] This condition is characterized by moderate to severe episodic pain that originates in the neck or suboccipital region and spreads to the head (Fig. 8-1). Pain attacks last from 3 weeks to 3 months, and may vary in frequency from occurring every 2 days to 2 months. People with cervicogenic headache describe symptoms that do not change sides during an attack,[16] and may also present with nausea, dizziness, and phonophobia or photophobia that is unresolved with migraine medications.

Background Information
Initial management includes amelioration of cervical spine musculoskeletal impairments. Nerve blockade may be effective in recalcitrant cases. A favorable response to this intervention also is pathognomic.[17] Typical management of cervicogenic headache involves rehabilitative interventions.

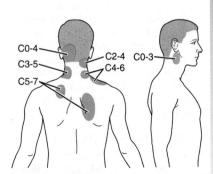

C0-4
C3-5
C5-7
C2-4   C0-3
C4-6

FIGURE 8-1 Referral patterns of the cervical facet joints. Cervical facet joints may refer pain to the jaw region, and these symptoms may be associated with suboccipital headaches.

■ Migraine

Chief Clinical Characteristics

This presentation typically includes a severe pulsating and throbbing unilateral headache with possible jaw pain that may switch sides, associated with nausea, vomiting, diarrhea, abdominal cramps, polyuria, sweating, facial pallor, photophobia, or phonophobia. This condition is a chronic condition of recurring attacks of transient focal neurological symptoms, headaches, or both.[18] This condition can also interfere with the function of other body systems, resulting in the characteristic associated symptoms such as nausea, vomiting, pallor, photophobia, and phonophobia.[19] Migraines are preceded by aura in 20% of cases.[20] Even in individuals who commonly experience them, auras may not accompany every headache. Auras can be visual, somatosensory, olfactory, or involve speech disturbances. The location of headache may switch sides from episode to episode.

Background Information

The pathophysiology of this condition is very complex. Current theories postulate that a cascade of events occurs that involve vasodilatation of meningeal blood vessels, irritation of perivascular sensory nerves, and stimulation of brainstem nuclei. Additionally, extrinsic factors such as hormonal fluctuations, fatigue, or anxiety may be triggers that initiate the pathophysiological cascade. This condition also has a strong familial tendency and begins at a young age, suggesting that genetic factors may predispose individuals to migraine attacks. The use of neuroimaging is not indicated in individuals with migraine symptoms and a normal neurological exam. Certain pharmaceutical agents, such as triptans and ergots, are effective in preventing migraine attacks from becoming too severe.[21] Other medications may be used to reduce the frequency of attacks.

■ Post-Traumatic Headache

Chief Clinical Characteristics

This presentation typically includes pain and dysfunction of the face and jaw. Concussion or vestibular system compromise may be caused by acute head injury, which also may clinically manifest in temporomandibular or facial pain.

Background Information

Computed tomography scan, magnetic resonance imaging, along with clinical assessment can confirm the diagnosis. Appropriate management of the head injury through surgical and medical intervention can resolve secondary temporomandibular joint and facial symptoms.

■ Tension-Type Headache

Chief Clinical Characteristics

This presentation typically includes a band-like distribution of nonthrobbing headache radiating from frontal region to occiput, associated with jaw pain, stress, anxiety, and neck tenderness.

Background Information

This condition is the most common headache presentation, accounting for more than two-thirds of all headache episodes and affecting 33% to 80% of the population.[22,23] Women are affected slightly more often than men.[22] Prevalence peaks in the 30- to 39-year-old age group[22] and is found to increase in incidence with increasing educational levels.[22] It is important to differentiate between the episodic type of tension headache and the more chronic form because the management of these two variations differs.[23] This differentiation is based entirely on the frequency and duration of occurrence. This condition lacks the IHS migraine-defining features of nausea, phonophobia, or photophobia.[22] Increased muscle hardness has been demonstrated in patients who experience chronic tension headaches, whether or not a headache is currently present.[24] Rehabilitative interventions, non-narcotic analgesics, and triptans may be used to manage this health condition.

■ Multiple Sclerosis

Chief Clinical Characteristics

This presentation typically includes weakness, incoordination, paresthesias, speech disturbance, visual complaints, and trigeminal neuralgia. Trigeminal nerve involvement in patients with multiple sclerosis is a distinct condition.

Background Information

The incidence of trigeminal neuralgia in individuals with this condition is higher than that in the general population. The differences in the two groups are younger onset of age and a preponderance of patients reporting bilateral symptoms in patients with multiple sclerosis.[25] The mechanism is possibly related to demyelination of the trigeminal entry root in the pons. Magnetic resonance imaging and computed tomography confirm the diagnosis. Typical management of trigeminal neuralgia related to multiple sclerosis involves options ranging from medication to surgery.

NEURALGIAS INVOLVING THE CRANIAL NERVES

■ Glossopharyngeal Nerve

Chief Clinical Characteristics
This presentation usually includes painful attacks on the tonsillar region and pharynx with possible radiation to the posterior auricular and jaw areas. Symptoms consist of painful attacks that are provoked with normal activities of speaking, swallowing, coughing, sneezing, or head rotation.

Background Information
In patients who report attacks during chewing and swallowing, it is not uncommon to observe striking weight loss. The cause is idiopathic in a majority of cases; potential causes include tumors of the brainstem region, morphological abnormalities of the stylohyoid process, and multiple sclerosis. Attacks are mainly unilateral; multiple sclerosis should be considered in the event of bilateral attacks. A comprehensive cranial evaluation through clinical examination, brain scan, and magnetic resonance imaging confirms the diagnosis and directs the most appropriate medical intervention. The diagnosis is confirmed with favorable response of lidocaine injections to trigger areas. Laryngeal electromyography also may be considered. In addition to lidocaine injections, treatment typically includes antiepileptic and antispasticity medications.[26]

■ Vagus Nerve

Chief Clinical Characteristics
This presentation typically includes pain that may radiate to the auricular or jaw regions, combined with hoarseness, breathy dysphonia, vocal fatigue, and effortful phonation.[27]

Background Information
The level of lesion may be determined based on the patient's symptoms and signs. The cause is usually idiopathic; however, tumors, trauma, and viruses may be contributory. Lesions affecting the proximal segment of the vagus nerve include oropharyngeal signs, such as absent gag reflex, uvular deviation, nasopharyngeal reflux, and absent cough reflex. Lesions affecting the distal segment will result in an unremarkable oropharyngeal examination.[28] A comprehensive cranial evaluation through clinical examination, brain scan, and magnetic resonance imaging confirms the diagnosis and directs the most appropriate medical intervention. Treatment typically includes antiepileptic and antispasticity medications.[26]

■ Osteoarthrosis/Osteoarthritis of the Cervical Spine

Chief Clinical Characteristics
This presentation typically includes neck pain, stiffness of the affected cervical joints, and tightness of the adjacent musculature. One resultant effect may be referred pain to the jaw and facial area. In addition, the cervical positioning that may result from altered cervical spine position in osteoarthrosis may cause primary local pathology of the temporomandibular joint.

Background Information
Biochemical processes adversely affect the bone, synovium, and articular cartilage. Over time, these processes affect the structure of all these tissues in concert, causing pain and the characteristic morphological changes of synovitis, subchondral sclerosis, bone marrow changes, and osteophyte formation.[29] Joint space narrowing, subchondral sclerosis, and osteophytes apparent on plain radiographs along with clinical examination maneuvers that result in downgliding or compression of the affected cervical functional spinal units confirm the diagnosis. Rehabilitative interventions and nonsteroidal anti-inflammatory medications can alleviate local cervical spine pain. Surgical decompression of the affected neural foramen may be indicated for individuals in whom neurologic involvement is clinically significant.

TEMPOROMANDIBULAR JOINT AND FACIAL PAIN

■ Otitis Media

Chief Clinical Characteristics

This presentation typically includes fever, pain in the ear and preaurical area, tinnitus, hearing loss, and vertigo.

Background Information

The most common cause of otitis is bacterial infection of the ear, including various strains. Physical examination confirms the diagnosis, including inspection of the acoustic canal for signs of infection, including redness and effusion. The natural history of most cases of otitis media without intervention is favorable; however, use of medications directed at the appropriate infective agent may be helpful to reduce symptoms and the potential for adverse effects of prolonged illness. In some cases, tympanocentesis may be considered as a diagnostic and therapeutic procedure.[30]

■ Systemic Lupus Erythematosus

Chief Clinical Characteristics

This presentation typically includes a characteristic "butterfly" skin rash over the maxillae, generalized body ache, fatigue, heart/lung/kidney involvement, and joint pain or swelling.

Background Information

This is a chronic, idiopathic autoimmune disorder that can affect virtually any organ in the body. The TMJ is often involved in this health condition. This health condition most often affects women of childbearing age. However, men also can be affected less frequently. Over 20% of individuals with this condition may develop fibromyalgia during the course of their illness.[31] Blood test, urine test, and skin and kidney biopsies confirm the diagnosis. Treatment includes medication, physical therapy, and management of associated complications of the skin, lungs, kidneys, joints, and nervous system.

TUMORS

■ Brain Tumor

Chief Clinical Characteristics

This presentation typically includes headaches, facial pain, and possible loss of motor function of one or more extremities.[32] A history of general malaise, nausea, vomiting, weight loss, fever, and headache that worsens with position changes with upper motor neuron signs such as seizures, personality changes, cognitive changes, clonus, spasticity, weakness, and incoordination is indicative of brain malignancy.

Background Information

Brain tumors account for 2% of all cancers annually. Brain tumors are classified according to their cellular origin and histological appearance, which helps to guide treatment, making a comprehensive neurosurgical evaluation potentially necessary. The most common brain primary metastatic tumor in adults is glioblastoma multiforme. Magnetic resonance imaging and brain scan confirm the diagnosis. Treatment may include surgical resection of the tumor, radiation, and chemotherapy.[33]

■ Nasopharyngeal Carcinoma

Chief Clinical Characteristics

This presentation may include facial pain combined with headaches, palpable mass in the head or neck, bloody nasal discharge, chronic unilateral nasal congestion, unilateral hearing loss or frequent ear infections, or cranial nerve signs.

Background Information

Nasopharyngeal tumors usually develop in the wall of the nasopharynx. The relatively large amount of space that can be occupied in this region of the body results in a late onset of presenting symptoms and diagnostic delay. This may result in a poorer prognosis related to advanced tumor development and increased potential for metastatic spread. The diagnosis is confirmed with fused positron emission tomography/computed tomography and head/neck magnetic resonance imaging. Treatment typically depends on cancer staging, ranging from surgical resection and radiation therapy to chemotherapy.

■ Oropharyngeal Carcinoma

Chief Clinical Characteristics

This presentation may involve facial pain combined with hoarseness, throat pain, change in the tongue, pain in the tongue, and lump in the neck region, dysphagia, dyspnea, coughing, or hemoptysis.

Background Information

Up to 90% of oropharyngeal carcinomas are squamous cell carcinomas, or abnormal collections of squamous cells on histological observation. Lower patient socioeconomic status, patient and clinician delay in recognizing the health condition, lack of indirect laryngoscopy performed on physical examination, failure to inspect the site of the tumor, and clinician failure to consider tumor or infection as potential causes of symptoms are associated with overlooking this disease process. In turn, overlooking this disease process results in reduced prognosis.[34] Computed tomography and magnetic resonance imaging can further confirm the diagnosis. Treatment typically depends on cancer staging, ranging from surgical resection and radiation therapy to chemotherapy.[35]

Local

■ Acute Viral Parotitis

Chief Clinical Characteristics
This presentation typically includes low-grade fever, malaise, and pain and swelling in the affected side of the face. The pain and swelling may last 3 to 10 days and subside gradually without sequelae.

Background Information
Inflammation of the parotid gland may be caused by viral infections, such as mumps, Epstein-Barr, and influenza A. Analgesics and cold compresses are helpful in relieving pain and swelling during the early stage of the condition. Supportive treatment of the underlying viral infection also may be indicated.

■ Adhesion of the Temporomandibular Joint

Chief Clinical Characteristics
This presentation typically includes a sudden onset of extremely limited mouth opening (between 10 and 30 mm), with deflection of the mandible toward the ipsilateral side (Fig. 8-2). There usually is no pain in the involved joint or the adjacent muscles.

Background Information
Temporomandibular joint overloading caused by macrotrauma (eg, injury) or microtrauma (eg, bruxing) may lead to damage of the joint lubrication system. The decrease in lubrication may cause increased friction between the articular disk and glenoid fossa. An adhesive force created by this condition may keep the disk from sliding down the slope of the articular eminence during normal month opening. This condition

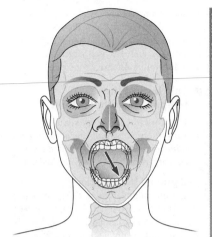

FIGURE 8-2 Deflection of the mandible with mouth opening.

is termed the anchored disk phenomenon. Magnetic resonance imaging that reveals the characteristic adherence of the disk to the glenoid fossa during the opening phase confirms the diagnosis. Treatment ranges from rehabilitative interventions to arthroscopic release.

■ Ankylosing Spondylitis

Chief Clinical Characteristics
This presentation typically includes temporomandibular joint (TMJ) and facial pain and limited TMJ range of motion, associated with a slowly progressive and significant loss of general spinal mobility. Symptoms may be worse in the morning and improve with light exercise.

Background Information
This condition is a progressive disease that affects primarily the axial joints of the spine and, eventually, the TMJ. It is more common in males, as well as people of American indigenous descent, less than 40 years of age, or who carry the human leukocyte antigen B27. It also may be associated with fever, malaise, and inflammatory bowel disease. The diagnosis is confirmed with plain radiographs of the sacroiliac joints and lumbar spine, which reveal characteristic findings of sacroiliitis and "bamboo spine." The TMJ dysfunction with this condition may be associated with TMJ ankylosis, which may be apparent on plain radiographs or computed tomography. Blood panels including erythrocyte

sedimentation rate are useful to track disease activity. Treatment includes various classes of nonsteroidal and biological anti-inflammatory medications and exercise. Surgery to correct joint deformities also may be indicated.

■ Ankylosis of the Temporomandibular Joint

Chief Clinical Characteristics

This presentation typically includes temporomandibular and facial pain, limited opening, and loss of vertical height of the involved ramus.

Background Information

Temporomandibular joint (TMJ) ankylosis can result from trauma, infection, growth defect, ankylosing spondylitis,[36] and inadequate surgical treatment of the condylar area. Myositis ossificans of the medial pterygoid muscle may also lead to ankylosis of the temporomandibular joint. It is important to determine the exact cause of the ankylosis for a successful treatment outcome.[37] Treatment depends on the underlying cause of ankylosis, and the main intervention is surgical reconstruction of the TMJ if rehabilitative measures are inadequate to restore functional opening.

■ Anteriorly Displaced Disk With or Without Reduction

Chief Clinical Characteristics

This presentation typically includes pain, joint noises, altered mandibular kinematics where the mandible deflects to the affected side during mouth opening (see Fig. 8-2), and limited mouth opening.

Background Information

When an anteriorly displaced disk is reduced during mouth closing, an opening click and a closing click will be present (reciprocal clicking). If the disk is completely displaced anteriorly without reduction, joint clicking is usually absent. This condition may be caused by direct macrotrauma to the joint or by microtrauma from daily clenching and bruxing. However, the patient may experience crepitus due to arthritic changes.[1] Clinical examination and dynamic magnetic resonance imaging of the temporomandibular joint confirm the diagnosis. Treatment typically involves rehabilitative interventions and splinting.

■ Atypical Facial Pain

Chief Clinical Characteristics

This presentation typically includes constant, boring pain primarily in the lower facial area.

Background Information

This is an idiopathic disorder. It is different from trigeminal neuralgia due to its atypical distribution, and its symptoms are not paroxysmal in nature. However, its pain pattern is similar to that caused by nasopharyngeal carcinoma, oropharyngeal carcinoma, or infection caused by tooth distraction. There is a high comorbidity between post-traumatic disorder syndrome and chronic orofacial pain. Psychometric questionnaires may be beneficial for assessment given the potential effect of affective causes or consequences of this health condition on treatment. Physical examination, plain radiographs, magnetic resonance imaging, and computed tomography confirm the diagnosis. Various classes of medications (eg, antidepressants and anti-seizure and narcotic agents) in combination with a biopsychosocial team approach to pain management are among usual interventions.

■ Avascular Necrosis

Chief Clinical Characteristics

This presentation typically includes temporomandibular joint arthropathy, headache, facial pain, and occlusal disturbance.

Background Information

Inflammatory internal derangement of the temporomandibular joint, sickle cell disease, and bisphosphonate medications may lead to avascular necrosis of the mandibular condyle. Magnetic resonance imaging is useful to confirm the diagnosis and monitor the condition's progression.[38] Intervention is directed at the underlying etiology. Reconstructive surgery for the affected portion of the mandible and teeth may be indicated depending on the extent of involvement.

■ Capsulitis of the Temporomandibular Joint

Chief Clinical Characteristics

This presentation typically includes pain in the temporomandibular joint and its immediate vicinity, limited opening, and other myofascial symptoms.

Background Information

Inflammation of the capsule of the temporomandibular joint results in capsulitis of the temporomandibular joint (TMJ). The cause of the inflammation can be either macrotrauma such as motor vehicle accident, or microtrauma, such as clenching and bruxing. Capsulitis may also be secondary to synovitis or retrodiscitis. Medical/dental history and physical examination can confirm the diagnosis. Treatment includes medication, modalities, and reeducation regarding proper oral habit. Symptoms usually improve when the inflammation is resolved, so nonsurgical interventions are directed at reducing the underlying inflammation of the TMJ capsule.

DENTAL INFECTION
■ Tooth Abscess
Chief Clinical Characteristics
This presentation typically includes sharp pain in the local area and often radiates to the jaw, cheek, eye, and ear of the side ipsilateral to the infection. Ingestion of cold drink or food usually worsens symptoms.

Background Information
If left untreated, usually uncomplicated gum boils and tooth decay may lead to a tooth abscess. In severe cases, soft tissue swelling of the involved jaw may be apparent on observation. Patients suspected of a dental abscess should be referred to a dentist for additional evaluation and management. Dental examination and radiographs can identify abscess. Treatment includes antimicrobial and analgesic medication.[39]

DENTAL TRAUMA
■ Edentulism and Denture Wear
Chief Clinical Characteristics
This presentation typically includes temporomandibular joint (TMJ) and facial pain, altered mandibular dynamics, and crepitus.

Background Information
It has been reported that approximately 15% to 20% of patients who wear complete dentures may present with this condition. Individuals with edentulism who do not wear dentures also may present with this condition, but to a much lesser degree. However, loss of posterior teeth may result in unilateral chewing patterns that result in overuse of the ipsilateral masticatory musculature and overload the contralateral TMJ. Positive correlations between poor denture fit and daytime clenching have also been reported. Clinical examination confirms the diagnosis. Adjustment of denture base to provide proper stability and retention can correct symptoms, and proper denture support is important in preventing further arthritic changes in the TMJ.[39]

■ Malocclusion
Chief Clinical Characteristics
This presentation typically includes pain in the facial area and dysfunction of the temporomandibular joint (TMJ).

Background Information
This condition encompasses several bite abnormalities, as shown in Figure 8-3: (A) crossbite, in which the lower tooth has a more buccal position than its opposing upper tooth; (B) open bite, in which the upper and lower incisors and canines are forced outward; (C) over bite, in which the upper incisors and canines protrude anteriorly excessively over their lower antagonist teeth; (D) under bite, in which the lower incisors and canines protrude anteriorly beyond their upper antagonist teeth; and other types of bite malalignments.

Clinical examination and dental x-ray confirm the diagnosis. Correction of the contributing malocclusion potentially can alleviate TMJ symptoms. However, inadequate orthodontic adjustment often causes increased symptoms in the TMJ region.

■ Tooth Injury
Chief Clinical Characteristics
This presentation typically includes pain in the jaw, face, and cheek area potentially associated with low-grade fever and general malaise.

Background Information
This condition can be external or iatrogenic. Tooth injuries that can cause facial pain include fractured teeth, a newly placed crown, impacted wisdom teeth, status post–endodontic surgery, and toothbrush-related tooth erosion are included in this category. These factors make dental history

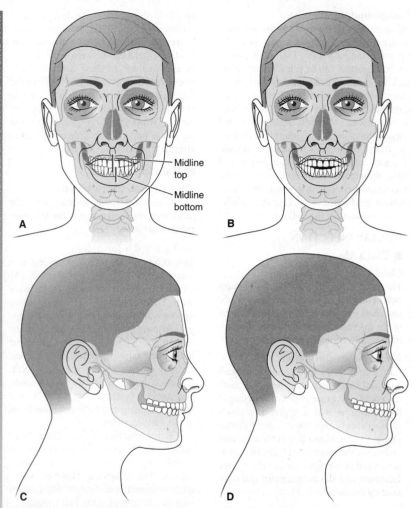

FIGURE 8-3 Bite abnormalities in malocclusion: (A) crossbite; (B) open bite; (C) over bite; (D) under bite.

important to solicit in assessing a patient's facial and TMJ pain. Clinical examination confirms the specific diagnosis. Referral to the dentist to correct the specific health condition can help relieve symptoms in a timely manner.

■ Developmental Defects of the Temporomandibular Joint

Chief Clinical Characteristics
This presentation may include pain in the facial and temporomandibular joint (TMJ) area, along with facial asymmetry.

Background Information
Congenital fusion of gums with ankylosis of the TMJ, flattening of the condylar head, bilateral zygomatic-mandibular fusion with mandibular hypoplasia, and hemimandibular hyperplasia are a few examples of congenital conditions. Clinical examination and diagnostic imaging modalities may be used to clarify the specific nature of developmental defect of the TMJ, and this directs appropriate surgical and nonsurgical management of specific defects.

DISLOCATIONS

■ Botulinum Toxin–Induced Dislocation

Chief Clinical Characteristics

This presentation can involve chewing difficulty, dysphasia, and recurrent temporomandibular joint dislocations following botulinum toxin injections.

Background Information

Botulinum toxin has been proven to be successful in treating various movement disorders and spastic masticatory musculature of patients with cerebral palsy. Recently, it has also been shown to be effective in treating excessive salivation in patients with Parkinson's disease, stroke, and amyotrophic lateral sclerosis. This health condition occurs when botulinum toxin diffuses into the surrounding masseter muscle, leading to jaw dislocation secondary to excessive muscle weakness. Medical history, clinical signs, and electromyography can confirm the diagnosis. Electrical activity of the masseter muscle typically returns to normal within 4 months of botulinum toxin injection.[40]

■ Dislocation of the Mandibular Condyle

Chief Clinical Characteristics

This presentation typically includes pain in the jaw area, excessive translation, deviation upon opening, and joint noises.

Background Information

This condition occurs when the condylar head is displaced beyond the mandibular tubercle (out of the glenoid fossa). Frequently, the condylar head remains within the joint capsule. Acute dislocation of the mandible may lead to secondary osteoarthritis of the temporomandibular joint due to fibrous adhesion and synovial inflammation. Early investigation of intra-articular injuries is important. Computed tomography and dynamic magnetic resonance imaging confirm the diagnosis and direct medical stabilization. Treatment includes reduction of the dislocation. Recurrent dislocations may be treated by the injection of sclerosing agents or autologous blood, intermaxillary fixation, or various surgical stabilization procedures.

■ Dislocation of the Mandibular Condyle into the Middle Cranial Fossa

Chief Clinical Characteristics

This presentation may include pain on mandibular movement, pain on preauricular palpation, preauricular depression, shortening of height of mandibular ramus, deviation of mandible to opposite site, and premature occlusion with open bite.

Background Information

This condition is rare, occurring when the mandibular condyle dislocates into the middle cranial fossa. The most common mechanism of injury is a direct blow to the mandible from a frontal or a lateral direction with an open-mouth position. The result is fracture of the condylar neck and possible neurological signs. Computed tomography confirms the diagnosis. Treatment involves reduction of the dislocation with surgical stabilization of the affected temporomandibular joint. Long-term follow-up in these individuals is important due to the potential development of craniofacial asymmetries and temporomandibular dysfunction.[41] Recurrent dislocations may be treated by the injection of sclerosing agents or autologous blood, intermaxillary fixation, or various surgical stabilization procedures.

■ Recurrent Neurological Dislocations of the Temporomandibular Joint

Chief Clinical Characteristics

This presentation typically includes pain and spasm in the temporomandibular joint area with involuntary open-lock of the jaw characteristic of dislocation.

Background Information

Nontraumatic dislocation of the temporomandibular joint has been described as a complication in a number of neurological diseases such as parkinsonism, multiple sclerosis, and amyotrophic lateral sclerosis. It is believed that increased tone in the lateral pterygoid muscles causes the recurrence of involuntary dislocation of the temporomandibular joint. The injection of botulinum toxin to the lateral pterygoid muscle can inhibit the release of acetylcholine at the neuromuscular junction, which results in its paresis and the decrease of mouth opening. This method is the treatment of choice for recurrent neurological dislocation.[10,42–44] Clinical examination confirms the diagnosis.

■ Effects of Radiation/ Chemotherapy

Chief Clinical Characteristics
This presentation involves severe pain and discomfort in the face and neck area, trismus, and difficulty swallowing.

Background Information
Radiation therapy and chemotherapy for carcinoma of the head and neck and regional lymphoma may lead to pain, mucositis, stomatitis, avascular necrosis, change in taste sensation, dry mouth, tooth decay, and gum disease. The soft tissue effects of radiation and chemotherapy can alter the normal tissue extensibility and flexibility that permits usual facial and jaw function. Rehabilitative interventions such as physical therapy modalities and exercise may help relieve symptoms and improve function.

■ Facial Nerve Palsy

Chief Clinical Characteristics
This presentation typically includes unilateral motor deficits of the muscles of facial expression that are innervated by the seventh cranial nerve, demonstrated by paralysis of ipsilateral facial muscles, drooping of eyelid, inability to close eyes tightly, deviation of mouth angle, and flaccid facial expression. Individuals with this condition often report pain in the facial area of the involved side.

Background Information
Changes to the muscles of facial expression that are responsible for these symptoms and signs often occur rapidly, such as over the course of 1 day. This condition, also called Bell's palsy, is caused by a viral infection. Clinical signs and symptoms confirm the diagnosis. Treatment includes steroid dose pack and pain medication.

FRACTURES
■ Mandible

Chief Clinical Characteristics
This presentation may include pain on mandibular movement, preauricular palpation, preauricular depression, possibly associated with shortening of the affected mandibular ramus, deviation of mandible to opposite site, and premature occlusion with open bite.

Background Information
Mandibular condylar fractures usually occur after trauma, and most often present in either condylar neck fracture or dislocation of the temporomandibular joint. Condylar fractures account for approximately 25% to 35% of all mandibular fractures. This diagnosis is confirmed with computed tomography. In children with this condition, the use of a functional appliance immediately after the trauma is recommended. It has been documented that the functional activation of the masticatory muscles can prevent mandibular asymmetries and facial malformation.[45]

■ Maxilla

Chief Clinical Characteristics
This presentation can involve pain and edema of the lips, midface, and eyes, possibly associated with sunken deformity of the involved side, diplopia, malocclusion, anterior open bite, and upper airway compromise.

Background Information
This condition may include compound fracture of the articular eminence and fracture of the glenoid fossa. This health condition may be caused by blunt trauma involving a direct blow to the maxilla, such as a motor vehicle accident. It may be associated with injuries to the orbit. Computed tomography confirms the diagnosis. Surgical repair of the fracture and correction of perifracture trauma to the upper airway, overlying soft tissues, and associated trauma to the orbit may be indicated in complicated cases.

■ Orbit

Chief Clinical Characteristics
This presentation typically involves orbital and cheek pain, vertical diplopia, orbital edema, enophthalmos, ecchymosis, tenderness of the orbital margin, and reduced cheek and upper gum sensation.

Background Information
A direct blow to the eye such as might occur in a motor vehicle accident or boxing match or with a ball may cause fracture of the orbit.

Enophthalmos may suggest herniation of the orbital contents into the maxillary sinus in large orbital fractures. Vertical diplopia may suggest entrapment of the optic musculature in the fracture site, and severe pain with eye movements might suggest significant orbital hemorrhage or edema. Computed tomography of the face and head confirms the diagnosis and guides appropriate management, which can include surgical repair of the fracture and correction of perifracture trauma to the orbital contents in complicated cases.[46]

■ Temporal Bone

Chief Clinical Characteristics
This presentation is characterized by pain and swelling of the cheek area and temporomandibular joint, fluid or bleeding from the ear on the affected side, unilateral facial paralysis, vertigo, or hearing changes.

Background Information
Temporal bone fractures are caused by significant blunt trauma to the skull base. A lateral blow to the temporal bone causes a longitudinal fracture pattern, which accounts for 80% of fractures. Significant blunt trauma to the frontal or occipital region causes a transverse fracture pattern that typically is more serious or fatal. Computed tomography confirms the diagnosis. Treatment usually involves a combination of surgical and nonsurgical stabilization of the fracture, as well as management of associated conditions.[47]

■ Zygomatic Arch

Chief Clinical Characteristics
This presentation typically involves pain and swelling of the cheek area, with possible indentation of the cheek on the affected side, numbness of the cheek and upper gum, and visual field disturbances. Painful temporomandibular joint movement, lower eyelid deformity, and paresthesia of the upper lip also may be present.

Background Information
Blunt trauma to the cheek is the main cause of this condition. Often soft tissue swelling can obscure deformities related to this injury. Visual field deficits may suggest traumatic optic neuropathy or concomitant orbital floor injury. Optic neuropathy should be suspected in the case of differing intensity of color perception between eyes, beginning with red. Computed tomography of the head and face confirms the diagnosis. Treatment usually involves a combination of surgical and nonsurgical stabilization of the fracture, as well as management of associated conditions.[48]

■ Gout of the Temporomandibular Joint

Chief Clinical Characteristics
This presentation involves abrupt, acute pain in the temporomandibular joint (TMJ), facial, and ear area. TMJ range of motion also may be limited and chewing usually aggravates pain.

Background Information
This health condition affects males predominantly. In addition, certain lifestyle factors predispose to the development of gout, such as a diet high in purines and protein and alcohol consumption. Gout is an acutely benign crystal deposition disease that rarely affects the temporomandibular joint alone. However, if left untreated, crystal deposition (tophi) can cause chronic disruption of joint morphology. Plain radiographs of the first metatarsophalangeal joint usually confirm the diagnosis. Management of the underlying etiology can resolve symptoms, including administration of medication and modification of potentially contributing lifestyle factors.

■ Herpes Zoster

Chief Clinical Characteristics
This presentation typically includes an exquisitely painful rash or blisters along the first division of the trigeminal nerve, potentially accompanied by flu-like symptoms. Individuals with this condition also demonstrate a previous history of varicella exposure or infection. Pain associated with this condition may be disproportionate to the extent of skin irritation. The presence of the rash, extreme pain, general malaise, and unclear association with neck or face movement aids in the differential diagnosis.

Background Information
The virus may remain dormant in the cranial nerve nuclei until its reactivation during a period of stress, infection, or physical

exhaustion. Treatment includes the administration of antiviral agents as soon as the zoster eruption is noted, ideally within 48 to 72 hours. If timing is greater than 3 days, treatment is aimed at controlling pain and pruritus and minimizing the risk of secondary infection.[49]

Internal Derangement of the Temporomandibular Joint

Chief Clinical Characteristics
This presentation is characterized by joint pain, headache and facial pain, joint noises, closed lock, and occlusal disturbance.[50]

Background Information
This condition involves disharmony of the disc–condyle relationship during mouth opening and closing. Disk displacement with or without reduction, masticatory muscle dysfunction, synovitis, and malocclusion are among causes of this condition. Advanced cases involve bone marrow edema, osteochondritis dissecans, and avascular necrosis. The microtrauma caused by functional and parafunctional activities leads to the release of free radicals that cause oxidative stress, which in turn reduces the effectiveness of synovial fluid. Over time, this process leads to osteoarthrosis/osteoarthritis of the temporomandibular joint.[2] Magnetic resonance imaging and laboratory findings of joint effusion, synovial hypertrophy, adhesion, and pathological synovial fluid confirm the diagnosis. Nonsteroidal anti-inflammatory medications and physical therapy modality treatment are beneficial for this condition.[51]

Mandibular Hypoplasia

Chief Clinical Characteristics
This presentation may include facial and temporomandibular joint (TMJ) pain associated with uneven growth of the mandibular rami, rotated facial appearance, overgrowth of mandibular alveolar bone, or malocclusion.

Background Information
This condition is commonly thought of as a congenital malformation of the maxillofacial structure, but it is possible blunt trauma also may result in this condition on an acquired basis. Often, congenital mandibular hypoplasia presents early in life. It may be present at birth or present during development. The patient should be referred to a craniofacial surgeon for diagnostic workup of the specific deformity, because this will guide management. In general, several different surgical procedures ordered in stages may be necessary to optimally address mandibular hypoplasia depending on the extent of involvement and functional compromise.[52]

Myofascial Pain Disorder Syndrome

Chief Clinical Characteristics
This presentation involves diffuse muscle pain with exquisite trigger points in the head, face, and neck area. Symptoms may also manifest in headaches, earaches, and tinnitus.

Background Information
This condition is the most prevalent cause of chronic orofacial pain and temporomandibular joint dysfunction. The etiology of this syndrome is multifactorial and includes chronic overuse, poor postural habits, and internal derangement of the temporomandibular joint. Individuals with chronic rheumatological conditions such as lupus, fibromyalgia, chronic fatigue syndrome, and irritable bowel syndrome have a higher incidence of this health condition. Brass and woodwind musicians, voice-over artists, and professional public speakers may also experience overuse syndrome due to the exaggeration of mandibular movements required by their professions. This diagnosis is confirmed by clinical examination primarily. To relieve symptoms, patients must be instructed in proper head and neck posture, frequent practice breaks, diaphragmatic breathing, relaxation, and stretching exercises for oral balance.

Osteoarthrosis/Osteoarthritis of the Temporomandibular Joint

Chief Clinical Characteristics
This presentation typically includes pain in the temporomandibular joint (TMJ) with crepitus during mouth opening and closing.

Background Information
This condition may be caused by acute, direct trauma to the jaw or chronic microtrauma from bruxism, tooth loss, and malocclusion.[39] Biochemical processes related to chronic trauma adversely affect the bone, synovium, and articular cartilage. Over time, these processes affect

the structure of all these tissues in concert, causing pain and characteristic morphological changes of synovitis, subchondral sclerosis, bone marrow changes, and osteophyte formation.[29] Joint space narrowing, subchondral sclerosis, and osteophytes may be apparent on plain radiographs of the TMJ, which confirms the diagnosis. Treatment can be accomplished by nonsteroidal anti-inflammatory medications, physical therapy modalities, and splinting. If malocclusion is involved in the etiology of this health condition, orthodontic management and/or orthognathic surgery may be indicated.[53]

■ **Osteomyelitis of the Mandible**

Chief Clinical Characteristics
This presentation can involve severe pain in the jaw and facial area, along with tinnitus, disk displacement, and limited mouth opening.

Background Information
This condition may be caused by tooth infection, iatrogenic trauma with dental procedure such as tooth extraction, and radiation exposure. Magnetic resonance imaging and computed tomography confirm the diagnosis; bone biopsy and culture may be used to differentiate this health condition from primary and metastatic tumors of the mandible and to determine the type of infective organism. High-dose antibiotic medication is indicated for this condition. Physical therapy modality treatment can provide palliative support. Hyperbaric chamber treatment can be beneficial in more serious cases, and surgical resection with reconstruction may be indicated.

PERIODONTAL DISEASE

■ **Alveolar Osteitis**

Chief Clinical Characteristics
This presentation typically involves a sharp increase in pain 2 to 5 days following tooth extraction, accompanied by facial or jaw pain with halitosis, unpleasant taste, an empty socket, and tenderness.

Background Information
This health condition is most common after excision of the lower molars than other teeth. Individuals suspected of this health condition should be referred to a dental professional for additional evaluation and

intervention. Treatment may include irrigation with warm saline or aqueous chlorhexidine, as well as administration of analgesic and antimicrobial agents.[54]

■ **Gingivitis**

Chief Clinical Characteristics
This presentation is characterized by gum swelling, bleeding, and halitosis potentially associated with jaw or facial tenderness.

Background Information
This health condition is present when bacterial adhesion occurs and coaggregation (plaque) becomes calcified (tartar), creating inflammation confined to the gums. This process creates a pocket around the tooth that becomes home to a variety of organisms that eventually may lead to periodontitis. Regular dental hygiene including checkup and cleaning are useful to prevent and treat this condition.[55]

■ **Periodontitis**

Chief Clinical Characteristics
This presentation may include by gum swelling, bleeding, and halitosis potentially associated with jaw or facial tenderness and tooth loosening or loss.

Background Information
This condition is considered a progression of gingivitis, in which the organisms that occupy the gum sulcus created by gum inflammation cause additional deepening of the sulcus and eventual destruction of periodontal tissue. Treatment of periodontitis involves resolution of the underlying gum infection and gum sulcus by a dental professional.

■ **Pseudogout of the Temporomandibular Joint**

Chief Clinical Characteristics
This presentation typically includes a sudden onset of deep stabbing hip pain, worsened with weight bearing and hip passive range of motion, and associated with tenderness, warmth, and redness of overlying soft tissues.

Background Information
This condition is more common in older males. It is less common in the temporomandibular joint. This health condition's presentation mimics gout; however, calcium

pyrophosphate dihydrate crystal deposits mediate its characteristic joint pain and articular cartilage destruction. Blood tests and microscopic examination of aspirated synovial fluid confirm the diagnosis.

■ Retrodiscitis of the Temporomandibular Joint

Chief Clinical Characteristics
This presentation may include preaurical pain, palpable tenderness in the external auditory meatus with the examiner's fifth finger, tinnitus, and altered mandibular dynamics during mouth opening and closing.

Background Information
Inflammation of the retrodiscal pad results in retrodiscitis of the temporomandibular joint. The inflammation may be caused by local trauma, overuse, or disk displacement. In addition, it also may occur secondary to systemic connective diseases. Biting down on a cotton roll with the back molars on the ipsilateral side can relieve pain because of the distraction of the temporomandibular joint. This maneuver can be used to confirm the diagnosis. Undiagnosed systemic disease or local infection can be further worked up by appropriate imaging and laboratory studies. Treatment of retrodiscitis is based on the etiology. Anti-inflammatory medication, modalities, a soft diet, and an intraoral appliance are usually effective.

■ Rheumatoid Arthritis of the Temporomandibular Joint

Chief Clinical Characteristics
This presentation typically is characterized by morning stiffness and generalized pain throughout multiple joints in a symmetric distribution, with possible tenderness and swelling of affected joints, as well as temporomandibular joint crepitus and limited mouth opening.

Background Information
Women are twice as likely as men to be affected. Symptoms associated with this progressive inflammatory joint disease are caused by synovial membrane thickening and cytokine production in synovial fluid. Articular cartilage erosion, synovial hypertrophy, and constant joint effusion[56] eventually cause bony erosions and joint deformities that have a significant impact on daily function. Younger age of onset is associated with a greater extent of disability later. Temporomandibular joint inflammation was found in 87% of the juvenile rheumatoid arthritis patients through the use of contrast-enhanced MRI.[57] The diagnosis is confirmed with the presence of rheumatoid factor in blood tests. A regimen of nonsteroidal, steroidal, or biological anti-inflammatory agents may be used to manage this health condition.

■ Sinusitis

Chief Clinical Characteristics
This presentation involves swollen maxillary, nasal, or paranasal sinuses, along with tenderness and pain in the paranasal and anterior facial area with possible fever. This condition also may be associated with sinus headaches, nasal congestion, facial pressure, nasal discharge, discolored postnasal drainage, fatigue, and tooth pain.

Background Information
Sinusitis is caused by infection of the sinuses. Important differential diagnosis includes migraine in individuals presenting with headache and tumor in individuals with chronic unilateral congestion. Differentiation between this condition and migraine without aura occurs based on lateralization and quality of symptoms. Computed tomography or nasal endoscopic examination is necessary to make an accurate diagnosis. Treatment includes antimicrobial agents directed at the specific infective agent.

■ Synovitis of the Temporomandibular Joint

Chief Clinical Characteristics
This presentation typically includes tenderness and pain in the temporomandibular joint and its immediate vicinity, possibly associated with headache, crepitus, clicking, or locking.

Background Information
This inflammatory temporomandibular joint arthropathy is defined by the inflammation of the synovium. If left untreated, this joint pathology may result in malocclusion, degeneration, osteochondritis dissecans, and avascular necrosis of the mandibular condyle. The characteristic joint effusion may be demonstrated on magnetic resonance imaging. Treatment

typically includes anti-inflammatory medication and rehabilitative interventions to restore range of motion and movement quality and to address pain.

■ Temporal Arteritis

Chief Clinical Characteristics

This presentation typically includes severe headache, unilateral or bilateral, over the scalp–temporal artery region. Jaw claudication presenting as pain or stiffness during chewing is highly suggestive of this condition due to ischemia of the muscles of mastication. Other nonspecific signs and symptoms of this disorder include malaise, myalgia, weight loss, fever, arthralgia, and possible blindness.

Background Information

This condition is caused by a subacute inflammation of the external carotid arterial system, affecting especially the superficial temporal artery and the vertebral artery. It appears either unilaterally or bilaterally. This condition rarely occurs before age 50 and it is twice as prevalent in women. The diagnosis is confirmed with biopsy of the temporal arteries. In individuals over 50 years old, 94.8% sensitivity and 100% sensitivity was obtained if a symptom cluster consisting of jaw claudication, new-onset headache and abnormal temporal arteries on examination was used to diagnose this condition compared with temporal arterial biopsy.[58] Ophthalmologic evaluation is vital because loss of vision is associated with this condition. Vision loss usually is characterized by sudden onset, and permanent blindness may result if left untreated. The therapy of choice for this condition is oral prednisone. Even though headaches and other clinical symptoms may subside within a few days of initiating treatment, prednisone should continue for 1 to 2 years due to the continued risk of blindness.

■ Trigeminal Neuralgia

Chief Clinical Characteristics

This presentation typically includes lightning-like momentary jabs of excruciating facial pain along the distribution of the second and third division of the trigeminal nerve. Pain may persist for a few minutes to weeks and then abate spontaneously. Excessive sensitivity to touch, cold, wind, talking, or chewing also may be present.

Background Information

This condition most commonly affects middle-aged and elderly individuals, females slightly more than males. The cause of trigeminal neuralgia is unknown, but it has been postulated that trigeminal nerve focal demyelination, tumor (eg, acoustic neuroma), or vascular compression may be the etiology. If upper motor neuron signs are present, the possibilities of multiple sclerosis and brainstem tumor should be considered. This is a condition that requires immediate referral for medical assessment. Magnetic resonance imaging and computed tomography are the methods of choice to confirm the diagnosis. Pharmacologic therapy is extremely important in this condition. In severe cases, surgical decompression and/or rhizotomy may be indicated.

■ Trismus

Chief Clinical Characteristics

This presentation typically includes severe spasm and pain in the masseter muscle, limited opening or closed lock, and earache with tinnitus.

Background Information

Trismus is defined as spasm of the masseter muscles due to the motor disturbance of the trigeminal nerve. Trismus can be caused by a variety of etiologies, such as dental infection, dental procedure (with superior/inferior nerve anesthesia), trauma to the jaw, nasopharyngeal/oropharyngeal tumors, adverse effect of medication (eg, tricyclic antidepressant, succinylcholine, phenothiazines), and radiotherapy/chemotherapy. Commonly, trismus is caused by overstretching of the masseter muscle while an individual's mouth is kept open during dental procedures over an extended period of time. Functional sequelae of this health condition may involve poor nutrition and oral hygiene. Clinical examination including limited mouth opening confirms the diagnosis in the absence of other contributing pathologies. Rehabilitative interventions are the treatment of choice for this health condition, including range-of-motion exercises and splinting. Treatment should begin as soon as possible to address functional impairment related to trismus.

TUMORS

■ Acoustic Neuroma

Chief Clinical Characteristics
This presentation typically includes facial pain or numbness, headache, hearing loss, tinnitus, and gait and balance disturbance.

Background Information
This condition is a benign tumor that grows on the vestibular division of the eighth cranial nerve in the internal auditory canal. Brainstem responsive audiometry is the main diagnostic test. The specificity is approximately 97%. Magnetic resonance imaging can further confirm the diagnosis. Commonly, surgical intervention is recommended. Surgical removal of the acoustic neuroma can sometimes cause delayed hearing loss. Postoperative medical treatment includes the use of vasoactive medication such as hydroxyethyl starch and nimodipine; these medications are effective to preserve hearing.[59]

■ External Auditory Canal Tumor

Chief Clinical Characteristics
This presentation typically includes pain, swelling, limited temporomandibular joint mobility, and hearing loss. Physical examination can usually confirm the diagnosis, including bloody ear discharge.

Background Information
Lack of response to topical or systemic medications to address more benign conditions that mimic this health condition may raise clinical suspicion and reduce diagnostic delay. The most common of this type of tumor is squamous cell carcinoma. A combination of preoperative radiation therapy and surgical resection of the tumor is effective and has fewer side effects than other interventions.[60]

■ Ganglion Cyst of the Temporomandibular Joint

Chief Clinical Characteristics
This presentation typically includes articular pain, preauricular swelling, limited temporomandibular joint mobility, and joint noises.

Background Information
This condition involves pseudocysts formed by connective tissue with a fibrous lining and filled with viscous fluid, which arises from the joint capsule. Palpation usually reveals a smooth, firm, and tender mass in the preaurical area. Computed tomography and magnetic resonance imaging confirm the diagnosis. Treatment may include surgical resection in recalcitrant cases that are characterized by significant symptoms or functional impairment.

■ Metastases from Adenocarcinoma of the Colon

Chief Clinical Characteristics
This presentation typically includes pain, swelling, trismus, dysphagia, paresthesia of the facial area, and progressive limitation of temporomandibular joint mobility. A thorough subjective assessment should include questioning about weight loss, night pain/sweats, fever and chills, bowel habits, blood in stools, and general malaise.

Background Information
This rare condition is the most common metastatic tumor to the temporomandibular joint. For individuals with a previous history of colon cancer, this metastatic process must be considered. The diagnosis is confirmed with biopsy, computed tomography, and magnetic resonance imaging. Needle biopsy has been advocated to be considered with all surgical procedures, even simple tooth extractions.[61] Treatment involves appropriate management of the underlying malignancy with a combination of chemotherapy, radiation therapy, and surgical resection of the primary or relevant metastatic tumors.

■ Metastases from Intracapsular Stomach Tumor

Chief Clinical Characteristics
This presentation typically includes progressive limitation of the temporomandibular joint function.

Background Information
Adenocarcinoma of the gastric cardia may metastasize to the temporomandibular joint.

This is a very rare condition. One case report showed that the condyle and disk were anteriorly displaced by the tumor, resulting in progressive crossbite. However, no destructive changes were noted on the radiography. Tumor staging indicated that this lesion was the only distant metastasis.[62] Treatment involves appropriate management of the underlying malignancy with a combination of chemotherapy, radiation therapy, and surgical resection of the primary or relevant metastatic tumors.

■ Neoplasm in the Temporomandibular Region

Chief Clinical Characteristics
This presentation typically includes pain in the epipharyngeal region, parotid gland, or the temporomandibular joint. Progressive worsening of limitation in mandibular movement and increasing pain suggest this health condition.

Background Information
Neoplasm of the oral cavity accounts for approximately 5% of all malignancies in the body.[61] Metastatic tumors of the oral cavity comprise 1% of all neoplasms. Confirmation by clinical signs and imaging studies is necessary for making a differential diagnosis.[63] Treatment depends on tumor staging, and may include surgical resection, chemotherapy, and radiation therapy.

■ Osteochondroma of the Mandibular Condyle

Chief Clinical Characteristics
This presentation typically includes pain, limited function of the temporomandibular joint, and crepitus.

Background Information
This condition is a benign tumor consisting of projecting adult bone capped by cartilage projecting from the lateral contours of endochondral bones. This is an uncommon health condition. Panoramic radiograph, magnetic resonance imaging, computed tomography, and arthroscopy confirm the diagnosis. Condylectomy with temporomandibular joint reconstruction may be considered as a form of clinical management for this health condition.

■ Parotid Gland Tumor

Chief Clinical Characteristics
This presentation typically includes pain and swelling in the masseter area, and facial nerve palsy ipsilateral to the side of symptoms.

Background Information
This health condition is usually benign. In rare cases, parotid gland tumor can be malignant in nature or referred from another organ such as the kidney.[64] Associated facial weakness increases the likelihood of malignancy. This diagnosis is confirmed with histopathological and immunohistochemical findings from parotid gland biopsy. Based on these findings, treatment may range from surgical resection of the tumor with or without parotidectomy, chemotherapy, or radiation therapy.[65]

■ Synovial Chondromatosis of the Temporomandibular Joint

Chief Clinical Characteristics
This presentation typically includes articular pain, preauricular swelling, occasional snapping with temporomandibular joint movement, and restricted joint movement.

Background Information
This is an uncommon disease of cartilaginous transformation of synovial membrane with formation of loose bodies in the joint space. The cause of this condition is unknown. Plain radiographs confirm the diagnosis when they reveal multiple loose bodies in the joint. Surgical resection of joint loose bodies and joint reconstructions are potential treatments for this health condition.

■ Synovial Cyst of the Temporomandibular Joint

Chief Clinical Characteristics
This presentation typically includes articular pain, preauricular tenderness and swelling, limited temporomandibular joint mobility, and joint noises. The clinical presentation of synovial cysts resembles those characteristics of the ganglion cysts.

Background Information
This health condition involves cysts lined by synovial cells that contain gelatinous fluid. It

may be caused by displacement of the synovial tissue during embryogenesis or herniation of the synovium into underlying bone due to trauma. Clinical imaging and biopsy confirm the diagnosis. Surgical resection may be considered for patients with significant functional compromise and symptoms.

■ Temporal Bone Chondroblastoma

Chief Clinical Characteristics

This presentation typically includes hearing loss, otalgia, otorrhea, and may be pain in the facial area referred from tumor mass in the external auditory canal.

Background Information

This condition usually is a benign tumor derived from immature cartilage cells, occurring primarily in the epiphyses of adolescents. It is extremely rare in the temporal bone. Computed tomography, magnetic resonance imaging, and biopsy confirm the diagnosis. Treatment typically involves resection of the tumor and reconstruction of bony structures. Intraoperatively, the temporomandibular joint (TMJ) may need to be dislocated or removed, causing postoperative complications regarding TMJ function.

References

1. Ho S. Temporomandibular joint. In: Shellock FG, Powers CM, eds. *Kinematics of the Joints.* Boca Raton, FL: CRC Press; 2001.
2. Nitzan DW, Goldfarb A, Gati I, Kohen R. Changes in the reducing power of synovial fluid from temporomandibular joints with "anchored disc phenomenon." *J Oral Maxillofac Surg.* Jul 2002;60(7):735–740.
3. Rosenberg H. Trismus is not trivial. *Anesthesiology.* Oct 1987;67(4):453–455.
4. Hinkle AJ, Dorsch JA. Maternal masseter muscle rigidity and neonatal fasciculations after induction for emergency cesarean section. *Anesthesiology.* Jul 1993;79(1):175–177.
5. Ferrari A. Headache: one of the most common and troublesome adverse reactions to drugs. *Curr Drug Saf.* Jan 2006;1(1):43–58.
6. American Psychiatric Association, American Psychiatric Association, Task Force on DSM-IV. *Diagnostic and statistical manual of mental disorders: DSM-IV-TR.* 4th ed. Text revision. Washington, DC: American Psychiatric Association; 2000.
7. Pallegama RW, Ranasinghe AW, Weerasinghe VS, Sitheeque MA. Anxiety and personality traits in patients with muscle related temporomandibular disorders. *J Oral Rehabil.* 2005;32(10):701–707.
8. Phillips JM, Gatchel RJ, Wesley AL, Ellis E. Clinical implications of sex in acute temporomandibular disorders. *J Am Dent Assoc.* Jan 2001;132(1):49–57.
9. Glaros AG. Emotional factors in temporomandibular joint disorders. *J Indiana Dent Assoc.* 2000;79(4):20–23.
10. Korszun A. Facial pain, depression and stress—connections and directions. *J Oral Pathol Med.* Nov 2002; 31(10):615–619.
11. Carruthers BM, Jain AK, DeMeirleir KL, et al. Myalgic encephalomyelitis/chronic fatigue syndrome: clinical working case definition, diagnostic and treatment protocols (a consensus document). *J Chronic Fatigue Syndr.* 2003;11(1):7–115.
12. Selaimen CM, Jeronymo JC, Brilhante DP, Grossi ML. Sleep and depression as risk indicators for temporomandibular disorders in a cross-cultural perspective: a case-control study. *Int J Prosthodont.* Mar–Apr 2006;19(2):154–161.
13. Yap AU, Tan KB, Chua EK, Tan HH. Depression and somatization in patients with temporomandibular disorders. *J Prosthet Dent.* Nov 2002;88(5):479–484.
14. McBeth J, Jones K. Epidemiology of chronic musculoskeletal pain. *Best Pract Res Clin Rheumatol.* Jun 2007;21(3):403–425.
15. Sjaastad O. Benign exertional headache. *Headache.* 2003;43:611–615.
16. D'Amico D, Leone M, Bussone G. Side locked unilaterality and pain localization in long lasting headaches: migraine, tension-type and cervicogenic headache. *Headache.* 1994;34:526–530.
17. Sjaastad O, Pfaffenrath V. Cervicogenic headache: diagnostic criteria. *Headache.* 1998;38:442–445.
18. Spierings ELH. Mechanisms of migraine and actions of antimigraine medications. *Med Clin North Am.* 2001; 85(4):943–958.
19. Ferrari MD. Migraine. *Lancet.* Apr 4 1998;351(9108): 1043–1051.
20. Marks DR, Rapoport AM. Diagnosis of migraine. *Semin Neurol.* 1997;17(4):303–306.
21. Maizels M. Headache evaluation and treatment by primary care physicians in an emergency department in the era of triptans. *Arch Intern Med.* 2001;161: 1969–1973.
22. Schwartz B. Epidemiology of tension-type headache. *JAMA.* 1998;279(5):381–383.
23. Walling AD. Tension-type headache: a challenge for family physicians. *Am Fam Physician.* 2002;66:728–730.
24. Ashina M. Muscle hardness in patients with chronic tension-type headache: relation to actual headache state. *Pain.* 1999;79:201–205.
25. Jensen TS, Rasmussen P, Reske-Nielsen E. Association of trigeminal neuralgia with multiple sclerosis: clinical and pathological features. *Acta Neurol Scand.* Mar 1982; 65(3):182–189.
26. De Simone R, Ranieri A, Bilo L, Fiorillo C, Bonavita V. Cranial neuralgias: from physiopathology to pharmacological treatment. *Neurol Sci.* May 2008;29(suppl 1): S69–78.
27. Amin MR, Koufman JA. Vagal neuropathy after upper respiratory infection: a viral etiology? *Am J Otolaryngol.* Jul–Aug 2001;22(4):251–256.
28. Jacobs CJ, Harnsberger HR, Lufkin RB, Osborn AG, Smoker WR, Parkin JL. Vagal neuropathy: evaluation with CT and MR imaging. *Radiology.* Jul 1987;164(1): 97–102.
29. Krasnokutsky S, Attur M, Palmer G, Samuels J, Abramson SB. Current concepts in the pathogenesis of osteoarthritis. *Osteoarthritis Cartilage.* 2008;16(suppl 3):S1–3.

30. Pichichero ME, Casey JR. Otitis media. *Expert Opin Pharmacother.* Aug 2002;3(8):1073–1090.
31. Wolfe F, Petri M, Alarcon GS, et al. Fibromyalgia, systemic lupus erythematosus (SLE), and evaluation of SLE activity. *J Rheumatol.* Jan 2009;36(1):82–88.
32. Marien M, Jr. Trismus: causes, differential diagnosis, and treatment. *Gen Dent.* Jul–Aug 1997;45(4):350–355.
33. Chandana SR, Movva S, Arora M, Singh T. Primary brain tumors in adults. *Am Fam Physician.* May 15 2008;77(10):1423–1430.
34. Alho OP, Teppo H, Mantyselka P, Kantola S. Head and neck cancer in primary care: presenting symptoms and the effect of delayed diagnosis of cancer cases. *CMAJ.* Mar 14 2006;174(6):779–784.
35. Beil CM, Keberle M. Oral and oropharyngeal tumors. *Eur J Radiol.* Jun 2008;66(3):448–459.
36. Dachowski MT, Dolan EA, Angelillo JC. Ankylosing spondylitis associated with temporomandibular joint ankylosis: report of a case. *J Craniomandib Disord.* Winter 1990;4(1):52–57.
37. Parkash H, Goyal M. Myositis ossificans of medial pterygoid muscle. A cause for temporomandibular joint ankylosis. *Oral Surg Oral Med Oral Pathol.* Jan 1992;73(1):27–28.
38. Schellhas KP, Wilkes CH, Baker CC. Facial pain, headache, and temporomandibular joint inflammation. *Headache.* Apr 1989;29(4):229–232.
39. Haskin CL, Milam SB, Cameron IL. Pathogenesis of degenerative joint disease in the human temporomandibular joint. *Crit Rev Oral Biol Med.* 1995; 6(3):248–277.
40. Tan EK, Lo YL, Seah A, Auchus AP. Recurrent jaw dislocation after botulinum toxin treatment for sialorrhoea in amyotrophic lateral sclerosis. *J Neurol Sci.* Sep 15, 2001;190(1–2):95–97.
41. Barron RP, Kainulainen VT, Gusenbauer AW, Hollenberg R, Sandor GK. Management of traumatic dislocation of the mandibular condyle into the middle cranial fossa. *J Can Dent Assoc.* Dec 2002;68(11):676–680.
42. Daelen B, Koch A, Thorwirth V. [Botulinum toxin treatment of neurogenic dislocation of the temporomandibular joint]. *Mund Kiefer Gesichtschir.* May 1998;2(suppl 1):S125–129.
43. Daelen B, Thorwirth V, Koch A. [Neurogenic temporomandibular joint dislocation. Definition and therapy with botulinum toxin]. *Nervenarzt.* Apr 1997;68(4): 346–350.
44. Sayama S, Fujimoto K, Shizuma N, Nakano I. [Habitual mandibular dislocation in two patients with Parkinson's disease]. *Rinsho Shinkeigaku.* Aug 1999;39(8):849–851.
45. Defabianis P. TMJ fractures in children: importance of functional activation of muscles in preventing mandibular asymmetries and facial maldevelopment. *Funct Orthod.* Summer 2002;19(2):34–42.
46. Harris GJ. Orbital blow-out fractures: surgical timing and technique. *Eye.* Oct 2006;20(10):1207–1212.
47. Gladwell M, Viozzi C. Temporal bone fractures: a review for the oral and maxillofacial surgeon. *J Oral Maxillofac Surg.* Mar 2008;66(3):513–522.
48. Kaufman Y, Stal D, Cole P, Hollier L, Jr. Orbitozygomatic fracture management. *Plast Reconstr Surg.* Apr 2008; 121(4):1370–1374.

49. Chen TM, George S, Woodruff CA, Hsu S. Clinical manifestations of varicella-zoster virus infection. *Dermatol Clin.* Apr 2002;20(2):267–282.
50. Friedman MH. Closed lock. A survey of 400 cases. *Oral Surg Oral Med Oral Pathol.* Apr 1993;75(4):422–427.
51. Nagai H, Kumamoto H, Fukuda M, Takahashi T. Inducible nitric oxide synthase and apoptosis-related factors in the synovial tissues of temporomandibular joints with internal derangement and osteoarthritis. *J Oral Maxillofac Surg.* Jul 2003;61(7):801–807.
52. Singh DJ, Bartlett SP. Congenital mandibular hypoplasia: analysis and classification. *J Craniofac Surg.* Mar 2005;16(2):291–300.
53. Ratcliffe A, Israel HA, Saed-Nejad F, Diamond B. Proteoglycans in the synovial fluid of the temporomandibular joint as an indicator of changes in cartilage metabolism during primary and secondary osteoarthritis. *J Oral Maxillofac Surg.* Feb 1998;56(2):204–208.
54. Roberts G, Scully C, Shotts R. ABC of oral health. Dental emergencies. *BMJ.* Sep 2 2000;321(7260):559–562.
55. Jain N, Jain GK, Javed S, et al. Recent approaches for the treatment of periodontitis. *Drug Discov Today.* Nov 2008;13(21–22):932–943.
56. Pincus T, Callahan LF. What is the natural history of rheumatoid arthritis? *Rheum Dis Clin North Am.* Feb 1993;19(1):123–151.
57. Kuseler A, Pedersen TK, Herlin T, Gelineck J. Contrast enhanced magnetic resonance imaging as a method to diagnose early inflammatory changes in the temporomandibular joint in children with juvenile chronic arthritis. *J Rheumatol.* Jul 1998;25(7):1406–1412.
58. Lee AG, Brazis PW. Temporal arteritis. *J Am Geriatr Soc.* 1999;47(11):1364–1370.
59. Strauss C, Bischoff B, Neu M, Berg M, Fahlbusch R, Romstock J. Vasoactive treatment for hearing preservation in acoustic neuroma surgery. *J Neurosurg.* Nov 2001;95(5):771–777.
60. Uchida N, Kuroda S, Kushima T, et al. Squamous cell carcinoma of the external auditory canal: two cases treated with high dose rate 192Ir remote afterloading system (RALS). *Radiat Med.* Nov–Dec 1999;17(6): 443–446.
61. Delfino JJ, Wilson TK, Rainero DM. Metastatic adenocarcinoma from the colon to the mandible. *J Oral Maxillofac Surg.* Mar 1982;40(3):188–190.
62. Smolka W, Brekenfeld C, Buchel P, Iizuka T. Metastatic adenocarcinoma of the temporomandibular joint from the cardia of the stomach: a case report. *Int J Oral Maxillofac Surg.* Oct 2004;33(7):713–715.
63. Trumpy IG, Lyberg T. Temporomandibular joint dysfunction and facial pain caused by neoplasms. Report of three cases. *Oral Surg Oral Med Oral Pathol.* Aug 1993;76(2):149–152.
64. Sist TC, Jr., Marchetta FC, Milley PC. Renal cell carcinoma presenting as a primary parotid gland tumor. *Oral Surg Oral Med Oral Pathol.* May 1982;53(5): 499–502.
65. Mohammed F, Asaria J, Payne RJ, Freeman JL. Retrospective review of 242 consecutive patients treated surgically for parotid gland tumours. *J Otolaryngol Head Neck Surg.* Jun 2008;37(3):340–346.

CHAPTER 9

Case Demonstration: Jaw Pain

■ *Jesus F. Dominguez, PT, PhD* ■ *Michael S. Simpson, PT, DPT*

NOTE: This case demonstration was developed using the diagnostic process described in Chapter 4 and demonstrated in Chapter 5. The reader is encouraged to use this diagnostic process in order to ensure thorough clinical reasoning.

THE DIAGNOSTIC PROCESS

Step 1 Identify the patient's chief concern.

Step 2 Identify *barriers to communication*.

Step 3 Identify *special concerns*.

Step 4 Create a symptom timeline and sketch the anatomy (if needed).

Step 5 Create a diagnostic hypothesis list considering all possible forms of *remote* and *local* pathology that could cause the patient's chief concern.

Step 6 Sort the diagnostic hypothesis list by epidemiology and specific case characteristics.

Step 7 Ask specific questions to rule specific conditions or pathological categories less likely.

Step 8 Re-sort the diagnostic hypothesis list based on the patient's responses to specific questioning.

Step 9 Perform tests to differentiate among the remaining diagnostic hypotheses.

Step 10 Re-sort the diagnostic hypothesis list based on the patient's responses to specific tests.

Step 11 Decide on a diagnostic impression.

Step 12 Determine the appropriate patient disposition.

Case Description

Mr. K.D. is a 57-year-old male accountant referred to physical therapy with a diagnosis of "jaw pain secondary to left temporomandibular joint dysfunction." He stated that the jaw

discomfort began about 8 months earlier after eating popcorn. There were several unpopped kernels in the bag and he felt the pain in his left lower jaw immediately after biting down on one. The discomfort occurred only with chewing for the next few days and he went to see his primary care physician who prescribed ibuprofen and a soft diet for 1 week. Mr. K.D. states that over the course of the next several weeks, the discomfort resolved completely.

Approximately 6 months ago, he again felt left lower jaw discomfort after helping his brother move heavy furniture. At the time, he thought that he had "strained some jaw muscles" because he remembers clenching his teeth during the strenuous lifting. He mentioned this in passing to his primary care physician who advised him to begin taking ibuprofen again and return in 2 weeks if the jaw discomfort did not resolve. Mr. K.D. stated that he did not find the ibuprofen helpful this time, but he did not return for a follow-up visit.

Over the course of the next 6 months, he noted that his jaw discomfort would come on when he would push his lawnmower or push trashcans to the curb, though these activities would not always provoke his symptoms. He described the severity of the symptoms as 4/10 on a visual analog scale (VAS), with 10 being the most unbearable discomfort that he could imagine. The symptom required 3 to 5 minutes to dissipate after stopping the activity, but he would be left with a dull ache that persisted for 10 minutes. At a yearly dental cleaning visit 2 months ago, he mentioned the symptoms to his dentist who noted that the left temporomandibular joint was mildly tender to palpation. Dental x-rays at the time did not reveal any evidence of dental abnormalities. The dentist then recommended the patient be evaluated by a physical therapist with a provisional diagnosis of temporomandibular dysfunction and instructed the patient to make an appointment within a week.

Beginning 3 weeks prior to his physical therapy evaluation, Mr. K.D. also began to notice shortness of breath associated with the jaw pain. He attributed this to a recent increase in smoking because of job-related stressors. The severity of the symptoms was now 6/10 on the VAS and would persist for more than 15 minutes after he sat down to "catch his breath." He also reported that the "quality" of the jaw discomfort was different than what he had felt 8 months prior. Although the jaw discomfort and the shortness of breath would resolve simultaneously, he was now experiencing these symptoms daily. He denied any concomitant nausea, vomiting, dizziness, or diaphoresis.

Past medical history was significant for hypertension, for which he took metoprolol, 100 mg daily, and smoking (64 pack-years). There was no known family history of coronary artery/peripheral vascular disease or diabetes. Mr. K.D. said that he did not engage in any regular exercise. He weighed 90 kg and was 168 cm tall. His body mass index (BMI) was calculated to be 31.9 kg/m², placing him in the "obese" category.

STEP #1: Identify the patient's chief concern.

Mr. K.D. reports his chief concern as left jaw pain.

STEP #2: Identify *barriers to communication.*

- **History of limited communication with health care professionals.** Mr. K.D. did not return to his primary care physician for a reassessment and waited 2 months to make an appointment with the physical therapist after being referred by his dentist. This pattern of behavior could most likely present a barrier to a timely diagnosis and effective treatment. He also demonstrated a limited understanding of the need to inform his physician of the change in the quality of the jaw discomfort, the associated symptoms, and the new pattern of provocation. Failure to inform a health care provider of new symptom patterns could significantly confound the diagnostic process and could lead to the development of ineffective treatment strategies.

STEP #3: Identify *special concerns.*

- **Unusual symptoms occurring with physical exertion.** Raises the index of clinical suspicion for contributory cardiovascular or pulmonary pathology.
- **Patient's age and a diagnosis of hypertension.** Raises the index of clinical suspicion for contributory cardiovascular or pulmonary pathology.
- **Smoking history, including a recent increase in smoking.** Raises the index of clinical suspicion for contributory cardiovascular or pulmonary pathology.
- **Unresponsive to previously effective treatment.** Raises the possibility of a different pathology presenting to create a similar previous chief concern.

STEP #4: Create a symptom timeline and sketch the anatomy (if needed).

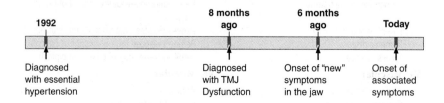

1992	8 months ago	6 months ago	Today
Diagnosed with essential hypertension	Diagnosed with TMJ Dysfunction	Onset of "new" symptoms in the jaw	Onset of associated symptoms

STEP #5: Create a diagnostic hypothesis list considering all possible forms of *remote* and *local* pathology that could cause the patient's chief concern.

Remote

T   Trauma

Poor posture
Whiplash

I   Inflammation

Aseptic
Chronic fatigue syndrome
Dental caries

Fibromyalgia
Sjögren's syndrome
Subacute granulomatous thyroiditis
Systemic lupus erythematosus

Septic
Dental abscess

Otitis media

Post-herpetic neuralgia
Rheumatoid arthritis
Septic arthritis
Sinus abscess
Sinus infection
Suppurative parotitis
Tetanus

M   Metabolic

Carnitine deficiency

Forbes' disease
Hypocalcemic tetany

McArdle's disease
Medication-induced dyskinesia

Mitochondrial myopathy

Paget's disease
Pompe's disease
Tarui's disease

Va   Vascular

Angina pectoris
Coronary insufficiency
Cranial/temporal arteritis

STEP #6: Sort the diagnostic hypothesis list by epidemiology and specific case characteristics.

Remote

T   Trauma

Poor posture
~~Whiplash~~ (absence of whiplash mechanism)

I   Inflammation

Aseptic
Chronic fatigue syndrome
~~Dental caries~~ (absence of positive findings on recent dental examination)
Fibromyalgia
~~Sjögren's syndrome~~ (gender not typical)
Subacute granulomatous thyroiditis
Systemic lupus erythematosus

Septic
~~Dental abscess~~ (absence of positive findings on recent dental examination)
~~Otitis media~~ (absence of ear pain or other associated symptoms)
Post-herpetic neuralgia
Rheumatoid arthritis
Septic arthritis
Sinus abscess
Sinus infection
Suppurative parotitis
~~Tetanus~~ (time course)

M   Metabolic

~~Carnitine deficiency~~ (age of onset not typical)
~~Forbes' disease~~ (age of onset not typical)
~~Hypocalcemic tetany~~ (age of onset not typical)
~~McArdle's disease~~ (age of onset not typical)
~~Medication-induced dyskinesia~~ (no history of Parkinson's medications)
~~Mitochondrial myopathy~~ (age of onset not typical)
~~Paget's disease~~ (age of onset not typical)
~~Pompe's disease~~ (age of onset not typical)
~~Tarui's disease~~ (age of onset not typical)

Va   Vascular

Angina pectoris
Coronary insufficiency
~~Cranial/temporal arteritis~~ (symptoms are intermittent, worse with exertion)

Dissecting aneurysm

~~Dissecting aneurysm~~ (time course, no associated abdominal or back pain)

Myocardial infarction

~~Myocardial infarction~~ (time course)

Sickle cell crisis pain

~~Sickle cell crisis pain~~ (age not typical)

De Degenerative

De Degenerative

Osteoarthritis of cervical spine

~~Osteoarthritis of cervical spine~~ (absence of neck pain not typical)

Tu Tumor

Tu Tumor

Acoustic neuroma

Acoustic neuroma

Co Congenital

Co Congenital

Hyperostosis cortical infantile

~~Hyperostosis cortical infantile~~ (age not typical)

Paroxysmal extreme pain disorder

~~Paroxysmal extreme pain disorder~~ (age not typical)

Ne Neurogenic/Psychogenic

Ne Neurogenic/Psychogenic

Depression
Gastroesophageal reflux disease
Hiatal hernia
Multiple sclerosis
Stress/anxiety

Depression
Gastroesophageal reflux disease
Hiatal hernia
Multiple sclerosis
Stress/anxiety

Local

Local

T Trauma

T Trauma

Barotrauma

~~Barotrauma~~ (no associated ear pain)

Bruxism

Bruxism

Dental trauma

~~Dental trauma~~ (absence of positive findings on recent dental examination)

Edentulism and denture wear

~~Edentulism and denture wear~~ (absence of positive findings on recent dental examination)

Ernest syndrome

~~Ernest syndrome~~ (absence of jaw trauma)

Malocclusion

~~Malocclusion~~ (absence of positive findings on recent dental examination)

Mandibular atrophy

~~Mandibular atrophy~~ (absence of positive findings on recent dental examination)

Onychophagia

~~Onychophagia~~ (worsened with prolonged physical exertion)

Pathological fracture

~~Pathological fracture~~ (absence of positive findings on recent dental examination)

Temporal tendinitis
Temporomandibular ankylosis
Temporomandibular dysfunction

Temporal tendinitis
Temporomandibular ankylosis
Temporomandibular dysfunction

Trismus

~~Trismus~~ (able to open mouth to speak and give history)

I Inflammation

I Inflammation

Aseptic

Aseptic

Capsulitis or synovitis

Capsulitis or synovitis

Dental ulcer

~~Dental ulcer~~ (absence of positive findings on recent dental examination)

Gingivitis

~~Gingivitis~~ (absence of positive findings on recent dental examination)

Impacted wisdom teeth

~~Impacted wisdom teeth~~ (absence of positive findings on recent dental examination)

Jaw cyst

~~Jaw cyst~~ (absence of positive findings on recent dental examination)

Rhabdomyolysis

~~Rhabdomyolysis~~ (no recent changes in physical training regimen)

Septic

Septic

Acute pulpitis or pulpal abscess

~~Acute pulpitis or pulpal abscess~~ (absence of positive findings on recent dental examination)

Acute suppurative sinusitis

Acute suppurative sinusitis

Gout

~~Gout~~ (unlikely as only joint affected)

Herpes zoster

~~Herpes zoster~~ (unlikely with absence of history of vesicular eruptions in the painful zone)

Lyme disease

Lyme disease

Osteomyelitis

Osteomyelitis

Pericoronitis

~~Pericoronitis~~ (age of onset not typical)

Pseudogout

~~Pseudogout~~ (unlikely as only joint affected)

M Metabolic

M Metabolic

Sialolithiasis

Sialolithiasis

Va Vascular

Va Vascular

Avascular necrosis

~~Avascular necrosis~~ (absence of positive findings on recent dental examination)

Microvascular compression

~~Microvascular compression~~ (absence of positive findings on recent dental examination)

De Degenerative

De Degenerative

Felty's syndrome

~~Felty's syndrome~~ (no long-standing history of rheumatoid arthritis)

Fibrous dysplasia

~~Fibrous dysplasia~~ (age not typical)

Osteoarthritis/osteoarthrosis of the temporomandibular joint

Osteoarthritis/osteoarthrosis of the temporomandibular joint

Tu Tumor

Tu Tumor

Ameloblastoma

Ameloblastoma

Ewing's sarcoma

~~Ewing's sarcoma~~ (age not typical)

Giant cell tumor

Giant cell tumor

Multiple myeloma

Multiple myeloma

Neoplasm/tumors of the mandible and maxilla

Neoplasm/tumors of the mandible and maxilla

Odontoma

Odontoma

Oropharyngeal cancer

Oropharyngeal cancer

Osteosarcoma

Osteosarcoma

Parotid (Warthin's) tumor

Parotid (Warthin's) tumor

Pathological fracture secondary to metastases

Pathological fracture secondary to metastases

Squamous cell carcinoma

Squamous cell carcinoma

Co	**Congenital**
	Not applicable
Ne	**Neurogenic/Psychogenic**
	Trigeminal neuralgia

Co	**Congenital**
	Not applicable
Ne	**Neurogenic/Psychogenic**
	Trigeminal neuralgia

STEP #7: Ask specific questions to rule specific conditions or pathological categories less likely.

- **Have you had any associated numbness or tingling in your face?** No, making less likely forms of pathology involving neurogenic pain.
- **Have you had congestion in the ear or nose?** No, ruling less likely sinus or ear pathology (ie, infection and acoustic neuroma). Fever? No, would also rule out (r/o) infection.
- **Have you experienced any unintentional weight gain or loss?** No, ruling less likely cancer as a contributory cause of the patient's symptoms.
- **Are your symptoms worsened or alleviated by eating?** No, ruling less likely upper gastrointestinal pathology as a cause of this patient's symptoms.
- **Do you feel fatigued or "out of it"?** No, ruling less likely systemic forms of aseptic inflammation (ie, rheumatoid arthritis and chronic fatigue syndrome) and neurogenic problems (ie, multiple sclerosis), which are associated with fatigue.

STEP #8: Re-sort the diagnostic hypothesis list based on the patient's responses to specific questioning.

Remote

T	**Trauma**
	Poor posture
I	**Inflammation**
	Aseptic
	~~Chronic fatigue syndrome~~ (no fatigue or malaise)
	~~Fibromyalgia~~ (no fatigue or malaise)
	~~Sjögren's syndrome~~ (no fatigue or malaise)
	~~Subacute granulomatous thyroiditis~~ (no fatigue or malaise)

	~~Systemic lupus erythematosus~~ (no fatigue or malaise)
	Septic
	~~Post-herpetic neuralgia~~ (no change in facial sensation)
	~~Rheumatoid arthritis~~ (no fatigue)
	~~Septic arthritis~~ (no fatigue)
	~~Sinus abscess~~ (no nasal congestion, fatigue)
	~~Sinus infection~~ (no nasal congestion, fatigue)
	~~Suppurative parotitis~~ (symptoms not worse with eating)
M	**Metabolic**
	Not applicable
Va	**Vascular**
	Angina pectoris
	Coronary insufficiency
De	**Degenerative**
	Not applicable
Tu	**Tumor**
	~~Acoustic neuroma~~ (no aural congestion)
Co	**Congenital**
	Not applicable
Ne	**Neurogenic/Psychogenic**
	Depression
	~~Gastroesophageal reflux disease~~ (no change in symptoms with eating)
	~~Hiatal hernia~~ (no change in symptoms with eating)
	~~Multiple sclerosis~~ (no fatigue or malaise)
	Stress/anxiety

Local

T	**Trauma**
	Bruxism
	Temporal tendinitis
	Temporomandibular ankylosis
	Temporomandibular dysfunction

I Inflammation

Aseptic
Capsulitis or synovitis

Septic
~~Acute suppurative sinusitis~~ (no nasal congestion)

~~Lyme disease~~ (no fatigue or malaise)

~~Osteomyelitis~~ (no fever)

M Metabolic

~~Sialolithiasis~~ (no change in perceived facial status)

Va Vascular

Not applicable

De Degenerative

Osteoarthritis/osteoarthrosis of the temporomandibular joint

Tu Tumor

~~Ameloblastoma~~ (no change in perceived facial status, fatigue/malaise, weight change)

~~Ewing's sarcoma~~ (no change in perceived facial status, fatigue/malaise, weight change)

~~Giant cell tumor~~ (no change in perceived facial status, fatigue/malaise, weight change)

~~Multiple myeloma~~ (no change in perceived facial status, fatigue/malaise, weight change)

~~Neoplasm/tumors of the mandible and maxilla~~ (no change in perceived facial status, fatigue/malaise, weight change)

~~Odontoma~~ (no change in perceived facial status, fatigue/malaise, weight change)

~~Oropharyngeal cancer~~ (no change in perceived facial status, fatigue/malaise, weight change)

~~Osteosarcoma~~ (no change in perceived facial status, fatigue/malaise, weight change)

~~Parotid (Warthin's) tumor~~ (no change in perceived facial status, fatigue/malaise, weight change)

~~Pathological fracture secondary to metastases~~ (no change in perceived facial status, fatigue/malaise, weight change)

~~Squamous cell carcinoma~~ (no change in perceived facial status, fatigue/malaise, weight change)

Co Congenital

Not applicable

Ne Neurogenic/Psychogenic

~~Trigeminal neuralgia~~ (no change in facial sensation)

STEP #9: Perform tests to differentiate among the remaining diagnostic hypotheses.

- **Cardiac and pulmonary auscultation.** Normal first (S_1) and second (S_2) heart sounds without murmurs. A fourth heart sound (S_4, often associated with long-standing hypertension) was also noted. Auscultation of the lungs revealed mild inspiratory crackles throughout both lower lung fields.

- **Temporomandibular examination.** Localized tenderness to palpation of the masseter and temporalis muscles. Mr. K.D. stated these symptoms were unlike his current chief concern. Mild and painless reciprocal click was noted.

STEP #10: Re-sort the diagnostic hypothesis list based on the patient's responses to specific tests.

Remote

T Trauma
Not applicable

I Inflammation

Aseptic
Not applicable

Septic
Not applicable

M Metabolic
Not applicable

Va Vascular
Angina pectoris
Coronary insufficiency

De Degenerative
Not applicable

Tu Tumor
Not applicable

Co Congenital
Not applicable

Ne Neurogenic/Psychogenic

Depression

Stress/anxiety

Local

T Trauma

~~Bruxism~~ (temporomandibular joint examination revealed symptoms that were inconsistent with chief concern)

~~Temporal tendinitis~~ (temporomandibular joint examination revealed symptoms that were inconsistent with chief concern)

~~Temporomandibular ankylosis~~ (temporomandibular joint examination revealed symptoms that were inconsistent with chief concern)

~~Temporomandibular dysfunction~~ (temporomandibular joint examination revealed symptoms that were inconsistent with chief concern)

I Inflammation

Aseptic

~~Capsulitis or synovitis~~ (temporomandibular joint examination revealed symptoms that were inconsistent with chief concern)

Septic

Not applicable

M Metabolic

Not applicable

Va Vascular

Not applicable

De Degenerative

~~Osteoarthritis/osteoarthrosis of the temporomandibular joint~~ (temporomandibular joint examination revealed symptoms that were inconsistent with chief concern)

Tu Tumor

Not applicable

Co Congenital

Not applicable

Ne Neurogenic/Psychogenic

Not applicable

STEP #11: Decide on a diagnostic impression.

- Rule out angina pectoris secondary to coronary insufficiency.

STEP #12: Determine the appropriate patient disposition.

- Refer the patient to a cardiologist by telephone for additional evaluation and treatment.
- Educate the patient about the urgency of the need for a cardiology appointment to take place.
- Inform the patient of symptoms and signs of an acute myocardial infarction, with instructions to activate the emergency medical system if these symptoms and signs take place.

Case Outcome

At the follow-up visit, the cardiologist ordered blood laboratory tests including a cardiac enzyme panel, a resting electrocardiogram, and an exercise tolerance test to aid in ruling cardiovascular disease less likely. The results of the blood work indicated that the patient had significantly elevated total and low-density lipoprotein cholesterol levels. The resting electrocardiogram was normal, but the exercise tolerance test demonstrated electrocardiographic changes consistent with myocardial ischemia. During the exercise tolerance test, Mr. K.D. also experienced his typical dull left jaw pain with shortness of breath and both resolved within 10 minutes of rest. He subsequently underwent a coronary angiogram that revealed 75% stenosis of the proximal left anterior descending artery. A balloon angioplasty with stent placement was performed and the patient was discharged 1 day after the procedure. Mr. K.D. subsequently returned 3 weeks later to the physical therapy clinic for treatment of his temporomandibular dysfunction.

CHAPTER 10

Neck Pain

■ *Larry Ho, PT, DPT, OCS* ■ *Shirley Wachi-See, PT, DPT, OCS*

Description of the Symptom

This chapter describes pathology that may lead to neck pain. **Local causes** of neck pain are defined as pathology occurring within the vertebral column from the occipital condyle to the seventh cervical vertebra, along with associated joint and soft tissue structures. **Remote causes** are defined as occurring outside this region. The chapter is divided between anterior and posterior/posterolateral neck pain.

Special Concerns
- Ataxia or other gait disturbances
- Clonus, positive Hoffman's and Babinski tests, or hyperreflexia
- Drop attacks
- Facial paresthesias or muscle paresis

- Horner's sign (ptosis, enophthalmos, anhidrosis, miosis, and facial flushing)
- Pain and stiffness associated with fever or recent illness
- Positive alar ligament test, Sharp-Purser test
- Radicular symptoms into bilateral upper extremities accompanied by lower extremity symptoms (eg, bilateral or quadrilateral paresthesias)
- Signs and symptoms of vertebral artery insufficiency including dizziness, dysphagia, dysarthria, dystonia, and disorientation
- Signs of upper cervical instability (eg, unwillingness to actively move head and neck, reports of dizziness, nausea, or paresthesias with neck flexion)
- Syncope

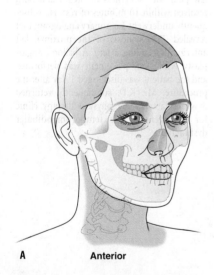

A   **Anterior**

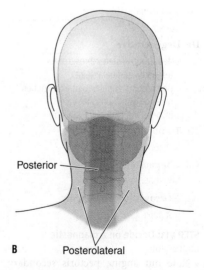

Posterior —

B   Posterolateral

CHAPTER PREVIEW: Conditions That May Lead to Neck Pain

T Trauma

REMOTE	LOCAL ANTERIOR	LOCAL POSTERIOR AND POSTEROLATERAL
COMMON		

Shoulder pathology 115
Thoracic outlet
  syndrome 116
	Blunt trauma to larynx or
	  trachea 118
		Brachial plexus/nerve root lesion 118
		Cervical disk herniation 120
		Cervical dystonia 120
		Cervical facet dysfunction 120
		Cervicogenic headache 121
		Coital neck pain 122
		Fractures:
		• Lower cervical spine (C3–C7) 124
		• Upper cervical spine (C0–C2) 124
		Muscle strain 125

UNCOMMON		

Internal organ injuries:
• Diaphragm
• Liver
• Lung
• Spleen
Spontaneous
  pneumomediastinum 115
T4 syndrome 116
	Digastric and stylohyoid
	  muscle strain 122
		Entrapments:
		• Greater occipital nerve (occipital
		  neuralgia) 123
		• Spinal accessory nerve 123

RARE		
Stylohyoid syndrome (Eagle's syndrome) 116	Not applicable	Subluxations/dislocations: • Congenital 128 • Degenerative 128 • Traumatic 128

I Inflammation

REMOTE	LOCAL ANTERIOR	LOCAL POSTERIOR AND POSTEROLATERAL
COMMON		

Not applicable	**Aseptic**
	Not applicable
	
	Septic
	Cervical lymphadenitis
	  121
		Aseptic
		Cervical lymphadenitis 121
		Fibromyalgia 123
		Rheumatoid arthritis of the cervical
		  spine 127
		
		Septic
		Not applicable

UNCOMMON		
Aseptic Not applicable	**Aseptic** Complex regional pain syndrome 122	**Aseptic** Ankylosing spondylitis 117 Chronic fatigue syndrome 122

(continued)

Inflammation *(continued)*

REMOTE	LOCAL ANTERIOR	LOCAL POSTERIOR AND POSTEROLATERAL
Septic Pericarditis 114 Pleurisy 115	**Septic** Abscess or cyst infection 117	Complex regional pain syndrome 122 Polymyalgia rheumatica 127 Systemic lupus erythematosus 129 **Septic** Bacterial meningitis 117
RARE		

Aseptic
Not applicable
 	
Septic
Submandibular space
  infection (Ludwig's
  angina) 116
	Aseptic
	Not applicable
	
	Septic
	Pharyngoesophageal
	  diverticulum 127
	Thyroiditis 129
		Aseptic
		Fibromyositis 124
		Lyme disease 125
		Meningismus (aseptic meningitis) 125
		Pachymeningitis cervicalis
		  hypertrophica 126
		Transverse myelitis 129
		
		Septic
		Cervical osteomyelitis 121

Ⓜ Metabolic

REMOTE	LOCAL ANTERIOR	LOCAL POSTERIOR AND POSTEROLATERAL
COMMON		
Not applicable	Not applicable	Osteomalacia 126 Osteoporosis 126
UNCOMMON		
Medication overuse headache 114	Not applicable	Crowned dens syndrome 122 Paget's disease 126
RARE		
Not applicable	Not applicable	Retropharyngeal calcific tendinitis 127

Ⓥ⒜ Vascular

REMOTE	LOCAL ANTERIOR	LOCAL POSTERIOR AND POSTEROLATERAL
COMMON		
Acute myocardial infarction 113	Not applicable	Not applicable
UNCOMMON		
Acute coronary insufficiency 113 Pericarditis 114	Arteritis 117 Hemorrhage 124	Not applicable

Vascular *(continued)*

REMOTE	LOCAL ANTERIOR	LOCAL POSTERIOR AND POSTEROLATERAL
RARE		
Dissecting aneurysm of the thoracic aorta 113	Dissection of the internal carotid artery 123	Arteritis 117 Epidural hematoma 123 Internal carotid arteritis 125 Subarachnoid hemorrhage 128 Subdural hematoma 128 Vertebral artery dissection 130

De Degenerative

REMOTE	LOCAL ANTERIOR	LOCAL POSTERIOR AND POSTEROLATERAL
COMMON		
Temporomandibular dysfunction 129	Not applicable	Cervical degenerative disk disease 118 Cervical degenerative joint disease 118 Cervical stenosis (bilateral and unilateral) 121
UNCOMMON		
Not applicable	Not applicable	Not applicable
RARE		
Riedel's struma 115	Not applicable	Subluxations/dislocations: • Congenital 128 • Degenerative 128 • Traumatic 128

Tu Tumor

REMOTE	LOCAL ANTERIOR	LOCAL POSTERIOR AND POSTEROLATERAL
COMMON		
Not applicable	Not applicable	Not applicable
UNCOMMON		
Malignant Primary, such as: • Breast tumor 116 • Pancoast tumor 117 *Malignant Metastatic:* Not applicable *Benign:* Not applicable	*Malignant Primary, such as:* • Anaplastic carcinoma 129 • Carcinoma of the esophagus 130 *Malignant Metastatic:* Not applicable *Benign:* Not applicable	Not applicable

(continued)

NECK PAIN

Tumor *(continued)*

REMOTE	LOCAL ANTERIOR	LOCAL POSTERIOR AND POSTEROLATERAL
RARE		
Not applicable	*Malignant Primary:* Not applicable *Malignant Metastatic, such as:* • Lymphoma 130 *Benign:* Not applicable	Not applicable

Co Congenital

REMOTE	LOCAL ANTERIOR	LOCAL POSTERIOR AND POSTEROLATERAL
COMMON		
Not applicable	Not applicable	Cervical stenosis 121
UNCOMMON		
Marfan's syndrome 114	Not applicable	Not applicable
RARE		
Not applicable	Not applicable	Subluxations/dislocations: • Congenital 128 • Degenerative 128 • Traumatic 128

Ne Neurogenic/Psychogenic

REMOTE	LOCAL ANTERIOR	LOCAL POSTERIOR AND POSTEROLATERAL
COMMON		
Not applicable	Not applicable	Not applicable
UNCOMMON		
Not applicable	Post-traumatic dysautonomic cephalgia 127	Not applicable
RARE		
Not applicable	Not applicable	Not applicable

Note: These are estimates of relative incidence because few data are available for the less common conditions.

Overview of Neck Pain

Pain in the cervical spine may involve any of the seven vertebral bodies, eight spinal nerves, 23 muscles, or three major vessels passing through the cervical region. In addition to the immediate involvement of the underlying structures, many of the structures and organs in other parts of the body can refer pain to the cervical spine because the cervical spine is an important conduit for innervation and vascularization to and from the rest of the body. Some systemic diseases such as rheumatoid arthritis, fibromyalgia, and lupus erythematosus can have profound effects and present with pain in the cervical spine.

Description of Conditions That May Lead to Neck Pain

Remote

■ Acute Coronary Insufficiency

Chief Clinical Characteristics
This presentation is mainly characterized by chest pain or tightness, but can present as pain radiating down one or both arms or as neck or jaw pain. This constellation of symptoms is similar to those experienced for myocardial infarction.

Background Information
Temporary occlusion or spasm of the coronary artery causes the onset of symptoms related to regional hypoxia of the myocardium. Symptoms may occur at rest or during activity. In contrast to acute myocardial infarction, pain is relieved by administration of nitroglycerin. This health condition merits urgent consultation with a physician, particularly during the first onset of symptoms or changes in symptom pattern, due to the risk for hypoxic myocardial damage.

■ Acute Myocardial Infarction

Chief Clinical Characteristics
This presentation often includes chest pain or tightness, but can present as pain radiating down one or both arms or as neck or jaw pain. This condition also may be associated with dyspnea, diaphoresis, pallor, weakness, and nausea.

Background Information
This health condition occurs when there is an acute disruption of blood flow to the myocardium. Women are more likely than men to report neck and jaw symptoms associated with this condition. Symptoms may be aggravated by exertion but also may occur at rest; symptoms are relieved neither by rest nor with administration of nitroglycerin.

This condition is a medical emergency due to the risk for significant myocardial damage and death.[1]

■ Dissecting Aneurysm of the Thoracic Aorta

Chief Clinical Characteristics
This presentation may involve severe tearing or crushing pain along the chest, anterior base of the neck, or interscapular region. Symptoms may include ischemic neuropathy.

Background Information
Dissecting aneurysms of the ascending aorta may manifest with symptoms of brain ischemia, whereas dissecting aneurysms of the descending aorta typically present with symptoms of spinal ischemia. Systolic blood pressure may drop below 100 mm Hg, and heart rate may increase to greater than 100 beats per minute. Risk factors include male sex, hypertension, lung disease, arteriosclerosis, and connective tissue disease. Abdominal computed tomography confirms the diagnosis.[2] This condition is a medical emergency.

INTERNAL ORGAN INJURIES

■ Diaphragm Injury

Chief Clinical Characteristics
The presentation of diaphragm injuries typically includes shoulder or lateral neck pain with chest pain.

Background Information
Diaphragm rupture can occur with blunt or penetrating trauma to the chest or abdomen. Deep breathing and changes in position also may aggravate the symptoms. The mechanism that causes shoulder pain may involve the phrenic nerve.[3] Chest radiographs confirm the diagnosis, with characteristic findings of irregular diaphragmatic contour or elevation, contralateral mediastinal shift, and gas collection in the hemithorax. This condition requires urgent referral for medical evaluation.

■ Liver Injury

Chief Clinical Characteristics
The presentation of liver injuries can include pain in the midepigastric region or right

upper quadrant, with referred pain to the superior shoulder, interscapular, and upper trapezius regions.

Background Information
Additional symptoms are right upper quadrant tenderness and guarding, and signs of blood loss such as shock and hypotension. Liver trauma accounts for 15% to 20% of blunt abdominal injuries. Common mechanisms of injury include motor vehicle accidents and receiving an abdominal blow while fighting. Abdominal computed tomography confirms the diagnosis.[4] This condition requires urgent referral for medical evaluation.

■ Lung Injury

Chief Clinical Characteristics
The presentation of lung injuries may involve sharp, pleuritic pain in the axilla, shoulder, or subscapular regions with possible referral pain to the neck.[5] Clinical findings may also include shoulder-arm pain, Horner's syndrome, and neurological deficits affecting the C8 and T1 nerve roots in the case of apical lung involvement.

Background Information
Chest radiographs or computed tomography confirm the diagnosis. This condition requires urgent referral for medical evaluation.

■ Spleen Injury

Chief Clinical Characteristics
The presentation of spleen injuries may be characterized by left shoulder pain possibly associated with neck pain. Symptoms are worse with coughing, deep breathing, and changes in position.

Background Information
Blunt trauma injury to the abdomen is the most common cause of this health condition, although delayed splenic rupture after colonoscopy is becoming a better recognized presentation. Abdominal distention and tenderness and hemodynamic instability may be associated signs. Abdominal computed tomography confirms the diagnosis.[6] This condition requires urgent referral for medical evaluation.

■ Marfan's Syndrome

Chief Clinical Characteristics
This presentation may include tall height, arachnodactyly, pectus excavatum, hypermobility, and skin stretch marks. It is potentially associated with anterior neck pain by way of characteristic cardiac pathology.

Background Information
Individuals with this rare congenital condition have a larger and more fragile aorta; aortic aneurysm, aortic dissection, aortic regurgitation, and mitral regurgitation are common. Defects and abnormalities of the heart valves can cause referred pain to the anterior aspect of the neck. This condition involves fibrillin protein deficiency that affects the mesodermal and ectodermal tissues, resulting in compromised form and function of the heart valves, blood vessels, lungs, kidneys, eyes, and skeleton.[7] Individuals with this condition require interdisciplinary management due to its cardiovascular, optic, and musculoskeletal manifestations.

■ Medication Overuse Headache

Chief Clinical Characteristics
This presentation typically involves progressively worsening daily headaches and neck pain that present on more than 15 days per month in the presence of regular overuse of a medication for greater than 3 months.[8]

Background Information
Headaches due to medication overuse resolve or revert to their previous pattern within 2 months of ceasing the overused medication. Inappropriate use of headache medications—such as ergotamine, triptans, opioids, and simple or combination analgesics—may contribute to the development of chronic daily headaches.[9] Medication overuse headache is a retrospective diagnosis made when the offending agent is withdrawn and the headache pattern ceases to be daily. This treatment should be undertaken with the advice of a physician.

■ Pericarditis

Chief Clinical Characteristics
This presentation typically involves sharp, stabbing anterior chest pain that may radiate to the

neck, back, left shoulder, or left supraclavicular region. Pain is worse with deep inspiration, coughing, trunk rotation or side-bending, and lying supine. It is alleviated by sitting up or leaning forward. This condition may be associated with a history of recent respiratory illness, fever, chills, neoplasm, or heart disease/myocardial infarction.

Background Information
Pericardial friction rub may be auscultated. This health condition commonly occurs in response to viral infection of the pericardium. Chest computed tomography and magnetic resonance imaging confirm the diagnosis.[10] This condition is a medical emergency due to the risk for cardiac tamponade.

■ Pleurisy

Chief Clinical Characteristics
This presentation is mainly characterized by pain in the chest over the affected site, short rapid breathing, coughing, dyspnea, and fever, with pain referred to the shoulder and neck regions. Aggravating factors include coughing, deep inspiration, and laughing.

Background Information
This condition involves inflammation of the pleura. Common causes of pleurisy include infection, trauma, rheumatoid arthritis, systemic lupus erythematosus, and tumor. Chest radiographs confirm the diagnosis.[11] Treatment commonly involves addressing the underlying infective agent with antibiotic medication.

■ Riedel's Struma

Chief Clinical Characteristics
This presentation includes anterior neck pain in association with a firm mass, hoarseness, or signs of tracheal compression. Women in the sixth decade of life are most commonly affected.

Background Information
This rare condition occurs due to an idiopathic autoimmune process that results in fibrosclerosis of the thyroid, impinging the recurrent pharyngeal nerve, trachea, and other adjacent structures. Individuals with this condition should be monitored for secondary hypothyroidism.[12] Common treatment for this health condition includes management with

corticosteroids, tamoxifen, and levothyroxine. Surgical resection of the affected thyroid may confirm the diagnosis and assist in the management of this health condition.

■ Shoulder Pathology

Chief Clinical Characteristics
This presentation typically involves shoulder pain, instability, and/or crepitus in combination with paracentral neck pain.

Background Information
A variety of conditions in the shoulder can lead to neck pain, usually through compensatory actions of the pectorals and upper trapezius. These actions also may cause cervicobrachial neural tissue provocation, resulting in pseudoradicular symptoms of the upper extremity. These conditions include upper trapezius strain, levator scapula strain, glenohumeral or sternoclavicular osteoarthrosis/osteoarthritis, rotator cuff tear, and subacromial impingement. Usual treatment for neck pain related to this condition involves addressing the underlying shoulder pathology through use of appropriate surgical or nonsurgical interventions.

■ Spontaneous Pneumomediastinum

Chief Clinical Characteristics
This presentation may involve moderate to severe pain in the anterior neck and chest, accompanied by shortness of breath, throat soreness, or dysphagia. Symptoms are aggravated by deep breathing, coughing, or lying supine, and they are alleviated by sitting up or leaning forward.

Background Information
This condition is most common in young men. It is caused by the presence of free air within the mediastinum due to alveolar rupture. Violent coughing, acute asthma, or inhalation of illicit drugs may contribute to the etiology of this condition.[13] Treatment includes analgesics and bed rest. Spontaneous resolution typically occurs within 3 to 5 days, but patients suspected of having this health condition should be referred for additional medical evaluation emergently to monitor for signs of serious complications.

Stylohyoid Syndrome (Eagle's Syndrome)

Chief Clinical Characteristics

This presentation can include pain in the upper region of the neck near the angle of the jaw. Symptoms may also occur in the ipsilateral side of the face, ears, throat, temple, and sternocleidomastoid. Pain may be aggravated by swallowing, talking, and turning the head toward the painful side.

Background Information

Stylohyoid syndrome can be caused by the styloid impinging on the carotid vessels. Scar tissue as a result of surgery also may be responsible. Lidocaine injection to the tip of the greater horn of the hyoid bone may be necessary. Surgical shortening or removal of the styloid may be necessary to alleviate the symptoms.[14]

Submandibular Space Infection (Ludwig's Angina)

Chief Clinical Characteristics

This presentation is mainly characterized by pain and edema of the mouth, submandibular, and anterior neck regions in association with sublingual firmness, excessive drooling, fever, malaise, and tachycardia. The significant swelling associated with this condition may impair breathing and swallowing rapidly.

Background Information

This condition is caused by dental disease or infection that progresses to the deep tissues of the anterior neck. Risk factors also include recent dental work, oral piercing, and mandibular fracture.[15] The diagnosis is made based on clinical examination. Treatments include antibiotic medication, surgical drainage, and airway access as needed to ensure adequate respiration.

T4 Syndrome

Chief Clinical Characteristics

This presentation involves pain in the cervical spine and upper extremities, associated with paresthesias and unremarkable reflex, sensation, and myotomal strength tests.

Background Information

T4 syndrome was first described by Maitland, when mobilization/manipulation of upper thoracic functional spinal units was observed to produce beneficial effects in individuals experiencing upper extremity pain.[16] This idiopathic health condition is considered to be rare. The mechanism of relief is still not clear, but it is believed that modulation of the autonomic nervous system may be involved.

Thoracic Outlet Syndrome

Chief Clinical Characteristics

This presentation is characterized by lateral neck pain that radiates into the arm and hand accompanied by paresthesias and numbness in the medial forearm and fourth and fifth fingers with possible weakness of the intrinsic hand muscles.

Background Information

This condition can result from a congenital cervical rib or other anatomical structure compressing the neurovascular structures between the cervical spine and axilla. It also can be the result of trauma. Thoracic outlet syndrome is broken down into three subcategories: arterial, venous, and neurogenic. Vascular forms of this condition are rare and account for fewer than 5% of all cases. The diagnosis is made clinically and usually requires a combination of tests for both the neurological and vascular components.[17] Although a variety of surgical and nonsurgical procedures are available to treat this health condition, the first intervention of choice is usually nonsurgical in patients without significant neurological and vascular compromise.

TUMORS

Breast Tumor

Chief Clinical Characteristics

This presentation involves a nonpainful, palpable, firm, irregular mass in the breast, and deep shoulder and neck pain, jaundice, or weight loss in individuals with advanced disease.

Background Information

The onset of aching pain in the shoulder with difficulty sleeping may be an indication of metastases to the lymph or osseous structures of the shoulder. Risk factors include personal and family history of cancer, late-onset pregnancy, and early menopause.

Screening breast radiographs may detect early disease. Blood tests for carcinoembryonic antigen, ferritin, and human chorionic gonadotropin confirm the diagnosis in individuals with metastasis. Treatment may include resection of the tumor and involved axillary lymph nodes, mastectomy, chemotherapy, or radiation.

■ Pancoast Tumor

Chief Clinical Characteristics
This presentation includes sharp, pleuritic pain in the axilla, shoulder, or subscapular regions with referral pain to the neck. Clinical findings also include shoulder-arm pain, Horner's syndrome, and neurological deficits affecting the C8 and T1 nerve roots.[18]

Background Information
True Pancoast tumors originate in the extrathoracic space. However, primary lung tumors and abscesses in the superior thoracic sulcus also may mimic this condition by invading or impinging the subclavian space. Risk factors include smoking, exposure to secondary smoke, prolonged asbestos exposure, and exposure to industrial elements. Cervical spine radiographs confirm the diagnosis.[19] Treatment may include a course of radiation therapy prior to surgical resection, along with medical management of pain and paraneoplastic syndromes.

Local

■ Abscess or Cyst Infection

Chief Clinical Characteristics
This presentation is mainly characterized by pain, tenderness, and swelling anteromedially to the sternocleidomastoid. Skin erythema is also common.

Background Information
CT scans may reveal an abscess or cyst in the deep soft tissues of the neck. Suppurative adenitis is the most common etiology. Other causes include puncture or perforation from a foreign body, thrombophlebitis, or osteomyelitis of the spine. This health condition is typically treated with antibiotics, and the abscess or cyst can be drained or excised.[20]

■ Ankylosing Spondylitis

Chief Clinical Characteristics
This presentation includes an insidious onset of spinal and symmetric posterior hip pain associated with a slowly progressive and significant loss of general spinal mobility. Symptoms may be worse in the morning and improve with light exercise.

Background Information
While lumbar spine involvement is classic, the cervical spine also may be involved. This condition is more common in males, as well as people of American indigenous descent, those less than 40 years of age, or those who carry the human leukocyte antigen B27. It also may be associated with fever, malaise, and inflammatory bowel disease. The diagnosis is confirmed with plain radiographs of the sacroiliac joints and lumbar spine, which reveal characteristic findings of sacroiliitis and "bamboo spine." Blood panels including erythrocyte sedimentation rate are useful to track disease activity. Individuals with this condition are encouraged to exercise to improve posture and maintain joint mobility in combination with a regimen of nonsteroidal, steroidal, or biological anti-inflammatory medications.

■ Arteritis

Chief Clinical Characteristics
This presentation typically involves pain and swelling of the carotid sheath and carotid artery, and is characterized by inflammation of the arterial wall that may result in occlusion or aneurysm formation. Symptoms may include general malaise and fever.

Background Information
Essential hypertension and atherosclerosis are risk factors. Carotid sheath infection may also present with Horner's syndrome and dysfunction of cranial nerves IX through XII. Rupture of an aneurysm may result in bleeding from the nose and mouth.[21,22] Individuals suspected of this condition require urgent medical evaluation.

■ Bacterial Meningitis

Chief Clinical Characteristics
This presentation may include neck pain and stiffness that is aggravated by flexion and

rotation movements, associated with headache, fever, nausea, vomiting, photophobia, and central nervous system dysfunction including altered mental status, seizures, gait disturbances, and paresis. Symptoms may progress rapidly or over a period of several days.

Background Information
Bacteria can enter the host via the upper airway and then invade the subarachnoid space. Lumbar puncture and obtaining cultures are important for correct diagnosis, as well as to guide medical management.[23] Usual treatment for meningitis includes antibiotics for causes other than viral etiology, antipyretic and antiseizure agents, and supportive interventions to maintain oxygen and fluids at homeostatic levels.

■ **Blunt Trauma to Larynx or Trachea**

Chief Clinical Characteristics
This presentation is mainly characterized by pain in the anterior neck/throat. Other symptoms can include hemoptysis, hoarseness of the voice when speaking, dysphagia, odynophagia, and obstruction of the airway.

Background Information
Hyperextension injuries or direct trauma to the larynx occur most commonly with motor vehicle accidents. Penetrating trauma injuries associated with violent crime are increasing in frequency. Other common mechanisms of injury are direct blows from a fist or other object and attempted strangulation. Physical examination may reveal laryngeal swelling with tenderness to palpation, tracheal shift or deviation, or subcutaneous emphysema. Depending on the mechanism of injury, radiographic findings may include pneumomediastinum or pneumothorax. Computed tomography, bronchoscopy, and indirect and flexible laryngoscopy can be used to assess the injury.[5,24,25] Surgical repair with or without placement of a stent may be required.

■ **Brachial Plexus/Nerve Root Lesion**

Chief Clinical Characteristics
This presentation may involve a traumatic onset of variable symptoms in the cervical spine and the upper extremities. Signs and symptoms of brachial plexus dysfunction may present as a constellation of sensory deficits, motor weakness, reflex changes, and the pattern may vary with the level of involvement and may present either unilaterally or bilaterally.

Background Information
Pain typically precedes motor and sensory signs in brachial plexus injuries. Up to 50% of patients with this condition will eventually present with central cord signs and symptoms. Horner's syndrome may be present if the stellate ganglion is affected. Computed tomography, electromyography, and cervical myelography confirm the diagnosis.[26] Treatment is palliative. Recovery is sometimes incomplete and may take months.

■ **Cervical Degenerative Disk Disease**

Chief Clinical Characteristics
This presentation can include pain in the posterior or posterolateral region of the neck with or without radiculopathy.

Background Information
This condition is associated with the degenerative changes of the cervical spine, and most commonly affects the C5–C6 and C6–C7 levels (Fig. 10-1). Patients may develop osteophytes, degenerative annular tears, loss of disk height, narrowing of the spinal canal, or compression of the spinal cord or nerve roots, resulting in radiculopathy. The diagnosis is confirmed with plain radiographs and magnetic resonance imaging. Treatment is variable; operative intervention may be required for individuals with extensive or rapidly progressing neurological symptoms, but nonsurgical intervention including rehabilitation is typically considered a primary treatment for most individuals with this health condition.

■ **Cervical Degenerative Joint Disease**

Chief Clinical Characteristics
This presentation is characterized by pain in the posterior or posterolateral aspect of the neck. This condition occurs in the older population and usually without radicular symptoms.

Background Information
Osteoarthritis of the zygapophyseal joints, hypertrophy of the ligamentum flavum, and

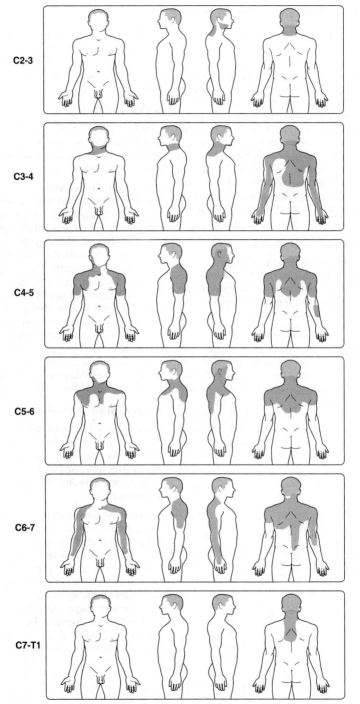

FIGURE 10-1 Reported referral patterns of the cervical intervertebral disks during discography.

C2-3

C3-4

C4-5

C5-6

C6-7

C7-T1

osteophyte formation around the intervertebral foramen can all contribute to symptoms (Fig. 10-2).[27] Plain radiographs and magnetic resonance imaging confirm the diagnosis, with joint space narrowing in the cervical facet or intervertebral joints, subchondral sclerosis of affected joints, and presence of periarticular osteophytes and articular hypertrophy. Treatment is variable; operative intervention may be required for individuals with extensive or rapidly progressing neurological symptoms, but nonsurgical intervention including rehabilitation is typically considered a primary treatment for most individuals with this health condition.

■ Cervical Disk Herniation

Chief Clinical Characteristics

This presentation involves pain in the posterior or posterolateral aspect of the neck with or without radicular symptoms down the arm or through the midthoracic region.

Background Information

A cervical disk herniation can result from trauma, occur spontaneously in midlife (between 30 and 40 years of age), or result from degenerative changes in the geriatric population (spondylosis). C5–C6 and C6–C7 are the most common levels of disk herniation in the cervical spine.[28] Magnetic resonance imaging best confirms the diagnosis. Treatment is variable; operative intervention may be required for individuals with extensive or rapidly progressing neurological symptoms, but nonsurgical intervention including rehabilitation is typically considered a primary treatment for most individuals with this health condition.

■ Cervical Dystonia

Chief Clinical Characteristics

This presentation is mainly characterized by anterior or lateral neck pain and rotational position of the head and neck.

Background Information

The sternocleidomastoid muscle is contracted or spastic, causing cervical spine ipsilateral side-bending and contralateral rotation to the side of involvement. This idiopathic condition also is known as torticollis. Congenital torticollis occurs in infants, whereas acquired (spastic) torticollis presents itself in adolescents and adults. Certain illicit drugs may cause temporary dystonia. Radiographic studies are important to rule out congenital anomalies and to detect unilateral atlantoaxial rotary subluxation. Medications, botulinum toxin, exercise, and cervical repositioning orthoses may be considered as treatment options for this health condition.

■ Cervical Facet Dysfunction

Chief Clinical Characteristics

This presentation involves sharp pain in the posterior or posterolateral aspect of the cervical spine accompanied by ipsilateral range-of-motion loss in the directions of side-bending and rotation.

Background Information

This condition is more common in younger and active individuals. Symptoms of this condition also may be referred to the shoulder and proximal brachium (see Fig. 10-2). Facet dysfunction implies injury that interrupts normal joint mobility, possibly associated with motor vehicle accidents, aggravating sleep positions, degenerative joint disease, and infection. The diagnosis is confirmed clinically with increased symptoms during movements that cause downgliding of the affected facets or with selective joint injections. Treatment for facet dysfunction includes mobilization or manipulation of the affected joints, exercise, and therapeutic modalities.

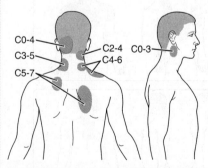

FIGURE 10-2 Referral patterns of the cervical facet joints. Cervical facet joints may refer pain to the jaw region, and these symptoms may be associated with suboccipital headaches.

■ Cervical Lymphadenitis

Chief Clinical Characteristics

This presentation typically includes pain along the sternocleidomastoid to the jaw with swelling and tenderness of the lymph nodes. Fever, sore throat, and pain with swallowing may also occur.

Background Information

Common causes are dental disease or infection, an oral ulceration, and an infection of the skin of the face or scalp. Most diagnoses can be made with a careful history and physical examination that reveals tenderness of involved lymph nodes (Fig. 10-3); however, ultrasonography or fine-needle biopsy may be necessary.[29,30] Treatment is directed at resolving the underlying infection, including antimicrobial and antipyretic agents where indicated.

■ Cervical Osteomyelitis

Chief Clinical Characteristics

This presentation includes posterior, midline neck pain and progresses to include radiculopathy/paresthesias and weakness into one or more extremities. Loss of bowel and bladder control follows. Symptoms may be aggravated by movement and accompanied by low-grade fever.

Background Information

Risk factors include diabetes mellitus, trauma, and infection outside the cervical spine. The diagnosis is confirmed with destruction of vertebral bodies and disks on plain radiographs, nuclear medicine scan, or magnetic resonance imaging. Typical treatment involves intravenous antibiotic therapy and may require surgical decompression with potential bone grafting or fusion to stabilize the spine.

■ Cervical Stenosis

Chief Clinical Characteristics

This presentation is characterized by pain in the posterior or posterolateral region of the neck with or without radiculopathy.

Background Information

Classically, symptoms increase with extension and decrease with flexion of the cervical spine. Symptoms can be bilateral as in central stenosis or unilateral in peripheral stenosis. This condition usually occurs in older individuals, but it may occur much earlier in individuals with congenital decrease in the central canal volume. This condition usually occurs in more than one spinal level. The multilevel involvement in a patient with stenosis results in a variable clinical presentation of neurological deficits.[27] The diagnosis is confirmed with magnetic resonance imaging. Nonsurgical treatment usually is successful to address this condition, with surgical intervention potentially indicated for patients with extensive or rapidly progressing neurological deficits.

■ Cervicogenic Headache

Chief Clinical Characteristics

This presentation typically includes unilateral head pain associated with neck movement; sustained or awkward cervical posture, restricted cervical range of motion; and ipsilateral neck, shoulder, or arm pain.[31] Cervicogenic headaches are characterized by moderate to severe episodic pain that originates in the neck or suboccipital region and spreads to the head. Pain attacks last from 3 weeks to 3 months, and may vary in frequency from occurring every 2 days to 2 months. People with cervicogenic headache describe symptoms that do not change sides during an attack,[32] and may also present with nausea, dizziness, and phonophobia or photophobia that is unresolved with migraine medications.

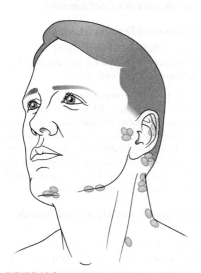

FIGURE 10-3 Cervical lymph nodes.

Background Information
Initial management includes amelioration of cervical spine musculoskeletal impairments. Nerve blockade may be effective in recalcitrant cases. A favorable response to this intervention also is pathognomic.[31]

■ Chronic Fatigue Syndrome

Chief Clinical Characteristics
This presentation is defined as a new onset of unexplained or persistent or recurrent physical or mental fatigue that substantially reduces activity level and is characterized by postexertional malaise, which requires an extended recovery period. Exclusion of other potentially explanatory medical or psychiatric conditions is required along with at least one symptom from two of the following categories: autonomic manifestations, neuroendocrine manifestations, and immune manifestations.[33]

Background Information
Other possible clinical features include joint and muscle pain (which may serve as the chief symptom that directs patients toward physical therapists for management), difficulty concentrating, tender lymph nodes, headaches, and sleep dysfunction. This health condition is diagnosed on the basis of clinical examination. There is significant diagnostic overlap with major depression, fibromyalgia, and systemic lupus erythematosus. Optimal treatment includes activity modification and stress management, anaerobic reconditioning, and medication for relief of associated symptoms.

■ Coital Neck Pain

Chief Clinical Characteristics
This presentation includes a sudden onset of severe neck and head pain on one or both sides during sexual intercourse. Pain may be accompanied by nausea, vomiting, and anxiety.

Background Information
This condition often mimics the symptoms of a subarachnoid hemorrhage without neck stiffness or photophobia, so this health condition must be excluded as an important differential diagnosis. This syndrome usually is benign, and may be addressed with a combination of avoidance or modification of aggravating activities in combination with nonsteroidal anti-inflammatory or beta-blocker medications.

■ Complex Regional Pain Syndrome

Chief Clinical Characteristics
This presentation can involve a traumatic onset of severe chronic neck and shoulder pain accompanied by allodynia, hyperalgesia, and trophic, vasomotor, and sudomotor changes in later stages.

Background Information
This idiopathic health condition is characterized by disproportionate responses to painful stimuli. It is a regional neuropathic pain disorder that presents either without direct nerve trauma (Type I) or with direct nerve trauma (Type II) in any region of the body.[34] Researchers hypothesize that the sympathetic nervous system and immune system may support the progressive increase in pain, sensitivity, and clinical signs that characterize this health condition. This health condition may precipitate due to an event distant to the affected area. Thermography may confirm associated sympathetic dysfunction. Treatment options are variable for this population, and include topical and oral analgesics, antidepressants, sympathetic nerve block, sympathectomy, and spinal cord stimulator.

■ Crowned Dens Syndrome

Chief Clinical Characteristics
This presentation typically includes moderate to severe neck pain and stiffness.

Background Information
This condition occurs when hydroxyapatite or calcium pyrophosphate dihydrate crystals form a halo or crown around the posterior and lateral regions of the dens. Computed tomography confirms the diagnosis. Neck pain usually resolves following treatment with nonsteroidal anti-inflammatory medications.

■ Digastric and Stylohyoid Muscle Strain

Chief Clinical Characteristics
This presentation is mainly characterized by anterior and/or posterior neck and jaw pain.

Background Information
This condition is commonly observed in patients with temporomandibular joint dysfunction, and associated with bruxism, teeth clenching, and grinding. Management consists of nonsteroidal anti-inflammatory medications, physical therapy, night splints, and relaxation therapy.

■ Dissection of the Internal Carotid Artery

Chief Clinical Characteristics
This presentation involves a sudden onset of knife-like, tearing, unilateral neck pain with headache and face pain. Horner's syndrome, cranial nerve palsy, hemicrania, and focal neurological abnormalities may follow the onset of pain. The blood pressure may be lower in one arm, and lying supine usually aggravates symptoms.

Background Information
Dissection may be caused by trauma or may occur idiopathically. The diagnosis is confirmed with Doppler ultrasound, computed tomographic angiography, or conventional angiography.[35,36] Individuals suspected of this condition should be referred for immediate medical evaluation.

ENTRAPMENTS

■ Greater Occipital Nerve (Occipital Neuralgia)

Chief Clinical Characteristics
This presentation includes unilateral or bilateral headache, pain, and paresthesia and hypoesthesia in the distribution of the greater or lesser suboccipital nerve with tenderness to palpation of the affected area. Nausea, dizziness, or visual disturbances also may be associated with this condition.

Background Information
Myofascial trigger points in the posterior neck and trapezius muscles are common clinical findings. Symptoms may occur following whiplash injury, head trauma, or with degenerative arthritis of the atlantoaxial joint.[37] The diagnosis is confirmed with selective injections to the suboccipital triangle. Administration of local anesthetic via injection resolves symptoms readily. In recalcitrant cases, sectioning of the inferior oblique muscle may be required.

■ Spinal Accessory Nerve

Chief Clinical Characteristics
This presentation typically involves unilateral neck and shoulder pain, associated with altered scapulohumeral mechanics during elevation and abduction.

Background Information
Injury to the nerve may occur during surgical procedures such as cervical lymph node biopsy or result from trauma such as gunshot or stab wounds. Entrapment can occur as the nerve travels through the posterior triangle. The diagnosis is confirmed with electromyography, which may demonstrate signs of chronic denervation.[38] Surgical exploration, neurolysis, grafting, or repair may be required for open injuries.[38]

■ Epidural Hematoma

Chief Clinical Characteristics
This presentation typically includes sudden onset of severe headache and/or severe localized neck pain with stiffness. A pattern of loss of consciousness, followed by lucidity/alertness, then another loss of consciousness is typical, though not present in all cases. Other symptoms include dizziness, nausea or vomiting, confusion, enlarged pupil, seizures, and focal neurological deficits. Delayed onset of radiating pain, weakness, and numbness into one or more extremities can occur and progress to bowel and bladder incontinence.

Background Information
Patients with ankylosing spondylitis, hypertension, coronary and peripheral vascular disease, and patients taking anticoagulant drugs are at higher risk for developing this condition. Individuals suspected of this condition require urgent referral for medical evaluation.

■ Fibromyalgia

Chief Clinical Characteristics
This presentation is mainly characterized by chronic widespread joint and muscle pain defined as bilateral upper body, lower body, and spine pain, associated with tenderness to palpation of 11 of 18 specific muscle-tendon sites.

Background Information

Individuals with this condition demonstrate lowered mechanical and thermal pain thresholds, high pain ratings for noxious stimuli, and altered temporal summation of pain stimuli.[39] The etiology of this condition is unclear; multiple body systems appear to be involved. Indistinct clinical boundaries between this condition and similar conditions (eg, chronic fatigue syndrome, irritable bowel syndrome, and chronic muscular headaches) pose a diagnostic challenge.[39] This condition is diagnosed by exclusion on the basis of clinical examination. Common pharmacologic interventions include antidepressants, opioids, nonsteroidal anti-inflammatory drugs, sedatives, muscle relaxants, and antiepileptics. Nonpharmacologic treatments can be helpful, including exercise, physical therapy, massage, acupuncture, and cognitive-behavioral therapy.[40]

■ Fibromyositis

Chief Clinical Characteristics
This presentation is characterized by pain in all areas of the cervical spine, associated with generalized body pain.

Background Information
The term *fibromyositis* is a combination of *fibrositis*—inflammation of the fibrous tissue—and *myositis*—inflammation in the muscular tissue.[41] Once the myofascial structure is inflamed, trigger points may develop. Trigger points can be quantified with thermography or measurement with pressure algometry or tissue compliance meters.[42] A combination of thermal therapeutic modalities, postural exercises, and manual therapy procedures is commonly used to address this health condition.

FRACTURES
■ Lower Cervical Spine (C3–C7)

Chief Clinical Characteristics
This presentation typically includes midline tenderness to palpation, neck pain with muscle spasm, crepitus, step-off deformity, and restricted and painful active range of motion. Common mechanisms of injury include motor vehicle accidents, falls, diving accidents, blunt trauma, and accidents that occur

during various recreational activities.[43] The diagnosis is confirmed with plain radiographs of the cervical spine.

Background Information
This condition is considered a medical emergency, and patients suspected of this health condition should be referred for immediate medical evaluation. All fractures in the lower cervical spine should be treated as unstable fractures until formally evaluated radiographically.

■ Upper Cervical Spine (C0–C2)

Chief Clinical Characteristics
This presentation includes suboccipital midline tenderness, muscle spasm, and neck pain that may or may not include neurological signs.

Background Information
Stable fractures may not present with neurological compromise, whereas fractures with concomitant ligamentous rupture may result in central or peripheral neural compression. Active range of motion is restricted and painful. Common mechanisms of injury include compression with flexion, distraction with flexion, and compression with extension. Compression fractures of the upper cervical spine include Jefferson fractures (burst fractures of the ring of C1), which are clinically significant because they are associated with neurological deficits. Distraction with hyperextension injuries of the upper cervical spine include hangman's fractures, which may be associated with cranial nerve, vertebral artery, and craniofacial injuries. Fractures of the dens are generally divided into three categories depending on the anatomical location of the break. Types I and II are stable and do not require surgical fusion. Type III fractures are unstable, and rupture of the transverse ligament may cause spinal cord compression. This condition is a medical emergency, and patients suspected of this health condition should be referred for immediate medical evaluation.[43]

■ Hemorrhage

Chief Clinical Characteristics
This presentation involves a rapid onset of unilateral neck pain and swelling.

Background Information

This health condition occurs when an artery ruptures, such as the sequel to an aneurysm. Arterial ruptures causing hemorrhage of the cervical spine may include the internal and external carotid, vertebral, and thyroid arteries. An elevated risk of hemorrhage is associated with hypertension, trauma, or thrombolytic therapy. Ultrasonography can be useful in determining the source of hemorrhage. This condition is a medical emergency, and patients suspected of this health condition should be referred for immediate medical evaluation.[23]

■ Internal Carotid Arteritis

Chief Clinical Characteristics

This presentation includes pain and swelling of the carotid sheath and carotid artery. Other symptoms include general malaise and fever.

Background Information

Carotid sheath infection may also present with Horner's syndrome and dysfunction of cranial nerves IX through XII. Advanced disease may result in bleeding from the nose and mouth or stroke.[21,23] Treatment typically involves administration of steroidal medications. Individuals who are suspected of this health condition should be referred for medical evaluation urgently to begin treatment and prevent the risks of advanced disease.

■ Lyme Disease

Chief Clinical Characteristics

This presentation can involve fatigue, headache, fever, neck stiffness, joint and muscle pain, anorexia, sore throat, and nausea.

Background Information

This condition is caused by a spirochete carried by ticks during the summer months in the Western Hemisphere. Neck pain occurs due to a local immune reaction in the cervical spine that produces both central and peripheral nervous system symptoms. One or more cervical, thoracic or lumbar nerve roots may also be involved. The diagnosis is confirmed by serologic testing for *Borrelia burgdorferi*, preferably by enzyme-linked immunosorbent assay followed by Western blot analysis.[44] Early treatment for Lyme disease is essential. Treatment usually includes a course of oral or intravenous antibiotics. Inadequate treatment may lead to chronic oligoarthritis and chronic disturbances.[26] Patients who are diagnosed later in the course of this health condition carry an elevated risk for neurological effects.

■ Meningismus (Aseptic Meningitis)

Chief Clinical Characteristics

This presentation is characterized by neck pain and stiffness, sore throat, headache, fever, nausea, vomiting, drowsiness, confusion, and myalgia.

Background Information

Viral vectors may infect the meninges, causing aseptic meningitis syndrome. Other causes include fungi and certain types of medication. Cerebrospinal fluid analysis and gadolinium-enhanced magnetic resonance imaging can confirm the diagnosis.[45,46] This condition is usually self-limiting, and supportive intervention is typically provided.

■ Muscle Strain

Chief Clinical Characteristics

This presentation typically includes local pain that may be present in various regions of the cervical spine dependent on the location of the injury.

Background Information

The mechanism of injury can range from sleep and postural dysfunction to sports activities and motor vehicle accidents. Causes of neck muscle strain include orthopedic shoulder pathologies (eg, rotator cuff injuries, impingement syndrome, bursitis, and tendinopathy) and temporomandibular joint dysfunction. These health conditions can affect the cervical spine through faulty posture, inadequate shoulder-scapular kinematics, dyskinesia of the shoulder and scapular musculatures, and abnormal tension on the cervical spinal nerves.[47] The diagnosis is confirmed clinically on palpation and resisted testing of the affected muscle. This health condition is addressed nonsurgically with a combination of exercise and anti-inflammatory or analgesic medications.

■ Osteomalacia

Chief Clinical Characteristics

This presentation often involves diffuse bone pain and tenderness of affected bones with progressive muscle weakness and fracture with minimal trauma.

Background Information

This condition is caused by a loss of calcium from the bones, and is common during pregnancy especially in regions where nutrition is suboptimal as well as in the urban population of elderly confined.[48] Deformity may follow mineral loss; bone deformation and fractures are the source of pain in this health condition. Pseudofractures on plain radiographs are pathognomonic.[26] Treatment depends on the underlying cause of the disorder and may include vitamin D, calcium, and phosphorous supplementation.[49]

■ Osteoporosis

Chief Clinical Characteristics

This presentation typically includes pain following a fracture of the cervical spine associated with limited bone mineral density in the affected region. Fractures due to this condition most frequently occur in the hip, spine, and wrist.[50]

Background Information

Women are four times more likely to be affected than men. Risk factors for primary osteoporosis include female sex, Caucasian or Asian descent, early menopause, family history, underweight, excessive drinking or smoking, and overuse of steroids. Fractures of the vertebrae due to osteoporosis can cause severe neck pain, loss of height, and spinal deformity. The diagnosis is confirmed with plain radiographs and a bone density test. Treatment includes calcium and vitamin D supplementation, bisphosphonates, calcitonin, estrogen, and parathyroid hormone. Exercise programs focus on increasing bone mineral density by loading the skeletal system using weight-bearing exercises and resistance training.[51] Improved strength, coordination, and balance may decrease the risk of other fractures by decreasing the likelihood of falls.

■ Pachymeningitis Cervicalis Hypertrophica

Chief Clinical Characteristics

This presentation includes posterior neck and arm pain with numbness and weakness in the affected extremity. Paresthesias usually involve three or more cervical nerve roots on the affected side and progress to bilateral upper extremity involvement.

Background Information

Severe cases can progress to spinal cord compression with paresthesias and weakness in the lower extremities as well. Symptoms occur secondary to the lack of filling of the dural sleeves surrounding the affected nerve roots, resulting in thickening of the dura surrounding the spinal cord and nerve root sheaths. Causes of this disorder include infection, trauma, injection of intrathecal steroids, and rheumatoid arthritis.[52] Surgical interventions including durotomy may be considered for individuals with this health condition.

■ Paget's Disease

Chief Clinical Characteristics

This presentation can include bone pain, bone deformity, fracture, and deafness.[53] Symptoms are described as continuous and, unlike osteoarthritis pain, pagetic bone pain usually increases with rest, on weight bearing, when the limbs are warmed, and at night.[54]

Background Information

Spinal pain is thought to be due to facet arthropathy, engorgement of the vertebral body caused by vascular processes, and hyperactive remodeling.[55] Complications of Paget's disease can include spinal stenosis or nerve root compression syndromes and fractures that can occur in 10% to 30% of individuals.[55] The diagnosis of Paget's disease is based on an elevated serum alkaline phosphatase in patients with radiographic findings of osteosclerosis, osteolysis, and bone expansion. Intervention usually includes a high-protein diet with vitamin C supplementation, bisphosphonates and calcitonin, and surgical interventions to address the consequences of bone deformation and fracture.

■ Pharyngoesophageal Diverticulum

Chief Clinical Characteristics

This presentation typically includes a sensation of a lump in the throat and may be accompanied by the presence of a gurgling sound when the patient drinks fluids.

Background Information

Pharyngoesophageal diverticulum occurs more frequently in women and the elderly. In this health condition, the esophageal mucosa herniates posteriorly, trapping food. This can lead to an infection that causes neck pain and odynophagia. Coughing may lead to aspiration, resulting in bronchitis or pneumonia. Diagnosis is confirmed with barium swallow or endoscopic studies. Surgical removal of the infected diverticulum may be necessary.[23]

■ Polymyalgia Rheumatica

Chief Clinical Characteristics

This presentation is mainly characterized by widespread muscle aching and stiffness in the neck and shoulder regions and the low back, hips, and thighs, possibly associated with weakness, fever, weight loss, stiffness, muscle tenderness, and anemia.

Background Information

The onset of pain can occur very suddenly with symptoms appearing overnight. This health condition typically affects people over the age of 50, and women are more frequently affected than men. This condition is regarded as a variant of giant cell arteritis, characterized by a subacute granulomatous inflammation that affects the external carotid arterial system.[26] Corticosteroids are considered among primary treatments for this health condition. This treatment course takes 1 to 2 years to resolve this pathology.[56]

■ Post-Traumatic Dysautonomic Cephalgia

Chief Clinical Characteristics

This presentation may involve headache and neck pain that resemble the classic migraine, but include signs of pupil dilation, sweating, and transient Horner's syndrome.

Background Information

The mechanism of injury is often postconcussion and may be caused by injury to the sympathetic fibers in the neck. Trauma to the carotid artery sheath in the anterior triangle of the neck also may be contributory. Beta-blocker medications such as propranolol are among primary treatments for this health condition.[57]

■ Retropharyngeal Calcific Tendinitis

Chief Clinical Characteristics

This presentation typically includes neck pain and stiffness often associated with dysphagia and odynophagia. Symptom onset may be spontaneous or associated with trauma such as whiplash. Aggravating factors include neck movements in any direction and swallowing.

Background Information

Plain radiographs reveal calcification anterior to the dens in the longus colli muscle, confirming the diagnosis.[58,59] Treatment includes nonsteroidal anti-inflammatory and analgesic medication.

■ Rheumatoid Arthritis of the Cervical Spine

Chief Clinical Characteristics

This presentation is mainly characterized by morning stiffness and generalized pain throughout multiple joints in a symmetric distribution, with possible tenderness and swelling of affected joints.

Background Information

Women are twice as likely to be affected as men. Symptoms associated with this progressive inflammatory joint disease are caused by synovial membrane thickening and cytokine production in synovial fluid. Articular cartilage erosion, synovial hypertrophy, and constant joint effusion[60] eventually cause bony erosions and joint deformities that have a significant impact on daily function. Younger age of onset is associated with a greater extent of disability later. Treatment typically includes a combination of nonsteroidal, steroidal, or biological anti-inflammatory medication and supportive rehabilitative intervention to maintain functional strength and joint motion.

■ Subarachnoid Hemorrhage

Chief Clinical Characteristics
This presentation includes severe headache and/or neck pain with nuchal rigidity. Passive and active flexion of the neck increase pain. Additional symptoms include nausea, vomiting, photophobia, drowsiness, confusion, dizziness, transient loss of consciousness, and enlarged pupils.

Background Information
Head trauma and intracranial aneurysms are the most common causes, and the incidence of nontraumatic hemorrhage increases linearly from the age of 25 to 64. Ruptured aneurysms and arteriovenous malformations can lead to this condition. Hypertension and diabetes mellitus are two significant risk factors,[61] and polycystic kidney disease, Ehlers-Danlos syndrome, systemic lupus erythematosus, and pregnancy are also known risk factors.[62] Polmear[63] reported that between 50% and 60% of patients with this condition described a previous history of an atypical headache days to weeks before the event. This warning sign is known as a *sentinel headache*. Computed tomography and lumbar puncture confirm the diagnosis. This condition is a medical emergency.[23]

■ Subdural Hematoma

Chief Clinical Characteristics
This presentation can involve neck pain and unilateral or occipital headache associated with a decline in level of consciousness and focal neurological deficits. Secondary symptoms include autonomic signs, vomiting, somnolence, or signs of personality change.[64]

Background Information
The location of headache depends on the location of hematoma. Symptoms develop within hours to weeks after the precipitating event. This condition may be caused by severe sneezing, coughing, strain from heavy lifting, and whiplash injury.[65] It is also a rare though well-documented sequela of lumbar punctures.[66] Predisposing factors include advanced age, alcoholism, and coagulation disorders.[64] Subdural hematomas form when bridging veins rupture and blood accumulates in the space between the arachnoid and the dura. This health condition is a medical emergency; individuals suspected of a subdural hematoma should be referred for computed tomography without contrast.

SUBLUXATIONS/DISLOCATIONS

■ Congenital

Chief Clinical Characteristics
This presentation is mainly characterized by neck pain with or without neurological deficits.

Background Information
Congenital abnormalities such as Chiari malformations and osteogenesis imperfecta can result in instability and subluxation. This condition is a medical emergency.[43,67] Treatment usually involves surgical stabilization of the affected region.

■ Degenerative

Chief Clinical Characteristics
This presentation may include neck pain with or without neurological deficits.

Background Information
Common causes of degenerative subluxation include transverse ligament rupture in patients with rheumatoid arthritis and Down syndrome. This condition is a medical emergency.[43,67] Treatment usually involves surgical stabilization of the affected region.

■ Traumatic

Chief Clinical Characteristics
This presentation typically includes neck pain with or without neurological deficits.

Background Information
Common causes of traumatic dislocation include motor vehicle accidents and diving. With traumatic injuries, concomitant disk herniation should be suspected and assessed.[43,67] This condition is a medical emergency. Treatment usually involves surgical stabilization of the affected region.

■ Systemic Lupus Erythematosus

Chief Clinical Characteristics

This presentation typically includes neck pain associated with fatigue and joint pain/ swelling affecting the hands, feet, knees, and shoulders.

Background Information

This condition affects mostly women of child-bearing age, but men also may be affected. This condition is a chronic autoimmune disorder that can affect virtually any organ system of the body, including skin, joints, kidneys, brain, heart, lungs, and blood. The diagnosis is confirmed by the presence of skin lesions; heart, lung, or kidney involvement; and laboratory abnormalities including low red or white cell counts, low platelet counts, or positive antinuclear antibody and anti-DNA antibody tests.[68] Blood test, urine test, and skin and kidney biopsies confirm the diagnosis. Treatment includes medication, physical therapy, and management of associated complications of the skin, lungs, kidneys, joints, and nervous system.

■ Temporomandibular Dysfunction

Chief Clinical Characteristics

This presentation may be characterized by headache radiating from the muscles of mastication, periauricular region, or the temporomandibular joint associated with abnormal jaw function, asymmetric chewing, bruxism, neck pain, tinnitus, and vertigo.

Background Information

Headache pain related to this condition may be caused by pathology of the temporomandibular joint or may be an associated symptom of another form of headache. This condition is believed to be an aggravating factor in headaches and only the cause if clearly related to the clinical signs and symptoms involving the masticatory system.[69] The typical management involves a combination of rehabilitative and pharmacologic interventions for headaches related to temporomandibular dysfunction.

■ Thyroiditis

Chief Clinical Characteristics

This presentation involves anterior neck pain, swelling, and tenderness to palpation of the thyroid. Subacutely, this presentation typically includes dull, aching paratracheal neck pain that radiates to one or both ears. Other symptoms include sore throat, thyroid enlargement and tenderness, and pain with swallowing.

Background Information

It is most commonly a result of infection in a cervical thymic cyst and is frequently accompanied by fever and dysphagia. Pharyngography or ultrasonography may identify the presence of thyroiditis.[23,70] Initial management involves antibiotic medications directed at the underlying infection.

■ Transverse Myelitis

Chief Clinical Characteristics

This presentation can include posterior neck pain with radiculopathy and paresthesias into the upper extremities followed by lower extremity weakness and paresthesias.

Background Information

Flaccid paresis of the extremities develops into spastic paresis. The pathogenesis of transverse myelitis is poorly understood; however, spontaneous recovery or improvement occurs in one-half of all cases. No effective medical intervention or therapy exists to act on the pathophysiology of this health condition, although corticosteroid medication and early mobilization is thought to reduce inflammation and enhance the likelihood of neurological return.[23]

TUMORS

■ Anaplastic Carcinoma

Chief Clinical Characteristics

This presentation may involve formation of a mass or nodule that is painful and tender to palpation along the lateral borders of the trachea. Airway compromise may result in stridor.

Background Information

This tumor is considered the most locally aggressive and fatal of thyroid tumors. Previous thyroid pathology and low iodine intake are among risk factors for development of this health condition. Positron emission tomography, computed tomography, and magnetic resonance imaging can be useful in detecting the presence of metastases.[23,41]

■ Carcinoma of the Esophagus

Chief Clinical Characteristics
This presentation typically includes sharp, burning, or stabbing substernal, anterior neck, and throat pain that can include radiating pain around the thorax to the middle of the back. Patients may report melena, odynophagia, and dysphagia.

Background Information
Dysphagia occurs initially with solid foods, but eventually progresses to include anything that is swallowed. Barium esophagraphy, contrast-enhanced computed tomography, magnetic resonance imaging, endoscopic ultrasonography, and positron emission tomography are powerful tools in the detection, diagnosis, and staging of this malignancy for determination of the most appropriate pharmacologic and surgical treatments.[23]

■ Lymphoma

Chief Clinical Characteristics
This presentation is mainly characterized by diffuse anterior neck pain with swelling and tenderness to palpation of the lymph nodes, combined with fatigue, fever, weight loss, night sweats, and itching without evidence of skin lesion.

Background Information
This tumor typically occurs in patients over 50 years of age. It stems from mutations in B cells. Lymphomas grow rapidly and can be diagnosed via needle biopsy of lymph nodes or bone marrow. Slow-growing lymphomas may be amenable to observation. A variety of treatments may be utilized to address this health condition, including chemotherapy, radiation therapy, immunotherapy, and stem cell implantation.

■ Vertebral Artery Dissection

Chief Clinical Characteristics
This presentation typically includes a rapid onset of severe unilateral or posterior neck pain with headache in the occipital region. Neurological phenomena also may be present, ranging from vertigo and focal neurological deficits to transient ischemic attacks or complete stroke.

Background Information
Lateral medullary syndrome is the most common neurological presentation, which includes ataxia, diplopia, dysphagia, Horner's syndrome, and nystagmus. Ultrasound, computed tomographic angiography, and magnetic resonance angiography can confirm the diagnosis.[71] Individuals suspected of this condition require urgent referral for medical evaluation to prevent the extension of neurological damage.

References

1. Chen W, Woods SL, Puntillo KA. Gender differences in symptoms associated with acute myocardial infarction: a review of the research. *Heart Lung.* Jul–Aug 2005; 34(4):240–247.
2. Klein DG. Thoracic aortic aneurysms. *J Cardiovasc Nurs.* Jul–Aug 2005;20(4):245–250.
3. Scawn ND, Pennefather SH, Soorae A, Wang JY, Russell GN. Ipsilateral shoulder pain after thoracotomy with epidural analgesia: the influence of phrenic nerve infiltration with lidocaine. *Anesth Analg.* Aug 2001; 93(2):260–264.
4. Goodman CC, Snyder TEK. *Differential diagnosis in physical therapy.* 3rd ed. Philadelphia: Saunders; 2000.
5. Werne C, Ulreich S. An unusual presentation of spontaneous pneumomediastinum. *Ann Emerg Med.* Oct 1985;14(10):1010–1013.
6. Taylor FC, Frankl HD, Riemer KD. Late presentation of splenic trauma after routine colonoscopy. *Am J Gastroenterol.* Apr 1989;84(4):442–443.
7. Francke U, Furthmayr H. Marfan's syndrome and other disorders of fibrillin. *N Engl J Med.* May 12, 1994; 330(19):1384–1385.
8. Society IH. The International Classification of Headache Disorders. *Cephalalgia.* 2004;24(suppl 1): 1–160.
9. Diener HC, Dahlof CG. Headache associated with chronic use of substances. In: Olesen J WK, ed. *The Headaches* (2nd ed.). Philadelphia, PA: Lippincott Williams & Wilkins; 2000:871–878.
10. Carter T, Brooks CA. Pericarditis: inflammation or infarction? *J Cardiovasc Nurs.* Jul–Aug 2005;20(4):239–244.
11. Sarwar A, Dellaripa PF, Beamis JF Jr. A 51-year-old man with fever, ulnar neuropathy, and bilateral pleural effusions. Lupus pleuritis. *Chest.* Oct 1999;116(4):1105–1107.
12. Schwaegerle SM, Bauer TW, Esselstyn CB Jr. Riedel's thyroiditis. *Am J Clin Pathol.* Dec 1988;90(6):715–722.
13. Koullias GJ, Korkolis DP, Wang XJ, Hammond GL. Current assessment and management of spontaneous pneumomediastinum: experience in 24 adult patients. *Eur J Cardiothorac Surg.* May 2004;25(5):852–855.
14. Fini G, Gasparini G, Filippini F, Becelli R, Marcotullio D. The long styloid process syndrome or Eagle's syndrome. *J Craniomaxillofac Surg.* Apr 2000;28(2): 123–127.
15. Cahill D. Ludwig angina. *Am J Nurs.* Oct 2002; 102(10):43–44.
16. Twomey LT, Taylor JR. *Physical therapy of the low back.* 3rd ed. New York, NY: Churchill Livingstone; 2000.

17. Leffert RD. Thoracic outlet syndrome. *J Am Acad Orthop Surg.* Nov 1994;2(6):317–325.

18. Vargo MM, Flood KM. Pancoast tumor presenting as cervical radiculopathy. *Arch Phys Med Rehabil.* Jul 1990;71(8):606–609.

19. Villas C, Collia A, Aquerreta JD, et al. Cervicobrachialgia and Pancoast tumor: value of standard anteroposterior cervical radiographs in early diagnosis. *Orthopedics.* Oct 2004;27(10):1092–1095.

20. Nusbaum AO, Som PM, Rothschild MA, Shugar JM. Recurrence of a deep neck infection: a clinical indication of an underlying congenital lesion. *Arch Otolaryngol Head Neck Surg.* Dec 1999;125(12):1379–1382.

21. Manabe S, Okura T, Watanabe S, Higaki J. Association between carotid haemodynamics and inflammation in patients with essential hypertension. *J Hum Hypertens.* Oct 2005;19(10):787–791.

22. Robinson WP 3rd, Detterbeck FC, Hendren RL, Keagy BA. Fulminant development of mega-aorta due to Takayasu's arteritis: case report and review of the literature. *Vascular.* May–Jun 2005;13(3):178–183.

23. Tintinalli J, Ruiz E, Krome R. *Emergency Medicine: A Comprehensive Study Guide.* 4th ed. New York, NY: McGraw-Hill; 1996.

24. Bhojani RA, Rosenbaum DH, Dikmen E, et al. Contemporary assessment of laryngotracheal trauma. *J Thorac Cardiovasc Surg.* Aug 2005;130(2):426–432.

25. Glinjongol C, Pakdirat B. Management of tracheobronchial injuries: a 10-year experience at Ratchaburi hospital. *J Med Assoc Thai.* Jan 2005;88(1):32–40.

26. Aminoff MJ, Greenberg DA, Simon RP, Greenberg DA. *Clinical Neurology.* 6th ed. New York, NY: Lange Medical Books/McGraw-Hill; 2005.

27. Rao R. Neck pain, cervical radiculopathy, and cervical myelopathy: pathophysiology, natural history, and clinical evaluation. *Instr Course Lect.* 2003;52:479–488.

28. Roh JS, Teng AL, Yoo JU, Davis J, Furey C, Bohlman HH. Degenerative disorders of the lumbar and cervical spine. *Orthop Clin North Am.* Jul 2005;36(3):255–262.

29. Ferrer R. Lymphadenopathy: differential diagnosis and evaluation. *Am Fam Physician.* Oct 15, 1998;58(6):1313–1320.

30. Rosario PW, de Faria S, Bicalho L, et al. Ultrasonographic differentiation between metastatic and benign lymph nodes in patients with papillary thyroid carcinoma. *J Ultrasound Med.* Oct 2005;24(10):1385–1389.

31. Sjaastad O. Benign exertional headache. *Headache.* 2003;43:611–615.

32. D'Amico D, Leone M, Bussone G. Side locked unilaterality and pain localization in long lasting headaches: migraine, tension-type and cervicogenic headaches. *Headache.* 1994;34:526–530.

33. Carruthers BM, Jain AK, DeMeirleir KL, et al. Myalgic encephalomyelitis/chronic fatigue syndrome: clinical working case definition, diagnostic and treatment protocols (a consensus document). *J Chronic Fatigue Syndr.* 2003;11(1):7–115.

34. Merskey H, Bogduk N. *Classification of Chronic Pain: Descriptions of Chronic Pain Syndromes and Definitions of Pain Terms.* Seattle, WA: IASP Press; 1994.

35. Benninger DH, Georgiadis D, Kremer C, Studer A, Nedeltchev K, Baumgartner RW. Mechanism of ischemic infarct in spontaneous carotid dissection. *Stroke.* Feb 2004;35(2):482–485.

36. Yang ST, Huang YC, Chuang CC, Hsu PW. Traumatic internal carotid artery dissection. *J Clin Neurosci.* Jan 2006;13(1):123–128.

37. Anthony M. Unilateral migraine or occipital neuralgia? In: Rose FC, ed. *New Advances in Headache Research: Proceedings of the 7th Migraine Trust International Symposium, London, September 1988.* London: Smith-Gordon and Company Ltd; 1989.

38. Blackwell KE, Landman MD, Calcaterra TC. Spinal accessory nerve palsy: an unusual complication of rhytidectomy. *Head Neck.* Mar–Apr 1994;16(2):181–185.

39. Goldenberg DL, Burckhardt C, Crofford L. Management of fibromyalgia syndrome [see comment]. *JAMA.* 2004;292(19):2388–2395.

40. Mease P. Fibromyalgia syndrome: review of clinical presentation, pathogenesis, outcome measures, and treatment. *J Rheumatol Suppl.* Aug 2005;75:6–21.

41. Ogawa M, Hori H, Hirayama M, et al. Anaplastic transformation from papillary thyroid carcinoma with increased serum CA19-9. *Pediatr Blood Cancer.* Jul 2005;45(1):64–67.

42. Graff-Radford SB. Myofascial pain: diagnosis and management. *Curr Pain Headache Rep.* Dec 2004;8(6):463–467.

43. Koval KJ, Zuckerman JD, Rockwood CA. *Rockwood, Green, and Wilkins' handbook of fractures.* 2nd ed. Philadelphia, PA: Lippincott Williams & Wilkins; 2001.

44. DePietropaolo DL, Powers JH, Gill JM, Foy AJ. Diagnosis of lyme disease. *Am Fam Physician.* Jul 15, 2005;72(2):297–304.

45. Ratzan KR. Viral meningitis. *Med Clin North Am.* Mar 1985;69(2):399–413.

46. Rossi R, Valeria Saddi M. Subacute aseptic meningitis as neurological manifestation of primary Sjögren's syndrome. *Clin Neurol Neurosurg.* 2005;108(7):688–691.

47. Sahrmann S. *Diagnosis and Treatment of Movement Impairment Syndromes.* St. Louis, MO: Mosby; 2002.

48. Reginato AJ, Coquia JA. Musculoskeletal manifestations of osteomalacia and rickets. *Best Pract Res Clin Rheumatol.* Dec 2003;17(6):1063–1080.

49. Simon RP, Aminoff MJ, Greenberg DA. *Clinical Neurology.* 4th ed. Stamford, CT: Appleton & Lange; 1999.

50. Parsons LC. Osteoporosis: incidence, prevention, and treatment of the silent killer. *Nurs Clin North Am.* Mar 2005;40(1):119–133.

51. Villareal DT, Binder EF, Yarasheski KE, et al. Effects of exercise training added to ongoing hormone replacement therapy on bone mineral density in frail elderly women. *J Am Geriatr Soc.* Jul 2003;51(7):985–990.

52. Ashkenazi E, Constantini S, Pappo O, Gomori M, Averbuch-Heller L, Umansky F. Hypertrophic spinal pachymeningitis: report of two cases and review of the literature. *Neurosurgery.* May 1991;28(5):730–732.

53. Langston AL, Ralston SH. Management of Paget's disease of bone. *Rheumatology (Oxford).* Aug 2004;43(8):955–959.

54. Giampietro PF, Peterson M, Schneider R, et al. Assessment of bone mineral density in adults and children with Marfan syndrome. *Osteoporos Int.* Jul 2003;14(7):559–563.

55. Hadjipavlou AG, Gaitanis IN, Kontakis GM. Paget's disease of the bone and its management. *J Bone Joint Surg Br.* Mar 2002;84(2):160–169.

56. Salvarani C, Cantini F, Boiardi L, Hunder GG. Polymyalgia rheumatica. *Best Pract Res Clin Rheumatol.* Oct 2004;18(5):705–722.

57. Vijayan N, Dreyfus PM. Posttraumatic dysautonomic cephalgia: clinical observations and treatment. *Trans Am Neurol Assoc.* 1974;99:260–262.

58. Herwig SR, Gluckman JL. Acute calcific retropharyngeal tendinitis. *Arch Otolaryngol.* Jan 1982;108(1):41–42.

59. Mihmanli I, Karaarslan E, Kanberoglu K. Inflammation of vertebral bone associated with acute calcific tendinitis of the longus colli muscle. *Neuroradiology.* Dec 2001;43(12):1098–1101.

60. Pincus T, Callahan LF. What is the natural history of rheumatoid arthritis? *Rheum Dis Clin North Am.* Feb 1993;19(1):123–151.

61. Simpson RK, et al. Epidemiological characteristics of subarachnoid hemorrhage in an urban population. *J Clin Epidemiol.* 1991;44(7):641–648.

62. Sawin PD, Loftus CM. Diagnosis of spontaneous subarachnoid hemorrhage. *Am Fam Physician.* 1997;55(1): 145–156.

63. Polmear A. Sentinel headaches in aneurysmal subarachnoid hemorrhage: what is the true incidence? *Cephalalgia.* 2003;23:935–941.

64. Nolte CH, Lehmann TN. Headache resulting from bilateral chronic hematoma after lumbar puncture. *Am J Emerg Med.* 2004;22(3):241–242.

65. Fukutake T. Roller coaster headache and subdural hematoma. *Neurology.* 2000;37:121.

66. Davies JM, et al. Subdural haematoma after dural puncture. *Br J Anaesthsia.* 2001;86(5):720–723.

67. Graber MA, Kathol M. Cervical spine radiographs in the trauma patient. *Am Fam Physician.* Jan 15, 1999;59(2): 331–342.

68. Katz R. Is it lupus or fibromyalgia? *Fibromyalgia Aware.* 2004;6:68–71.

69. Grath-Radford S. Oromandibular disorders. In: Olesen J HP, Welch K, ed. *The Headaches.* 2nd ed. Philadelphia, PA: Lippincott Williams & Wilkins; 2000.

70. Ozaki O, Sugimoto T, Suzuki A, Yashiro T, Ito K, Hosoda Y. Cervical thymic cyst as a cause of acute suppurative thyroiditis. *Jpn J Surg.* Sep 1990;20(5):593–596.

71. Tay KY, U-King-Im JM, Trivedi RA, et al. Imaging the vertebral artery. *Eur Radiol.* Jul 2005;15(7): 1329–1343.

CHAPTER **11**

Shoulder Pain

■ *Chris A. Sebelski, PT, DPT, OCS, CSCS*

Description of the Symptom

This chapter describes pathology that may lead to shoulder pain. **Local causes** of shoulder pain include pathology that occurs within the humerus, scapula, and clavicle; acromioclavicular joint, glenohumeral joint, and sternoclavicular joint; and associated soft tissue structures. **Remote causes** are defined as occurring outside this region.

Special Concerns

■ Asymmetry in shoulder contour between sides, or change in contour of the affected shoulder, with loss of rotation range of motion

■ Abnormal sensorimotor status of the affected upper extremity
■ Warmth and erythema of the shoulder region
■ Constitutional symptoms associated with onset of shoulder pain
■ History of trauma or recent seizure
■ Unremitting pain not associated with direct movement of the shoulder
■ Severe sharp, stabbing pain of several minutes in duration
■ Trauma associated with high irritability and inability to move the shoulder

LOCAL LATERAL	LOCAL POSTERIOR	LOCAL SUPERIOR
Dislocations: • Acromioclavicular dislocation 157 • Glenohumeral dislocation 157 Fractures: • Proximal humerus 159 Glenoid labrum tears 159 Impingement syndromes: • Subacromial impingement 161 Joint injuries: • Acromioclavicular sprain 161 • Glenohumeral sprain/subluxation 161 Rotator cuff tear 167	Fractures: • Scapula 159 Glenoid labrum tears 159 Impingement syndromes: • Internal impingement (posterior glenoid impingement) 160 Joint injuries: • Glenohumeral sprain/subluxation 161 Muscle strains 162	Dislocations: • Acromioclavicular dislocation 157 • Glenohumeral dislocation 157 Glenoid labrum tears 159 Joint injuries: • Acromioclavicular sprain 161 • Glenohumeral sprain/subluxation 161 Muscle strains 162
Nerve injuries: • Axillary nerve injury 162	Nerve injuries: • Suprascapular nerve injury 163	Nerve injuries: • Suprascapular nerve injury 163
Not applicable	Nerve injuries: • Spinal accessory nerve trauma 163	Not applicable

LOCAL LATERAL	LOCAL POSTERIOR	LOCAL SUPERIOR
Aseptic Adhesive capsulitis (frozen shoulder) 155 Bursitis (subdeltoid/subacromial) 156 Complex regional pain syndrome (CRPS; also reflex sympathetic dystrophy, algodystrophy, Sudeck's atrophy) 157 Myofascial pain syndrome 162	**Aseptic** Adhesive capsulitis (frozen shoulder) 155 Bursitis (subdeltoid/subacromial) 156 Complex regional pain syndrome (CRPS; also reflex sympathetic dystrophy, algodystrophy, Sudeck's atrophy) 157 Myofascial pain syndrome 162	**Aseptic** Bursitis (subdeltoid/subacromial) 156 Complex regional pain syndrome (CRPS; also reflex sympathetic dystrophy, algodystrophy, Sudeck's atrophy) 157 Myofascial pain syndrome 162 Rheumatoid arthritis 165 Tendinopathies: • Biceps long tendinitis 167 *(continued)*

Inflammation *(continued)*

REMOTE	LOCAL GENERALIZED	LOCAL ANTERIOR
COMMON		
	Myofascial pain syndrome 162 Rheumatoid arthritis 165 **Septic** Osteomyelitis 164 Septic arthritis 167	Tendinopathies: • Biceps long tendinitis 167 • Calcific tendinopathy 168 **Septic** Not applicable
UNCOMMON		

Aseptic
Acute cholecystitis 143
Costochondritis 148
Gaseous distention of the
  stomach 149
Rheumatoid arthritis–like
  diseases of the cervical
  spine:
• Crohn's disease
  (regional enteritis) 151
• Psoriatic arthritis 152
• Scleroderma 152
• Systemic lupus
  erythematosus 152
• Ulcerative colitis 152
Tietze's syndrome 153
 	
Septic
Acute viral/idiopathic
  pericarditis 144
	Aseptic
	Ankylosing spondylitis 155
	Chronic fatigue syndrome 156
	Neuralgic amyotrophy
	  (Parsonage-Turner
	  syndrome) 163
	Polymyalgia rheumatica 164
	Rheumatoid–like health
	  conditions:
	• Dermatomyositis 166
	• Polymyositis 166
	• Psoriatic arthritis 166
	• Scleroderma 166
	• Systemic lupus
	  erythematosus 167
	
	Septic
	Not applicable
		Not applicable

RARE		

Aseptic
Not applicable
 	
Septic
Cat-scratch disease 144
Cervical epidural
  abscess 145
Cervical lymphadenitis 145
Perihepatitis (Fitz-Hugh–
  Curtis syndrome) 150
Subphrenic abscess 153
	Aseptic
	Reiter's syndrome 165
	
	Septic
	Ankylosing spondylitis 155
	Skeletal tuberculosis (Pott's
	  disease) 167
		Not applicable

M Metabolic

REMOTE	LOCAL GENERALIZED	LOCAL ANTERIOR
COMMON		
Not applicable	Not applicable	Not applicable

LOCAL LATERAL	LOCAL POSTERIOR	LOCAL SUPERIOR
Tendinopathies: • Calcific tendinopathy 168 • Rotator cuff tendinitis 168 **Septic** Osteomyelitis 164 Septic arthritis 167	Tendinopathies: • Calcific tendinopathy 168 • Rotator cuff tendinitis 168 **Septic** Osteomyelitis 164	• Calcific tendinopathy 168 • Rotator cuff tendinitis 168 **Septic** Osteomyelitis 164
Aseptic Neuralgic amyotrophy (Parsonage-Turner syndrome) 163 Polymyalgia rheumatica 164 Rheumatoid arthritis 165 Rheumatoid–like health conditions: • Dermatomyositis 166 • Polymyositis 166 • Psoriatic arthritis 166 • Scleroderma 166 • Systemic lupus erythematosus 167 **Septic** Not applicable	**Aseptic** Neuralgic amyotrophy (Parsonage-Turner syndrome) 163 **Septic** Not applicable	**Aseptic** Neuralgic amyotrophy (Parsonage-Turner syndrome) 163 Polymyalgia rheumatica 164 **Septic** Not applicable
Aseptic Not applicable **Septic** Skeletal tuberculosis (Pott's disease) 167	**Aseptic** Not applicable **Septic** Skeletal tuberculosis (Pott's disease) 167	**Aseptic** Not applicable **Septic** Skeletal tuberculosis (Pott's disease) 167
LOCAL LATERAL	**LOCAL POSTERIOR**	**LOCAL SUPERIOR**
Not applicable	Not applicable	Not applicable

(continued)

Metabolic *(continued)*

REMOTE	LOCAL GENERALIZED	LOCAL ANTERIOR
UNCOMMON		
Osteomalacia 150	Hereditary neuralgic amyotrophy 160 Heterotopic ossification/ myositis ossificans 160	Hereditary neuralgic amyotrophy 160
RARE		
Ectopic pregnancy 148	Amyloid arthropathy 155 Gout 160 Pseudogout (calcium pyrophosphate dihydrate deposition disease) 165	Not applicable

Va   Vascular

REMOTE	LOCAL GENERALIZED	LOCAL ANTERIOR
COMMON		
Acute myocardial infarction 144 Coronary artery insufficiency 148	Not applicable	Not applicable
UNCOMMON		
Not applicable	Avascular necrosis of the humeral head 156 Quadrilateral space syndrome 165	Not applicable
RARE		
Aneurysm 144 Pulmonary embolus 151 Upper extremity deep venous thrombosis (UEDVT; includes Paget-Schroetter syndrome) 154	Aneurysm 155 Upper extremity deep venous thrombosis (UEDVT; includes Paget-Schroetter syndrome) 154	Aneurysm 155 Upper extremity deep venous thrombosis (UEDVT; includes Paget-Schroetter syndrome) 154

De   Degenerative

REMOTE	LOCAL GENERALIZED	LOCAL ANTERIOR
COMMON		
Cervical osteoarthrosis/ osteoarthritis 146	Osteoarthrosis/osteoarthritis: • Acromioclavicular joint 164 • Glenohumeral joint 164 Rotator cuff tear 167	Osteoarthrosis/osteoarthritis: • Acromioclavicular joint 164 • Glenohumeral joint 164 Tendinopathies: • Biceps long tendinosis 168 • Calcific tendinopathy 168

LOCAL LATERAL	LOCAL POSTERIOR	LOCAL SUPERIOR
Not applicable	Heterotopic ossification/ myositis ossificans 160	Hereditary neuralgic amyotrophy 160 Heterotopic ossification/ myositis ossificans 160
Not applicable	Not applicable	Not applicable

LOCAL LATERAL	LOCAL POSTERIOR	LOCAL SUPERIOR
Not applicable	Not applicable	Not applicable
Avascular necrosis of the humeral head 156	Avascular necrosis of the humeral head 156 Quadrilateral space syndrome 165	Not applicable
Aneurysm 155 Upper extremity deep venous thrombosis (UEDVT; includes Paget-Schroetter syndrome) 154	Aneurysm 155 Upper extremity deep venous thrombosis (UEDVT; includes Paget-Schroetter syndrome) 154	Aneurysm 155 Upper extremity deep venous thrombosis (UEDVT; includes Paget-Schroetter syndrome) 154

LOCAL LATERAL	LOCAL POSTERIOR	LOCAL SUPERIOR
Osteoarthrosis/osteoarthritis: • Acromioclavicular joint 164 • Glenohumeral joint 164 Rotator cuff tear 167 Tendinopathies: • Rotator cuff tendinosis 168	Osteoarthrosis/osteoarthritis: • Glenohumeral joint 164 Rotator cuff tear 167 Tendinopathies: • Rotator cuff tendinosis 168	Rotator cuff tear 167 Tendinopathies: • Biceps long tendinosis 168 • Calcific tendinopathy 168 • Rotator cuff tendinosis 168

(continued)

Degenerative *(continued)*

REMOTE	LOCAL GENERALIZED	LOCAL ANTERIOR
UNCOMMON		
Not applicable	Osteoarthrosis/osteoarthritis: • Sternoclavicular 164	Osteoarthrosis/osteoarthritis: • Sternoclavicular 164
RARE		
Not applicable	Not applicable	Not applicable

Tu Tumor

REMOTE	LOCAL GENERALIZED	LOCAL ANTERIOR
COMMON		
Not applicable	Not applicable	Not applicable
UNCOMMON		
Malignant Primary, such as: • Breast tumor 153 • Pancoast tumor 154 *Malignant Metastatic:* Not applicable *Benign:* Not applicable	*Malignant Primary, such as:* • Chondrosarcoma 169 • Lung tumor 169 • Osteosarcoma 170 *Malignant Metastatic, such as:* • Metastases, including from primary breast, kidney, lung, prostate, and thyroid disease 169 *Benign, such as:* • Enchondroma 169 • Lipoma 169 • Osteoblastoma 169 • Osteochondroma 170 • Osteoid osteoma 170 • Unicameral bone cyst 170	*Malignant Primary, such as:* • Chondrosarcoma 169 • Lung tumor 169 • Osteosarcoma 170 *Malignant Metastatic, such as:* • Metastases, including from primary breast, kidney, lung, prostate, and thyroid disease 169 *Benign, such as:* • Enchondroma 169 • Lipoma 169 • Osteoblastoma 169 • Osteochondroma 170 • Osteoid osteoma 170 • Unicameral bone cyst 170
RARE		
Not applicable	Not applicable	Not applicable

Co Congenital

REMOTE	LOCAL GENERALIZED	LOCAL ANTERIOR
COMMON		
Not applicable	Not applicable	Not applicable
UNCOMMON		
Not applicable	Not applicable	Not applicable
RARE		
Not applicable	Not applicable	Not applicable

LOCAL LATERAL	LOCAL POSTERIOR	LOCAL SUPERIOR
Osteoarthrosis/osteoarthritis: • Sternoclavicular 164	Not applicable	Not applicable
Not applicable	Not applicable	Not applicable

LOCAL LATERAL	LOCAL POSTERIOR	LOCAL SUPERIOR
Not applicable	Not applicable	Not applicable
Malignant Primary, such as: • Chondrosarcoma 169 • Lung tumor 169 • Osteosarcoma 170 *Malignant Metastatic, such as:* • Metastases, including from primary breast, kidney, lung, prostate, and thyroid disease 169 *Benign, such as:* • Enchondroma 169 • Lipoma 169 • Osteoblastoma 169 • Osteochondroma 170 • Osteoid osteoma 170 • Unicameral bone cyst 170	*Malignant Primary, such as:* • Chondrosarcoma 169 • Lung tumor 169 • Osteosarcoma 170 *Malignant Metastatic, such as:* • Metastases, including from primary breast, kidney, lung, prostate, and thyroid disease 169 *Benign, such as:* • Enchondroma 169 • Lipoma 169 • Osteoblastoma 169 • Osteochondroma 170 • Osteoid osteoma 170 • Unicameral bone cyst 170	*Malignant Primary, such as:* • Chondrosarcoma 169 • Lung tumor 169 • Osteosarcoma 170 *Malignant Metastatic, such as:* • Metastases, including from primary breast, kidney, lung, prostate, and thyroid disease 169 *Benign, such as:* • Enchondroma 169 • Lipoma 169 • Osteoblastoma 169 • Osteochondroma 170 • Osteoid osteoma 170 • Unicameral bone cyst 170
Not applicable	Not applicable	Not applicable

LOCAL LATERAL	LOCAL POSTERIOR	LOCAL SUPERIOR
Not applicable	Not applicable	Not applicable
Not applicable	Not applicable	Not applicable
Not applicable	Not applicable	Not applicable

(continued)

Ne Neurogenic/Psychogenic

REMOTE	LOCAL GENERALIZED	LOCAL ANTERIOR
COMMON		
Not applicable	Not applicable	Not applicable
UNCOMMON		
Not applicable	Erb's palsy 158 Neuropathic arthropathy (Charcot-Marie-Tooth disease) 163	Erb's palsy 158
RARE		
Not applicable	Not applicable	Not applicable

Note: These are estimates of relative incidence because few data are available for the less common conditions.

Overview of Shoulder Pain

The shoulder girdle is composed of the clavicle, acromion process of the scapula, and the proximal humerus. These bones form the acromioclavicular, sternoclavicular, and glenohumeral joints. A physiological articulation between the scapula and thorax also exists. The position of the shoulder girdle as the first major set of articulations of the upper extremity distal to the cervical spine makes cervical spine pathology an important remote source of symptoms that should be considered in each patient presenting with shoulder pain. Its relatively proximal position within the body, proximity to lung and breast tissue, and rich blood supply place it at particularly elevated risk for health conditions that are characterized by hematogenous spread, such as metastatic tumors and infection. Certain anatomical characteristics of the shoulder girdle place a special premium on muscular activity and passive restraint provided by ligaments to the overall stability and optimal function of this region:

1. The only articular connection between the shoulder girdle and axial skeleton is the sternoclavicular joint.
2. The head of the humerus also is disproportionably large compared to the glenoid fossa.

These same anatomical characteristics also make the shoulder girdle uniquely susceptible to pathology secondary to microtrauma, macrotrauma, and degeneration that should be considered if health conditions in other pathological categories are ruled less likely.

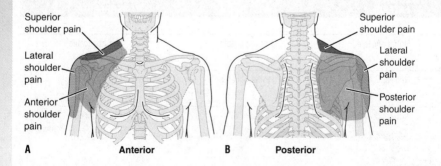

A   **Anterior**   **B**   **Posterior**

LOCAL LATERAL	LOCAL POSTERIOR	LOCAL SUPERIOR
Not applicable	Not applicable	Not applicable
Not applicable	Not applicable	Not applicable
Not applicable	Not applicable	Not applicable

Description of Conditions That May Lead to Shoulder Pain

Remote

■ Acute Cholecystitis

Chief Clinical Characteristics

This presentation involves a gradual onset of pain that progresses to a very severe level, which is mainly located in the right upper quadrant of the abdomen. Pain in the interscapular or scapular region may be associated with this health condition without compromise of shoulder motion (Fig. 11-1). Fever is typically present, as well as vomiting, nausea, or visible jaundice in some cases.

Background Information

Radiation of pain to the area of the right acromioclavicular joint or tip of the shoulder is not as common. On abdominal examination, subcostal tenderness or guarding in the right upper quadrant that increases with respiration or thoracic movement (Murphy's sign)

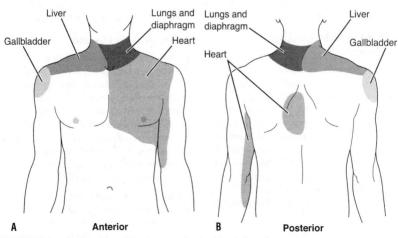

A **Anterior** **B** **Posterior**

FIGURE 11-1 Referral patterns of the viscera to the shoulder girdle region.

may be present. Surgical removal of the gallbladder may be indicated. Although biliary calculi are considered common, they become symptomatic in 1% to 4% of patients annually. The prevalence of gallstones is higher in women; however, attacks tend to be more prevalent and severe in men. Individuals with diabetes mellitus appear at elevated risk for this health condition.[1] The main symptom is caused by obstruction of the gallbladder neck by a stone. Abdominal sonography or hepatobiliary scintigraphy confirms the diagnosis. Shoulder pain is a common sequela to this surgical procedure that may be addressed effectively with injection of a short-term anesthetic agent into the gallbladder.[2]

■ Acute Myocardial Infarction

Chief Clinical Characteristics

This presentation includes crushing, strangling, or stabbing pressure across the chest, which also may be present in the anterior or lateral left shoulder that radiates to one or both arms in the T1 dermatome, neck, or jaw (see Fig. 11-1). Associated symptoms include diaphoresis, dyspnea, weakness, palpitations, and dizziness.

Background Information

This severe paroxysmal pain may or may not be associated with a recent increase of activity. It may not be changed by rest, body position, breathing pattern, or with the administration of nitroglycerin. This condition is a medical emergency due to the risk for significant myocardial damage.[3]

■ Acute Viral/Idiopathic Pericarditis

Chief Clinical Characteristics

This presentation is mainly characterized by sharp and stabbing anterior chest pain that may radiate to the neck, back, left shoulder, or left supraclavicular region with worsening pain with deep inspiration, coughing, trunk rotation or side-bending, and lying supine. The presentation closely mimics that of an acute myocardial infarction with a similar referral pattern to the left shoulder and in the T1 dermatome (see Fig. 11-1). This condition is more common in young males.

Background Information

This condition is typically associated with cough, fever, and pain usually 10 to 12 days after presumed viral illness. Alleviating positions include kneeling with hands on floor, leaning forward, or sitting upright. Pericardial friction rub may be auscultated. Episodes are longer in duration than that of an acute myocardial infarction or anginal pain. Pericarditis may be due to an acute viral infection or it may be idiopathic in nature. Chest computed tomography and magnetic resonance imaging confirm the diagnosis.[4] This condition is a medical emergency due to the risk for cardiac tamponade.

■ Aneurysm

Chief Clinical Characteristics

This presentation can include localized shoulder pain and neuropathic or myopathic symptoms either with or without functional limitations; the distribution of symptoms depends on the affected artery.[5,6] Aortic and carotid artery aneurysms have been documented to give rise to shoulder pain. Secondary signs may include warmth, redness, and swelling.

Background Information

The potential compression of the brachial plexus or cervical nerve roots or vascular compromise may elicit these associated signs and symptoms. Aneurysms or pseudoaneurysms may be present due to recent surgery, trauma, or iatrogenic complications.[7] The diagnosis is confirmed with arteriography or Doppler ultrasound. This condition typically is managed with surgical procedures such as stent placement, the goal of which is to reinforce the structural integrity of the arterial wall.

■ Cat-Scratch Disease

Chief Clinical Characteristics

This presentation typically involves a unilateral, painless, subacute granulomatous lymphadenopathy that is most common in the axillary lymph nodes but may present in the cervical or inguinal lymph nodes. Constitutional symptoms such as prolonged fever, headache, and malaise may be present. A slow to heal scratch may also be present with a history of recent cat scratch within the past several months.[8]

Background Information

Though less frequent in adults, this health condition often may be initially misdiagnosed as breast cancer.[9] The diagnosis is confirmed with lymph node biopsy, blood culture, or imaging of the local soft tissues. Treatment may include antibiotic agents with surgical excision reserved for the most severe cases.

■ Cervical Disk Herniation

Chief Clinical Characteristics

This presentation involves pain in the posterior or posterolateral aspect of the neck with or without radicular symptoms down the arm or through the midthoracic region. Aching pain, burning, numbness, or tingling radicular pain at the supraclavicular area (C4; Fig. 11-2A), the anterior shoulder (C5, Fig. 11-2B), superior-posterior shoulder into the lateral brachium (C6, Fig. 11-2C), posterior shoulder (C7-C8; Fig. 11-2D and E) or the axilla (T1) also may be present. Location of the signs and symptoms may be seen to correlate to the dermatome, myotome, or sclerotome of the nerve root or adjacent root. Other signs may include muscle weakness, muscle wasting, or diminution or loss of reflex response. Aggravating factors could include neck rotation or compression.

Background Information

Cervical disk herniation can result from trauma, occur spontaneously in midlife (between 30 and 40 years of age), or result from degenerative changes in the geriatric population (spondylosis). C5–C6 and C6–C7 are the most common levels of disk herniation in the cervical spine.[10] Magnetic resonance imaging best confirms the diagnosis. Treatment is variable; surgical intervention may be required for individuals with extensive or rapidly progressing neurological symptoms, but nonsurgical intervention including rehabilitation is considered a primary treatment for most individuals with this health condition.

■ Cervical Epidural Abscess

Chief Clinical Characteristics

This presentation often may include pain in the axial or appendicular region corresponding to the segmental level of involvement in the cervical spine and an elevated white cell count. A fever may be present in up to 50% of cases.[11] Sensorimotor signs including potential bowel and bladder disturbances may be present.

Background Information

The abscess is usually an infection that generates a pus-filled sac in the epidural space. The most common risk factor is hematogenous

spreading of an infectious organism, such as *Staphylococcus aureus*, due to an untreated infection of a skin lesion or intravenous drug abuse. This diagnosis is confirmed with magnetic resonance imaging, which reveals an abnormal region of high signal on T2-weighted images in the epidural space within the affected region of the cervical spine. Treatment typically includes some combination of intravenous antibiotic medication and surgical decompression of the abscess.

■ Cervical Lymphadenitis

Chief Clinical Characteristics

This presentation may involve a supraclavicular mass with neck pain radiating to the shoulder. The presence of a draining fistula is possible. Masses also may appear at other locations including the posterior neck and the submandibular area.[12]

Background Information

Cervical lymphadenitis is an infection of the cervical lymph nodes that results in formation of a mass. In adults, the mass may be secondary to tuberculosis or other form of bacterial infection. The bacterial infection may not present with the usual constitutional

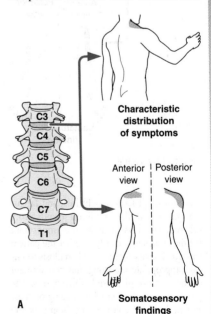

A

FIGURE 11-2 Patterns of cervical radiculopathy.

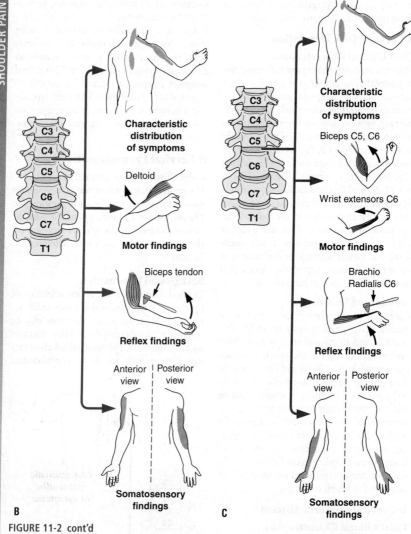

B

FIGURE 11-2 cont'd

symptoms, but fever, weight loss, and fatigue are possible if the condition results from tuberculosis. This suggests the importance for the clinician to clarify whether the patient was previously exposed to tuberculosis to ensure appropriate reporting and containment in the presence of possible tuberculosis. The diagnosis is confirmed with imaging of chest and neck, blood cultures, and biopsy of the mass itself. A combination of surgical and pharmacologic management provides optimal outcomes.[13]

■ Cervical Osteoarthrosis/ Osteoarthritis

Chief Clinical Characteristics

This presentation is characterized by pain in the posterior or posterolateral aspect of the neck, which may be related with aching pain, burning, numbness, or tingling radicular pain at the

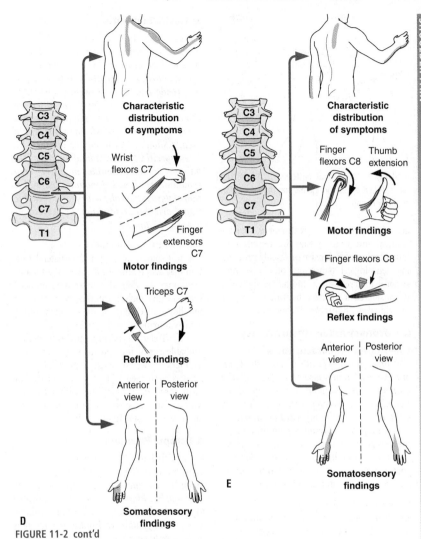

D

E

FIGURE 11-2 cont'd

supraclavicular area (C4), the anterior shoulder (C5), superior-posterior shoulder into the lateral brachium (C6), posterior shoulder (C7), or the axilla (see Fig. 11-2A to E). Location of the signs and symptoms may be seen to correlate to the dermatome, myotome, or sclerotome of the nerve root or adjacent root. Other signs may include muscle weakness, muscle wasting, or diminution or loss of reflex response. This condition occurs in the older population and usually without radicular symptoms.

Background Information

Osteoarthrosis/osteoarthritis of the zygapophyseal joints, hypertrophy of the ligamentum flavum, and osteophyte formation around the intervertebral foramen can all contribute to symptoms (Fig. 11-3).[14] Plain radiographs and magnetic resonance imaging confirm the diagnosis, with joint space narrowing in the cervical facet or intervertebral joints, subchondral sclerosis of affected joints, and presence of periarticular osteophytes and

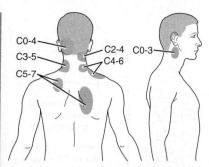

FIGURE 11-3 Referral patterns of the cervical facet joints. Cervical facet joints may refer pain to the shoulder region.

articular hypertrophy. Treatment is variable; surgical intervention may be required for individuals with extensive or rapidly progressing neurological symptoms; otherwise, nonsurgical intervention including rehabilitation is considered a primary treatment for most individuals with this health condition.

■ Coronary Artery Insufficiency

Chief Clinical Characteristics

This presentation typically involves chest pain or tightness, but may also present as radiating pain into the shoulder or shoulder girdle. Episodes may be accompanied by anginal type symptoms similar to myocardial infarction, such as diaphoresis, dyspnea, palpitations, and presyncope. Women are more greatly affected than men, especially when older than 50 years, postmenopausal on hormone replacement therapy, and with diabetes mellitus.[15]

Background Information

Shoulder movement will not be specifically restricted. This health condition occurs due to occlusion or spasm of the coronary artery.[3] In contrast to acute myocardial infarction, pain from coronary artery insufficiency is relieved by administration of nitroglycerin. This health condition is a progressive disorder with more severe cardiac disease to be expected without treatment. The diagnosis is confirmed with response to stress testing and cardiac imaging. Treatment may include prevention for those with the greatest risk factors, in combination with pharmacologic and surgical management to reduce symptoms and ensure adequate cardiac perfusion.

■ Costochondritis

Chief Clinical Characteristics

This presentation commonly includes dull pain with anterior chest wall tenderness that is frequently perceived at the anterior shoulder. Tenderness without swelling typically is focused along the third, fourth, or fifth costochondral joints with possible corresponding deeper pain at the posterior midscapular area.[16] Shoulder pain may be bilateral but is less specific. Provocation of anterior chest pain occurs with shoulder mobility versus shoulder pain limiting mobility. Reproduction of pain is typically with shoulder abduction, horizontal adduction, or movements against resistance.

Background Information

Cervical spine extension and ipsilateral rotation may also reproduce the pain. Costochondritis may be idiopathic or trauma induced, such as with coughing or other overexertion of the chest wall. Costochondritis is often considered synonymous with Tietze's syndrome, although Tietze's syndrome presents with a probable aseptic inflammatory etiology with a hallmark of swelling in the area.[16] Each diagnosis is confirmed with clinical examination. Most cases are self-limiting with resolution within 1 year of onset or cortisone injection into effected costochondral joint.

■ Ectopic Pregnancy

Chief Clinical Characteristics

This presentation may involve pain that extends from the superior shoulder to the proximal brachium or axilla, accompanied by hypotensive symptoms including nausea, dizziness, fainting, pallor, weak pulse, or other signs of shock or hemorrhage.[17]

Background Information

This health condition occurs when an ectopic pregnancy ruptures or becomes large enough that it disrupts surrounding tissues. Some cases of ectopic pregnancy present with unilateral or bilateral shoulder pain due to irritation of the diaphragm from bleeding. A patient with an as-yet unruptured ectopic pregnancy may report having vague abdominal pains for several weeks prior to the rupture. Other possible symptoms include missed menstruation and vaginal spotting. Treatment of this health condition typically includes surgical excision; a ruptured ectopic pregnancy is a medical emergency.

■ **Gaseous Distention of the Stomach**

Chief Clinical Characteristics
This presentation can be characterized by midepigastric abdominal pain, associated with unilateral axilla or anterolateral chest wall pain that is unrelated to activity or mobility. Alleviating factors may involve belching and antacids.

Background Information
This health condition occurs when excessive gastric gases cause distention of the stomach to the extent that it irritates the inferior portion of the diaphragm. In turn, diaphragm irritation may result in referred pain to the shoulder. Common risk factors for shoulder pain related to excessive stomach gas include constipation, lactose intolerance, and status post–laparoscopy procedure. Association of pain with meal habits and diet are important clinical considerations. Typical treatment is directed at the underlying cause of excessive gastric gases, including antacid and antibiotic agents.

■ **Hepatitis**

Chief Clinical Characteristics
This presentation commonly involves tenderness and pain in the right upper abdominal quadrant, scapular region, and right shoulder, possibly associated with headaches, myalgias, arthralgias, fatigue, anorexia, nausea, jaundice, and fever.

Background Information
Hepatitis refers to a family of pathological conditions that is related to inflammation of the liver, consisting of five main types. Patients presenting with hepatitis-related shoulder or midback pain may be clinically undiagnosed and appear healthy (see Fig. 11-1). There is also an acutely progressive type of hepatitis in which the patient may be extremely ill within 2 to 8 weeks of exposure. Each type of hepatitis, named for the infectious agent, has specific epidemiological characteristics. Treatment varies by type and involves pharmacologic therapy. Depending on the type, hepatitis may be contracted via personal or sexual contact, food, as well as airborne or fecal–oral transmission. Assessing the patient history regarding the extent of alcohol use/abuse, intravenous drug use/

abuse, and recent blood transfusions may assist typing of hepatitis. In turn, typing of hepatitis guides clinical management.

INTERNAL ORGAN INJURIES
See Figure 11-1.

■ **Diaphragm Injury**

Chief Clinical Characteristics
This presentation typically includes lateral neck or shoulder pain with chest pain.

Background Information
Diaphragm rupture can occur with blunt or penetrating trauma to the chest or abdomen. Deep breathing and changes in position also may aggravate the symptoms. The mechanism that causes shoulder pain may involve the phrenic nerve.[18] Chest radiographs confirm the diagnosis, with characteristic findings of irregular diaphragmatic contour or elevation, contralateral mediastinal shift, and gas collection in the hemithorax. This condition requires urgent referral for medical evaluation.

■ **Liver Injury**

Chief Clinical Characteristics
This presentation may be characterized by pain in the midepigastric region or right upper quadrant, with referred pain to the superior shoulder, interscapular, and upper trapezius regions. Additional symptoms are right upper quadrant tenderness and guarding, and signs of blood loss such as shock and hypotension.

Background Information
Liver trauma accounts for 15% to 20% of blunt abdominal injuries. Common mechanisms of injury include motor vehicle accidents and fighting. Abdominal computed tomography confirms the diagnosis.[19] This condition requires urgent referral for medical evaluation.

■ **Lung Injury**

Chief Clinical Characteristics
This presentation can involve sharp, pleuritic pain in the axilla, shoulder, or subscapular regions with possible referral pain to the neck.[20] Clinical findings may also include shoulder-arm pain, Horner's syndrome, and neurological deficits affecting the C8

and T1 nerve roots in the case of apical lung involvement.

Background Information
Chest radiographs or computed tomography confirm the diagnosis. This condition requires urgent referral for medical evaluation.

■ Spleen Injury

Chief Clinical Characteristics
This presentation may include left shoulder pain associated with at least one of the following: unilateral neck pain, upper left abdomen pain and tenderness, nausea, vomiting, dizziness, and syncope. Symptoms are worse with coughing, deep breathing, and changes in position and may be provoked via lying in the Trendelenburg position.

Background Information
Symptoms may be delayed. Splenic rupture after colonoscopy is becoming more recognized as a potential consequence. Abdominal computed tomography confirms the diagnosis.[21] This condition requires urgent referral for medical evaluation.

■ Osteomalacia

Chief Clinical Characteristics
This presentation can involve an initial clinical picture of diffuse, general aching and global fatigue. Typically affecting the axial skeleton and lower extremities, the patient rarely may report generalized shoulder region discomfort. Symptoms should be present with the following risk factors: advanced age, cold geographic area, vitamin D deficiency, gastrectomy, and intestinal malabsorption pathology

Background Information
This diagnosis is rarely made quickly due to the vague initial presentation. A thorough history should query other risk factors including use of medications such as anticonvulsants, tranquilizers, sedatives, muscle relaxants, diuretics, and antacids and a medical history of hyperparathyroidism, chronic renal failure, and renal tubular defects. Bone and articular tenderness may occur in the spine, ribs, pelvis, and proximal extremities including the humerus.[22] As the disease progresses one might notice postural deformities, which result from the muscular weakness and softening of the bone, such as increased thoracic kyphosis,

bowing of the lower quadrant, and a heart-shaped pelvis. Presentation of shoulder pain in isolation of any of the other factors is rare. Treatment is directed at the underlying etiology and therefore a consultation with other health care professionals is necessary for appropriate management of a patient with this health condition.

■ Perihepatitis (Fitz-Hugh–Curtis Syndrome)

Chief Clinical Characteristics
This presentation may involve an insidious onset of general shoulder pain that may extend into the area of the clavicle. The pain may progress to "sharp" in nature over the course of a few days versus months. This condition presents almost exclusively in females, with concurrent symptoms that may include right upper quadrant pain, reports of vague abdominal symptoms, and reproduction of right shoulder pain with palpation of the right upper quadrant of the abdomen. Aggravating movements include right side-lying, deep breathing, or reports of shortness of breath.

Background Information
Limitations of shoulder range of motion or tenderness to palpation at the shoulder will not be present. In case studies, procedures involving the liver have produced right shoulder pain that may be of viscerosomatic referral.[23] This condition is an infectious type of perihepatitis and has been noted to be associated with pelvic inflammatory disorders,[24] gonococcus, and *Chlamydia* infections. Treatment typically includes pharmacologic management.

■ Pleurisy

Chief Clinical Characteristics
This presentation is mainly characterized by a moderate aching pain focused in the chest over the affected site. Associated symptoms include short rapid breathing, coughing, dyspnea, and fever with pain referred to the shoulder and neck regions. Aggravating factors include coughing, deep inspiration, and laughing. Alleviating factors include side-lying on the affected side.

Background Information
After several hours, this condition may progress to a constant pain with any movement

of shoulder/neck. This condition involves inflammation of the pleura. Common causes of pleurisy include infection, trauma, rheumatoid arthritis, systemic lupus erythematosus, and tumor. Chest radiographs confirm the diagnosis.[25] Pleurisy is treated by the underlying cause; a bacterial infection is treated via antibiotics and a viral-based infection is typically monitored without pharmacologic interference.

■ Pneumonia

Chief Clinical Characteristics
This presentation may involve severe shoulder pain at the tip of the acromioclavicular joint that is associated with chest pain, cough, sputum production, or breathlessness.

Background Information
The referred pain to the shoulder is theorized to be due to irritation of the diaphragm and the C4 sensory axons of the phrenic nerve. Diagnosis is via clinical presentation, radiography, and blood cultures with the causative agent typically being bacterial. Treatment is via antibiotics and as the pneumonia resolves, shoulder function should return.

■ Pulmonary Embolus

Chief Clinical Characteristics
This presentation may involve crushing pain that may mimic myocardial infarction or angina-type pain. Typically, the symptoms are substernal but may present anywhere in the trunk including the shoulder. It is associated with dyspnea, wheezing, and a marked drop in blood pressure.[26]

Background Information
This condition occurs when an embolus of clotted blood or less commonly cholesterol plaque becomes lodged in the pulmonary vascular tree, resulting in reduced oxygen exchange. Risk factors include immobilization or recent surgery. Treatment commonly involves anticoagulant medications, and this condition is considered a medical emergency.

■ Rheumatoid Arthritis of the Cervical Spine

Chief Clinical Characteristics
This presentation involves an onset of transitory pain and stiffness in the shoulder. Long-duration stiffness is especially prevalent in the morning.

Background Information
Involvement of the cervical spine as the first site of pathology is rare. Protective posturing of the upper extremity in internal rotation held against the stomach is common. Females are more affected than males with a peak age of 35 to 45 years old. Criteria for diagnosis of this condition includes prolonged morning stiffness (greater than 60 to 90 minutes), soft tissue swelling, symmetric arthritis, subcutaneous nodules, positive rheumatoid factor, or radiographic evidence. Treatment should be tailored to the patient and his or her specific symptoms, but typically involves steroidal, nonsteroidal, and biological anti-inflammatory medications.

INFLAMMATORY DISEASES

■ Crohn's Disease (Regional Enteritis)

Chief Clinical Characteristics
This presentation may be characterized by generalized aching pain in the shoulder. This symptom is infrequently the initial presenting symptom but may be an associated arthralgia during an acute episode of Crohn's disease. Other associated issues may include erythema nodosum, fever, weight loss, arthritis, and complications from long-term corticosteroid use.[27]

Background Information
Intestinal symptoms may vary according to the involved area of the gastrointestinal tract but may include nausea, cramping, anorexia, and diarrhea without blood in the stool. This condition is a subcategory of inflammatory bowel disease where the inflammation and ulceration occur primarily in the terminal ileum and colon, although any portion of the intestinal tract can be affected.[26] The etiology has not been identified though it is suspected to include genetic, microbial, inflammatory, immune, and permeability abnormalities.[26] Treatment of the disease process focuses on pharmacologic, homeopathic, or surgical management. Management of the pathophysiology of this condition decreases the extraintestinal presentations. Therefore, the

therapist should advocate a multidisciplinary approach.

■ Psoriatic Arthritis

Chief Clinical Characteristics

This presentation may involve an insidious onset of lumbopelvic and hip pain associated with psoriasis. The severity of arthritis is uncorrelated with the extent of skin involvement.[28] Pitting nail lesions occur in 80% of individuals with this condition. Dactylitis, tenosynovitis, and peripheral arthritis also are common.

Background Information

Radiographs of the distal phalanges may reveal a characteristic "pencil in cup" deformity. Blood panels including erythrocyte sedimentation rate are useful to track disease activity.

■ Scleroderma

Chief Clinical Characteristics

This presentation typically includes myalgia, arthralgia, fatigue, weight loss, limited mobility, and hardened skin about the hands, knees, or elbows. This condition occurs in individuals between 25 and 55 years of age, and is four to five times more likely in women than men. Additional symptoms may include dry mouth and eyes, as well as Raynaud's phenomenon.

Background Information

This rare and progressive autoimmune disorder affects blood vessels and many internal organs, including the lungs and the gastrointestinal system. Overproduction of collagen in this condition eventually leads to poor blood flow in the extremities, which can cause ulcers in the fingers, changes in skin color, and a disappearance of creases in the skin. Continued damage to small-diameter vasculature leads to scar tissue production that impairs joint range of motion. Blood tests confirm the diagnosis. Treatment includes both steroidal and nonsteroidal anti-inflammatory medications and gentle exercise.

■ Systemic Lupus Erythematosus

Chief Clinical Characteristics

This presentation can include lower back pain radiating to the hip and groin pain. It is associated with fatigue and joint pain/swelling affecting the hands, feet, knees, and shoulders.

Background Information

This condition affects mostly women of childbearing age. It is a chronic autoimmune disorder that can affect any organ system, including skin, joints, kidneys, brain, heart, lungs, and blood. The diagnosis is confirmed by the presence of skin lesions; heart, lung, or kidney involvement; and laboratory abnormalities including low red or white cell counts, low platelet counts, or positive antinuclear antibody and anti-DNA antibody tests.[29]

■ Ulcerative Colitis

Chief Clinical Characteristics

This presentation may include generalized aching pain. This condition is infrequently the initial presenting symptom but may be an associated arthralgia during an acute episode or progression of ulcerative colitis. Other associated symptoms may include fever, weight loss, arthritis, hepatobiliary disease, and complications from long-term corticosteroid use.[27]

Background Information

Intestinal symptoms include blood in the stool, abdominal cramping especially during bowel movements, and episodic diarrhea.[27] Ulcerative colitis is a subcategory of inflammatory bowel disease in which the inflammation and ulceration that occur are confined to the colon. The etiology is unknown but is suspected to include genetic, microbial, inflammatory, immune, and permeability abnormalities.[26] Treatment of the disease process focuses on pharmacologic, homeopathic, or surgical management. Management of the pathophysiology of this condition decreases the extraintestinal presentations. Therefore, the therapist should advocate a multidisciplinary approach.

■ Status Post–Laparoscopic Procedure

Chief Clinical Characteristics

This presentation can include moderate to severe shoulder pain that escalates 1 to 3 days following a surgical procedure.[27]

Background Information

Theoretically, the pain is generated from phrenic nerve irritation. Prevention and resolution of the pain into the shoulder is dependent on the surgical procedure and management postsurgically.

■ Subphrenic Abscess

Chief Clinical Characteristics

This presentation involves aching and persistent pain at the "tip" of the shoulder (see Fig. 11-1). Further specific location may depend on the area inferior to the diaphragm that is affected. Abdominal guarding or pain will be present.[30] Patient may or may not have a fever, recent trauma, or surgical intervention.

Background Information

This condition is an area of localized pus inferior to the diaphragm. It may be diagnosed via imaging. Early intervention by way of surgical or nonsurgical management gives the best outcomes.

■ Thoracic Outlet Syndrome

Chief Clinical Characteristics

This presentation may be characterized by diffuse pain in the shoulder or axilla, neck, arm, or chest. Symptoms may also include paresthesias, discoloration, numbness, weakness, nonpitting edema, and/or fatigue.[31]

Background Information

Postural abnormalities, macrotrauma, or microtrauma from repetitive overhead activities are possible contributors. These may result in a variety of syndromes in which the name of the syndrome is derived from the hypothetical source of neurovascular entrapment, such as cervical rib syndrome, scalenus anticus syndrome, pectoralis minor syndrome, or first thoracic rib syndrome. This is a clinical diagnosis with neurological, vascular, or nonspecific symptoms that may be secondary to either upper or lower trunk compression of the brachial plexus and vasculature. Multiple clinical exam measures have been developed though few are sensitive or specific to diagnose this condition. The 90-degree abduction test with external rotation appears to have the best predictive value.[32] Surgical intervention is indicated for those with symptoms that do not respond to nonoperative treatments.

■ Tietze's Syndrome

Chief Clinical Characteristics

This presentation may be associated with an insidious and rapid onset of dull pain with anterior chest wall tenderness that may be perceived at the anterior shoulder.[33] An inflammatory reaction with noted swelling is present at the second and third costochondral joints with concomitant irritation at the chondrosternal, sternoclavicular, or manubriosternal areas. Tietze's is aggravated by a history of prolonged coughing or overexertion. It is bilateral in 30% of cases. Provocation of anterior chest pain occurs with shoulder mobility versus shoulder pain that limits mobility. Reproduction of pain is typically with shoulder abduction, horizontal adduction, or movements against resistance.

Background Information

This syndrome is similar to costochondritis and the two are often considered to be synonymous conditions. However, Tietze's may involve an aseptic inflammatory etiology. This condition is equally common in both sexes, and commonly presents within the second to fourth decades of life. The diagnosis is confirmed with clinical examination. The cases are self-limiting with a relapsing, remitting presentation.[16] Case studies[34,35] now support the view that malignancy should be considered when Tietze's is considered in the differential diagnosis.

TUMORS

■ Breast Tumor

Chief Clinical Characteristics

This presentation is usually characterized by initial report of a nonpainful palpable firm, irregular mass in the breast, which is the most common presentation of breast cancer. Reports of shoulder pain, deep bone pain, and jaundice or weight loss are less commonly seen as the initial presentation.

Background Information

The onset of aching pain in the shoulder with difficulty sleeping may be an indication of metastases to the lymph or osseous structures of the shoulder. Upper extremity edema is rarely seen as an initial sign. Blood tests for the markers (carcinoembryonic antigen, ferritin, and human chorionic gonadotropin) have been noted as elevated in as many as 70% of patients with metastasis. Risk factors include female with age greater than 40, personal and family history of cancer, late-onset pregnancy, and early menopause. Breast cancer treatments include needle biopsy, lumpectomy, mastectomy, and lymph node removal. Radiation and chemotherapy with continued and monitored oral medications follow surgical intervention. Early range of motion is recommended to prevent limitations on the involved side during the postsurgical phase.

■ Pancoast Tumor

Chief Clinical Characteristics

This presentation may involve diffuse, sharp pleuretic pain reported in the ipsilateral axillary, shoulder, or subscapular region with possible referred pain to the neck. Each of these symptoms may be the initial presenting symptom. Clinical findings also include shoulder-arm pain, Horner's syndrome, and neurological deficits affecting the C8 and T1 nerve roots.[36] Risk factors include smoking, exposure to secondary smoke, prolonged asbestos exposure, and exposure to industrial elements.[37] Absence of breath sounds over the affected lung and absence of pulmonary air in the lobe of the affected lung via radiograph are primary methods of diagnosis.

Background Information

True Pancoast tumors originate in the extrathoracic space with lysis at the ribs evident via anteroposterior cervical radiographs.[38] The tumor typically also invades the apex of the affected lung, lower brachial plexus, first ribs, vertebrae, and vessels.[39] However, primary lung tumors and abscesses in the superior thoracic sulcus also may mimic this condition by invading or impinging the subclavian space.[38] Palliative radiotherapy may produce pain relief at the shoulder.[40] Preoperative radiation, chemotherapy with excision, and follow-up treatment are typical.

ULCERS

■ Duodenal Ulcer

Chief Clinical Characteristics

This presentation can involve gnawing, dull, or aching pain in the supraclavicular area on the right (see Fig. 11-1). Similar pain may also be present in the midscapular region or in the epigastric region.[41]

Background Information

An ulcer may become more symptomatic, that is, with greater incidence of referred pain to the shoulder, following perforation into the subdiaphragmatic region. Ulcers develop when the lining of the digestive tract is exposed to acids. Specifically, duodenal ulcers are caused by *Helicobacter pylori* bacteria in the stomach. The onset of symptoms will coincide when the stomach is empty and will temporarily resolve with eating or taking of antacids. The reproduction of symptoms will not be demonstrated through range of motion in the shoulder or scapula. Treatment is typically pharmacologic.

■ Gastric Ulcer

Chief Clinical Characteristics

This presentation may most commonly involve aching pain at the "tip" of the on the left shoulder,[42] although this symptom is rare as an initial presentation (see Fig. 11-1). Pain also may be present in the interscapular region, anterior chest, or into the facial region.[41] The onset of symptoms differs from duodenal ulcers in that with a gastric ulcer symptoms may coincide with when the stomach is full rather than empty. The reproduction of symptoms will not be demonstrated through range of motion in the shoulder or scapula.

Background Information

An ulcer may become more symptomatic, that is, with greater incidence of referred pain to the shoulder, following perforation into the subdiaphragmatic region. Ulcers develop when the lining of the digestive tract is exposed to acids. This condition may be secondary to bacteria or due to malignancy. Treatment is typically pharmacologic after exploring the underlying etiology.

■ Upper Extremity Deep Venous Thrombosis (UEDVT; Includes Paget-Schroetter Syndrome)

Chief Clinical Characteristics

This presentation may include pain in the shoulder, neck, or upper extremity. Swelling, discoloration, tenderness, and venous distention may be present. It may mimic a muscular strain or it may be completely asymptomatic.[43]

Background Information

Subclavian vessels are the most commonly affected with axillary and brachial vessels next in the order of frequency.[43] Primary forms of this condition include idiopathic and Paget-Schroetter syndrome or "effort" thrombosis. "Effort" thrombosis is typically seen in healthy young men with overdeveloped scalene musculature,[43] which compresses the subclavian vein during overexertion, leading to thrombosis development. Secondary forms of this condition account for the majority of episodes. Age greater than 50, diseased state, and a slightly elevated risk for females may be included in the epidemiology.[43] Risk factors include cancer, central venous catheters, anatomical abnormalities, recent trauma, acquired hypercoagulable states, and spontaneous events. Diagnosis is via noninvasive techniques. One serious complication is pulmonary embolus. Suspicion of thrombosis should be considered an emergent referral.

Local

■ Adhesive Capsulitis (Frozen Shoulder)

Chief Clinical Characteristics

This condition presents as insidious and painful loss of both active and passive range of motion in a capsular pattern. There are two types: if not associated with a traumatic event, then it is considered primary adhesive capsulitis; if associated with a traumatic or surgical event, then it is considered secondary adhesive capsulitis. Initial presentation mimics subacromial impingement syndrome.

Background Information

Females are more affected than males with the dominant arm most involved. Other associated factors include age greater than 40, trauma, prolonged immobilization, diabetes, thyroid disorders, autoimmune disorders, and stroke/myocardial infarction.[44] Diagnosis may include imaging, exploratory arthroscopic procedure, and blood panel. Pathology of the midshaft of the humerus has been known to be associated and must be excluded.[45] Etiology remains unknown. Staging of the condition is important for determination of treatment though both operative and nonoperative treatment remain controversial.

■ Amyloid Arthropathy

Chief Clinical Characteristics

This presentation involves the presence of the "shoulder pad" sign, which is localized anterior swelling at the shoulder. This sign is pathognomic for the rare disorder of amyloidosis. There may be associated shoulder pain and functional limitation with systemic signs and symptoms of fatigue, edema, and weight loss.

Background Information

Amyloidosis is a deposit of insoluble fragments of a protein in tissues and may affect nerves, muscles, and ligaments. Underlying disease processes may include renal insufficiency, cardiomyopathy, hepatomegaly, peripheral neuropathy, and autonomic failure.[46] Biochemical analysis of blood is required for diagnosis.

■ Aneurysm

Chief Clinical Characteristics

This presentation can include localized shoulder pain and neuropathic or myopathic symptoms either with or without functional limitations; the distribution of symptoms depends on the affected artery.[5,6] Axillary and subclavian artery aneurysms have been documented to give rise to shoulder pain. Secondary signs may include warmth, redness, and swelling.

Background Information

The potential compression of the brachial plexus or cervical nerve roots or vascular compromise may elicit these associated signs and symptoms. Aneurysms or pseudoaneurysms may be present due to recent surgery, trauma, or iatrogenic complications.[7] The diagnosis is confirmed with arteriography or Doppler ultrasound. This condition typically is managed with surgical procedures such as stenting, the goal of which is to reinforce the structural integrity of the arterial wall.

■ Ankylosing Spondylitis

Chief Clinical Characteristics

This presentation typically includes an insidious onset of shoulder pain associated with a slowly progressive and significant loss of general spinal mobility. Low back symptoms may be worse in the morning and improve with light exercise.

Background Information

This condition is more common in males, as well as people of American indigenous descent, those less than 40 years of age, or those who carry the human leukocyte antigen B27. It also may be associated with fever, malaise, and inflammatory bowel disease. Shoulder joint arthritis may develop during the later stages of the disease in up to 60% of patients.[47] The diagnosis is confirmed with plain radiographs of the sacroiliac joints and lumbar spine, which reveal characteristic findings of sacroiliitis and "bamboo spine." Blood panels including erythrocyte sedimentation rate are useful to track disease activity.

■ Avascular Necrosis of the Humeral Head

Chief Clinical Characteristics

This presentation may include limited motion at the glenohumeral joint, deep joint pain, and increasing pain with motion and time of weight bearing. Such symptoms should lead to suspicion of osteonecrosis. Reports of difficulty sleeping and pain at rest are common.[48] Patients are typically asymptomatic at the shoulder until the later stages of the disease.[49]

Background Information

Associated nontraumatic and traumatic pathologies include proximal humerus trauma, sickle cell disease, history of radiation, Gaucher's disease, dysbaric disorders, alcohol intake, corticosteroid use, or a history of systemic lupus erythematosus. The presence of avascular necrosis in other joints, especially of the hip, are common.[49] Complete blood screen and plain radiographs assist with diagnosis. Nonsurgical treatment is often difficult due to the delayed presentation of the patient for treatment. However, with early diagnosis, rest, immobilization, nonsteroidal anti-inflammatory medication, and therapy are recommended. Surgical management depends on the severity of the destruction.[48,49]

■ Biceps Long Tendon Tear/Rupture

Chief Clinical Characteristics

This presentation may be characterized by pain in the anterior shoulder in middle-aged to older males following heavy lifting or quick onset of an eccentric load. A "pop" may be heard with weakness of supination and elbow flexion noted. Observable distal muscle convexity may be seen due to retraction of the muscle toward the remaining attachment.[50]

Background Information

Risk factors include recurrent biceps tendinitis, anabolic steroid use, age, and heavy lifting.[51] Partial ruptures are rare. Glenohumeral instability and anterior shoulder swelling resulting from complete rupture making the diagnosis more difficult. Ultrasound and magnetic resonance imaging may be utilized to assist with diagnosis. Objective exam techniques such as Speed's test are utilized but are nonspecific.[52] Questions regarding activity level and sport participation may be helpful in determining management. Nonsurgical management is successful for optimizing the surrounding structures for compensation. Surgical management is repair of the tendon.

■ Bursitis (Subdeltoid/ Subacromial)

Chief Clinical Characteristics

This presentation typically includes an insidious onset of pain at the anterior or lateral shoulder. Passive movements are painful especially at the end range of motion into abduction, internal rotation, and horizontal adduction. Active movements typically present with pain during flexion and abduction.

Background Information

Secondary bursitis as a sign of underlying shoulder pathologies is more common than primary. For primary bursitis, typical treatment is a course of local anesthetic injections. For secondary bursitis, treatment consists of treatment of the underlying contributing shoulder pathology.

■ Chronic Fatigue Syndrome

Chief Clinical Characteristics

This presentation is defined as a new onset of unexplained, persistent, or recurrent physical or mental fatigue that substantially reduces activity level, postexertional malaise, and exclusion of other potentially explanatory medical or psychiatric conditions; also requires at least one symptom from two of the following categories: autonomic manifestations, neuroendocrine manifestations, and immune manifestations.[53]

Background Information

Other possible clinical features include pain, which may serve as the chief symptom that directs patients toward physical therapists for management, and sleep dysfunction. This health condition is diagnosed on the basis of clinical examination. There is significant diagnostic overlap with major depression, fibromyalgia, and systemic lupus erythematosus. Optimal treatment includes activity modification and stress management, anaerobic reconditioning, and medication for relief of associated symptomatology.

■ Complex Regional Pain Syndrome (CRPS; Also Reflex Sympathetic Dystrophy, Algodystrophy, Sudeck's Atrophy)

Chief Clinical Characteristics
This presentation may include a "burning or throbbing pain." Symptoms typically manifest in the distal extremity including escalated pain pattern, swelling, autonomic vasomotor dysfunction, and impaired upper extremity function.[54]

Background Information
There are two types of CRPS. Type I is precipitated by a noxious event and Type II occurs specifically from a peripheral nerve injury. The noxious event or nerve injury may occur in the shoulder.[55] Staging of the disorder is according to skin changes, pain response, and edema. The diagnosis is one of exclusion; therefore, competing differential diagnoses must be ruled out. Treatment is nonsurgical for type I; for type II, identification of the underlying peripheral nerve pathology may indicate surgical intervention.[55]

DISLOCATIONS
■ Acromioclavicular Dislocation

Chief Clinical Characteristics
This presentation can involve acute onset of superior lateral shoulder pain with sharp reproduction during attempts of movement. Observable deformity at the acromioclavicular joint and/or clavicle will assist with grading the severity of injury. Mechanisms may include traumatic high-velocity injury in younger patients or older patients with low to moderate velocity injury, such as a fall on an outstretched hand.

Background Information
Grades of injury are from I to VI with progressive involvement of ligamentous, capsular, muscular, bony, and neural structures.

Radiographs are required to confirm the presence of fracture and grade of injury. Grades I and II require immobilization and physical therapy. Grade III may require operative or nonoperative treatment with immobilization and therapy. Grades IV through VI require operative management due to disruption of muscular structures and severity of displacement of the clavicle.

■ Glenohumeral Dislocation

Chief Clinical Characteristics
This presentation may include patients, typically male and in their 20s, who may experience mechanical symptoms along with pain from soft tissue disruption in overhead activities.

Background Information
The injury can occur across the life span, though the soft tissues injured differ. In the adolescent age group, injuries to the glenohumeral ligament and capsular avulsions are more common. In the middle-aged group, rotator cuff pathology is more common.[56] Up to 96% of all dislocations are due to acute trauma to the shoulder.[57] Typically the mechanism is in the anterior direction (98%) secondary to the mechanism of forceful abduction and external rotation.[58] Other mechanisms include a fall on an outstretched arm, traction, or some form of wrenching. Diagnosis is dependent on history exam due to intolerance by the patient for many of the clinical exam procedures following an acute trauma.[59] Imaging may be necessary to detect associated lesions, such as impaction fractures of the humeral head or inferior glenoid surface. Complications include axillary nerve injury or supraspinatus injury. Outcomes of nonsurgical management of unilateral-direction traumatic dislocation in adolescents are typically poor, so surgical intervention is often recommended. Multidirectional instability may be managed nonsurgically initially.[57]

■ Sternoclavicular Dislocation

Chief Clinical Characteristics
This presentation typically involves anterior shoulder pain coupled with the patient's preference toward placing his or her affective upper extremity in a protective posture to avoid

medial clavicle pain. The neck may be postured toward the affected side. Swelling and/or a lump over the joint region is palpated.[60] The patient may have difficulty with lying supine and on the affected shoulder. Atraumatic dislocations typically occur in young females with generalized joint laxity.[61]

Background Information
The mechanism is typically from an acute injury such as a sports injury or motor vehicle accident. Though both are rarely seen, anterior dislocation is of greater prevalence than posterior. Posterior dislocation must be treated as an emergent situation due to the proximity to neurovasculature structures. Once effectively diagnosed via imaging, intervention for a mild to moderate displacement is typically a sling and protective rest. For dislocations, the decision of closed reduction versus surgical intervention may be dependent on the direction of the dislocation.

■ Erb's Palsy
Chief Clinical Characteristics
This presentation may involve shoulder pain secondary to a known neurological injury, possibly occurring at birth, resulting in significant weakness of the shoulder musculature. Adaptive posturing will be present typically of 30 degrees of abduction, flexion, 60 degrees of humeral internal rotation, and potential elbow flexion contracture.[62] Pain and limited function will be present due to secondary osteoarthritis.

Background Information
Resolution of deteriorating function via shoulder arthrodesis is common.

■ Fibromyalgia
Chief Clinical Characteristics
This presentation involves chronic widespread joint and muscle pain defined as bilateral upper body, lower body, and spine pain, associated with tenderness to palpation of 11 of 18 specific muscle-tendon sites.

Background Information
Individuals with this condition will demonstrate lowered mechanical and thermal pain thresholds, high pain ratings for noxious stimuli, and altered temporal summation of pain stimuli.[63] The etiology of this condition is unclear; multiple body systems appear to be involved. Indistinct clinical boundaries between this condition and similar conditions (eg, chronic fatigue syndrome, irritable bowel syndrome, and chronic muscular headaches) pose a diagnostic challenge.[63] This condition is diagnosed by exclusion. Treatment will often include polypharmacy and elements to improve self-efficacy, physical training, and cognitive-behavioral techniques.[64]

FRACTURES
■ Bankart Lesion
Chief Clinical Characteristics
This presentation may be asymptomatic or minimally symptomatic with overhead motions. The patient more typically presents with symptoms of glenohumeral instability secondary to repetitive microtrauma or dislocation.

Background Information
Bankart lesion is a capsular avulsion of the anterior and inferior portions of the labrum. It is strongly associated with traumatic dislocations. A "bony" Bankart lesion is a disruption of the bone of the inferior glenoid rim following a dislocation.[56] Imaging is necessary to diagnose this condition. Repair is considered if surgical intervention is necessary for the treatment of the shoulder dislocation or instability.

■ Bennett Lesion
Chief Clinical Characteristics
This presentation more commonly presents in patients who are male, long-term throwers (ie, baseball pitchers) with posterior shoulder pain during forced extension or with full external rotation and abduction. Pain is absent in daily activities.

Background Information
Failure of nonsurgical management is typical. Diagnosis is difficult because this lesion may be asymptomatic. Etiology is unknown but the biomechanics and mechanical stresses of the throwing arm are suspected. A local anesthetic test with lidocaine injection into the lesion via fluoroscope is assistive in determining symptomatic contribution of the lesion to the shoulder pain. Surgical management with full return to sports should be expected.[65]

■ Clavicle

Chief Clinical Characteristics

This presentation includes immediate pain, inability to move shoulder and possibly the neck with swelling, and observable deformity. Tenting of the skin is commonly seen.[66]

Background Information

In adults, clavicle fractures account for ~10% of all trauma. Grading of the severity of a clavicle fractures is dependent on the degree of displacement, number and severity of the involved ligaments, and the presence of acromioclavicular joint involvement. Open clavicle fractures are uncommon with the risk of pneumothorax at ~3% with high-energy mechanisms of injury. Radiographs are necessary for appropriate diagnosis. Treatment is dependent on the grade of the fracture with complications including delayed healing and nonunion. The majority of clavicle fractures are nondisplaced and managed nonsurgically via a sling or figure-eight harness with therapy to follow the period of immobilization.

■ Hills-Sachs Lesion

Chief Clinical Characteristics

This presentation involves shoulder instability; the lesion itself is typically asymptomatic. Poorly localized shoulder pain, either anterior or posterior, is present, especially with late-phase cocking or the early acceleration phases of throwing or overhead activities.

Background Information

Occurring in approximately 80% of traumatic dislocations, this condition is a compression fracture of the posterolateral corner of the humeral head created when the humeral head passes over the lip of the glenoid.[56] The lesion contributes to instability if greater than 30% of the articular surface is involved.[57] If nonsurgical management fails, then several surgical options are available.

■ Proximal Humerus

Chief Clinical Characteristics

This presentation may be characterized by pain and bony tenderness in the axilla, crepitus, and significant limitation of range of motion. The mechanism of injury is typically

that of a fall.[67] *Incidence increases with age, and women are more affected than men.*[68]

Background Information

Dependent on the severity of the fracture, there may not be observable deformity, necessitating plain radiographs for diagnosis. Neer's classification system assists with determining severity of injury and therefore the appropriate nonsurgical or surgical management.[69] Complications include neurovascular-associated injuries.

■ Scapula

Chief Clinical Characteristics

This condition commonly presents as posterior shoulder pain in patients who hold their involved upper extremity in adduction with severely restricted motion. Weak rotator cuff function may be present, yet tenderness is localized to the scapula. Edema and ecchymosis may be absent. Pain may be present with inspiration due to respiratory muscular attachments. A flattened shoulder is typical of a displaced glenoid neck or acromial fracture.[70]

Background Information

These uncommon injuries are typically seen in males from 20 to 40 years of age due to direct trauma with considerable energy. This condition is often overlooked on initial evaluation, but clinicians are advised that the presence of a scapular fracture should raise the suspicion of associated injuries if not already evident.[70] Complications include pneumothorax, which may be delayed up to 3 days,[65] and associated fractures including of the skull and brachial plexus. Nonsurgical treatment is still preferred despite the advances with open reduction internal fixation procedures.

■ Glenoid Labrum Tears

Chief Clinical Characteristics

This presentation may include poorly localized anterior or posterior pain in the shoulder that may range from constant to episodic and sharp.[51] *It is typically activity-related shoulder pain that increases with overhead motion.*

Background Information

The most common is a superior labrum anteroposterior tear of the labrum. History from the patient should include a description of compressive or traction force on the shoulder. A history of trauma or repetitive overhead motion also may be indicated as the mechanism of injury. The labrum demonstrates increasing degenerative changes with advancing age.[51] It is speculated that there is a strong relationship between underlying glenohumeral instability and labral tears. A variety of clinical examination procedures have been reported but an ideal test remains elusive. Imaging is utilized to assist with diagnosing labral tears. Nonsurgical treatment is successful with the identification of the underlying associated pathologies. Surgical intervention is common if nonsurgical management is unsuccessful.

■ Gout

Chief Clinical Characteristics

This presentation may include mechanical impingement signs, such as sharp pain at the anterior shoulder with movement from 90 to 120 degrees humeral abduction, limited overhead movement, and possible associated rotator cuff tendinitis.[66] Typical patient presentation: male, 40 to 60 years old, obese, probable excessive alcohol intake, with history of gout attacks in other joints. Fever is infrequently present. Local warmth and edema may be present.

Background Information

Gout is the presence of monosodium crystals within the joint or soft tissue. Synovial fluid analysis is critical for an intra-articular differential diagnosis. Diagnosis of a soft tissue lesion is more challenging and may require imaging. This is an unusual presentation of shoulder pain because tophaceous gout is more common in the finger, carpal tunnel, and spine. Management is through urate lowering therapy which includes pharmacology, diet modifications, and treatment of associated impairments due to pain and secondary shoulder impingement.[71]

■ Hereditary Neuralgic Amyotrophy

Chief Clinical Characteristics

This presentation may involve recurrent sudden episodes of pain and weakness in the shoulder girdle. Patients with this condition are typically ages 20 to 40 years. Episodes may be brought on by physical exertion, viral illness, or extreme stress.

Background Information

This condition is a rare autosomal dominant disorder that may affect entire families.[72] Full recovery is expected between episodes; however, it is not uncommon to see residual weakness and atrophy. Two types of this condition have been reported: "classic" relapsing-remitting or chronic undulating with exacerbations. Symptoms may be bilateral or unilateral lasting up to 6 months. Treatment involves self-monitoring.

■ Heterotopic Ossification/Myositis Ossificans

Chief Clinical Characteristics

This presentation may commonly include pain with limited passive and active range of motion with a history of trauma and/or immobilization.

Background Information

Development at the proximal humerus is not atypical following shoulder arthroplasty, but there is significantly less risk than that which is found after lower extremity total joint surgery.[73] Risk factors for development following arthroplasty may include rotator cuff tears.[73] The development of clavicle heterotopic ossification after acromioplasty or resection is associated with patients with a history of chronic pulmonary disease.[74] Surgical management is dependent on level of functional limitation.

IMPINGEMENT SYNDROMES

■ Internal Impingement (Posterior Glenoid Impingement)

Chief Clinical Characteristics

This presentation includes posterior shoulder pain and less commonly joint line pain associated with repetitive positioning of the shoulder into an abducted and externally rotated position. Patients are typically athletes under the age of 40; though there are case reports of internal impingement in the non-athletic population.[75] Progression of symptoms may be acute onset (more common with non-throwers) or insidious (more common with throwers). Jobe[76] classified three stages for presentation: Stage I, reports of stiffness with pain occurring specifically during the late cocking and early acceleration phases; stage II, progression to significant posterior joint-line pain with activity; and stage III, failure to improve with conservative means.

Background Information

The etiology of pain is theorized as being multifactorial and complex with impingement of the undersurface (deep layer) of the posterior supraspinatus tendon and/or the anterior infraspinatus tendon by the posterosuperior glenoid margin. Differential diagnosis should include cervical radiculopathy, neurological conditions, tendinopathy of rotator cuff musculature, and shoulder instability.[77]

■ Subacromial Impingement

Chief Clinical Characteristics

This presentation may be characterized in the earliest stages as sharp episodic pain at the anterolateral acromion with radiating pain to the midlateral humerus. In the later stages, the pain is "toothache like" and the limitations in physical activity are more apparent.[77] Affected demographics are variable for age, severity of functional limitations, and pain reports.

Background Information

With any stage, mechanism is typically of an insidious onset though traumatic onset is possible. Resting pain is not common. Night pain is exacerbated by lying on the shoulder or sleeping with arm overhead and is alleviated by position changes. Overhead activities especially with movements into the frontal plane are commonly limited with an impingement arc present: pain is experienced during 70 to 120 degrees of humeral motion. Pain is generated when the structures beneath the subacromial arch become compressed within the subacromial space. Causative factors may include rotator cuff pathology, degenerative changes of the acromioclavicular joint, or improper temporal sequencing of the scapulothoracic musculature. Differential diagnosis should include cervical radiculopathy, neurological conditions, tendinopathy of rotator cuff musculature, and shoulder instability.[77] Nonsurgical treatment is commonly successful.

JOINT INJURIES

■ Acromioclavicular Sprain

Chief Clinical Characteristics

This presentation involves an acute onset of superior lateral shoulder pain with sharp reproduction during attempts at movement. Observable deformity at the acromioclavicular joint and/or clavicle will assist with grading the severity of injury. Mechanisms may include traumatic high-velocity injury in younger patients or older patients with low- to moderate-velocity injury, such as a fall on an outstretched hand.

Background Information

Grades of injury are from I to VI with progressive involvement of ligamentous, capsular, muscular, bony, and neural structures. Radiographs are required to confirm the presence of fracture and grade of injury. Grades I and II require immobilization and physical therapy. Grade III may be operative or nonoperative treatment with immobilization and therapy. Grades IV through VI require operative management due to disruption of muscular structures and severity of displacement of the clavicle.

■ Glenohumeral Sprain/ Subluxation

Chief Clinical Characteristics

This presentation may involve vague shoulder pain, especially with overhead activities, due to the disruption of the soft tissue structures. If the mechanism is secondary to neurological injury, then the presentation may be of generalized shoulder pain, even at rest.

Background Information

Subluxation is described as minor disruption of the joint where the articular surface remains intact and soft tissues are disrupted.[56] Mechanisms may include trauma to the joint in the younger athletic population or from sustained hemiplegia or spasticity after a stroke. Differential diagnosis should include dislocation, labral pathology, axillary nerve injury, and rotator cuff pathology. Imaging is utilized to exclude associated pathologies including Bennett, Bankart, or superior labrum anterior to posterior lesions. Treatment is determined by the underlying mechanism of the subluxation and may vary significantly from neuromuscular stimulation to the neurologically impaired shoulder to strengthening activities overhead for the athletic shoulder.

■ Sternoclavicular Sprain

Chief Clinical Characteristics

This presentation may include acute onset of medial clavicular pain with possible production of sharp pain with attempts at ipsilateral shoulder girdle motion, sidelying on the affected side, and lying supine. The neck may be postured toward the affected side. Swelling and/or a lump over the joint region may be palpated.[60]

Background Information

The mechanism is typically a sports injury. Once effectively diagnosed via imaging, intervention for a mild to moderate displacement is typically a sling and protective rest.

■ Muscle Strains

Chief Clinical Characteristics

This presentation involves localized pain that is dependent on the location of the muscle affected. Limited active range of motion will be present and may be correlated with the action of the injured muscle. Tenderness with palpation and muscular inhibition upon isometric contraction may be present.

Background Information

The mechanisms of injury include postural dysfunction, repetitive motion, sports activities, or motor vehicle accidents. Examination of proximal structures is necessary to ensure a thorough comprehension of the etiology due to the association between the axial and the scapular musculature. Occurrence in any age group is possible in the event of a recent, finite mechanism of injury. Common sites of muscle strain include the levator scapula, pectoralis major and minor, rotator cuff, and upper trapezius. The diagnosis is confirmed clinically on palpation and resistance testing of the affected muscle. This health condition is addressed nonsurgically with a combination of exercise and anti-inflammatory or analgesic medications.

■ Myofascial Pain Syndrome

Chief Clinical Characteristics

This presentation may include diffuse, deep aching or soreness in the axioscapular muscles. Also included in the presentation are palpable tender taut bands in the muscles and trigger points, paresthesias in the area of trigger points, and weakness of the affected axioscapular muscle.

Background Information

Affected muscles may be sensitive to prolonged activation or passive stretching, creating adaptive shortening over the course of the pathology.[78] Differential diagnosis should include fibromyalgia. Treatment is injection of saline, anesthetic, or Botox into the offending trigger point.[79]

NERVE INJURIES

■ Axillary Nerve Injury

Chief Clinical Characteristics

This presentation can involve shoulder pain with abduction and external rotation or low endurance with overhead activities.[80] Denervation to the teres minor and the deltoid and sensation to the lateral shoulder may or may not be spared.

Background Information

The axillary nerve is most commonly injured during an anterior dislocation of the glenohumeral joint, via fracture of the proximal humerus, due to blunt trauma to the anterolateral deltoid or as a complication of shoulder surgery.[81] Neurological injury is more common in patients greater than 50 years of age or if the shoulder remains dislocated for greater than 12 hours.[82] The axillary nerve is one of the structures implicated in quadrilateral space syndrome secondary to proposed fibrous bands constricting the axillary nerve or less commonly from a space-occupying lesion.[80] Differential diagnosis should include neuralgic amyotrophy, quadrilateral space syndrome, and cervical radiculopathy. For atraumatic injury of the axillary nerve, nonsurgical management should be attempted for 3 months while awaiting the return of muscle function.[80] If there is no clinical or electromyographic evidence of axillary nerve recovery by 3 to 6 months, then surgical intervention is recommended.[82]

■ Spinal Accessory Nerve Trauma

Chief Clinical Characteristics
This presentation may commonly involve shoulder pain, scapular winging, depressed shoulder girdle, and limitations in shoulder range of motion. These characteristics are typical following traumatic disruption of the spinal accessory nerve affecting the function of the trapezius.[83]

Background Information
Mechanisms of injury include direct trauma to the nerve, shoulder, or neck or neurapraxia from surgical intervention. Manual muscle testing and electromyographic testing of the trapezius muscle will reveal weakness. Associated symptoms may include subacromial impingement, neck pain, and tendinopathy due to the inadequate scapulothoracic muscular sequencing of the shoulder. Identification of muscular weakness and determination of its cause guide treatment and prognosis.

■ Suprascapular Nerve Injury

Chief Clinical Characteristics
This presentation may include deep, poorly localized shoulder pain with muscular wasting of the infraspinatus or supraspinatus.

Background Information
Patient will demonstrate inadequate strength into abduction and external rotation of the shoulder. Irritation or compression of the nerve most frequently occurs at the suprascapular foramen, affecting the supraspinatus and the infraspinatus. However, isolated muscle involvement may occur via impingement at the spinoglenoid notch or various presentations from microtrauma, repetitive trauma, or distal trauma to the upper extremity. The injury may be due to a compression lesion, trauma, the presence of a lipoma, or neuritis. Electromyographic studies may be used to determine the extent of the injury and the potential for recovery.[84] Anterior lesions most commonly affect the supraspinatus, and the posterior lesions affect the infraspinatus. The etiology must be determined for the best outcomes.

■ Neuralgic Amyotrophy (Parsonage-Turner Syndrome)

Chief Clinical Characteristics
This presentation can involve sudden acute onset of burning and severe pain at the shoulder and into the upper arm with unknown etiology. This pain resolves and precedes the weakness in the shoulder and shoulder girdle due to denervation of the muscles.[85]

Background Information
The deltoid, infraspinatus, and supraspinatus are typically affected with serratus anterior involvement as noted by scapular winging. Progression of symptoms may be within days or weeks. Relatively uncommon, this health condition affects males more often than females and occurs primarily between 20 and 60 years of age. Acute brachial neuritis is of unknown etiology, although hereditary, viral, infectious, and immune causes are being investigated.[85] It is often misdiagnosed and cervical spine radiculopathy must be considered as a differential diagnosis. Electrodiagnostic testing will be assistive in localizing to the brachial plexus, and magnetic resonance imaging may reveal edema within the involved musculature.[86] Gradual improvement occurs over 3 to 4 months with pharmacologic management and physical therapy.

■ Neuropathic Arthropathy (Charcot-Marie-Tooth Disease)

Chief Clinical Characteristics
This presentation may be characterized by generalized pain, burning, paresthesia, swelling, and functional limitation of the involved joint. The symptoms may progress over several months or years.

Background Information
Typical onset of symptoms is a benign or unrelated mechanism of injury. Neuropathic arthropathy is a destructive joint disease with decreased sensory innervation and proprioception to the involved joint. Pathogenesis remains controversial, involving potential neurovascular, neurotrophic, or central nervous system pathology. Syringomyelia with or without complication of Arnold-Chiari malformation is a likely underlying contribution to neuropathic arthropathy at the shoulder and elbow.[87] Diagnosis requires imaging and follow-up for the destruction of the joint. Treatment is based

on the discovery of the underlying causative factor of the destruction of the joint.

OSTEOARTHROSIS/ OSTEOARTHRITIS

■ Acromioclavicular Joint

Chief Clinical Characteristics
This presentation involves localized tenderness, pain, or aching in the lateral deltoid region with overhead activities and/or shoulder adduction. There may be reports of difficulty lying in an ipsilateral side-lying position. A history of heavy lifting or repetitive overhead activity may be present.

Background Information
Radiographic evidence may not match the clinical picture.[88] Treatment focuses on resolution of impairments such as posture, including shoulder girdle position and axioscapular strength.

■ Glenohumeral Joint

Chief Clinical Characteristics
This presentation may include insidious onset of shoulder pain and progressive loss of range of motion, most commonly in an older individual. Marked loss of external rotation typically is present. Disuse atrophy of the rotator cuff may also be present.

Background Information
Radiographs provide evidence of the destructive pattern of posterior glenoid erosion and central baldness of the humeral cartilage.[89] Nonsurgical and surgical treatments exist for this health condition.

■ Secondary Osteoarthritis/ Osteoarthrosis of the Glenohumeral Joint

Chief Clinical Characteristics
This presentation commonly involves shoulder pain ranging from mild to severe in the presence of a contributory event, such as a history of significant trauma and/or surgical intervention. This health condition is typically associated with a younger patient population than primary osteoarthritis/ osteoarthrosis. As is true in primary osteoarthritis/osteoarthrosis, significant stiffness and the loss of active/passive range of motion is seen on physical exam.[89]

Background Information
Nonsurgical and surgical treatments exist for this health condition.

■ Sternoclavicular

Chief Clinical Characteristics
This presentation may commonly range from absence of pain to possible localized tenderness to mild aching pain typically of insidious onset with female patients age 40 or older. Swelling may be present over the joint and may go unnoticed by the patient. Aggravating factors may be ipsilateral shoulder motion. Other joints will not be affected and radiographic evidence may not match the clinical picture.[33]

Background Information
Treatment focuses on resolution of impairments such as posture, including shoulder girdle position.

■ Osteomyelitis

Chief Clinical Characteristics
This presentation involves pain, as well as limited motion of the shoulder with or without warmth or swelling. Up to 50% of patients with this health condition may present with nausea, anorexia, and night sweats.[90]

Background Information
Though primarily a condition in childhood, it may affect drug abusers or adults with sickle cell disease or may follow intensive surgery. Diagnosis may be delayed for several months.[90] Blood tests, aspiration biopsies, and imaging assist with diagnosis. Treatment is dependent on the offending organism and may include pharmacologic or operative intervention.

■ Polymyalgia Rheumatica

Chief Clinical Characteristics
This presentation typically includes aching and stiffness at the bilateral shoulder joints with radiating pain distally into the elbows. Patients with this condition are typically over the age of 50 years with a peak incidence at age 70 to 80 years. Involvement of the pelvis and hips is typical with similar symptoms of aching/ stiffness with radiation of pain into the knees. Distal pitting edema and asymmetric peripheral arthritis are less typical.

Background Information
The stiffness will require greater than 1 hour to resolve and is typical in the morning. Both

passive and active range of motion will be restricted at the involved shoulder(s) due to pain. Imaging studies reveal a greater appearance of subacromial or subdeltoid bursitis rather than synovitis of the glenohumeral joint. This is an inflammatory condition of unknown etiology with a suspicion of environmental and genetic causes. An erythrocyte sedimentation rate greater than 40 mm/hr, imaging studies to detect the synovitis, and a rapid response to corticosteroids combined with the clinical presentation above assist with the differential diagnosis.[91]

■ Pseudogout (Calcium Pyrophosphate Dihydrate Deposition Disease)

Chief Clinical Characteristics
This presentation may involve episodic aching and limited mobility of the shoulder without a specific mechanism of injury. This condition is most common in women and with advancing age.

Background Information
The shoulder may be the first affected joint. Causes for the contributory calcium pyrophosphate crystal deposition in synovial joints are unknown. Diagnosis is based on the clinical presentation, the pattern of joints involved, radiographic intra-articular and periarticular involvement, and aspiration of calcium pyrophosphate crystals in the joint fluid.[92] Anti-inflammatory medication comprises the usual treatment for this condition. Unlike gout, uric acid–lowering medications are not used.

■ Quadrilateral Space Syndrome

Chief Clinical Characteristics
This presentation will include poorly localized shoulder pain with paresthesias in the involved extremity in a nondermatomal pattern. Weakness may be of sudden onset with episodic history of shoulder pain. Commonly, abduction and external rotation of the shoulder are the actions affected.

Background Information
The proposed etiology of quadrilateral space syndrome is vascular occlusion or compression of the posterior circumflex humeral artery and the axillary nerve possibly due to fibrous bands, scarring, or adhesions. This results in atrophy and denervation of the teres minor with or without deltoid involvement.[81] This uncommon injury is difficult to diagnose clinically and is frequently misdiagnosed as rotator cuff pathology or impingement syndrome. Electromyography and magnetic resonance imaging are the recommended diagnostic tests. Nonsurgical treatment is the initial plan of care with surgical intervention recommended only for those with long-term pathology.[81]

■ Reiter's Syndrome

Chief Clinical Characteristics
This presentation may involve acute onset with pain and swelling in an asymmetric multiple-joint pattern. Prolonged stiffness following inactivity is a common complaint for any of the involved joints.

Background Information
This condition is rarely present in the shoulder, except possibly in the advanced stages of the disease. This syndrome is a combination of four syndromes: peripheral arthritis syndrome, painful bone syndrome, back and pelvis pain, and intestinal and/or genitourinary symptoms. Asymmetrical arthritis of the lower extremity with urethritis and conjunctivitis often occurs early in the disease. Typically males are affected more commonly than females. A history of infection (venereal or dysenteric) is associated with increased risk. Range-of-motion exercises and stretching are emphasized along with nonsteroidal anti-inflammatory medications. Rest/immobilization is discouraged.[93]

■ Rheumatoid Arthritis

Chief Clinical Characteristics
This presentation is characterized by an insidious onset of transitory pain and stiffness in the shoulder. Long-duration stiffness is especially prevalent in the morning. Shoulder pain is rarely the first report of pain in individuals presenting with this condition.

Background Information
Protective posturing of the upper extremity in internal rotation held against the stomach is common. Females are more affected than males with a peak age of 35 to 45 years. Criteria for diagnosis of this condition include prolonged morning stiffness, soft tissue swelling,

symmetric arthritis, subcutaneous nodules, positive rheumatoid factor, and/or radiographic evidence. The four types of shoulder involvement in rheumatoid arthritis are dry, wet, resorptive, and bursal. Treatment should be tailored to the patient and their symptoms, but usually includes steroidal, nonsteroidal, or biological anti-inflammatory medications.

RHEUMATOID–LIKE HEALTH CONDITIONS

■ Dermatomyositis

Chief Clinical Characteristics
This presentation involves myalgia coupled with a significant decline in function such as difficulty standing from a chair, stepping off curbs, and performing overhead activities of daily living. A skin rash most commonly precedes the muscular manifestations and may be present on the eyelids, in a V sign or a shawl sign.[94] The heliotrope rash is present in 25% of cases, and in 30% of cases, lesions appear on the metacarpophalangeal, proximal, and distal interphalangeal joints.[95] Sensation remains normal and deep tendon reflexes are rarely affected early in the disease.

Background Information
This condition affects women more frequently than men. Though considered rare, dermatomyositis is the most common of the idiopathic inflammatory diseases. It is a multisystem autoimmune disease characterized by inflammation of the muscles and the skin and is similar in presentation to polymyositis. Diagnosis may be via several different tests such as electromyographic studies, laboratory tests, and muscle biopsy.[95] Treatment is pharmacologic.

■ Polymyositis

Chief Clinical Characteristics
This presentation includes a gradual onset of mild muscle pain in the shoulder girdle and other proximal muscles, associated with proximal muscle weakness that causes difficulty with daily activities such as walking, ascending and descending stairs, and rising from chairs.

Background Information
Although proximal extremity weakness is a classic finding, up to 50% also demonstrate distal weakness that may be equally as severe.[96] Blood panels help confirm the diagnosis and track disease activity, revealing elevated serum levels of creatine phosphokinase. Treatment typically involves steroidal, nonsteroidal, and biological anti-inflammatory medications.

■ Psoriatic Arthritis

Chief Clinical Characteristics
This presentation may involve an insidious onset of lumbopelvic and hip pain associated with psoriasis. The severity of arthritis is uncorrelated with the extent of skin involvement.[28] Pitting nail lesions occur in 80% of individuals with this condition. Dactylitis, tenosynovitis, and peripheral arthritis also are common.

Background Information
Radiographs of the distal phalanges may reveal a characteristic "pencil in cup" deformity. Blood panels including erythrocyte sedimentation rate are useful to track disease activity.

■ Scleroderma

Chief Clinical Characteristics
This presentation typically includes myalgia, arthralgia, fatigue, weight loss, limited mobility, and hardened skin about the hands, knees, or elbows. This condition occurs in individuals between 25 and 55 years of age, and is four to five times more likely in women than men. Additional symptoms may include dry mouth and eyes, as well as Raynaud's phenomenon.

Background Information
This rare and progressive autoimmune disorder affects blood vessels and many internal organs, including the lungs and the gastrointestinal system. Overproduction of collagen in this condition eventually leads to poor blood flow in the extremities, which can cause ulcers in the fingers, changes in skin color, and a disappearance of creases in the skin. Continued damage to small-diameter vasculature leads to scar tissue production that impairs joint range of motion. Blood tests confirm the diagnosis. Treatment includes both steroidal

and nonsteroidal anti-inflammatory medications and gentle exercise.

■ Systemic Lupus Erythematosus

Chief Clinical Characteristics
This presentation can include lower back pain radiating to the hip and groin and is associated with fatigue and joint pain/swelling affecting the hands, feet, knees, and shoulders.

Background Information
This condition affects mostly women of childbearing age. It is a chronic autoimmune disorder that can affect any organ system, including skin, joints, kidneys, brain, heart, lungs, and blood. The diagnosis is confirmed by the presence of skin lesions; heart, lung, or kidney involvement; and laboratory abnormalities including low red or white cell counts, low platelet counts, or positive antinuclear antibody and anti-DNA antibody tests.[29]

■ Rotator Cuff Tear

Chief Clinical Characteristics
This presentation may involve weakness, posterior atrophy over the involved muscle, and pain at the lateral brachium with attempts at movement. Night pain, mechanical impingement signs, and crepitus are common.

Background Information
Reaching overhead in the frontal plane and with a long lever arm may be most significantly affected. Age-related changes in the tissue predispose the rotator cuff to tears on the articular side. Severity of involvement may be noted via radiographs or computed tomography. Nonsurgical management may return full patient function. Surgical management and preferred technique are dependent on surgeon skill and number of tendons involved.

■ Septic Arthritis

Chief Clinical Characteristics
This presentation may involve a primary report of limited range of motion at the shoulder because an absence of pain as the primary complaint is not uncommon. Local signs of infection will be present. A low-grade or transient fever may occur in anywhere from 40% to 90% of the cases. During the acute phase, the patient might note incapacitating shoulder pain with fever and chills.

Background Information
This is the most common of the septic inflammatory causes of shoulder pain. A blood culture will be positive in 50% of the cases. This infection can be caused by dissemination from a different organ system with such examples including skin breakdown, urinary tract infection, or pneumonia. Comorbidities that may be associated with spontaneous septic arthritis include a prosthetic joint, cancer, cirrhosis, rheumatoid arthritis, impaired immune system, diabetes, or the presence of indwelling intravenous or catheter lines. This is typically a disease of the older patient with primary shoulder sepsis occurring in between 10% and 15% of all joint infections. Clinical presentation and subjective questioning must assist with differentiating a soft tissue lesion from infection.

■ Skeletal Tuberculosis (Pott's Disease)

Chief Clinical Characteristics
This presentation is characterized by limited range of motion, pain, and the presence of a soft tissue abscess. Typically there is an absence of constitutional symptoms.[97]

Background Information
Erythrocyte sedimentation levels may be elevated, although the tuberculosis skin test may be negative. A history of trauma may be present. Osteomyelitis and osteoarticular forms of this condition are seldom separated in the literature. Peripheral referral is uncommon though if affected the shoulder is more common than other joints of the upper extremity. Diagnosis is accomplished via blood value tests, chest x-ray, and local imaging. Surgical management includes debridement.[97]

TENDINOPATHIES

■ Biceps Long Tendinitis

Chief Clinical Characteristics
This presentation can involve aggravating activities of lifting, pulling, and reaching with pain and tenderness to palpation at the anterior shoulder at the level of the bicipital groove.

Background Information

This inflammatory condition typically results from repetitive activities and may be associated with poor mechanics. This condition is often diagnosed as subacromial impingement syndrome. Diagnosis is typically based on the clinical exam including special orthopedic tests that have a low specificity. The nonoperative management of this condition focuses on optimizing shoulder function and decreasing the local inflammatory response.

■ Biceps Long Tendinosis

Chief Clinical Characteristics

This presentation may include aggravating activities of lifting, pulling, and reaching with pain and tenderness to palpation at the anterior shoulder at the level of the bicipital groove. Patient may report a history of episodic discomfort with waxing/waning periods increasing in frequency. Physical exam will not reveal local warmth or swelling over the tendon.

Background Information

This condition is often diagnosed as subacromial impingement syndrome. Diagnosis is based on the clinical exam including special orthopedic tests that have a low specificity, especially in determination of tendinosis versus tendinitis. The goal of nonsurgical management is optimization of shoulder function and a decrease in the local inflammatory response.

■ Calcific Tendinopathy

Chief Clinical Characteristics

This presentation may commonly include pain and limited range of motion. These characteristics are present in approximately 50% of the patients affected by calcific tendinitis in the shoulder. This condition typically occurs in the fourth decade.

Background Information

The supraspinatus tendon is theorized to be primarily affected by hypoperfusion of the musculotendinous junction. Differential diagnosis should include rotator cuff pathology. Evidence does support the use of ultrasound as a successful therapeutic treatment.[98]

■ Rotator Cuff Tendinitis

Chief Clinical Characteristics

This presentation may involve weakness, atrophy, palpatory tenderness over the involved tendon, and pain at the lateral brachium, night pain, painful arc of movement between 80 and 120 degrees of upper extremity elevation, and crepitus.[99]

Background Information

Functional overhead activities are often difficult and lead to increased pain. Tenderness to palpation is most frequently over the supraspinatus musculotendinous junction. Athletes or manual laborers in the fourth to seventh decade of life are most commonly affected. Imaging studies are helpful to determine if a tear is present. Limitation in motion may be present, although strength may be preserved or inhibited by pain. Underlying laxity should be ruled out in the younger population. Initially, nonsurgical management is attempted. Failure following 6 to 9 months of treatment may suggest the need to evaluate the patient for surgical management.[100]

■ Rotator Cuff Tendinosis

Chief Clinical Characteristics

This presentation can include weakness, atrophy, pain at the lateral brachium, night pain, painful arc of movement between 80 and 120 degrees of upper extremity elevation, crepitus, and less frequently tenderness to palpation of the involved tendon.[99]

Background Information

Functional overhead activities are often limited with reports of pain or weakness. Athletes or manual laborers in the fourth to seventh decade of life are most commonly affected. Imaging studies are helpful to determine if a tear is present. Limitation in motion may be present, although strength may be preserved or inhibited by pain. Underlying laxity should be ruled out in the younger population. Initially, nonsurgical management is attempted. Failure following 6 to 9 months of treatment may suggest the need to evaluate the patient for surgical management.[100]

TUMORS

■ Chondrosarcoma

Chief Clinical Characteristics

This presentation may involve shoulder pain and restricted motion located in various areas of the proximal humerus in a middle-aged patient. A nonpainful mass may be the initial presenting sign.

Background Information

Tapping along the bone appears to be sensitive to prediction of neoplasm along with a more significant score for fatigue and low energy.[101] This condition is caused by a slow growing and destructive primary bone tumor. Abnormal findings in radiographic images should increase suspicion. Intra-articular invasion should be suspected until proven otherwise. Preoperative chemotherapy and radiation are used to reduce tumor size with resection afterward.

■ Enchondroma

Chief Clinical Characteristics

This presentation may involve pain that is unassociated with the lesion itself, since the lesion is typically asymptomatic. Yet association of pain with this type of lesion needs to be explored for potential malignancy. Loss of range of motion and night pain are not consistently present.

Background Information

This condition is most common during the third decade of life. Treatment involves surgical excision after detection.

■ Lipoma

Chief Clinical Characteristics

This presentation can include a small, mobile, and palpable mass if superficial; however, these are typically intramuscular, smaller than 5 cm, and asymptomatic.

Background Information

Lipomas are commonly present in the trunk, shoulder, and upper arm.[102] Any lack of range of motion or production of pain may be due to invasion of the joint space or extra-articular block of motion. Surgical removal is successful as a treatment; however, these lesions may recur.

■ Lung Tumor

Chief Clinical Characteristics

This presentation may be characterized by shoulder pain associated with changes in function, shortness of breath, and probable Horner's sign.

Background Information

Symptoms may be associated with direct extension of the tumor into the ribs and soft tissues or bones of the shoulder girdle; however, there are some reports of shoulder pain without evidence of direct extension of the tumor into the shoulder region.[40] Typical treatment includes a combination of radiation, chemotherapy, and surgical excision of the tumor.

■ Metastases, Including From Primary Breast, Kidney, Lung, Prostate, and Thyroid Disease

Chief Clinical Characteristics

This presentation typically includes unremitting pain in individuals with the risk factors of previous history of cancer, age 50 years or older, failure to improve with conservative therapy, and unexplained weight change of more than 10 pounds in 6 months.[103]

Background Information

The skeletal system is the third most common site of metastatic disease.[104] Symptoms also may be related to pathological fracture in affected sites. Common primary sites causing metastases to bone include breast, prostate, lung, and kidney. Bone scan confirms the diagnosis.

■ Osteoblastoma

Chief Clinical Characteristics

This presentation may include pain and limited shoulder range of motion. Night pain is typically present.

Background Information

Often termed a *giant osteoid osteoma*, this is a rare primary bone tumor that may reoccur after treatment. Differential diagnosis is difficult to distinguish from a low-grade osteosarcoma until surgical excision and biopsy confirm the diagnosis.[105] Surgical management is typical.

■ Osteochondroma

Chief Clinical Characteristics

This presentation may involve shoulder pain, limited range of motion, and crepitus in skeletally immature and young adults with presentation of an enlarging mass. Pain may be present with palpation.

Background Information

Onset of neuropathic symptoms preceded by upper extremity exercise have been reported in case studies as the precipitating event of discovery of the osteochondroma.[106] Though most typical in the proximal humerus, it is the most common tumor of the scapula.[107] Surgical interventions have been successful in resolution of patient symptoms.

■ Osteoid Osteoma

Chief Clinical Characteristics

This presentation involves shoulder pain and limited motion. Night pain is typically present (80% of time) and is alleviated by salicylates. Soft tissue edema and effusion may also be present.[108]

Background Information

Osteoid osteomas are typically found in the long bones of the lower extremities, but may be found in the shoulder including the flat bone of the scapula, though their presence is rare.[108] Imaging should detect the presence of the nidus in the majority of patients. The diagnosis may be confused with nonspecific arthritis if the nidus is not detected on the imaging.[109] Surgical management is typical.

■ Osteosarcoma

Chief Clinical Characteristics

This presentation typically involves generalized shoulder pain, tenderness along bone shaft, and advanced patient age with limited shoulder motion. A nonpainful mass may be initial presenting sign.

Background Information

Of greatest significance is the tenderness along the bone and the age of the patient for the possibility of malignancy.[110] Though seen in the scapula and distal clavicle, osteosarcomas are more commonly seen in the proximal humerus. Abnormal findings in radiographic images should increase

suspicion. Intra-articular invasion should be suspected until proven otherwise. Preoperative chemotherapy and radiation are used to reduce tumor size with resection afterward.

■ Unicameral Bone Cyst

Chief Clinical Characteristics

This presentation may include an acute onset of arm pain with inadequate range of motion secondary to the pain. A mass or tenderness to palpation may not be present.[110]

Background Information

This condition is defined as a fluid-filled lesion in the proximal humerus that is generally considered benign despite typical reoccurrence following surgical removal. Radiographs and biopsy of tissue are necessary to confirm diagnosis and rule out more aggressive forms of cancer. Surgical removal is typically recommended.

References

1. Strasberg SM. Clinical practice. Acute calculous cholecystitis. *N Engl J Med.* Jun 26, 2008;358(26):2804–2811.
2. Gharaibeh KI, Al-Jaberi TM. Bupivacaine instillation into gallbladder bed after laparoscopic cholecystectomy: does it decrease shoulder pain? *J Laparoendosc Adv Surg Tech A.* Jun 2000;10(3):137–141.
3. Chen W, Woods SL, Puntillo KA. Gender differences in symptoms associated with acute myocardial infarction: a review of the research. *Heart Lung.* Jul–Aug 2005; 34(4):240–247.
4. Carter T, Brooks CA. Pericarditis: inflammation or infarction? *J Cardiovasc Nurs.* Jul–Aug 2005;20(4): 239–244.
5. Azzarone M, Cento M, Gobbi S, Tecchio T, Piazza P, Salcuni PF. Neuropathy as the only symptom of common carotid artery spontaneous rupture. Case report. *J Cardiovasc Surg (Torino).* Dec 2003;44(6):767–769.
6. Gupta S, Lee DC, Goldstein RS, Villani R. Axillary artery aneurysm. *J Emerg Med.* Feb 2005;28(2):215–216.
7. Tripp HF, Cook JW. Axillary artery aneurysms. *Mil Med.* Sep 1998;163(9):653–655.
8. McEwan J, Basha S, Rogers S, Harkness P. An unusual presentation of cat-scratch disease. *J Laryngol Otol.* Oct 2001;115(10):826–828.
9. Garvey J, Joyce MR, Khan F, et al. Axillary lymphadenopathy secondary to cat-scratch disease. *Ir Med J.* Sep 2005;98(8):243–244.
10. Roh JS, Teng AL, Yoo JU, Davis J, Furey C, Bohlman HH. Degenerative disorders of the lumbar and cervical spine. *Orthop Clin North Am.* Jul 2005;36(3):255–262.
11. Curry WT, Jr., Hoh BL, Amin-Hanjani S, Eskandar EN. Spinal epidural abscess: clinical presentation, management, and outcome. *Surg Neurol.* Apr 2005;63(4): 364–371; discussion 371.
12. Penfold CN, Revington PJ. A review of 23 patients with tuberculosis of the head and neck. *Br J Oral Maxillofac Surg.* Dec 1996;34(6):508–510.

13. Kanlikama M, Mumbuc S, Bayazit Y, Sirikci A. Management strategy of mycobacterial cervical lymphadenitis. *J Laryngol Otol*. Apr 2000;114(4):274–278.

14. Rao R. Neck pain, cervical radiculopathy, and cervical myelopathy: pathophysiology, natural history, and clinical evaluation. *Instr Course Lect*. 2003;52:479–488.

15. Chiamvimonvat V, Sternberg L. Coronary artery disease in women. *Can Fam Physician*. Dec 1998;44:2709–2717.

16. Gregory PL, Biswas AC, Batt ME. Musculoskeletal problems of the chest wall in athletes. *Sports Med*. 2002;32(4):235–250.

17. Bildik F, Demircan A, Keles A, Pamukcu G, Biri A, Bildik E. Heterotopic pregnancy presenting with acute left chest pain. *Am J Emerg Med*. Sep 2008;26(7):835 e831–832.

18. Scawn ND, Pennefather SH, Soorae A, Wang JY, Russell GN. Ipsilateral shoulder pain after thoracotomy with epidural analgesia: the influence of phrenic nerve infiltration with lidocaine. *Anesth Analg*. Aug 2001;93(2): 260–264.

19. Goodman CC, Snyder TEK. *Differential Diagnosis in Physical Therapy*. 3rd ed. Philadelphia, PA: Saunders; 2000.

20. Werne C, Ulreich S. An unusual presentation of spontaneous pneumomediastinum. *Ann Emerg Med*. Oct 1985;14(10):1010–1013.

21. Taylor FC, Frankl HD, Riemer KD. Late presentation of splenic trauma after routine colonoscopy. *Am J Gastroenterol*. Apr 1989;84(4):442–443.

22. Reginato AJ, Falasca GF, Pappu R, McKnight B, Agha A. Musculoskeletal manifestations of osteomalacia: report of 26 cases and literature review. *Semin Arthritis Rheum*. Apr 1999;28(5):287–304.

23. Eisenberg E, Konopniki M, Veitsman E, Kramskay R, Gaitini D, Baruch Y. Prevalence and characteristics of pain induced by percutaneous liver biopsy. *Anesth Analg*. May 2003;96(5):1392–1396.

24. Piscaglia F, Vidili G, Ugolini G, et al. Fitz-Hugh–Curtis-syndrome mimicking acute cholecystitis: value of new ultrasound findings in the differential diagnosis. *Ultraschall Med*. Jun 2005;26(3):227–230.

25. Sarwar A, Dellaripa PF, Beamis JF, Jr. A 51-year-old man with fever, ulnar neuropathy, and bilateral pleural effusions. *Chest*. Oct 1999;116(4): 1105–1107.

26. Head K, Jurenka JS. Inflammatory bowel disease. Part II: Crohn's disease—pathophysiology and conventional and alternative treatment options. *Altern Med Rev*. Dec 2004;9(4):360–401.

27. Hendrickson BA, Gokhale R, Cho JH. Clinical aspects and pathophysiology of inflammatory bowel disease. *Clin Microbiol Rev*. Jan 2002;15(1):79–94.

28. Kataria RK, Brent LH. Spondyloarthropathies. *Am Fam Physician*. Jun 15, 2004;69(12):2853–2860.

29. Fauci AS, Haynes B, Katz P. The spectrum of vasculitis: clinical, pathologic, immunologic and therapeutic considerations. *Ann Intern Med*. Nov 1978;89(5, pt 1): 660–676.

30. Johnson JD, Raff MJ, Barnwell PA, Chun CH. Splenic abscess complicating infectious endocarditis. *Arch Intern Med*. May 1983;143(5):906–912.

31. Karas SE. Thoracic outlet syndrome. *Clin Sports Med*. Apr 1990;9(2):297–310.

32. Huang JH, Zager EL. Thoracic outlet syndrome. *Neurosurgery*. Oct 2004;55(4):897–902; discussion 902–893.

33. Hiramuro-Shoji F, Wirth MA, Rockwood CA, Jr. Atraumatic conditions of the sternoclavicular joint. *J Shoulder Elbow Surg*. Jan–Feb 2003;12(1):79–88.

34. Fioravanti A, Tofi C, Volterrani L, Marcolongo R. Malignant lymphoma presenting as Tietze's syndrome. *Arthritis Rheum*. Jun 15, 2002;47(3):229–230.

35. Uthman I, El-Hajj I, Traboulsi R, Taher A. Hodgkin's lymphoma presenting as Tietze's syndrome. *Arthritis Rheum*. Oct 15, 2003;49(5):737.

36. Vargo MM, Flood KM. Pancoast tumor presenting as cervical radiculopathy. *Arch Phys Med Rehabil*. Jul 1990;71(8):606–609.

37. Yang P, Allen MS, Aubry MC, et al. Clinical features of 5,628 primary lung cancer patients: experience at Mayo Clinic from 1997 to 2003. *Chest*. Jul 2005;128(1): 452–462.

38. Villas C, Collia A, Aquerreta JD, et al. Cervicobrachialgia and pancoast tumor: value of standard anteroposterior cervical radiographs in early diagnosis. *Orthopedics*. Oct 2004;27(10):1092–1095.

39. Pitz CC, de la Riviere AB, van Swieten HA, Duurkens VA, Lammers JW, van den Bosch JM. Surgical treatment of Pancoast tumours. *Eur J Cardiothorac Surg*. Jul 2004;26(1):202–208.

40. Khaw PY, Ball DL. Relief of non-metastatic shoulder pain with mediastinal radiotherapy in patients with lung cancer. *Lung Cancer*. Apr 2000;28(1):51–54.

41. Valenzuela GA, Mittal RK, Shaffer HA, Jr., Hanks J. Shoulder pain: an unusual presentation of gastric ulcer. *South Med J*. Nov 1989;82(11):1446–1447.

42. Kewalramani LS. Neurogenic gastroduodenal ulceration and bleeding associated with spinal cord injuries. *J Trauma*. Apr 1979;19(4):259–265.

43. Prandoni P, Bernardi E. Upper extremity deep vein thrombosis. *Curr Opin Pulm Med*. Jul 1999;5(4): 222–226.

44. Hannafin JA, Chiaia TA. Adhesive capsulitis. A treatment approach. *Clin Orthop Relat Res*. Mar 2000;(372):95–109.

45. Smith CR, Binder AI, Paice EW. Lesions of the mid-shaft of the humerus presenting as shoulder capsulitis. *Br J Rheumatol*. Oct 1990;29(5):386–388.

46. Gertz MA, Kyle RA. Primary systemic amyloidosis—a diagnostic primer. *Mayo Clin Proc*. Dec 1989;64(12): 1505–1519.

47. Baek HJ, Shin KC, Lee YJ, et al. Clinical features of adult-onset ankylosing spondylitis in Korean patients: patients with peripheral joint disease (PJD) have less severe spinal disease course than those without PJD. *Rheumatology (Oxford)*. Dec 2004;43(12):1526–1531.

48. Loebenberg MI, Plate AM, Zuckerman JD. Osteonecrosis of the humeral head. *Instr Course Lect*. 1999;48:349–357.

49. Hasan SS, Romeo AA. Nontraumatic osteonecrosis of the humeral head. *J Shoulder Elbow Surg*. May–Jun 2002;11(3):281–298.

50. Aldridge JW, Bruno RJ, Strauch RJ, Rosenwasser MP. Management of acute and chronic biceps tendon rupture. *Hand Clin*. Aug 2000;16(3):497–503.

51. Harwood MI, Smith CT. Superior labrum, anterior-posterior lesions and biceps injuries: diagnostic and treatment considerations. *Prim Care*. Dec 2004;31(4): 831–855.

52. Bennett WF. Specificity of the Speed's test: arthroscopic technique for evaluating the biceps tendon at the level of the bicipital groove. *Arthroscopy*. Nov–Dec 1998;14(8): 789–796.

SHOULDER PAIN

53. Carruthers BM, Jain AK, DeMeirleir KL, et al. Myalgic encephalomyelitis/chronic fatigue syndrome: clinical working case definition, diagnostic and treatment protocols (a consensus document). *J Chronic Fatigue Syndr.* 2003;11(1):7–115.

54. Alvarez-Lario B, Aretxabala-Alcibar I, Alegre-Lopez J, Alonso-Valdivielso JL. Acceptance of the different denominations for reflex sympathetic dystrophy. *Ann Rheum Dis.* Jan 2001;60(1):77–79.

55. Placzek JD, Boyer MI, Gelberman RH, Sopp B, Goldfarb CA. Nerve decompression for complex regional pain syndrome type II following upper extremity surgery. *J Hand Surg [Am].* Jan 2005;30(1):69–74.

56. Johnson R, Lehnert S, Moser B, Juenemann S. Shoulder instability. *Prim Care.* Dec 2004;31(4):867–886, viii.

57. Walton J, Paxinos A, Tzannes A, Callanan M, Hayes K, Murrell GA. The unstable shoulder in the adolescent athlete. *Am J Sports Med.* Sep–Oct 2002;30(5):758–767.

58. Rodeo SA, Suzuki K, Yamauchi M, Bhargava M, Warren RF. Analysis of collagen and elastic fibers in shoulder capsule in patients with shoulder instability. *Am J Sports Med.* Sep–Oct 1998;26(5):634–643.

59. Paxinos A, Walton J, Tzannes A, Callanan M, Hayes K, Murrell GA. Advances in the management of traumatic anterior and atraumatic multidirectional shoulder instability. *Sports Med.* 2001;31(11):819–828.

60. Jaggard MK, Gupte CM, Gulati V, Reilly P. A comprehensive review of trauma and disruption to the sternoclavicular joint with the proposal of a new classification system. *J Trauma.* Feb 2009;66(2):576–584.

61. Rockwood CA Jr, Odor JM. Spontaneous atraumatic anterior subluxation of the sternoclavicular joint. *J Bone Joint Surg Am.* Oct 1989;71(9):1280–1288.

62. Gosens T, Neumann L, Wallace WA. Shoulder replacement after Erb's palsy: a case report with ten years' follow-up. *J Shoulder Elbow Surg.* Sep–Oct 2004;13(5):568–572.

63. Goldenberg DL, Burckhardt C, Crofford L. Management of fibromyalgia syndrome [see comment]. *JAMA.* 2004;292(19):2388–2395.

64. Nampiaparampil DE, Shmerling RH. A review of fibromyalgia. *Am J Manag Care.* 2004;10(11, pt 1):794–800.

65. McLennan JG, Ungersma J. Pneumothorax complicating fracture of the scapula. *J Bone Joint Surg Am.* Apr 1982;64(4):598–599.

66. O'Leary ST, Goldberg JA, Walsh WR. Tophaceous gout of the rotator cuff: a case report. *J Shoulder Elbow Surg.* Mar–Apr 2003;12(2):200–201.

67. Court-Brown CM, Garg A, McQueen MM. The epidemiology of proximal humeral fractures. *Acta Orthop Scand.* Aug 2001;72(4):365–371.

68. Kristiansen B, Kofoed H. Transcutaneous reduction and external fixation of displaced fractures of the proximal humerus. A controlled clinical trial. *J Bone Joint Surg Br.* Nov 1988;70(5):821–824.

69. Handoll HH, Gibson JN, Madhok R. Interventions for treating proximal humeral fractures in adults. *Cochrane Database Syst Rev.* 2003(4): CD000434.

70. McKoy BE, Bensen CV, Hartsock LA. Fractures about the shoulder: conservative management. *Orthop Clin North Am.* Apr 2000;31(2):205–216.

71. Wallace SL, Singer JZ. Therapy in gout. *Rheum Dis Clin North Am.* Aug 1988;14(2):441–457.

72. Watts GD, O'Briant KC, Borreson TE, Windebank AJ, Chance PF. Evidence for genetic heterogeneity in hereditary neuralgic amyotrophy. *Neurology.* Mar 13 2001;56(5):675–678.

73. Boehm TD, Wallace WA, Neumann L. Heterotopic ossification after primary shoulder arthroplasty. *J Shoulder Elbow Surg.* Jan–Feb 2005;14(1):6–10.

74. Berg EE, Ciullo JV. Heterotopic ossification after acromioplasty and distal clavicle resection. *J Shoulder Elbow Surg.* May–Jun 1995;4(3):188–193.

75. Heyworth BE, Williams RJ 3rd. Internal impingement of the shoulder. *Am J Sports Med.* May 2009;37(5):1024–1037.

76. Jobe CM. Superior glenoid impingement. Current concepts. *Clin Orthop Relat Res.* Sep 1996(330):98–107.

77. Henrichs J, Stone D. Shoulder impingement syndrome. *Prim Care.* Dec 2004;31(4):789–805, vii.

78. Davidoff RA. Trigger points and myofascial pain: toward understanding how they affect headaches. *Cephalalgia.* Sep 1998;18(7):436–448.

79. Ojala T, Arokoski JP, Partanen J. The effect of small doses of botulinum toxin a on neck-shoulder myofascial pain syndrome: a double-blind, randomized, and controlled crossover trial. *Clin J Pain.* Jan 2006;22(1):90–96.

80. Steinmann SP, Moran EA. Axillary nerve injury: diagnosis and treatment. *J Am Acad Orthop Surg.* Sep–Oct 2001;9(5):328–335.

81. Hoskins WT, Pollard HP, McDonald AJ. Quadrilateral space syndrome: a case study and review of the literature. *Br J Sports Med.* Feb 2005;39(2):e9.

82. Perlmutter GS. Axillary nerve injury. *Clin Orthop Relat Res.* Nov 1999(368):28–36.

83. McNeely ML, Parliament M, Courneya KS, et al. A pilot study of a randomized controlled trial to evaluate the effects of progressive resistance exercise training on shoulder dysfunction caused by spinal accessory neurapraxia/neurectomy in head and neck cancer survivors. *Head Neck.* Jun 2004;26(6):518–530.

84. Antoniou J, Tae SK, Williams GR, Bird S, Ramsey ML, Iannotti JP. Suprascapular neuropathy. Variability in the diagnosis, treatment, and outcome. *Clin Orthop Relat Res.* May 2001(386):131–138.

85. Miller JD, Pruitt S, McDonald TJ. Acute brachial plexus neuritis: an uncommon cause of shoulder pain. *Am Fam Physician.* Nov 1, 2000;62(9):2067–2072.

86. Bredella MA, Tirman PF, Fritz RC, Wischer TK, Stork A, Genant HK. Denervation syndromes of the shoulder girdle: MR imaging with electrophysiologic correlation. *Skeletal Radiol.* Oct 1999;28(10):567–572.

87. Jones J, Wolf S. Neuropathic shoulder arthropathy (Charcot joint) associated with syringomyelia. *Neurology.* Mar 1998;50(3):825–827.

88. Montellese P, Dancy T. The acromioclavicular joint. *Prim Care.* Dec 2004;31(4):857–866.

89. Parsons IM, Weldon EJ 3rd, Titelman RM, Smith KL. Glenohumeral arthritis and its management. *Phys Med Rehabil Clin N Am.* May 2004;15(2):447–474.

90. Pfeiffenberger J, Meiss L. Septic conditions of the shoulder—an up-dating of treatment strategies. *Arch Orthop Trauma Surg.* 1996;115(6):325–331.

91. Michet CJ, Matteson EL. Polymyalgia rheumatica. *BMJ.* Apr 5 2008;336(7647):765–769.

92. Cassetta M, Gorevic PD. Crystal arthritis. Gout and pseudogout in the geriatric patient. *Geriatrics.* Sep 2004;59(9):25–30; quiz 31.

93. Amor B, Dougados M, Khan MA. Management of refractory ankylosing spondylitis and related spondy

loarthropathies. *Rheum Dis Clin North Am.* Feb 1995;21(1):117–128.

94. Dalakas MC, Hohlfeld R. Polymyositis and dermatomyositis. *Lancet.* Sep 20, 2003;362(9388):971–982.

95. Zampieri S, Ghirardello A, Iaccarino L, et al. Polymyositis-dermatomyositis and infections. *Autoimmunity.* May 2006;39(3):191–196.

96. Lotz BP, Engel AG, Nishino H, Stevens JC, Litchy WJ. Inclusion body myositis. Observations in 40 patients. *Brain.* Jun 1989;112(pt 3):727–747.

97. Monach PA, Daily JP, Rodriguez-Herrera G, Solomon DH. Tuberculous osteomyelitis presenting as shoulder pain. *J Rheumatol.* Apr 2003;30(4):851–856.

98. Harris GR, Susman JL. Managing musculoskeletal complaints with rehabilitation therapy: summary of the Philadelphia Panel evidence-based clinical practice guidelines on musculoskeletal rehabilitation interventions. *J Fam Pract.* Dec 2002;51(12):1042–1046.

99. Mehta S, Gimbel JA, Soslowsky LJ. Etiologic and pathogenetic factors for rotator cuff tendinopathy. *Clin Sports Med.* Oct 2003;22(4):791–812.

100. McConville OR, Iannotti JP. Partial-thickness tears of the rotator cuff: evaluation and management. *J Am Acad Orthop Surg.* Jan 1999;7(1):32–43.

101. Robinson D, Halperin N, Agar G, Alk D, Rami K. Shoulder girdle neoplasms mimicking frozen shoulder syndrome. *J Shoulder Elbow Surg.* Sep–Oct 2003;12(5):451–455.

102. Rydholm A, Berg NO. Size, site and clinical incidence of lipoma. Factors in the differential diagnosis of lipoma and sarcoma. *Acta Orthop Scand.* Dec 1983;54(6):929–934.

103. Joines JD, McNutt RA, Carey TS, Deyo RA, Rouhani R. Finding cancer in primary care outpatients with low back pain: a comparison of diagnostic strategies. *J Gen Intern Med.* 2001;16(1):14–23.

104. Holman PJ, Suki D, McCutcheon I, Wolinsky JP, Rhines LD, Gokaslan ZL. Surgical management of metastatic disease of the lumbar spine: experience with 139 patients. *Journal of Neurosurgery Spine.* 2005;2(5):550–563.

105. Bilkay U, Erdem O, Ozek C, et al. A rare location of benign osteoblastoma: review of the literature and report of a case. *J Craniofac Surg.* Mar 2004;15(2):222–225.

106. Yamamoto T, Tanaka K, Nagira K, et al. Intermittent radial nerve palsy caused by a humeral osteochondroma: a case report. *J Shoulder Elbow Surg.* Jan–Feb 2002;11(1):92–94.

107. Tomo H, Ito Y, Aono M, Takaoka K. Chest wall deformity associated with osteochondroma of the scapula: a case report and review of the literature. *J Shoulder Elbow Surg.* Jan–Feb 2005;14(1):103–106.

108. Ishikawa Y, Okada K, Miyakoshi N, et al. Osteoid osteoma of the scapula associated with synovitis of the shoulder. *J Shoulder Elbow Surg.* May–Jun 2005;14(3):329–332.

109. Swee RG, McLeod RA, Beabout JW. Osteoid osteoma. Detection, diagnosis, and localization. *Radiology.* Jan 1979;130(1):117–123.

110. Cleeman E, Auerbach JD, Springfield DS. Tumors of the shoulder girdle: a review of 194 cases. *J Shoulder Elbow Surg.* Sep–Oct 2005;14(5):460–465.

SHOULDER PAIN

CHAPTER 12

Elbow Pain

■ *Julia L. Burlette, PT, DPT, OCS* ■ *John M. Itamura, MD*

Description of the Symptom

This chapter describes pathology that may lead to elbow pain. **Local causes** of elbow pain include the distal one-third of the humerus, proximal one-third of the radium and ulna, and the corresponding articular and periarticular structures. **Remote causes** are defined as occurring outside these regions.

Special Concerns
■ Decreased pulses
■ Marked swelling and paresthesias
■ Recent change of status from previous status
■ Skin breakdown or wound problems
■ Warmth and swelling associated with a fever

CHAPTER PREVIEW: Conditions That May Lead to Elbow Pain

T Trauma

REMOTE	LOCAL GENERALIZED	LOCAL ANTERIOR
COMMON		
Cervical radiculopathies: • C6 radiculopathy 182	Elbow dislocation 184	Muscle strains: • Flexor/pronator muscle strain 190
UNCOMMON		
Cervical radiculopathies: • C8 radiculopathy 182	Fractures: • Intercondylar fracture of the humerus 185 • Monteggia fracture-dislocation 186 • Supracondylar fracture of the humerus 188 • Transolecranon fracture-dislocation 188 Post-traumatic osteoarthrosis/osteoarthritis 193 Terrible triad 196	Biceps tendon distal rupture 182 Nerve entrapments: • Median nerve compression in the proximal forearm 191

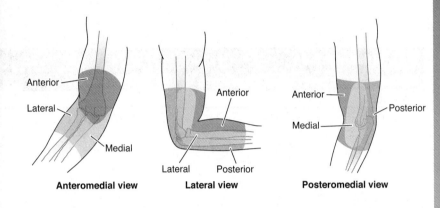

| Anteromedial view | Lateral view | Posteromedial view |

LOCAL LATERAL	LOCAL POSTERIOR	LOCAL MEDIAL
Fractures: • Radial head fracture 187 Muscle strains: • Extensor muscle strain 190	Bursitis: • Traumatic aseptic olecranon bursitis 183 Fractures: • Olecranon fracture 186 Nerve entrapments: • Ulnar neuropathy/neuritis 192	Ligament injuries: • Medial collateral ligament insufficiency 189 Muscle strains: • Flexor/pronator muscle strain 190 Nerve entrapments: • Ulnar neuropathy/neuritis 192
Ligament injuries: • Lateral ulnar collateral ligament insufficiency (posterolateral rotatory instability) 189 Nerve entrapments: • Deep radial nerve entrapment (posterior interosseous nerve paralysis, supinator syndrome, radial tunnel syndrome) 190 Posterior interosseous nerve injury postsurgical 192	Valgus extension overload syndrome 198	Ligament injuries: • Medial collateral ligament insufficiency 189

(continued)

ELBOW PAIN

Trauma *(continued)*

REMOTE	LOCAL GENERALIZED	LOCAL ANTERIOR
RARE		
Not applicable	Snapping triceps syndrome 194	Biceps muscle tear 182 Fractures: • Coronoid fracture 185

I Inflammation

REMOTE	LOCAL GENERALIZED	LOCAL ANTERIOR
COMMON		
Not applicable	**Aseptic** Rheumatoid arthritis 193 **Septic** Not applicable	Not applicable
UNCOMMON		

Not applicable	**Aseptic**
	Not applicable
	
	Septic
	Osteomyelitis of the distal
	  humerus, proximal radius,
	  and ulna 192
	Septic arthritis 193
		Not applicable

RARE		
Not applicable	Not applicable	**Aseptic** Tendinopathies: • Distal biceps tendinitis 194 **Septic** Not applicable

M Metabolic

REMOTE	LOCAL GENERALIZED	LOCAL ANTERIOR
COMMON		
Not applicable	Not applicable	Not applicable
UNCOMMON		
Not applicable	Gout 189 Heterotopic ossification 189	Not applicable
RARE		
Not applicable	Pseudogout 193	Not applicable

LOCAL LATERAL	LOCAL POSTERIOR	LOCAL MEDIAL
Fractures: • Capitellar fracture 184 Nerve entrapments: • Musculocutaneous or lateral antebrachial cutaneous nerve entrapment 191	Triceps rupture 196	Nerve entrapments: • Median nerve compression in the supracondylar tunnel 191 Snapping triceps syndrome 194

LOCAL LATERAL	LOCAL POSTERIOR	LOCAL MEDIAL
Aseptic Tendinopathies: • Lateral epicondylitis (tennis elbow) 194 **Septic** Not applicable	**Aseptic** Tendinopathies: • Triceps tendinitis 195 **Septic** Not applicable	**Aseptic** Tendinopathies: • Medial epicondylitis (golfer's elbow) 195 **Septic** Not applicable
Not applicable	**Aseptic** Bursitis: • Chronic aseptic olecranon bursitis 183 **Septic** Bursitis: • Septic olecranon bursitis 183	Not applicable
Not applicable	Not applicable	Not applicable

LOCAL LATERAL	LOCAL POSTERIOR	LOCAL MEDIAL
Not applicable	Not applicable	Not applicable
Not applicable	Not applicable	Not applicable
Not applicable	Not applicable	Not applicable

Va Vascular

REMOTE	LOCAL GENERALIZED	LOCAL ANTERIOR
COMMON		
Not applicable	Not applicable	Not applicable
UNCOMMON		
Not applicable	Arterial injury 182 Compartment syndrome 183	Superficial thrombophlebitis of the cephalic or basilic veins 194
RARE		
Not applicable	Not applicable	Not applicable

De Degenerative

REMOTE	LOCAL GENERALIZED	LOCAL ANTERIOR
COMMON		
Not applicable	Not applicable	Not applicable
UNCOMMON		
Not applicable	Primary osteoarthrosis/ osteoarthritis 193	Not applicable
RARE		
Not applicable	Not applicable	Tendinopathies: • Distal biceps tendinosis 194

Tu Tumor

REMOTE	LOCAL GENERALIZED	LOCAL ANTERIOR
COMMON		
Not applicable	Not applicable	Not applicable
UNCOMMON		
Not applicable	Not applicable	Not applicable
RARE		
Not applicable	*Malignant Primary, such as:* • Malignant lymphoma 197 • Osteosarcoma 198 • Synovial sarcoma 198 *Malignant Metastatic:* Not applicable	Not applicable

LOCAL LATERAL	LOCAL POSTERIOR	LOCAL MEDIAL
Not applicable	Not applicable	Not applicable
Not applicable	Not applicable	Not applicable
Not applicable	Not applicable	Not applicable

LOCAL LATERAL	LOCAL POSTERIOR	LOCAL MEDIAL
Tendinopathies: • Lateral epicondylosis 195	Tendinopathies: • Triceps tendinosis 196	Tendinopathies: • Medial epicondylosis 195
Not applicable	Not applicable	Not applicable
Not applicable	Not applicable	Not applicable

LOCAL LATERAL	LOCAL POSTERIOR	LOCAL MEDIAL
Not applicable	Not applicable	Not applicable
Not applicable	Not applicable	Not applicable
Not applicable	Not applicable	Not applicable

(continued)

Tumor *(continued)*

REMOTE	LOCAL GENERALIZED	LOCAL ANTERIOR
RARE		
	Benign, such as:	
	• Ganglion cyst 196	
	• Giant cell tumor 197	
	• Lipoma 197	
	• Osteoblastoma 197	
	• Osteochondroma 197	
	• Osteoid osteoma 197	
	• Synovial chondromatosis 198	

Co Congenital

REMOTE	LOCAL GENERALIZED	LOCAL ANTERIOR
COMMON		
Not applicable	Not applicable	Not applicable
UNCOMMON		
Not applicable	Not applicable	Not applicable
RARE		
Not applicable	Not applicable	Not applicable

Ne Neurogenic/Psychogenic

REMOTE	LOCAL GENERALIZED	LOCAL ANTERIOR
COMMON		
Not applicable	Not applicable	Not applicable
UNCOMMON		
Not applicable	Not applicable	Not applicable
RARE		
Not applicable	Not applicable	Not applicable

Note: These are estimates of relative incidence because few data are available for the less common conditions.

Overview of Elbow Pain

Successful management of elbow injuries requires a thorough screening and detailed history. Fractures can be misdiagnosed or the extent of the injury and associated injuries may not be recognized. Obtaining the operative notes following surgery and communication with the physician are paramount. It may be useful to review the radiology reports. Certain fracture patterns are more difficult to stabilize and the surgical incision may not necessarily indicate the areas of fixation. Often the incision is posterior and then skin flaps are made to approach posterior, medial, or lateral regions. The bone and tissue quality will also determine the appropriate interventions and progression.

Early range of motion following injury and surgery is indicated to prevent loss of motion; however, aggressive mobilization may cause increased inflammation and contribute to the development of heterotopic ossification. Static versus dynamic splints are more beneficial and should be used to assist in achieving elbow range of motion. While functional elbow

LOCAL LATERAL	LOCAL POSTERIOR	LOCAL MEDIAL

LOCAL LATERAL	LOCAL POSTERIOR	LOCAL MEDIAL
Not applicable	Not applicable	Not applicable
Not applicable	Not applicable	Not applicable
Not applicable	Not applicable	Not applicable

LOCAL LATERAL	LOCAL POSTERIOR	LOCAL MEDIAL
Not applicable	Not applicable	Not applicable
Not applicable	Not applicable	Not applicable
Not applicable	Not applicable	Not applicable

range is considered to be 30 degrees of extension to 130 degrees of flexion, the patients' individual goals and range needed to return to their prior level of function should be considered. Certain occupations and extracurricular activities require greater ranges of elbow motion.

Overuse injuries at the elbow are common. Tendinitis is an acute inflammatory process characterized by the presence of inflammatory cells. Tendinosis is a degenerative process resulting in incomplete/failed tendon healing characterized by disorganized collagen fibers and the lack of inflammatory cells. Because of common usage of tendinitis to describe any tendon condition the literature is difficult to interpret. The term *tendinopathy* has been suggested to encompass both the inflammatory and degenerative conditions. Treatment of overuse injuries at the elbow necessitates addressing proximal areas of weakness and decreased flexibility to restore alignment and improve mechanics at the elbow, thereby decreasing stress at the elbow. Focusing treatment interventions solely on the elbow will lead to less than optimal outcomes and will not assist in

ELBOW PAIN

preventing recurrence of the injury and chronic tendon symptoms.

Description of Conditions That May Lead to Elbow Pain

Remote

CERVICAL RADICULOPATHIES

■ C6 Radiculopathy

Chief Clinical Characteristics
This presentation, while variable, typically includes pain in the neck, shoulder, medial border of the scapula, radial side of the upper arm and forearm, thumb, and index finger. Pain is increased with cervical movement and use of the extremity. Coughing or sneezing may also increase symptoms. Sensory changes may be present in the thumb and index finger and the radial aspect of the hand and forearm.

Background Information
In severe cases, the brachioradialis or biceps reflexes may be absent and motor loss evident in the muscles innervated by the C6 nerve. Cervical radiculopathy may occur from cervical disk herniation or other lesions (space-occupying, infection, hemorrhage). A test item cluster consisting of an upper limb tension test, Spurling test, distraction test, and cervical rotation ipsilateral to the side of involvement less than 60 degrees is useful to identify this condition.[1] The diagnosis is confirmed with magnetic resonance imaging. Treatment includes inflammation control, restoration of mobility, and strengthening. Severe or progressive neurological deficits may require surgical intervention.

■ C8 Radiculopathy

Chief Clinical Characteristics
This presentation may be characterized by pain in the neck, scapula, ulnar aspect of the upper arm and forearm, and fourth and fifth fingers. Pain is increased with cervical movement and use of the extremity. Coughing or sneezing may also increase symptoms. Sensory disturbances may be reported in the fourth and fifth fingers as well as the medial aspect of the forearm.

Background Information
The presentation may also include motor loss in the muscles innervated by the C8 nerve. Cervical disk herniation, infection, hemorrhage, or other space-occupying lesions may cause cervical radiculopathy. C8 radiculopathy is uncommon.[2] The diagnosis is confirmed with magnetic resonance imaging. Treatment includes inflammation control, restoration of mobility, and strengthening. Surgical intervention may be necessary in cases with severe or progressive neurological deficits.

Local

■ Arterial Injury

Chief Clinical Characteristics
This presentation includes pain out of proportion to the injury, decreased or absent pulses, decreased skin temperature, and pallor. Pain increases with passive stretching of the involved muscles.

Background Information
The presentation may also include weakness and hypoesthesia. The mechanism of injury is usually traumatic. Arteriography confirms the diagnosis. Operative repair may be required.

■ Biceps Muscle Tear

Chief Clinical Characteristics
This presentation includes distal upper arm or anterior elbow pain, tenderness, swelling, and ecchymosis. The muscle defect in the distal biceps may be palpable. Elbow flexion and forearm supination strength are impaired. The patient may report a tearing or popping sensation above the anterior elbow.[3]

Background Information
This injury is rare and is reported most frequently by military parachutists.[3] It may also be associated with anabolic steroid use. Clinical examination and magnetic resonance imaging or ultrasonography confirm the diagnosis.

■ Biceps Tendon Distal Rupture

Chief Clinical Characteristics
This presentation typically includes local tenderness in the antecubital fossa and ecchymosis in the antecubital fossa and medial elbow. The defect may be palpated and visible during active elbow flexion with the biceps muscle retracted

up in the proximal upper arm. The retracted tendon may be a palpable mass. Decreased flexion, supination, and grip strength occur in varying degrees with supination most impacted. Patients typically report a sharp or tearing pain in the antecubital fossa. Patients may report an inability to perform activities of daily living.

Background Information
The mechanism of injury is typically flexion of the elbow against resistance with the elbow in flexion but may also occur with repetitive heavy use of the elbow.[4] Abuse of anabolic steroids and preexisting degenerative changes in the tendon predispose it to rupture. Distal biceps tendon rupture is uncommon.[5] Tendon avulsion from the radial tuberosity is the most common distal biceps tendon injury. A complete avulsion is more common than a partial tear. The clinical presentation of a partial distal biceps tendon tear is more subtle than a complete rupture and the injury may be misdiagnosed. Magnetic resonance imaging has been found to be useful in accurately diagnosing this injury.[4] Complete ruptures are managed surgically for the most optimal outcomes. Partial tears can be managed nonsurgically but if conservative therapy is ineffective surgical intervention can provide good results.

BURSITIS
■ Chronic Aseptic Olecranon Bursitis

Chief Clinical Characteristics
This presentation includes a distended olecranon bursa and may include tenderness. The patient will report a gradual onset of symptoms and may report pain with elbow movement. Fever and axillary adenopathy are not present, differentiating it from septic olecranon bursitis.

Background Information
The mechanism of injury is repeated trauma. Chronic bursitis typically coexists with chronic inflammation of adjacent tissues.[6] Treatment includes compression dressing, elbow pad, and icing. Eliminating the repetitive trauma to the region is necessary to prevent continued inflammation. Surgical excision may be needed in cases that do not respond to nonoperative treatment.

■ Septic Olecranon Bursitis

Chief Clinical Characteristics
This presentation is characterized by pain and swelling over the tip of the olecranon and a palpable bursa. The area is often warm and erythematous. The patient may have a fever and axillary or epitrochlear adenopathy. Cellulitis overlying the bursa may be present.[7] End-range elbow flexion may be limited.

Background Information
Onset can occur from a laceration or injection or from hematogenous seeding. Traumatic aseptic olecranon bursitis can develop into septic olecranon bursitis and occurs more frequently in immunocompromised patients. Clinical examination and culture of bursal fluid aspirate confirm the diagnosis. Treatment includes bursectomy and antibiotic therapy.

■ Traumatic Aseptic Olecranon Bursitis

Chief Clinical Characteristics
This presentation includes pain and swelling over the tip of the olecranon and a large palpable bursa. Warmth and redness may also be present in the same region.

Background Information
The mechanism of injury is either a direct blow or acute overexertion. It can also develop following surgical procedures utilizing a posterior approach. The bursa may require aspiration if elbow motion is limited or in recalcitrant cases. Clinical examination and resolution of symptoms with conservative management confirms the diagnosis. Blood tests and cultures of aspirated fluid may be indicated. In the presence of diabetes or renal failure, aseptic olecranon bursitis may develop into septic olecranon bursitis. Immunosuppressant and anti-inflammatory medications may mask signs and symptoms, making assessment difficult. Treatment includes icing, compression dressing, and an elbow pad.

■ Compartment Syndrome
Chief Clinical Characteristics
This presentation includes pain, feelings of increased pressure, tense compartment, weakness,

numbness, and swelling. Pain is out of proportion to that expected for injury and increases with passive stretching of the muscles.

Background Information

Immobilization does not relieve the pain. Peripheral pulses are usually intact except if there has been arterial injury. The mechanisms of injury include fracture, crush injury, burns, and vascular injury. Prolonged external pressure from a compressive cast or bandage may also cause compartment syndrome. Clinical examination and compartmental pressure measurement confirm the diagnosis. Immediate identification of compartment syndrome is critical to prevent muscle ischemia. If compartment syndrome is suspected, an immediate referral to an emergency department should be made. A decompressive fasciotomy is required to alleviate the pressure. The major complication of compartment syndrome is a Volkmann contracture.

■ Elbow Dislocation

Chief Clinical Characteristics

This presentation includes pain, swelling, ecchymosis, and deformity.

Background Information

The mechanism of injury is typically a fall onto the outstretched hand. Motor vehicle accidents and direct trauma can also cause elbow dislocation. In adults, the elbow joint is the second most commonly dislocated joint. Simple elbow dislocation can result in injury to the medial and lateral collateral ligaments, and anterior and posterior capsule. Other associated injuries are common including radial head and neck fractures, coronoid fractures, osteochondral fractures, avulsion fragments from the medial and lateral epicondyles, and wrist and shoulder injuries. Triceps avulsion can also occur but is rare. Dislocation with associated fractures can lead to instability and poor outcomes. Complications include contracture, instability, heterotopic ossification, neurovascular injury, and compartment syndrome. Clinical examination, history, and plain radiographs confirm the diagnosis. If the elbow has relocated, plain radiographs may not be helpful because there may only be ligamentous injury. However, even if the patient

has studies documenting reduction follow-up radiographs are necessary to identify any residual instability. Treatment options range from surgical to nonsurgical forms of management, depending on the associated injuries and the patient's lifestyle.

FRACTURES

■ Capitellar Fracture

Chief Clinical Characteristics

This presentation includes pain and swelling at the lateral elbow and antecubital fossa, and crepitus during motion, especially flexion and extension. Pain is increased during forearm rotation.[8]

Background Information

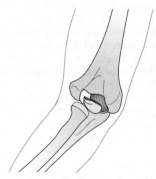

Capitellar fracture

The mechanism of injury is typically a fall onto an outstretched hand, with the elbow partially flexed and the forearm pronated. Capitellar fractures account for less than 1% of all elbow fractures and are more common in females.[9,10] The fracture can involve the osseous and cartilaginous portions of the capitellum or less frequently present as a shearing off of the articular cartilage and a thin layer of subchondral bone. This condition may occur in isolation but may also be associated with other injuries. Medial joint line tenderness would suggest a medial collateral ligament injury. Identification of a ligament injury is important to prevent future instability. Plain radiographs confirm the diagnosis. Capitellar fractures typically require surgical intervention.

■ Coronoid Fracture

Chief Clinical Characteristics

This presentation may include pain and swelling at the antecubital fossa and instability. Crepitus may occur with end-range elbow extension.

Background Information

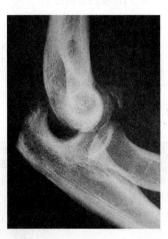

This injury rarely occurs in isolation and is associated with other injuries including elbow dislocation or olecranon fractures.[11] Coronoid fractures are commonly unrecognized and may be the cause of continued instability following elbow trauma.[12] The size and location of the coronoid fracture will implicate what other structures may be involved (capsule versus ulnar collateral ligament) and the severity of the injury.[13] Plain radiographs confirm the diagnosis; however, computerized tomography and/or magnetic resonance imaging may be indicated to identify all injured structures. Nondisplaced fractures that do not have instability may be managed nonsurgically, while comminuted fractures or those associated with dislocation are typically managed with surgical stabilization.

■ Intercondylar Fracture of the Humerus

Chief Clinical Characteristics

This presentation includes pain, swelling, paresthesias, and tenderness.

Background Information

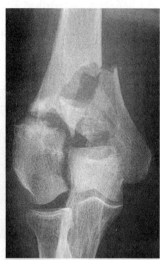

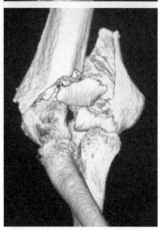

The fracture usually occurs from forces against the posterior aspect of the flexed elbow or from a fall on the outstretched hand. The diagnosis is confirmed with traction films and possibly a computerized tomography scan. This fracture is managed surgically. Certain fracture patterns are easily addressed but others, especially the low-H pattern, are difficult to stabilize, necessitating extreme caution during postsurgical rehabilitation, particularly in patients with osteoporotic bone.

ELBOW PAIN

■ **Monteggia Fracture-Dislocation**

Chief Clinical Characteristics

This presentation includes pain, swelling, tenderness, angulation of the ulna, and impaired supination and pronation.

Background Information

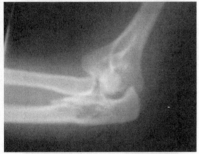

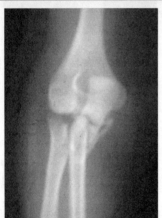

The dislocated radial head can be palpated. Radial nerve injury may also occur, resulting primarily in weakness. A Monteggia lesion involves a fracture of the proximal third of the ulna and dislocation of the radial head. It is classified according to the direction of the radial head dislocation and the trauma to the ulna. The mechanism of injury is typically a fall onto the outstretched hand with the forearm pronated or direct trauma to the ulna. The most commonly reported associated nerve injury is dysfunction of the posterior interosseous nerve (Fig. 12-1).[14] Monteggia fracture-dislocation is managed surgically. Plain radiographs confirm the diagnosis. Stable, anatomical fixation of the ulnar fracture including any associated coronoid fracture results in satisfactory outcomes in most adults.[15] Impaired rotation postsurgically may indicate instability of the proximal radioulnar joint or radiocapitellar joint secondary to malreduction of the ulna.

■ **Olecranon Fracture**

Chief Clinical Characteristics

This presentation includes posterior elbow pain, swelling, tenderness, and ecchymosis. The bone may have a palpable defect. An inability to actively extend the elbow occurs with a displaced fracture.

Background Information

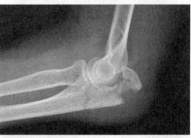

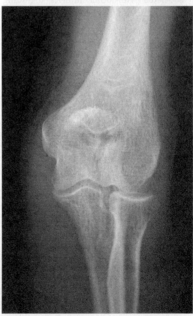

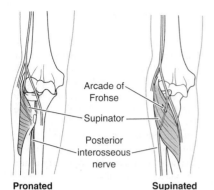

FIGURE 12-1 Anatomical course of the posterior interosseous nerve.

Pronated   Supinated

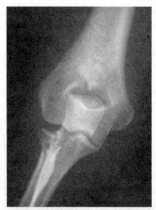

The mechanism of injury is typically either a direct impact with the tip of the elbow or a strong contraction of the triceps at the time of a fall on the extended arm. Plain radiographs confirm the diagnosis. Nondisplaced fractures are usually managed nonsurgically and displaced fractures are managed surgically. Complications include failure of fixation, loss of motion, heterotopic ossification, and ulnar neuropathy.[16]

■ Radial Head Fracture

Chief Clinical Characteristics
This presentation includes pain, swelling, and tenderness on the lateral side of the elbow over the radial head. Supination and pronation may be limited secondary to pain or a mechanical block.

Background Information

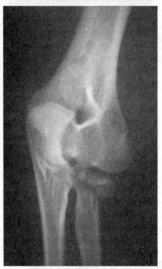

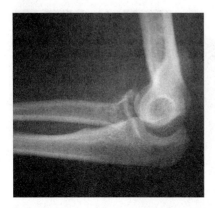

Ecchymosis and tenderness on the medial side of the elbow are suggestive of medial collateral ligament involvement. Radial head fracture usually results from a fall onto the outstretched hand with the elbow partially flexed and pronated or directly onto the lateral elbow. Plain radiographs confirm the diagnosis. Associated injuries are common and include dislocation, capitellum fracture, Essex-Lopresti injury, and medial and/ or lateral collateral ligament disruption. The incidence of associated concomitant osseous, osteochondral, and ligamentous injuries has been demonstrated to be high.[17] Nondisplaced fractures may be managed nonsurgically, but must be closely monitored for delayed fracture displacement. Early range of motion for patients with nondisplaced fractures is necessary to prevent contracture but can increase the risk of displacement. A loss of motion, an increase in pain, or the occurrence of crepitus would indicate a need for imaging. The physician may routinely order radiographs to monitor the fracture during the healing stage. Displaced fractures are usually managed surgically.

■ Supracondylar Fracture of the Humerus

Chief Clinical Characteristics

This presentation is mainly characterized by pain, swelling, visible deformity, ecchymosis, and tenderness of the distal humerus.

Background Information

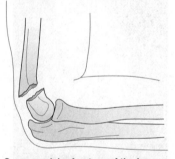

Supracondylar fracture of the humerus

This fracture occurs with a fall on the outstretched hand with the elbow extended or with a force against the posterior aspect of the flexed elbow.[18] Supracondylar fracture of the humerus is uncommon in adults, although it can occur during manipulation of a stiff osteoporotic joint. The neurovascular status must be evaluated thoroughly because the median, ulnar, and radial nerves and the brachial artery may be injured with this fracture. Plain radiographs confirm the diagnosis. Displaced supracondylar fractures are managed surgically.

■ Transolecranon Fracture-Dislocation

Chief Clinical Characteristics

This presentation includes pain, swelling, and tenderness at the elbow joint.

Background Information

This injury typically results from a high-energy trauma.[19] A transolecranon fracture-dislocation is an anterior fracture-dislocation of the olecranon and is associated with fracture of the coronoid process. The olecranon fracture is often comminuted.[16] The injury may be misdiagnosed as a Monteggia fracture but usually has more chondral injury and a poorer prognosis. Plain radiographs confirm the diagnosis. Transolecranon fracture-dislocations require surgical intervention. Despite the complexity of the injury, good results are obtained in most cases

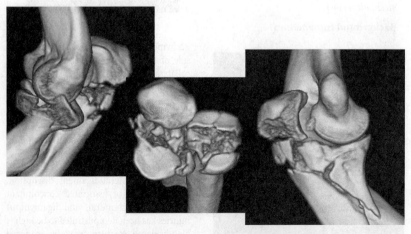

Transolecranon fracture-dislocation

if stable, anatomical reconstruction is achieved.[19] Active and active-assisted range-of-motion exercises should be initiated immediately postsurgically if stable fixation is achieved.

■ Gout

Chief Clinical Characteristics
This presentation involves a sudden onset of pain, swelling, redness of the superficial tissues, and tenderness of the joint or bursal cavity. Advanced cases may have palpable firm tophi.

Background Information
Gout commonly manifests as acute olecranon bursitis. The olecranon bursa is a common location for tophi. The toes should also be assessed for metatarsal joint involvement. Gout is usually associated with elevated uric acid levels. Increased prevalence is associated with advanced age, male gender, and regular alcohol consumption. Polarized microscopic examination of aspirated synovial fluid confirms the diagnosis. Treatment includes inflammation control, medication, and diet modification.

■ Heterotopic Ossification

Chief Clinical Characteristics
This presentation typically includes loss of range of motion, swelling, and local warmth. The patient may report pain.

Background Information

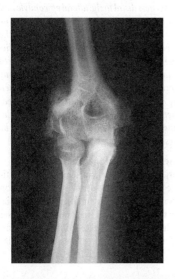

Heterotopic bone development around the elbow has been associated with severe trauma with extensive soft tissue injury, infected fracture, closed head or spinal cord injury, burn injury, and genetic conditions such as fibrodysplasia ossificans progressiva and history of ectopic bone formation.[20,21] It manifests clinically 3 to 4 weeks following injury or surgery but may occur earlier. Plain radiographs and sometimes computerized tomography scan confirm the diagnosis. Resection of the heterotopic bone may be necessary to restore functional motion, but frequently recurs.

LIGAMENT INJURIES

■ Lateral Ulnar Collateral Ligament Insufficiency (Posterolateral Rotatory Instability)

Chief Clinical Characteristics
This presentation mainly involves pain and reports of catching, clicking, and locking. The patient may report slipping of the elbow joint. Apprehension with the elbow supinated and fully extended may occur.

Background Information
Lateral ulnar collateral ligament injury can result from dislocation, fracture, or surgery to the lateral aspect of the elbow including lateral epicondyle revision. Injections for lateral epicondylitis may also weaken the ligament. The most sensitive clinical test is the overhead lateral pivot-shift test performed with the patient supine.[22] Magnetic resonance imaging or fluoroscopic examination confirms the diagnosis. Active patients will require surgery to restore the stability. Sedentary patients may be able to modify their activities and be managed nonsurgically.

■ Medial Collateral Ligament Insufficiency

Chief Clinical Characteristics
This presentation can include medial elbow pain, tenderness, instability to valgus stress, and possible ecchymosis (Fig. 12-2). The patient commonly reports symptoms with reaching out and back during activities of daily living. Chronic cases may present with ulnar nerve involvement.

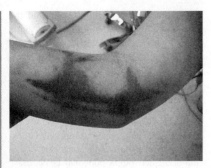

FIGURE 12-2 Elbow ecchymosis in a patient with medial collateral ligament insufficiency.

Background Information
This condition usually occurs from a valgus force on the extended arm, which may occur from a fall on the outstretched hand with a valgus force at the elbow or with throwing sports. It may be associated with a flexor/pronator avulsion. Commonly a history of repetitive overhead throwing activities will be reported. The moving valgus stress test is highly sensitive for medial elbow pain arising from the medial collateral ligament.[23] Stress radiographs and often magnetic resonance imaging assist in confirming the diagnosis. A throwing athlete returning to competition will usually require surgery, however, nonoperative treatment has been successful in returning athletes to throwing competitively.[24] It is important to obtain the operative notes to determine if the flexor/pronator mass was taken down or split during repair of the ligament.

MUSCLE STRAINS
■ Extensor Muscle Strain
Chief Clinical Characteristics
This presentation can include muscle soreness and tenderness at the wrist extensor muscle group. Reproduction of symptoms occurs with active wrist extension, with increased symptoms when resistance is applied. Symptoms may be produced with passive wrist flexion.

Background Information
Extensor muscle strain is commonly associated with increased use of the forearm,

specifically the wrist extensors, 1 to 2 days prior to the onset of symptoms. Clinical examination confirms the diagnosis. Symptoms typically resolve within 1 to 3 days with avoidance of aggravating activities.

■ Flexor/Pronator Muscle Strain
Chief Clinical Characteristics
This presentation involves muscle soreness and tenderness at the wrist flexor/pronator muscle group. Symptoms are reproduced with active wrist flexion and forearm pronation, with symptoms greater when resistance is provided. Passive wrist extension and forearm supination may reproduce symptoms.

Background Information
This condition is commonly associated with increased forearm use 1 to 2 days prior to the onset of symptoms. Clinical examination confirms the diagnosis. Symptoms will resolve within 1 to 3 days with avoidance of aggravating activities.

NERVE ENTRAPMENTS
■ Deep Radial Nerve Entrapment (Posterior Interosseous Nerve Paralysis, Supinator Syndrome, Radial Tunnel Syndrome)
Chief Clinical Characteristics
This presentation may involve minimal to severe aching pain in the lateral forearm and tenderness distal to the lateral epicondyle and in the supinator region.[25] Symptoms may be reproduced with resisted supination of the forearm or resisted wrist extension with the elbow extended. Passive wrist flexion with ulnar deviation and the elbow extended may reproduce symptoms that are increased when the shoulder is depressed and abducted. Partial or complete paralysis of the muscles innervated by the deep radial nerve may be present. Sensation is not impaired.

Background Information
Patients may report participating in repetitive forearm pronation and supination prior to onset of symptoms. Deep radial nerve compression has multiple causes including trauma, space-occupying lesions, inflammation, and excessive muscular

activity. Compression at the arcade of Frohse (the proximal edge of the supinator) occurs most frequently (see Fig. 12-1).[26] Isolated entrapment is rare. This condition is often difficult to differentiate from lateral epicondylitis; they may occur independently or simultaneously. Tennis elbow straps may cause increased symptoms in a patient with deep radial nerve entrapment. It is essential to rule out cervical radiculopathy and other potential sites of compression. Clinical examination and selective injections confirm the diagnosis. Treatment should initially focus on rest and inflammation control. Surgical interventions are rarely indicated.

■ Median Nerve Compression in the Proximal Forearm

Chief Clinical Characteristics
This presentation typically includes nonlocalized aching pain in the anterior forearm and pain with palpation to the forearm along the course of the nerve. Symptoms may be associated with weakness in the muscles innervated by the median nerve and numbness in the hand, primarily the first and second digits. Reproduction of symptoms may vary depending on the site of compression.

Background Information
The mechanism of injury may be acute trauma or chronic, repetitive microtrauma. Common sites of entrapment include the pronator teres, flexor superficialis arch, and the bicipital aponeurosis.[25] Symptoms with resisted forearm, elbow, or finger motions may implicate the structures involved in the entrapment.[27] Activities that require repetitive, resisted pronation and supination of the forearm may play a role in this entrapment. It is important to rule out cervical radiculopathy and other potential sites of compression. Clinical examination and selective injections confirm the diagnosis. Median nerve entrapment should initially be managed with inflammation control and activity modification. Stretching and strengthening should be initiated once the initial symptoms have decreased. Surgical intervention may be necessary for patients who do not

respond to the above treatment or who demonstrate progressive weakness.

■ Median Nerve Compression in the Supracondylar Tunnel

Chief Clinical Characteristics
This presentation includes deep pain in the region of the supracondylar tunnel (comprised of the supracondylar process, the medial epicondyle, and the ligament of Struthers) and pain and paresthesias in the median nerve dermatome. Pain is typically worse at night. Weakness of the muscles innervated by the median nerve may be present.

Background Information
The supracondylar process is rare, occurring in 0.3% to 2.7% of individuals.[25] The mechanism of injury is typically a fracture of the supracondylar process but may occur from surgical treatment of an intra-articular distal humerus fracture. Clinical examination and plain radiographs to assess for a supracondylar process confirm the diagnosis. Treatment initially consists of inflammation control and avoidance of aggravating positions. Surgical decompression to remove the supracondylar process may be indicated if the patient is not responsive to conservative treatment.

■ Musculocutaneous or Lateral Antebrachial Cutaneous Nerve Entrapment

Chief Clinical Characteristics
This presentation is mainly characterized by pain and tenderness in the anterolateral elbow and forearm. Symptoms may be aggravated with full elbow extension and forearm pronation. Acute compression may cause burning pain. Chronic irritation of the nerve results in hypoesthesia in the wrist and forearm and pain.[25]

Background Information
The mechanism of injury may be acute or chronic trauma to the elbow involving forced elbow extension and pronation. Chronic trauma may occur from repetitive pronation and supination of the forearm. Elbow flexor hypertrophy may also be a contributing factor in compression of the nerve.

Clinical examination and electrodiagnostic evaluation confirm the diagnosis.[28] Selective injections may also be helpful to confirm the diagnosis. Treatment includes avoidance of aggravating activities and inflammation control. Stretching and strengthening should be initiated when the inflammatory stage resolves. Surgical decompression may be indicated if symptoms do not respond to nonoperative measures.

■ Ulnar Neuropathy/Neuritis

Chief Clinical Characteristics
This presentation initially includes paresthesias in the sensory distribution of the ulnar nerve. Aching pain may occur in the medial elbow and forearm. Less commonly, pain may occur in the posterior elbow. Tinel's sign over the ulnar sulcus or distally may reproduce symptoms. Weakness of the muscles innervated by the ulnar nerve and atrophy may be found if the nerve compression is severe or continues for an extended period.

Background Information
The mechanism of injury may be acute trauma (elbow dislocation, fracture, direct blow, direct pressure for extended period), chronic nerve microtrauma, or ulnar nerve entrapment. Activities that involve repetitive elbow flexion and extension, leaning on the elbow, and ulnar nerve subluxation may contribute to microtrauma of the nerve. Ulnar nerve entrapment at the elbow can occur at the medial intermuscular septum, arcade of Struthers, the cubital tunnel, and under the transverse fascia of the flexor carpi ulnaris.[27] The cubital tunnel is the most common compression site. Decreased volume of the cubital tunnel and compression of the ulnar nerve have been found to occur with increasing elbow flexion.[29] The intraneural pressure of the ulnar nerve within the cubital tunnel and proximal to it also increases as the elbow is flexed 120 degrees or more.[29] Entrapment of the ulnar nerve at the cubital tunnel has also been associated with medial elbow ganglia and osteoarthritis.[30] Clinical examination and electrodiagnostic tests confirm the diagnosis. Treatment should initially include soft bracing, night splinting, and avoidance of aggravating activities and positions. Strengthening and stretching to improve trunk and upper extremity alignment should be included to prevent recurrence. Surgical intervention, although controversial, may be indicated if conservative treatment does not provide relief or the weakness is progressing.

■ Osteomyelitis of the Distal Humerus, Proximal Radius, and Ulna

Chief Clinical Characteristics
This presentation involves local pain, tenderness, swelling, warmth, and axillary and/or epitrochlear adenopathy. The elbow may be held in flexion.

Background Information
Gentle passive range of motion is tolerated. Bone infection occurs hematogenously, after surgery or open fracture, or by spread from a local process.[31] It should be suspected in any postoperative case directly involving osseous structures. An increased prevalence is observed in individuals with a history of immunocompromise and rheumatoid arthritis. The diagnosis is confirmed with blood work. An indium-labeled white blood cell scan and magnetic resonance imaging may also be indicated. Early diagnosis and surgical treatment with adjuvant antibiotic therapy improve outcomes.

■ Posterior Interosseous Nerve Injury Postsurgical

Chief Clinical Characteristics
This presentation includes partial or complete paralysis of the muscles innervated by the posterior interosseous nerve. This is differentiated from radial nerve palsy by the ability to extend the wrist (see Fig. 12-1).

Background Information
Iatrogenic radial nerve injury may result from arthroscopic surgery or surgery utilizing a dorsal or volar approach. Electromyographic and nerve conduction studies are indicated if return of function has not occurred 4 to 6 weeks following injury. Initially the extremity should be protected and monitored for recovery. Neurapraxia may take several months to resolve. Surgical intervention may be indicated for restoring function.

Post-Traumatic Osteoarthrosis/Osteoarthritis

Chief Clinical Characteristics

This presentation typically includes pain and loss of elbow motion, most commonly extension.

Background Information

Post-traumatic osteoarthrosis of the elbow can occur following dislocation or intra-articular fracture. Inadequate stabilization or restoration of the joint following injury contributes to increased arthrosis.[32] Plain radiographs typically show osteophytes and joint space narrowing with this condition. Nonoperative treatment should include activity modification, stretching, and strengthening. Significant post-traumatic arthrosis may require surgical interventions, such as debridement and interpositional arthroplasty.

Primary Osteoarthrosis/Osteoarthritis

Chief Clinical Characteristics

This presentation may include pain at terminal elbow flexion and/or extension but may also occur throughout the range or at rest. A loss of elbow extension and reports of locking are common findings.

Background Information

Ulnar nerve irritation may be present. Primary degenerative arthrosis of the elbow is an uncommon disorder reported primarily in middle-aged men.[33] The mechanism of injury is repetitive use of the upper extremity. Plain radiographs that show olecranon and coronoid osteophytes and intra-articular loose bodies confirm the diagnosis.[33] Nonoperative treatment should include activity modification, stretching, and strengthening. Surgical intervention may be necessary to restore functional motion and eliminate locking.

Pseudogout

Chief Clinical Characteristics

This presentation includes a sudden onset of pain, swelling, tenderness, and redness of the superficial tissues. The elbow commonly lacks full extension.

Background Information

This condition's presentation is often indistinguishable from gout; however, the acute synovitis is caused by deposition of calcium pyrophosphate dihydrate crystals. The onset typically occurs during the sixth and seventh decade. Pseudogout occurs less commonly in the elbow compared to the knees and wrists. Polarized microscopic examination of aspirated synovial fluid confirms the diagnosis. Treatment includes inflammation control and medication directed at the underlying pathophysiological process responsible for crystal deposition.

Rheumatoid Arthritis

Chief Clinical Characteristics

This presentation, while variable, can involve joint pain, swelling, and tenderness. Inflammatory symptoms are episodic. Morning stiffness, decreased stiffness with use of the involved joint, and symmetrical joint involvement are common findings. The earliest finding with elbow involvement is loss of elbow extension. With progression of the disease process, joint deformity and loss of function occur.

Background Information

Loss of rotation may be observed secondary to radial head subluxation and involvement of the distal radioulnar joint. The onset may be acute or insidious. The elbow is frequently involved in patients with rheumatoid arthritis.[34] Plain radiographs indicating the lack of osteophytes and blood tests confirm the diagnosis. Treatment includes medication, activity modification, and general conditioning. Psychosocial support groups are beneficial. Surgical intervention may be necessary to improve joint function. Advancements in total elbow arthroplasty have resulted in improved outcomes.[35,36]

Septic Arthritis

Chief Clinical Characteristics

This presentation includes severe aching pain, swelling, warmth, axillary adenopathy, and fever. The fever may be low grade. The elbow is typically held in about 80 degrees of flexion and passive motion is painful.[37]

Background Information

Common risk factors include rheumatoid arthritis, immunodeficiency, intravenous drug use, and joint replacement. Clinical examination, blood tests, fluid cell count, polarized microscopic analysis, and culture of the aspirated synovial fluid confirm the diagnosis. The treatment includes antibiotic therapy and aspiration. Surgical intervention may be necessary in cases that do not respond to aspiration.

■ Snapping Triceps Syndrome

Chief Clinical Characteristics

This presentation includes a snapping sensation over the medial epicondyle, and may occur with concomitant chronic ulnar neuritis. The snapping may be painless.

Background Information

The most common etiology is subluxation of the medial head of the triceps over the medial epicondyle.[38] The diagnosis is confirmed by magnetic resonance imaging or computed tomography.[39] Selective injections may be helpful in diagnosis when the snapping is painful. If conservative measures fail, treatment involves rerouting the medial head laterally and, if needed, ulnar nerve management.

■ Superficial Thrombophlebitis of the Cephalic or Basilic Veins

Chief Clinical Characteristics

This presentation may involve aching pain in the antecubital region and/or forearm. A raised, warm, red, tender cord will be palpable along the course of the involved vein.[40]

Background Information

This condition is associated with chronic intravenous treatment.[41] Although rare, the potential exists for pulmonary embolization or extension to deep veins. Clinical examination and Doppler ultrasonography confirm the diagnosis. Treatment includes control of local pain and inflammation. Anticoagulants may be utilized in some cases; rarely, thrombectomy is indicated.

TENDINOPATHIES

■ Distal Biceps Tendinitis

Chief Clinical Characteristics

This presentation includes pain and tenderness deep in the anterior elbow. Symptoms may occur with resisted elbow flexion and forearm supination.

Background Information

Distal biceps tendinitis is a rare injury and occurs most often in power athletes and workers who carry heavy loads with flexed elbows.[6] Chronic cases or a history of intermittent symptoms should be classified as distal biceps tendinosis. Treatment for distal biceps tendinitis includes activity modification and inflammation control. Any strength deficits should be addressed when the acute inflammatory stage has resolved.

■ Distal Biceps Tendinosis

Chief Clinical Characteristics

This presentation may include pain and tenderness deep in the anterior elbow. Reproduction of symptoms may occur with resisted elbow flexion and forearm supination.

Background Information

Symptoms result from forceful and repetitive elbow flexion movements. It is a rare injury and occurs most often in power athletes and workers who carry heavy loads with flexed elbows.[6] It may be a factor in spontaneous distal biceps ruptures. Treatment is similar to that for distal biceps tendinitis but there may not be an acute inflammatory stage. Eccentric strengthening may be beneficial for distal biceps tendinosis.

■ Lateral Epicondylitis (Tennis Elbow)

Chief Clinical Characteristics

This presentation is characterized by pain and point tenderness at the lateral epicondyle and the involved tendon(s), most commonly the extensor carpi radialis brevis. Pain is worse with use of the arm. Reproduction of symptoms will occur with resisted wrist extension and passive wrist flexion with increased symptoms when the elbow is extended.

Background Information

This condition is also called tennis elbow, but symptoms can result from any excessive forearm use including gardening, gripping a heavy briefcase, and using a screwdriver. Infrequently, acute onset may be associated with a direct blow to the lateral elbow. Posterolateral rotatory instability may mimic or be associated with lateral epicondylitis.[42,43] Lateral epicondylitis occurs most commonly between the ages of 30 and 55 years.[44] If symptoms are long-standing or the patient has a history of excessive forearm use, the classification should be lateral epicondylosis. Treatment includes inflammation control, stretching, postural training, bracing, and strengthening when the acute inflammatory phase has resolved. Avoidance of painful activities, modification of provoking activities that cannot be avoided, and environmental adaptations (at work and leisure) are an integral part of successfully treating lateral epicondylitis. Infrequently, surgical treatment is utilized to treat patients who have not responded to nonoperative intervention.

■ Lateral Epicondylosis

Chief Clinical Characteristics
This presentation may include pain and point tenderness at the lateral epicondyle. Symptoms will be reproduced with resisted wrist extension and passive wrist flexion with increased symptoms when the elbow is extended.

Background Information
This condition occurs in response to repetitive microtrauma from excessive use of the wrist extensors and forearm supinators. It can be work induced or sports induced. Degeneration of tendons is very common and may be initially asymptomatic. Lateral epicondylosis is associated with aging but is seen most commonly between the ages of 30 and 55 years. Treatment is similar to that for lateral epicondylitis but may not have an acute inflammatory phase. Eccentric strengthening may be beneficial in the treatment of lateral epicondylosis.

■ Medial Epicondylitis (Golfer's Elbow)

Chief Clinical Characteristics
This presentation may include pain, point tenderness at the common flexor origin, and inflammation. Tenderness may also occur distal to the medial epicondyle in the proximal flexor and pronator mass. Reproduction of symptoms will occur with resisted wrist flexion, resisted forearm pronation, and passive wrist extension with the elbow extended. Making a tight fist increases pain.

Background Information
Also called golfer's elbow, pain may result from throwing, tennis, golf, or any other excessive forearm use. Medial epicondylitis is only 15% to 20% as common as lateral epicondylitis.[45] It occurs most commonly between the ages of 30 and 59 years and twice as often in males. Ulnar nerve symptoms have been associated in up to 50% of cases.[45] It is important to differentiate from medial collateral ligament rupture and instability. Treatment includes activity modification, inflammation control, postural training, stretching, and strengthening when the acute inflammatory phase has resolved. Chronic symptoms or a history of intermittent symptoms would indicate medial epicondylosis. Surgical intervention is used in cases where symptoms have lasted for longer than 1 year and have not responded to the above interventions.

■ Medial Epicondylosis

Chief Clinical Characteristics
This presentation may include pain and point tenderness at the medial epicondyle. Symptoms will be reproduced with resisted wrist flexion, resisted forearm pronation, and passive wrist extension with the elbow extended. Symptoms may also occur when making a tight fist. Mild extension loss at the elbow may occur with chronic cases.

Background Information
Microtrauma results from repetitive valgus stress on the medial elbow and wrist flexors and pronators. It can be work induced or sports induced. Degeneration of tendons may be initially asymptomatic. Medial epicondylosis is seen most commonly between the ages of 30 and 59 years. Treatment is similar to that for medial epicondylitis. Eccentric strengthening may be beneficial in the treatment of medial epicondylosis.

■ Triceps Tendinitis

Chief Clinical Characteristics
This presentation includes pain and tenderness at the insertion of the triceps. Symptoms will occur with resisted elbow extension. Symptoms may be produced with full passive elbow flexion. Elbow motion is typically not affected.

Background Information
Also called posterior tennis elbow, triceps tendinitis is uncommon as an isolated event and is usually associated with other posterior

elbow disorders (loose bodies and synovitis).[44] It is seen more commonly in throwers but can occur with any repetitive elbow extension movements. Chronic cases or a history of intermittent symptoms should be classified as triceps tendinosis. Treatment for triceps tendinitis includes activity modification and inflammation control. When the acute inflammatory stage has resolved, treatment should also include strengthening.

■ Triceps Tendinosis

Chief Clinical Characteristics
This presentation may be characterized by pain and tenderness at the tip at the triceps insertion. Reproduction of symptoms will occur with resisted elbow extension.

Background Information
Symptoms result from forceful and repetitive elbow extension movements. It is seen more commonly in throwers and is associated with loose bodies and synovitis of the elbow.[44] Radiographs may demonstrate insertional calcifications. Treatment includes activity modification, stretching, and strengthening. Inflammation control may also be necessary. Rarely, chronic cases may require surgical excision of the degenerated tissue.

■ Terrible Triad

Chief Clinical Characteristics
This presentation can be characterized by pain, swelling, ecchymosis, tenderness, and deformity.

Background Information
The terrible triad is a combination of injuries including posterior dislocation of the ulnohumeral joint, fracture of the radial head, and fracture of the coronoid. A comminuted radial head fracture should be assumed a triad injury until proven otherwise. The mechanism of injury is typically a fall onto the outstretched hand or direct trauma. This injury pattern is uncommon and difficult to manage. Inadequate fixation results in redislocation or chronic subluxation, and ulnohumeral arthrosis develops quickly in most patients.[46] Loss of motion is common with this condition. External fixation following surgical management of the radial head and coronoid fractures and lateral collateral ligament allows early motion without compromising stability. A historical

account of the injury and plain radiographs confirm the diagnosis.

■ Triceps Rupture

Chief Clinical Characteristics
This presentation includes pain and tenderness at the site of the osseous tendon insertion. Swelling and ecchymosis will be observed, as well as an inability to extend the elbow against gravity.

Background Information
A palpable defect may be present above the elbow. The mechanism of injury is typically a fall on the outstretched hand, but may also result from direct trauma or elbow dislocation or it may occur spontaneously or following surgical release and reattachment. The rupture is not always obvious when the injury is acute and may be misdiagnosed.[47] Spontaneous ruptures may be associated with chronic diseases such as renal osteodystrophy and secondary hyperthyroidism.[48] Clinical examination and magnetic resonance imaging or ultrasonography confirm the diagnosis. Complete triceps rupture is managed surgically (Fig. 12-3); partial tendon rupture can be treated nonoperatively.[47]

TUMORS

■ Ganglion Cyst

Chief Clinical Characteristics
This presentation includes a small, tender mass in the elbow region.

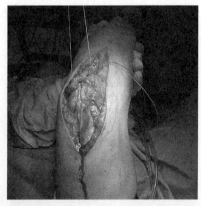

FIGURE 12-3 Surgical approach for surgical repair of a triceps tendon rupture.

Background Information

Ganglion cysts are single or multilobulated structures that are idiopathic mucin-filled outgrowths of tendon sheaths. Usually they are asymptomatic, but they may become painful and limit joint range of motion in some individuals. Elbow ganglions are more common postsurgically, especially following arthroscopic procedures. The diagnosis is confirmed with clinical examination and aspiration. Surgical excision may be indicated for symptom relief.

■ Giant Cell Tumor

Chief Clinical Characteristics

This presentation may include pain and tenderness but the tumor is typically asymptomatic.

Background Information

Pain may occur from the associated inflammatory response. Giant cell tumor is rare in the upper extremity. It affects females more commonly than males and occurs most often in persons over 20 years of age.[49] The tumor typically occurs in the epiphyseal region and may extend to the articular surface of the bone. Biopsy confirms the diagnosis. Surgical excision is required.

■ Lipoma

Chief Clinical Characteristics

This presentation typically involves a small, asymptomatic soft tissue mass. Occasionally the lipoma may grow and become symptomatic.

Background Information

Lipoma is a benign soft tissue neoplasm comprised of a localized collection of adipose tissue. It is the most common tumor in the elbow region.[50] Biopsy or magnetic resonance imaging confirms the diagnosis. Surgical excision may be indicated if the lipoma increases in size, becomes symptomatic, or interferes with function.

■ Malignant Lymphoma

Chief Clinical Characteristics

This presentation typically includes pain and sometimes swelling in the region of the lesion.

Background Information

Malignant lymphoma is a malignant bone tumor. The tumor may extend into the soft tissues. It occurs more frequently in middle-aged or elderly adults. Diagnosis is confirmed with biopsy. Treatment is dependent on the stage of the disease process but generally includes radiation therapy.

■ Osteoblastoma

Chief Clinical Characteristics

This presentation is characterized by pain and loss of elbow motion. The pain is less severe than with an osteoid osteoma.

Background Information

Osteoblastoma is an uncommon, benign tumor. It is histologically similar to an osteoid osteoma but typically greater than 2 cm in diameter. There is equal incidence of this condition between sexes, usually between the ages of 10 to 35 years.[49] Plain radiographs and computerized tomography scan confirm the diagnosis. The tumor requires surgical intervention.

■ Osteochondroma

Chief Clinical Characteristics

This presentation includes pain and may impair elbow motion. Symptoms are caused by pressure on neighboring structures.

Background Information

Osteochondroma is the most common benign bone tumor but is rare in the elbow. The tumor can occur at any age but growth usually ceases when skeletal maturity is achieved. The tumor develops from the surface of the bone and tends to extend away from the joint. Plain radiographs confirm the diagnosis. Surgical excision may be necessary to relieve symptoms and/or restore motion.

■ Osteoid Osteoma

Chief Clinical Characteristics

This presentation may include sharp, unremitting pain that is worse at night and relieved significantly with aspirin. The pain often increases with alcohol intake. The patient may have a progressive loss of elbow flexion or extension motion.

Background Information

Osteoid osteoma is a benign tumor, usually no greater than 1 cm in diameter. It typically affects persons 5 to 25 years of age, with a greater occurrence in males. Plain radiographs and computerized tomography scan confirm the diagnosis. The tumor typically requires surgical excision.

■ Osteosarcoma

Chief Clinical Characteristics
This presentation can involve pain with progressing severity and eventual swelling. The overlying skin may be warm. Loss of elbow motion may occur secondary to swelling. The patient may report weight loss.

Background Information
Osteosarcoma is one of the most common bone malignancies but is uncommon in the elbow. The tumor frequently metastasizes. Osteosarcoma is more common in males and usually occurs between the ages of 10 and 20 years of age. Diagnosis is confirmed with biopsy. Treatment usually consists of surgical ablation and chemotherapy.

■ Synovial Chondromatosis

Chief Clinical Characteristics
This presentation includes pain, swelling, and limited elbow motion. Patients may report locking or catching.[51] The patient may report symptoms lasting several years.

Background Information
Synovial chondromatosis is benign and involves the subsynovial connective tissue of joints, tendon sheaths, or bursa. It can occur at any joint. The tumor typically occurs in adults in their 20s to 40s, with males affected more commonly than females.[49] Clinical examination and plain radiographs confirm the diagnosis. The treatment includes surgical removal of the involved synovium and loose osteochondromatous bodies. Longstanding synovial chondromatosis may contribute to secondary osteoarthritis.

■ Synovial Sarcoma

Chief Clinical Characteristics
This presentation may include a tender, firm mass. Symptoms may be present for many years before a diagnosis is made. The mass may initially be painless.

Background Information
Synovial sarcoma is a malignant soft tissue tumor. It is more common in the lower extremity, but it does occur in the elbow region. The tumor is more common in young or middle-aged adults. Biopsy confirms the diagnosis. The most optimal prognosis is achieved with wide excision or radical surgery. Radiation therapy may be combined with the surgery.

■ Valgus Extension Overload Syndrome

Chief Clinical Characteristics
This presentation includes posterior elbow pain, tenderness of the olecranon, flexion contracture, and pain with passive elbow extension. Increased valgus laxity and painful locking may also occur. Reproduction of symptoms will occur with the valgus extension snap maneuver in which a firm valgus stress is placed on the elbow and the elbow is then snapped into extension.[52]

Background Information
This syndrome occurs most commonly in athletes who do a lot of overhead throwing. The repetitive hyperextension stress combined with medial elbow laxity results in impingement of the olecranon in the olecranon fossa. The impingement results in osteophytes and loose bodies. Valgus extension overload syndrome is almost always progressive. Clinical examination and radiographs confirm the diagnosis. Treatment includes inflammation control and activity modification. Once the inflammatory stage has resolved, stretching, strengthening, and a gradual return to throwing are indicated. Surgical intervention may be necessary for patients who do not respond to nonoperative treatment.

References
1. Wainner RS, Fritz JM, Irrgang JJ, Boninger ML, Delitto A, Allison S. Reliability and diagnostic accuracy of the clinical examination and patient self-report measures for cervical radiculopathy. *Spine.* Jan 1, 2003;28(1):52–62.
2. Murphy DR, Gruder MI, Murphy LB. Cervical radiculopathy and pseudo radiculopathy syndrome. In: Murphy DR, ed. *Conservative Management of Cervical Spine Syndromes.* New York, NY: McGraw-Hill; 2000:189–219.
3. Weiner S. *Differential Diagnosis of Acute Pain by Body Region.* New York, NY: McGraw-Hill; 1993.
4. Kelly EW, Steinmann S, O'Driscoll SW. Surgical treatment of partial distal biceps tendon ruptures through a single posterior incision. *J Shoulder Elbow Surg.* Sep–Oct 2003;12(5):456–461.
5. Ly JQ, Sanders TG, Beall DP. MR imaging of the elbow: a spectrum of common pathologic conditions. *Clin Imaging.* Jul–Aug 2005;29(4):278–282.

6. Jozsa L, Kannus P. *Human Tendons Anatomy, Physiology and Pathology.* Champaign, IL: Human Kinetics; 1997.

7. Raddatz DA, Hoffman GS, Franck WA. Septic bursitis: presentation, treatment and prognosis. *J Rheumatol.* Dec 1987;14(6):1160–1163.

8. Kozin SH. Capitellum fractures. In: Mirzayan R, Itamura JM, eds. *Shoulder and Elbow Trauma.* New York, NY: Thieme Medical Publishers; 2004:36–51.

9. Grantham SA, Norris TR, Bush DC. Isolated fracture of the humeral capitellum. *Clin Orthop Relat Res.* Nov–Dec 1981(161):262–269.

10. McKee MD, Jupiter JB, Bamberger HB. Coronal shear fractures of the distal end of the humerus. *J Bone Joint Surg Am.* Jan 1996;78(1):49–54.

11. Regan W, Morrey B. Fractures of the coronoid process of the ulna. *J Bone Joint Surg Am.* Oct 1989;71(9):1348–1354.

12. Sanchez-Sotelo J, O'Driscoll SW, Morrey BF. Medial oblique compression fracture of the coronoid process of the ulna. *J Shoulder Elbow Surg.* Jan–Feb 2005;14(1):60–64.

13. O'Driscoll SW, Jupiter JB, Cohen MS, Ring D, McKee MD. Difficult elbow fractures: pearls and pitfalls. *Instr Course Lect.* 2003;52:113–134.

14. Ristic S, Strauch RJ, Rosenwasser MP. The assessment and treatment of nerve dysfunction after trauma around the elbow. *Clin Orthop Relat Res.* Jan 2000(370):138–153.

15. Ring D, Jupiter JB, Simpson NS. Monteggia fractures in adults. *J Bone Joint Surg Am.* Dec 1998;80(12):1733–1744.

16. Harness N, Ring D, Jupiter JB. Olecranon fractures. In: Mirzayan R, Itamura J, eds. *Shoulder and Elbow Trauma.* New York, NY: Thieme Medical Publishers; 2004:53–66.

17. Itamura J, Roidis N, Mirzayan R, Vaishnav S, Learch T, Shean C. Radial head fractures: MRI evaluation of associated injuries. *J Shoulder Elbow Surg.* Jul–Aug 2005;14(4):421–424.

18. Early SD, Tolo VT. Pediatric elbow fractures. In: Mirzayan R, Itamura J, eds. *Shoulder and Elbow Trauma.* New York, NY: Thieme Medical Publishers; 2004:115–131.

19. Ring D, Jupiter JB, Sanders RW, Mast J, Simpson NS. Transolecranon fracture-dislocation of the elbow. *J Orthop Trauma.* Nov 1997;11(8):545–550.

20. Morrey BF. Ectopic ossification about the elbow. In: Morrey BF, ed. *The Elbow and Its Disorders.* 3rd ed. Philadelphia, PA: Saunders; 2000:437–446.

21. Chen FS, Mirzayan R, Itamura JM. The post-traumatic stiff elbow: overview and management. In: Mirzayan R, Itamura JM, eds. *Shoulder and Elbow Trauma.* New York: Thieme Medical Publishers; 2004:99–114.

22. O'Driscoll SW. Classification and evaluation of recurrent instability of the elbow. *Clin Orthop Relat Res.* Jan 2000(370):34–43.

23. O'Driscoll SW, Lawton RL, Smith AM. The "moving valgus stress test" for medial collateral ligament tears of the elbow. *Am J Sports Med.* Feb 2005;33(2):231–239.

24. Rettig AC, Sherrill C, Snead DS, Mendler JC, Mieling P. Nonoperative treatment of ulnar collateral ligament injuries in throwing athletes. *Am J Sports Med.* Jan–Feb 2001;29(1):15–17.

25. Pecina MM, Krmpotic-Nemanic J, Markiewitz AD. *Tunnel Syndromes Peripheral Nerve Compression Syndromes.* 2nd ed. Boca Raton, FL: CRC Press; 1997.

26. Ritts GD, Wood MB, Linscheid RL. Radial tunnel syndrome. A ten-year surgical experience. *Clin Orthop Relat Res.* Jun 1987(219):201–205.

27. Mazurek MT, Shin AY. Upper extremity peripheral nerve anatomy: current concepts and applications. *Clin Orthop Relat Res.* Feb 2001(383):7–20.

28. Naam NH, Massoud HA. Painful entrapment of the lateral antebrachial cutaneous nerve at the elbow. *J Hand Surg [Am].* Nov 2004;29(6):1148–1153.

29. Gelberman RH, Yamaguchi K, Hollstien SB, et al. Changes in interstitial pressure and cross-sectional area of the cubital tunnel and of the ulnar nerve with flexion of the elbow. An experimental study in human cadavera. *J Bone Joint Surg Am.* Apr 1998;80(4):492–501.

30. Kato H, Hirayama T, Minami A, Iwasaki N, Hirachi K. Cubital tunnel syndrome associated with medial elbow Ganglia and osteoarthritis of the elbow. *J Bone Joint Surg Am.* Aug 2002;84-A(8):1413–1419.

31. Perry CR. *Bone and Joint Infections.* St. Louis, MO: Mosby; 1996.

32. Doornberg J, Ring D, Jupiter JB. Effective treatment of fracture-dislocations of the olecranon requires a stable trochlear notch. *Clin Orthop Relat Res.* Dec 2004(429):292–300.

33. Antuna SA, Morrey BF, Adams RA, O'Driscoll SW. Ulnohumeral arthroplasty for primary degenerative arthritis of the elbow: long-term outcome and complications. *J Bone Joint Surg Am.* Dec 2002;84-A(12):2168–2173.

34. Lems WF, Dijkmans BAC. Rheumatoid arthritis: clinical picture and its variants. In: Firestein GS, Panayi GS, Wollheim FA, eds. *Rheumatoid Arthritis: New Frontiers in Pathogenesis and Treatment.* Oxford, UK: Oxford University Press; 2000.

35. Hargreaves D, Emery R. Total elbow replacement in the treatment of rheumatoid disease. *Clin Orthop Relat Res.* Sep 1999(366):61–71.

36. Gill DR, Morrey BF. The Coonrad-Morrey total elbow arthroplasty in patients who have rheumatoid arthritis. A ten to fifteen-year follow-up study. *J Bone Joint Surg Am.* Sep 1998;80(9):1327–1335.

37. Butters KP, Morrey BF. Septic arthritis. In: Morrey BF, ed. *The Elbow and Its Disorders.* 3rd ed. Philadelphia, PA: Saunders; 2000:809–817.

38. Dreyfuss U, Kessler I. Snapping elbow due to dislocation of the medial head of the triceps. A report of two cases. *J Bone Joint Surg Br.* Feb 1978;60(1):56–57.

39. Spinner RJ, Goldner RD. Snapping of the medial head of the triceps and recurrent dislocation of the ulnar nerve. Anatomical and dynamic factors. *J Bone Joint Surg Am.* Feb 1998;80(2):239–247.

40. Goodman CC, Snyder TEK. *Differential diagnosis in physical therapy.* 2nd ed. Philadelphia, PA: Saunders; 1995.

41. De Sanctis MT, Cesarone MR, Incandela L, Belcaro G, Griffin M. Treatment of superficial vein thrombophlebitis of the arm with Essaven gel—a placebo-controlled, randomized study. *Angiology.* Dec 2001;52 (suppl 3):S63–67.

42. Baker CLJ, Nirschl RP. Lateral tendon injury: open and arthroscopic treatment. In: Altchek DW, Andrews JR, eds. *The Athlete's Elbow.* Philadelphia, PA: Lippincott Williams & Wilkins; 2001:91–103.

43. Kalainov DM, Cohen MS. Posterolateral rotatory instability of the elbow in association with lateral epicondylitis. A report of three cases. *J Bone Joint Surg Am.* May 2005;87(5):1120–1125.

44. Nirschl RP. Muscle and tendon trauma: tennis elbow tendinosis. In: Morrey BF, ed. *The Elbow and Its Disorders.* 3rd ed. Philadelphia, PA: Saunders; 2000:523–535.

45. Gabel GT, Morrey BF. Medial Epicondylitis. In: Morrey BF, ed. *The Elbow and Its Disorders*. 3rd ed. Philadelphia, PA: Saunders; 2000:537–542.

46. Ring D, Jupiter JB, Zilberfarb J. Posterior dislocation of the elbow with fractures of the radial head and coronoid. *J Bone Joint Surg Am*. Apr 2002;84-A(4): 547–551.

47. van Riet RP, Morrey BF, Ho E, O'Driscoll SW. Surgical treatment of distal triceps ruptures. *J Bone Joint Surg Am*. Oct 2003;85-A(10):1961–1967.

48. Pina A, Garcia I, Sabater M. Traumatic avulsion of the triceps brachii. *J Orthop Trauma*. Apr 2002;16(4):273–276.

49. Levesque J, Marx R, Bell RS, Wunder JS, Kandel R, White LM. *A Clinical Guide to Primary Bone Tumors*. Baltimore, MD: Williams & Wilkins; 1998.

50. Pritchard DJ, Unni KK. Neoplasms of the elbow. In: Morrey BF, ed. *The Elbow and Its Disorders*. 3rd ed. Philadelphia, PA: Saunders; 2000:873–889.

51. Kamineni S, O'Driscoll SW, Morrey BF. Synovial osteochondromatosis of the elbow. *J Bone Joint Surg Br*. Sep 2002;84(7):961–966.

52. Wilk K, Andrews JA. Elbow injuries. In: Brotzman SB, Wilk K, eds. *Clinical Orthopedic Rehabilitation*. Philadelphia, PA: Mosby; 2003:85–123.

CHAPTER 13

Wrist and Hand Pain

■ *Robin I. Burks, PT, DPT, CHT* ■ *Stephen Schnall, MD*

Description of the Symptom

Wrist and hand pain, as discussed in this chapter, includes diffuse/general wrist and hand pain, central wrist pain, radial wrist pain, ulnar wrist pain, dorsal hand pain, palmar hand pain, and digit pain. **Local causes** of wrist and hand pain are defined as pathology that occurs within the distal one-quarter of the radius and ulna, carpals, metacarpals, and phalanges; component articulations of the wrist and hand; and associated soft tissue structures. **Remote causes** are defined as those occurring outside this region.

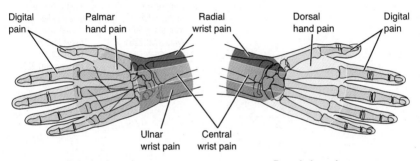

Palmar ulnar view   **Dorsal ulnar view**

Special Concerns
- Decreased pulses
- Fracture with suspected skin break
- Pain in bilateral hands provoked with cervical movements
- Pain out of proportion to the injury
- Severe edema following trauma in areas with fascial muscle compartments
- Skin break and fever
- Sudden or progressive paresthesia or loss of sensation associated with trauma
- Warmth and swelling associated with a fever or purulent drainage

CHAPTER PREVIEW: Conditions That May Lead to Wrist and Hand Pain

T Trauma

REMOTE	LOCAL DIFFUSE/ GENERAL WRIST AND HAND	LOCAL CENTRAL WRIST	LOCAL RADIAL WRIST
COMMON			
Radiculopathies: • C6 radiculopathy 214 Ulnar nerve compression at the elbow (cubital tunnel syndrome) 218	Not applicable	Fractures: • Capitate and lunate fractures 221 • Distal radioulnar joint fracture/ dislocation 221 Lunate dislocation 225 Nerve injuries: • Median nerve compression at the wrist (carpal tunnel syndrome) 226 Scapholunate ligament sprain 231	Fractures: • Distal radius fracture 222 • Scaphoid fracture 223 • Thumb metacarpal base fracture (Bennett's or Rolando's fracture) 224 Nerve injuries: • Radial sensory nerve injury (without entrapment) 227
UNCOMMON			
Pronator syndrome 214 Radiculopathies: • C7 radiculopathy 214 • C8 radiculopathy 215 Thoracic outlet syndrome 216	Not applicable	Not applicable	Nerve injuries: • Radial sensory nerve entrapment (Wartenberg's syndrome) 226
RARE			
Not applicable	Not applicable	Not applicable	Not applicable

LOCAL ULNAR WRIST	LOCAL DORSAL HAND	LOCAL PALMAR HAND	LOCAL DIGITS
Fractures: • Distal radioulnar joint fracture/ dislocation 221 • Distal radius fracture 222 • Distal ulna fracture 222 • Hamate fracture (non-hook) 222 • Pisiform fracture 223 • Triquetrum fracture 224 Lunotriquetral ligament tear (and lunotriquetral dissociation) 226	Fractures: • Metacarpal fractures (including Boxer's fracture) 223 Nerve injuries: • Radial sensory nerve entrapment (Wartenberg's syndrome) 226 • Radial sensory nerve injury (without entrapment) 227	Fractures: • Hamate fracture (hook) 222 Nerve injuries: • Median nerve compression at the wrist (carpal tunnel syndrome) 226	Acute central slip rupture (Boutonnière deformity) 218 Flexor digitorum profundus avulsion/rupture (jersey finger) 221 Fractures: • Phalangeal fracture 223 • Thumb metacarpal base fracture (Bennett's or Rolando's fracture) 224 Interphalangeal joint dislocation 225 Nerve injuries: • Median nerve compression at the wrist (carpal tunnel syndrome) 226 • Radial sensory nerve injury (without entrapment) 227 Terminal extensor tendon rupture (Mallet finger) 234 Ulnar collateral ligament tear (Gamekeeper's or Skier's thumb) 237
Nerve injuries: • Ulnar nerve compression at the wrist (Guyon's canal) 227 Triangular fibrocartilage complex tear 234	Not applicable	Not applicable	Nerve injuries: • Ulnar digital nerve compression (Bowler's thumb) 227 Subungual hematoma 232
Not applicable	Not applicable	Not applicable	Not applicable (continued)

I Inflammation

REMOTE	LOCAL DIFFUSE/ GENERAL WRIST AND HAND	LOCAL CENTRAL WRIST	LOCAL RADIAL WRIST
COMMON			
Aseptic Trigger points 216 **Septic** Not applicable	Not applicable	**Aseptic** Tendinopathies: • Extensor digitorum communis tendinitis 233 **Septic** Not applicable	**Aseptic** Tendinopathies: • Extensor pollicis longus tendinitis 233 • First dorsal compartment (De Quervain's) tenosynovitis 234 **Septic** Not applicable
UNCOMMON			
Aseptic Not applicable **Septic** Herpes zoster/ post-herpetic neuralgia 213	**Aseptic** Complex regional pain syndrome 220 Inflammatory arthritis (including rheumatoid, psoriatic, scleroderma, and systemic lupus erythematosus) 225 **Septic** Septic arthritis 231	**Aseptic** Not applicable **Septic** Osteomyelitis: • Wrist and hand 229 Septic arthritis 231	**Aseptic** Flexor carpi radialis tunnel syndrome 220 **Septic** Osteomyelitis: • Wrist and hand 229 Septic arthritis 231
RARE			
Aseptic Not applicable **Septic** Cervical epidural abscess 213 Cervical osteomyelitis 213	**Aseptic** Arthritis associated with inflammatory bowel disease 218 Reiter's syndrome 231 **Septic** Cellulitis 219 Lyme disease 226	**Aseptic** Arthritis associated with inflammatory bowel disease 218 Foreign body reaction 221 **Septic** Not applicable	**Aseptic** Arthritis associated with inflammatory bowel disease 218 Foreign body reaction 221 Intersection syndrome 225 **Septic** Not applicable

LOCAL ULNAR WRIST	LOCAL DORSAL HAND	LOCAL PALMAR HAND	LOCAL DIGITS
Aseptic Tendinopathies: • Extensor carpi ulnaris tendinitis 232 • Flexor carpi ulnaris tendinitis 234 **Septic** Not applicable	**Aseptic** Tendinopathies: • Extensor digitorum communis tendinitis 233 **Septic** Not applicable	**Aseptic** Stenosing tenosynovitis (trigger finger/thumb) 231 **Septic** Not applicable	**Aseptic** Stenosing tenosynovitis (trigger finger/thumb) 231 **Septic** Paronychia 230
Aseptic Ulnocarpal impaction/abutment syndrome 237 **Septic** Osteomyelitis: • Wrist and hand 229 Septic arthritis 231	**Aseptic** Not applicable **Septic** Osteomyelitis: • Wrist and hand 229 Septic arthritis 231	**Aseptic** Not applicable **Septic** Osteomyelitis: • Wrist and hand 229 Septic arthritis 231	**Aseptic** Inflammatory arthritis (including rheumatoid, psoriatic, scleroderma, and systemic lupus erythematosus) 225 **Septic** Animal bite infections 218 Felon 220 Human bite infections 224 Osteomyelitis: • Wrist and hand 229 Septic arthritis 231 Suppurative digital flexor tenosynovitis 232
Aseptic Arthritis associated with inflammatory bowel disease 218 Foreign body reaction 221 **Septic** Not applicable	**Aseptic** Arthritis associated with inflammatory bowel disease 218 Foreign body reaction 221 **Septic** Not applicable	**Aseptic** Arthritis associated with inflammatory bowel disease 218 Foreign body reaction 221 **Septic** Not applicable	**Aseptic** Arthritis associated with inflammatory bowel disease 218 Foreign body reaction 221 **Septic** Not applicable

(continued)

M Metabolic

REMOTE	LOCAL DIFFUSE/ GENERAL WRIST AND HAND	LOCAL CENTRAL WRIST	LOCAL RADIAL WRIST
COMMON			
Not applicable	Gout 224 Pseudogout 230	Gout 224 Pseudogout 230	Gout 224 Pseudogout 230
UNCOMMON			
Not applicable	Not applicable	Not applicable	Not applicable
RARE			
Not applicable	Not applicable	Not applicable	Not applicable

Va Vascular

REMOTE	LOCAL DIFFUSE/ GENERAL WRIST AND HAND	LOCAL CENTRAL WRIST	LOCAL RADIAL WRIST
COMMON			
Not applicable	Not applicable	Not applicable	Not applicable
UNCOMMON			
Myocardial infarction 214	Vascular malformation 238	Avascular necrosis: • Avascular necrosis of the lunate (Kienböck's disease) 219 Vascular malformation 238	Vascular malformation 238
RARE			
Not applicable	Compartment syndrome 219 Emboli 220	Not applicable	Avascular necrosis: • Avascular necrosis of the scaphoid (Preiser's disease) 219

De Degenerative

REMOTE	LOCAL DIFFUSE/ GENERAL WRIST AND HAND	LOCAL CENTRAL WRIST	LOCAL RADIAL WRIST
COMMON			
Not applicable	Not applicable	Osteoarthrosis/ osteoarthritis: • Intercarpal osteoarthrosis/ osteoarthritis 228 Tendinopathies: • Extensor digitorum communis tendinosis 233	Osteoarthrosis/ osteoarthritis: • Intercarpal osteoarthrosis/ osteoarthritis 228 • Radioscaphoid osteoarthrosis/ osteoarthritis 228

LOCAL ULNAR WRIST	LOCAL DORSAL HAND	LOCAL PALMAR HAND	LOCAL DIGITS
Gout 224 Pseudogout 230	Gout 224 Pseudogout 230	Gout 224 Pseudogout 230	Gout 224 Pseudogout 230
Not applicable	Not applicable	Not applicable	Not applicable
Not applicable	Not applicable	Not applicable	Not applicable

LOCAL ULNAR WRIST	LOCAL DORSAL HAND	LOCAL PALMAR HAND	LOCAL DIGITS
Not applicable	Not applicable	Not applicable	Not applicable
Vascular malformation 238	Vascular malformation 238	Vascular malformation 238	Hypothenar hammer syndrome 224 Peripheral vascular disease 230 Raynaud's phenomenon/ disease 230 Vascular malformation 238
Not applicable	Not applicable	Not applicable	Emboli 220

LOCAL ULNAR WRIST	LOCAL DORSAL HAND	LOCAL PALMAR HAND	LOCAL DIGITS
Osteoarthrosis/ osteoarthritis: • Distal radioulnar joint osteoarthrosis/ osteoarthritis 227 • Intercarpal osteoarthrosis/ osteoarthritis 228	Tendinopathies: • Extensor digitorum communis tendinosis 233	Not applicable	Osteoarthrosis/ osteoarthritis: • Distal interphalangeal joint osteoarthrosis/ osteoarthritis 227 • Metacarpophalangeal joint osteoarthrosis/ osteoarthritis 228

(continued)

Degenerative *(continued)*

REMOTE	LOCAL DIFFUSE/ GENERAL WRIST AND HAND	LOCAL CENTRAL WRIST	LOCAL RADIAL WRIST
COMMON			
			• Thumb carpometacarpal joint osteoarthrosis/ osteoarthritis (basilar joint or CMC arthrosis) 229
UNCOMMON			
Cervical degenerative disk disease 212 Cervical degenerative joint disease 213	Osteoarthrosis/ osteoarthritis: • Scapholunate advanced collapse (SLAC) wrist 229	Osteoarthrosis/ osteoarthritis: • Distal radioulnar joint osteoarthrosis/ osteoarthritis 227	Not applicable
RARE			
Not applicable	Not applicable	Not applicable	Not applicable

Tu Tumor

REMOTE	LOCAL DIFFUSE/ GENERAL WRIST AND HAND	LOCAL CENTRAL WRIST	LOCAL RADIAL WRIST
COMMON			
Not applicable	Not applicable	Not applicable	Not applicable
UNCOMMON			
Not applicable	Not applicable	*Malignant Primary:* Not applicable *Malignant Metastatic:* Not applicable *Benign, such as:* • Ganglion cyst 235	*Malignant Primary:* Not applicable *Malignant Metastatic:* Not applicable *Benign, such as:* • Ganglion cyst 235
RARE			
Malignant Primary, such as: • Pancoast tumor 217 *Malignant Metastatic, such as:* • Metastases to the cervical spine or other tissue adjacent to nerves to the upper extremity 217	*Malignant Primary:* Not applicable *Malignant Metastatic, such as:* • Metastases to the wrist and hand, including from primary breast, kidney, lung, prostate, and thyroid disease 236	*Malignant Primary:* Not applicable *Malignant Metastatic, such as:* • Metastases to the wrist and hand, including from primary breast, kidney, lung, prostate, and thyroid disease 236	*Malignant Primary:* Not applicable *Malignant Metastatic, such as:* • Metastases to the wrist and hand, including from primary breast, kidney, lung, prostate, and thyroid disease 236

LOCAL ULNAR WRIST	LOCAL DORSAL HAND	LOCAL PALMAR HAND	LOCAL DIGITS
• Pisotriquetral osteoarthrosis/ osteoarthritis 228 Tendinopathies: • Extensor carpi ulnaris tendinosis 232			• Proximal interphalangeal joint osteoarthrosis/ osteoarthritis 228 • Sesamoid osteoarthrosis/ osteoarthritis (thumb) 229 • Thumb carpometacarpal joint osteoarthrosis/ osteoarthritis (basilar joint or CMC arthrosis) 229
Tendinopathies: • Flexor carpi ulnaris tendinosis 234	Not applicable	Not applicable	Not applicable
Not applicable	Not applicable	Not applicable	Not applicable

LOCAL ULNAR WRIST	LOCAL DORSAL HAND	LOCAL PALMAR HAND	LOCAL DIGITS
Not applicable	Not applicable	Not applicable	Not applicable
Malignant Primary: Not applicable *Malignant Metastatic:* Not applicable *Benign, such as:* • Ganglion cyst 235	*Malignant Primary:* Not applicable *Malignant Metastatic:* Not applicable *Benign, such as:* • Ganglion cyst 235	*Malignant Primary:* Not applicable *Malignant Metastatic:* Not applicable *Benign, such as:* • Ganglion cyst 235	*Malignant Primary:* Not applicable *Malignant Metastatic:* Not applicable *Benign, such as:* • Ganglion cyst 235
Malignant Primary: Not applicable *Malignant Metastatic, such as:* • Metastases to the wrist and hand, including from primary breast, kidney, lung, prostate, and thyroid disease 236	*Malignant Primary, such as:* • Chondrosarcoma 235 • Epithelioid sarcoma 235 • Osteosarcoma 237 • Sarcoidosis 231 • Squamous cell carcinoma 237	*Malignant Primary, such as:* • Chondrosarcoma 235 • Osteosarcoma 237	*Malignant Primary, such as:* • Chondrosarcoma 235 • Epithelioid sarcoma 235 • Osteosarcoma 237 • Squamous cell carcinoma 237

(continued)

Tumor *(continued)*

REMOTE	LOCAL DIFFUSE/ GENERAL WRIST AND HAND	LOCAL CENTRAL WRIST	LOCAL RADIAL WRIST
RARE			
Benign, such as: • Meningioma 217 • Syringomyelia 217	*Benign, such as:* • Sarcoidosis 231	*Benign, such as:* • Osteoblastoma 236 • Osteoid osteoma 237 • Sarcoidosis 231	*Benign, such as:* • Osteoblastoma 236 • Osteoid osteoma 237 • Sarcoidosis 231

Co   Congenital

REMOTE	LOCAL DIFFUSE/ GENERAL WRIST AND HAND	LOCAL CENTRAL WRIST	LOCAL RADIAL WRIST
COMMON			
Not applicable	Not applicable	Not applicable	Not applicable
UNCOMMON			
Not applicable	Not applicable	Not applicable	Not applicable
RARE			
Not applicable	Not applicable	Not applicable	Not applicable

Ne   Neurogenic/Psychogenic

REMOTE	LOCAL DIFFUSE/ GENERAL WRIST AND HAND	LOCAL CENTRAL WRIST	LOCAL RADIAL WRIST
COMMON			
Not applicable	Not applicable	Not applicable	Not applicable
UNCOMMON			
Somatoform disorders: • Hypochondriasis 215 • Malingering 215 • Pain disorder 216	Not applicable	Not applicable	Not applicable

LOCAL ULNAR WRIST	LOCAL DORSAL HAND	LOCAL PALMAR HAND	LOCAL DIGITS
Benign, such as: • Osteoblastoma 236 • Sarcoidosis 231	*Malignant Metastatic, such as:* • Metastases to wrist and hand, including from primary breast, kidney, lung, prostate, and thyroid disease 236 *Benign, such as:* • Enchondroma 235 • Epithelial inclusion cyst 235 • Osteoblastoma 236	*Malignant Metastatic, such as:* • Metastases to the wrist and hand, including from primary breast, kidney, lung, prostate, and thyroid disease 236 *Benign, such as:* • Enchondroma 235 • Epithelial inclusion cyst 235 • Giant cell tumor of the tendon sheath 235 • Osteoblastoma 236 • Sarcoidosis 231	*Malignant Metastatic, such as:* • Metastases to the wrist and hand, including from primary breast, kidney, lung, prostate, and thyroid disease 236 *Benign, such as:* • Enchondroma 235 • Epithelial inclusion cyst 235 • Giant cell tumor of the tendon sheath 235 • Glomus tumor 236 • Mucous cyst 236 • Osteochondroma 236 • Osteoid osteoma 237 • Sarcoidosis 231

LOCAL ULNAR WRIST	LOCAL DORSAL HAND	LOCAL PALMAR HAND	LOCAL DIGITS
Not applicable	Not applicable	Not applicable	Not applicable
Not applicable	Not applicable	Not applicable	Not applicable
Not applicable	Not applicable	Not applicable	Not applicable

LOCAL ULNAR WRIST	LOCAL DORSAL HAND	LOCAL PALMAR HAND	LOCAL DIGITS
Not applicable	Not applicable	Not applicable	Not applicable
Not applicable	Not applicable	Not applicable	Not applicable

(continued)

Neurogenic/Psychogenic *(continued)*

REMOTE	LOCAL DIFFUSE/ GENERAL WRIST AND HAND	LOCAL CENTRAL WRIST	LOCAL RADIAL WRIST
RARE			
Somatoform disorders: • Factitious disorder 215 • Somatization disorder 216	Not applicable	Not applicable	Not applicable

Note: These are estimates of relative incidence because few data are available for the less common conditions.

Overview of Wrist and Hand Pain

Due to the delicacy of structures in the hand, both examination and treatment of the wrist and hand should be performed with great care. A partial ligament or tendon rupture that could have been treated conservatively may become a complete injury requiring surgery following an overly vigorous examination. Plain radiographs should be taken after any injury to the hand to rule out fractures, dislocations, foreign bodies, or other pathology. Injuries with fractures or suspected tendon or ligament injuries should be referred to a hand surgeon for further consultation. Splinting is an essential part of treatment for many hand problems (Box 13-1). Some can be treated with prefabricated splints, but many require splints to be custom-made by the therapist. Therapists unfamiliar with splinting should consider referring these cases to a colleague, at least for the splint fabrication.

Description of Conditions That May Lead to Wrist and Hand Pain

Remote

■ Cervical Degenerative Disk Disease

Chief Clinical Characteristics
This presentation typically includes pain in the posterior or posterolateral region of the neck with or without radiculopathy.

Background Information
This condition is associated with advanced age and most commonly affects the C5–C6 and C6–C7 levels. Patients may develop osteophytes,

degenerative annular tears, loss of disk height, narrowing of the spinal canal, or compression of the spinal cord or nerve roots, resulting in radiculopathy. Upper extremity symptoms occur when pathology progresses to the point of encroachment on the neural foramina. The diagnosis is confirmed with plain radiographs that reveal decreased disk height and osteophyte formation along the anterior and posterior margins of the intervertebral joint.[1] Surgery may be necessary in severe and resistant cases that do not respond to nonoperative treatment, including severe or worsening neurological deficits.

BOX 13-1 Conditions of the Wrist and Hand That May Require Splinting

- Acute central slip rupture (Boutonnière deformity)
- Extensor carpi ulnaris tendinitis/tendinosis
- Extensor digitorum communis tendinitis/ tendinosis
- Extensor pollicis longus tendinitis/tendinosis
- First dorsal compartment (De Quervain's) tenosynovitis
- Flexor carpi radialis tunnel syndrome
- Flexor carpi ulnaris tendinitis/tendinosis
- Interphalangeal joint dislocation
- Median nerve compression at the wrist (carpal tunnel syndrome)
- Ulnar collateral ligament tear (gamekeeper's or skier's thumb)
- Ulnar nerve compression at the elbow (cubital tunnel syndrome)

LOCAL ULNAR WRIST	LOCAL DORSAL HAND	LOCAL PALMAR HAND	LOCAL DIGITS
Not applicable	Not applicable	Not applicable	Not applicable

■ Cervical Degenerative Joint Disease

Chief Clinical Characteristics

This presentation can involve pain in the posterior or posterolateral aspect of the neck with possible radiation to the upper extremity, possibly associated with dermatomal sensory loss and myotomal weakness.

Background Information

This condition becomes more common with advancing age. Osteoarthrosis (osteoarthritis) of the facet joints, hypertrophy of the ligamentum flavum, and osteophyte formation around the intervertebral foramen can contribute to symptoms. It usually presents without radicular symptoms; upper extremity symptoms occur when pathology progresses to the point of encroachment on the neural foramina. Plain radiographs and magnetic resonance imaging confirm the diagnosis.[2] Surgery may be necessary in severe and resistant cases that do not respond to nonoperative treatment, especially those that involve severe or progressing neurological deficits.

■ Cervical Epidural Abscess

Chief Clinical Characteristics

This presentation may include neck pain and fever. Extremity pain develops a few days later due to nerve root irritation or compression. Symptoms may be unilateral or bilateral, involving single or multiple dermatomes depending on the specific location of the infection.

Background Information

This condition is often associated with immune suppressive conditions such as acquired immunodeficiency syndrome or diabetes mellitus. This condition is caused by an infection that usually results from bloodborne spread of bacteria from an infection site elsewhere in the body. It also may be associated with intravenous drug use. The diagnosis is confirmed with magnetic resonance imaging.[3] This condition is a medical emergency.

■ Cervical Osteomyelitis

Chief Clinical Characteristics

This presentation typically includes upper extremity pain, sensory loss, and weakness possibly associated with fever and neck pain. Fever may or may not be present. Extremity symptoms may occur in single or multiple dermatomal patterns.

Background Information

Cervical osteomyelitis is often associated with immune suppression (acquired immunodeficiency syndrome, diabetes mellitus, liver failure), intravenous drug abuse, or infection in other areas. Epidural abscess, discitis, segmental deformity, or instability may develop as a result of this condition. The diagnosis is confirmed with plain radiographs or magnetic resonance imaging of the cervical spine.[4,5] Individuals suspected of having this condition must be referred to a physician for medical management, which includes antibiotics and surgery.

■ Herpes Zoster/Post-Herpetic Neuralgia

Chief Clinical Characteristics

This presentation is characterized by hypersensitivity and pain in a unilateral dermatomal distribution, associated with a vivid red skin rash that is distinguished by small vesicles filled with clear fluid. Pain may persist for up to a year following resolution of the rash (post-herpetic neuralgia), although the typical duration of symptoms is a few months.

Background Information

This condition occurs when varicella virus is latently reactivated in a spinal ganglion. This condition may present initially without the rash, leading to an incorrect diagnosis of radiculopathy due to the distribution of symptoms. The presence of the rash, extreme pain, unilateral involvement, general malaise, and unclear association with spinal movement aids in differential diagnosis.[6] Treatment with antiviral and anti-inflammatory medications is most effective if started as soon as possible.

■ Myocardial Infarction

Chief Clinical Characteristics

This presentation typically involves pain and pressure in the chest or between shoulder blades that may radiate to upper extremities, neck, torso, or jaw. Infrequently, symptoms may refer distally to the wrist and hand. Pain may be worsened by physical exertion.

Background Information

Other findings include diaphoresis, dyspnea, dizziness, loss of consciousness, pallor, and tachycardia. Blood pressure may be normal, decreased, or elevated. Symptoms are responsive to nitroglycerin.[7] This health condition occurs when occlusion of a coronary artery results in myocardial ischemia. Echocardiography, serial blood tests, and angiogram confirm the diagnosis. This condition is a medical emergency.

■ Pronator Syndrome

Chief Clinical Characteristics

This presentation typically includes pain, tingling, and numbness in the volar aspect of the thumb, index, and middle and the radial half of the ring fingers, as well as pain in the anterior surface of the distal arm and proximal forearm and weakness of the flexor pollicis longus and the flexor digitorum profundus to the index and middle fingers.

Background Information

This condition involves compression of the median nerve in the antecubital area. Negative Phalen's and Tinel's tests at the wrist will help distinguish this condition from carpal tunnel syndrome.[8] Diagnosis is usually made based on clinical findings; electromyogram/nerve conduction studies are used to confirm the diagnosis. Surgical release at the site of compression is generally indicated if symptoms are severe.

RADICULOPATHIES

■ C6 Radiculopathy

Chief Clinical Characteristics

This presentation typically includes pain, paresthesia, and numbness of the neck, shoulder, upper arm, radial forearm and wrist, entire surface of the thumb, and possibly index finger. Weakness of forearm pronation or wrist extension, or changes in the biceps or brachioradialis reflex may be noted. Arm and hand use may worsen symptoms.

Background Information

This condition may be caused by cervical disk protrusion, arthritic spurs on the cervical facet joints, and tumors or other space-occupying lesions in the spine.[9] A negative upper limb tension test is useful in ruling out the condition. The combination of positive upper limb tension test, cervical rotation toward the involved side less than 60 degrees, decreased symptoms with cervical distraction, and positive Spurling's test increases the likelihood of cervical radiculopathy to 90%.[10] Cervical spine magnetic resonance imaging confirms the diagnosis. Depending on the etiology, cervical radiculopathy can often be managed nonsurgically, but must be monitored for worsening symptoms, especially constant numbness and developing weakness.

■ C7 Radiculopathy

Chief Clinical Characteristics

This presentation typically includes pain, paresthesia, and numbness of the neck, shoulder, upper arm, dorsal forearm and wrist, and the entire surface of the middle finger. Weakness with elbow extension, wrist flexion, and finger extension or changes in the triceps reflex may be noted. Arm and hand use may worsen symptoms.

Background Information

This condition may be caused by cervical disk protrusion, arthritic spurs on the cervical facet joints, and tumors or other space-occupying lesions in the spine.[9] A negative upper limb tension test is useful in ruling out the condition. The combination of positive upper limb tension test, cervical rotation toward the involved side less than 60 degrees, decreased symptoms with cervical distraction, and positive Spurling's test increases the likelihood of cervical radiculopathy to 90%.[10] Cervical spine magnetic resonance imaging confirms the diagnosis. Depending on the etiology, cervical radiculopathy can often be managed nonsurgically, but must be monitored for worsening symptoms, especially constant numbness and developing weakness.

■ C8 Radiculopathy

Chief Clinical Characteristics
This presentation typically includes pain, numbness, and tingling throughout the small finger, ulnar border of the hand, and medial aspect of the forearm. There may be weakness of extensor indicis, flexor pollicis longus, and hand intrinsics. Arm and hand use may worsen symptoms.

Background Information
This condition may be caused by cervical disk protrusion, arthritic spurs on the cervical facet joints, and tumors or other space-occupying lesions in the spine.[9] A negative upper limb tension test is useful in ruling out the condition. The combination of positive upper limb tension test, cervical rotation toward the involved side less than 60 degrees, decreased symptoms with cervical distraction, and positive Spurling's test increases the likelihood of cervical radiculopathy to 90%.[10] Cervical spine magnetic resonance imaging confirms the diagnosis. Depending on the etiology, cervical radiculopathy can often be managed nonsurgically, but must be monitored for worsening symptoms, especially constant numbness and developing weakness.

SOMATOFORM DISORDERS

Psychological factors may contribute to a patient's perception or report of pain and other symptoms in the hand and wrist. These factors should be considered when a patient's symptoms do not seem to conform to recognized pathologies or when they fail to respond to treatment. Psychological issues can affect the patient's perception of physical well-being and lead to exaggeration or misrepresentation of symptoms. This can complicate the diagnostic process. Clinical psychiatric disorders may, in addition, be a primary cause of perceived wrist and hand pain. Somatoform disorders involve psychiatric problems that manifest as apparent physical symptoms.

■ Factitious Disorder

Chief Clinical Characteristics
This presentation is characterized by intentional production or feigning of physical symptoms that could include wrist and hand symptoms. These patients are motivated by a desire to assume the sick role. When perceived as being sick, these patients derive emotional rewards such as increased tolerance, attention, or compassion from family, friends, or coworkers.

Background Information
External motivation (eg, obtaining narcotic medication, financial gain through litigation or disability payments) to assume the sick role is absent in this condition. Evaluation by a clinical psychologist or psychiatrist is necessary to confirm the diagnosis.[11] This health condition may be amenable to a combination of pharmacologic and cognitive-behavioral management.

■ Hypochondriasis

Chief Clinical Characteristics
This presentation typically involves fear of having a serious medical condition despite its absence and reassurance that one does not exist; this may include wrist and hand disorders. The fear associated with this condition causes clinically significant distress or impairment in social, occupational, or other important areas of functioning lasting greater than 6 months.

Background Information
Individuals with this condition either may or may not recognize that their behavior is excessive or dysfunctional. Evaluation by a clinical psychologist or psychiatrist is necessary to confirm the diagnosis.[11]

■ Malingering

Chief Clinical Characteristics
This presentation typically involves intentionally producing or feigning physical

symptoms. These complaints could include wrist and hand symptoms.

Background Information
Patients with this condition are motivated to assume the sick role to achieve external rewards such as financial gain, narcotic medication, or decreased demands to function in the home or workplace. Evaluation by a clinical psychologist or psychiatrist is necessary to confirm the diagnosis.[11]

■ Pain Disorder

Chief Clinical Characteristics
This presentation typically involves reports of pain in one or more areas (which may occur in the wrist or hand) that is not faked or intentionally produced, but in which psychological factors are felt to play a contributory role in the intensity, beginning, worsening, or continuation of the pain. The pain must result in a significant loss of function.

Background Information
Evaluation by a clinical psychologist or psychiatrist is necessary to confirm the diagnosis.[11] A combination of pharmacologic and cognitive-behavioral management may be necessary.

■ Somatization Disorder

Chief Clinical Characteristics
This presentation may include reports of pain in one or more areas (which may occur in the wrist or hand), as well as a variety of other physical symptoms such as gastrointestinal dysfunction, balance disorders, and sexual dysfunction in addition to pain. These symptoms are not adequately explained by a physical diagnosis.

Background Information
There must be a history of multiple complaints beginning before the fourth decade of life. Complaints must involve several areas or organ symptoms, and must have resulted in impairment of function or in the seeking of treatment. They must not be intentionally produced or faked. Evaluation by a clinical psychologist or psychiatrist is necessary to confirm the diagnosis.[11] This health condition may be amenable to a combination of pharmacologic and cognitive-behavioral management.

■ Thoracic Outlet Syndrome

Chief Clinical Characteristics
This presentation typically includes aching, throbbing pain and limited numbness in the hand, especially on the ulnar side. There may be atrophy of the intrinsic muscles of the hand. Fine-motor dexterity in the hand may be decreased.

Background Information
Circulatory changes including edema, Raynaud's phenomenon, and pallor may be noted. This condition can result from compression of the brachial plexus at several points along its course, including between the anterior and middle scalene muscles and against the first rib. Contributing factors may include a cervical rib, clavicular fracture malunion or callus, neck trauma, poor posture, or abnormal breathing patterns that utilize muscles of deep inspiration for normal breathing.[8] The diagnosis is confirmed with the clinical examination, although its diagnostic accuracy is controversial. Imaging modalities also may implicate involved structures. Surgery is indicated if symptoms do not respond to nonsurgical treatment.

■ Trigger Points

Chief Clinical Characteristics
This presentation involves variable, poorly localized, and mobile symptoms in the wrist and hand that may be associated with severe local tenderness of muscles distant to the site of wrist and hand pain.

Background Information
Tenderness at the trigger point will be intense, but may not always reproduce the hand symptoms. Tenderness to palpation in the hand, if present, is generally less intense than would be anticipated based on patient reports. Trigger points in muscles throughout the upper quarter may produce pain in the wrist and hand.[12] This diagnosis should only be accepted after other more serious pathologies are rejected. The diagnosis is confirmed through the clinical examination, and management involves options ranging from rehabilitation interventions to injections.

TUMORS

■ Meningioma

Chief Clinical Characteristics

This presentation typically includes variable symptoms, including upper extremity radicular symptoms.

Background Information

This condition involves a benign tumor of the meninges, and symptoms depend on the specific nerve roots affected. Onset is usually in the second to third decade of life.[13] Despite the benign nature of the tumor, this condition may involve significant morbidity. The diagnosis is confirmed with magnetic resonance imaging of the cervical spine. Surgery, radiation, or chemotherapy may be necessary to address this health condition.

■ Metastases to the Cervical Spine or Other Tissue Adjacent to Nerves to the Upper Extremity

Chief Clinical Characteristics

This presentation can include unremitting pain in individuals with these risk factors: previous history or cancer, age 50 years or older, failure to improve with conservative therapy, and unexplained weight change of more than 10 pounds in 6 months.[14]

Background Information

The skeletal system is the third most common site of metastatic disease.[15] Symptoms also may be related to pathological fracture in affected sites. Metastatic tumors may develop in the cervical spine or near the brachial plexus or radial, median, or ulnar nerves. Common primary sites causing metastases to bone include breast, prostate, lung, and kidney. Nerve symptoms not explained by other diagnoses, or symptoms accompanied by palpable tumors along the path of the nerve, should be referred to a physician for further workup. Bone scan confirms the diagnosis in the event of bony metastases. Electromyogram/nerve conduction studies can be useful in localizing nerve compression; plain radiography, computed tomography, and magnetic resonance imaging are also useful for assessing etiology. Intervention may involve options such as chemotherapy, radiation therapy, and surgical resection.

■ Pancoast Tumor

Chief Clinical Characteristics

This presentation typically involves sharp, pleuritic pain in the axilla, shoulder, or subscapular regions with referral pain to the neck. Clinical findings also include shoulder-arm pain, Horner's syndrome, and neurological deficits affecting the C8 and T1 nerve roots.[16] Neck movements, and cervical compression or distraction may not change symptoms. Symptoms may be similar to thoracic outlet syndrome. Pain is severe and constant; patients often support the involved elbow with the opposite hand to relieve pressure.

Background Information

Because of their location at the extreme apex of the lung, much of the mass of Pancoast tumors is located in the extrathoracic space.[17] Risk factors for lung tumors include smoking, exposure to secondary smoke, prolonged asbestos exposure, and exposure to industrial elements. Chest radiographs confirm the diagnosis.[17–19] Surgery, chemotherapy, and radiation therapy are all possible options for treatment.

■ Syringomyelia

Chief Clinical Characteristics

This presentation may involve bilateral but asymmetrical loss of pain and temperature sensation in the upper extremity, possibly associated with pain. Weakness may also develop, especially in the hand intrinsic muscles; this can produce a clawing deformity of the fingers.

Background Information

Upper extremity deep tendon reflexes may be absent. Painless ulcers may occur on the hands. Hyperhidrosis and edema may develop. This condition usually is caused by trauma to the cervical spine. Patients with bilateral upper extremity symptoms, especially weakness, should be referred to a physician to rule out possible spinal cord pathology. This diagnosis is confirmed with magnetic resonance imaging of the cervical spine.[20] Surgical decompression of the characteristic lesion (syrinx) may be indicated.

WRIST AND HAND PAIN

■ Ulnar Nerve Compression at the Elbow (Cubital Tunnel Syndrome)

Chief Clinical Characteristics

This presentation can include pain, numbness, and tingling in the small and ulnar half of the ring fingers, and in the ulnar half of the dorsum of the hand (this is differentiated from ulnar nerve compression at the wrist, which does not include symptoms on the dorsum of the hand). Weakness may be present in the flexor digitorum profundus to the ring and small fingers, the thumb adductor, the interosseous muscles, the lumbricals to the ring and small fingers, and the hypothenar muscles.

Background Information

If there is severe compression, the ring and small fingers may be held in a "claw deformity," with the metacarpophalangeal joints hyperextended and the interphalangeal joints flexed; the patient will be unable to simultaneously flex the metacarpophalangeal joints and extend the interphalangeal joints. The condition may begin acutely following a blow to the posterior elbow, or develop chronically due to prolonged positioning in elbow flexion or weight bearing on the elbow. Diagnosis is usually made based on clinical findings; electromyogram/nerve conduction studies are used to confirm the diagnosis. Nonoperative treatment consists of splinting and activity modification to decrease pressure on the nerve. Surgery is indicated if numbness is constant or if significant weakness is noted.

Local

■ Acute Central Slip Rupture (Boutonnière Deformity)

Chief Clinical Characteristics

This presentation typically includes pain, edema, and bruising over the dorsum of the proximal interphalangeal joint and inability to actively extend the proximal interphalangeal joint.

Background Information

This injury usually results from a blow to the dorsum of the middle phalanx that forces the proximal interphalangeal (PIP) joint to flex during attempted active extension, or from a volar dislocation of the PIP joint that may have spontaneously reduced. With dislocation, there may also be collateral ligament injury. If the central slip tear is not properly treated acutely, permanent deformity can develop as the central slip retracts proximally, the triangular ligament attenuates, and the lateral bands slip volarly to become PIP flexors.[21] Plain radiographs are useful to rule out fractures that may be associated with this health condition. This condition may be managed nonoperatively with splinting of the PIP in extension while allowing distal interphalangeal joint flexion. Surgery is indicated if a large bone fragment is avulsed.

■ Animal Bite Infections

Chief Clinical Characteristics

Animal bite infections involve a variable clinical presentation, depending on the depth of bite, organism introduced, and tissue affected.

Background Information

Animal bites produce complex wounds. They must be thoroughly assessed to determine the involved structures, and tendon or nerve injuries or fractures must be treated appropriately. These wounds are prone to infection; a physician must prescribe proper antibiotics. Cat bites may be deep without much bleeding and introduce bacteria deep into the affected tissue due to the slenderness of their teeth. Therefore infection in the joint, flexor sheath, or other anatomical space can result from a seemingly insignificant wound. If not treated promptly, the developing infection can lead to extensive tissue damage and may threaten the viability of the finger or even the limb. All bite wounds should be referred to a physician for evaluation. Treatment involves systemic antibiotics as soon as possible, even if no signs of infection have developed.

■ Arthritis Associated with Inflammatory Bowel Disease

Chief Clinical Characteristics

This presentation may include asymmetrical migratory polyarthritis associated with a history of inflammatory bowel disease (IBD).

Background Information

Although lower extremity joints are affected more frequently, the upper extremity may be involved as well. Flare-ups tend to last 2 to 3 months, although recurrence and chronic arthritis are possible. About 20% of patients with IBD develop arthritis.[22] Patients with IBD and arthritic symptoms should be referred for medical management. Medical management may include palliative medication, as well as corticosteroids or immune modifying agents, in combination with dietary advice.

AVASCULAR NECROSIS

■ Avascular Necrosis of the Lunate (Kienböck's Disease)

Chief Clinical Characteristics

This presentation typically includes dorsal central wrist pain worsened with activity, tenderness to palpation over the lunate (Fig. 13-1), decreased wrist range of motion and grip strength, and dorsal wrist edema.

Background Information

Onset is usually in the second or third decade of life. The cause of this condition is unclear. It is associated with negative ulnar variance (ulna shorter than radius) and may accompany lunate fracture. Plain radiographs confirm this diagnosis. Kienböck's may be initially managed nonoperatively with cast immobilization, but must be closely monitored for improvement. Surgery is indicated if degeneration continues, or if lunate collapse has occurred. Complications may include lunate collapse and wrist osteoarthrosis/osteoarthritis.

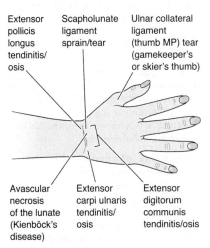

Extensor pollicis longus tendinitis/osis

Scapholunate ligament sprain/tear

Ulnar collateral ligament (thumb MP) tear (gamekeeper's or skier's thumb)

Avascular necrosis of the lunate (Kienböck's disease)

Extensor carpi ulnaris tendinitis/osis

Extensor digitorum communis tendinitis/osis

FIGURE 13-1 Palpation guide: causes of dorsal hand pain.

■ Avascular Necrosis of the Scaphoid (Preiser's Disease)

Chief Clinical Characteristics

This presentation can involve pain in the radial side of the wrist and tenderness to palpation over the scaphoid, especially at the anatomical snuffbox. Edema may be present. Pain may be worse with wrist extension and radial deviation, or with end-range pronation and supination.

Background Information

This condition usually results from a fall on the extended, radially deviated wrist, leading to a scaphoid fracture. It also may develop idiopathically.[23] Plain radiographs confirm the diagnosis. Surgery is indicated in all cases to prevent degenerative changes in the wrist.

■ Cellulitis

Chief Clinical Characteristics

This presentation typically involves swelling, pain, and erythema. The edges are usually not clearly demarcated. As the infection progresses, blisters may develop in the central portion of the affected tissue. Fever and/or serous or purulent drainage may be present.

Background Information

This health condition results from an acute infection of the skin and subdermal tissues. This secondary infection may result from a nearby contaminated wound, or through the bloodstream from a remote site of infection. This condition occurs more frequently among individuals with immune compromise.[24] Individuals suspected of cellulitis should be referred immediately for medical treatment.

■ Compartment Syndrome

Chief Clinical Characteristics

This presentation typically includes swelling (often producing tissue rigidity) and pain at initial presentation, with increasing pain and numbness as the condition progresses.

Background Information

Passive stretching may increase pain; active contraction of involved muscles may be too painful to perform. Palpable distal pulses do not preclude a diagnosis of compartment syndrome since blood pressure in the large arteries may be higher than compartment pressure.

This condition may follow a closed injury to the wrist and hand, especially a crush injury. It develops when pressure due to edema or bleeding in the fascial compartments exceeds the perfusion pressure of muscle and nerve tissue in the compartment; this produces ischemia. This condition is more likely in the presence of multiple fractures. It also may result from external pressure such as an overly restrictive cast or bandage, high-pressure injection injuries (such as with a paint or grease gun), extravasated intravenous lines, and pressure due to an unconscious or inebriated patient lying on the affected arm for a prolonged period. Anticoagulant use increases risk. The diagnosis is made based on clinical findings, confirmed by tonometer measurement of compartment pressures. This condition is a medical emergency, typically treated by fasciotomy. Complications of delayed fasciotomy may include Volkmann's ischemic contracture (irreversible fibrotic changes and contracture of involved muscles) and renal damage (resulting from the toxic by-products of muscle necrosis).[25]

■ Complex Regional Pain Syndrome

Chief Clinical Characteristics
This presentation can involve a traumatic onset of severe chronic wrist and hand pain accompanied by allodynia, hyperalgesia, as well as trophic, vasomotor, and sudomotor changes in later stages.

Background Information
This condition is characterized by disproportionate responses to painful stimuli. It is a regional neuropathic pain disorder that presents either without direct nerve trauma (type I) or with direct nerve trauma (type II) in any region of the body.[26] This condition may precipitate as a result of an event distant to the affected area. Thermography may confirm associated sympathetic dysfunction. Plain radiographs may reveal associated osteopenia.[27,28]

■ Emboli

Chief Clinical Characteristics
This presentation may include pain, pallor, and coldness in the involved tissues.

Background Information
This condition occurs when small blood clots travel through the larger vessels of the arterial system until they occlude a smaller vessel. This condition can occur anywhere in the hand, but is more likely to result from blockage of arteries supplying the fingers due to the redundancy of more proximal circulation. Loss of blood flow can eventually lead to cell death, chronic wounds, and dry gangrene. The diagnosis is confirmed by vascular studies and laser Doppler. This condition is a medical emergency.

■ Felon

Chief Clinical Characteristics
This presentation typically includes deep aching or throbbing pain, accompanied by erythema and tense swelling of the tip and extreme tenderness to touch. Individuals with this condition will avoid using the involved digit.

Background Information
This is an infection of the distal pulp space; it results from introduction of commonly occurring skin bacteria into the deep compartments of the finger tip via a puncture wound; bacteria can also enter this space from an untreated paronychia. A felon differs from a paronychia in that the erythema and swelling are throughout the finger tip, rather than just near the nail. This condition may progress to osteomyelitis of the distal phalanx or infection of the distal interphalangeal joint if left untreated.[29] Diagnosis is based on clinical findings. Treatment consists of irrigation, debridement, and systemic antibiotics.

■ Flexor Carpi Radialis Tunnel Syndrome

Chief Clinical Characteristics
This presentation may be characterized by pain on the volar/radial aspect of the wrist, from the proximal pole of the scaphoid up the forearm 1 to 4 cm. The pain will worsen with resisted wrist flexion and radial deviation.

Background Information
This condition usually results from overuse and awkward hand postures, especially with constant active wrist flexion. The diagnosis is based on clinical findings.[30] This health condition is usually managed nonoperatively with anti-inflammatory medications and splinting/casting. Surgery is indicated if conservative measures fail.

■ Flexor Digitorum Profundus Avulsion/Rupture (Jersey Finger)

Chief Clinical Characteristics

This presentation involves edema and ecchymosis over the volar aspect of the distal interphalangeal (DIP) joint, associated with an inability to actively flex the DIP.

Background Information

There may be a tender, palpable mass on the volar aspect of the DIP joint, the proximal interphalangeal joint, or in the distal palm. Onset is usually in the second to third decade of life, but may occur at any age. This injury usually results from forcible extension of the DIP during active flexion, as when a football player attempts to grab an opponent's jersey and slips off. When the tendon is avulsed, plain radiographs may reveal a bone fragment drawn proximally as the tendon retracts. Otherwise, diagnosis is based on clinical findings. Complications may result from late or absent repair, including more complicated surgery with little likelihood of full recovery of range of motion. If the flexor digitorum profundus is not repaired, a boutonnière deformity may develop.[21] Surgical repair is always indicated, and should be performed within 10 days of injury.

■ Foreign Body Reaction

Chief Clinical Characteristics

This presentation includes localized pain. Signs include local redness, swelling, and tenderness. An entrance wound may be noted, but it already may have healed.

Background Information

Hands are especially susceptible to penetration by foreign bodies due to their functional role in manipulating objects. Slivers of wood, metal, or glass, cactus or other plant spines and thorns, and fish spines are frequently involved. Individuals with this condition do not always remember the initial injury. Foreign body penetration may introduce a variety of organisms into the wound, leading to infection; however, a foreign body reaction is aseptic. If the foreign body can be visualized, it is within the scope of physical therapy practice to remove it using clean technique and sterile instruments. However, if the object is not apparent from the surface, or if infection is suspected, referral to a physician is necessary. If not removed, the foreign body can produce a granuloma that can compress surrounding structures and produce ongoing pain and stiffness.[31]

FRACTURES

■ Capitate and Lunate Fractures

Chief Clinical Characteristics

This presentation may involve pain, swelling, and bruising throughout the wrist, especially centered dorsally and volarly. There is tenderness to palpation over these bones. Wrist movement is markedly limited due to pain.

Background Information

Bleeding into the carpal tunnel, or edema resulting from the injury, may produce symptoms of median nerve compression. These fractures are uncommon in isolation; due to their relatively protected position in the hand, an injury with sufficient force to fracture these bones will also produce other injuries such as distal radius fracture, ligament tears, and carpal dislocations. The diagnosis is confirmed by plain radiographs.[32] These injuries require cast immobilization or surgical repair.

■ Distal Radioulnar Joint Fracture/Dislocation

Chief Clinical Characteristics

This presentation is characterized by pain, swelling, and bruising along the central dorsal aspect of the distal forearm. The area may be tender to palpation. Deformity may be present if the ulna is dislocated out of the sigmoid notch of the radius. Pain is worse with forearm movement, especially supination, and range of motion will be limited.

Background Information

Fracture may be due to a fall on an outstretched hand, especially with a rotation force. The fracture/dislocation may also be associated with tears of the triangular fibrocartilage complex, dorsal radioulnar ligaments, or fracture of the ulnar styloid. The diagnosis is confirmed by plain radiographs.[32] Following fracture healing, therapy may be indicated to restore motion and function.

■ Distal Radius Fracture

Chief Clinical Characteristics

This presentation may include pain throughout the wrist, edema, tenderness to palpation, bruising, and deformity. Wrist movements may be especially painful. Deformity may be apparent if there is significant displacement of fracture fragments.

Background Information

This fracture usually results from a fall on an outstretched hand. Fractures of the scaphoid and ulnar styloid and tears of wrist ligaments can occur concurrently. Complications include nonunion, malunion (eg, radial shortening and altered radial palmar tilt), and median nerve compression. A fracture involving Lister's tubercle may lead to later rupture of the extensor pollicis longus tendon. The diagnosis is confirmed by plain radiographs.[32] This condition may be managed with closed reduction and casting but must be closely monitored for loss of anatomical reduction. Surgery is indicated if stable reduction cannot be achieved.

■ Distal Ulna Fracture

Chief Clinical Characteristics

This presentation can involve pain throughout the wrist, edema, tenderness to palpation, bruising, and deformity. Pronation and supination may be especially painful.

Background Information

This fracture usually results from a fall on an outstretched wrist. This condition may be associated with distal radius fracture, tear of the triangular fibrocartilage complex, or dislocation of the distal radioulnar joint. Complications include ulnar shortening (which can lead to Kienböck's disease).[32] The diagnosis is confirmed by plain radiographs. This condition may be managed with closed reduction and casting but must be closely monitored for loss of anatomical reduction. Surgery is indicated if stable reduction cannot be achieved.

■ Hamate Fracture (Hook)

Chief Clinical Characteristics

This presentation may include pain and tenderness to localized deep palpation in the

proximal hypothenar area (Fig. 13-2). If the ulnar nerve is compressed, there may be numbness, tingling, or pain in the palmar aspect of the small and ulnar aspect of the ring fingers.

Background Information

This condition usually results from impact with a held object (golf club, tennis racket, or baseball bat) or fall on an outstretched hand. Complications may include rupture of the flexor tendons to the ring and small fingers due to abrasion on rough fracture edges.[32] The fracture may be visible on plain radiographs (carpal tunnel view), but CT scan is necessary to rule out fracture when plain radiographs are negative. This condition may be managed nonoperatively with cast immobilization as long as ulnar nerve compression is not present. Surgery is indicated if there is displacement, if nonunion occurs, or if the ulnar nerve is involved.

■ Hamate Fracture (Non-Hook)

Chief Clinical Characteristics

This presentation typically includes pain, swelling, and bruising along the ulnar border of the hand with localized tenderness to palpation over the hamate.

Background Information

This condition is uncommon in isolation; a blow to the ulnar side of the hand may

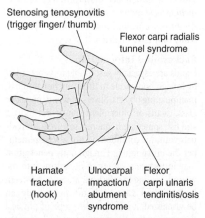

FIGURE 13-2 Palpation guide: causes of palmar pain.

fracture the hamate in addition to the bases of the fourth and fifth metacarpals or the triquetrum.[32] The diagnosis is confirmed by plain radiographs or computed tomography. These injuries require cast immobilization or surgical repair.

■ Metacarpal Fractures (Including Boxer's Fracture)

Chief Clinical Characteristics
This presentation typically includes pain, tenderness, ecchymosis, and swelling over the fractured metacarpal. There may be visible or palpable deformity if the fracture is sufficiently angulated, usually on the dorsum of the hand.

Background Information
These fractures usually result from impact to the hand, frequently from punching a hard object such as a wall. Onset is usually in the second or third decades of life.[32] A boxer's fracture is specifically a fracture of the fifth metacarpal neck. Fractures sustained in a fight may also be associated with tooth punctures of the metacarpophalangeal joint; infection should be assumed in these cases. Complications may include rotational malalignment; the finger may appear normal in extension, but cross over an adjacent finger when the patient attempts to make a fist. The diagnosis is confirmed by plain radiographs. Surgical correction is required if rotational malalignment is functionally and cosmetically unacceptable.

■ Phalangeal Fracture

Chief Clinical Characteristics
This presentation may involve pain, tenderness, and swelling in the involved digit; ecchymosis or bony deformity may be visible, but significant redness or heat is unlikely.

Background Information
These injuries may result from falls, crush injuries, or other impact to the digit. Fractures near the joints may also be associated with dislocations or tendon avulsions.[32] The diagnosis is confirmed by plain radiographs. Management of these fractures is determined by characteristics of the individual fracture including stability, degree of comminution,

amount and type of displacement, and whether the fracture is intra-articular.

■ Pisiform Fracture

Chief Clinical Characteristics
This presentation typically includes local pain and tenderness to palpation over the pisiform, and edema in the proximal hypothenar area.

Background Information
This uncommon fracture can result from a blow to the palm or a fall on an outstretched hand.[32] Plain radiographs or CT scan confirm the diagnosis. Treatment involves casting for 6 weeks.

■ Scaphoid Fracture

Chief Clinical Characteristics
This presentation can include pain in the radial side of the wrist and tenderness to palpation over the scaphoid, especially at the anatomical snuffbox (Fig. 13-3). Edema may be present. Pain may be worse with wrist extension and radial deviation, or with end-range thumb movements, pronation, and supination.

Background Information
Onset is usually in the second or third decade of life, but can occur at any age. This condition usually results from a fall on the extended, radially deviated wrist. Nonunion of the fracture can result in necrosis of one of the fragments; this leads to severe degeneration of the wrist joints.[32] The diagnosis is

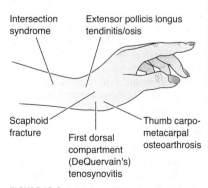

FIGURE 13-3 Palpation guide: causes of radial wrist and hand pain.

confirmed by plain radiographs; however, fractures are often difficult to identify on plain films immediately after injury. If clinical signs of scaphoid fracture are present, a cast should be applied to the affected hand and imaging repeated in 2 weeks.

■ Thumb Metacarpal Base Fracture (Bennett's or Rolando's Fracture)

Chief Clinical Characteristics
This presentation mainly includes pain, tenderness, and swelling at the base of the thumb; ecchymosis or bony deformity may be visible, but significant redness or heat is unlikely.

Background Information
This fracture usually results from axial loading of a partially flexed thumb. A Bennett's fracture is extra-articular, whereas a Rolando's fracture is intra-articular.[32] The diagnosis is confirmed by plain radiographs. A variety of treatment options are available depending on the characteristics of the particular fracture. Physical therapy may be beneficial in restoring range and function following fracture healing.

■ Triquetrum Fracture

Chief Clinical Characteristics
This presentation includes pain, swelling, and tenderness to palpation on the ulnar border of the wrist.

Background Information
Ecchymosis may be present with this condition. This fracture is uncommon in isolation. A blow to the ulnar side of the hand may fracture the triquetrum in addition to the bases of the fourth and fifth metacarpals or the hamate.[32] The diagnosis is confirmed by plain radiographs. Isolated injuries require cast immobilization; injuries that are more complex may need surgical repair.

■ Gout

Chief Clinical Characteristics
This presentation can involve a red, swollen, acutely painful joint. As this condition progresses, subcutaneous deposits of white pasty material (tophi) may develop and occasionally erupt through the skin. Advanced cases may include deforming arthritic changes at multiple joints.

Background Information
Initial onset is typically in middle age or later, and 95% of cases occur in men. Initial presentation in the hand is uncommon, so a history of involvement in other joints, especially the great toe metatarsophalangeal joint, may help guide the diagnosis. This condition results from overproduction of uric acid, resulting in sodium urate crystal deposition in affected tissues. This condition is commonly mistaken for an infection. Microscopic examination of aspirated synovial joint fluid confirms the diagnosis.[31] Treatment involves medication to correct the metabolic disorder. Surgery is indicated in cases with advanced joint destruction.

■ Human Bite Infections

Chief Clinical Characteristics
This presentation may involve minor pain associated with a small laceration over the metacarpophalangeal joint of one of the fingers, and increasing erythema and swelling at the joint. Range of motion will become limited and painful.

Background Information
This injury results from impact of the knuckle with a tooth; it is not uncommon for the tooth to penetrate the joint capsule, introducing bacteria into the joint space. Onset is usually in the second to third decade of life. Eventually, septic arthritis and osteomyelitis may result if left untreated. Clinical examination confirms the diagnosis. Treatment includes irrigation, debridement, and systemic antibiotics.

■ Hypothenar Hammer Syndrome

Chief Clinical Characteristics
This presentation includes burning pain in the proximal hypothenar area, numbness in the palmar aspect of the small finger and ulnar-palmar aspect of the ring finger, cold intolerance, and ischemia to the fingers.

Background Information
This condition occurs with trauma to the ulnar artery in the area of Guyon's canal, which may produce thrombosis, vasospasm, or aneurysm. The ulnar nerve may be compressed by the enlarged vascular structures.

Clinically, there may be a positive finding of occlusion of the ulnar artery on an Allen's test. An arteriogram confirms the diagnosis. This condition usually results from isolated or repeated trauma to the hypothenar area where the heel of the hand is used as a hammer, such as in karate or in workplace activities.[30] The injury may be managed nonoperatively in mild cases, and the use of padded gear may allow return to previous activity. Injury that is more serious requires surgery to repair or reconstruct the vascular damage.

■ Inflammatory Arthritis (Including Rheumatoid, Psoriatic, Scleroderma, and Systemic Lupus Erythematosus)

Chief Clinical Characteristics

Inflammatory arthritides typically present with pain in multiple joints in the wrists and hands; symptoms are usually symmetrical in rheumatoid arthritis, systemic lupus erythematosus (SLE), and scleroderma, but may not be in other diseases. In addition to pain, there may be swelling, stiffness, and erythema.

Background Information

These diseases produce progressive deformity in the wrist and digital joints. These conditions are often associated with Raynaud's phenomenon. They may be managed nonoperatively with medication and splinting; paraffin baths often provide temporary relief of pain. Surgery is often valuable to correct deformity and repair damaged structures; joint replacements are performed for metacarpophalangeal joints and, less often, for the wrist.[33] Therapy may increase range and strength and help to reduce pain. Complications differ for specific diseases, but may include joint erosion, deformity (ulnar drift at the metacarpophalangeal joints, boutonnière and swan neck deformities), and attritional tendon ruptures.

■ Interphalangeal Joint Dislocation

Chief Clinical Characteristics

This presentation typically includes edema, tenderness, and possibly ecchymosis at the involved joint. The affected joint may be visibly dislocated, but more often either spontaneous or deliberate reduction of the dislocation may be reported.

Background Information

This injury can result from a variety of forces across the joint including impact, traction, torsion, and linear forces pushing the joint beyond physiological limits. Complications include residual joint stiffness, especially proximal interphalangeal joint flexion contractures.[34] Fractures also may accompany a dislocation, so plain radiographs are generally indicated. These injuries are usually managed nonoperatively with a brief period of splinting followed by buddy taping and active range of motion. Surgery is indicated if soft tissue or fracture injuries require repair.

■ Intersection Syndrome

Chief Clinical Characteristics

This presentation mainly involves sharp pain in the radial aspect of the distal forearm about 1 to 2 inches proximal to the radial styloid (see Fig. 13-3). Pain may be reproduced with resisted wrist extension. Edema may be present.

Background Information

There will be tenderness to palpation where the tendons of the extensor carpi radialis longus and brevis pass deep to the extensor pollicis brevis and abductor pollicis longus.[30] Diagnosis is made based on clinical findings. Intersection syndrome is usually managed nonoperatively with corticosteroid injections or iontophoresis, oral anti-inflammatory medication, splinting to limit wrist movement, and thermal modalities.

■ Lunate Dislocation

Chief Clinical Characteristics

This presentation is characterized by pain and swelling in the wrist and hard volar bulge of the lunate in the area of the carpal tunnel. There may be decreased finger flexion due to pressure on the flexor tendons, or pressure on the median nerve may produce pain, numbness, and weakness in a median distribution.

Background Information

This injury usually results from a fall on an outstretched hand. Complications may include nerve injury and loss of range of motion in the wrist. The diagnosis is confirmed by plain radiographs.[34] A surgeon should manage this injury; if nerve compression is suspected, the referral should be urgent.

◼ Lunotriquetral Ligament Tear (and Lunotriquetral Dissociation)

Chief Clinical Characteristics

This presentation typically includes pain in the ulnar wrist and tenderness over the lunotriquetral joint. The ligaments supporting the joint may be merely sprained; however, a painful click with ulnar and radial deviation may indicate complete rupture.

Background Information

This injury usually results from a fall on an outstretched hand, or from forceful twisting of the wrist. The diagnosis is confirmed by plain radiographs. Sprains may be managed nonoperatively. Surgery is indicated if instability is present. Complications may develop if instability is not addressed; abnormal lunate movement can eventually lead to degenerative osteoarthrosis/osteoarthritis requiring salvage surgery.[35]

◼ Lyme Disease

Chief Clinical Characteristics

This presentation involves myalgia and migratory joint pain associated with a characteristic "bull's-eye" shaped rash (erythema migrans), fever, chills, and lymphadenopathy.

Background Information

This condition results from infection with *Borrelia burgdorferi* bacteria following a tick bite. One to 4 months following inoculation, neurological symptoms including radiculoneuritis may develop, as well as conjunctivitis, cardiac abnormalities, and myocarditis. Long-standing disease (greater than 6 months) may result in chronic synovitis, chronic arthritis, chronic fatigue, and encephalopathy. This diagnosis is confirmed with the clinical examination in early stages, and serologic tests in later stages.[36,37] Individuals with multijoint pain should always be referred for medical workup.

NERVE INJURIES

◼ Median Nerve Compression at the Wrist (Carpal Tunnel Syndrome)

Chief Clinical Characteristics

This presentation mainly includes pain, paresthesia, or numbness in the volar aspect of the thumb, index and middle fingers, and radial

aspect of the ring finger. Pain may be present in the wrist, and may radiate up the arm to the shoulder. In advanced cases, atrophy of the thenar muscles may be noted. Reproduction of symptoms when holding a full fist suggests that the lumbrical attachment on the flexor digitorum profundus (FDP) tendon may be too proximal, causing the muscle bellies to be drawn into the tunnel with full FDP contraction. Patients will often report difficulty manipulating small objects such as buttons or earrings. Symptoms are frequently worse at night.

Background Information

This condition may result from repetitive activity or from frequent exposure to vibration. It can also occur due to sustained wrist flexion in sleep, pregnancy, and hypothyroidism. Diagnosis is through clinical examination, and may be confirmed by electromyogram/nerve conduction studies. Worsening symptoms or symptoms that do not respond to nonsurgical treatment within 6 weeks also indicate a need for surgical referral.[30,38]

◼ Radial Sensory Nerve Entrapment (Wartenberg's Syndrome)

Chief Clinical Characteristics

This presentation involves pain, tingling, and numbness over the dorsoradial aspect of the wrist, index finger, and thumb.

Background Information

With this condition a positive Tinel's sign is often seen in the distal third of the forearm. This syndrome results from compression of the radial sensory nerve as it passes between the brachioradialis and extensor carpi radialis longus. Acute injury or chronic overuse may contribute to the development of this condition.[30] Diagnosis is made based on clinical findings and confirmed by electromyogram/nerve conduction studies. This condition may be managed nonoperatively with corticosteroid injection or iontophoresis, splinting to hold the wrist in a neutral position, and removal of sources of compression such as jewelry or tight clothing. Surgery is indicated if nonsurgical treatment is unsuccessful.

■ Radial Sensory Nerve Injury (Without Entrapment)

Chief Clinical Characteristics

This presentation includes pain (frequently described as burning), tingling, and numbness in the radial dorsal aspect of the hand and the dorsum of the thumb and index finger.

Background Information

The radial sensory nerve can be injured at any point along its course, from just distal to the elbow to the dorsoradial aspect of the hand. This nerve is easy to irritate and slow to heal. This injury (contusion or stretch) can result from impact, prolonged pressure (including from an overly tight cast or splint), surgery to the radial wrist, or placement of an external fixator.[32] Diagnosis is made based on clinical findings, and may be confirmed by electromyogram/nerve conduction studies or injection of local anesthetic. This injury is generally managed without intervention. However, recovery can be very slow. Iontophoresis with dexamethasone via a low-current (24-hour) delivery system may help reduce recovery time.

■ Ulnar Digital Nerve Compression (Bowler's Thumb)

Chief Clinical Characteristics

This presentation can involve pain and numbness in the ulnar side of the thumb from the metacarpophalangeal joint to the tip.

Background Information

This results from compression of the nerve, frequently against the edge of the hole in the bowling ball.[39] Diagnosis is based on history and clinical findings. Protective splinting of the thumb and redrilling of the bowling ball to relieve pressure and allow return to sport.

■ Ulnar Nerve Compression at the Wrist (Guyon's Canal)

Chief Clinical Characteristics

This presentation mainly involves pain, numbness, and tingling in the small and ulnar half of the ring fingers, but not in the ulnar half of the dorsum of the hand. This is differentiated from ulnar nerve compression at the elbow, which includes dorsal symptoms. There may be weakness in the adductor pollicis, the

interosseous muscles, the lumbricals to the ring and small fingers, and the hypothenar muscles.

Background Information

If there is severe compression, the ring and small fingers may be held in a "claw deformity," with the metacarpophalangeal joints hyperextended and the IP joints flexed; the patient will be unable to flex the MPs with the IPs extended. The condition may begin acutely following a blow to the wrist, or result from ulnar artery thrombosis or aneurysm or a ganglion cyst in Guyon's canal.[35] Diagnosis is based on clinical findings and confirmed with electromyogram/nerve conduction studies. Nonsurgical treatment following direct trauma consists of splinting and activity modification to decrease pressure on the nerve. Surgery is indicated if imaging reveals a mass in the tunnel, if numbness is constant, or if significant weakness is noted.

OSTEOARTHROSIS/ OSTEOARTHRITIS

■ Distal Interphalangeal Joint Osteoarthrosis/Osteoarthritis

Chief Clinical Characteristics

This presentation typically includes pain, swelling, stiffness, and palpable crepitus with movement at the distal interphalangeal joint.

Background Information

The condition usually develops after the fourth decade of life. The underlying pathology in distal interphalangeal joint degeneration is usually osteoarthrosis/osteoarthritis, but similar changes also may occur with psoriatic arthritis.[8] The diagnosis is confirmed with plain radiographs that reveal subchondral sclerosis and osteophyte formation about the affected joints. It may be managed nonsurgically, or the joint may be fused if pain is debilitating.

■ Distal Radioulnar Joint Osteoarthrosis/Osteoarthritis

Chief Clinical Characteristics

This presentation can involve pain and swelling along the central dorsal aspect of the distal forearm.

Background Information

The area may be tender to palpation. Pain is worse with forearm movement, especially at the end of range. This osteoarthrosis/osteoarthritis can develop following trauma, but may occur without prior injury.[35] The diagnosis is confirmed with plain radiographs that reveal subchondral sclerosis and osteophyte formation about the affected joints. Nonsurgical treatments include physical therapy and nonsteroidal anti-inflammatory medication. Surgery may be indicated if nonoperative measures are inadequate.

■ Intercarpal Osteoarthrosis/Osteoarthritis

Chief Clinical Characteristics

This presentation is mainly characterized by aching pain that is worse in the morning and improved with heat, such as after bathing.

Background Information

This condition may occur in any joint of the wrist and usually affects older individuals. It may be associated with recent or past injury to the area, but symptoms can begin without identifiable cause. A history of heavy physical labor or avid participation in vigorous sports or hobbies may increase the likelihood of developing osteoarthrosis/osteoarthritis.[35] The diagnosis is confirmed with plain radiographs. Intercarpal osteoarthrosis is usually managed nonsurgically with anti-inflammatory medication, activity modification, and splinting.

■ Metacarpophalangeal Joint Osteoarthrosis/Osteoarthritis

Chief Clinical Characteristics

This presentation can involve pain, swelling, stiffness, and palpable crepitus with movement at the metatarsophalangeal joint.

Background Information

A history of isolated or repetitive trauma is frequently reported. Metacarpophalangeal joint osteoarthrosis/osteoarthritis may be associated with hemochromatosis.[8] This condition is uncommon; rheumatoid arthritis should be considered as a contributing pathology when arthritic changes in this joint are noted, especially if multiple joints are involved. The diagnosis is confirmed by plain radiographs. It may be managed

nonoperatively as long as adequate pain control and functional ability are maintained. Joint replacement is indicated if deformity, pain, and loss of function are unacceptable.

■ Pisotriquetral Osteoarthrosis/Osteoarthritis

Chief Clinical Characteristics

This presentation is characterized by pain and tenderness in the area of the pisiform; crepitus may be present.

Background Information

The flexor carpi ulnaris tendon will not be tender. Osteoarthrosis/osteoarthritis in this joint usually develops insidiously as the result of chronic bearing of the weight of the hand through the joint (eg, using a computer mouse).[35] Plain radiographs confirm the diagnosis. It may be managed nonsurgically with anti-inflammatory medication, or the pisiform may be excised.

■ Proximal Interphalangeal Joint Osteoarthrosis/Osteoarthritis

Chief Clinical Characteristics

This presentation typically includes pain, swelling, stiffness, and palpable crepitus with movement at the proximal interphalangeal joint.

Background Information

Degeneration at this joint can result from either rheumatoid arthritis or osteoarthrosis/osteoarthritis.[8] The diagnosis is confirmed with plain radiographs, which reveal reduced joint space, subchondral sclerosis, and osteophyte formation about affected joints. It is usually managed nonsurgically. Surgery is indicated if symptoms are severe; joint fusion is more common than arthroplasty.

■ Radioscaphoid Osteoarthrosis/Osteoarthritis

Chief Clinical Characteristics

This presentation is characterized by aching to sharp pain in the radial side of the wrist with all movements.

Background Information

Ulnar deviation may be less painful. Pain may be worse early in the morning and with cold, wet weather. This condition may result from abnormal joint forces following a number of traumatic injuries including distal radius fracture malunion, scaphoid fracture nonunion, or scapholunate ligament rupture. It may develop because of chronic overuse. Plain radiographs, which are used to confirm the diagnosis, reveal reduced joint space, osteophyte formation, and subchondral sclerosis within affected joints. This condition may be managed nonsurgically with anti-inflammatory medication, splints, heat modalities, and activity modification. Surgery generally involves salvage procedures such as proximal row carpectomy or scaphoid resection and four-corner fusion if nonoperative treatment fails.

■ **Scapholunate Advanced Collapse (SLAC) Wrist**

Chief Clinical Characteristics
This presentation typically includes pain throughout the wrist, which may be worse on the ulnar side. There will be a generalized decrease in wrist range of motion. There may be palpable crepitus in the radiocarpal and intercarpal joints with active movement or compressive testing.

Background Information
This condition is the result of inadequate treatment for scapholunate dissociation. Rupture of the scapholunate ligament causes instability and altered mechanics throughout the wrist, leading to arthritic changes.[40] Plain radiographs confirm the diagnosis with findings of osteoarthritis/osteoarthrosis. It may be managed nonoperatively with anti-inflammatory medication, and surgery is indicated if nonoperative measures are inadequate.

■ **Sesamoid Osteoarthrosis/ Osteoarthritis (Thumb)**

Chief Clinical Characteristics
This presentation typically includes pain over the volar surface of the thumb metacarpophalangeal joint worsened by compression or resisted thumb flexion, and tenderness to palpation.

Background Information
This condition usually results from overuse. It may also be associated with a direct blow. Clinical findings suggest the diagnosis, which can be confirmed with plain radiographs.

This condition may be managed nonsurgically with steroid injection, protective splinting, and activity modification.

■ **Thumb Carpometacarpal Joint Osteoarthrosis/Osteoarthritis (Basilar Joint or CMC Arthrosis)**

Chief Clinical Characteristics
This presentation can involve pain in the base of the thumb, just distal to the scaphoid (see Fig. 13-3). Symptoms may radiate distally into the thumb. Pain is typically worst with pinching activities such as turning a key, and with activities involving grip and turn such as opening jars and door knobs.

Background Information
This condition usually develops insidiously, although it can follow specific joint trauma. This condition is frequently bilateral and its incidence is higher among women. Pantrapezial osteoarthrosis/osteoarthritis—degenerative changes to the articulations of the trapezium with the trapezoid and scaphoid—shares a similar presentation.[8] Plain radiographs confirm the diagnosis. Surgery is indicated if nonoperative management does not provide acceptable relief.

OSTEOMYELITIS

■ **Digit**

Chief Clinical Characteristics
This presentation involves redness, swelling, and pain over the involved bone, stiffness at adjacent joints, and signs of systemic illness such as fever and malaise.

Background Information
This condition commonly results from a fracture with an open wound. However, contaminated small cutaneous wounds may provide a sufficient portal of entry for bacteria, and distant infection can seed the site via the bloodstream. Individuals with compromised immune responses are more susceptible to this condition. Plain radiographs confirm the diagnosis.[31] This condition requires urgent medical attention.

■ **Wrist and Hand**

Chief Clinical Characteristics
This presentation typically includes redness, swelling, and pain over the involved bone,

stiffness at adjacent joints, and signs of systemic illness such as fever and malaise.

Background Information
This condition commonly results from a fracture with an open wound. However, contaminated small cutaneous wounds may provide a sufficient portal of entry for bacteria, and distant infection can seed the site via the bloodstream. Individuals with compromised immune responses are more susceptible to this condition. Plain radiographs confirm the diagnosis.[31] This condition requires urgent medical evaluation and management.

■ **Paronychia**

Chief Clinical Characteristics
This presentation typically involves erythema around the nail, perhaps with a central whitening of the skin, associated with exquisite tenderness, disuse of the affected digit, and a palpable core of pus that also may drain from the nail fold.

Background Information
This infection results from the introduction of common skin bacteria beneath the nail fold by a minor trauma such as a torn hangnail, nail biting, or a puncture wound. In acute infections, the responsible organism is usually *Staphylococcus aureus*; in chronic infections a variety of bacteria and fungi may be involved. This condition may develop into a felon or osteomyelitis if left untreated.[29] Diagnosis is based on clinical findings. Depending on how far the infection has progressed, management options for paronychia include warm soaks and oral antibiotics. Infections that do not respond to these measures may require lancing to drain the pus.

■ **Peripheral Vascular Disease**

Chief Clinical Characteristics
This presentation can include cold intolerance, pain, and impaired wound healing, associated with pale and cold digits, Raynaud's phenomenon, and chronic ulceration; dry gangrene can develop in severe cases.

Background Information
This condition results from arteriosclerosis in the arteries supplying the hand. Doppler ultrasonography confirms the diagnosis. This condition may be managed nonoperatively, but must be closely monitored for worsening symptoms and tissue necrosis. Tobacco use is a major contributing factor. Smoking cessation, maintaining local warmth, and avoidance of constrictive garments should be recommended. Medication may enhance tissue perfusion. Surgery may be useful in restoring circulation in cases of discrete blockage or to amputate nonviable structures.

■ **Pseudogout**

Chief Clinical Characteristics
This presentation may include uni- or multiarticular joint pain in the wrists, knees, and hips, although any joint may be affected. Pain develops over a period of days, and is accompanied by redness, swelling, warmth, and tenderness to palpation. Fever may be present.

Background Information
The presentation is similar to gout or septic arthritis. This condition is uncommon in patients younger than 50 years of age, and becomes increasingly common with increasing age. Pseudogout results from calcium pyrophosphate crystal deposits that mediate its characteristic joint pain and articular cartilage destruction. Microscopic examination of aspirated synovial joint fluid confirms the diagnosis.[41] Treatment involves medication to correct the underlying metabolic disorder.

■ **Raynaud's Phenomenon/Disease**

Chief Clinical Characteristics
This presentation typically includes painful blanching of the fingers, toes, nose, and ears in response to cold, vibration, or stress.

Background Information
This condition results from vasospasm in the digital arteries. It usually occurs as a complication of collagen vascular diseases or thoracic outlet syndrome (Raynaud's phenomenon), but can occur in isolation (Raynaud's disease). Diagnosis is based on history and clinical findings. Treatment generally involves smoking cessation if applicable, and avoidance of triggering stimuli. Patients may find wearing warm gloves particularly helpful. Digital sympathectomy may be indicated if pain is unremitting or if tissue necrosis is developing.

▪ Reiter's Syndrome

Chief Clinical Characteristics

This presentation involves asymmetric joint pain and enthesitis at multiple sites in the spine and extremities. A triad of symptoms characterizes Reiter's syndrome: joint pain, urethritis, and conjunctivitis.

Background Information

Musculoskeletal symptoms usually begin 1 to 4 weeks following a gastrointestinal or genitourinary tract infection. Diagnosis is confirmed by hematologic studies including erythrocyte sedimentation rate, C-reactive protein, rheumatoid factor, antibody to nuclear antigens, and human leucocyte antigen B27.[33] Individuals with this triad of symptoms should be referred to a physician for medical management. Nonsteroidal anti-inflammatory agents are commonly used to address joint symptoms.

▪ Sarcoidosis

Chief Clinical Characteristics

This presentation mainly includes symmetric, migratory, and intermittent joint and periarticular pain and swelling.

Background Information

There may also be associated flexor and extensor tendinitis, which can produce median nerve compression if located in the carpal tunnel. Although onset can occur at any age, it is most common in the second through fourth decades of life.[42–44] This condition can produce granulomatous lesions in any tissue, although the primary involvement is in the lungs. Bone involvement occurs in 5% and joint involvement occurs in 25% to 50% of patients, most often in the hands and feet. Individuals suspected of this diagnosis should be referred to a hand surgeon. Hand manifestations of this condition are generally managed symptomatically with nonsteroidal anti-inflammatory medications.

▪ Scapholunate Ligament Sprain

Chief Clinical Characteristics

This presentation is characterized by pain and edema in the area of the anatomical snuffbox (see Fig. 13-1). There may be limited wrist range of motion.

Background Information

The degree of ligament injury varies, from partial tear of a single ligament to complete rupture of all three ligaments (dorsal scapholunate, volar radioscapholunate, and interosseous). This injury usually results from a fall on an outstretched hand; however, the trauma may be remote, having been initially dismissed as a trivial sprain. Left untreated, complete tears produce instability in the carpus. Over time, this leads to osteoarthrosis/osteoarthritis in the radiocarpal and intercarpal joints, and eventually to erosion of the carpals and a scapholunate advanced collapse (SLAC) wrist. Plain radiographs may help to distinguish this injury from scaphoid fracture, but should be repeated 2 weeks following injury if initially negative.[34] Partial tears can be managed with casting; complete tears require surgery.

▪ Septic Arthritis

Chief Clinical Characteristics

This presentation can involve joint redness, pain, swelling, and stiffness. Fever may be present, and a tract to the surface may develop, allowing purulent or serous fluid to drain.

Background Information

This condition usually results from a penetrating wound by a contaminated object near the joint, such as from a nail, fish hook, thorn, or tooth. The underlying infection may originate in or spread to other tissues producing osteomyelitis or cellulitis. Complications may include degenerative changes in the joint and significant residual pain stiffness and loss of function.[45] This diagnosis is confirmed with a blood test to detect the responsible infective agent. Antibiotic therapy should be initiated immediately, and the joint will often require surgical exploration.

▪ Stenosing Tenosynovitis (Trigger Finger/Thumb)

Chief Clinical Characteristics

This presentation may involve pain over the volar aspect of the metacarpophalangeal joints of the involved digit(s) (see Fig. 13-2) that is worse with active flexion and frequently worse on waking. Pain may refer distally into the digit. There may be reports of the finger "getting stuck" in flexion, requiring passive extension with the other hand.

Background Information

The volar aspect of the MP will be tender to palpation, and a mobile nodule may be felt to move proximally with contraction of the flexor muscles. This condition results when a thickening of the tendon sheath moves through the lumen of the A1 pulley in the palm. It may develop because of isolated trauma to the area or from chronic overuse.[30] Diagnosis is based on history and clinical findings. This condition may be managed nonoperatively with anti-inflammatory medication and splinting. Surgery to release the A1 pulley is indicated if these measures fail or if the condition recurs.

■ Subungual Hematoma

Chief Clinical Characteristics

This presentation involves purple or black coloration deep to the finger or thumbnail. There may be excruciating, often throbbing, pain.

Background Information

This injury usually results from a crushing blow to the tip of the finger. If the discoloration involves half or more of the nailbed, a nailbed tear or distal phalanx fracture should be suspected. A melanoma under the nail can be similar in appearance to a subungual hematoma, although there will not be a history of trauma. To differentiate between the two, a line may be scratched in the nail with a nail file at the proximal margin of the darkened area. A hematoma will move distally as the nail grows out, so the scratch will not cross it. A melanoma will be stationary under the nail, and the scratch will move across the darkened area as the nail grows. Plain radiographs are indicated if fracture is suspected. Subungual hematomas may be managed nonoperatively by draining the accumulated blood to relieve pressure.

■ Suppurative Digital Flexor Tenosynovitis

Chief Clinical Characteristics

This presentation typically includes tenderness over the volar aspect of the finger, flexed posture of the finger, severe edema, and pain with passive extension of the finger (the classic "four signs of Kanavel").[46]

Background Information

The infection responsible for this condition can result from a bite wound or other puncture that introduces bacteria into the flexor tendon sheath. Diagnosis is based on clinical findings. Scarring in the tendon sheath following these infections may permanently limit range of motion. Patients suspected of this condition should be referred to a hand surgeon on an emergent basis. Delayed treatment can result in loss of the digit or occasionally the hand.[29]

TENDINOPATHIES

■ Extensor Carpi Ulnaris Tendinitis

Chief Clinical Characteristics

This presentation can include pain localized to the ulnar/dorsal aspect of the wrist, frequently near the ulnar styloid. Pain may be worse with resisted wrist extension or ulnar deviation. A "popping" may be reported and palpated during resisted pronation and supination if the tendon is subluxing out of its groove on the distal ulna; these movements may also be painful. This condition frequently results from overuse. It also may be associated with ulnar styloid fractures and rheumatoid arthritis.[35]

Background Information

Diagnosis is based on clinical findings. It may be managed nonoperatively with splinting/casting and corticosteroid injection. Surgery is indicated if these measures fail, but may increase the tendency for the tendon to sublux. Over time, this condition can develop into a tendinosis.

■ Extensor Carpi Ulnaris Tendinosis

Chief Clinical Characteristics

This presentation typically includes pain localized to the ulnar/dorsal aspect of the wrist (see Figures 13-1 and 13-4), frequently near the ulnar styloid. Pain may be worse with resisted wrist extension or ulnar deviation. A "popping" may be reported and palpated during resisted pronation and supination if the tendon is subluxing out of its groove on the distal ulna; these movements may also be painful. This condition frequently results from

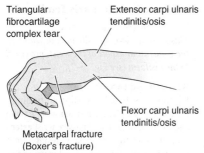

Triangular fibrocartilage complex tear

Extensor carpi ulnaris tendinitis/osis

Flexor carpi ulnaris tendinitis/osis

Metacarpal fracture (Boxer's fracture)

FIGURE 13-4 Palpation guide: causes of ulnar wrist and hand pain.

overuse. It also may be associated with ulnar styloid fractures and rheumatoid arthritis.[35]

Background Information
Diagnosis is based on clinical findings. It may be managed nonoperatively with splinting/casting and corticosteroid injection. Surgery is indicated if these measures fail, but may increase the tendency for the tendon to sublux.

■ **Extensor Digitorum Communis Tendinitis**

Chief Clinical Characteristics
This presentation mainly involves pain over the dorsum of the wrist and hand. Pain will be worse with resisted MP extension. There may be edema and tenderness to palpation over the fourth dorsal compartment. This condition usually results from overuse involving prolonged finger extension such as keyboarding with the keyboard positioned too low. It may also occur following trauma of the dorsum of the hand. Individuals with rheumatoid arthritis may develop extensor digitorum communis tendinitis as a result of abrasion over roughened areas on the carpus.[30]

Background Information
The diagnosis is generally made based on clinical findings. This condition may be managed nonoperatively with physical therapy, nonsteroidal anti-inflammatory medication, and corticosteroid injection, but must be closely monitored for worsening symptoms in rheumatoid patients, in whom it may indicate impending tendon rupture. Surgery is indicated if symptoms do not respond to conservative treatment. Over time, this condition can develop into a tendinosis.

■ **Extensor Digitorum Communis Tendinosis**

Chief Clinical Characteristics
This presentation can include pain over the dorsum of the wrist and hand (see Fig. 13-1).

Background Information
This condition usually results from overuse involving prolonged finger extension such as keyboarding with the keyboard positioned too low. It may also occur following trauma to the dorsum of the hand. Individuals with rheumatoid arthritis may develop extensor digitorum communis tendinosis as a result of abrasion over roughened areas on the carpus.[30] The diagnosis is generally made based on clinical findings. Pain will be worse with resisted MP extension. Edema and tenderness to palpation may be present over the fourth dorsal compartment. This condition may be managed nonoperatively with physical therapy, nonsteroidal anti-inflammatory medication, and corticosteroid injection, but must be closely monitored for worsening symptoms in rheumatoid patients, in whom it may indicate impending tendon rupture. Surgery is indicated if symptoms do not respond to conservative treatment.

■ **Extensor Pollicis Longus Tendinitis**

Chief Clinical Characteristics
This presentation involves pain on the dorsum of the wrist at and just ulnar to Lister's tubercle (see Fig. 13-3).

Background Information
Diagnosis is based on clinical findings. Pain will be worse with resisted thumb extension, especially interphalangeal joint extension, or with active and passive thumb flexion. This condition usually results from chronic overuse in situations requiring thumb extension; it may also be associated with a distal radius fracture when malunion creates a roughened area in the tendon's path. Surgery is mandatory due to a high risk of tendon rupture, especially following a distal radius fracture. Rupture of the tendon produces a condition known as drummer's palsy, characterized by

inability to actively extend the thumb interphalangeal joint.

First Dorsal Compartment (De Quervain's) Tenosynovitis

Chief Clinical Characteristics

This presentation can involve sharp pain in the radial aspect of the wrist (see Fig. 13-3) with thumb flexion, wrist ulnar deviation, and (less often) thumb radial abduction. The pain will be worse with resistance to thumb metacarpophalangeal joint extension, but little or no pain is evoked with resisted isolated interphalangeal joint extension.

Background Information

There will be tenderness to palpation in this area; there may be swelling or crepitus. The patient may report difficulty with grasping activities. This diagnosis is based on clinical findings, and most notably a positive Finkelstein's test.[30] This condition usually results from overuse of the abductor pollicis longus and extensor pollicis brevis. Treatment may include steroid injection or iontophoresis, oral anti-inflammatory medications, and splinting with a thumb spica splint to prevent ulnar deviation and thumb use. Activity modification is essential. Surgery to release the first dorsal compartment is indicated if the condition does not respond to conservative treatment.

Flexor Carpi Ulnaris Tendinitis

Chief Clinical Characteristics

This presentation typically includes pain on the volar/ulnar aspect of the wrist, proximal to the pisiform (see Figures 13-2 and 13-4).

Background Information

Diagnosis is based on clinical findings. Provocative actions are resisted wrist flexion and ulnar deviation, and passive wrist extension. This condition usually results from overuse, especially with awkward hand postures.[35] This condition is usually managed nonoperatively with anti-inflammatory medications and splinting/casting. Surgery is indicated if nonoperative measures fail. Over time, this condition can develop into a tendinosis.

Flexor Carpi Ulnaris Tendinosis

Chief Clinical Characteristics

This presentation typically includes pain on the volar/ulnar aspect of the wrist, proximal to the pisiform (see Fig. 13-2).

Background Information

Diagnosis is based on clinical findings. Provocative actions are resisted wrist flexion and ulnar deviation, and passive wrist extension. This condition usually results from overuse, especially with awkward hand postures.[35] This condition is usually managed nonoperatively with anti-inflammatory medications and splinting/casting. Surgery is indicated if nonoperative measures fail.

Terminal Extensor Tendon Rupture (Mallet Finger)

Chief Clinical Characteristics

This presentation includes pain, edema, and bruising over the dorsum of the distal interphalangeal (DIP) joint and inability to actively extend the DIP.

Background Information

This usually results from a direct blow to the tip of the finger, forcing the dip into flexion during active extension. Onset is usually in the second to third decade of life. Diagnosis is based on clinical findings. It may be managed nonsurgically by splinting the DIP in constant full extension for at least 6 weeks.[21]

Triangular Fibrocartilage Complex Tear

Chief Clinical Characteristics

This presentation typically involves ulnar-sided wrist pain (see Fig. 13-4) that is worse with pronation, supination, and possibly wrist flexion.

Background Information

Through careful palpation of the extensor carpi ulnaris tendon, a painful click or snap may be noted with pronation or supination. This injury results from a fall on an outstretched hand, especially with a rotation force component. Chronic tears may be associated with ulnocarpal abutment.[35] The diagnosis is confirmed with magnetic resonance imaging, arthrography, or diagnostic arthroscopy.

Initially, these injuries may be managed with casting or splinting. Arthroscopic surgery is indicated if symptoms persist.

TUMORS

■ Chondrosarcoma

Chief Clinical Characteristics
This presentation may include a gradually enlarging mass on the metacarpals or proximal phalanx that is usually painless.

Background Information
Pain may result from impingement of surrounding structures or pathological fracture. Onset is usually in the fourth to fifth decades of life. Diagnosis is confirmed by plain radiographs and biopsy.[47] Individuals suspected of this condition should be referred to a hand surgeon for additional evaluation and management, which may include surgical excision.

■ Enchondroma

Chief Clinical Characteristics
This presentation typically includes wrist and hand pain following pathological fracture. Onset is most often in the second to third decades of life.

Background Information
Although usually benign, this condition can rarely undergo malignant transformation. The diagnosis is confirmed by plain radiographs.[47] Individuals suspected of this diagnosis should be referred to a hand surgeon. Treatment of pathological fracture associated with this condition consists of immobilization to allow fracture healing, followed by surgery to address the tumor.

■ Epithelial Inclusion Cyst

Chief Clinical Characteristics
This presentation is mainly characterized by a firm, mobile, pain-free mass on the wrist and hand.

Background Information
Trauma or medical procedures may transport epithelial cells into deeper tissue, typically in the palm, that eventually produce this tumor. Diagnosis is based on clinical findings and history; biopsy is definitive.[31] Individuals suspected of this health condition should be referred to a hand surgeon for potential excision and drainage.

■ Epithelioid Sarcoma

Chief Clinical Characteristics
This presentation can involve a slow-growing, firm, pain-free subcutaneous lump on the palm or palmar surface of the digits. Pain may result from impingement of the tumor on surrounding structures. These tumors eventually may develop draining ulcers.

Background Information
Onset is usually in the second to fourth decades of life. The rate of metastasis with epithelioid sarcoma is high, in part because the tumor is often overlooked or misdiagnosed as a benign lesion. Following metastasis, there is a high mortality rate. Diagnosis is confirmed by biopsy.[48,49] Any lump that presents the possibility of epithelioid sarcoma should be referred to a hand surgeon.

■ Ganglion Cyst

Chief Clinical Characteristics
This presentation involves a lump on the wrist and hand, most commonly on the dorsum of the wrist although it can also occur on the volar wrist or at any other joint in the hand.

Background Information
On palpation, the lump will be firm but not rigid. This cyst may increase and decrease in size over time. Pain may be present or absent; if present, it usually results from irritation to adjacent structures. The etiology of this condition is unclear, although trauma or irritation may be involved. Onset is usually in the second to third decades of life, but the patient may not seek treatment at initial onset if pain is not present. Magnetic resonance imaging confirms the diagnosis.[31] Individuals suspected of this diagnosis should be referred to a hand surgeon. Surgery is indicated if pain, functional interference, or cosmesis is unacceptable for the patient.

■ Giant Cell Tumor of the Tendon Sheath

Chief Clinical Characteristics
This presentation typically includes a mobile benign tumor found on the volar aspect of

the fingers, associated with tenderness to impact and pressure.

Background Information

Onset is usually in the fourth to fifth decades of life. Diagnosis is made based on clinical findings, confirmed by biopsy.[50] Individuals suspected of this diagnosis should be referred to a hand surgeon. The tumor is generally managed with excisional biopsy.

■ Glomus Tumor

Chief Clinical Characteristics

This presentation mainly involves a painful, tender soft tissue mass that is sensitive to cold. It may occur throughout the hand, but is most common in the fingertip and nailbed.

Background Information

It can develop at any age, but is more likely in adults.[51] Diagnosis is based on clinical findings and history, especially a report of exquisite pain with cold exposure. Individuals suspected of this diagnosis should be referred to a hand surgeon. Surgical excision is indicated.

■ Metastases to the Wrist and Hand, Including from Primary Breast, Kidney, Lung, Prostate, and Thyroid Disease

Chief Clinical Characteristics

This presentation typically includes unremitting pain in individuals with these risk factors: previous history or cancer, age 50 years or older, failure to improve with conservative therapy, and unexplained weight change of more than 10 pounds in 6 months.[14]

Background Information

The skeletal system is the third most common site of metastatic disease,[15] although metastasis to the wrist and hand is rare. Symptoms also may be related to pathological fracture in affected sites. Common primary sites causing metastases to bone include breast, prostate, lung, and kidney. Bone scan, plain radiographs, or magnetic resonance imaging confirms the diagnosis. Individuals suspected of this diagnosis should be referred to a hand surgeon.

■ Mucous Cyst

Chief Clinical Characteristics

This presentation may involve localized digit pain and limited joint range of motion, associated with possible nail growth distortion.

Background Information

This tumor can appear translucent when transilluminated with a penlight. The cyst may deform the fingernail through pressure on or deformation of the germinal matrix.[8] Onset is usually after the fifth decade of life. It is a ganglion cyst arising from the distal interphalangeal (DIP) joint, generally located on the dorsum of the finger. The tumor is usually associated with an osteophyte on the DIP joint. Plain radiographs may confirm the osteophyte. Complications may include rupture and infection. Individuals suspected of this diagnosis should be referred to a hand surgeon. Surgical excision (including the underlying osteophyte) is indicated.

■ Osteoblastoma

Chief Clinical Characteristics

This presentation is characterized by a painful swollen area over a carpal, primarily the scaphoid.

Background Information

Onset is usually in the second to third decades of life. These tumors are rare in the hand. The diagnosis is confirmed by plain radiographs. Diagnosis is made following plain radiograph, computed tomography, or magnetic resonance imaging.[52] Individuals suspected of this diagnosis should be referred to a hand surgeon. Surgical options include curettage with or without bone graft, or wider excision. If excessive bone destruction has occurred, surgical reconstruction of the bone may be necessary.

■ Osteochondroma

Chief Clinical Characteristics

This presentation typically includes a hard prominence on bone that may produce pain in the surrounding soft tissues.

Background Information

Onset is most common in the second decade of life.[47] Solitary lesions are rare, and assessment for multiple lesions is warranted. Pathological fractures may occur, but malignant transformation is rare. The diagnosis is confirmed by plain radiographs. Individuals suspected of this diagnosis should be referred to a hand surgeon. Surgical excision is indicated for pain or pathological fracture.

■ Osteoid Osteoma

Chief Clinical Characteristics
This presentation may include a focal area of painful bone with possible swelling that is often worse at night and substantially relieved by aspirin or other nonsteroidal anti-inflammatories.

Background Information
There frequently is tenderness to palpation. Joint effusion and loss of range of motion may be present if the lesion is within the joint capsule. Any bone in the hand or wrist may be involved. Onset is usually in the second or third decade of life.[52,53] The diagnosis is confirmed by plain radiographs. Individuals suspected of this diagnosis should be referred to a hand surgeon. Although they may be self-limiting, osteoid osteomas are usually surgically excised.

■ Osteosarcoma

Chief Clinical Characteristics
This presentation involves pain and swelling over the metacarpals and digits. A palpable tender mass is often present. Symptoms may have been present for several months, and may be associated with a pathological fracture.

Background Information
This tumor is rare in the hand. Onset of osteosarcoma in the hand is in the fifth to seventh decades of life. Plain radiographs and magnetic resonance images may be helpful, but definitive diagnosis is made following biopsy.[52] Individuals suspected of this diagnosis should be referred to a hand surgeon for potential surgical excision.

■ Squamous Cell Carcinoma

Chief Clinical Characteristics
This presentation mainly involves patches of pink, red, gray, tan, or brown scaly skin on areas of the skin frequently exposed to the sun, such as the dorsum of the hand.

Background Information
This condition also may appear as horn-like protrusions from the skin or disruptions of the nailbed. Individuals with lighter skin pigmentation are at greater risk, and incidence increases with amount of lifetime sun exposure of the skin. Onset is progressively more likely with age, and is most common in the seventh decade of life or later.[54] Tentative diagnosis is made based on appearance and confirmed by biopsy. Individuals suspected of this diagnosis should be referred to a hand surgeon.

■ Ulnar Collateral Ligament Tear (Gamekeeper's or Skier's Thumb)

Chief Clinical Characteristics
This presentation mainly includes pain, swelling, tenderness to palpation, and possibly ecchymosis on the ulnar aspect of the thumb metacarpophalangeal joint (see Fig. 13-1). With a partial tear, radially directed force distal to the metacarpophalangeal joint will increase pain but not demonstrate laxity as compared to the uninjured side. If the tear is complete, radially directed force may not increase pain, but will produce radial deviation at the metacarpophalangeal joint that is at least 30 degrees greater than that on the uninjured side.

Background Information
Stress testing should be done very cautiously to avoid worsening a partial or nondisplaced complete tear. This injury results from forceful radial deviation at the metacarpophalangeal joint, such as when a skier falls on a ski pole held in the first web space. It also can develop following repeated radial stress. This condition may be associated with volar plate or radial collateral ligament injuries; a fragment of the articular surface of the proximal phalanx may be avulsed. The diagnosis is confirmed with clinical examination. A partial or nondisplaced complete tear can be managed nonoperatively with splinting or casting. Displaced complete lesions will not heal, and require surgical repair.

■ Ulnocarpal Impaction/Abutment Syndrome

Chief Clinical Characteristics
This presentation typically includes pain in the central to ulnar aspects of the wrist

(see Fig. 13-2) that is worse with active or passive ulnar deviation, possibly associated with a mechanical limitation to ulnar deviation.

Background Information

This condition results when an excessively long ulna (ulnar positive variance) contacts the lunate or triquetrum during movement. Ulnocarpal abutment may occur following malunion of a distal radius fracture with shortening, or when developmental anomalies lead to excessive ulnar length.[35] The diagnosis is confirmed with plain radiographs and magnetic resonance imaging. Surgery is indicated to correct the length discrepancy between the radius and ulna.

■ Vascular Malformation

Chief Clinical Characteristics

This presentation may involve one or more soft, compressible masses in the wrist and hand that may be tender or produce pain.

Background Information

These structures may penetrate and destroy bone, leading to pathological fractures. The condition is usually present at birth, but is usually diagnosed in the first decade of life.[55] The diagnosis is usually made through clinical exam, in particular, the finding of palpable thrills and bruits. This condition may be managed nonoperatively with splinting and pressure garments. Surgery is indicated if pain is excessive or if bone destruction occurs.

References

1. Furman MB, Simon J. Cervical disc disease. http://www.emedicine.com/pmr/topic25.htm. Accessed March 4, 2006.
2. Baron EM, Young WF. Cervical spondylosis: diagnosis and management. http://www.emedicine.com/neuro/topic564.htm. Accessed March 4, 2006.
3. Huff JS. Spinal epidural abscess. http://www.emedicine.com/neuro/topic349.htm. Accessed March 4, 2006.
4. Acosta FL, Jr., Chin CT, Quinones-Hinojosa A, Ames CP, Weinstein PR, Chou D. Diagnosis and management of adult pyogenic osteomyelitis of the cervical spine. *Neurosurg Focus.* Dec 15, 2004;17(6):E2.
5. Barnes B, Alexander JT, Branch CL, Jr. Cervical osteomyelitis: a brief review. *Neurosurg Focus.* Dec 15, 2004;17(6):E11.
6. Stankus SJ, Dlugopolski M, Packer D. Management of herpes zoster (shingles) and postherpetic neuralgia. *Am Fam Physician.* Apr 15, 2000;61(8):2437–2444, 2447–2448.
7. Garas S, Zafari AM. Myocardial infarction. http://www.emedicine.com/med/topic1567.htm. Accessed March 8, 2006.
8. Jebson PJL, Kasdan ML. *Hand Secrets.* 2nd ed. Philadelphia, PA: Hanley & Belfus; 2002.
9. Malanga GA. Cervical radiculopathy. http://www.emedicine.com/sports/topic21.htm. Accessed March 4, 2006.
10. Wainner RS, Fritz JM, Irrgang JJ, Boninger ML, Delitto A, Allison S. Reliability and diagnostic accuracy of the clinical examination and patient self-report measures for cervical radiculopathy. *Spine.* Jan 1, 2003;28(1):52–62.
11. American Psychiatric Association, American Psychiatric Association, Task Force on DSM-IV. *Diagnostic and Statistical Manual of Mental Disorders: DSM-IV-TR.* 4th ed. Washington, DC: American Psychiatric Association; 2000.
12. Simons DG, Travell JG, Simons LS, Travell JG. *Travell & Simons' Myofascial Pain and Dysfunction: The Trigger Point Manual.* 2nd ed. Baltimore, MD: Williams & Wilkins; 1999.
13. Zee C-S, Xu M. Meningiomas, spine. http://www.emedicine.com/radio/topic440.htm. Accessed February 4, 2006.
14. Joines JD, McNutt RA, Carey TS, Deyo RA, Rouhani R. Finding cancer in primary care outpatients with low back pain: a comparison of diagnostic strategies. *J Gen Intern Med.* 2001;16(1):14–23.
15. Holman PJ, Suki D, McCutcheon I, Wolinsky JP, Rhines LD, Gokaslan ZL. Surgical management of metastatic disease of the lumbar spine: experience with 139 patients. *J Neurosurg Spine.* 2005;2(5):550–563.
16. Vargo MM, Flood KM. Pancoast tumor presenting as cervical radiculopathy. *Arch Phys Med Rehabil.* Jul 1990;71(8):606–609.
17. Bhimji S. Pancoast tumor. http://www.emedicine.com/med/topic3576.htm. Accessed March 4, 2006.
18. Villas C, Collia A, Aquerreta JD, et al. Cervicobrachialgia and Pancoast tumor: value of standard anteroposterior cervical radiographs in early diagnosis. *Orthopedics.* Oct 2004;27(10):1092–1095.
19. Guerrero M, Williams SC. Pancoast tumor. http://www.emedicine.com/radio/topic515.htm. Accessed March 4, 2006.
20. Galhom AA, Wagner FC. Syringomyelia. http://www.emedicine.com/NEURO/topic359.htm. Accessed March 4, 2006.
21. Aronowitz ER, Leddy JP. Closed tendon injuries of the hand and wrist in athletes. *Clin Sports Med.* Jul 1998;17(3):449–467.
22. De Keyser F, Elewaut D, De Vos M, et al. Bowel inflammation and the spondyloarthropathies. *Rheum Dis Clin North Am.* Nov 1998;24(4):785–813, ix–x.
23. Kalainov DM, Cohen MS, Hendrix RW, Sweet S, Culp RW, Osterman AL. Preiser's disease: identification of two patterns. *J Hand Surg [Am].* Sep 2003;28(5):767–778.
24. Swartz MN. Clinical practice. Cellulitis. *N Engl J Med.* Feb 26 2004;350(9):904–912.
25. Paula R. Compartment syndrome, extremity. http://www.emedicine.com/EMERG/topic739.htm. Accessed March 4, 2006.
26. Merskey H, Bogduk N. *Classification of Chronic Pain: Descriptions of Chronic Pain Syndromes and Definitions of Pain Terms.* Seattle, WA: IASP Press; 1994.
27. Kasdan ML, Johnson AL. Reflex sympathetic dystrophy. *Occup Med.* Jul–Sep 1998;13(3):521–531.

28. Stanton-Hicks M, Baron R, Boas R, et al. Complex regional pain syndromes: guidelines for therapy. *Clin J Pain*. Jun 1998;14(2):155–166.

29. Stein JH. *Internal Medicine*. 5th ed. St. Louis, MO: Mosby; 1998.

30. Rettig AC. Wrist and hand overuse syndromes. *Clin Sports Med*. Jul 2001;20(3):591–611.

31. Shapiro PS, Seitz WH, Jr. Non-neoplastic tumors of the hand and upper extremity. *Hand Clin*. May 1995;11(2):133–160.

32. Katarincic JA. Fractures of the wrist and hand. *Occup Med*. Jul–Sep 1998;13(3):549–568.

33. Kataria RK, Brent LH. Spondyloarthropathies. *Am Fam Physician*. Jun 15 2004;69(12):2853–2860.

34. Maupin BK. Ligament injuries of the hand and wrist. *Occup Med*. Jul–Sep 1998;13(3):533–547.

35. Shin AY, Deitch MA, Sachar K, Boyer MI. Ulnar-sided wrist pain: diagnosis and treatment. *Instr Course Lect*. 2005;54:115–128.

36. Keenan GF. Lyme disease: diagnosis & management. *Compr Ther*. Mar 1998;24(3):147–152.

37. Sigal LH. Musculoskeletal manifestations of Lyme arthritis. *Rheum Dis Clin North Am*. May 1998;24(2):323–351.

38. Pratt N. Anatomy of nerve entrapment sites in the upper quarter. *J Hand Ther*. Apr–Jun 2005;18(2):216–229.

39. Dobyns JH, O'Brien ET, Linscheid RL, Farrow GM. Bowler's thumb: diagnosis and treatment. A review of seventeen cases. *J Bone Joint Surg Am*. Jun 1972;54(4):751–755.

40. Danikas D, Lee S. Scapholunate advanced collapse. http://www.emedicine.com/orthoped/topic553.htm. Accessed March 4, 2006.

41. Saadeh C, Malacara J. Calcium pyrophosphate deposition disease. http://www.emedicine.com/med/topic1938.htm. Accessed June 5, 2005.

42. Awada H, Abi-Karam G, Fayad F. Musculoskeletal and other extrapulmonary disorders in sarcoidosis. *Best Pract Res Clin Rheumatol*. Dec 2003;17(6):971–987.

43. Khan AN, Aird M. Thoracic sarcoidosis. http://www.emedicine.com/radio/topic618.htm. Accessed February 20, 2006.

44. Wu JJ, Schiff KR. Sarcoidosis. *Am Fam Physician*. Jul 15 2004;70(2):312–322.

45. Berendt T, Byren I. Bone and joint infection. *Clin Med*. Nov–Dec 2004;4(6):510–518.

46. Kanavel AB. *Infections of the Hand; A Guide to the Surgical Treatment of Acute and Chronic Suppurative Processes in the Fingers, Hand and Forearm*. Philadelphia and New York: Lea & Febiger; 1912.

47. O'Connor MI, Bancroft LW. Benign and malignant cartilage tumors of the hand. *Hand Clin*. Aug 2004;20(3):317–323, vi.

48. Bryan RS, Soule EH, Dobyns JH, Pritchard DJ, Linscheid RL. Primary epithelioid sarcoma of the hand and forearm. A review of thirteen cases. *J Bone Joint Surg Am*. Apr 1974;56(3):458–465.

49. Murray PM. Soft tissue sarcoma of the upper extremity. *Hand Clin*. Aug 2004;20(3):325–333, vii.

50. Verheyden JR, Damron T. Giant cell tumor of the tendon sheath. http://www.emedicine.com/orthoped/topic121.htm. Accessed February 1, 2006.

51. Reynolds MB, Sangueza OP. Glomus tumor. http://www.emedicine.com/derm/topic167.htm. Accessed February 20, 2006.

52. Sforzo CR, Scarborough MT, Wright TW. Bone-forming tumors of the upper extremity and Ewing's sarcoma. *Hand Clin*. Aug 2004;20(3):303–315, vi.

53. Bednar MS, Weiland AJ, Light TR. Osteoid osteoma of the upper extremity. *Hand Clin*. May 1995;11(2):211–221.

54. Goldman GD. Squamous cell cancer: a practical approach. *Semin Cutan Med Surg*. Jun 1998;17(2):80–95.

55. Walsh JJ, Eady JL. Vascular tumors. *Hand Clin*. Aug 2004;20(3):261–268, v–vi.

CHAPTER 14

Anterior Thorax Pain

■ *Yogi Matharu, PT, DPT, OCS*

Description of the Symptom

This chapter describes pathology that may lead to anterior thorax pain. **Local causes** are defined as pathology occurring within the chest wall structures. **Remote causes** are defined as pathology occurring outside this region, most notably deep to the parietal pleura.

Special Concerns

■ Acute chest pain with nausea, pallor, anxiety, vomiting, or diaphoresis
■ Severe fatigue or shortness of breath
■ Pain unresolved by rest or change in position, or worse at night
■ Pain that worsens following meals or while inhaling
■ Fainting, dizziness, or vertigo
■ Persistent cough that is dry in the presence of limited medical follow-up, productive, or includes blood

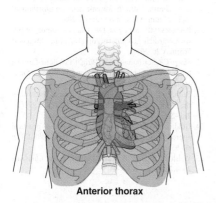

Anterior thorax

CHAPTER PREVIEW: Conditions That May Lead to Anterior Thorax Pain

T Trauma	
REMOTE	**LOCAL**
COMMON	
Not applicable	Delayed-onset muscle soreness 254
	Dorsal nerve root irritation 254
	Fracture of the rib or sternum 255
UNCOMMON	
Not applicable	Not applicable
RARE	
Pneumothorax 250	Not applicable

I Inflammation

REMOTE	LOCAL
COMMON	
Aseptic Gastroesophageal reflux disease 246	**Aseptic** Costochondritis 253
Septic Bronchitis 245	**Septic** Not applicable
UNCOMMON	
Aseptic Pleuritis secondary to rheumatic disease 250	**Aseptic** Fibromyalgia 255 Galactocele 255 Rheumatoid arthritis–like diseases: • Dermatomyositis 257
Septic Pericarditis 249 Pleurisy/pleurodynia 250 Pneumonia 250 Tracheobronchitis 251 Tuberculosis 252	**Septic** *Candida* breast infection 253 Herpes zoster 256 Mastitis 256 Vertebral osteomyelitis 258
RARE	
Aseptic Esophageal rupture 246	**Aseptic** Precordial catch syndrome 256 Rheumatoid arthritis–like diseases: • Inclusion body myositis 257 • Polymyositis 257
Septic Infectious esophagitis 247 Infectious esophagitis (secondary): • *Candida* species infection 247 • Cytomegalovirus 247 • Herpes simplex virus 247 Subdiaphragmatic abscess 251	**Septic** Breast abscess 253 Septic mediastinitis 258

M Metabolic

REMOTE	LOCAL
COMMON	
Not applicable	Cyclic breast pain 254 Early pregnancy 254
UNCOMMON	

Medication or stimulant use/abuse:
• Illicit substances:
  • Amphetamine, cocaine, or "crack" use/abuse 248
  • Ecstasy/3,4-methylenedioxymethamphetamine (MDMA) use/abuse 248
• Over-the-counter substances:
  • Caffeine use/abuse 248
  • Monosodium glutamate intake 248
  • Pseudoephedrine (allergy/cold medicine) use/abuse 249
	Iatrogenic muscle pain 256

(continued)

ANTERIOR THORAX PAIN

Metabolic *(continued)*

REMOTE	LOCAL
UNCOMMON	
• Prescription substances: • Beta-agonist use 249 • Bronchodilators/nonspecific beta-agonist use 249 • Withdrawal from beta blockers 249	
RARE	
Not applicable	Not applicable

Va Vascular

REMOTE	LOCAL
COMMON	
Angina: • Stable angina 244 • Unstable angina/acute coronary insufficiency 244 • Variant angina 244 Myocardial infarction 249 Pulmonary embolism/infarction 251	Not applicable
UNCOMMON	
Aortic dissection (ascending aorta or thoracic descending aorta) 245	Not applicable
RARE	
Sickle cell pain crisis 251	Mondor's disease 256

De Degenerative

REMOTE	LOCAL
COMMON	
Not applicable	Not applicable
UNCOMMON	
Not applicable	Thoracic disk herniation 258
RARE	
Not applicable	Not applicable

Tu Tumor

REMOTE	LOCAL
COMMON	
Not applicable	Not applicable
UNCOMMON	
Not applicable	*Malignant Primary, such as:* • Breast adenocarcinoma (women) 253 *Malignant Metastatic:* Not applicable *Benign, such as:* • Fibrocystic breast disease 254

Tumor *(continued)*

REMOTE	LOCAL
RARE	
Malignant Primary, such as:	*Malignant Primary, such as:*
• Esophageal tumor 252	• Breast adenocarcinoma (men) 253
• Lung tumor 252	*Malignant Metastatic:*
• Mesothelioma 252	Not applicable
Malignant Metastatic:	*Benign*
Not applicable	Not applicable
Benign:	
Not applicable	

Co Congenital

REMOTE	LOCAL
COMMON	
Not applicable	Not applicable
UNCOMMON	
Not applicable	Not applicable
RARE	
Not applicable	Not applicable

Ne Neurogenic/Psychogenic

REMOTE	LOCAL
COMMON	
Hyperventilation 246	Not applicable
UNCOMMON	
Chest pain with panic attack 245	Not applicable
Chest pain without panic attack 245	
RARE	
Hypochondriasis 246	Not applicable
Malingering 247	

Note: These are estimates of relative incidence because few data are available for the less common conditions.

Overview of Anterior Thorax Pain

Physical therapists often come into contact with patients reporting anterior thorax pain. In some cases, this may be their chief concern. More likely, it will be a concern that may be reported during treatment of another diagnosis. Recent studies reveal that myocardial infarctions are unrecognized in 20% to 60% of the population.[1] Because the consequence of untreated cardiopulmonary disease is severe, physical therapists have historically been well trained to identify acute and dangerous conditions. However, making a sound judgment in less dangerous, although still urgent, conditions can be difficult. As the diagnosis list demonstrates, many conditions are amenable to physical therapy intervention if correctly identified and may not require physician intervention. Others may benefit from physical therapy after a physician has begun treatment. If there is any doubt in the clinician's mind about the diagnosis, signs, or symptoms, urgent referral to a physician is indicated, particularly in the presence of risk factors for cardiovascular disease, such as cigarette smoking, hypertension, hypercholesterolemia, diabetes, family history, obesity, and prolonged exposure to stress. Finally, when the patient is in the office, a physical therapist must decide if the emergency medical system must be activated (Box 14-1), if the physician should be contacted immediately, or if the patient can wait until his or her next scheduled physician visit.

Description of Conditions That May Lead to Anterior Thorax Pain

Remote

ANGINA

■ Stable Angina

Chief Clinical Characteristics
This presentation typically includes pain and pressure in the chest or between shoulder blades that may or may not radiate to arms, neck, torso, or jaw with symptoms lasting 2 to 10 minutes. Symptoms are aggravated by activity, emotional distress, or large meals.

Background Information
The diagnosis is made with echocardiography, serial blood tests (cardiac troponin T or I, or CK-MB),[2–4] angiogram,[2] symptom provocation during a cardiac stress test, and symptom relief following nitroglycerin administration. Symptoms are consistently present at a certain rate–pressure product. If an individual with this condition develops symptoms, a physical therapist should

---

BOX 14-1   Conditions Requiring Activation of Emergency Medical Services

- Angina
- Aortic dissection
- Esophageal rupture
- Medication or stimulant use/abuse
- Myocardial infarction
- Pneumothorax
- Pulmonary embolism/infarction

---

request that the individual stop activity, sit down, and use his or her prescribed nitroglycerin spray or pills. If symptoms fail to resolve or this is the first presentation of symptoms, the physical therapist should activate the emergency medical service.

■ Unstable Angina/Acute Coronary Insufficiency

Chief Clinical Characteristics
This presentation is usually characterized by pain and pressure in the chest and intrascapular region with possible radiation to the arms, neck, torso, or jaw with symptoms lasting 20 to 30 minutes or occurring at rest.

Background Information
Individuals suspected of this condition may be unable to relieve their symptoms with nitroglycerin. Often the individual has a clot or spasm superimposed on a region of existing coronary artery plaque.[2,5] The diagnosis is confirmed with echocardiography,[1] serial blood tests (cardiac troponin T or I or CK-MB),[2–4] and angiogram.[2] Infarction is not present. This condition is defined as new onset, angina at rest, recent increase in frequency, duration, or intensity of angina.[2,3,5] Initial management by physical therapists involves activation of the emergency medical service.

■ Variant Angina

Chief Clinical Characteristics
This presentation involves pain and pressure in the chest or between shoulder blades that may or may not radiate to arms, neck, torso, or jaw that occurs spontaneously, often in the morning hours, causing the patient to be awakened with pain.[2,5] Symptoms are variable and do not always occur at the same activity level.

Background Information
Symptoms may not be resolved with nitroglycerin. Diagnosis is made by echocardiography, echocardiographic changes or symptom provocation during a cardiac stress test, angiogram,[2,4,5] serial blood tests (cardiac troponin T or I or CK-MB),[2–4] or symptom provocation with use of medication that produces artery spasm. Initial management by physical therapists involves activating the emergency medical service.

■ Aortic Dissection (Ascending Aorta or Thoracic Descending Aorta)

Chief Clinical Characteristics

This presentation typically includes sudden "tearing" or "ripping" pain in the anterior chest with radiation to the intrascapular region, accompanied by diaphoresis, syncope, or weakness. Pain may migrate into abdomen and lower back as dissection progresses. Symptoms peak immediately and are not affected by change in position.

Background Information

Other findings include hypertension or hypotension, loss of pulses, and pulmonary edema. Individuals most at risk for this diagnosis are those with Marfan's syndrome, Ehlers-Danlos syndrome, systemic hypertension, congenital aortic anomalies, and women in their third trimester of pregnancy. This condition most commonly occurs in people between 60 and 70 years of age. Men are twice more likely to be affected than women. Compression of surrounding structures and/or ischemia may cause neurological findings (compression of nerves or cord ischemia) or other complications. Chest plain radiographs are usually the first examination performed, followed by computed tomography or magnetic resonance imaging to clarify location and extent of damage. Abdominal examination is usually ineffective to determine if an aortic aneurysm is present.[6] The "Ritter Rules," named for the actor John Ritter, were created for patients to recognize, treat, and prevent this condition. Emergent surgical correction is the typical treatment for dissections. Physical therapists should activate the emergency medical service so that individuals suspected of this condition can be taken immediately to an emergency room for evaluation and treatment.

■ Bronchitis

Chief Clinical Characteristics

This presentation typically involves chest tightness and burning anterior chest pain that is worsened by a dry cough that later becomes productive. Patient may also develop a fever or bronchospasm as the disease progresses. These symptoms may be associated with muscular and joint dysfunctions related to increased coughing and pressure on the chest. Individuals with this

condition may also have exertional dyspnea and difficulty sleeping.

Background Information

Acute cases may be treated with antibiotics[7]; therefore, physical therapists should refer acute cases to a physician for initial management. Treatment includes use of medications such as bronchodilators, glucocorticoids, supplemental oxygen, transplantation, and surgery to decrease lung volume. Chronic cases of bronchitis, as well as associated issues such as decreased bone mass secondary to prolonged glucocorticoid use or airway clearance, can be addressed through physical therapy intervention after the disease process has been evaluated by a physician.

■ Chest Pain With Panic Attack

Chief Clinical Characteristics

This presentation may include pain in the left anterior chest of a sharp, stabbing nature. In addition, patient may have palpitations, sweating, light-headedness, gastrointestinal distress, nausea, chills or hot flushes, vomiting, shortness of breath, and restlessness or a feeling of nervousness.

Background Information

Tachycardia, elevated blood pressure, and moist palms may be present. Diagnosis is confirmed by negative tests for cardiac disease such as echocardiography and blood tests, although some patients may present with echocardiographic changes. Individuals with recurrent attacks are advised to seek counseling, avoid stimulants, and may be prescribed medication. Thyroid disease and hypoglycemia must also be ruled out as causes. Physical therapists can assist as part of a team-based approach by prescribing an exercise program to address anxiety and mood disorder. Physical therapists may be treating an individual for a different condition when the chest pain presents. Individuals who experienced recurrent medical workup may be reluctant to seek additional medical assessment when symptoms recur; individuals suspected of this condition should be encouraged to follow up with a physician when symptoms are noted.

■ Chest Pain Without Panic Attack

Chief Clinical Characteristics

This presentation can involve pain in the left anterior chest of a sharp, stabbing nature. Pain may be sporadic, lasting only for a few seconds, but recurring several times per minute for extended periods of time. Often pain is a constant ache lasting for hours or days. Another presentation is a subjective description of pressure in throat and chest. Pain and paresthesias may radiate to arm.

Background Information
Diagnosis is confirmed by negative tests for cardiac disease such as echocardiography and blood tests, although some patients may present with echocardiographic changes. Patients with chest pain should be referred to a physician for a complete cardiac examination.

■ Esophageal Rupture

Chief Clinical Characteristics
This presentation includes anterior chest pain in the retrosternal region. Depending on the location of rupture, the pain may be severe or mild. Often pain will worsen with swallowing or breathing.

Background Information
Patients with this condition may present with dyspnea and cyanosis. Air entering the mediastinum may cause crackling sounds on auscultation and pneumothorax. A mediastinal shift may also occur. The rupture may be caused by an instrument during endoscopy, external trauma, increased pressure during forceful vomiting or weight lifting, or by diseases of the esophagus (ulcer, esophagitis, and neoplasm). The diagnosis is confirmed with plain radiographs of the chest or barium swallowing study. Depending on the severity of the injury, surgical intervention may be required.[8] Physical therapists should facilitate immediate evaluation by a physician including activation of the emergency medical service depending on the severity of the presenting symptoms.

■ Gastroesophageal Reflux Disease

Chief Clinical Characteristics
This presentation may be characterized by a dull anterior chest pain usually in the region of the lower sternum. The pain may radiate and is often associated with food intake, especially large meals. Symptoms may be worsened by bending forward or lying down. Some patients may report flatulence, hoarseness, sleep apnea, dyspnea, halitosis, difficulty swallowing, and (rarely) hematemesis.[9,10]

Background Information
Symptoms are caused by acid reflux into the esophagus. This may be related to acid hypersecretion, hiatal hernia, obesity, decreased lower esophageal tone, and/or presence of *Helicobacter pylori* bacteria in the stomach. Intragastric and intraesophageal pH monitoring (>4), endoscopy (only effective if erosive changes are present), or trial treatment with proton pump inhibitors confirms the diagnosis.[9–14] Patients should avoid large meals, caffeine, alcohol, chocolate, fatty foods, citrus foods, and excessive use of nonsteroidal antiinflammatory medications. Physical therapists should consider whether development of this disorder may be related to nonsteroidal antiinflammatory medication use prescribed for other inflammation or pain disorders and recommend (to patient and physician) alternative means for treating pain and inflammation.

■ Hyperventilation

Chief Clinical Characteristics
This presentation can include chest pain, abdominal pain, rapid or deep breathing, lightheadedness, and arm/face tingling.

Background Information
Echocardiography may be altered, resulting in ST-T wave abnormalities. Clinical tests include deep breathing (as deep and fast as possible) for 2 minutes. If symptoms are reproduced, patient may be having symptoms secondary to hyperventilation. Diagnosis is confirmed with negative cardiac tests. Treatment includes having the patient breathe into a paper bag that covers the mouth and nose. This will increase the partial pressure of carbon dioxide in the inspired air. Recurrent symptoms are treated with psychotherapy. Physical therapists should encourage individuals suspected of this condition to have a physician evaluate all new episodes of symptoms.

■ Hypochondriasis

Chief Clinical Characteristics
This presentation may include a variety of chest pain complaints and the belief that these symptoms are related to a very severe medical illness despite medical evaluation and reassurance.

Background Information

The patient reports somatic symptoms that cannot be explained by a known medical condition. Often, individuals with this condition have a history of inappropriate and inadequate medical treatment. Physical therapy intervention should be coordinated within a team approach to care in order to ensure that the individual is not given conflicting information, because conflicting data may fuel a perception that inappropriate care is being provided. Individuals suspected of this condition should be referred to a mental health professional to confirm the diagnosis.

■ Infectious Esophagitis

Chief Clinical Characteristics

This presentation may involve anterior chest pain with possible dysphasia, painful swallowing, and weight loss.

Background Information

Individuals with carcinoma related to acquired immunodeficiency syndrome, diabetes mellitus, acid suppression, gastric surgery, or steroid use (oral or inhaled) are at increased risk. The diagnosis is confirmed with a barium swallowing examination, endoscopy with brush specimens of tissue, or biopsy. Infectious esophagitis has several etiologies, and treatment is directed at the identified organism. Patients suspected of having infectious esophagitis or anyone with swallowing difficulty or pain should be referred to a physician. If very difficult or unable to swallow, contact physician immediately.

INFECTIOUS ESOPHAGITIS (SECONDARY)

■ Candida Species Infection

Chief Clinical Characteristics

This presentation can include anterior chest pain and may include dysphagia, painful swallowing, oral thrush, or bleeding.

Background Information

This condition is the most common cause of esophagitis; therefore, a trial treatment is often given rather than subjecting the patient to endoscopy. Further examination is reserved for individuals with persistent discomfort. Endoscopy reveals whitish plaques and exudates. Most individuals suspected

of this condition will have some degree of immunodeficiency.[15–18] Treatment includes the appropriate antifungal agents.

■ Cytomegalovirus

Chief Clinical Characteristics

This presentation may be characterized by anterior chest pain, painful swallowing, hematemesis, nausea, and vomiting.

Background Information

Most individuals suspected of this condition will have some degree of immunodeficiency, such as with human immunodeficiency virus or patients who received transplants.[15,17] Transmission occurs by way of multiple routes, such as droplets, sexual contact, and blood transfusions. Sites of infection may include the eye, brain, and gastrointestinal tract. Several antiviral agents have shown efficacy against this health condition.

■ Herpes Simplex Virus

Chief Clinical Characteristics

This presentation may include anterior chest pain, painful swallowing, dysphasia, vomiting, fever, and chills.[15,19]

Background Information

Outbreaks may be caused by herpes simplex virus 1, which is classically associated with mouth sores, or herpes simplex virus 2, which is classically associated with genital herpes. Blisters usually heal within 6 to 10 days. Over time, outbreaks are thought to become less severe and may change from sores to a scar-like presentation as immunity against the virus improves. This condition is self-limiting and often untreated. Initial occurrence or new symptoms should be evaluated by a physician.

■ Malingering

Chief Clinical Characteristics

This presentation may involve consciously and intentionally produced physical symptoms in order to obtain some external reward.

Background Information

The reward is often secondary gain such as disability payments, free medical treatment at an emergency department, narcotic medication, or compensation via a lawsuit. Symptoms are not always "faked"; an individual suspected of this condition may deliberately exacerbate an actual physical condition. Because chest pain is alarming to medical personnel and is sufficient to secure immediate access to an emergency department, this may be a presenting symptom. Individuals suspected of this condition should be referred to a mental health professional to confirm the diagnosis.

MEDICATION OR STIMULANT USE/ABUSE

Chief Clinical Characteristics
This presentation may include nonspecific chest pain after prescriptive or recreational use of stimulant medication. The patient may be of any age group, ethnicity, or sex.

Background Information
Many illicit, over-the-counter, and prescription drugs can cause chest pain, tachycardia, pulmonary changes, and cardiac palpitations of sufficient severity that a patient may seek medical care.[20] Individuals suspected of this condition may come to the clinic because of these symptoms or they may develop during treatment for another condition. It is difficult to differentiate drugs based on clinical signs and symptoms because intoxication often results in tachycardia, dilated pupils, marked confusion, bizarre and sometimes violent behavior, psychosis, and hallucinations. Emergency medical service should be activated.

Illicit Substances

■ Amphetamine, Cocaine, or "Crack" Use/Abuse

Chief Clinical Characteristics
This presentation can involve chest pain, palpitations, hypertension, faintness, panic attacks, loss of consciousness, seizures, and heart failure.[21]

Background Information
Up to 25% of acute myocardial infarction cases in 18- to 45-year-old patients are related to cocaine use. Many cases of cocaine-related chest pain are from cardiac causes such as heart failure, angina, arrhythmias, and palpitations.[22] However, there is evidence that the inhalation of amphetamines and crack cocaine can also directly cause cardiopulmonary

dysfunction.[23,24] This condition is thought to be related to coronary artery vasospasm secondary to noradrenaline release associated with the drugs' main effect. Because most cases of chest pain induced by illicit stimulants do not progress into myocardial infarction, individuals suspected of having this condition are usually observed for 9 to 12 hours and then released.[22,25]

■ Ecstasy/3,4-Methylene-dioxymethamphetamine (MDMA) Use/Abuse

Chief Clinical Characteristics
This presentation may be characterized by chest pain in adolescents and young adults in a broad range of ethnic groups.[26]

Background Information
Ecstasy/MDMA may cause chest pain, palpitations, hypertension, faintness, panic attacks, loss of consciousness, seizures, and heart failure.

Over-the-Counter Substances

■ Caffeine Use/Abuse

Chief Clinical Characteristics
This presentation has been inconsistently correlated to an increase in angina pectoris and acute coronary syndromes.[27]

Background Information
The stimulant effects of caffeine may cause palpitations that could alarm an individual enough that he or she would seek medical treatment. It would be difficult for a physical therapist to make this determination in their office so it should be treated as if it were true angina.

■ Monosodium Glutamate Intake

Chief Clinical Characteristics
This presentation may be characterized by acute chest pain, burning, pressure, and shortness of breath.

Background Information
Symptoms mimic an acute myocardial infarction. Laboratory tests, echocardiography, and imaging are negative. Individuals with this condition report a recent history of eating a meal high in monosodium glutamate, which is a common ingredient in Chinese food and a variety of other ethnic and

processed foods. This is a benign condition that resolves spontaneously.[28]

■ Pseudoephedrine (Allergy/Cold Medicine) Use/Abuse

Chief Clinical Characteristics
This presentation may involve sufficient chest pain in adults and adolescents to cause the patient to seek emergency care.[29]

Background Information
The Centers for Disease Control and Prevention have received reports of adverse cardiac effects, including death, secondary to pseudoephedrine use. Pseudoephedrine is contained in dietary supplements and allergy/ cold medicines. Many individuals will take these drugs without awareness of the side effects. These conditions should be treated as angina.

Prescription Substances
■ Beta-Agonist Use

Chief Clinical Characteristics
This presentation may include chest pain in pregnant women.

Background Information
This substance is sometimes used during pregnancy to prevent preterm labor. It is estimated that 5% of the total obstetrics population will take a beta agonist during their pregnancy. Although serious adverse reactions are rare, pregnant patients presenting with chest pain should immediately contact their physician or present to an emergency room.

■ Bronchodilators/Nonspecific Beta-Agonist Use

Chief Clinical Characteristics
This presentation typically involves an increase in heart rate and palpitations that may be associated with chest pain in an individual with asthma who recently used an inhaler or handheld nebulizer.[30,31]

Background Information
One substance, Proventil (albuterol), also may cause paradoxical bronchospasm.

■ Withdrawal From Beta Blockers

Chief Clinical Characteristics
The presentation of this condition typically involves a rebound increase in angina in an individual who recently ceased taking beta-blocker medication.

Background Information
Angina may be associated with ischemic activity, which can result in serious cardiovascular injury.[32] Physical therapists should screen individuals suspected of this condition to ensure they are taking their medication as prescribed.

■ Myocardial Infarction

Chief Clinical Characteristics
This presentation typically includes pain and pressure in the chest or between shoulder blades that may or may not radiate to arms, neck, torso, or jaw. Pain may be slightly eased by flexing the shoulders and worsened by deep breaths and/or activity.

Background Information
Other findings include diaphoresis, dyspnea, dizziness, loss of consciousness, pallor, and tachycardia. Blood pressure may be normal, decreased, or elevated.[2,5] Symptoms are unremitting to nitroglycerin. Echocardiography,[1] serial blood tests (cardiac troponin T or I, or CK-MB),[2–4] and angiogram[2] confirm the diagnosis. Physical therapists should activate the emergency medical services for patients with symptoms of acute chest pain as described above lasting for more than 2 minutes. Recognition of this disease is imperative, because immediate medical intervention improves prognosis.[33,34]

■ Pericarditis

Chief Clinical Characteristics
This presentation can be characterized by anterior chest pain, which may radiate up toward the neck, that is relieved with sitting up, standing, and leaning forward; the pain is worsened with lying supine. Pain also may be worsened with deep breathing or coughing.

Background Information
A friction rub is audible during cardiac auscultation. In 9 out of 10 cases, the cause is undetermined but may include viral, bacterial, trauma, and post-transmural myocardial infarction.[35] Viral and idiopathic causes may be accompanied by a fever starting at approximately the same time as the pain. Bacterial causes may involve a fever that precedes the

pain by several days. Tuberculosis-related pericarditis may be accompanied by chest pain, productive or nonproductive cough, malaise, and dyspnea. Fluid in the lungs may be noted on the radiographs and a tuberculin skin test is positive. Physical therapists should refer patient to a physician and facilitate immediate evaluation.

■ Pleurisy/Pleurodynia

Chief Clinical Characteristics

This presentation typically includes sharp and stabbing pain in the anterior or lateral chest (unilateral or bilateral) that is made worse by deep inspiration, by movements, and in some cases by lying down. Pain may be constant or intermittent, lasting 2 to 10 hours at a time. Fever may or may not be present.

Background Information

Individuals with this condition may be sensitive to palpation of the chest wall in the area of pain and may present with myalgias, dyspnea, and fatigue. Pleuritic rub or crackles may be heard on auscultation. Negative lung perfusion scan and plain radiographs showing small effusion confirm the diagnosis.[36] Physical therapists should refer individuals suspected of this condition to a physician for evaluation.

■ Pleuritis Secondary to Rheumatic Disease

Chief Clinical Characteristics

This presentation may involve pain in the anterior or lateral chest (unilateral or bilateral), typically in an individual with a history of rheumatoid arthritis or systemic lupus erythematosus. Pain is sharp and stabbing in nature. It is made worse by deep inspiration, by movements, and in some cases by lying down. Pain may be constant or intermittent, lasting 2 to 10 hours at a time.

Background Information

Fever may or may not be present. The patient may demonstrate tenderness with palpation of the chest wall in area of pain and may present with myalgias, dyspnea, and fatigue. Pleuritic rub or crackles may be heard on auscultation. The diagnosis is confirmed with negative lung perfusion scan, and plain radiographs showing small effusion.[36] Physical therapists should refer individuals suspected of this condition for evaluation by a physician, usually a rheumatologist.

■ Pneumonia

Chief Clinical Characteristics

This presentation typically involves "stabbing" or "sharp" unilateral or bilateral anterior chest pain that may radiate to the shoulders; it is worsened with arm and neck movements or deep inspiration. Onset may be gradual or sudden, beginning with a dry cough and often other symptoms such as myalgias, headache, or gastrointestinal distress.

Background Information

Local tenderness may be present at the shoulder, neck, or chest wall. Fever, chills, and vomiting may or may not be present. Disease is caused by bacterial or viral infections that are believed to be aspirated from oropharynx. Consequently, people with impaired consciousness, such as individuals who abuse alcohol and drugs, individuals fed with nasogastric or endotracheal tubes, and individuals with neurological impairments are at an elevated risk for developing this condition. Aspiration pneumonia may follow an episode of vomiting or occur because of poor swallowing function. Chest plain radiographs, sputum examination, and blood cultures confirm the diagnosis. In cases with radiographic changes that are unresolved with treatment after 4 to 8 weeks, bronchoscopic evaluation is recommended to exclude the presence of unusual infections or a noninfectious process.[37] Physical therapists should refer individuals suspected of having this condition to a physician for evaluation, but can often assist with managing the symptoms and disease process.

■ Pneumothorax

Chief Clinical Characteristics

This presentation typically includes sudden, sharp unilateral chest pain in the anterior or lateral chest, worsened with deep inspiration and potentially accompanied by shortness of breath or rapid breathing.

Background Information

Tracheal deviation contralateral to the side of the pneumothorax and jugular venous distension may be observed (Fig. 14-1). Tachycardia, hypotension, and tachypnea may be present, and breath sounds may be absent. Spontaneous pneumothorax occurs most commonly in people 20 to 40 years of age often preceded

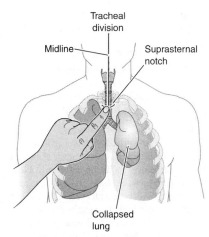

Tracheal division

Midline

Suprasternal notch

Collapsed lung

FIGURE 14-1 Characteristic midline shift of mediastinum with pneumothorax.

by strenuous activity, coughing, or prolonged Valsalva maneuver (as is common during cocaine use). Tension pneumothorax may also be a result of blunt trauma, penetrating trauma (knife, bullet, or iatrogenic puncture during placement of central lines), use of mechanical ventilators, or CPR. Plain radiographs confirm diagnosis when they reveal the characteristic finding of a visceral pleural line with absence of distal lung markings.[38] Physical therapists should activate emergency medical service for immediate management of the condition.

■ Pulmonary Embolism/Infarction

Chief Clinical Characteristics
This presentation may be characterized by chest and throat pain often accompanied by dyspnea and worsened by thoracic spine movements and deep breathing.

Background Information
Evaluation may reveal tachycardia, cough, fever, diaphoresis, cyanosis, and clubbing of fingernails. There may be local tenderness on the rib cage. Pulmonary embolus is a complication of calf deep venous thrombosis, so physical therapists should screen all at-risk patients for this pathology. The diagnosis is confirmed with plain radiographs, negative echocardiography, and lung perfusion scan. Immediate physical therapy intervention is activation of the emergency medical service.

■ Sickle Cell Pain Crisis

Chief Clinical Characteristics
This presentation may involve diffuse pain that progresses to pain in limbs and in the chest and sometimes back. The pain is aggravated by movement and deep breathing.

Background Information
The chest wall may be tender to palpation especially along the ribs and intercostal region. Pain is often caused by rib infarctions.[39] Dyspnea and fever also may be present. Auscultation of lungs sounds may reveal atelectasis. The diagnosis is confirmed with history of sickle cell disease and absence of other causes of pain. Treatment includes analgesics, intravenous fluids, and incentive spirometry to prevent pneumonia and mitigate atelectasis. Episodes resolve spontaneously in approximately 1 week, but may recur. Individuals suspected of this condition should be referred to a physician for evaluation and management.

■ Subdiaphragmatic Abscess

Chief Clinical Characteristics
This presentation includes chest and shoulder pain that is made worse by movement, breathing, coughing, and sneezing. Upper abdomen may be tender and patient may have a fever.

Background Information
This condition may occur secondary to abdominal surgery or perforation of the bowel or gallbladder. Computed tomography confirms the diagnosis. Physical therapists should refer individuals suspected of having this condition to an emergency medical service for evaluation.

■ Tracheobronchitis

Chief Clinical Characteristics
This presentation involves anterior chest pain that may be increased by cough or breathing, productive cough, fever, and sometimes bronchospasm.

Background Information
This condition is often caused by viral or bacterial infection. Crackles, rhonchi, and wheezes may be heard to auscultation in midline position. Physical therapists should refer individuals suspected of having this condition to a physician for evaluation and initial management.

■ Tuberculosis

Chief Clinical Characteristics

This presentation typically is characterized by chest pain, productive or nonproductive cough, malaise, and dyspnea. Chest pain is caused by irritation of the pleura.

Background Information

A friction rub can often be heard during auscultation. This condition is most common in patients under 30 years of age. Chest plain radiographs confirm the diagnosis. Fluid in the lungs may be noted on radiographs and a tuberculin skin test is positive. Individuals with this condition may have active pulmonary lesions and present with pericarditis as part of this disease process. Physical therapists should refer any individuals with chronic cough for physician evaluation, especially if chest pain is present. Precautions should be taken when working with individuals who demonstrate active pulmonary lesions to prevent disease spread.

TUMORS

■ Esophageal Tumor

Chief Clinical Characteristics

This presentation involves anterior chest pain with possible dysphagia, painful swallowing, and weight loss.

Background Information

Pain is caused by irritation of the esophagus similar to that of esophagitis. Painful swallowing and dysphagia are caused by the tumor blocking the path of swallowed food. Late symptoms include hoarseness, hiccups, pneumonia, and high blood calcium levels. Risk factors include age greater than 70 years old, male sex, African American race, history of Barrett's esophagus or gastroesophageal reflux disease, tobacco use, long-term heavy alcohol use, obesity, drinking very hot liquids, a diet lacking fruits and vegetables, occupational exposure to chemicals used in dry cleaning, and history of lye ingestion. Diagnosis is confirmed by barium swallow studies and endoscopy. Biopsies are taken during endoscopy to confirm cancer. Computed tomography is sometimes used to stage the cancer and plan for surgical intervention. Physical therapists should refer individuals suspected of having this condition to a physician for evaluation.

■ Lung Tumor

Chief Clinical Characteristics

This presentation includes chest pain, arm pain, dyspnea, hoarseness, and cough, sometimes with blood-tinged sputum.

Background Information

Pain may be caused by pleural irritation or may be caused my pressure of the tumor on local structures such as a nerve root. Pleuritic pain includes sharp and stabbing pain in the anterior or lateral chest (unilateral or bilateral) that is made worse by deep inspiration, by movements, and in some cases by lying down. Pain may be constant or intermittent, lasting 2 to 10 hours at a time. Some individuals with this condition may also describe weight loss, shortness of breath, or loss of appetite. A Pancoast tumor may also cause shoulder pain. Diagnosis is made by plain radiographs, with computed tomography, magnetic resonance imaging, and biopsy used to determine extent of lesion and the occurrence of metastasis. Physical therapists should refer individuals suspected of having this condition to a physician for evaluation, because early detection can improve odds of recovery.[40]

■ Mesothelioma

Chief Clinical Characteristics

This presentation typically includes dull, aching pain in the anterior chest unchanged by coughing or inspiration/expiration. In some cases, pleuritic pain may be present.

Background Information

Pleuritic pain includes sharp and stabbing pain in the anterior or lateral chest (unilateral or bilateral) that is made worse by deep inspiration, by movements, and in some cases by lying down. Pain may be constant or intermittent, lasting 2 to 10 hours at a time. Individuals with this condition may also describe joint pain, cough, and dyspnea. They also may display clubbing of the fingers, bone tenderness, and swelling. This disorder is related to an exposure to asbestos 20 to 50 years prior to onset of symptoms. The diagnosis is confirmed with plain radiographs that demonstrate irregular thickening of the pleura, calcium deposits on the pleura, or fluid in the pleural space.[41] Computed tomography or magnetic resonance imaging may be used to determine extent of disease. The prognosis for individuals with this type of malignancy is poor, often resulting in death.

Local

■ Breast Abscess

Chief Clinical Characteristics
This presentation may include nipple pain, burning, itching, radiating pain toward the chest wall, and redness around the nipple and areola, a mass in the affected area of the breast, and fever.

Background Information
Axillary nodes may be enlarged. Abscess occurs in 5% to 11% of women with mastitis.[42] Most cases occur within 8 weeks postpartum and are more common in women over 30 years old or who give birth postmaturely.[43] Breast abscess in a woman who is not lactating may be associated with pituitary neoplasm. Needle aspiration confirms the diagnosis. Initial treatment is directed at the underlying infection. Physical therapists should refer individuals suspected of having this condition to a physician (most likely a gynecologist) for evaluation.

■ Breast Adenocarcinoma

Chief Clinical Characteristics
This presentation involves localized, unilateral breast pain of an aching nature. Symptoms may be aggravated by pressure to the breast.

Background Information
Individuals may experience generalized swelling of part of a breast, skin irritation, nipple pain, redness of the nipple or breast skin, or a discharge. A lump may be palpable, which is significant because most breast cancer initially presents as a nonpainful mass in the breast. This condition is rare in men but does occur. The diagnosis is confirmed with the combination of palpation, mammogram, and biopsy; all three tests are usually performed. Ultrasound and magnetic resonance imaging may also be used to differentiate a breast mass from a cyst if the mammogram is positive.[44]

Physical therapists should refer individuals suspected of having this condition to a physician (most likely a gynecologist) for evaluation.

■ Candida Breast Infection

Chief Clinical Characteristics
This presentation can be characterized by nipple pain, burning, itching, radiating pain toward the chest wall, and redness around the nipple and areola.[42]

Background Information
Risk factors include steroid or antibiotic use, diabetes, immune deficiency, yeast infections elsewhere in body, breast-feeding, and nipple trauma. Diagnosis is made based on analysis of the history and risk factors. In some cases, milk and skin cultures are used to determine the presence of fungus. Treatment includes topical medications, cleaning items that have touched the breast, and topical medications to baby's mouth if the individual is breast-feeding. Oral antifungal medication such as fluconazole may be given for persistent cases. Physical therapists should refer individuals suspected of having this condition to a physician (most likely a gynecologist) for evaluation.

■ Costochondritis

Chief Clinical Characteristics
This presentation typically includes "aching" pain in the upper anterior thorax, either centrally or in the parasternal region, episodically worsened to a "sharp, jabbing pain" with activity, sneezing, coughing, and deep breaths.[45,46]

Background Information
People over the age of 40 years and women are most commonly affected. The costal cartilage is often tender to palpation. Pain may be reproduced with activities that require deep breathing and or upper extremity movement. Resisted horizontal abduction, resisted shoulder abduction or adduction, or hugging self may also reproduce symptoms. During another provocation test, the patient is instructed to take a deep breath, extend the arms, retract the shoulders, and extend the neck. Then the examiner applies traction to the extended arms. In Tietze's syndrome, the costal cartilage will also present as swollen and red in addition to being painful. Cardiac testing, radiographs, and echocardiograms are usually normal in

costochondritis. It is important for the physical therapist to educate the patient that all future episodes of chest pain should be evaluated as independent conditions.[45] This will prevent future potentially life-threatening disease processes such as cardiovascular disease from being attributed to this relatively benign condition. Physical therapists may begin treatment, but should refer individuals suspected of having this condition to a physician to rule out comorbid cardiovascular disease.

■ Cyclic Breast Pain

Chief Clinical Characteristics

This presentation may involve bilateral recurrent breast pain that may be aggravated by movement and pressure but is not tender at a focal point. Pain resolves after onset of menstruation.

Background Information

Diet may have an influence on the degree of symptoms. Diagnosis is made by exclusion, history of recurrent nature, and blood tests that reveal the occurrence of pain during the late luteal phase of menstruation.[46] Physical therapists should refer individuals suspected of this condition to a physician (most likely a gynecologist) to verify this relatively benign cause of pain.

■ Delayed-Onset Muscle Soreness

Chief Clinical Characteristics

This presentation may include pain in the upper thorax with occasional referral to the upper extremities. Pain may be described as aching, burning, or pulling.

Background Information

This type of muscle soreness is often preceded by an abrupt increase in physical activity approximately 12 to 48 hours prior to onset of pain. The symptoms usually occur in the muscles that were most active during exercise. While the pain is not usually severe enough to seek medical attention, a person who is currently under treatment for another condition may present with these symptoms. Blood tests and imaging usually are negative. Clinical examination confirms the diagnosis. Physical therapists may begin treatment but should reevaluate the patient after 48 hours to confirm that the symptoms have resolved.

■ Dorsal Nerve Root Irritation

Chief Clinical Characteristics

This presentation involves sharp, lancinating pain that starts in the back and shoots through to the anterior chest in the midthoracic region. The pain is aggravated by any spinal movement, coughing, and sneezing.

Background Information

A history of previous back pain may be present. Sensory changes may be present as may be a description of a burning sensation. This irritation may occur because of disk herniation, osteophyte formation, degeneration of the intervertebral disk space, tumor, tuberculosis, or osteomyelitis. The diagnosis is confirmed with magnetic resonance imaging and plain radiographs when they demonstrate the characteristic degenerative changes in the spine. Physical therapists may begin treatment, but should refer the patient to a physician to determine what other medical interventions may be available.

■ Early Pregnancy

Chief Clinical Characteristics

This presentation includes bilateral breast ache, associated with swelling, chest wall pain, nausea, vomiting, and light-headedness.

Background Information

Urine or blood pregnancy tests confirm the diagnosis. Physical therapists should refer individuals suspected of being pregnant to a physician and emphasize the need for prenatal care.

■ Fibrocystic Breast Disease

Chief Clinical Characteristics

This presentation typically includes lateral breast pain in one breast, tenderness, and palpable mass. There is a focal region of pain at the site of the mass.

Background Information

Diagnosis is made by mammogram, ultrasonography, and/or breast biopsy.[46] Generally, all three tests are done to verify that this is not a manifestation of breast cancer. Needle aspiration will remove the fluid and relieve the pain, and aspirate fluid may be analyzed by a pathologist to confirm the benign nature of this condition. Physical therapists should refer individuals suspected of having this condition to a physician (most likely a gynecologist) for evaluation.

■ Fibromyalgia

Chief Clinical Characteristics
This presentation may be characterized by pain in the anterior and posterior neck, upper chest, arms, lower back, and legs. Pain is described as aching and burning, or as soreness and stiffness. Individuals will describe fatigue, difficulty sleeping, and pain increase with even mild activity.

Background Information
Some patients will also present with psychological dysfunctions such as depression and anxiety disorders. Fibromyalgia is more common in women than men in a ratio of approximately 8:1. The prevalence increases with age. Because laboratory tests and imaging are usually normal, patients are most commonly diagnosed using the criteria established by the American College of Rheumatology.[47] These criteria include widespread pain for at least 3 months, pain (not tenderness) to digital palpation in 11 of 18 points, fatigue, insomnia, joint pain, headaches, and mood disorders.[47] Sleep disorders and deficiencies in growth hormone, serotonin, and cortisol response have been implicated in the pathogenesis, but the disease is still poorly understood. Clinical examination confirms the diagnosis. Physical therapists may begin treatment, but should refer patient to a physician (most likely a rheumatologist) to rule out autoimmune disease and to determine what other medical interventions may be available.

■ Fracture of the Rib or Sternum

Chief Clinical Characteristics
This presentation involves chest wall pain following blunt trauma. Pain may be worsened with trunk movements that move the fracture site or when taking a deep breath.

Background Information
Typically, low-velocity impacts (ie, sports participation) can cause unilateral and isolated rib fractures, whereas high-velocity impacts (ie, deceleration against a steering wheel during a motor vehicle accident) and crushes cause more extensive, bilateral fractures that also may involve the sternum. Complex fractures may result in a flail segment, in which a portion of the chest wall paradoxically moves inward on inspiration and compromises tidal volume. Approximately 150 mL of blood loss occurs with each rib fracture and fracture lines are associated with sharp edges that may further damage surrounding tissues. Therefore, concern for excessive blood loss increases as the number of rib fractures increases. Metastases and other disease processes also may predispose individuals to this condition. All individuals with rib fractures should be evaluated for potential pneumothorax or hemothorax by way of plain radiographs. In individuals with fewer than five rib fractures, treatment usually involves analgesics and physical therapy. Individuals with more than five rib fractures or a flail segment may also require surgery to fixate fracture segments and aspirate secretions.[48] Physical therapists should refer individuals suspected of having this condition to a physician for evaluation but may begin treatment for comfort and body mechanics training to protect the region.

■ Galactocele

Chief Clinical Characteristics
This presentation can involve sometimes painful, unilateral, tender breast mass. Onset is gradual and the patient will usually report a recent episode of breast-feeding.

Background Information
Fever is not usually present. This is caused by a blocked duct and usually resolves spontaneously.[42] Women who wear tight or restrictive clothing may be at increased risk for this disorder. This is a diagnosis of exclusion, although needle aspiration may reveal milky fluid, and mammography may identify a fluid in the lesion. Mammography is usually reserved for individuals with recurrent lesions. Physical therapists should refer individuals suspected of having this condition to a physician (most likely a gynecologist) for evaluation. In addition, physical therapists may advise regarding infant feeding positions, avoidance of restrictive clothing, and application of heat to breast prior to breast-feeding.

■ Herpes Zoster

Chief Clinical Characteristics

This presentation includes unilateral, sharp, and shooting pain in the anterior chest similar to that of myocardial infarction, accompanied by a nodular skin rash several days after onset.

Background Information

Skin nodules are usually small, red, and oval. As the pathology progresses, the pain may change to a burning nature. Individuals with this condition may have fever, malaise, or sensory changes in the region of symptoms. Wrestlers sometimes develop infections on the thorax because of skin trauma. This condition can also cause viral esophagitis, characterized by retrosternal chest pain. Clinical examination confirms the diagnosis. Treatment includes the administration of antiviral agents as soon as the zoster eruption is noted, ideally within 48 to 72 hours. If timing is greater than 3 days, treatment is aimed at controlling pain and pruritus and minimizing the risk of secondary infection.[49] Physical therapists should refer individuals suspected of having this condition to a physician for evaluation. After antiviral medications are initiated, the physical therapist can participate in developing pain management strategies.

■ Iatrogenic Muscle Pain

Chief Clinical Characteristics

This presentation may involve generalized or specific region muscle pain or "soreness" without apparent cause. Symptoms do not resolve as would be expected with delayed-onset muscle soreness.

Background Information

"Muscle soreness" is a predominant symptom in certain myalgias resulting from medication use such as with cholesterol-lowering drugs. Individuals using these medications who have symptoms that do not resolve or improve within a few days should consult with their physician regarding these pains, because they can be a sign of a serious side effect.

■ Mastitis

Chief Clinical Characteristics

This presentation typically includes unilateral pain in the breast, accompanied by fever and flu-like symptoms. The affected breast will have an area of redness, swelling, tenderness, and warmth.

Background Information

This occurs most commonly in women who are breast-feeding and may be accompanied by visible breaks in the skin.[42] In persistent cases, milk cultures will be taken to identify the specific bacteria to determine the most appropriate intravenous antibiotics. Because this condition is caused by a bacterial infection, it is usually treated with oral antibiotic medication. Physical therapists should refer individuals suspected of having this condition to a physician (most likely a gynecologist) for evaluation.

■ Mondor's Disease

Chief Clinical Characteristics

This presentation can involve pain on one side of the anterior chest that is made worse by deep inspiration. Individuals with this condition may describe a trauma to this region that causes the superficial chest wall vein rupture characteristic of this pathology.

Background Information

Palpation may reveal a tender cord-like structure with topical redness. Symptoms resolve spontaneously in 1 to 4 weeks. Clinical examination confirms the diagnosis; imaging, blood tests, and urinalysis are usually unhelpful.

■ Precordial Catch Syndrome

Chief Clinical Characteristics

This presentation can be characterized by severe, sharp, nonradiating pain in the central chest at rest or after mild exertion.[50,51] This pain may last only a few seconds but may be followed by a short period of residual ache.

Background Information

There is usually no tenderness and it is not possible to reproduce symptoms. Radiographs and electrocardiograms are usually normal. Clinical examination confirms the diagnosis. Treatment consists of instructing the individuals about how to alleviate symptoms by standing upright or taking a deep breath.

RHEUMATOID ARTHRITIS–LIKE DISEASES

■ Dermatomyositis

Chief Clinical Characteristics

This presentation typically includes pain with movement in any direction and muscle tenderness, aching, and weakness. The weakness often results in increasing functional deficits particularly in tasks requiring the use of proximal musculature.

Background Information

This condition affects children and adults, but women more commonly than men. It is identified by a blue-purple rash on the upper eyelids, red rash on the face and trunk, and erythema of the knuckles. Scaly eruptions are also common. The rash may also be present on other areas of the body and may worsen with sun exposure. Muscle weakness may be absent or may occur after the rash appears. Extramuscular symptoms include fever, malaise, dysphagia, cardiac disturbances, pulmonary dysfunction, and subcutaneous calcifications. It is associated with the presence of a malignancy in 20% of all cases. Other connective tissue diseases may be also be present. Diagnosis is most commonly confirmed by the presence of an elevated serum creatine kinase level and pathology findings on muscle biopsy. Needle electromyography may be useful to demonstrate affected muscles. Physical therapists should refer individuals suspected of having these conditions to a physician (most likely a rheumatologist) for evaluation.

■ Inclusion Body Myositis

Chief Clinical Characteristics

This presentation includes pain with movement in any direction and muscle tenderness, aching, and weakness. The weakness often results in increasing functional deficits particularly in tasks requiring the use of proximal musculature.

Background Information

This disease is the most common myopathy in persons over 50 years of age. It is three times more common in men than in women, and is more common in Caucasians than African Americans. Dysphagia is present in 60% of the patients. In this condition, unlike polymyositis and dermatomyositis, it is common for distal extremity weakness to be more pronounced than proximal weakness. Extramuscular symptoms include fever, malaise, dysphagia, cardiac disturbances, pulmonary dysfunction, and subcutaneous calcifications. Other connective tissue diseases also may be present. Diagnosis is confirmed by the presence of an elevated serum creatine kinase level and pathology findings on muscle biopsy. Needle electromyography may be useful to demonstrate affected muscles. Physical therapists should refer individuals suspected of having these conditions to a physician (most likely a rheumatologist) for evaluation.

■ Polymyositis

Chief Clinical Characteristics

This presentation involves pain with movement in any direction and muscle tenderness, aching, and weakness. The weakness often results in increasing functional deficits particularly in tasks requiring the use of proximal musculature.

Background Information

This disease is rare and is predominantly a disease of adults. This disease is overdiagnosed in patients presenting with multiple regions of myalgia[52,53] and is the subject of considerable medical debate. Generalized proximal muscle weakness in multiple regions of the body is the most common symptom. Dysphagia and facial weakness are uncommon. Extramuscular symptoms include fever, malaise, dysphagia, cardiac disturbances, pulmonary dysfunction, and subcutaneous calcifications. Other connective tissue diseases may be also be present. Elevated serum creatine kinase level and pathology findings on muscle biopsy confirm the diagnosis. Needle electromyography may be useful to demonstrate affected muscles. Physical therapists should refer individuals suspected of having these conditions to a physician (most likely a rheumatologist) for evaluation.

Septic Mediastinitis

Chief Clinical Characteristics

This presentation may be characterized by chest pain and shortness of breath. Pain may radiate to back or shoulder and become worse with deep breathing, coughing, or sneezing.

Background Information

Individuals with this condition may also have fever or difficulty swallowing. This condition is usually caused by esophageal rupture or infection related to recent chest or sternal surgery.[54] Diagnosis is confirmed with mediastinal needle aspiration and computed tomography, and plain radiographs may not be accurate enough for diagnosis.[54] Physical therapists should refer suspected cases to an emergency department immediately, because the mortality rate for individuals with this condition is 20% even with appropriate medical intervention.

Thoracic Disk Herniation

Chief Clinical Characteristics

This presentation typically includes sharp, lancinating pain that starts in the back and shoots through to the anterior chest in the midthoracic region. The condition is aggravated by any spinal movement, coughing, and sneezing.

Background Information

Individuals with this condition may report a long history of discomfort, but then one movement or activity that caused symptoms to appear. Sensory changes may be present as may be a description of a burning sensation. Magnetic resonance imaging and plain radiographs confirm the diagnosis, revealing a disk herniation that compresses a spinal nerve root and spinal degenerative changes, respectively. Physical therapists may begin treatment but should refer the individual to a physician to determine what other medical interventions may be available.

Vertebral Osteomyelitis

Chief Clinical Characteristics

This presentation involves pain in the neck or back along with anterior chest pain. The condition is aggravated by any movement of the spine.

Background Information

Chest pain or extremity pain is present in about 15% of individuals with vertebral osteomyelitis. Percussion over the involved segment spinous process elicits tenderness. Muscle spasm and decreased motion in the paraspinal region are often noted. Fever is often absent. Infections often originate from bacteremia caused by organisms in the urinary tract, contaminated intravenous lines, intravenous drug use, penetrative injuries, or spinal surgery. The diagnosis is confirmed with plain radiographs that show erosions in the vertebral endplate, magnetic resonance imaging or computed tomography that shows spinal abscesses, and an elevated erythrocyte sedimentation rate. Magnetic resonance imaging is considered the best test for diagnosis. Physical therapists should refer suspected cases to a physician as soon as possible to prevent further bone erosion.

References

1. Ammar KA, Yawn BP, Urban L, et al. Identification of optimal electrocardiographic criteria for the diagnosis of unrecognized myocardial infarction: a population-based study. *Ann Noninvasive Electrocardiol.* Apr 2005;10(2):197–205.
2. Achar SA, Kundu S, Norcross WA. Diagnosis of acute coronary syndrome. *Am Fam Physician.* Jul 1, 2005; 72(1):119–126.
3. Findlay IN, Cunningham AD. Definition of acute coronary syndrome. *Heart.* Jul 2005;91(7):857–859.
4. Gibler WB, Cannon CP, Blomkalns AL, et al. Practical implementation of the Guidelines for Unstable Angina/Non-ST-Segment Elevation Myocardial Infarction in the emergency department. *Ann Emerg Med.* Aug 2005;46(2):185–197.
5. Wiviott SD, Braunwald E. Unstable angina and non-ST-segment elevation myocardial infarction: part I. Initial evaluation and management, and hospital care. *Am Fam Physician.* Aug 1, 2004;70(3):525–532.
6. Lynch RM. Accuracy of abdominal examination in the diagnosis of non-ruptured abdominal aortic aneurysm. *Accid Emerg Nurs.* Apr 2004;12(2):99–107.
7. Smucny J, Fahey T, Becker L, Glazier R. Antibiotics for acute bronchitis. *Cochrane Database Syst Rev.* 2004(4):CD000245.
8. Duncan M, Wong RK. Esophageal emergencies: things that will wake you from a sound sleep. *Gastroenterol Clin North Am.* Dec 2003;32(4):1035–1052.
9. Gomez JE. Typical and atypical presentations of gastroesophageal reflux disease and its management. *Bol Assoc Med P R.* Sep–Dec 2004;96(4):264–269.
10. Wang WH, Huang JQ, Zheng GF, et al. Is proton pump inhibitor testing an effective approach to diagnose gastroesophageal reflux disease in patients with noncardiac

chest pain?: a meta-analysis. *Arch Intern Med.* Jun 13, 2005;165(11):1222–1228.

11. Delaney BC, Moayyedi P, Forman D. Initial management strategies for dyspepsia. *Cochrane Database Syst Rev.* 2003(2):CD001961.

12. Demir H, Ozen H, Kocak N, Saltik-Temizel IN, Gurakan F. Does simultaneous gastric and esophageal pH monitoring increase the diagnosis of gastroesophageal reflux disease? *Turk J Pediatr.* Jan–Mar 2005;47(1):14–16.

13. Katz PO. Use of intragastric pH monitoring in gastroesophageal reflux disease. *Gastrointest Endosc Clin N Am.* Apr 2005;15(2):277–287.

14. Madan K, Ahuja V, Gupta SD, Bal C, Kapoor A, Sharma MP. Impact of 24-h esophageal pH monitoring on the diagnosis of gastroesophageal reflux disease: defining the gold standard. *J Gastroenterol Hepatol.* Jan 2005;20(1):30–37.

15. Bini EJ, Micale PL, Weinshel EH. Natural history of HIV-associated esophageal disease in the era of protease inhibitor therapy. *Dig Dis Sci.* Jul 2000;45(7):1301–1307.

16. Mimidis K, Papadopoulos V, Margaritis V, et al. Predisposing factors and clinical symptoms in HIV-negative patients with Candida oesophagitis: are they always present? *Int J Clin Pract.* Feb 2005;59(2):210–213.

17. Monkemuller KE, Wilcox CM. Diagnosis of esophageal ulcers in acquired immunodeficiency syndrome. *Semin Gastrointest Dis.* Jul 1999;10(3):85–92.

18. Underwood JA, Williams JW, Keate RF. Clinical findings and risk factors for Candida esophagitis in outpatients. *Dis Esophagus.* 2003;16(2):66–69.

19. Ramanathan J, Rammouni M, Baran J Jr, Khatib R. Herpes simplex virus esophagitis in the immunocompetent host: an overview. *Am J Gastroenterol.* Sep 2000;95(9):2171–2176.

20. Brugada P, Gursoy S, Brugada J, Andries E. Investigation of palpitations. *Lancet.* May 15 1993;341(8855):1254–1258.

21. Lan KC, Lin YF, Yu FC, Lin CS, Chu P. Clinical manifestations and prognostic features of acute methamphetamine intoxication. *J Formos Med Assoc.* Aug 1998;97(8):528–533.

22. Keller KB, Lemberg L. The cocaine-abused heart. *Am J Crit Care.* Nov 2003;12(6):562–566.

23. Khalsa ME, Tashkin DP, Perrochet B. Smoked cocaine: patterns of use and pulmonary consequences. *J Psychoactive Drugs.* Jul–Sep 1992;24(3):265–272.

24. Tashkin DP, Khalsa ME, Gorelick D, et al. Pulmonary status of habitual cocaine smokers. *Am Rev Respir Dis.* Jan 1992;145(1):92–100.

25. Weber JE, Shofer FS, Larkin GL, Kalaria AS, Hollander JE. Validation of a brief observation period for patients with cocaine-associated chest pain. *N Engl J Med.* Feb 6 2003;348(6):510–517.

26. National Institute on Drug Abuse. MDMA (Ecstasy) abuse. In: *Research Report Series.* National Clearinghouse on Alcohol and Drug Information; 2006.

27. Stensvold I, Tverdal A. The relationship of coffee consumption to various self-reported cardiovascular events in middle-aged Norwegian men and women. *Scand J Soc Med.* Jun 1995;23(2):103–109.

28. Walker R. The significance of excursions above the ADI. Case study: monosodium glutamate. *Regul Toxicol Pharmacol.* Oct 1999;30(2 Pt 2):S119–121.

29. James LP, Farrar HC, Komoroski EM, et al. Sympathomimetic drug use in adolescents presenting to a pediatric emergency department with chest pain. *J Toxicol Clin Toxicol.* 1998;36(4):321–328.

30. Newton GE, Azevedo ER, Parker JD. Inotropic and sympathetic responses to the intracoronary infusion of a beta₂-receptor agonist: a human in vivo study. *Circulation.* May 11, 1999;99(18):2402–2407.

31. Perry KG, Jr., Morrison JC, Rust OA, Sullivan CA, Martin RW, Naef RW 3rd. Incidence of adverse cardiopulmonary effects with low-dose continuous terbutaline infusion. *Am J Obstet Gynecol.* Oct 1995;173(4):1273–1277.

32. Chiladakis JA, Alexopoulos D. Autonomic antecedents to variant angina exacerbation after beta-blockade withdrawal. *J Electrocardiol.* Jan 2005;38(1):82–84.

33. Bett JH, Tonkin AM, Thompson PL, Aroney CN. Failure of current public educational campaigns to impact on the initial response of patients with possible heart attack. *Intern Med J.* May 2005;35(5):279–282.

34. Ross AM, Coyne KS, Moreyra E, et al. Extended mortality benefit of early postinfarction reperfusion. GUSTO-I Angiographic Investigators. Global Utilization of Streptokinase and Tissue Plasminogen Activator for Occluded Coronary Arteries Trial. *Circulation.* Apr 28, 1998;97(16):1549–1556.

35. Lange RA, Hillis LD. Clinical practice. Acute pericarditis. *N Engl J Med.* Nov 18, 2004;351(21):2195–2202.

36. Rahman NM, Chapman SJ, Davies RJ. Pleural effusion: a structured approach to care. *Br Med Bull.* 2004; 72:31–47.

37. Low DE, Mazzulli T, Marrie T. Progressive and nonresolving pneumonia. *Curr Opin Pulm Med.* May 2005;11(3):247–252.

38. O'Connor AR, Morgan WE. Radiological review of pneumothorax. *BMJ.* Jun 25, 2005;330(7506):1493–1497.

39. Ballas SK. Complications of sickle cell anemia in adults: guidelines for effective management. *Cleve Clin J Med.* Jan 1999;66(1):48–58.

40. American Cancer Society. How is lung cancer diagnosed? http://www.cancer.org. Accessed September 11, 2005.

41. American Cancer Society. How is malignant mesothelioma diagnosed? http://www.cancer.org. Accessed September 25, 2005.

42. Mass S. Breast pain: engorgement, nipple pain and mastitis. *Clin Obstet Gynecol.* Sep 2004;47(3):676–682.

43. Kvist LJ, Rydhstroem H. Factors related to breast abscess after delivery: a population-based study. *BJOG.* Aug 2005;112(8):1070–1074.

44. American Cancer Society. How is breast cancer diagnosed? http://www.cancer.org. Accessed September 25, 2005.

45. Freeston J, Karim Z, Lindsay K, Gough A. Can early diagnosis and management of costochondritis reduce acute chest pain admissions? *J Rheumatol.* Nov 2004; 31(11):2269–2271.

46. Santen RJ, Mansel R. Benign breast disorders. *N Engl J Med.* Jul 21, 2005;353(3):275–285.

47. Wolfe F, Smythe HA, Yunus MB, et al. The American College of Rheumatology 1990 Criteria for the Classification of Fibromyalgia. Report of the Multicenter

Criteria Committee. *Arthritis Rheum.* Feb 1990;33(2): 160–172.

48. Westaby S, Brayley N. ABC of major trauma. Thoracic trauma—I. *BMJ.* Jun 23, 1990;300(6740):1639–1643.

49. Chen TM, George S, Woodruff CA, Hsu S. Clinical manifestations of varicella-zoster virus infection. *Dermatol Clin.* Apr 2002;20(2):267–282.

50. Miller AJ, Texidor TA. Precordial catch, a neglected syndrome of precordial pain. *J Am Med Assoc.* Dec 3, 1955;159(14):1364–1365.

51. Miller AJ, Texidor TA. The "precordial catch," a syndrome of anterior chest pain. *Ann Intern Med.* Sep 1959;51:461–467.

52. Hilton-Jones D. Diagnosis and treatment of inflammatory muscle diseases. *J Neurol Neurosurg Psychiatry.* Jun 2003;74(Suppl 2):ii25–ii31.

53. Troyanov Y, Targoff IN, Tremblay JL, Goulet JR, Raymond Y, Senecal JL. Novel classification of idiopathic inflammatory myopathies based on overlap syndrome features and autoantibodies: analysis of 100 French Canadian patients. *Medicine (Baltimore).* Jul 2005; 84(4):231–249.

54. Akman C, Kantarci F, Cetinkaya S. Imaging in mediastinitis: a systematic review based on aetiology. *Clin Radiol.* Jul 2004;59(7):573–585.

CHAPTER 15

Case Demonstration: Chest Pain

▨ *Amy B. Pomrantz, PT, DPT, OCS, ATC* ▨ *Chris A. Sebelski, PT, DPT, OCS, CSCS*

NOTE: This case demonstration was developed using the diagnostic process described in Chapter 4 and demonstrated in Chapter 5. The reader is encouraged to use this diagnostic process in order to ensure thorough clinical reasoning. If additional elaboration is required on the information presented in this chapter, please consult Chapters 4 and 5.

THE DIAGNOSTIC PROCESS

Step 1 Identify the patient's chief concern.
Step 2 Identify *barriers to communication.*
Step 3 Identify *special concerns.*
Step 4 Create a symptom timeline and sketch the anatomy (if needed).
Step 5 Create a diagnostic hypothesis list considering all possible forms of *remote* and *local* pathology that could cause the patient's chief concern.
Step 6 Sort the diagnostic hypothesis list by epidemiology and specific case characteristics.
Step 7 Ask specific questions to rule specific conditions or pathological categories less likely.
Step 8 Re-sort the diagnostic hypothesis list based on the patient's responses to specific questioning.
Step 9 Perform tests to differentiate among the remaining diagnostic hypotheses.
Step 10 Re-sort the diagnostic hypothesis list based on the patient's responses to specific tests.
Step 11 Decide on a diagnostic impression.
Step 12 Determine the appropriate patient disposition.

Case Description

OS was a 24-year-old Egyptian female who had been enrolled in a master's degree communications program in the United States for the past 8 months. Her chief concern was left anterior chest pain located immediately lateral to her sternum and distal to the clavicle, deep to her breast tissue at approximately the T3–T5 region. The onset of pain was 12 days prior, while the patient was lying in a semi-reclined position on the couch. She could not recall any specific mechanism of injury or movements she made before the pain began. At the onset of symptoms, the pain was described as sharp with an intensity of 8 to 10 on the 10-point verbal numeric pain scale. At that time, the pain was constant, but was aggravated by sitting in a slumped position, inspirations during her breathing cycle, and general movement. She did not experience shortness of breath.

No position of comfort could be found in the supine, side-lying, or prone positions. Easing factors included heat, Advil, sitting up with lumbar and thoracic spine in extended positions, and unloading of left shoulder.

When her symptoms did not change after 3 days, OS visited the Student Health Center. Plain radiographs of the chest obtained by her referring physician were unremarkable and she was referred to physical therapy. Two days later, the pain was significantly decreased and by the morning of the initial physical therapy visit, symptoms at the chest region were only aggravated with palpation or weight bearing through her left upper extremity. Easing factors had not changed. Despite her symptoms, the patient was attending classes.

OS denied a personal history of cardiac disease, respiratory pathology, and cancer. She denied alcohol or recreational drug use and was a nonsmoker. Current medications included Advil and Tylenol. She had no past surgical history and stated that she was not pregnant. OS reported her general health as good, with her last physical performed before starting graduate school 8 months before the onset of current symptoms. She reported experiencing symptoms of a cold approximately 1 month ago that were now resolved.

STEP #1: Identify the patient's chief concern.

- Left anterolateral chest pain

STEP #2: Identify *barriers to communication*.

- **English is the patient's second language.** Although the patient demonstrated proficiency in English to enter graduate school, the therapist was sensitive to the fact that certain terminology and colloquialisms may have been unfamiliar to the patient, even though an interpreter was not required.

STEP #3: Identify *special concerns*.

- **Recent illness.** This report was determined to require further exploration to determine its potential relationship to the patient's current symptoms.

> **Teaching Comments:** A thorough examination should include an exploration of the relationship of any illness with the onset of pain. This will appropriately increase the breadth and depth of the examination.

STEP #4: Create a symptom timeline and sketch the anatomy (if needed).

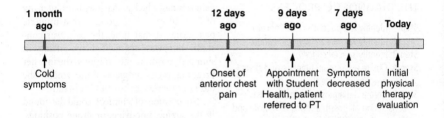

1 month ago	12 days ago	9 days ago	7 days ago	Today
↑ Cold symptoms	↑ Onset of anterior chest pain	↑ Appointment with Student Health, patient referred to PT	↑ Symptoms decreased	↑ Initial physical therapy evaluation

STEP #5: Create a diagnostic hypothesis list considering all possible forms of *remote* and *local* pathology that could cause the patient's chief concern.

STEP #6: Sort the diagnostic hypothesis list by epidemiology and specific case characteristics.

Remote	Remote
T Trauma	**T Trauma**
Esophageal rupture	~~Esophageal rupture~~ (no trauma)
Pneumothorax	~~Pneumothorax~~ (no trauma, no shortness of breath)
Thoracic disk lesion	Thoracic disk lesion
I Inflammation	**I Inflammation**
Aseptic	*Aseptic*
Gastroesophageal reflux disease	~~Gastroesophageal reflux disease~~ (symptom location, report of mechanical aggravating factors)
Pleuritis secondary to rheumatic disease	~~Pleuritis secondary to rheumatic disease~~ (plain radiographs unremarkable)
Septic	*Septic*
• Bronchitis	• Bronchitis

Infectious esophagitis secondary to:
- Candida
- Cytomegalovirus
- Herpes simplex virus

Pericarditis
- Bacterial
- Idiopathic
- Viral

Pleurisy/pleurodynia

Pneumonia

Subdiaphragmatic abscess

Tracheobronchitis
Tuberculosis

Infectious esophagitis secondary to:
- Candida
- Cytomegalovirus
- Herpes simplex virus

Pericarditis
- Bacterial
- Idiopathic
- Viral

~~Pleurisy/pleurodynia~~ (plain radiographs unremarkable)

~~Pneumonia~~ (plain radiographs unremarkable)

~~Subdiaphragmatic abscess~~ (time course of symptoms)

Tracheobronchitis
~~Tuberculosis~~ (plain radiographs unremarkable)

M   Metabolic

Medication or stimulant use/abuse, such as:
- Illicit substances
  - Amphetamines, cocaine, or "crack"

  - Ecstasy
- Over-the-counter substances
  - Caffeine
  - Monosodium glutamate

  - Pseudoephedrine

- Prescription drugs
  - Beta agonists

  - Bronchodilators/nonspecific beta agonists
  - Withdrawal from beta blockers

M   Metabolic

~~Medication or stimulant use/abuse, such as:~~
- ~~Illicit substances~~ (time course of symptoms)
  - ~~Amphetamines, cocaine, or crack~~ (time course of symptoms)
  - ~~Ecstasy~~ (time course of symptoms)
- ~~Over-the-counter substances~~
  - ~~Caffeine~~ (time course of symptoms)
  - ~~Monosodium glutamate~~ (time course of symptoms)
  - ~~Pseudoephedrine~~ (time course of symptoms)
- ~~Prescription drugs~~
  - ~~Beta agonists~~ (no medications per report)
  - ~~Bronchodilators/nonspecific beta agonists~~ (no medications per report)
  - ~~Withdrawal from beta blockers~~ (no medications per report)

Va   Vascular

Angina:
- Stable angina
- Unstable angina
- Variant angina

Aortic dissection
Cardiac disease
Myocardial infarction

Pulmonary embolism
Sickle cell pain crisis

Va   Vascular

Angina:
- Stable angina
- Unstable angina
- Variant angina

~~Aortic dissection~~ (time course)
Cardiac disease
~~Myocardial infarction~~ (patient age, time course)

~~Pulmonary embolism~~ (time course)
~~Sickle cell pain crisis~~ (patient age, patient sex, time course)

De   Degenerative

Not applicable

De   Degenerative

Not applicable

Tu Tumor

Malignant Primary, such as:
- Esophageal tumor
- Lung tumor

Malignant Metastatic:
Not applicable
Benign:
Not applicable

Co Congenital

Not applicable

Ne Neurogenic/Psychogenic

Chest pain with panic attack
Chest pain without panic attack
Hypochondriasis
Hyperventilation
Malingering

Local

T Trauma

Delayed-onset muscle soreness

Fracture of costal cartilage, rib, sternum, or vertebra

Intercostal muscle strain
Subluxation of rib

I Inflammation

Aseptic
Costochondritis
Fibromyalgia
Galactocele
Inflammatory muscle diseases:
- Dermatomyositis

- Inclusion body myositis

- Polymyositis

Intercostal neuritis
Pectoral myositis
Precordial catch syndrome

Tietze's syndrome

Septic
Breast abscess
Candida breast infection
Herpes zoster
Mastitis

Tu Tumor

Malignant Primary, such as:
- ~~Esophageal tumor~~ (symptom behavior)
- ~~Lung tumor~~ (plain radiographs unremarkable)

Malignant Metastatic:
Not applicable
Benign:
Not applicable

Co Congenital

Not applicable

Ne Neurogenic/Psychogenic

Chest pain with panic attack
Chest pain without panic attack
Hypochondriasis
~~Hyperventilation~~ (symptom behavior)
~~Malingering~~ (no apparent secondary gain)

Local

T Trauma

~~Delayed-onset muscle soreness~~ (symptom onset)

~~Fracture of costal cartilage, rib, sternum, or vertebra~~ (no trauma, plain radiographs unremarkable)

Intercostal muscle strain
~~Subluxation of rib~~ (no trauma, plain radiographs unremarkable)

I Inflammation

Aseptic
Costochondritis
Fibromyalgia
Galactocele
~~Inflammatory muscle diseases:~~
- ~~Dermatomyositis~~ (patient age, symptom location)

- ~~Inclusion body myositis~~ (patient age, symptom location)

- ~~Polymyositis~~ (patient age, symptom location)

Intercostal neuritis
Pectoral myositis
~~Precordial catch syndrome~~ (report of mechanical aggravating factors)

Tietze's syndrome

Septic
Breast abscess
Candida breast infection
Herpes zoster
Mastitis

Septic mediastinitis	~~Septic mediastinitis~~ (symptom location and behavior)
Vertebral osteomyelitis	~~Vertebral osteomyelitis~~ (plain radiographs unremarkable)

M Metabolic

Cyclic breast pain
Early pregnancy

M Metabolic

Cyclic breast pain
~~Early pregnancy~~ (patient report, which may require additional objective confirmation)

Va Vascular

Mondor's disease

Va Vascular

~~Mondor's disease~~ (symptom behavior)

De Degenerative

Not applicable

De Degenerative

Not applicable

Tu Tumor

Malignant Primary, such as:
• Breast adenocarcinoma
• Chondrosarcoma

• Mesothelioma

• Osteosarcoma of sternum or ribs

Malignant Metastatic:
Not applicable
Benign, such as:
• Fibrocystic breast disease

Tu Tumor

Malignant Primary, such as:
• Breast adenocarcinoma
• ~~Chondrosarcoma~~ (plain radiographs unremarkable)
• ~~Mesothelioma~~ (plain radiographs unremarkable)
• ~~Osteosarcoma of sternum or ribs~~ (plain radiographs unremarkable)

Malignant Metastatic:
Not applicable
Benign, such as:
• Fibrocystic breast disease

Co Congenital

Not applicable

Co Congenital

Not applicable

Ne Neurogenic/Psychogenic

Not applicable

Ne Neurogenic/Psychogenic

Not applicable

STEP #7: Ask specific questions to rule specific conditions or pathological categories less likely.

• **Have you been ill recently?** Yes, the patient reported having nasal congestion and a cough with mucous secretions in her throat and chest. She confirmed symptoms of fatigue, nausea, and loss of appetite, but denied vomiting. She also denied having a fever during this illness, but had no thermometer to confirm her body temperature. The response to this question rules more likely septic and aseptic forms of inflammation associated with systemic illness.

• **Have you noticed any rashes?** Yes, approximately 1 week before the onset of pain, the patient reported that she developed a rash in the same location of current pain. She visited the Student Health Center at that time and the rash was diagnosed by the physician as an allergic reaction. This finding raises the index of clinical suspicion for septic and aseptic forms of inflammation.

• **Do symptoms vary at different points in your menstrual cycle?** No, the patient denied changes in symptoms with her menstrual cycle, excluding pathology that may be sensitive to menstruation.

STEP #8: Re-sort the diagnostic hypothesis list based on the patient's responses to specific questioning.

Remote

T   Trauma

~~Thoracic disk lesion~~ (onset not associated with illness and rash, plain radiographs unremarkable)

I   Inflammation

Aseptic
Not applicable

Septic
Bronchitis
Infectious esophagitis secondary to:
• Candida
• Cytomegalovirus
• Herpes simplex virus
Pericarditis
• Bacterial
• Idiopathic
• Viral
Tracheobronchitis

M   Metabolic
Not applicable

Va   Vascular

Angina:
• ~~Stable angina~~ (onset not associated with illness and rash)
• ~~Unstable angina~~ (onset not associated with illness and rash)
• ~~Variant angina~~ (onset not associated with illness and rash)
~~Cardiac disease~~ (onset not associated with illness and rash)

De   Degenerative
Not applicable

Tu   Tumor
Not applicable

Co   Congenital
Not applicable

Ne   Neurogenic/Psychogenic
Chest pain with panic attack
Chest pain without panic attack
Hypochondriasis

Local

T   Trauma
Intercostal muscle strain

I   Inflammation

Aseptic
Costochondritis
~~Fibromyalgia~~ (onset not associated with illness and rash)
~~Galactocele~~ (onset not associated with illness and rash)
Intercostal neuritis
Pectoral myositis
Tietze's syndrome

Septic
Breast abscess
Candida breast infection
Herpes zoster
Mastitis

M   Metabolic
~~Cyclic breast pain~~ (symptoms do not vary with menstruation)

Va   Vascular
Not applicable

De   Degenerative
Not applicable

Tu   Tumor
Malignant Primary, such as:
• Breast adenocarcinoma
Malignant Metastatic:
Not applicable
Benign, such as:
• Fibrocystic breast disease

Co   Congenital
Not applicable

Ne   Neurogenic/Psychogenic
Not applicable

STEP #9: Perform tests to differentiate among the remaining diagnostic hypotheses.

• **Observation.** The demeanor of the patient was observed to be calm during questioning, helping to rule less likely the contribution of panic or anxiety disorders.

• **Temperature.** Normal, reducing the likelihood of current pyrogenic conditions.

• **Palpation.** Breast tissue, intercostal spaces in the affected area, and the pectoral muscles were unremarkable. These findings help exclude pathology that affects these tissues. Palpation of the costochondral joints of ribs 3, 4, and 5 reproduced symptoms, increasing the possibility of symptoms related to these structures.

- **Anteroposterior rib spring manual technique.** Negative for reproduction of symptoms, reducing the likelihood of costochondral joint structural involvement.

Teaching Comments: Examination of the indicated region in this case included the breast tissue, because it covers the costosternal joints and identification of the spacing between the ribs. A therapist must be sensitive to the cultural implications of such an examination. Education of the patient on the importance of the exam procedure and enlisting the patient's assistance for setting appropriate boundaries will ensure patient comfort with the procedure.

STEP #10: Re-sort the diagnostic hypothesis list based on the patient's responses to specific tests.

Remote

T Trauma

Not applicable

I **Inflammation**

Aseptic

Not applicable

Septic

~~Bronchitis~~ (no fever)

~~Infectious esophagitis secondary to:~~

- ~~Candida~~ (no fever)
- ~~Cytomegalovirus~~ (no fever)
- ~~Herpes simplex virus~~ (no fever)

~~Pericarditis:~~

- ~~Bacterial~~ (no fever, aggravating and alleviating factors)
- ~~Idiopathic~~ (no fever, aggravating and alleviating factors)
- ~~Viral~~ (no fever, aggravating and alleviating factors)

~~Tracheobronchitis~~ (no fever)

M **Metabolic**

Not applicable

Va **Vascular**

Not applicable

De **Degenerative**

Not applicable

Tu **Tumor**

Not applicable

Co **Congenital**

Not applicable

Ne **Neurogenic/Psychogenic**

~~Chest pain with panic attack~~ (observation negative for anxiety)

~~Chest pain without panic attack~~ (observation negative for anxiety)

~~Hypochondriasis~~ (observation negative for anxiety)

Local

T **Trauma**

~~Intercostal muscle strain~~ (no tenderness of intercostals)

I **Inflammation**

Aseptic

Costochondritis

Intercostal neuritis

~~Pectoral myositis~~ (no tenderness of pectoral musculature)

Tietze's syndrome

Septic

~~Breast abscess~~ (no tenderness of breast tissue)

~~Candida breast infection~~ (no tenderness of breast tissue)

Herpes zoster

~~Mastitis~~ (no tenderness of breast tissue)

M **Metabolic**

Not applicable

Va **Vascular**

Not applicable

De **Degenerative**

Not applicable

Tu **Tumor**

Malignant Primary, such as:

- ~~Breast adenocarcinoma~~ (no tenderness of breast tissue)

Malignant Metastatic:

Not applicable

Benign, such as:

- ~~Fibrocystic breast disease~~ (no tenderness of breast tissue)

Co **Congenital**

Not applicable

Ne **Neurogenic/Psychogenic**

Not applicable

STEP #11: Decide on a diagnostic impression.

- Rule out herpes zoster (and potentially related intercostals neuritis) vs. costochondritis and Tietze's syndrome.

Teaching Comments: The patient's presentation, in conjunction with the presence of a rash (previously diagnosed as an allergic reaction), would be consistent with herpes zoster and related intercostal neuritis. The illness reported by the patient approximately a week before the onset of the rash could be considered part of a prodrome, which often accompanies herpes zoster. Due to the limited time course (less than 1 month since onset of the rash), the diagnosis would not be considered post-herpetic neuralgia.[1] The current absence of an active rash indicates the patient is no longer contagious; however, referral to a physician for a medical screening would be appropriate for antiviral intervention and application of an anti-inflammatory cream in the region. Physical therapy intervention would not be indicated.

STEP #12: Determine the appropriate patient disposition.

- Refer OS back to her physician urgently for additional evaluation.

Case Outcome

OS was managed by her primary care provider with a combination of topical corticosteroid ointment and oral acyclovir. Her symptoms subsequently resolved without need for physical therapy intervention.

Reference

1. Dworkin RH, Portenoy RK. Pain and its persistence in herpes zoster. *Pain.* 1996;67:241-251.

CHAPTER 16

Posterior Thorax Pain

■ *Kathy Doubleday, PT, DPT, OCS*

Description of the Symptom

This chapter describes pathology that may lead to posterior thorax pain. **Local causes** are defined as pathology occurring within the spine and posterior chest wall structures. **Remote causes** are defined as occurring outside this region, most notably deep to the parietal pleura.

Special Concerns

■ Acute chest pain with nausea, pallor, anxiety, vomiting, or diaphoresis
■ Coughing up blood, blood in stool
■ Fainting, dizziness, or vertigo
■ Pain unresolved by rest or change in position, or worse at night
■ Pain that worsens following meals or while inhaling
■ Severe fatigue or shortness of breath

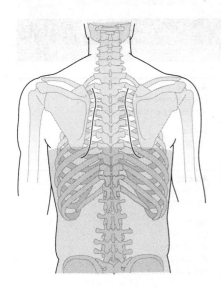

CHAPTER PREVIEW: Conditions That May Lead to Posterior Thorax Pain

T   Trauma

REMOTE	LOCAL
COMMON	
Cervical facet joint dysfunction 274	Costovertebral or costotransverse joint dysfunction 277
	Fractures:
	• Compression fracture 279
	• Rib fracture 279
	Thoracic facet joint dysfunction 281
UNCOMMON	
Not applicable	T4 syndrome 281
RARE	
Pneumothorax 276	Fractures:
	• Vertebral fracture/dislocation 279

I   Inflammation

REMOTE	LOCAL
COMMON	
Aseptic	**Aseptic**
Gastroesophageal reflux disease 274	Delayed-onset muscle soreness 278
	Myofascial pain disorder 280
Septic	
Peptic ulcer disease 275	**Septic**
	Not applicable
UNCOMMON	
Aseptic	**Aseptic**
Not applicable	Ankylosing spondylitis 277
	Fibromyalgia 278
Septic	
Gallstones and biliary disease 274	**Septic**
Pancreatitis 275	Discitis 278
Pneumonia 276	Herpes zoster 279
	Meningitis 280
	Vertebral osteomyelitis 284
RARE	
Aseptic	**Aseptic**
Not applicable	Transverse myelitis 282
Septic	**Septic**
Pleurisy/empyema 275	Epidural abscess 278
Pyelonephritis 276	Tuberculosis of the spine (Pott's disease) 282

M   Metabolic

REMOTE	LOCAL
COMMON	
Not applicable	Osteoporosis 280

Metabolic *(continued)*

REMOTE	LOCAL
UNCOMMON	
Not applicable	Paget's disease 281
RARE	
Not applicable	Cushing's syndrome 277 Osteomalacia 280

Va **Vascular**

REMOTE	LOCAL
COMMON	
Angina: • Stable angina 273 • Unstable angina/acute coronary insufficiency 273 • Variant angina 273	Not applicable
UNCOMMON	
Myocardial infarction/acute coronary insufficiency 275	Dissecting aortic aneurysm 278
RARE	
Not applicable	Not applicable

De **Degenerative**

REMOTE	LOCAL
COMMON	
Cervical degenerative disk disease 274	Not applicable
UNCOMMON	
Not applicable	Thoracic degenerative disk disease 281 Thoracic osteoarthrosis/osteoarthritis 282
RARE	
Not applicable	Not applicable

Tu **Tumor**

REMOTE	LOCAL
COMMON	
Not applicable	Not applicable
UNCOMMON	
Not applicable	*Malignant Primary:* Not applicable *Malignant Metastatic, such as:* • Metastases, including from primary breast, kidney, lung, prostate, and thyroid disease 283 *Benign:* Not applicable

(continued)

Tumor *(continued)*

REMOTE	LOCAL
RARE	
Malignant Primary, such as:	*Malignant Primary, such as:*
• Esophageal adenocarcinoma 276	• Leukemias 282
• Gastric adenocarcinoma 277	• Multiple myeloma 283
• Pancreatic carcinoma 277	• Primary bone tumors 284
Malignant Metastatic:	*Malignant Metastatic:*
Not applicable	Not applicable
Benign:	*Benign, such as:*
Not applicable	• Neurogenic tumors 283
	• Osteoblastoma 283
	• Osteoid osteoma 283

Co Congenital

REMOTE	LOCAL
COMMON	
Not applicable	Not applicable
UNCOMMON	
Not applicable	Not applicable
RARE	
Not applicable	Not applicable

Ne Neurogenic/Psychogenic

REMOTE	LOCAL
COMMON	
Not applicable	Not applicable
UNCOMMON	
Not applicable	Not applicable
RARE	
Not applicable	Not applicable

Note: These are estimates of relative incidence because few data are available for the less common conditions.

Overview of Posterior Thorax Pain

Physical therapists commonly treat the thoracic spine as a critical mobility segment in movement dysfunction. The structural architecture of the spine and adjoining rib cage give protection to vital organs and as a result give stiffness to this spinal region. The central location of the thoracic spine and proximity of these organs and the adjacent cervical spine require consideration as possible sources of thoracic pain. The organs most posterior in the cavity are most likely to refer to the posterior thoracic region (ie, lungs, esophagus, aorta, kidneys, gallbladder, and pancreas), but any of the structures in the visceral cavities may feature thoracic pain as one component of their clinical presentation. This chapter discusses many diagnoses outside the scope of physical therapy, a few of them are emergent, and many require referral to other specialists for diagnosis.

Remote

ANGINA

■ Stable Angina

Chief Clinical Characteristics

This presentation can include pain and pressure in the chest or between shoulder blades that may or may not radiate to arms, neck, torso, or jaw with symptoms lasting 2 to 10 minutes (Fig. 16-1). Symptoms are aggravated by activity, emotional distress, or large meals.

Background Information

The diagnosis is made with echocardiography, serial blood tests (cardiac troponin T or I, or CK-MB),[1–3] angiogram,[1] symptom provocation during a cardiac stress test, and symptom relief following nitroglycerin administration. Symptoms are consistently present at a certain rate–pressure product. If an individual with this condition develops symptoms, a physical therapist should request

that the individual stop activity, sit down, and use his or her prescribed nitroglycerin spray or pills. If symptoms fail to resolve or this is the first presentation of symptoms, the physical therapist should activate the emergency medical services.

■ Unstable Angina/Acute Coronary Insufficiency

Chief Clinical Characteristics

This presentation may include pain and pressure in the chest and intrascapular region with possible radiation to the arms, neck, torso, or jaw with symptoms lasting 20 to 30 minutes or occurring at rest (see Fig. 16-1).

Background Information

Individuals suspected of this condition may be unable to relieve their symptoms with nitroglycerin. Often the individual has a clot or spasm superimposed on a region of existing coronary artery plaque.[1,4] The diagnosis is confirmed with echocardiography,[5] serial blood tests (cardiac troponin T or I or CK-MB),[1–3] and angiogram.[1] Infarction is not present. This condition is defined as new onset, angina at rest, recent increase in frequency, duration, or intensity of angina.[1,2,4] Initial management by physical therapists involves activation of the emergency medical services.

■ Variant Angina

Chief Clinical Characteristics

This presentation can involve pain and pressure in the chest or between shoulder blades that may or may not radiate to arms, neck, torso, or jaw that occurs spontaneously, often in the morning hours, causing the patient to be awakened with pain (see Fig. 16-1).[1,4] Symptoms are variable and do not always occur at the same activity level.

Background Information

Symptoms may not be resolved with nitroglycerin. Diagnosis is made by echocardiography, echocardiographic changes, or symptom provocation during a cardiac stress test, angiogram,[1,3,4] serial blood tests (cardiac troponin T or I or CK-MB),[1–3] or symptom provocation with use of medication that produces artery spasm. Initial management by physical therapists involves activating the emergency medical services.

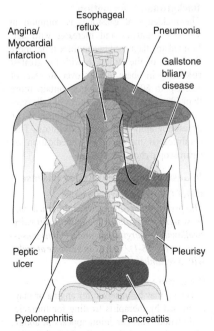

Angina/ Myocardial infarction — Esophageal reflux — Pneumonia — Gallstone biliary disease — Peptic ulcer — Pleurisy — Pyelonephritis — Pancreatitis

FIGURE 16-1 Visceral referral patterns to the posterior thorax.

Cervical Degenerative Disk Disease

Chief Clinical Characteristics

This presentation can be characterized by unilateral thoracic and posterior neck pain, limited neck motion, or upper extremity symptoms.

Background Information

Palpation of the cervical spine may reveal altered mobility, and pain with possible reproduction of upper extremity and thoracic symptoms. Trapezius and interscapular pain patterns exist depending on the level of involvement.[6] Associated symptoms such as arm paresthesias, weakness, or loss of reflexes in a radicular pattern will help to identify level of involvement. This condition is associated with a history of trauma, family history of degenerative changes, smoking, nutrition deficits, and high-impact physical activities. The C5–C6 then C6–C7 and C4–C5 disks are the most frequently affected levels.[7] Cervical radiographs confirm the diagnosis. Advancing radiculopathy or myelopathy may require surgical decompression or stabilization.

Cervical Facet Joint Dysfunction

Chief Clinical Characteristics

This presentation may include unilateral and medial scapular border pain with or without neck pain along with marked motion deficits in the neck or shoulder.

Background Information

Extension or ipsilateral rotation may exacerbate symptoms. Palpation of the cervical spine will reveal limited joint motion, pain and tenderness, and occasionally reproduction of referred symptoms. This condition is prevalent during the second to fourth decade and may not show any signs of disk disease on imaging studies but may have a history of cervical trauma. It has been suggested that cervical facet joint pain may contribute to cervical pain in up to 63% of nonradicular neck pain patients.[8] Facets C4–C5 to C7–T1 have been shown to have pain referral patterns that extend to the upper scapula or to the lower and medial scapular border (Fig. 16-2).[9–12] The treatment of choice for this condition is physical therapy. However, facet joint injections may be used if treatments do not sufficiently

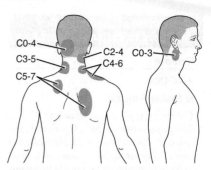

FIGURE 16-2 Referral patterns of the cervical facet joints.

resolve symptoms; relief with facet joint injections also may be pathognomonic.

Gallstones and Biliary Disease

Chief Clinical Characteristics

This presentation involves rapid onset of severe pain in the right epigastrium, and referred pain to the upper thoracic spine, shoulder, and scapula. An acute attack may be associated with fever, chills, and vomiting (see Fig. 16-1).

Background Information

The incidence of gallstones is common in Western countries and increases with age. Women are diagnosed two to three times more than men of the same age, with the greatest risk being in obese females over 40 years of age. Up to 80% of gallstones contain more than 50% cholesterol. Two-thirds of gallstones are asymptomatic.[13] Cholecintigraphy or ultrasonography confirms the diagnosis. This condition is managed with medication or laparoscopic cholecystectomy.[13]

Gastroesophageal Reflex Disease

Chief Clinical Characteristics

This presentation can involve midthoracic and chest pain postprandial along with difficulty swallowing, regurgitation, and a globus sensation (see Fig. 16-1).[14] Pain can be worse at night with a recumbent position.

Background Information

This pain may be mistaken for angina or may be missed by therapists treating for thoracic dysfunction. This condition appears in about 20% of the population in the United States, who report episodes at least once weekly.[15]

Increasing age does not seem to lead to increased prevalence. Short-term utilization of proton pump inhibitor medications can be used to rule in reflux prior to undergoing an upper gastrointestinal endoscopy, which can identify histopathological changes in the mucosa.[16] Pharmacologic management with antacids or H_2 blockers and diet modification is usually needed to control symptoms.

■ Myocardial Infarction/Acute Coronary Insufficiency

Chief Clinical Characteristics
This presentation typically includes an acute onset of mild to severe substernal chest, interscapular, and shoulder pain with possible associated atypical symptoms including nausea, vomiting, diaphoresis, dyspnea, or lightheadedness (see Fig. 16-1).

Background Information
One out of every five deaths in adults can be attributed to this condition. Risk factors include male sex, obesity, diabetes mellitus, hypertension, heredity, and elevated fibrinogen, homocysteine, and C-reactive protein levels.[17,18] Individuals who are older, female, hypertensive, and have diabetes are at risk for atypical symptoms.[19] Patients without chest pain presenting with atypical or minimal symptoms are less likely to seek care or receive a correct diagnosis. This condition is a medical emergency. Treatment within the first 4 hours should include thrombolytic therapy, cardiac drug therapy, or angioplasty to improve myocardial perfusion.

■ Pancreatitis

Chief Clinical Characteristics
This presentation involves severe diffuse abdominal pain in the epigastric region, upper quadrants, and mid to low back (see Fig. 16-1). This pain will be constant and may have an abrupt onset associated with nausea, vomiting, fever, and dizziness.

Background Information
Eating and alcohol intake will exacerbate their symptoms. There may be palpable tenderness and postural guarding in the epigastric area. Mobility and positional change will not change symptoms. More than 50% of acute cases of pancreatitis are related to gallstone disease and 90% of chronic cases are secondary to alcohol abuse.[13] Acute pancreatitis is usually evaluated with contrast-enhanced computed tomography in order to judge the severity of the inflammation. Treatment usually requires hospitalization for treatment of hypovolemia with close fluid regulation and packed cells if severe anemia is present.[20]

■ Peptic Ulcer Disease

Chief Clinical Characteristics
This presentation may involve deep, gnawing, constant pain in the midthoracic to low thoracic spine and right upper abdominal quadrant and epigastric regions. This pain is relieved with antacids, H_2 blockers, or food (see Fig. 16-1). Pain is worse on an empty stomach and symptoms may be worse at night.

Background Information
It is estimated that around 10% of the population of Western countries has peptic ulcer dysfunction. Peak incidence is between the ages of 30 and 60 years. The peak damage to the mucosa of the duodenum is caused primarily by infection with *H. pylori* bacteria, whereas ulcers induced by nonsteroidal anti-inflammatory ulcers usually affect the stomach.[21] Utilization of anti-inflammatories, heavy smoking, or alcohol abuse increases the likelihood of developing ulcerations. Endoscopy can be used to diagnose gastrointestinal disorders, as well as to repair ulcers that do not heal and continue to bleed.[22]

■ Pleurisy/Empyema

Chief Clinical Characteristics
This presentation includes sharp stabbing lateral chest wall, scapular, neck, and abdominal pain and is exacerbated by deep inspiration (see Fig. 16-1). Pain will gradually increase over minutes to hours, and when the condition is severe, breathing may become shallow or labored and is accompanied with cough, fever, and chills.

Background Information
Movement may agitate the pain, but splinting with holding a breath and lying down may give temporary relief. Pleurisy is inflammation of the pleura caused by infection or injury and irritation of the parietal pleura is the pain generator. When fluid collects between the parietal and visceral pleura around the lungs

and pus forms, this is called *empyema*. Pleural effusions can be diagnosed by physical exam and subjective complaints and often a pleural friction rub or decreased breath sounds can be auscultated. Children and older adults (more than 65 years old) are at highest risk for developing an empyema. Individuals with this condition are hospitalized and treated with thoracocentesis and antibiotics.[23,24]

■ Pneumonia

Chief Clinical Characteristics

This presentation can involve sharp and stabbing pain in the interscapular region that worsens with a deep breath and may be associated with a cough and fever, chills, rigors, or general malaise (see Fig. 16-1).

Background Information

In older patients, altered mentation or confusion may be the first signs of infection. There is an increased risk of developing a respiratory infection in smokers and in patients with organ transplants, sickle cell anemia, chronic organ diseases, or immunosuppressed conditions.[25] Symptoms frequently follow a viral upper respiratory tract infection in which secretions proliferate resident bacteria and transport them into the alveoli. The diagnosis can be confirmed with plain chest radiographs. Gram stain and culture of sputum allows for treatment of bacterial causes with appropriate antibiotic therapy.[26,27] Approximately 20% of community-acquired pneumonia requires hospitalization and the fatality rate can be near 9%.

■ Pneumothorax

Chief Clinical Characteristics

This presentation may include rapid onset of chest pain, as well as possible abrupt upper and lateral thoracic wall pain that is aggravated by movement and coughing.

Background Information

Sitting upright may be the most comfortable position and will be associated with shortness of breath and rapid breathing. Traumatic pneumothorax can be caused by multiple types of trauma or penetrating injury and iatrogenic causes like biopsy or treatment with a mechanical ventilator. Spontaneous pneumothorax can occur with underlying pulmonary disease

or no identifiable pathology. The incidence has been reported to be six times greater in males, 85% of whom are under the age of 40. Plain chest radiographs confirm the diagnosis. Minor cases may resolve themselves in a few days, whereas when larger regions are affected, aspiration of the air from the pleural cavity or chest tube placement may be required. This situation is considered a medical emergency.[28]

■ Pyelonephritis

Chief Clinical Characteristics

This presentation typically includes dull, constant pain in the flank, interscapular, lumbar, or groin regions accompanied by fever, chills, and dysuria (see Fig. 16-1). Tenderness and rigor can be palpated in the flank or abdomen with percussion.

Background Information

Painful urination with hematuria, frequency, and urgency are common with recurrent or untreated bladder infections subsequently leading to bacterial infection of the kidney. The incidence is highest in women under 50 years old with uncomplicated cases.[29] Urinalysis confirms the diagnosis and is treated with appropriate antibiotic therapy.

TUMORS

■ Esophageal Adenocarcinoma

Chief Clinical Characteristics

This presentation can be characterized by painful dysphagia, anorexia, persistent thorax pain, and chronic cough. Barrett's esophagus (gastric epithelium) and prolonged persistent gastroesophageal reflux disease may be possible precursors to this malignancy.[30]

Background Information

Positive risk factors are excessive alcohol consumption; cigarette smoking; diets lacking fresh fruits, vegetables, and animal proteins; and esophageal abnormalities.[25] Diagnosis is made with endoscopic evaluation and endoscopic ultrasonography, and positron emission tomography is needed for appropriate staging of the lesion. Surgical resection of the tumor is the primary direction for treatment but palliative care to maintain the esophageal lumen may be used with nonsurgical candidates.

▪ Gastric Adenocarcinoma

Chief Clinical Characteristics
This presentation involves epigastric or back pain and frequently the first symptom is weight loss associated with nausea.

Background Information
Early gastric cancer is usually asymptomatic and may already be metastatic to lymph nodes by the time it is detected, resulting in a poor outcome.[25] Symptoms may be alleviated with H_2-receptor antagonists but they no longer assist with dyspepsia as the disease advances. Men are twice as likely as women to develop these carcinomas. Diagnosis can be confirmed with endoscopy or double-contrast studies of the upper gastrointestinal tract. Surgical treatment with a transhiatal approach has been shown to have the fewest respiratory complications and least thoracic pain.[31] Stent placement can be used to decrease obstruction in nonsurgical candidates.

▪ Pancreatic Carcinoma

Chief Clinical Characteristics
This presentation may include left epigastrium and left shoulder pain along with middle to low back pain. The early signs of this tumor are weight loss, epigastric pain (usually postprandial), and jaundice.

Background Information
Mean age of diagnosis was reported to be 64 with a ratio of men to women at 1.27:1.[32] The lack of symptoms early in the progression of this tumor delays diagnosis and contributes to a poor prognosis. Early and more liberal diagnostic testing may allow for diagnosis before it becomes nonoperable. The diagnosis is confirmed with ultrasound, which has 95% specificity and 70% sensitivity for detecting pancreatic carcinoma.[32]

Local

▪ Ankylosing Spondylitis

Chief Clinical Characteristics
This presentation typically includes an insidious onset of low-back and symmetric posterior hip pain associated with a slowly progressive and significant loss of general spinal mobility. Symptoms may be worse in the morning and improve with light exercise.

Background Information
This condition is more common in males, as well as people of American indigenous descent, less than 40 years of age, or who carry the human leukocyte antigen B27.[33] It also may be associated with fever, malaise, and inflammatory bowel disease. The diagnosis is confirmed with plain radiographs of the sacroiliac joints and lumbar spine, which reveal characteristic findings of sacroiliitis and "bamboo spine." Blood panels including erythrocyte sedimentation rate are useful to track disease activity. Treatment may involve use of steroidal, nonsteroidal, and biological anti-inflammatory agents directed to the underlying inflammation of this disease process, as well as physical therapy to ensure optimal posture and body mechanics.

▪ Costovertebral or Costotransverse Joint Dysfunction

Chief Clinical Characteristics
This presentation can be characterized by posterior thorax pain that may extend to the shoulder, arm, and chest and is unilaterally worsened by respiration.

Background Information
The upper half of the thoracic spine is affected most frequently and can show signs of joint locking and may be associated with spasm of the multisegmental paraspinal muscles. Costovertebral joints have innervation of the synovium adequate to produce thoracic pain.[34] Plain radiograph findings may be normal or may show marked joint degeneration. This diagnosis is localized with the clinical examination but definitive diagnosis can be made with a local joint nerve block.

▪ Cushing's Syndrome

Chief Clinical Characteristics
This presentation may include kyphosis, back pain secondary to bone loss of the spine, along with muscle wasting and weakness, slow wound healing, easy bruising, and memory deficits.

Background Information
This condition is associated with thoracic hyperkyphosis due to a fatty hump at the cervicothoracic junction. Patients often present with a large pendulous abdomen, thin legs, increased facial hair, and purple and red striations on the

skin. This condition is associated with chronic corticosteroid treatment such as prednisone or pituitary and adrenal tumors, which lead to increased cortisol levels. Urine, blood, and saliva tests are done to detect elevated levels of cortisol. Treatment includes determining the source for the increased cortisol levels and using medication modification or tumor management with surgical resection and/or radiation.

■ Delayed-Onset Muscle Soreness

Chief Clinical Characteristics
This presentation can involve mild to severe muscle soreness in the first 12 to 48 hours after strenuous exercise or resistance activities. It can be felt in any muscle group.

Background Information
Eccentric loads most commonly result in this condition; self-limiting upper back and scapular symptoms may be reported after lifting and pulling loads.[35] This diagnosis is confirmed by clinical examination.[36]

■ Discitis

Chief Clinical Characteristics
This presentation may include mild to excruciating, constant low back pain, localized at the level of the disk involved, which is associated with fever and unrelieved by rest.

Background Information
This condition is associated with tenderness over the affected segment with associated muscle spasm and limited motion. As symptoms worsen, pain may radiate to adjacent areas and into the lower extremities. Adult onset usually follows spinal surgery but may occur following bacteremia from urinary tract infection in older patients. Magnetic resonance imaging is the most sensitive and specific imaging modality for diagnosis of discitis. Variable organisms have been responsible for these infections requiring blood and biopsy cultures to establish appropriate antibiotic treatment.[37]

■ Dissecting Aortic Aneurysm

Chief Clinical Characteristics
This presentation involves excruciating, severe radiating pain to the neck, interscapular region, shoulders, low back, or abdomen. The pain is often described as hot searing or throbbing in nature. Aneurysms can be silent or cause

gnawing pain. This condition also may be associated with syncope, dyspnea, aphasia, hemiparesis, and a sudden drop in blood pressure.

Background Information
One-time ultrasonography screening has been shown to be 95% sensitive and nearly 100% specific in men 65 to 75 years old who have smoked.[38] Physical examination may reveal a pulsatile abdominal mass but this exam has low accuracy and if found is a severe medical emergency because it can lead to myocardial infarction and death.

■ Epidural Abscess

Chief Clinical Characteristics
This presentation typically includes midthoracic back pain associated with fever and variable motor weakness. This condition is associated with alcohol and intravenous drug abuse or a concurrent nonspinal infection site.

Background Information
Multiple organisms can cause this condition. Screening should occur in the presence of fever, elevated erythrocyte sedimentation rate, and increased white blood cell count in an individual with spinal pain. The diagnosis is confirmed with magnetic resonance imaging with contrast.[39,40] Individuals with progressive neurological weakness require emergent surgical decompression and long-term antimicrobial treatment for the specific organism identified.

■ Fibromyalgia

Chief Clinical Characteristics
This presentation may involve chronic widespread joint and muscle pain defined as bilateral upper body, lower body, and spine pain, associated with tenderness to palpation of 11 of 18 specific muscle-tendon sites.

Background Information
Individuals with this condition will demonstrate lowered mechanical and thermal pain thresholds, high pain ratings for noxious stimuli, and altered temporal summation of pain stimuli.[41] The etiology of this condition is unclear; multiple body systems appear to be involved. Indistinct clinical boundaries between this condition and similar conditions (eg, chronic fatigue syndrome, irritable bowel syndrome, and chronic

muscular headaches) pose a diagnostic challenge.[41] This condition is diagnosed by exclusion. Treatment may include aerobic exercise, manual therapy, and behavior modification for chronic pain and sleep disorders.

FRACTURES

■ Compression Fracture

Chief Clinical Characteristics

This presentation typically involves traumatic or relative insidious onset of sharp midline back pain, limited tolerance for movement, especially flexion, and decreased sitting tolerance. Local tenderness and muscle spasm may also be present.

Background Information

Percussion over the affected vertebral spinous processes while the spine is flexed may reproduce symptoms. Compression fractures are the most common thoracic spine fracture, usually resulting from hyperflexion injuries and, in the case of pathological fractures, more moderate activities or falls. Stability of the rib cage causes most thoracic compression fractures to occur in the lower thoracic and thoracolumbar regions. The diagnosis is confirmed with thoracic spine plain radiographs. Depending on severity, extension bracing may be required to limit flexion forces and allow the anterior vertebral body to heal. Persistent pain may be treated with minimally invasive percutaneous spinal augmentation.[42]

■ Rib Fracture

Chief Clinical Characteristics

This presentation involves chest wall pain following blunt trauma. Pain may be worsened with trunk movements that move the fracture site.

Background Information

Typically, low-velocity impacts (ie, sports participation) can cause unilateral and isolated rib fractures, whereas high-velocity impacts (ie, deceleration against a steering wheel during a motor vehicle accident) and crushes cause more extensive, bilateral fractures that also may involve the sternum. Complex fractures may result in a flail segment, in which a portion of the chest wall paradoxically moves inward on inspiration

and compromises tidal volume. Approximately 150 mL of blood loss occurs with each rib fracture, and fracture lines are associated with sharp edges that may further damage surrounding tissues. Therefore, concern for excessive blood loss increases as the number of rib fractures increases. Metastases and other disease processes also may predispose individuals to this condition. All individuals with rib fractures should be evaluated for potential pneumothorax or hemothorax by way of plain radiographs. In individuals with fewer than five rib fractures, treatment usually involves analgesics and physical therapy. Individuals with more than five rib fractures or a flail segment may also require surgery to fixate fracture segments and aspirate secretions.[43] Physical therapists should refer individuals suspected of having this condition to a physician for evaluation but may begin treatment for comfort and body mechanics training to protect the region.

■ Vertebral Fracture/Dislocation

Chief Clinical Characteristics

This presentation can include severe trauma with excruciating pain, tenderness, and severe muscle splinting in the spinal region of injury. Up to 80% of thoracic fracture dislocations result in complete paralysis.[44] Thoracic pain may also be associated with extremity pain and paresthesias when nerve roots or the spinal cord is involved.

Background Information

Acceleration or deceleration injuries commonly encountered in automobile accidents and falls from height can cause a variety of osseous structure injuries. Mechanisms of injury include axial loading (resulting in burst fractures) and hyperextension (resulting in posterior element shear injuries).[45] This diagnosis is confirmed with plain radiographs or computed tomography of the thoracic spine. In cases of posterior element disruption or dislocation, surgical stabilization is required.

■ Herpes Zoster

Chief Clinical Characteristics

This presentation may involve burning interscapular pain that wraps around one side of the thorax to the anterior chest associated with itching, hyperesthesias, paresthesia, dysesthesia, or a painful red vesicle.

Background Information
The prodromal phase of this condition involves itching and sensory changes that last 2 to 3 days, followed by eruption of painful red vesicles up to 3 weeks later. Vesicles may burst, leaving brown crusts over the skin lesions. T5 and T6 are the most common dermatomes affected.[46] Individuals with this condition demonstrate a previous history of varicella exposure or infection. The virus remains dormant in spinal ganglia until its reactivation during a period of stress, infection, or physical exhaustion. Pain associated with this condition may be disproportionate to the extent of skin irritation. Risk factors for this condition include decreased immune function. The primary complication is post-herpetic neuralgia or persistent pain for longer than 1 to 3 months following the vesicles.[47] This diagnosis is confirmed clinically. Treatment typically includes oral antiviral agents, which appear most effective if initiated within 72 hours of an outbreak. If treatment is initiated later than 3 days after outbreak, treatment is aimed at controlling pain and pruritus and minimizing the risk of secondary infection.

■ Meningitis
Chief Clinical Characteristics
This presentation may include acute severe neck and thoracic pain that is worsened with neck flexion and associated with headache, vomiting, fever, rash, severe fatigue, and possible altered consciousness. Symptoms may last several weeks with bacterial meningitis, whereas severity of symptoms will be less with viral infection and usually will last 5 to 7 days.

Background Information
This condition is most commonly caused by meningococcal or pneumococcal bacteria. Fungal infection presents with more mild chronic symptoms and occurs in individuals with immunosuppression. Meningitis affects children under the age of 5 more often than adults. Clinical exam should include meningeal tests such as Kernig's or Brudzinski's sign. These tests may be remarkable,[48] where active neck flexion results in hip and knee flexion secondary to pain response. Lumbar puncture confirms the diagnosis.[49] This condition is a medical emergency; early diagnosis and treatment are essential for optimal outcome. Treatment includes an intravenously administered antibiotic or antiviral agents as appropriate, along with other supportive medical therapies.

■ Myofascial Pain Disorder
Chief Clinical Characteristics
This presentation typically involves soreness, tightness, and tenderness in the neck and upper back musculature following chronic sustained postural positions or a single overloading episode.

Background Information
These muscles are described to be abnormally shortened and have palpable firm nodules called trigger points along with hypercontracted extrafusal muscle fibers called the *taut band*.[50] These entities are thought to be reverberating spinal reflex loops of sustained neural activity.[51] This diagnosis is confirmed by clinical examination. Physical therapy interventions are the treatment of choice for this condition.

■ Osteomalacia
Chief Clinical Characteristics
This presentation can include back pain, fractures, bone tenderness to palpation, muscle weakness, kyphoscoliosis, bowing of the lower extremities, and enlarged costochondral junctions. These patients may have difficulty with getting up from sitting or negotiating stairs.

Background Information
This condition is caused by bone weakening secondary to vitamin D deficiency or altered biotransformation of vitamin D, resulting in limited calcium uptake into bone. It can be caused by anticonvulsant medications, renal disease, or intestinal disorders. Plain radiographs reveal the characteristic transverse fracture-like lines in affected bone and areas of demineralization in the matrix. Treatment usually involves oral vitamin D and treatment of underlying disorders that may result in altered vitamin D metabolism.

■ Osteoporosis
Chief Clinical Characteristics
This presentation includes low thoracic or high lumbar back pain associated with characteristic

thoracic kyphosis, loss of height, and a recent history of fracture, which causes pain. Fracture pain may be the first symptom experienced by individuals with this condition.

Background Information
Porous bone develops secondary to decreased deposition or increased resorption rates, leading to an imbalance and gradual loss of bone mass.[52] This loss is most common in postmenopausal women who experience decreasing estrogen levels, but men are at risk in the seventh to eighth decade of life as testosterone levels decline. The diagnosis is confirmed with dual x-ray absorptiometry. Treatment may include resistance exercise, bisphosphonates, and dietary supplements of calcium.

■ Paget's Disease

Chief Clinical Characteristics
This presentation may involve deep, aching pain that is worse at night and associated with fatigue, headaches, hearing loss, and often a pronounced kyphosis.

Background Information
Men are affected more than women in a 3:2 ratio. Long-bone deformities occur and lead to adjacent joint osteoarthrosis. Bones of the pelvis, lumbar spine, sacrum, thoracic spine, and ribs also are commonly affected by deformity. Vertebral collapse may occur in the thoracic region and compression neuropathies may develop. Its incidence increases by age 50 with peak incidence after 70 years of age.[53] Deformities are a result of haphazard resorption of bone that then fills in with fibrous tissue. Subsequent attempts to form bone lead to large, less compact, more vascular bone susceptible to fracture.[54] Diagnosis is confirmed with radiographs and treated with bisphosphonates.

■ T4 Syndrome

Chief Clinical Characteristics
This presentation can include some localized thoracic pain and stiffness with palpation. Commonly the presentation also includes a glove-like distribution of paresthesias in one or both of the arms and is associated with headache. Symptoms usually occur at night or wake the patient in the early morning.

Background Information
This condition often is associated with prior thoracic and cervical symptoms that tend to increase in frequency and intensity. It is most common in women between the ages of 20 and 50 years.[55] Functional spinal units adjacent to T4 may also be involved.[56] Clinical examination confirms this diagnosis, and physical therapy interventions are the initial treatments of choice.

■ Thoracic Degenerative Disk Disease

Chief Clinical Characteristics
This presentation can be characterized by thoracic pain described as coming through to the chest from the back and may include a dull ache, spasm, or burning or may be lancinating in nature. Compression of the T1 nerve root will cause symptoms in the axilla and the ulnar border of the arm and hand. For lesions below T6, patients may show signs and symptoms in the lower extremities.

Background Information
Pain may increase with a cough or sneeze and worsen with neck flexion or rotation. This diagnosis is confirmed with magnetic resonance imaging. Large lesions characterized by progressive weakness or upper motor neuron signs should be referred to a surgeon immediately for additional evaluation. Delay in referral may reduce the prognosis for neurological and functional recovery.

■ Thoracic Facet Joint Dysfunction

Chief Clinical Characteristics
This presentation may involve a horizontal band of symptoms across the posterior thorax at the level of the dysfunction.

Background Information
Symptoms can be reproduced and dysfunction localized with combined thoracic motions of side-bending, rotation, with flexion or extension. Injection studies found the pain to be one to two segments lower than the tested level and share several overlapping patches along the spine.[57] Definitive diagnosis can be made with a facet joint nerve block. While physical therapy interventions are the primary treatment of choice for this condition, facet joint

nerve blockade also may be considered in individuals who do not respond favorably to physical therapy.

■ Thoracic Osteoarthrosis/ Osteoarthritis

Chief Clinical Characteristics
This presentation includes a focal region of pain unilaterally along the thoracic spine or pain centrally between the scapula that worsens with prolonged positions and chronic postures of the neck and back. Symptoms are usually worse during the morning and warming up with motion or a hot shower improves function.

Background Information
Postural deformity may be identified and can lead to movement and palpation findings that can identify the source of symptoms. Arthrosis of the thoracic vertebral column is more likely at the lower thoracic regions.[58] Lateral thoracic plain radiographs will show degenerative joint and disk changes. Physical therapy interventions are the primary treatment of choice for this condition.

■ Transverse Myelitis

Chief Clinical Characteristics
This presentation may be characterized by severe sharp localized midthoracic pain that may be combined with a dull constant ache and low-grade fever. Progressive motor loss and hypoesthesia will occur in the first 72 hours up to 1 week.[59]

Background Information
Inflammation causes sensory loss at a transverse sensory level on the lower trunk and motor loss may proceed to full paraplegia. Lumbar puncture testing and magnetic resonance imaging of the spine with contrast can be used to differentiate this disorder from multiple sclerosis, tumor, abscess, herniated disk, or hematoma.[60] High-dose corticosteroids are used in treatment but prognosis is inconsistent for full recovery.

■ Tuberculosis of the Spine (Pott's Disease)

Chief Clinical Characteristics
This presentation includes spinal pain, segmental bone tenderness, weakness, and in rare cases spastic paraplegia that may be associated with fever, chills, weight loss, and fatigue during active disease.

Background Information
Airborne transmission of *Mycobacterium tuberculosis* causes infection of the lungs that can spread through the circulatory system to spinal structures. Lower thoracic spinal segments are the most likely to be infected. This condition is becoming more prevalent secondary to drug-resistant strains of tuberculosis and an increasing population of immunocompromised individuals. The diagnosis is confirmed by bacteriological and histological studies of biopsy samples and standard radiographs of the spine.[61] Appropriate antibiotic treatment must be followed through a full course of the prescription to ensure that the organism does not become resistant. Anterior spinal stabilization has been recommended for spinal deformities, progressive neurological compromise, or significant paravertebral or epidural abcess.[62]

TUMORS
■ Leukemias

Chief Clinical Characteristics
This presentation involves a variety of symptoms including vague back pain, bone and joint pains, malaise, fatigue, excessive bruising or bleeding, night sweats, and weight loss. Acute disorders have a more rapid onset with illness, with thoracic and lumbar pain being one of the first symptoms experienced in children, teens, and adults.[63] Chronic leukemias may go undiagnosed with few symptoms until a routine blood test identifies them.

Background Information
Acute myelogenous leukemias constitute 85% of adult acute leukemias. Chronic lymphocytic leukemia is responsible for 30% of all leukemias with the median age of onset in the seventh decade.[25] A proliferation of abnormal and dysfunctional blood cells originates in the bone marrow and then progresses into the peripheral circulation, lymph, spleen, and liver. Diagnosis is made with aspiration or biopsy of bone marrow and complete blood cell examination and chemistry.

■ **Metastases, Including From Primary Breast, Kidney, Lung, Prostate, and Thyroid Disease**

Chief Clinical Characteristics

This presentation may include unremitting pain in individuals with these risk factors: previous history or cancer, age 50 years or older, failure to improve with conservative therapy, and weight change of more than 10 pounds in 6 months.[64,65]

Background Information

The prevalence of metastatic disease in primary care patients is less than 1%. Symptoms also may be related to pathological fracture in affected sites. Involvement of the costovertebral joints has been shown to be the greatest factor for predicting vertebral collapse in the thoracic spine.[66] Common primary sites causing metastases to bone include breast, prostate, lung, and kidney. Bone scan confirms the diagnosis. Treatment may include chemotherapy, radiation, surgical resection, and/or palliative care depending on the type of tumor and extent of metastases.

■ **Multiple Myeloma**

Chief Clinical Characteristics

This presentation can include bone pain in the vertebrae and ribs. Aching pain in the spine may be the first sign of this disease following pathological vertebral fracture and vertebral collapse.

Background Information

This condition is a destructive cancer of the immune system plasma cells that leads to tumor formation in the bone marrow and interference with normal blood cell formation. Diagnosis requires several steps including protein and immunofixation electrophoresis, plain radiographs, and bone marrow aspiration and biopsy. Precaution must be taken during exercise prescription with areas of fracture and bone demineralization for individuals treated while recovering from this condition. Treatment will depend on the stage and severity and may include chemotherapy, radiation, stem cell transplantation, or plasmapheresis.[67]

■ **Neurogenic Tumors**

Chief Clinical Characteristics

This presentation typically includes symptoms arising from the thoracic spine producing back pain, intercostal neuralgia, and central canal location, upper motor neuron signs and gait disturbances.

Background Information

The location rather than the histology of neurogenic tumors is critical because these lesions are space occupying. Neural foramen encroachment and spinal cord compression is common with intrathoracic and intraspinal tumors.[68] Schwannomas originate from the neural sheath as benign encapsulated dumbbell-shaped tumors, whereas neurofibromas are nonencapsulated fusiform enlargements of the parent peripheral nerve root. Meningiomas arise from arachnoid matter and have a dural attachment. Diagnosis can be confirmed with computed tomography and magnetic resonance imaging. Early surgical exploration with resection is optimal.

■ **Osteoblastoma**

Chief Clinical Characteristics

This presentation may involve an insidious onset of deep and aching pain, typically in males under 30 years of age. Pain associated with this condition is not usually worse at night.

Background Information

Primary osteoblastomas are rare primary bone tumors, but they occur more commonly in the thoracic region than other spinal segments.[69] This condition involves abnormal production of osteoid and primitive bone, although its specific etiology remains unclear. Biopsy and plain radiographs confirm the diagnosis. Computed tomography is necessary to define the tumor margins when surgical resection is considered. Other forms of treatment may include radiation and chemotherapy, although the use of these interventions is considered controversial.

■ **Osteoid Osteoma**

Chief Clinical Characteristics

This presentation can be characterized by focal bone pain at the site of the tumor that is associated with tenderness and warmth to palpation, with significant increase in pain with activity and at night, as well as substantial and immediate relief of pain with anti-inflammatory medication.

Background Information
This condition is more common in males than females and in the 20- to 40-year-old age groups. Its pathology includes abnormal production of osteoid and primitive bone. Pain associated with this condition is self-limiting, but in many cases needs surgical resection to relieve symptoms.[69,70]

■ Primary Bone Tumors

Chief Clinical Characteristics
This presentation may include severe and abrupt or low-grade aching pain in the posterior thorax, fatigue, malaise, and pain that can awaken individuals from a sound sleep.

Background Information
Osteosarcoma and chondrosarcoma are the two most common types of malignant primary bone tumors. Osteosarcoma is more commonly present in individuals during the second and third decade and in older adults it is usually secondary to Paget's disease or radiation exposure. The blastic nature of this lesion differs from the lytic nature of most chondrosarcomas. Chondrosarcoma is more common during the fifth and sixth decades and most often found in the thoracic spine and ribs. Plain radiographs and computed tomography help to identify skeletal lesions and soft tissue extension can be seen with magnetic resonance imaging.[71] Needle biopsy may be needed to confirm a diagnosis. Complete surgical resection is optimal but outcome differs depending on location and stage; chemotherapy and radiation may be adjunctive.

■ Vertebral Osteomyelitis

Chief Clinical Characteristics
This presentation typically involves local back pain that may improve with rest and may have positive signs of radiculopathy. These symptoms mimic many other normal musculoskeletal disorders and often lack classic signs of infection, which makes this diagnosis difficult.

Background Information
This condition is increasingly common in younger populations due to the increased incidence of immunosuppression, and also may be associated with recent surgery, intravenous cauterization, or drug abuse.[72] Pathogens infect the vertebrae via a penetrating trauma or through the circulatory system from an infection elsewhere in the body. This condition is most common in elderly patients following urinary tract infections or diabetes mellitus. Elevated white blood cells, increased erythrocyte sedimentation rate, and increased C-reactive protein will be detected in blood work. Radiographs are used to determine the level of bony destruction, and magnetic resonance imaging or computed tomography may be used to locate any paravertebral abscess. Biopsy determines the type of pathogen. Appropriate antibiotic therapy may be used with surgical management of the infected bone depending on severity.[62]

References
1. Achar SA, Kundu S, Norcross WA. Diagnosis of acute coronary syndrome. *Am Fam Physician.* Jul 1, 2005;72(1):119–126.
2. Findlay IN, Cunningham AD. Definition of acute coronary syndrome. *Heart.* Jul 2005;91(7):857–859.
3. Gibler WB, Cannon CP, Blomkalns AL, et al. Practical implementation of the Guidelines for Unstable Angina/Non-ST-Segment Elevation Myocardial Infarction in the emergency department. *Ann Emerg Med.* Aug 2005;46(2):185–197.
4. Wiviott SD, Braunwald E. Unstable angina and non-ST-segment elevation myocardial infarction: part I. Initial evaluation and management, and hospital care. *Am Fam Physician.* Aug 1, 2004;70(3):525–532.
5. Ammar KA, Yawn BP, Urban L, et al. Identification of optimal electrocardiographic criteria for the diagnosis of unrecognized myocardial infarction: a population-based study. *Ann Noninvasive Electrocardiol.* Apr 2005;10(2):197–205.
6. Slipman CW, Plastaras C, Patel R, et al. Provocative cervical discography symptom mapping. *Spine J.* Jul–Aug 2005;5(4):381–388.
7. Murphey F. Sources and patterns of pain in disc disease. *Clin Neurosurg.* 1968;15:343–351.
8. Aprill C, Bogduk N. The prevalence of cervical zygapophyseal joint pain. A first approximation. *Spine.* Jul 1992;17(7):744–747.
9. Aprill C, Dwyer A, Bogduk N. Cervical zygapophyseal joint pain patterns. II: a clinical evaluation. *Spine.* Jun 1990;15(6):458–461.
10. Connell MD, Wiesel SW. Natural history and pathogenesis of cervical disk disease. *Orthop Clin North Am.* Jul 1992;23(3):369–380.

11. Dwyer A, Aprill C, Bogduk N. Cervical zygapophyseal joint pain patterns. I: a study in normal volunteers. *Spine.* Jun 1990;15(6):453–457.

12. Fukui S, Ohseto K, Shiotani M, et al. Referred pain distribution of the cervical zygapophysial joints and cervical dorsal rami. *Pain.* Nov 1996;68(1):79–83.

13. Kalloo AN, Kantsevoy SV. Gallstones and biliary disease. *Prim Care.* Sep 2001;28(3):591–606, vii.

14. Locke GR 3rd, Talley NJ, Fett SL, Zinsmeister AR, Melton LJ 3rd. Prevalence and clinical spectrum of gastroesophageal reflux: a population-based study in Olmsted County, Minnesota. *Gastroenterology.* May 1997;112(5):1448–1456.

15. Malfertheiner P, Hallerback B. Clinical manifestations and complications of gastroesophageal reflux disease (GERD). *Int J Clin Pract.* Mar 2005;59(3):346–355.

16. Mones J. Diagnostic value of potent acid inhibition in gastro-oesophageal reflux disease. *Drugs.* 2005;65(suppl 1):35–42.

17. Culic V, Miric D, Eterovic D. Correlation between symptomatology and site of acute myocardial infarction. *Int J Cardiol.* Feb 2001;77(2–3):163–168.

18. Patel H, Rosengren A, Ekman I. Symptoms in acute coronary syndromes: does sex make a difference? *Am Heart J.* Jul 2004;148(1):27–33.

19. Brieger D, Eagle KA, Goodman SG, et al. Acute coronary syndromes without chest pain, an underdiagnosed and undertreated high-risk group: insights from the Global Registry of Acute Coronary Events. *Chest.* Aug 2004;126 (2):461–469.

20. Mayerle J, Simon P, Lerch MM. Medical treatment of acute pancreatitis. *Gastroenterol Clin North Am.* Dec 2004;33(4):855–869, viii.

21. Bytzer P, Teglbjaerg PS. *Helicobacter pylori*-negative duodenal ulcers: prevalence, clinical characteristics, and prognosis—results from a randomized trial with 2-year follow-up. *Am J Gastroenterol.* May 2001;96(5): 1409–1416.

22. Kuipers EJ. Review article: exploring the link between *Helicobacter pylori* and gastric cancer. *Aliment Pharmacol Ther.* Mar 1999;13 Suppl 1:3–11.

23. Storm HK, Krasnik M, Bang K, Frimodt-Moller N. Treatment of pleural empyema secondary to pneumonia: thoracocentesis regimen versus tube drainage. *Thorax.* Oct 1992;47(10):821–824.

24. Cham CW, Haq SM, Rahamim J. Empyema thoracis: a problem with late referral? *Thorax.* Sep 1993;48(9): 925–927.

25. Rubin E, Farber JL, eds. *Pathology.* 3rd ed. Philadelphia, PA: Lippincott-Raven; 1999.

26. Lamping DL, Schroter S, Marquis P, Marrel A, Duprat-Lomon I, Sagnier PP. The community-acquired pneumonia symptom questionnaire: a new, patient-based outcome measure to evaluate symptoms in patients with community-acquired pneumonia. *Chest.* Sep 2002;122(3):920–929.

27. Marston BJ, Plouffe JF, File TM, Jr., et al. Incidence of community-acquired pneumonia requiring hospitalization. Results of a population-based active surveillance Study in Ohio. The Community-Based Pneumonia Incidence Study Group. *Arch Intern Med.* Aug 11–25 1997;157(15):1709–1718.

28. Baumann MH, Noppen M. Pneumothorax. *Respirology.* Jun 2004;9(2):157–164.

29. Gujral S, Bell CR, Dare L, Smith PJ, Persad RA. A prospective evaluation of the management of acute pyelonephritis in adults referred to urologists. *Int J Clin Pract.* Apr 2003;57(3):238–240.

30. Shaheen NJ. Advances in Barrett's esophagus and esophageal adenocarcinoma. *Gastroenterology.* May 2005;128(6):1554–1566.

31. Di Martino N, Izzo G, Cosenza A, et al. Adenocarcinoma of gastric cardia in the elderly: surgical problems and prognostic factors. *World J Gastroenterol.* Sep 7, 2005;11(33):5123–5128.

32. Elli M, Piazza E, Franzone PC, Isabella L, Poliziani D, Taschieri AM. Considerations on early diagnosis of carcinoma of the pancreas. *Hepatogastroenterology.* Nov–Dec 2003;50(54):2205–2207.

33. Goie The HS, Steven MM, van der Linden SM, Cats A. Evaluation of diagnostic criteria for ankylosing spondylitis: a comparison of the Rome, New York and modified New York criteria in patients with a positive clinical history screening test for ankylosing spondylitis. *Br J Rheumatol.* Aug 1985;24(3):242–249.

34. Erwin WM, Jackson PC, Homonko DA. Innervation of the human costovertebral joint: implications for clinical back pain syndromes. *J Manipulative Physiol Ther.* Jul–Aug 2000;23(6):395–403.

35. Weerakkody NS, Whitehead NP, Canny BJ, Gregory JE, Proske U. Large-fiber mechanoreceptors contribute to muscle soreness after eccentric exercise. *J Pain.* Aug 2001;2(4):209–219.

36. Hilbert JE, Sforzo GA, Swensen T. The effects of massage on delayed onset muscle soreness. *Br J Sports Med.* Feb 2003;37(1):72–75.

37. Honan M, White GW, Eisenberg GM. Spontaneous infectious discitis in adults. *Am J Med.* Jan 1996;100(1): 85–89.

38. Fleming C, Whitlock EP, Beil TL, Lederle FA. Screening for abdominal aortic aneurysm: a best-evidence systematic review for the U.S. Preventive Services Task Force. *Ann Intern Med.* Feb 1 2005;142(3):203–211.

39. Curry WT, Jr., Hoh BL, Amin-Hanjani S, Eskandar EN. Spinal epidural abscess: clinical presentation, management, and outcome. *Surg Neurol.* Apr 2005;63(4): 364–371; discussion 371.

40. Soehle M, Wallenfang T. Spinal epidural abscesses: clinical manifestations, prognostic factors, and outcomes. *Neurosurgery.* Jul 2002;51(1):79–85; discussion 86–87.

41. Wolfe F, Smythe HA, Yunus MB, et al. The American College of Rheumatology 1990 Criteria for the Classification of Fibromyalgia. Report of the Multicenter Criteria Committee. *Arthritis Rheum.* Feb 1990;33(2): 160–172.

42. Frankel BM, Monroe T, Wang C. Percutaneous vertebral augmentation: an elevation in adjacent-level fracture risk in kyphoplasty as compared with vertebroplasty. *Spine J.* Sep–Oct 2007;7(5):575–582.

43. Westaby S, Brayley N. ABC of major trauma. Thoracic trauma—I. *BMJ.* Jun 23 1990;300(6740):1639–1643.

44. Shapiro S, Abel T, Rodgers RB. Traumatic thoracic spinal fracture dislocation with minimal or no cord injury. Report of four cases and review of the literature. *J Neurosurg.* Apr 2002;96(3 suppl):333–337.

45. Chen JF, Wu CT, Lee ST. Percutaneous vertebroplasty for the treatment of burst fractures. Case report. *J Neurosurg Spine.* Sep 2004;1(2):228–231.

46. Stankus SJ, Długopolski M, Packer D. Management of herpes zoster (shingles) and postherpetic neuralgia. *Am Fam Physician.* Apr 15, 2000;61(8):2437–2444, 2447–2448.

47. Carmichael JK. Treatment of herpes zoster and postherpetic neuralgia. *Am Fam Physician.* Jul 1991;44(1): 203–210.

48. Verghese A, Gallemore G. Kernig's and Brudzinski's signs revisited. *Rev Infect Dis.* Nov–Dec 1987;9(6): 1187–1192.

49. Brivet FG, Guibert M, Dormont J. Acute bacterial meningitis in adults. *N Engl J Med.* Jun 10, 1993;328(23):1712–1713.

50. Simons DG, Travell JG, Simons LS, Travell JG. *Travell & Simons' Myofascial Pain and Dysfunction: The Trigger Point Manual.* 2nd ed. Baltimore, MD: Williams & Wilkins; 1999.

51. Wheeler AH. Myofascial pain disorders: theory to therapy. *Drugs.* 2004;64(1):45–62.

52. Barr JD, Barr MS, Lemley TJ, McCann RM. Percutaneous vertebroplasty for pain relief and spinal stabilization. *Spine.* Apr 15, 2000;25(8):923–928.

53. Dell'Atti C, Cassar-Pullicino VN, Lalam RK, Tins BJ, Tyrrell PN. The spine in Paget's disease. *Skeletal Radiol.* Jul 2007;36(7):609–626.

54. Langston AL, Ralston SH. Management of Paget's disease of bone. *Rheumatology (Oxford).* Aug 2004;43(8): 955–959.

55. Grieve GP, Boyling JD, Jull GA. *Grieve's Modern Manual Therapy: The Vertebral Column.* 3rd ed. Edinburgh and New York: Churchill Livingstone; 2004.

56. DeFranca GG, Levine LJ. The T4 syndrome. *J Manipulative Physiol Ther.* Jan 1995;18(1):34–37.

57. Dreyfuss P, Tibiletti C, Dreyer SJ. Thoracic zygapophyseal joint pain patterns. A study in normal volunteers. *Spine.* Apr 1994;19(7):807–811.

58. Nathan H. Osteophytes of the spine compressing the sympathetic trunk and splanchnic nerves in the thorax. *Spine.* Jul–Aug 1987;12(6):527–532.

59. Kim KK. Idiopathic recurrent transverse myelitis. *Arch Neurol.* Sep 2003;60(9):1290–1294.

60. Krishnan C, Kerr DA. Idiopathic transverse myelitis. *Arch Neurol.* Jun 2005;62(6):1011–1013.

61. Almeida A. Tuberculosis of the spine and spinal cord. *Eur J Radiol.* Aug 2005;55(2):193–201.

62. Christodoulou AG, Givissis P, Karataglis D, Symeonidis PD, Pournaras J. Treatment of tuberculous spondylitis with anterior stabilization and titanium cage. *Clin Orthop Relat Res.* Mar 2006;444:60–65.

63. Beckers R, Uyttebroeck A, Demaerel P. Acute lymphoblastic leukaemia presenting with low back pain. *Eur J Paediatr Neurol.* 2002;6(5):285–287.

64. Joines JD, McNutt RA, Carey TS, Deyo RA, Rouhani R. Finding cancer in primary care outpatients with low back pain: a comparison of diagnostic strategies. *J Gen Intern Med.* 2001;16(1):14–23.

65. Deyo RA, Diehl AK. Cancer as a cause of back pain: frequency, clinical presentation, and diagnostic strategies. *J Gen Intern Med.* May–Jun 1988;3(3):230–238.

66. Taneichi H, Kaneda K, Takeda N, Abumi K, Satoh S. Risk factors and probability of vertebral body collapse in metastases of the thoracic and lumbar spine. *Spine.* Feb 1997;22(3):239–245.

67. Rule S. Managing cancer-related skeletal events with bisphosphonates. *Hosp Med.* Jun 2004;65(6): 355–360.

68. Shamji FM, Todd TR, Vallieres E, Sachs HJ, Benoit BG. Central neurogenic tumours of the thoracic region. *Can J Surg.* Oct 1992;35(5):497–501.

69. Kan P, Schmidt MH. Osteoid osteoma and osteoblastoma of the spine. *Neurosurg Clin N Am.* Jan 2008;19 (1):65–70.

70. Crist BD, Lenke LG, Lewis S. Osteoid osteoma of the lumbar spine. A case report highlighting a novel reconstruction technique. *J Bone Joint Surg Am.* Feb 2005; 87(2):414–418.

71. Shives TC, McLeod RA, Unni KK, Schray MF. Chondrosarcoma of the spine. *J Bone Joint Surg Am.* Sep 1989;71(8):1158–1165.

72. Rath SA, Neff U, Schneider O, Richter HP. Neurosurgical management of thoracic and lumbar vertebral osteomyelitis and discitis in adults: a review of 43 consecutive surgically treated patients. *Neurosurgery.* May 1996;38(5):926–933.

CHAPTER 17

Case Demonstration: Infrascapular Pain

■ *Todd E. Davenport, PT, DPT, OCS* ■ *Hugh G. Watts, MD*

NOTE: This case demonstration was developed using the diagnostic process described in Chapter 4 and demonstrated in Chapter 5. The reader is encouraged to use this diagnostic process in order to ensure thorough clinical reasoning. If additional elaboration is required on the information presented in this chapter, please consult Chapters 4 and 5.

THE DIAGNOSTIC PROCESS

Step 1 Identify the patient's chief concern.
Step 2 Identify *barriers to communication.*
Step 3 Identify *special concerns.*
Step 4 Create a symptom timeline and sketch the anatomy (if needed).
Step 5 Create a diagnostic hypothesis list considering all possible forms of *remote* and *local* pathology that could cause the patient's chief concern.
Step 6 Sort the diagnostic hypothesis list by epidemiology and specific case characteristics.
Step 7 Ask specific questions to rule specific conditions or pathological categories less likely.
Step 8 Re-sort the diagnostic hypothesis list based on the patient's responses to specific questioning.
Step 9 Perform tests to differentiate among the remaining diagnostic hypotheses.
Step 10 Re-sort the diagnostic hypothesis list based on the patient's responses to specific tests.
Step 11 Decide on a diagnostic impression.
Step 12 Determine the appropriate patient disposition.

Case Description

Robert is a 41-year-old male, tall and slender, who presents without notable physical distress. His chief concern is of pain in the right infrascapular region. He is an avid weekend basketball player. He reports that his symptoms began about 1 month ago when he was struck from behind while attempting to rebound a missed shot. He denies falling to the ground and continued to play that day. His symptoms have worsened overall since their onset, which led him to seek physical therapy. He is currently not participating in his exercise program due to the pain. Robert is very anxious about returning to his exercise routine in order to control his work-related stress. Robert is the chief financial officer of a local television production company. He started taking 800 mg ibuprofen twice daily beginning the day after his injury, which was prescribed by his internist. However, he stopped 4 days following his injury secondary to no effect on symptoms. In general, Robert reports he has been healthy without history of recent illness.

STEP #1: Identify the patient's chief concern.

• Pain in the right infrascapular region

STEP #2: Identify *barriers to communication.*

• **Inability to collect diagnostically relevant information due to the patient's eagerness to return to recreational basketball.** The patient may be less willing to share the full extent of symptoms or demonstrate a bias against musculoskeletal causes of pain secondary to the level of his desire to return to activity.

• **Presence of trauma.** May lead the physical therapist to deprioritize atraumatic causes of symptoms in this patient too early in the process.

STEP #3: Identify *special concerns.*
None identified.

STEP #4: Create a symptom timeline and sketch the anatomy (if needed).

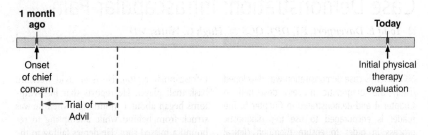

STEP #5: Create a diagnostic hypothesis list considering all possible forms of *remote* and *local* pathology that could cause the patient's chief concern.

Remote

T   Trauma

Cervical facet joint dysfunction (C6–T1)
Pneumothorax

I   Inflammation

Aseptic

Gastroesophageal reflux disease

Septic

Gallstones (biliary disease, cholecystitis)
Pancreatitis
Peptic ulcer
Pleurisy/empyema
Pneumonia
Pyelonephritis

M   Metabolic

Cushing's syndrome
Renal calculus

Va   Vascular

Angina:
• Stable angina
• Unstable angina
• Variant angina
Myocardial infarction/acute coronary
   insufficiency

De   Degenerative

Cervical degenerative disk disease

Tu   Tumor

Malignant Primary, such as:
• Esophageal adenocarcinoma

STEP #6: Sort the diagnostic hypothesis list by epidemiology and specific case characteristics.

Remote

T   Trauma

Cervical facet joint dysfunction (C6–T1)
~~Pneumothorax~~ (time course)

I   Inflammation

Aseptic

Gastroesophageal reflux disease

Septic

Gallstones (biliary disease, cholecystitis)
Pancreatitis
Peptic ulcer
~~Pleurisy/empyema~~ (time course)
~~Pneumonia~~ (no recent illness)
Pyelonephritis

M   Metabolic

Cushing's syndrome
Renal calculus

Va   Vascular

Angina:
• Stable angina
• Unstable angina
• Variant angina
~~Myocardial infarction, acute coronary
   insufficiency~~ (time course)

De   Degenerative

Cervical degenerative disk disease

Tu   Tumor

Malignant Primary, such as:
• ~~Esophageal adenocarcinoma~~ (no recent
   illness)

- Gastric adenocarcinoma

- Pancreatic carcinoma
Malignant Metastatic:
Not applicable
Benign:
Not applicable

Co Congenital

Not applicable

Ne Neurogenic/Psychogenic

Anxiety disorder
Hypochondriasis

Local

T Trauma

Compression fracture of rib or scapula
Costovertebral or costotransverse joint
  dysfunction
T4 syndrome
Thoracic facet joint dysfunction
Vertebral fracture/dislocation

I Inflammation

Aseptic

Ankylosing spondylitis

Costochondritis
Delayed-onset muscle soreness

Fibromyalgia
Hepatitis
Myofascial pain disorder

Transverse myelitis

Septic

Discitis
Epidural abscess
Herpes zoster

Meningitis
Tuberculosis of the spine (Pott's disease)

Vertebral osteomyelitis

M Metabolic

Osteomalacia
Osteoporosis
Paget's disease

Va Vascular

Dissecting aortic aneurysm

- ~~Gastric adenocarcinoma~~ (no recent
  illness)
- ~~Pancreatic carcinoma~~ (no recent illness)
Malignant Metastatic:
Not applicable
Benign:
Not applicable

Co Congenital

Not applicable

Ne Neurogenic/Psychogenic

Anxiety disorder
Hypochondriasis

Local

T Trauma

Compression fracture of rib or scapula
Costovertebral or costotransverse joint
  dysfunction
~~T4 syndrome~~ (distribution of symptoms)
Thoracic facet joint dysfunction
Vertebral fracture/dislocation

I Inflammation

Aseptic

~~Ankylosing spondylitis~~ (no relief with
  ibuprofen)
~~Costochondritis~~ (no relief with ibuprofen)
~~Delayed-onset muscle soreness~~ (time
  course of symptoms)
~~Fibromyalgia~~ (pattern of symptoms)
~~Hepatitis~~ (no recent illness)
~~Myofascial pain disorder~~ (pattern of
  symptoms)
~~Transverse myelitis~~ (time course)

Septic

Discitis
Epidural abscess
~~Herpes zoster~~ (distribution of symptoms
  across multiple dermatomes)
~~Meningitis~~ (no recent illness)
~~Tuberculosis of the spine (Pott's disease)~~
  (no recent illness)
~~Vertebral osteomyelitis~~ (no recent illness)

M Metabolic

Osteomalacia
~~Osteoporosis~~ (age)
~~Paget's disease~~ (location of symptoms)

Va Vascular

~~Dissecting aortic aneurysm~~ (time course)

De Degenerative

Thoracic degenerative disk disease
Thoracic osteoarthrosis

Tu Tumor

Malignant Primary, such as:
• Leukemias
• Multiple myeloma
• Primary bone tumors
Malignant Metastatic, such as:
• Metastatic tumors
Benign, such as:
• Neurogenic tumors

• Osteoblastoma
• Osteoid osteoma

Co Congenital

Not applicable

Ne Neurogenic/Psychogenic

Not applicable

De Degenerative

Thoracic degenerative disk disease
Thoracic osteoarthrosis

Tu Tumor

Malignant Primary, such as:
• Leukemias
• Multiple myeloma
• Primary bone tumors
Malignant Metastatic, such as:
• Metastatic tumors
Benign, such as:
• ~~Neurogenic tumors~~ (pattern of
  symptoms)
• ~~Osteoblastoma~~ (age)
• ~~Osteoid osteoma~~ (no ready relief with
  Advil)

Co Congenital

Not applicable

Ne Neurogenic/Psychogenic

Not applicable

STEP #7: Ask specific questions to rule specific conditions or pathological categories less likely.

• Do you have a fever? No.
• Is your pain worsened with moving or exercising? No.
• Do you have a pinkish tinge to your urine? Yes.

Teaching Comments: Questioning of the effect of the gastric system on symptoms may require several follow-up or clarification questions to ensure that if a pattern exists, it can be explored. Clarifying questions may include 24-hour behavior of pain, association with meals and/or mealtimes, alcohol consumption, and diet.

STEP #8: Re-sort the diagnostic hypothesis list based on the patient's responses to specific questioning.

~~**Remote**~~

T Trauma

~~Cervical facet joint dysfunction (C6–T1)~~
(pain unrelated to movement)

I Inflammation

Aseptic

~~Gastroesophageal reflux disease~~ (pain
unrelated to eating)

Septic

~~Gallstones (biliary disease, cholecystitis)~~
(blood in urine)
~~Pancreatitis~~ (blood in urine)
~~Peptic ulcer~~ (blood in urine)
~~Pleurisy/empyema~~ (blood in urine)
~~Pneumonia~~ (blood in urine)
Pyelonephritis

M Metabolic

~~Cushing's syndrome~~ (blood in urine)
Renal calculus

Va Vascular

Angina:
• ~~Stable angina~~ (pain not associated with
  exercising)
• ~~Unstable angina~~ (pain not associated
  with exercising)
• ~~Variant angina~~ (pain not associated with
  exercising)

De Degenerative

~~Cervical degenerative disk disease~~ (pain
unrelated to movement)

Tu Tumor

Malignant Primary:
Not applicable
Malignant Metastatic:
Not applicable
Benign:
Not applicable

Co Congenital

Not applicable

Ne Neurogenic/Psychogenic

Not applicable

Local

T Trauma

~~Compression fracture of rib or scapula~~
(pain unrelated to movement)
~~Costovertebral or costotransverse joint dysfunction~~ (pain unrelated to movement)
~~T4 syndrome~~ (pain unrelated to movement)
~~Thoracic facet joint dysfunction~~ (pain unrelated to movement)
~~Vertebral fracture/dislocation~~ (pain unrelated to movement)

I Inflammation

Aseptic
Not applicable

Septic
~~Discitis~~ (no fevers)
~~Epidural abscess~~ (blood in urine)

M Metabolic
~~Osteomalacia~~ (blood in urine)

Va Vascular
Not applicable

De Degenerative

~~Thoracic degenerative disk disease~~ (less likely as it is not related to motion)
~~Thoracic osteoarthrosis~~ (less likely as it is not related to motion)

Tu Tumor

Malignant Primary, such as:
• ~~Leukemias~~ (no fever)
• ~~Multiple myeloma~~ (no fever)
• ~~Primary bone tumors~~ (no fever)
Malignant Metastatic, such as:
• ~~Metastatic tumors~~ (no fever)
Benign:
Not applicable

Co Congenital

Not applicable

Ne Neurogenic/Psychogenic

Not applicable

STEP #9: Perform tests to differentiate among the remaining diagnostic hypotheses.

• **Percussion over the costovertebral angle.** Positive for reproduction of symptoms, making more likely primary renal pathology.
• **Urinalysis with culture.** Requested from the physician; positive for blood in urine, but negative for bacteria. This finding makes pyelonephritis less likely.

STEP #10: Re-sort the diagnostic hypothesis list based on the patient's responses to specific tests.

I Inflammation

Septic
Pyelonephritis

M Metabolic
Renal calculus

STEP #11: Decide on a diagnostic impression.

A thorough history combined with physical exam techniques such as percussion over the costovertebral angle accurately reflects renal involvement in the presenting symptoms.[1] From the physical therapist's perspective, this cluster of findings is sufficient to suggest that referral to a physician is warranted. Given the range of pathology remaining most likely after history and physical examination, the definitive test to differentiate the remaining pathologies is urinalysis with culture. This test will help differentiate between kidney infection and renal calculus, which then can be appropriately managed by the physician.

STEP #12: Determine the appropriate patient disposition.

• Refer patient to a physician for consultation.

Case Outcome

After excluding infection as a cause of the patient's symptoms, the patient was to follow up with his primary care physician at an appointment 36 hours after intake to physical therapy. While awaiting his appointment, the patient passed the kidney stone and experienced resolution of infrascapular symptoms.

Reference

1. Eskelinen M, Ikonen J, Lipponen P. Usefulness of history-taking, physical examination and diagnostic scoring in acute renal colic. *Eur Urol.* 1998;34(6):467–473.

CHAPTER **18**

Lumbar Pain

Michael A. Andersen, PT, DPT, OCS ■ *J. Raul Lona, DPT, OCS, ATC*

Description of the Symptom

This chapter describes pathology that may lead to lumbar pain, including thoracolumbar pain. **Local causes** of lumbar pain are defined as pathology occurring within anatomical structures posterior to the abdominal aorta. **Remote causes** are defined as originating from structures anterior to and including the abdominal aorta.

Special Concerns

■ Abdominal pulsating mass
■ Bilateral lower extremity pain/numbness or weakness
■ Bowel and bladder changes
■ First episode of back pain in individuals younger than age 20 or older than age 55
■ Pain at rest or at night
■ Previous history of cancer
■ Previous history of prolonged use of steroidal medication, diabetes, human immune deficiency virus, or organ transplant
■ Rapid progression of neurological symptoms
■ Recent significant trauma
■ Saddle anesthesia

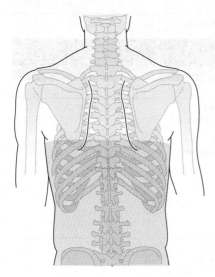

CHAPTER PREVIEW: Conditions That May Lead to Lumbar Pain

T Trauma

REMOTE	LOCAL
COMMON	
Not applicable	Acute lumbar sprain/strain 305
	Disk disruption (with or without disk herniation) 306
	Facet syndrome 307
	Fractures:
	• Burst fracture 307
	• Compression fracture 307
	• Pars interarticularis fracture (spondylolysis) 308
	• Traumatic spondylolisthesis 308
	Myofascial pain (quadratus lumborum syndrome, piriformis syndrome) 308
UNCOMMON	
Not applicable	Not applicable
RARE	
Not applicable	Not applicable

I Inflammation

REMOTE	LOCAL
COMMON	
Aseptic	**Aseptic**
Not applicable	Fibromyalgia 307
Septic	**Septic**
Acute appendicitis 297	Not applicable
Acute cholecystitis 298	
Acute pelvic inflammatory disease 298	
Acute renal or urinary tract disease 298	
Diverticulitis of the colon 299	
Urinary tract infection 303	
UNCOMMON	
Aseptic	**Aseptic**
Not applicable	Abscesses:
	• Epidural abscess 303
Septic	• Paraspinal muscle abscess 304
Acute prostatitis 298	• Psoas muscle abscess 304
Crohn's disease 299	• Subdural abscess 304
Duodenal ulcer 300	Ankylosing spondylitis 305
Herpes zoster 300	Complex regional pain syndrome 306
	Reiter's syndrome 309
	Rheumatoid arthritis of the lumbar spine 310
	Septic
	Meningitis 308

Inflammation *(continued)*

REMOTE	LOCAL
RARE	
Aseptic Not applicable	**Aseptic** Polymyalgia rheumatica 309 Psoriatic arthritis 309
Septic Bacterial endocarditis 299 Pancreatitis 301 Pleuritis 301 Splenic abscess 302	**Septic** Arachnoiditis 305 Septic discitis 310 Spinal osteomyelitis 310 Transverse myelitis 311 Tuberculosis of the spine (Pott's disease) 311

M Metabolic

REMOTE	LOCAL
COMMON	
Not applicable	Not applicable
UNCOMMON	
Ectopic pregnancy 300 Endometriosis 300	Osteoporosis 308 Paget's disease 309
RARE	
Not applicable	Not applicable

Va Vascular

REMOTE	LOCAL
COMMON	
Not applicable	Not applicable
UNCOMMON	
Aortic or iliac aneurysm 298 Aortic or iliac arteriosclerosis 299	Not applicable
RARE	
Infarctions: • Kidney 301 • Spinal cord/conus medullaris 301 • Spleen 301	Arteriovenous malformation of spinal cord 305 Epidural hematoma 306

De Degenerative

REMOTE	LOCAL
COMMON	
Not applicable	Degenerative spondylolisthesis 306 Disk degeneration 306 Spinal stenosis 310
UNCOMMON	
Not applicable	Not applicable

(continued)

Degenerative *(continued)*

REMOTE	LOCAL
RARE	
Not applicable	Not applicable

Tu Tumor

REMOTE	LOCAL
COMMON	
Malignant Primary: Not applicable *Malignant Metastatic:* Not applicable *Benign, such as:* • Uterine fibroids 303	Not applicable
UNCOMMON	
Malignant Primary: Not applicable *Malignant Metastatic:* Not applicable *Benign, such as:* • Ovarian cysts 303	*Malignant Primary:* Not applicable *Malignant Metastatic, such as:* • Metastases, including from primary breast, kidney, lung, prostate, and thyroid disease 311 *Benign:* Not applicable
RARE	
Malignant Primary, such as: • Carcinoma of the colon 302 • Multiple myeloma 302 • Retroperitoneal tumor 303 *Malignant Metastatic, such as:* • Metastases, including from primary breast, kidney, lung, prostate, and thyroid disease 302 *Benign:* Not applicable	*Malignant Primary, such as:* • Primary bone tumor (eg, osteosarcomas, Ewing's sarcoma, fibrosarcoma, and chondrosarcoma) 312 • Spinal cord tumor 312 *Malignant Metastatic:* Not applicable *Benign, such as:* • Intraspinal lipoma 311 • Osteoblastoma 312

Co Congenital

REMOTE	LOCAL
COMMON	
Not applicable	Not applicable
UNCOMMON	
Not applicable	Not applicable
RARE	
Not applicable	Tethered spinal cord 311

(continued)

Ne Neurogenic/Psychogenic	
REMOTE	**LOCAL**
COMMON	
Not applicable	Not applicable
UNCOMMON	
Not applicable	Not applicable
RARE	
Not applicable	Not applicable

Note: These are estimates of relative incidence because few data are available for the less common conditions.

Overview of Lumbar Pain

Lower back and thoracolumbar pain is a major public health concern because it causes significant functional disability, emotional distress, and annual treatment costs. The causes of lower back pain are often difficult to identify. As a result, referral diagnoses from physicians describing lumbar and thoracolumbar pain are often nonspecific. Physical therapists' expertise and the large amount of time they spend with each patient place them in a unique position to provide information to a physician that may lead to a more specific diagnosis. Pertinent information for appropriate medical management may include additional details about the patient's presentation or changes in the patient's status. The purpose of this chapter is to serve as a building block to help clinicians develop a system of differential diagnosis in patients with lumbar and/or thoracolumbar pain.

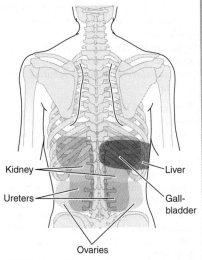

Kidney — — Liver
Ureters — — Gall-
bladder
Ovaries

FIGURE 18-1 Referred pain patterns from abdominal and pelvic viscera.

Description of Conditions That May Lead to Lumbar Pain

Remote

■ Acute Appendicitis

Chief Clinical Characteristics
This presentation can involve pain in the right lower abdominal and lumbar regions with local right iliac and/or lumbar direct tenderness. Reports of vague periumbilical pain followed by anorexia, nausea, and vomiting are common (Fig. 18-1).[1]

Background Information
Other physical findings include mild tachycardia, low-grade fever, hypoactive bowel sounds, and tenderness in the right lower quadrant at McBurney's point.[1] The duration of pain is shorter in individuals with appendicitis than with other disorders. The diagnosis is confirmed with clinical examination or computed tomography scanning. This condition is a medical emergency. Patients presenting to physical therapy with signs and

symptoms of this condition should be referred to the emergency department for immediate treatment.

■ Acute Cholecystitis

Chief Clinical Characteristics

This presentation typically includes back pain associated with abdominal right upper quadrant and/or right infrascapular pain, fever, and signs of local peritoneal irritation including right upper quadrant pain and tenderness (see Fig. 18-1). The characteristic abdominal pain commonly begins after eating a large or fatty meal. Constant pain in the right upper quadrant (>12 hours) and Murphy's sign (inspiration is inhibited by pain on palpation) are used to help diagnose acute cholecystitis.[2] The pain may radiate to the upper and lower back, as well as the right shoulder.[3] Some patients with acute cholecystitis may also report nausea vomiting, fever, and chills.

Background Information

Most patients with chronic cholecystitis will also report a similar previous episode that resolved spontaneously. In 90% of cases, cholecystitis is caused by gallstones that obstruct the neck of the gallbladder or the cystic duct. Other less common causes of cholecystitis include alcoholism, severe illness, and tumors.[4] The diagnosis is confirmed with ultrasound scanning. Individuals with signs of this condition should be referred to the emergency department immediately.

■ Acute Pelvic Inflammatory Disease

Chief Clinical Characteristics

This presentation may include lumbosacral pain associated with dull, constant, and poorly localized abdominal pain (see Fig. 18-1), abnormal vaginal discharge, fever, painful intercourse, and irregular menstrual bleeding.

Background Information

Acute pelvic inflammatory disease is most prevalent in women between 15 and 23 years of age.[5] Bacterial infection in the upper genital tract causes this condition, most commonly associated with gonorrhea and chlamydia. Urinalysis confirms the diagnosis. Treatment includes aggressive antibiotics and

hospitalization. If left untreated, this condition often leads to infertility, ectopic pregnancy, and chronic pelvic pain.[5]

■ Acute Prostatitis

Chief Clinical Characteristics

This presentation may be characterized by pain in the central lower back, rectal, and/or perineal region associated with fever, chills, and painful urination. Other initial symptoms may include malaise, arthralgia, and myalgia. As the disease progresses, prostatic inflammation produces symptoms of dysuria, frequency, urgency, and urine retention.

Background Information

Prostatitis is usually caused by a bacterial infection in the prostate gland. Prostatitis commonly accompanies or follows a urinary tract infection, urethritis, or epididymitis.[6] The diagnosis is confirmed by urinalysis. Treatment usually includes intravenous antibiotics, which are specific to the infective agent.

■ Acute Renal or Urinary Tract Disease

Chief Clinical Characteristics

This presentation includes pain in the central lower back (see Fig. 18-1), flank, and groin, associated with fever, nausea, and vomiting. Other common symptoms include urgent, frequent, and painful urination, abdominal bloating, and pain upon palpation of the kidney.[6]

Background Information

Renal or urinary tract disease may follow streptococcal infection of the upper respiratory tract or skin within 8 to 21 days. Blood and urine tests are necessary for a definitive diagnosis. Treatment typically includes an appropriate antibiotic, and hospitalization for monitoring.

■ Aortic or Iliac Aneurysm

Chief Clinical Characteristics

This presentation typically involves vague abdominal pain, usually located in the epigastrium that may radiate to the low back, flank, or groin.[7] Other symptoms include early satiety, nausea, vomiting, gastrointestinal bleeding, and lower extremity ischemia.[7]

Background Information

Sixty-six to 75% of abdominal aortic aneurysms are asymptomatic. This condition can be diagnosed during a routine physical examination by palpation of a pulsatile abdominal mass above the umbilicus in the epigastrium.[7] Patients are considered for elective repair of aneurysm when the risk of rupture exceeds the risk of surgery, which is typically an open repair for the aneurysm.[7]

■ Aortic or Iliac Arteriosclerosis

Chief Clinical Characteristics

This presentation may involve generalized low back pain and symptoms consistent with lumbar disk degeneration.[8]

Background Information

Studies have correlated the occurrence of aortic arteriosclerosis and disk degeneration.[8,9] The first to fourth lumbar arteries leave the aorta in front of the corresponding vertebral body supplying that vertebra and the adjacent intervertebral disk via diffusion through the vertebral end plate.[8] Findings suggest that calcific lesions in the upper part of the abdominal aorta predict disk deterioration at any lumbar level.[8] The link between arteriosclerosis and low back pain can be explained by the common risk factors between the two pathologies, including age and smoking. The diagnosis is confirmed with radiographs or computed tomography. Surgical techniques for treatment of occlusive disease of the artery include endovascular stented-graft treatment.[10]

■ Bacterial Endocarditis

Chief Clinical Characteristics

This presentation may include generalized arthralgia in large proximal joints, low back pain, neck pain, and myalgia in the presence of fever, chills, weight loss, and weakness.[11] Musculoskeletal symptoms present early during the course of the disease.

Background Information

This condition is an infectious disease of the endothelial lining of the heart and/or valves. As the pathology progresses clinical symptoms will include chest pain, dyspnea, and edema, which if left untreated will lead to heart failure.[6] Early diagnosis is confirmed by blood culture and is crucial in order to prevent the cardiac sequelae that occur. Treatment may include hospitalization with specific intravenous bactericidal antibiotics.[6]

■ Crohn's Disease

Chief Clinical Characteristics

This presentation can involve abdominal pain, bowel obstruction, weight loss, fever, chronic or nocturnal diarrhea, or night sweats.[12]

Background Information

Symptoms of back pain occur in up to 20% of bowel-related spondyloarthropathies.[13] Crampy, intermittent abdominal right lower quadrant pain is common in patients with ileal Crohn's disease and is exacerbated by eating. Arthralgia and arthritis may also be associated with this condition. The arthritis usually affects the lower extremities in an asymmetrical fashion and has a migratory pattern.[13] The diagnosis is confirmed with endoscopy. Depending on the severity of the pathology, medical management includes use of salicylates, corticosteroids, antibiotics, and immunosuppressants.[12]

■ Diverticulitis of the Colon

Chief Clinical Characteristics

This presentation typically includes left lower quadrant tenderness.[14,15] Back pain can be a clinical symptom, representing the varied disposition of the sigmoid colon. Signs of localized peritoneal inflammation including involuntary guarding, localized percussion tenderness, and fever may also be present.[14] Anorexia, nausea, and vomiting may occur as well as dysuria and urinary frequency due to an irritated bladder from the sigmoid colon.[15]

Background Information

A palpable, tender cylindrical mass may be present with guarding and rebound tenderness.[15] This condition is caused by fecal material that becomes lodged in the diverticulum.[14,15] The diagnosis is confirmed with colonoscopy. Minimal symptoms are treated by placing the patient on a clear liquid diet for 7 to 10 days. Patients with signs of more significant diverticulitis are typically hospitalized for bowel rest, intravenous fluids, and broad-spectrum intravenous antibiotics.[14,15] Elective surgery is recommended following a recurrent episode because the chance for a third episode is greater than 50%.[14]

■ Duodenal Ulcer

Chief Clinical Characteristics

This presentation involves midline thoracolumbar pain with or without abdominal epigastric pain (see Fig. 18-1). Symptoms are typically episodic, lasting for weeks or months at a time before resolution.[16] Pain associated with this condition is usually absent in the morning, but occurs 1 to 3 hours after meals. This symptom is usually relieved by the ingestion of food or antacids.

Background Information

There are no specific physical findings but an individual with a duodenal ulcer may present with epigastric tenderness or fecal occult blood.[16] *Helicobacter pylori* and use of nonsteroidal anti-inflammatory medications are two major causes of ulcers.[16,17] The diagnosis is confirmed by endoscopy. Treatment of duodenal ulcers includes the use of medications to neutralize gastric acids resulting in up to 80% to 90% ulcer healing.[18] Standard medical therapy also includes the use of antibiotics designed to eradicate *H. pylori* colonization.[18] Patients who exhibit acute duodenal ulcer perforation or other complication may require surgical management.

■ Ectopic Pregnancy

Chief Clinical Characteristics

This presentation can be characterized by pelvic pain and abdominal pain with spotting that occurs 6 to 8 weeks following last normal menstrual period. Sharp, stabbing low-back pain with possible pain referral to the shoulder or neck may be another indication of this condition.

Background Information

Other physical findings can include an enlarged uterus, a palpable adnexal mass, abdominal tenderness with guarding, and rebound tenderness. There are numerous risk factors for this condition, including pelvic inflammatory disease, previous ectopic pregnancy, and endometriosis. The reported incidence of this condition is approximately 19.7 cases per 1,000 pregnancies, and it is detected more often in females over 35 years of age.[19] The diagnosis is confirmed with abdominal or transvaginal ultrasonography. Although most ectopic pregnancies (68% to 77%) will resolve without intervention, treatment may include medication and surgical intervention if necessary.[19]

■ Endometriosis

Chief Clinical Characteristics

This presentation may include dysmenorrhea, dyspareunia, and low back pain that worsens with menses.[20] Rectal pain and painful defecation can also be present.[20]

Background Information

This condition is the presence of tissues that are histologically similar to endometrium at sites outside the endometrial cavity. Causes include retrograde menstruation and peritoneal epithelium transformation to endometrial tissue, as well as possible genetic causes.[20] Pelvic ultrasonography, computed tomography, magnetic resonance imaging, and laparoscopy are commonly used to confirm the diagnosis.[20] Treatment in cases of women with few symptoms can include oral contraceptives or progestins for pain relief.[20] Surgery may be required in more advanced stages to remove endometrial lesions.[20]

■ Herpes Zoster

Chief Clinical Characteristics

This presentation may involve an exquisitely painful rash or blisters along a specific dermatomal pattern of the lumbar region accompanied by flu-like symptoms.

Background Information

Individuals with this condition also demonstrate a previous history of varicella exposure or infection. The virus remains dormant in the spinal ganglia until its reactivation during a period of stress, infection, or physical exhaustion. Pain associated with this condition may be disproportionate to the extent of skin irritation. The initial presentation of this condition may be confused with radiculopathy due to the distribution of symptoms. The presence of the rash, extreme pain, general malaise, and an unclear association with spinal movement aid in differential diagnosis. Treatment includes the administration of antiviral agents as soon as the zoster eruption is noted, ideally within 48 to 72 hours. If timing is greater than 3 days, treatment is aimed at controlling pain and pruritus and minimizing the risk of secondary infection.[21]

INFARCTIONS

■ Kidney

Chief Clinical Characteristics
This presentation typically involves persistent low back, abdominal, and flank pain (see Fig. 18-1).[22] Accompanying nausea and vomiting are common as well.

Background Information
Diagnosis is often delayed or missed due to its nonspecific clinical presentation.[22] Clinical diagnosis is typically made based on these nonspecific clinical findings and patients with an increased risk for thromboembolism.[22] Risk factors for renal infarction include atrial fibrillation, previous embolism, and valvular or ischemic heart disease.[22] The diagnosis is confirmed with contrast-enhanced computed tomography. Treatment involves thrombolysis, anticoagulation, or embolectomy.[22]

■ Spinal Cord/Conus Medullaris

Chief Clinical Characteristics
This presentation can involve neurological symptoms depending on the artery involved and the level of the infarction.[23] Initial symptoms can include lower thoracic and lumbar pain.

Background Information
Spinal infarction is typically located in the anterior spinal artery area.[23] Neurological symptoms can include para- or tetraparesis, bladder dysfunction, and pain and temperature loss below the level of infarction in cases of anterior spinal artery involvement.[23] The diagnosis is confirmed with magnetic resonance imaging. Treatment is usually palliative, with rehabilitation necessary to recover function and strength after paralysis.

■ Spleen

Chief Clinical Characteristics
This presentation typically includes a sudden onset of pain in the left upper abdomen, flank, and shoulder (see Fig. 18-1).[24] Pain is typically sharp and increased by deep respiration or jarring.

Background Information
Common physical findings include fever and left pleural effusion. Splenic artery occlusion due to torsion, tumor invasion, compression, thrombosis, or thromboembolism causes this condition.[24] Infarction of the spleen frequently occurs in patients with myeloproliferative disorders, endocarditis, and sickle cell anemia.[24] The diagnosis is confirmed with ultrasonography. There is a high self-healing tendency in acute splenic infarction.[24]

■ Pancreatitis

Chief Clinical Characteristics
This presentation may include central low back pain occurring with pain in the middle to left upper abdominal quadrant that is worse after eating (see Fig. 18-1).

Background Information
Pain associated with pancreatitis also may be exacerbated by supine positions and alleviated by flexing forward or assuming a fetal position.[6] Nausea and vomiting may also be associated with this condition. This condition may be painless. It commonly is associated with diabetes mellitus, weight loss and nutritional insufficiencies, anemia, and jaundice. Major causes include chronic alcohol abuse and cholelithiasis. The diagnosis is confirmed with pancreas function lab tests followed by computed tomography if necessary. Treatment is usually supportive and includes fluid resuscitation, oxygen supplementation, and pain control.

■ Pleuritis

Chief Clinical Characteristics
This presentation can be characterized by bilateral lower back pain in association with chest or bilateral shoulder pain (see Fig. 18-1). It can be worsened by deep inspiration.

Background Information
This condition arises from multiple etiologies. Fever in the presence of chest pain is suggestive of active pneumonia. Weight loss and malaise in the presence of chest pain may be suggestive of a malignancy or tuberculosis. Severe cases also may lead to pulmonary compromise, resulting in a cough or dyspnea.[6] Auscultation of the chest wall will reveal a pleural friction rub, which is a constant grating sound during inspiration and expiration. The diagnosis is confirmed with

chest plain radiographs or ultrasonography. Treatment is directed toward the underlying cause.

■ Splenic Abscess

Chief Clinical Characteristics
This presentation can include generalized abdominal pain, left upper quadrant tenderness, and fever.[25],[26] Other less common symptoms include left-sided chest pain, left shoulder pain, and generalized weakness.[26]

Background Information
Pain can also be reported at the base of the left thorax.[26] This condition usually is observed in individuals with underlying disorders including infection, emboli, trauma, recent surgery, malignant hematologic conditions, and immunosuppression. The diagnosis is confirmed with abdominal ultrasound and computed tomography. Treatment may involve the use of appropriate antibiotics followed by splenectomy in all patients who are reasonable anesthetic risks.[25] Percutaneous drainage guided by computed tomography also has gained favor as a viable first-line treatment option with success rates ranging between 51% and 72%.[27]

TUMORS

■ Carcinoma of the Colon

Chief Clinical Characteristics
This presentation includes abdominal pain, as well as tenderness and infrequent distention of the lower abdomen. Leakage from a perforated carcinoma can cause pain in the left lumbar and iliac region (see Fig. 18-1).[6] Most cases of early colon cancer are asymptomatic; however, patients displaying the following symptoms may lead the clinician to suspect colon cancer: change in bowel habits (diarrhea or constipation), rectal bleeding or blood in the stool, unexplained anemia, unexplained weight loss, and stools narrower than usual.

Background Information
Digital rectal examination may reveal a mass if the malignancy is in the rectum. Carcinomas of the colon arise from the lining of the large intestine as polyps, which over a period of several years develop into cancer. Definitive diagnosis of colon cancer is made with a sigmoidoscopy or colonoscopy. Treatment depends on the stage of the cancer and may include surgical resection and colostomy, chemotherapy, and radiation.[6]

■ Metastases, Including From Primary Breast, Kidney, Lung, Prostate, and Thyroid Disease

Chief Clinical Characteristics
This presentation can include unremitting low back pain due to referral from abdominal sites of metastases. The four clinical findings with the highest likelihood ratios for predicting cancer are a previous history of cancer, age 50 years or older, failure to improve with conservative therapy, and unexplained weight loss of more than 10 pounds in 6 months.

Background Information
Radiotherapy is the most common treatment for metastases, with surgical decompression and stabilization required if spinal instability or neurological compromise exists[28],[29] or if the tumor is relatively radioresistant.[29]

■ Multiple Myeloma

Chief Clinical Characteristics
This presentation typically involves low back pain, dermatomal sensation loss, and possible weakness and numbness of the lower extremities.[30]

Background Information
Presentation is typically insidious and nonspecific. Approximately two-thirds of patients present with back[30–32] and/or rib pain that is exacerbated by movement.[30] Weakness and fatigue are also common.[30] Pathological fracture is the presenting feature in approximately 30% of cases.[31] A high index of suspicion should be assigned to individuals with low back pain who are over 50 years of age and have pain that is worse in the supine position, occurs at night or awakens patient, is located in a band-like distribution around the body, is unrelieved with conventional methods, and is associated with constitutional symptoms or progressive neurological deficits.[31] Diagnostic tests include serum and urine immunoelectrophoresis.[30]

Radiographic findings include classic punched-out lesions of the skull and long bones with diffuse osteopenia and vertebral compression fractures.[30,31]

■ Ovarian Cysts

Chief Clinical Characteristics

This presentation includes ipsilateral pain in the lumbar and thigh regions and lower quadrant of the abdomen, with possible nausea and vomiting, abnormal vaginal bleeding, and difficulty urinating completely (see Fig. 18-1).

Background Information

Ovarian cysts are fluid-filled sacs that develop adjacent to the ovary in the fallopian tube. Most cysts are asymptomatic remnants of normal ovulation.[33] Enlarged cysts may lead to torsion or distention of the fallopian tube. The diagnosis is confirmed with clinical pelvic examination and pelvic ultrasound. Prescribed hormones may be utilized to shrink the cyst. If the cysts persists or symptoms progress, laparoscopic examination is required and surgical removal may be indicated.[6]

■ Retroperitoneal Tumor

Chief Clinical Characteristics

This presentation typically includes abdominal pain with radiation into the flank or lumbar region, groin, and anterior thighs.[34] If the tumor extends into the spinal canal, radiating pain and numbness into the lower extremities may also be present.[35]

Background Information

Retroperitoneal masses also may present as cysts, or benign versus malignant tumors. If the tumor is malignant, symptoms may be associated with malaise, weight loss, and night pain. Retroperitoneal tumors often reach a large size and may be palpable over the abdominal cavity or compress other vital structures. The diagnosis is confirmed with abdominal computed tomography or magnetic resonance imaging. Treatment includes aggressive and complete laparoscopic removal of the tumor.

■ Uterine Fibroids

Chief Clinical Characteristics

This presentation may include pelvic pain and pressure, with possible neurogenic pain in the thighs and lower legs due to impingement of the lumbosacral plexus (see Fig. 18-1). Symptoms and signs also may include abdominal distention, palpable evidence of a pelvic mass, heavy prolonged menstrual cycles, bladder pressure leading to constant urinary urgency, and constipation or bloating due to pressure on the bowels.[36]

Background Information

These are common benign tumors that develop in the muscular walls of the uterus. First detection usually occurs during routine gynecological examination because most are asymptomatic. Abdominal ultrasound confirms the diagnosis. If the fibroids are large enough to cause significant symptoms, treatment options will include surgical embolization or resection (myomectomy), as well as hysterectomy in severe cases.[36]

■ Urinary Tract Infection

Chief Clinical Characteristics

This presentation can involve dysuria, frequency, hematuria, and back pain (see Fig. 18-1). These symptoms significantly increase the probability of an individual having this condition.[37]

Background Information

Acute cases account for 7 million office visits annually in the United States and can affect half of all women at least once during their lifetime.[37] Three well-established risk factors for this condition in young women are recent sexual intercourse, use of spermicide during sexual intercourse, and previous history.[37] A urine culture is the most common diagnostic tool for all types of this condition. Treatment typically involves an oral antibiotic medication directed against the infective agent.

Local

ABSCESSES

■ Epidural Abscess

Chief Clinical Characteristics

This presentation typically includes fever and malaise and is associated with local low back pain and tenderness, with or without neurological deficits.[38,39]

Background Information

Pain is the most consistent symptom and occurs in virtually all patients presenting with a spinal epidural abscess. Neurological deficits may be due to cord and nerve root compression from the extradural mass within the spinal canal.[38] Compromise of the spinal cord vasculature is thought to be the cause of neurological compromise rather than direct compression. Posterior abscesses originate from a distant area, such as a skin infection, pharyngitis, or dental abscess.[38,40] Anterior epidural abscesses are associated with discitis or vertebral osteomyelitis.[38] Predisposing factors include a compromised immune system as in patients with diabetes mellitus, acquired immune deficiency syndrome, chronic renal failure, alcoholism, or cancer, or following epidural anesthesia, spinal surgery, or trauma.[38] Leukocytosis may be the only abnormal laboratory value.[38,39] The diagnosis is confirmed with magnetic resonance imaging. Surgical decompression with a follow-on course of antibiotic medication comprises the primary treatment for spinal epidural abscess.

■ Paraspinal Muscle Abscess

Chief Clinical Characteristics

This presentation can involve severe progressive back pain, hip pain, and possible neurological symptoms following progress of the infecting mass causing spinal cord compromise.[41]

Background Information

Regional lumbar soft tissue swelling, or fluctuance, may be palpated in association with increased regional temperature. Case reports in the literature of paraspinal abscesses have been shown following lumbar injections, such as epidural anesthesia for women in labor.[41] This condition is associated with the possibility of systemic infection, so urgent referral to a physician is necessary if this condition is suspected. Magnetic resonance imaging has been supported as the method of choice for confirming the diagnosis.[41] Treatment includes surgically guided drainage and irrigation followed by appropriate antibiotic treatment.

■ Psoas Muscle Abscess

Chief Clinical Characteristics

This presentation involves fever, lateral lumbar or abdominal pain, and limp. The classical triad of symptoms (ie, fever, back pain, and limping) is present in approximately 30% of patients with a psoas abscess.[42] Other symptoms include malaise, weight loss, or presentation with a mass. Physical findings include an externally rotated hip, flank tenderness, and fullness in the lateral lumbar region.

Background Information

Psoas abscesses may be primary, due to hematogenous spread, or secondary due to such pathologies as Crohn's disease, appendicitis, diverticulitis, ulcerative colitis, osteomyelitis, neoplasm, disk infection, renal infections, and trauma.[42,43] Computed tomography of the abdomen with contrast is the most effective imaging study to confirm the diagnosis. Treatment usually begins with a course of antibiotics, with surgical or radiologically guided percutaneous drainage essential to effective treatment.[42,43]

■ Subdural Abscess

Chief Clinical Characteristics

This presentation may be characterized by fever, pain over the involved segment(s), progressive neurological weakness, and numbness in the lower extremities. Depending on the severity of neural compression, fecal and urinary incontinence may be present.[44]

Background Information

These symptoms appear in stages with an unpredictable rate of progression. The first stage is fever with or without spinal pain; the second stage consists of neurological symptoms such as motor deficits, sensory loss, and sphincter dysfunction; and the third is paralysis and complete sensory loss.[44] This condition results from the spread of a distant or local infection, most commonly *Staphylococcus aureus*, following a neurosurgical procedure or spinal puncture. Diagnosis is confirmed with magnetic resonance imaging.[3] Due to its potentially devastating consequences, this condition is treated with immediate surgical decompression, drainage, and follow-up with the appropriate antibiotics.[3]

■ Acute Lumbar Sprain/Strain

Chief Clinical Characteristics

This presentation involves pain, muscle spasm, edema, and increased temperature of the local tissues. Pain may radiate into the buttocks and rarely into the thighs or lower legs.

Background Information

Pain may increase with extension (contraction) or flexion (stretch). Sprains are limited to ligaments, and strains affect muscle-tendon units. This condition often is caused by excessive physical demands on the back, including repetitive lifting, excessive flexion, extension, or rotation movements with or without load.[45] The diagnosis is confirmed with clinical examination. Treatment generally involves nonsurgical interventions, such as lumbar mobilization and manipulation, trunk and proximal lower extremity exercises, activity modification, and physical modalities.

■ Ankylosing Spondylitis

Chief Clinical Characteristics

This presentation may involve an insidious onset of low back and symmetric posterior hip pain associated with a slowly progressive and significant loss of general spinal mobility.

Background Information

Symptoms may be worse in the morning and improve with light exercise. This condition is more common in males, as well as people of American indigenous descent, less than 40 years of age, or who carry the human leukocyte antigen B27. It also may be associated with fever, malaise, and inflammatory bowel disease. The diagnosis is confirmed with plain radiographs of the sacroiliac joints and lumbar spine, which reveal characteristic findings of sacroiliitis and "bamboo spine." Blood panels including erythrocyte sedimentation rate are useful to track disease activity. Treatment typically includes a combination of steroidal, nonsteroidal, and biological anti-inflammatory medications combined with physical therapy to address postural and movement considerations associated with changing spinal position.

■ Arachnoiditis

Chief Clinical Characteristics

This presentation typically includes severe lower back or thoracic pain, depending on the location of the spine that is affected. Pain usually is described as burning and stinging, and can be very debilitating in nature. Symptoms of this condition also may include bilateral asymmetric radiating lower leg pain and accompanying neurological symptoms such as numbness and tingling (sciatica).

Background Information

This condition is caused by an inflammation of the arachnoid layer of the central nervous system due to trauma during surgery, lumbar punctures during epidural anesthesia, chemicals such as myelographic contrast dye, and infection.[46] This inflammation causes constant irritation, scarring, and binding of nerve roots and blood vessels.[3] The disease can progress to cause bowel/bladder dysfunctions, sexual dysfunction, and spinal cord cysts. The diagnosis is confirmed with computed tomography, magnetic resonance imaging, and/or myelograms. There is no cure for this condition. Treatments are often aimed at controlling the severe pain that results and include transcutaneous electrical nerve stimulation, steroidal/nonsteroidal pain medications, antispasmodic medications, and spinal cord stimulators.

■ Arteriovenous Malformation of Spinal Cord

Chief Clinical Characteristics

This presentation involves back pain, progressive paraparesis, paresthesias of the lower extremities, and possible urinary incontinence.

Background Information

This condition is divided into dural arteriovenous fistulas and intradural medullary spinal cord angiomas.[47] Intradural arteriovenous malformations are seen in patients less than 30 years old with acute onset of symptoms, subarachnoid hemorrhage, a spinal bruit, and symptoms affecting the arms. Patients with dural arteriovenous malformations are usually greater than 40 years of age, have gradual onset and progressive worsening of symptoms, experience exacerbation of symptoms by a change in posture or activity, and the lesions are always in the lower half of the spinal cord, affecting the legs.[48] Magnetic resonance imaging is typically used to search for vascular abnormalities of the spinal cord with gadolinium increasing the sensitivity of the detection of arteriovenous malformation.[47] Embolization using microcatheters has been suggested as a primary treatment especially for dural fistulas.[47,49]

■ Complex Regional Pain Syndrome

Chief Clinical Characteristics

This presentation may include a traumatic onset of severe chronic lower back pain accompanied by allodynia, hyperalgesia, as well as trophic, vasomotor, and sudomotor changes in later stages.

Background Information

This condition is characterized by disproportionate responses to painful stimuli. It is a regional neuropathic pain disorder that presents either without direct nerve trauma (Type I) or with direct nerve trauma (Type II) in any region of the body.[50] This condition may precipitate due to an event distant to the affected area. Thermography may confirm associated sympathetic dysfunction. Treatment may include physical therapy interventions to improve patient and client functioning, biofeedback, analgesic or anti-inflammatory medication, transcutaneous or spinal electrical nerve stimulation, and surgical or pharmacologic sympathectomy.

■ Degenerative Spondylolisthesis

Chief Clinical Characteristics

This presentation involves low back pain with concurrent symptoms of spinal stenosis, involving unilateral or bilateral hip or lower extremity pain, and chronic nerve root compression.

Background Information

Degenerative spondylolisthesis is the result of prolonged instability of the spinal motion segment. Spondylolisthesis can be caused by facet joint dysplasia, elongation or fracture of the pars interarticularis, degeneration and secondary instability of the facet joints, trauma, or pathologies including bone tumor, osteogenesis imperfecta, or primary bone disorders.[51] Plain radiographs confirm the diagnosis. Nonsurgical treatment is a common first approach. Surgical treatment typically includes discectomy or spinal fusion for individuals with progressive neurological symptoms.[52]

■ Disk Degeneration

Chief Clinical Characteristics

This presentation can be characterized by an individual's report of low back pain with possible radiation to the hips, with or without neurological symptoms.

Background Information

Disk degeneration can alter disk height leading to symptoms of sciatica or neurological compression, change the mechanics of the spinal column affecting spinal muscles and ligaments, and limit lumbar range of motion. The incidence of disk degeneration increases sharply with age. Failure of the nutrient supply to the disk, abnormal mechanical loading of the disks, and genetic factors have been implicated.[52] Magnetic resonance imaging confirms the diagnosis. Nonsurgical treatment is a common initial approach. Surgical treatment typically includes discectomy or spinal fusion for individuals with progressive neurological symptoms.[52]

■ Disk Disruption (With or Without Disk Herniation)

Chief Clinical Characteristics

This presentation involves an individual's reports of pain deep in the lumbar region with occasional buttock pain. Usually symptoms are preceded by a traumatic event such as lifting a heavy object or other forceful movement. Pain is aggravated with lumbar rotation, flexion, and side-bending, and sitting tolerance is typically diminished.

Background Information

Individuals with true internal disk disruption lack symptoms of radiculopathy; when present, leg pain follows a nondermatomal pattern.[53] Magnetic resonance imaging and discography confirm the diagnosis. Nonsurgical treatment is a common first approach. Surgical treatment typically includes discectomy or spinal fusion for individuals with progressive neurological symptoms.[52]

■ Epidural Hematoma

Chief Clinical Characteristics

This presentation may involve the acute onset of back (or neck) pain followed by rapidly progressive sensory and/or motor deficits. Less frequently, this condition is associated with slowly progressive, chronic or relapsing symptoms or with neurological signs and symptoms that mimic an acute intervertebral disk prolapse.[54]

Background Information

Epidural bleeding could be the result of a ruptured epidural vein caused by either a sudden increase in intra-abdominal pressure or by mild trauma. This condition is confirmed with magnetic resonance imaging. It is a medical emergency, so individuals suspected of this condition should be referred to an emergency department immediately.[54]

■ Facet Syndrome

Chief Clinical Characteristics

This presentation includes pain in the lumbar region with referral to the buttocks and upper thigh. The majority of pain referral for the L1–L2 through L4–L5 joints includes the lumbar spinal region. Other referral areas include the gluteal region (L3–L4 to L5–S1), the lateral upper thigh (L2–L3 to L5–S1), and the posterior thigh (L2–L3 to L5–S1).[55]

Background Information

Causes of facet-mediated pain include systemic inflammatory arthritidies, microtrauma, and osteoarthritis. The etiology of this condition may include meniscoid entrapment, synovial impingement, joint subluxation, chondromalacia facetiae, capsular and synovial inflammation, mechanical injury to the joint capsule, and restriction of normal articular motion.[56] This diagnosis is confirmed by controlled diagnostic blocks of the joint or its nerve supply.[56] Nonsurgical treatment is a common initial approach to management of this condition

■ Fibromyalgia

Chief Clinical Characteristics

This presentation involves chronic widespread joint and muscle pain defined as bilateral upper body, lower body, and spine pain, associated with tenderness to palpating 11 of 18 specific muscle-tendon sites.

Background Information

Individuals with this condition will demonstrate lowered mechanical and thermal pain thresholds, high pain ratings for noxious stimuli, and altered temporal summation of pain stimuli.[57] The etiology of this condition is unclear; multiple body systems appear to be involved. Indistinct clinical boundaries between this condition and similar conditions (eg, chronic fatigue syndrome, irritable bowel syndrome, and chronic muscular headaches) pose a diagnostic challenge.[57] This condition is diagnosed by exclusion. Treatment will often include polypharmacy and elements to improve self-efficacy, physical training, and cognitive-behavioral techniques.[58]

FRACTURES

■ Burst Fracture

Chief Clinical Characteristics

This presentation typically involves severe debilitating low back pain and, depending on the extent of the injury, neurological symptoms, including complete paralysis and loss of bowel and bladder control.

Background Information

Most burst fractures result from high-energy axial trauma (eg, motor vehicle accidents and falls), although pathological burst fractures could result from bone tumors.[59] Burst fractures are most common in the thoracolumbar region of the spine and involve damage to the anterior and middle columns of the body of a spinal vertebra. This injury is confirmed with plain radiographs of the spine, and is considered a medical emergency.

■ Compression Fracture

Chief Clinical Characteristics

This presentation of can involve severe debilitating low back pain, which usually worsens with walking, as well as other potential sequelae of secondary symptoms.[60]

Background Information

Radiating pain into the leg is highly unlikely with vertebral compression fractures.[3] This condition usually is associated with osteoporotic changes within the vertebral body, usually in the lower thoracic and upper lumbar spine. The loss of vertebral height may lead to reduction in abdominal space with associated loss of appetite and secondary sequelae related to poor nutrition. Most notably, this condition leads to chronic pain with an associated loss of sleep, decreased

LUMBAR PAIN

mobility, and depression.[60] The diagnosis is confirmed with plain radiographs of the spine. Treatment usually includes rest, narcotic analgesics, and spinal orthoses.[60]

Pars Interarticularis Fracture (Spondylolysis)

Chief Clinical Characteristics

This presentation may involve low back pain following severe trauma with possible radiation to the thigh depending on affected level, neurological deficits, and cauda equina syndrome.[61] Symptoms may begin following an acute injury or gradually after an initiating event. The neurological examination should be normal.

Background Information

This condition may lead to spondylolisthesis, which involves local tenderness, swelling, and a palpable step-off between L5 and S1. Radiographic findings can include dislocated and locked facets with the inferior facets of L5 anterior to the S1 facets. This condition is considered rare and may occur following extreme hyperflexion, axial rotation, and application of compression forces. Indications for surgical interventions, including decompressive laminectomy and fusion, include progressive segmental instability, intractable pain, and development of neurological deficits.[62,63]

Traumatic Spondylolisthesis

Chief Clinical Characteristics

This presentation can be characterized by low back pain following severe trauma with possible radiation to the thigh depending on affected level, neurological deficits, and cauda equina syndrome.[61]

Background Information

Local tenderness, swelling, and a palpable step-off between L5 and S1 are also reported. Radiographic findings for diagnosis can include dislocated and locked facets with the inferior facets of L5 anterior to the S1 facets. Traumatic spondylolisthesis is considered rare and may occur following extreme hyperflexion, axial rotation, and application of compression forces. Surgical treatment may be warranted due to the frank instability of the injury.[61]

Meningitis

Chief Clinical Characteristics

This presentation may involve high body temperature, poor feeding, vomiting, lethargy, and irritability. The infection can also present as a meningoradiculitis with its initial presentation as low back pain.[64] More classical signs also can include neck stiffness, headache, and photophobia as well as signs of nuchal stiffness.

Background Information

Progression of this presentation can include neurological signs such as weakness and loss of reflexes.[64] This condition occurs when an organism crosses the blood-brain barrier and becomes isolated from the immune system. It can occur following lumbar punctures as a diagnostic tool or for spinal anesthesia for pelvic and intra-abdominal surgery,[65] following corticosteroid injections, and after diagnostic myelograms.[65] The diagnosis is confirmed with magnetic resonance imaging, blood serum level, and cerebrospinal fluid culture. Treatment of meningitis includes antibiotics directed against the causative agent with treatment time depending on the offending agent as well (10 to 21 days).[66]

Myofascial Pain (Quadratus Lumborum Syndrome, Piriformis Syndrome)

Chief Clinical Characteristics

This presentation typically includes low back pain with reports of a regional, persistent pain with the presence of one of more trigger points.

Background Information

Trigger points within the iliocostalis lumborum, longissimus thoracis, multifidus, quadratus lumborum, gluteus medius, and piriformis have been implicated. Trigger points typically include localized tenderness, referred pain, a taut, palpable band in the muscle, and limited stretch range of motion.[67] Clinical examination confirms the diagnosis. Common initial nonsurgical interventions include physical therapy to improve patient functioning and also injections.

Osteoporosis

Chief Clinical Characteristics

This presentation includes midline spinal pain and deformity over the involved thoracolumbar spinal segments. Radiating leg pain or radicular symptoms are very uncommon.

Background Information
Symptoms relate to fractures of the hip and vertebrae. Vertebral compression fractures result from the collapse of columns within the vertebral bodies. This condition is a disease of decreased bone mass density, in which bone resorption exceeds bone formation. Dual-energy x-ray absorptiometry confirms the diagnosis.[3] Treatment of osteoporosis is geared toward prevention of future bone loss in younger women. Women postmenopause can be treated with hormone replacement therapy to slow the rate of bone loss.[68]

■ Paget's Disease

Chief Clinical Characteristics
This presentation is characterized by deep, aching pain that is worse at night and associated with fatigue, headaches, hearing loss, and likely a pronounced kyphosis.

Background Information
Men are affected more than women in a 3:2 ratio. Long bone deformities occur and lead to adjacent joint osteoarthrosis. Bones of the pelvis, lumbar spine, sacrum, thoracic spine, and ribs also are commonly affected by deformity. Vertebral collapse may occur in the thoracic region and compression neuropathies may be identified. Deformities are a result of haphazard resorption of bone that then fills in with fibrous tissue. Subsequent attempts to form bone lead to large, less compact, more vascular bone susceptible to fracture. This condition is the second-most common skeletal disorder. Its incidence increases by age 50 with peak incidence after 70 years of age. The diagnosis of this condition is based on an elevated serum alkaline phosphatase in patients with x-ray findings of osteosclerosis, osteolysis, and bone expansion.[69] Treatment includes the use of osteoclast-inhibiting and antiresorptive medications.[69]

■ Polymyalgia Rheumatica

Chief Clinical Characteristics
This presentation typically includes the acute onset of proximal myalgias and stiffness involving the neck, shoulders, pelvic girdle, and hips that is worse at night and with movement and associated with fatigue, weight loss, fever, and sweats.

Background Information
Pelvic girdle involvement usually causes pain that radiates to the knee.[70] Diagnosis is confirmed with blood panels that demonstrate an elevated erythrocyte sedimentation rate.[70] This condition is associated with temporal arteritis, which can cause blindness if untreated, so urgent referral to a physician is necessary if this condition is suspected. Treatment of this condition mainly includes the use of low-dose oral prednisone in the morning.[70,71]

■ Psoriatic Arthritis

Chief Clinical Characteristics
This presentation can be characterized by an insidious onset of spinal pain associated with psoriasis. Pitting nail lesions occur in 80% of individuals with this condition. Dactylitis, tenosynovitis, and peripheral arthritis also are common.

Background Information
The severity of arthritis is uncorrelated with the extent of skin involvement.[13] Radiographs of the distal phalanges may reveal a characteristic "pencil and cup" deformity. Blood panels including erythrocyte sedimentation rate are useful to track disease activity. Psoriatic arthritis is treated using patient education, nonsteroidal anti-inflammatory medications, and disease-modifying drugs.[13,72]

■ Reiter's Syndrome

Chief Clinical Characteristics
This presentation typically includes pain and stiffness in the low back, sacroiliac, and posterior hip regions in the presence of conjunctivitis and urethritis.[73] Dactylitis may be present.[72] Weight loss and fever are common in the acute phase as well.[13]

Background Information
This condition is a reactive arthritis that includes the clinical triad of nongonococcal urethritis, conjunctivitis, and arthritis.[13,72] It typically begins after an infection of the genitourinary or gastrointestinal tract[72] and usually involves more than one joint, preferentially affecting the joints of the lower extremities.[13] Onset of symptoms is acute with two to

four joints becoming painful within a few days.[13] There is usually an asymmetrical involvement of the distal interphalangeal joint and asymmetrical sacroiliitis with skin lesions frequently seen on the palms and soles of the feet.[72] The diagnosis is confirmed by blood panel and radiographs. Symptomatic treatment is used including nonsteroidal anti-inflammatory medications, sulfasalazine, and intra-articular corticosteroid injections.[13]

■ Rheumatoid Arthritis of the Lumbar Spine

Chief Clinical Characteristics
This presentation involves low back pain that radiates to the hips and lower extremities with positions that involve spinal loading, as well as possible cauda equina symptoms. Leg pain (18%) and leg numbness (14%) have been reported in people with this condition.[74]

Background Information
This condition affects women twice as often as men. Symptoms associated with this progressive inflammatory joint disease are caused by synovial membrane thickening and cytokine production in synovial fluid. Blood tests confirm the diagnosis if rheumatoid factor is detected. Typical radiographic findings include disk space narrowing, facet erosion, and endplate erosion.[74] Various steroidal, nonsteroidal, and biological anti-inflammatory medications have been widely used in the treatment of this condition.[74]

■ Septic Discitis

Chief Clinical Characteristics
This presentation may include fever, chills, sweats, and intractable lower back pain with possible radiation to the hip or groin, worsened by movement and not easily alleviated even with narcotic analgesia.

Background Information
From most to least common etiology, discitis may occur following spinal surgery during or after an infection, following spine or skin punctures, or spontaneously.[75] The diagnosis is confirmed by aspiration of the affected disk guided by computed tomography. Early diagnosis is critical to prevent infection of the surrounding tissues. Treatment of septic discitis is usually successful with specific intravenous antibiotics and external mobilization; surgery is rarely needed.[76]

■ Spinal Osteomyelitis

Chief Clinical Characteristics
This presentation can include low back pain and tenderness that is not relieved by rest and tends to be the primary complaint.[77–79] Various neurological impairments may be associated with this condition, including lower extremity weakness, bowel/bladder incontinence, or even paraplegia. Approximately one-third of patients also may present with fever.[78]

Background Information
This condition can be caused by direct extension of an infection or through hematogenous seeding from a distant sight of infection.[78] Risk factors for osteomyelitis include the use of central venous catheters, immunosuppression, surgery, and placement of a urinary catheter.[78] The diagnosis is confirmed with magnetic resonance imaging followed by microbiological tests. Treatment generally includes medication for the particular infecting agent. Some individuals with this condition will undergo combined medical and surgical treatment, which consists of extensive debridement, bone grafting, decompression, and stabilization of the vertebral column.[77–79]

■ Spinal Stenosis

Chief Clinical Characteristics
This presentation typically involves a prolonged history of low back pain in older individuals that is aggravated with standing, walking, or other positions of lumbar spinal extension and alleviated with spinal flexion or no weight bearing. Chronic nerve root compression can lead to radicular pain and sensory, motor, and reflex changes in one or both lower extremities, most commonly affecting the L3–L4 and L4–L5 segments.[80] Unilateral or bilateral leg pain is reported in up to 90% of cases with a more recent onset than low back pain, and walking tolerance is often diminished due to neurogenic claudication.[81]

Background Information
Causes of symptoms involve spinal cord and nerve root impingement due to spinal canal narrowing. Plain radiographs and magnetic resonance imaging confirm the diagnosis.

Indications for surgery have not been clearly defined and serve as elective procedures to improve quality of life in persons with disabling low back pain.[81] Therefore, nonsurgical options such as physical therapy to improve patient functioning and injections are the initial treatments of choice.

■ Tethered Spinal Cord

Chief Clinical Characteristics
This presentation typically includes back pain, associated with neurological deficits, and bowel and bladder dysfunction.[82] The most common manifestations of this condition are reduced motor function of the lower extremities (and upper extremities, although less likely), changes in muscle tone and deep tendon reflexes, progressive loss of articular dexterity, progressively worsening scoliosis or kyphosis, and back or leg pain.[83]

Background Information
This condition occurs commonly in children, but can present in undiagnosed adults as well. Magnetic resonance imaging confirms the diagnosis, with a low-lying (caudally positioned) conus medullaris present. Surgical resection of a thickened filum terminale is a common treatment.

■ Transverse Myelitis

Chief Clinical Characteristics
This presentation typically includes low back pain associated with acute or subacute motor, sensory, and autonomic neurological deficits.[84,85] At maximal level of deficits (within 4 hours to 21 days), approximately 50% of individuals with this condition lose all movements of their legs, virtually all have bladder dysfunction, and 80% to 94% have numbness, paresthesias, or band-like dysesthesias.[84]

Background Information
This condition is associated with various viral and bacterial infections as well as systemic autoimmune diseases. The etiology of this condition is unclear. Magnetic resonance imaging combined with lumbar puncture confirms the diagnosis. Treatment includes the use of multiple medications typically directed against an autoimmune response even when this condition cannot be attributed to a particular etiology.[86]

■ Tuberculosis of the Spine (Pott's Disease)

Chief Clinical Characteristics
This presentation typically includes insidious onset of stiffness with pain over the involved vertebrae radiating into the buttock or lower extremity, low-grade fever, chills, weight loss, and nonspecific constitutional symptoms of varying duration.[87] Weakness, nerve root compression, and sensory involvement can be present to varying degrees.

Background Information
This condition usually results from spread of pulmonary or other primary infection involving *Mycobacterium tuberculosis*. If the disease affects one vertebral body, the intervertebral disk may be spared. However, collapse of the affected segment could occur due to impaired disk nutrition. Magnetic resonance imaging confirms the diagnosis. Treatment consists of antituberculosis medications, which are effective 90% of the time, with surgery in more advanced cases.[88]

TUMORS

■ Intraspinal Lipoma

Chief Clinical Characteristics
This presentation includes lumbosacral pain and skin stigmata.[89] Symptoms depend on the location of the lipoma and proximity to neurological tissue; this condition may be associated with spinal cord tethering and progressive neurological symptoms.

Background Information
If the lipoma is impinging on neurological tissue, sphincter disturbance and incontinence will occur.[89] This condition is characterized by slow-growing, fatty cells.[89] This condition often is associated with spina bifida. Computed tomography and magnetic resonance imaging confirm the diagnosis. Treatment consists of surgical exploration and resection of the tumor.

■ Metastases, Including from Primary Breast, Kidney, Lung, Prostate, and Thyroid Disease

Chief Clinical Characteristics
This presentation involves unremitting pain in individuals with these risk factors:

previous history of cancer, age 50 years or older, failure to improve with conservative therapy, and unexplained weight change of more than 10 pounds in 6 months.[90]

Background Information

Cauda equina symptoms or nerve root compression of the spinal canal can be caused by vertebral collapse or infiltration of the tumor.[28] The skeletal system is the third most common site of metastatic disease; lumbar metastases account for 20% of cases.[29] Symptoms also may be related to pathological fracture in affected sites. Common primary sites causing metastases to bone include breast, prostate, lung, and kidney. Bone scan confirms the diagnosis. Common treatments for metastases include surgical resection, chemotherapy, radiation treatment, and palliation, depending on the tumor type and extent of metastasis.

■ Osteoblastoma

Chief Clinical Characteristics

This presentation can involve an insidious onset of deep and aching pain, typically in males under 30 years of age. Pain associated with this condition is not usually worse at night. This condition may rarely affect the pelvic bones, and the proximal femoral epiphysis is even less commonly affected.

Background Information

This condition involves abnormal production of osteoid and primitive bone, although its specific etiology remains unclear. Biopsy and plain radiographs confirm the diagnosis. Computed tomography is necessary to define the tumor margins if surgical resection is considered.

■ Primary Bone Tumor (eg, Osteosarcomas, Ewing's Sarcoma, Fibrosarcoma, and Chondrosarcoma)

Chief Clinical Characteristics

This presentation can include an insidious onset of pain in the buttock, pelvis, hip, lower back, and along the sciatic nerve distribution,[91] particularly in an individual older than 45 years with symptoms for more than 1 month, progressive pain that fails conservative

therapy, and the presence of anorexia, malaise, or night pain.[92]

Background Information

Diagnosis of a malignant bone tumor may be delayed due to the similarity in clinical presentation to other musculoskeletal disorders. Definitive diagnosis is made using appropriate imaging, blood tests (elevated alkaline phosphatase), and tumor biopsy. Depending on the location and stage, treatment of this condition may include surgical resection, radiation therapy, or chemotherapy.

■ Spinal Cord Tumor

Chief Clinical Characteristics

This presentation may involve low back pain, sciatica, saddle and perianal hypesthesia or analgesia, decreased rectal tone, absent patellar and Achilles reflexes, bowel and bladder dysfunction, and lower extremity weakness. Other symptoms may include unexplained weight loss, spontaneous onset of symptoms, failure to improve with prior medical care, and duration of symptoms longer than 1 month.[93] A long history of back pain and paresthesias as well as occasional urinary difficulties is common in patients with this condition.[94]

Background Information

Primary tumors common to the lumbar spine include myxopapillary ependymomas, schwannomas, paragangliomas, astrocytomas, and chordomas.[94] Common metastases to the lumbar spine occur in lung, breast, renal cell, and colorectal carcinomas and lymphoma.[93,94] Magnetic resonance imaging confirms the diagnosis.[93] Primary treatment includes surgical excision with possible radiotherapy and/or chemotherapy.[95] Treatment of spinal cord tumors causing cauda equina includes immediate surgical decompression.[94]

References

1. Shelton T, McKinlay R, Schwartz RW. Acute appendicitis: current diagnosis and treatment. *Curr Surg.* Sep–Oct 2003;60(5):502–505.
2. Indar AA, Beckingham IJ. Acute cholecystitis. *BMJ.* Sep 21, 2002;325(7365):639–643.
3. Braunwald E, Harrison TR. *Harrison's Principles of Internal Medicine.* 11th ed. New York: McGraw-Hill; 1987.
4. Ransohoff DF, Gracie WA. Treatment of gallstones [see comment]. *Ann Intern Med.* 1993;119(7 Pt 1):606–619.

5. Igra V. Pelvic inflammatory disease in adolescents. *AIDS Patient Care & Stds.* 1998;12(2):109–124.

6. Harwood-Nuss A, ed. *The Clinical Practice of Emergency Medicine.* Philadelphia, PA: Lippincott; 1991.

7. Anderson LA. Abdominal aortic aneurysm. *J Cardiovasc Nurs.* Jul 2001;15(4):1–14.

8. Kauppila LI, McAlindon T, Evans S, Wilson PW, Kiel D, Felson DT. Disc degeneration/back pain and calcification of the abdominal aorta. A 25-year follow-up study in Framingham. *Spine.* Aug 15, 1997;22(14):1642–1647; discussion 1648–1649.

9. Kurunlahti M, Tervonen O, Vanharanta H, Ilkko E, Suramo I. Association of atherosclerosis with low back pain and the degree of disc degeneration. *Spine.* Nov 15, 1999;24(20):2080–2084.

10. Gravereaux EC, Marin ML. Endovascular repair of diffuse atherosclerotic occlusive disease using stented grafts. *Mt Sinai J Med.* Dec 2003;70(6):410–417.

11. Churchill MA Jr, Geraci JE, Hunder GG. Musculoskeletal manifestations of bacterial endocarditis. *Ann Intern Med.* Dec 1977;87(6):754–759.

12. Knutson D, Greenberg G, Cronau H. Management of Crohn's disease—a practical approach. *Am Fam Physician.* Sep 15, 2003;68(4):707–714.

13. Kataria RK, Brent LH. Spondyloarthropathies. *Am Fam Physician.* Jun 15, 2004;69(12):2853–2860.

14. Place RJ, Simmang CL. Diverticular disease. *Baillieres Best Pract Res Clin Gastroenterol.* Feb 2002;16(1):135–148.

15. Stollman NH, Raskin JB. Diverticular disease of the colon. *J Clin Gastroenterol.* Oct 1999;29(3):241–252.

16. Shiotani A, Graham DY. Pathogenesis and therapy of gastric and duodenal ulcer disease. *Med Clin North Am.* Nov 2002;86(6):1447–1466, viii.

17. Dore MP, Graham DY. Pathogenesis of duodenal ulcer disease: the rest of the story. *Baillieres Best Pract Res Clin Gastroenterol.* Feb 2000;14(1):97–107.

18. Kauffman GL Jr. Duodenal ulcer disease: treatment by surgery, antibiotics, or both. *Adv Surg.* 2000;34:121–135.

19. Tenore JL. Ectopic pregnancy [see comment]. *Am Fam Physician.* 2000;61(4):1080–1088.

20. Wellbery C. Diagnosis and treatment of endometriosis [see comment]. *Am Fam Physician.* 1767;60(6):1753–1762. [Erratum appears in *Am Fam Physician.* May 1, 2000;61(9):2614.]

21. Chen TM, George S, Woodruff CA, Hsu S. Clinical manifestations of varicella-zoster virus infection. *Dermatol Clin.* Apr 2002;20(2):267–282.

22. de la Iglesia F, Asensio P, Diaz A, Darriba M, Nicolas R, Diz-Lois F. Acute renal infarction as a cause of low-back pain. *South Med J.* May 2003;96(5):497–499.

23. Weidauer S, Nichtweiss M, Lanfermann H, Zanella FE. Spinal cord infarction: MR imaging and clinical features in 16 cases. *Neuroradiology.* 2002;44(10):851–857.

24. Gorg C, Seifart U, Gorg K. Acute, complete splenic infarction in cancer patient is associated with a fatal outcome. *Abdom Imaging.* Mar–Apr 2004;29(2):224–227.

25. Teich S, Oliver GC, Canter JW. The early diagnosis of splenic abscess. *Am Surg.* Jun 1986;52(6):303–307.

26. Freund R, Pichl J, Heyder N, Rodl W, Riemann JF. Splenic abscess-clinical symptoms and diagnostic possibilities. *Am J Gastroenterol.* Jan 1982;77(1):35–38.

27. Thanos L, Dailiana T, Papaioannou G, Nikita A, Koutrouvelis H, Kelekis DA. Percutaneous CT-guided drainage of splenic abscess. *Am J Roentgenol.* Sep 2002;179(3):629–632.

28. Hatrick NC, Lucas JD, Timothy AR, Smith MA. The surgical treatment of metastatic disease of the spine. *Radiother Oncol.* 2000;56(3):335–339.

29. Holman PJ, Suki D, McCutcheon I, Wolinsky JP, Rhines LD, Gokaslan ZL. Surgical management of metastatic disease of the lumbar spine: experience with 139 patients. *J Neurosurg Spine.* 2005;2(5):550–563.

30. Sparkes JM, Kingston R, O'Flanagan SJ, Keogh P. Multiple myeloma in young persons. *Ir Med J.* Jun 2002;95(5):149.

31. George ED, Sadovsky R. Multiple myeloma: recognition and management. *Am Fam Physician.* May 1, 1999; 59(7):1885–1894.

32. Burton CH, Fairham SA, Millet B, DasGupta R, Sivakumaran M. Unusual aetiology of persistent back pain in a patient with multiple myeloma: infectious discitis. *J Clin Pathol.* Sep 1998;51(8):633–634.

33. anonymous. Case records of the Massachusetts General Hospital. Weekly clinicopathological exercises. Case 27–1996. A 31-year-old woman with lumbar and abdominal pain, hypertension, and a retroperitoneal mass. *N Engl J Med.* 1996;335(9):650–655.

34. Kaya M, Aydin F. Pancreatic mass lesion mimicking carcinoma: Initial presentation of retroperitoneal fibrosis. *Turk J Gastroenterol.* Sep 2005;16(3):156–159.

35. Kao TH, Shen CC, Chen CC, Kwan PH. "Primary" benign retroperitoneal and intraspinal dumbbell-shaped cystic teratoma: case report. *Spine.* Aug 1, 2005;30(15): E439–443.

36. Umezurike C, Feyi-Waboso P. Successful myomectomy during pregnancy: a case report. *Reprod Health.* Aug 16 2005;2(1):6.

37. Bent S, Nallamothu BK, Simel DL, Fihn SD, Saint S. Does this woman have an acute uncomplicated urinary tract infection? [see comment]. *JAMA.* 2002;287(20): 2701–2710.

38. Chao D, Nanda A. Spinal epidural abscess: a diagnostic challenge. *Am Fam Physician.* Apr 1, 2002;65(7):1341–1346.

39. Tang HJ, Lin HJ, Liu YC, Li CM. Spinal epidural abscess—experience with 46 patients and evaluation of prognostic factors. *J Infect.* Aug 2002;45(2):76–81.

40. Okano K, Kondo H, Tsuchiya R, Naruke T, Sato M, Yokoyama R. Spinal epidural abscess associated with epidural catheterization: report of a case and a review of the literature. *Jpn J Clin Oncol.* Jan 1999;29(1):49–52.

41. Hill JS, Hughes EW, Robertson PA. A Staphylococcus aureus paraspinal abscess associated with epidural analgesia in labour. *Anaesthesia.* 2001;56(9):873–878.

42. Mallick IH, Thoufeeq MH, Rajendran TP. Iliopsoas abscesses. *Postgrad Med J.* 2004;80(946):459–462.

43. Agrawal SN, Dwivedi AJ, Khan M. Primary psoas abscess. *Dig Dis Sci.* 2002;47(9):2103–2105.

44. Wu AS, Griebel RW, Meguro K, Fourney DR. Spinal subdural empyema after a dural tear. Case report. *Neurosurg Focus.* Dec 15, 2004;17(6):E10.

45. Magee DJ. *Orthopedic Physical Assessment.* 3rd ed. Philadelphia, PA: W. B. Saunders; 1997.

46. Rice I, Wee MY, Thomson K. Obstetric epidurals and chronic adhesive arachnoiditis [see comment]. *Br J Anaesthesia.* 2004;92(1):109–120.

47. Kahara VJ, Seppanen SK, Kuurne T, Laasonen EM. Diagnosis and embolizing of spinal arteriovenous malformations. *Ann Med.* Oct 1997;29(5):377–382.

48. Oldfield EH, Doppman JL. Spinal arteriovenous malformations. *Clin Neurosurg.* 1988;34:161–183.

49. Caragine LP Jr, Halbach VV, Ng PP, Dowd CF. Vascular myelopathies-vascular malformations of the spinal

cord: presentation and endovascular surgical management. *Semin Neurol.* Jun 2002;22(2):123–132.

50. Merskey H, Bogduk N. *Classification of Chronic Pain: Descriptions of Chronic Pain Syndromes and Definitions of Pain Terms.* Seattle, WA: IASP Press; 1994.

51. Berven S, Tay BB, Colman W, Hu SS. The lumbar zygapophyseal (facet) joints: a role in the pathogenesis of spinal pain syndromes and degenerative spondylolisthesis. *Semin Neurol.* Jun 2002;22(2):187–196.

52. Urban JP, Roberts S. Degeneration of the intervertebral disc. *Arthritis Res Ther.* 2003;5(3):120–130.

53. Biyani A, Andersson GB, Chaudhary H, An HS. Intradiscal electrothermal therapy: a treatment option in patients with internal disc disruption. *Spine.* 2003;28(15 suppl):S8–14.

54. Groen RJ. Non-operative treatment of spontaneous spinal epidural hematomas: a review of the literature and a comparison with operative cases. *Acta Neurochir (Wien).* Feb 2004;146(2):103–110.

55. Fukui S, Ohseto K, Shiotani M, Ohno K, Karasawa H, Naganuma Y. Distribution of referred pain from the lumbar zygapophyseal joints and dorsal rami. *Clin J Pain.* 1997;13(4):303–307.

56. Dreyfuss PH, Dreyer SJ, Nass. Lumbar zygapophysial (facet) joint injections. *Spine.* 2003;3(3 Suppl):50S–59S.

57. Goldenberg DL, Burckhardt C, Crofford L. Management of fibromyalgia syndrome [see comment]. *JAMA.* 2004;292(19):2388–2395.

58. Nampiaparampil DE, Shmerling RH. A review of fibromyalgia. *Am J Managed Care.* 2004;10(11 Pt 1): 794–800.

59. Meves R, Avanzi O. Correlation between neurological deficit and spinal canal compromise in 198 patients with thoracolumbar and lumbar fractures. *Spine.* Apr 1, 2005;30(7):787–791.

60. Garfin SR, Yuan HA, Reiley MA. New technologies in spine: kyphoplasty and vertebroplasty for the treatment of painful osteoporotic compression fractures. *Spine.* 2001;26(14):1511–1515.

61. Roche PH, Dufour H, Graziani N, Jolivert J, Grisoli F. Anterior lumbosacral dislocation: case report and review of the literature. *Surg Neurol.* 1998;50(1):11–16.

62. Bono CM. Low-back pain in athletes. *J Bone Joint Surg Am.* Feb 2004;86A(2):382–396.

63. Standaert CJ, Herring SA. Spondylolysis: a critical review. *Br J Sports Med.* Dec 2000;34(6):415–422.

64. Demaerel P, Crevits I, Casteels–Van Daele M, Baert AL. Meningoradiculitis due to borreliosis presenting as low back pain only. *Neuroradiology.* 1998;40(2):126–127.

65. Pandian JD, Sarada C, Radhakrishnan VV, Kishore A. Iatrogenic meningitis after lumbar puncture—a preventable health hazard. *J Hosp Infect.* 2004;56(2):119–124.

66. El Bashir H, Laundy M, Booy R. Diagnosis and treatment of bacterial meningitis. *Arch Dis Child.* 2003;88(7):615–620.

67. Njoo KH, Van der Does E. The occurrence and interrater reliability of myofascial trigger points in the quadratus lumborum and gluteus medius: a prospective study in non-specific low back pain patients and controls in general practice [see comment]. *Pain.* 1994; 58(3):317–323.

68. Grinspoon S, Miller K, Coyle C, et al. Severity of osteopenia in estrogen-deficient women with anorexia nervosa and hypothalamic amenorrhea. *J Clin Endocrinol Metab.* Jun 1999;84(6):2049–2055.

69. Langston AL, Ralston SH. Management of Paget's disease of bone. *Rheumatology (Oxford).* Aug 2004;43(8): 955–959.

70. Salvarani C, Cantini F, Boiardi L, Hunder GG. Polymyalgia rheumatica and giant-cell arteritis. *N Engl J Med.* Jul 25, 2002;347(4):261–271.

71. Mandell BF. Polymyalgia rheumatica: clinical presentation is key to diagnosis and treatment. *Cleve Clin J Med.* Jun 2004;71(6):489–495.

72. Gladman DD. Clinical aspects of the spondyloarthropathies. *Am J Med Sci.* Oct 1998;316(4): 234–238.

73. Klippel JH, Weyand CM, Crofford LJ, Stone JH, Arthritis Foundation. *Primer on the Rheumatic Diseases.* 12th ed. Atlanta, GA: Arthritis Foundation; 2001.

74. Kawaguchi Y, Matsuno H, Kanamori M, Ishihara H, Ohmori K, Kimura T. Radiologic findings of the lumbar spine in patients with rheumatoid arthritis, and a review of pathologic mechanisms. *J Spinal Disord Tech.* 2003;16(1):38–43.

75. Honan M, White GW, Eisenberg GM. Spontaneous infectious discitis in adults. *Am J Med.* 1996;100(1): 85–89.

76. Friedman JA, Maher CO, Quast LM, McClelland RL, Ebersold MJ. Spontaneous space infections in adults. *Surg Neurol.* 2002;57(2):81–86.

77. Seravalli L, Van Linthoudt D, Bernet C, et al. Candida glabrata spinal osteomyelitis involving two contiguous lumbar vertebrae: a case report and review of the literature. *Diagn Microbiol Infect Dis.* Feb 2003;45(2): 137–141.

78. Miller DJ, Mejicano GC. Vertebral osteomyelitis due to Candida species: case report and literature review. *Clin Infect Dis.* Aug 15 2001;33(4):523–530.

79. Babinchak TJ, Riley DK, Rotheram EB Jr. Pyogenic vertebral osteomyelitis of the posterior elements. *Clin Infect Dis.* Aug 1997;25(2):221–224.

80. Arbit E, Pannullo S. Lumbar stenosis: a clinical review. *Clin Orthop.* Mar 2001(384):137–143.

81. Fritz JM, Delitto A, Welch WC, Erhard RE. Lumbar spinal stenosis: a review of current concepts in evaluation, management, and outcome measurements. *Arch Phys Med Rehabil.* Jun 1998;79(6):700–708.

82. Iskandar BJ, Fulmer BB, Hadley MN, Oakes WJ. Congenital tethered spinal cord syndrome in adults [see comment]. *Journal of Neurosurgery.* 1998;88(6): 958–961.

83. Di Rocco C, Peter JC. Management of tethered spinal cord. *Surgical Neurology.* 1997;48(4):320–322.

84. Transverse Myelitis Consortium Working G. Proposed diagnostic criteria and nosology of acute transverse myelitis [see comment]. *Neurology.* 2002;59(4):499–505.

85. Harzheim M, Schlegel U, Urbach H, Klockgether T, Schmidt S. Discriminatory features of acute transverse myelitis: a retrospective analysis of 45 patients. *J Neurol Sci.* 2004;217(2):217–223.

86. Banit DM, Wheeler AH, Darden BV, 2nd. Recurrent transverse myelitis after lumbar spine surgery: a case report. *Spine.* 2003;28(9):E165–168.

87. Gorse GJ, Pais MJ, Kusske JA, Cesario TC. Tuberculous spondylitis. A report of six cases and a review of the literature. *Medicine.* 1983;62(3):178–193.

88. Dass B, Puet TA, Watanakunakorn C. Tuberculosis of the spine (Pott's disease) presenting as "compression fractures." *Spinal Cord.* 2002;40(11):604–608.

89. Sakho Y, Badiane SB, Kabre A, et al. Les lipomes intra-rachidiens lombo-sacres associes ou non a un syndrome de la moelle attachee (serie de 8 cas). *Dakar Medical.* 1998;43(1):13–20.

90. Joines JD, McNutt RA, Carey TS, Deyo RA, Rouhani R. Finding cancer in primary care outpatients with low back pain: a comparison of diagnostic strategies. *J Gen Intern Med.* 2001;16(1):14–23.

91. Wurtz LD, Peabody TD, Simon MA. Delay in the diagnosis and treatment of primary bone sarcoma of the pelvis. *J Bone Joint Surg Am.* 1999;81(3):317–325.

92. Thompson RC Jr, Berg TL. Primary bone tumors of the pelvis presenting as spinal disease. *Orthopedics.* 1996;19(12):1011–1016.

93. Slipman CW, Patel RK, Botwin K, et al. Epidemiology of spine tumors presenting to musculoskeletal physiatrists. *Arch Phys Med Rehabil.* Apr 2003;84(4):492–495.

94. Bagley CA, Gokaslan ZL. Cauda equina syndrome caused by primary and metastatic neoplasms. *Neurosurg Focus.* Jun 15 2004;16(6):e3.

95. Guerrero D. The management of primary spinal cord tumours. *Nurs Times.* Oct 21–27 2003;99(42):28–31.

CHAPTER 19

Hip Pain

■ *Kyle F. Baldwin, PT, DPT* ■ *Todd E. Davenport, PT, DPT, OCS*

■ *Michael A. Andersen, PT, DPT, OCS*

Description of the Symptom

This chapter describes pathology that may lead to hip pain, including anterior, buttock, inguinal/ medial thigh, and lateral pain. **Local causes** of hip pain are defined as pathology occurring within the intra- and extra-articular structures of the hip joint. **Remote causes** are defined as originating from sites external to this region.

Special Concerns

■ Acute inability to bear weight through the affected lower extremity or pelvis secondary to pain
■ Decreased pulses in the lower extremities
■ Skin break and fever
■ Sudden loss of motor or sensory function associated with trauma
■ Warmth and swelling in the legs associated with a fever

CHAPTER PREVIEW: Conditions That May Lead to Hip Pain

REMOTE	LOCAL INGUINAL/ MEDIAL THIGH
COMMON	
Acute lumbar sprain/strain 324	Hernias:
Disk disruption (with or without herniation) 326	• Femoral hernia 340
Facet syndrome 327	• Inguinal hernia 340
Lumbar compression fracture 328	Labral tear 343
Lumbar radiculopathies:	Muscle strains:
• L1–L3 radiculopathy 328	• Adductor strain 343
• L4 radiculopathy 328	• Iliopsoas strain 343
• L5 radiculopathy 330	
• S1 radiculopathy 330	
UNCOMMON	
Not applicable	Fractures:
	• Intracapsular femur fracture 339
	• Stress fracture of the femoral neck 339
	Hernias:
	• Sports hernia 340
	Nerve entrapments/neuropathy:
	• Femoral neuropathy 344

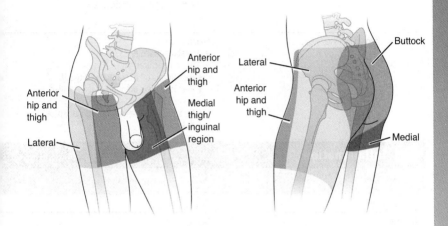

LOCAL LATERAL	LOCAL BUTTOCK	LOCAL ANTERIOR HIP/THIGH
Iliotibial band friction syndrome 343 Trochanteric contusion (hip pointer) 350	Fractures: • Avulsion fractures: 　◦ Hamstrings off ischial tuberosity 338 Gluteal contusion 339 Muscle strains: • Hamstring strain 343 Sacroiliac joint dysfunction 349	Labral tear 343 Muscle strains: • Iliopsoas strain 343 • Quadriceps muscle strain 344
Iliac crest apophysitis 342 Nerve entrapments/neuropathy: • Meralgia paresthetica 345	Bursitis: • Ischiogluteal bursitis 336 Nerve entrapments/neuropathy: • Piriformis syndrome 345	Fractures: • Extracapsular femur fracture 338 • Femoral shaft fracture 339 Hernias: • Sports hernia 340

(continued)

HIP PAIN

Trauma *(continued)*

REMOTE	LOCAL INGUINAL/ MEDIAL THIGH
UNCOMMON	
	• Genitofemoral nerve entrapment 344 • Iliohypogastric nerve entrapment 344 • Ilioinguinal nerve entrapment 345 • Obturator nerve entrapment 345 Sacroiliac joint dysfunction 349
RARE	

Traumatic spondylolisthesis 335	Fractures:
	• Acetabular fracture 337
	• Avulsion fractures:
	  • Hamstrings off ischial tuberosity 338
	  • Rectus femoris off anterior inferior iliac spine 338
	  • Sartorius off anterior superior iliac spine 338
	Hip dislocation 341

I Inflammation

REMOTE	LOCAL INGUINAL/ MEDIAL THIGH
COMMON	
Aseptic Not applicable	Not applicable
Septic Appendicitis 326	
UNCOMMON	
Aseptic Rheumatoid arthritis–like diseases of the lumbar spine: • Scleroderma 333 • Systemic lupus erythematosus 333	**Aseptic** Complex regional pain syndrome 337 Iliopsoas tendinitis 342 Osteitis pubis 345 Reiter's syndrome 347 Rheumatoid arthritis of the hip 348 Rheumatoid arthritis–like diseases: • Scleroderma 348 • Systemic lupus erythematosus 348
Septic Brucellosis of the lumbar spine 326 Pelvic inflammatory disease 331 Prostatitis 331 Renal or urinary tract infection 332 Septic arthritis of the sacroiliac joint 334	**Septic** Herpes zoster 340

Chapter 19 **Hip Pain** **319**

LOCAL LATERAL	LOCAL BUTTOCK	LOCAL ANTERIOR HIP/THIGH
		Nerve entrapments/ neuropathy: • Femoral neuropathy 344 • Meralgia paresthetica 345
Hip dislocation 341	Hip dislocation 341	Hip dislocation 341

LOCAL LATERAL	LOCAL BUTTOCK	LOCAL ANTERIOR HIP/THIGH
Aseptic Bursitis: • Ischiogluteal bursitis 336 • Trochanteric bursitis 336 Fibromyalgia 337 **Septic** Not applicable	**Aseptic** Fibromyalgia 337 **Septic** Not applicable	Not applicable
Aseptic Complex regional pain syndrome 337 Polymyalgia rheumatica 347 Reiter's syndrome 347 Rheumatoid arthritis of the hip 348 Rheumatoid arthritis–like diseases: • Scleroderma 348 • Systemic lupus erythematosus 348 **Septic** Herpes zoster 340	**Aseptic** Ankylosing spondylitis 336 Complex regional pain syndrome 337 Polymyalgia rheumatica 347 **Septic** Herpes zoster 340	**Aseptic** Complex regional pain syndrome 337 Iliopsoas tendinitis 342 Rheumatoid arthritis of the hip 348 Rheumatoid arthritis–like diseases: • Scleroderma 348 • Systemic lupus erythematosus 348 **Septic** Herpes zoster 340

Inflammation *(continued)*

REMOTE	LOCAL INGUINAL/ MEDIAL THIGH
RARE	

REMOTE	LOCAL INGUINAL/ MEDIAL THIGH
Aseptic Reiter's syndrome of the lumbar spine 331 Rheumatoid arthritis of the lumbar spine 332 Rheumatoid arthritis–like diseases of the spine: • Inflammatory bowel disease 332 • Inflammatory muscle diseases 333 • Psoriatic arthritis 333 **Septic** Psoas muscle abscess 331 Retrocecal appendicitis 332 Retroperitoneal abscess 332 Septic discitis 334 Systemic fungal infection of the lumbar spine 335 Tuberculosis of the lumbar spine (Pott's disease) 335	**Aseptic** Rheumatoid arthritis–like diseases: • Inflammatory muscle diseases 348 • Psoriatic arthritis 348 **Septic** Brucellosis of the hip 336 Iliopsoas abscess 342 Septic arthritis of the hip 349 Systemic fungal infection 349 Tuberculosis of the hip 350

M   Metabolic

REMOTE	LOCAL INGUINAL/ MEDIAL THIGH
COMMON	
Not applicable	Not applicable
UNCOMMON	
Endometriosis 327	Heterotopic ossification 341 Myositis ossificans 344 Osteomalacia 346 Transient osteoporosis of the hip 350
RARE	
Not applicable	Gout 339 Pseudogout 347

Va   Vascular

REMOTE	LOCAL INGUINAL/ MEDIAL THIGH
COMMON	
Not applicable	Not applicable
UNCOMMON	
Not applicable	Not applicable
RARE	
Aortic artery aneurysm 325 Aortic or iliac arteriosclerosis 325 Epidural hematoma 327	Avascular necrosis of the hip 336 Greater saphenous vein thrombophlebitis 340 Iliac artery aneurysm 341 Iliofemoral venous thrombosis 342 Sickle cell crisis 349

LOCAL LATERAL	LOCAL BUTTOCK	LOCAL ANTERIOR HIP/THIGH
Aseptic	**Aseptic**	**Aseptic**
Herpes zoster 340	Reiter's syndrome 347	Gout 339
Rheumatoid arthritis–like	Rheumatoid arthritis–like	Pseudogout 347
diseases:	diseases:	Reiter's syndrome 347
• Inflammatory muscle	• Inflammatory muscle	Rheumatoid arthritis–like
diseases 348	diseases 348	diseases:
• Psoriatic arthritis 348	• Psoriatic arthritis 348	• Inflammatory muscle
		diseases 348
Septic	**Septic**	• Psoriatic arthritis 348
Cellulitis 337	Brucellosis of the hip 336	
Systemic fungal infection 349	Cellulitis 337	**Septic**
	Systemic fungal infection 349	Brucellosis of the hip 336
	Tuberculosis of the hip 350	Iliopsoas abscess 342
		Tuberculosis of the hip 350

LOCAL LATERAL	LOCAL BUTTOCK	LOCAL ANTERIOR HIP/THIGH
Not applicable	Not applicable	Not applicable
Not applicable	Transient osteoporosis of the hip 350	Transient osteoporosis of the hip 350
Not applicable	Not applicable	Not applicable

LOCAL LATERAL	LOCAL BUTTOCK	LOCAL ANTERIOR HIP/THIGH
Not applicable	Not applicable	Not applicable
Not applicable	Not applicable	Not applicable
Not applicable	Not applicable	Iliac artery aneurysm 341

(continued)

De Degenerative

REMOTE	LOCAL INGUINAL/ MEDIAL THIGH
COMMON	
Degenerative spondylolisthesis 326 Disk degeneration 326 Spinal stenosis 334 Spondylolysis 334	Hip osteoarthrosis/ osteoarthritis 341
UNCOMMON	
Not applicable	Iliopsoas tendinosis 342
RARE	
Not applicable	Not applicable

Tu Tumor

REMOTE	LOCAL INGUINAL/ MEDIAL THIGH
COMMON	
Malignant Primary: Not applicable *Malignant Metastatic:* Not applicable *Benign, such as:* • Ovarian cysts 331 • Uterine fibroids 335	Not applicable
UNCOMMON	
Not applicable	*Malignant Primary, such as:* • Primary bone tumor of the acetabulum or proximal femur: • Ewing's sarcoma 347 • Osteosarcoma 347 *Malignant Metastatic, such as:* • Metastases, including from primary breast, kidney, lung, prostate, and thyroid disease 343 *Benign:* Not applicable
RARE	
Malignant Primary, such as: • Spinal cord tumor 334 *Malignant Metastatic, such as:* • Leukemia 327 *Benign, such as:* • Osteoblastoma of the spine 331	*Malignant Primary, such as:* • Primary bone tumor of the acetabulum or proximal femur: • Ewing's sarcoma 347 • Osteosarcoma 347 *Malignant Metastatic:* Not applicable *Benign, such as:* • Osteoblastoma of the hip 346 • Osteochondroma 346 • Osteoid osteoma 346 • Pigmented villonodular synovitis 346

LOCAL LATERAL	LOCAL BUTTOCK	LOCAL ANTERIOR HIP/THIGH
Hip osteoarthrosis/ osteoarthritis 341	Hip osteoarthrosis/ osteoarthritis 341	Not applicable
Not applicable	Not applicable	Iliopsoas tendinosis 342
Not applicable	Not applicable	Not applicable

LOCAL LATERAL	LOCAL BUTTOCK	LOCAL ANTERIOR HIP/THIGH
Not applicable	Not applicable	Not applicable

Malignant Primary, such as:
• Primary bone tumor of the acetabulum or proximal femur:
  • Ewing's sarcoma 347
  • Osteosarcoma 347
Malignant Metastatic, such as:
• Metastases, including from primary breast, kidney, lung, prostate, and thyroid disease 343
Benign:
Not applicable
	Malignant Primary, such as:
	• Primary bone tumor of the acetabulum or proximal femur:
	  • Ewing's sarcoma 347
	  • Osteosarcoma 347
	Malignant Metastatic, such as:
	• Metastases, including from primary breast, kidney, lung, prostate, and thyroid disease 343
	Benign:
	Not applicable
		Malignant Primary, such as:
		• Primary bone tumor of the acetabulum or proximal femur:
		  • Ewing's sarcoma 347
		  • Osteosarcoma 347
		Malignant Metastatic, such as:
		• Metastases, including from primary breast, kidney, lung, prostate, and thyroid disease 343
		Benign:
		Not applicable

Malignant Primary, such as:
• Primary bone tumor of the acetabulum or proximal femur:
  • Ewing's sarcoma 347
  • Osteosarcoma 347
Malignant Metastatic:
Not applicable
Benign:
Not applicable
	Not applicable	*Malignant Primary, such as:*
		• Primary bone tumor of the acetabulum or proximal femur:
		  • Ewing's sarcoma 347
		  • Osteosarcoma 347
		Malignant Metastatic:
		Not applicable
		Benign, such as:
		• Pigmented villonodular synovitis 346

(continued)

Co Congenital

REMOTE	LOCAL INGUINAL/ MEDIAL THIGH
COMMON	
Not applicable	Not applicable
UNCOMMON	
Not applicable	Not applicable
RARE	
Not applicable	Not applicable

Ne Neurogenic/Psychogenic

REMOTE	LOCAL INGUINAL/ MEDIAL THIGH
COMMON	
Not applicable	Not applicable
UNCOMMON	
Not applicable	Not applicable
RARE	
Not applicable	Not applicable

Note: These are estimates of relative incidence because few data are available for the less common conditions.

Overview of Hip Pain

The diagnosis of hip pain is complex because precise symptom localization often is confusing for the patient and clinician. Patients may associate their hip within the region extending anywhere between the lateral midlumbar spine and lateral thigh. Pain referral patterns also may serve as diagnostic pitfalls in the hip region. Lumbar, sacroiliac, and hip causes of pain may be difficult to differentiate, particularly in individuals with long-standing pain. In addition, primary hip pathology may present as inguinal, medial thigh, or medial knee pain. A careful history should elicit the patient's own anatomical definition of the hip region in order to clarify the location of pain, due to the importance of this information to accurate diagnosis in the hip region.

Description of Conditions That May Lead to Hip Pain

Remote

■ Acute Lumbar Sprain/Strain

Chief Clinical Characteristics
This presentation may involve pain, muscle spasm, edema, and increased temperature with radiation into the buttocks and rarely into the thighs or lower legs. Pain may increase with contraction or stretching of affected musculature.

Background Information
Sprains and strains involve ligamentous and musculotendinous damage, respectively. This condition often results from excessive physical demands on the low back, such as repetitive lifting, excessive flexion, extension, or rotation movements with or without load.[1] Treatment

LOCAL LATERAL	LOCAL BUTTOCK	LOCAL ANTERIOR HIP/THIGH
Not applicable	Not applicable	Not applicable
Not applicable	Not applicable	Not applicable
Not applicable	Not applicable	Not applicable

LOCAL LATERAL	LOCAL BUTTOCK	LOCAL ANTERIOR HIP/THIGH
Not applicable	Not applicable	Not applicable
Not applicable	Not applicable	Not applicable
Not applicable	Not applicable	Not applicable

typically includes lumbar mobilization/manipulation, activity modification, exercise for the trunk and proximal lower extremities, and physical modalities.

■ Aortic Artery Aneurysm

Chief Clinical Characteristics
This presentation typically includes vague abdominal pain, usually located in the epigastrium, that may radiate to the low back, flank, or groin. Other symptoms include early satiety, nausea, vomiting, gastrointestinal bleeding, and lower extremity ischemia.[2] The problem arises in that 66% to 75% of abdominal aortic aneurysms are asymptomatic.[2]

Background Information
Aneurysms can be diagnosed during a routine physical examination by palpation of a pulsatile abdominal mass above the umbilicus, which may be associated with erythema nodosum. This condition occurs when the tunica intima, tunica media, and tunica adventitia become structurally compromised due to various acquired factors (eg, hypertension, cigarette smoking) and congenital factors (eg, Marfan's syndrome). Most often, this condition is asymptomatic prior to rupture. The abdominal aorta is most commonly involved due to its morphology. Elective open surgical repair may be considered when the risk of rupture exceeds that of surgery.[2]

■ Aortic or Iliac Arteriosclerosis

Chief Clinical Characteristics
This presentation may be characterized by generalized low back and hip pain, and symptoms consistent with lumbar disk degeneration.[3]

Background Information
Studies have correlated the occurrence of aortic arteriosclerosis and disk degeneration.[3,4]

The first to fourth lumbar arteries leave the aorta in front of the corresponding vertebral body supplying that vertebra and the adjacent intervertebral disk via diffusion through the vertebral end plate.[3] Findings suggest that calcific lesions in the upper part of the abdominal aorta predict disk deterioration at any lumbar level.[3] The link between arteriosclerosis and low back/hip pain can be explained by the common risk factors between the two pathologies, including age and smoking. The diagnosis is confirmed with radiographs or computed tomography. Surgical techniques for treatment of occlusive disease of the artery include endovascular stented-graft treatment.[5]

■ Appendicitis

Chief Clinical Characteristics
This presentation typically includes pain in the right lower abdominal and lumbar regions with local right iliac and/or lumbar direct tenderness. Reports of vague periumbilical pain followed by anorexia, nausea, and vomiting are common. Other physical findings include tachycardia, low-grade fever, hypoactive bowel sounds, and tenderness in the right lower quadrant at McBurney's point.[6]

Background Information
This condition involves septic inflammation of the appendix, involving obstruction of the appendix lumen. The end result of this disease process is rupture of contents into the abdominal cavity and the corresponding potential for systemic infection. Therefore, individuals suspected of this condition should be referred to an emergency department for immediate treatment.

■ Brucellosis of the Lumbar Spine

Chief Clinical Characteristics
This presentation can be characterized by a gradual onset of nonspecific myalgias, fever, malaise, and generalized lumbopelvic, hip, or sacroiliac joint pain.

Background Information
This uncommon condition in the United States results from ingestion of bacteria that are found in nonpasteurized milk or other infected animal products. It is associated with sacroiliac joint effusions that produce some arthritic changes over time if left untreated. Treatment includes antibiotics.

■ Degenerative Spondylolisthesis

Chief Clinical Characteristics
This presentation may involve low back pain with concurrent symptoms of spinal stenosis, involving unilateral or bilateral hip or lower extremity pain, and chronic nerve root compression.

Background Information
Degenerative spondylolisthesis is the result of prolonged instability of the spinal motion segment. Spondylolisthesis can be caused by facet joint dysplasia, elongation or fracture of the pars interarticularis, degeneration and secondary instability of the facet joints, trauma, or pathologies including bone tumor, osteogenesis imperfecta, or primary bone disorders.[7] Plain radiographs confirm the diagnosis. Nonsurgical intervention may be considered for individuals without progressive neurological deficits. Surgical treatment typically includes discectomy or spinal fusion for individuals with neurological symptoms.[8]

■ Disk Degeneration

Chief Clinical Characteristics
This presentation typically includes reports of low back pain with possible radiation to the hips, with or without neurological symptoms.

Background Information
The incidence of disk degeneration increases sharply with age. Disk degeneration can alter disk height leading to symptoms of sciatica or neurological compression, change the mechanics of the spinal column affecting spinal muscles and ligaments, and limit lumbar range of motion. Failure of the nutrient supply to the disk, abnormal mechanical loading of the disks, and genetic factors have been implicated.[8] Plain radiographs and magnetic resonance imaging confirm the diagnosis. Surgical treatment typically includes discectomy or spinal fusion for individuals with neurological symptoms.[8]

■ Disk Disruption (With or Without Disk Herniation)

Chief Clinical Characteristics
This presentation involves an individual's reports of pain deep in the lumbar region with occasional buttock pain. Usually symptoms are preceded by a traumatic event such as lifting a heavy object or other forceful movement. Pain is

aggravated with lumbar rotation, flexion, and side-bending, and sitting tolerance is typically diminished.

Background Information
Individuals with true internal disk disruption lack symptoms of radiculopathy; when present, leg pain follows a nondermatomal pattern.[9] Magnetic resonance imaging and discography confirm the diagnosis. Nonsurgical treatment is a common first approach. Surgical treatment typically includes discectomy or spinal fusion for individuals with progressive neurological symptoms.[8]

■ **Endometriosis**

Chief Clinical Characteristics
This presentation may include dysmenorrhea, dyspareunia, and low back pain that worsens with menses.[10] Rectal pain and painful defecation can also be present.[10]

Background Information
This condition is the presence of tissues that are histologically similar to endometrium at sites outside the endometrial cavity. Causes include retrograde menstruation and peritoneal epithelium transformation to endometrial tissue, as well as possible genetic causes.[10] Pelvic ultrasonography, computed tomography, magnetic resonance imaging, and laparoscopy are commonly used to confirm the diagnosis.[10] Treatment in cases of women with few symptoms can include oral contraceptives or progestins for pain relief.[10] Surgery may be required in more advanced stages to remove endometrial lesions.[10]

■ **Epidural Hematoma**

Chief Clinical Characteristics
This presentation typically includes the acute onset of back (or neck) pain with possible referral to the hip, followed by rapidly progressive sensory and/or motor deficits. Less frequently, patients may present with slowly progressive, chronic or relapsing symptoms or with neurological signs and symptoms that mimic an acute intervertebral disk prolapse.

Background Information
Epidural bleeding could be the result of a ruptured epidural vein caused by either a sudden increase in intra-abdominal pressure or by mild trauma.[11] Magnetic resonance imaging confirms the diagnosis. An epidural hematoma is a medical emergency that requires surgical management.

■ **Facet Syndrome**

Chief Clinical Characteristics
This presentation includes pain in the lumbar region with referral to the buttocks and upper thigh. The majority of pain referral for the L1–L2 through L4–L5 joints includes the lumbar spinal region. Other referral areas include the gluteal region (L3–L4 to L5–S1), the lateral upper thigh (L2–L3 to L5–S1), and the posterior thigh (L2–L3 to L5–S1).[12]

Background Information
Causes of facet-mediated pain include systemic inflammatory arthritides, microtrauma, and osteoarthritis. The etiology of this condition may include meniscoid entrapment, synovial impingement, joint subluxation, chondromalacia facetiae, capsular and synovial inflammation, mechanical injury to the joint capsule, and restriction of normal articular motion.[13] This diagnosis is confirmed by controlled diagnostic blocks of the joint or its nerve supply.[13] Nonsurgical treatment is a common initial approach to management of this condition.

■ **Leukemia**

Chief Clinical Characteristics
This presentation typically includes lumbopelvic and hip pain, malaise, fatigue, excessive bruising or bleeding, night sweats, and weight loss. Acute disorders have a more rapid onset with illness.[14]

Background Information
Leukemic cells will accumulate in the bone marrow and replace the normal hematopoietic cells, which may then infiltrate any other organ. Acute myelogenous leukemias constitute 85% of adult acute leukemias. Chronic lymphocytic leukemia is responsible for 30% of all leukemias in Western countries and the median age of onset in the seventh decade, whereas acute lymphoblastic leukemia is responsible for 80% of childhood cases.[15] Lower back pain may result from reactive arthritis, as well as metastatic disease. The diagnosis is confirmed with the presence of disabling bone pain, night pain, hematologic findings in the blood tests, leukopenia, or positive findings in a bone marrow biopsy.[16–18]

■ Lumbar Compression Fracture

Chief Clinical Characteristics

This presentation can involve severe debilitating low back pain that is usually worse with walking, as well as other potential sequelae of secondary symptoms.[19]

Background Information

Radiating pain into the leg is highly unlikely with vertebral compression fractures.[20] This condition usually is associated with osteoporotic changes within the vertebral body; usually in the lower thoracic and upper lumbar spine. The loss of vertebral height may lead to reduction in abdominal space with associated loss of appetite and secondary sequelae related to poor nutrition. Most notably, this condition leads to chronic pain with an associated loss of sleep, decreased mobility, and depression.[19] The diagnosis is confirmed with plain radiographs of the spine. Treatment usually includes rest, narcotic analgesics, and spinal orthoses.[19]

LUMBAR RADICULOPATHIES (Fig. 19-1A to E)

■ L1–L3 Radiculopathy

Chief Clinical Characteristics

This presentation typically includes pain in the lumbar spine and paresthesias in the anteromedial aspect of the hip and knee. Depending on severity, the presentation may also include a decreased or absent patellar tendon reflex and motor loss in the muscles innervated by the L2 or L3 nerve. The prone knee bend test may reproduce symptoms.

Background Information

A lumbar disk herniation is the most common cause for this condition; however, compression of the L2 and L3 nerve roots is relatively uncommon. The diagnosis is confirmed with magnetic resonance imaging. Surgical intervention may be indicated in severe cases of lower extremity pain accompanied by neurological signs.

■ L4 Radiculopathy

Chief Clinical Characteristics

This presentation typically includes pain in the lumbar spine and paresthesias radiating from the anterior aspect of the hip, thigh, and knee, sometimes extending anteromedially from the knee to the foot. Depending on the severity, the presentation may also include a decreased or absent patellar tendon reflex and motor loss in the muscles innervated by the L4 nerve. The prone knee bend test may reproduce symptoms.

Background Information

A lumbar disk herniation is the most common cause for this condition. The diagnosis is confirmed with magnetic resonance imaging. Surgical intervention may be indicated in severe cases of lower extremity pain accompanied by neurological signs.

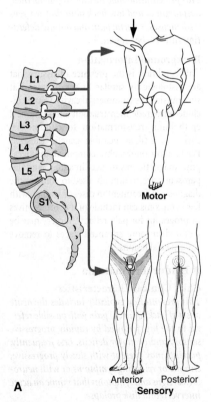

FIGURE 19-1 Lumbar radiculopathy creates characteristic reflex, motor, and sensory findings including (A) L1–L2 radiculopathy;

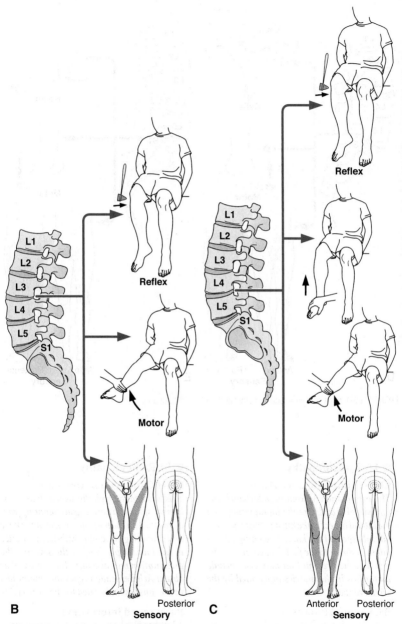

FIGURE 19-1 cont'd (B) L3 radiculopathy; (C) L4 radiculopathy;

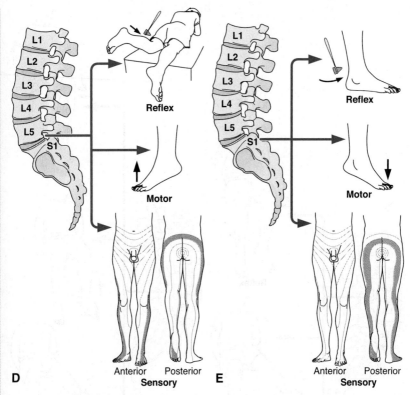

FIGURE 19-1 cont'd (D) L5 radiculopathy; and (E) S1 radiculopathy.

■ L5 Radiculopathy

Chief Clinical Characteristics

This presentation typically includes pain in the lumbar spine and paresthesias radiating from the lateral aspect of the hip and buttock to the lateral aspect of the knee, extending antero-laterally down to the foot. Depending on the severity, the presentation may also include motor loss in the muscles innervated by the L5 nerve root.

Background Information

A lumbar disk herniation is the most common cause for this condition. The diagnosis is confirmed with magnetic resonance imaging. Surgical intervention may be indicated in severe cases of lower extremity pain accompanied by neurological signs.

■ S1 Radiculopathy

Chief Clinical Characteristics

This presentation typically includes pain in the lumbar spine and paresthesias radiating from the buttock to the posterior aspect of the knee and extending posterolaterally from the knee to the foot. Depending on the severity, the presentation may also include a decreased or absent Achilles tendon reflex and motor loss in the muscles innervated by the S1 nerve.

Background Information

A lumbar disk herniation is a common cause for this condition. The diagnosis is confirmed with magnetic resonance imaging. Surgical intervention may be indicated in severe cases of lower extremity pain accompanied by neurological signs.

Osteoblastoma of the Spine

Chief Clinical Characteristics

This presentation typically includes deep and aching pain of insidious onset that is not worse at night, most commonly in males under 30 years of age. Approximately 40% of these tumors are found in the spine, so a number of these lesions may refer pain into the hip region depending on their exact location around the spinal column.

Background Information

Biopsy is necessary to determine the nature of the tumor. Surgical excision is required, particularly in cases that involve neurological signs.

Ovarian Cysts

Chief Clinical Characteristics

This presentation includes ipsilateral pain in the lumbar and thigh region, and the lower quadrant of the abdomen, with possible nausea and vomiting, abnormal vaginal bleeding, and difficulty urinating completely.

Background Information

Ovarian cysts are fluid-filled sacs that develop adjacent to the ovary in the fallopian tube. Most cysts are asymptomatic remnants of normal ovulation.[21] Enlarged cysts may lead to torsion or distention of the fallopian tube. The diagnosis is confirmed with clinical examination and pelvic ultrasonography. Prescribed hormones may be utilized to shrink the cyst. If the cysts persist or symptoms progress, laparoscopic examination is required and surgical removal may be indicated.[22]

Pelvic Inflammatory Disease

Chief Clinical Characteristics

This presentation may involve lumbosacral and hip pain associated with dull, constant, and poorly localized abdominal pain, abnormal vaginal discharge, fever, painful intercourse, and irregular menstrual bleeding.

Background Information

Pelvic inflammatory disease is most prevalent in women between 15 and 23 years of age. Gonorrhea and chlamydia infections of the upper genital tract are common causes. This condition may lead to infertility, ectopic pregnancy, and chronic pelvic pain if left untreated.[23] Blood and urine tests confirm the diagnosis. Treatment typically includes an aggressive course of antibiotic medication.

Prostatitis

Chief Clinical Characteristics

This presentation involves pain in the central lower back, hip, rectal, or perineal region associated with fever, chills, and painful urination. Other initial symptoms may include malaise, arthralgia, and myalgia. As this condition progresses, prostatic inflammation produces dysuria, frequency, urgency, and urine retention.

Background Information

Prostatitis is usually caused by a bacterial infection of the prostate gland, commonly associated with urinary tract infection, urethritis, or epididymitis.[22] Blood and urine tests confirm the diagnosis. Treatment for this condition includes intravenous antibiotics, which are specific to the infecting organism.

Psoas Muscle Abscess

Chief Clinical Characteristics

This presentation involves fever, lateral lumbar or abdominal pain, and limp. The classical triad of symptoms (ie, fever, back pain, and limping) is present in approximately 30% of patients with a psoas abscess.[24] Other symptoms include malaise, weight loss, or presentation with a mass. Physical findings include an externally rotated hip, flank tenderness, and fullness in the lateral lumbar region.

Background Information

Psoas abscesses may be primary, due to hematogenous spread, or secondary due to such pathologies as Crohn's disease, appendicitis, diverticulitis, ulcerative colitis, osteomyelitis, neoplasm, disk infection, renal infections, and trauma.[24,25] Computed tomography of the abdomen with contrast is the most effective imaging study to confirm the diagnosis. Treatment usually begins with a course of antibiotics, with surgical or radiologically guided percutaneous drainage essential to effective treatment.[24,25]

Reiter's Syndrome of the Lumbar Spine

Chief Clinical Characteristics

This presentation can include pain and stiffness in the low back, sacroiliac, and posterior hip regions in the presence of conjunctivitis and urethritis.[26] These patients will have asymmetric distribution of pain between the hips and will most certainly have some form of spinal discomfort associated with this condition.

Background Information

This condition also has been called a reactive arthritis because it may present after other infections. Clinical examination confirms the diagnosis. Symptomatic treatment is used including nonsteroidal anti-inflammatory medications, sulfasalazine, and intra-articular corticosteroid injections.[27]

■ Renal or Urinary Tract Infection

Chief Clinical Characteristics

This presentation may involve pain in the central lower back, flank, and groin, associated with fever, nausea, and vomiting. Other common symptoms include urgent, frequent, and painful urination, abdominal bloating, and pain upon palpation of the kidney.[22] Renal or urinary tract disease may follow streptococcal infection of the upper respiratory tract or skin within 8 to 21 days.[28]

Background Information

Blood and urine tests confirm the diagnosis. Treatment typically includes an appropriate antibiotic medication and possible hospitalization for monitoring.

■ Retrocecal Appendicitis

Chief Clinical Characteristics

This presentation can be characterized by groin, anterior thigh, or lower back pain, associated with fever, nausea, and vomiting. Only mild abdominal symptoms are usually present with this condition because of the retrocecal orientation of the infected appendix.

Background Information

Abdominal computed tomography confirms the diagnosis. This condition involves septic inflammation of the appendix, involving obstruction of the appendix lumen. The end result of this disease process is rupture of contents into the abdominal cavity and the corresponding potential for systemic infection. Therefore, individuals suspected of this condition should be referred to an emergency department for immediate treatment.

■ Retroperitoneal Abscess

Chief Clinical Characteristics

This presentation can include constant groin and low back pain associated with a fever. The patient may choose to rest with the hip in 20 to 30 degrees of flexion to slacken the psoas muscle. Individuals with this condition also may present with quadriceps weakness and decreased knee jerk secondary to compression on the femoral nerve as it courses through the iliopsoas muscle.

Background Information

Magnetic resonance imaging or abdominal computed tomography confirms the diagnosis. Surgical management involving percutaneous drainage may be indicated, and individuals suspected of having this condition should be referred for emergent medical attention due to the high risk for mortality related to systemic infection in individuals with a retroperitoneal abscess.

■ Rheumatoid Arthritis of the Lumbar Spine

Chief Clinical Characteristics

This presentation may involve low back pain that radiates to the hips and lower extremities with positions that involve spinal loading, as well as possible cauda equina symptoms. Leg pain (18%) and leg numbness (14%) have been reported in people with this condition.[29]

Background Information

This condition affects women twice as often as men. Symptoms associated with this progressive inflammatory joint disease are caused by synovial membrane thickening and cytokine production in synovial fluid. Blood tests confirm the diagnosis if rheumatoid factor is detected. Typical radiographic findings include disk space narrowing, facet erosion, and end-plate erosion.[29] A variety of steroidal, nonsteroidal, and biological anti-inflammatory medications have been widely used in the treatment of this condition.[29]

RHEUMATOID ARTHRITIS–LIKE DISEASES OF THE LUMBAR SPINE

■ Inflammatory Bowel Disease

Chief Clinical Characteristics

This presentation may involve abdominal pain, bowel obstruction, weight loss, fever, chronic or nocturnal diarrhea, night sweats, and rectal bleeding, as well as asymmetric and migratory arthralgia/arthritis that may affect the hip. Crampy, intermittent abdominal right lower quadrant pain is common in patients with ileal disease and is exacerbated by eating.[30]

Background Information
Inflammatory bowel disease refers to Crohn's disease and ulcerative colitis.[31] The etiology of these conditions is unclear, but immune system abnormalities seem to cause inflammation of the small intestine. Colonoscopy confirms the diagnosis. Management usually includes use of salicylates, corticosteroids, antibiotics, and immunosuppressants depending on the severity of the pathology.[30]

■ Inflammatory Muscle Diseases

Chief Clinical Characteristics
This presentation includes a gradual onset of mild muscle pain associated with proximal muscle weakness that causes difficulty with daily activities such as walking, ascending and descending stairs, and rising from chairs.

Background Information
This condition describes a group of pathologically, histologically, and clinically distinct disorders: polymyositis, dermatomyositis, and inclusion body myositis. They may be associated with other collagen, vascular, and immune disorders. Although proximal extremity weakness is a classic finding, up to 50% also demonstrate distal weakness that may be equally as severe.[32] Blood panels help confirm the diagnosis and track disease activity, revealing elevated serum levels of creatine phosphokinase. Management usually includes use of salicylates, corticosteroids, antibiotics, and immunosuppressants depending on the severity of the pathology.[30]

■ Psoriatic Arthritis

Chief Clinical Characteristics
This presentation can be characterized by an insidious onset of lumbopelvic and hip pain associated with psoriasis. The severity of arthritis is uncorrelated with the extent of skin involvement.[27] Pitting nail lesions occur in 80% of individuals with this condition.

Dactylitis, tenosynovitis, and peripheral arthritis also are common.

Background Information
Radiographs of the distal phalanges may reveal a characteristic "pencil in cup" deformity. Blood panels including erythrocyte sedimentation rate are useful to track disease activity. Management usually includes use of salicylates, corticosteroids, antibiotics, and immunosuppressants depending on the severity of the pathology.[30]

■ Scleroderma

Chief Clinical Characteristics
This presentation typically includes myalgia, arthralgia, fatigue, weight loss, limited mobility, and hardened skin about the hands, knees, or elbows. This condition occurs in individuals between 25 and 55 years of age, and is four to five times more likely in women than men. Additional symptoms may include dry mouth and eyes, as well as Raynaud's phenomenon.

Background Information
This rare and progressive autoimmune disorder affects blood vessels and many internal organs, including the lungs and the gastrointestinal system. Overproduction of collagen in this condition eventually leads to poor blood flow in the extremities, which can cause ulcers in the fingers, changes in skin color, and a disappearance of creases in the skin. Continued damage to small-diameter vasculature leads to scar tissue production that impairs joint range of motion. Blood tests confirm the diagnosis. Treatment includes both steroidal and nonsteroidal anti-inflammatory medications and gentle exercise.

■ Systemic Lupus Erythematosus

Chief Clinical Characteristics
This presentation may involve low back pain radiating to the hip and groin pain, associated with fatigue and joint pain/swelling affecting the hands, feet, knees, and shoulders.

Background Information
This condition affects mostly women of childbearing age. It is a chronic autoimmune disorder that can affect any organ system, including skin, joints, kidneys, brain, heart,

lungs, and blood. The diagnosis is confirmed by the presence of skin lesions; heart, lung, or kidney involvement; and laboratory abnormalities including low red or white cell counts, low platelet counts, or positive ANA and anti-DNA antibody tests.[33]

■ Septic Arthritis of the Sacroiliac Joint

Chief Clinical Characteristics
This presentation can include an insidious onset of buttock, hip, and groin pain with weight bearing and movement, accompanied by possible fever and malaise. Overlying tissue is usually swollen and inflamed, and this may extend to the anterior and lateral thigh.

Background Information
Septic arthritis of the sacroiliac joint occurs by way of bacterial, yeast, fungal, or viral infection of the hip joint. The infection also can damage articular cartilage, leading to osteoarthritis later in life. Culture of aspirated synovial fluid confirms the diagnosis and directs medical management, which consists of a regimen of antibiotic medication directed to the infective agent.

■ Septic Discitis

Chief Clinical Characteristics
This presentation may include fever, chills, sweats, and intractable lower back pain with possible radiation to the hip or groin, worsened by movement and not easily alleviated even with narcotic analgesia.

Background Information
From most to least common etiology, discitis may occur following spinal surgery during or after an infection, following spine or skin punctures, or spontaneously.[34] The diagnosis is confirmed by aspiration of the affected disk guided by computed tomography. Early diagnosis is critical to prevent infection of the surrounding tissues. Treatment of septic discitis is usually successful with specific intravenous antibiotics and external mobilization; surgery is rarely needed.[35]

■ Spinal Cord Tumor

Chief Clinical Characteristics
This presentation typically includes a long history of insidious back and lower extremity pain that may involve the hip region. Symptoms may include slowly progressive paresis, sensory deficits, and difficulty walking.

Background Information
This condition is rare. However, spinal paragangliomas demonstrate a particular affinity for the cauda equina and filum terminale, so they may cause sciatic symptoms.[36] Biopsy and magnetic resonance imaging confirm the diagnosis. Primary treatment of spinal cord neoplasms includes surgical excision with possible radiotherapy and/or chemotherapy.[37] Treatment of spinal cord tumors causing cauda equina includes immediate surgical decompression.[38]

■ Spinal Stenosis

Chief Clinical Characteristics
This presentation typically involves a prolonged history of low back pain, typically in older individuals, that is aggravated with standing, walking, or other positions of lumbar spinal extension and alleviated with spinal flexion or no weight bearing. Chronic nerve root compression can lead to radicular pain and sensory, motor, and reflex changes in one or both lower extremities, most commonly affecting the L3–L4 and L4–L5 segments.[39] Unilateral or bilateral leg pain is reported in up to 90% of cases with a more recent onset than low back pain, and walking tolerance is often diminished due to neurogenic claudication.[40]

Background Information
Causes of symptoms involve spinal cord and nerve root impingement due to spinal canal narrowing. Plain radiographs and magnetic resonance imaging confirm the diagnosis. Indications for surgery have not been clearly defined and serve as elective procedures to improve quality of life in persons with disabling low back pain.[40] Therefore, nonsurgical options such as physical therapy to improve patient functioning and injections are the initial treatments of choice.

■ Spondylolysis

Chief Clinical Characteristics
This presentation typically includes low back pain with possible radiation to the buttock or proximal lower extremity that is worsened with positions and activities involving spinal extension and rotation. Symptoms may begin

following an acute injury or gradually prior to an initiating event. The neurological examination should be normal.

Background Information

This condition is a defect in the pars interarticularis due to repetitive loading. It is most common in young athletes.[41] This condition can progress to spondylolisthesis, particularly before skeletal maturity.[41] Plain radiographs confirm the diagnosis; computed tomography and magnetic resonance imaging demonstrate higher diagnostic accuracy. Indications for surgical interventions, such as decompressive laminectomy and fusion, include progressive segmental instability, intractable pain, and development of neurological deficits.[41,42]

■ Systemic Fungal Infection of the Lumbar Spine

Chief Clinical Characteristics

This presentation can be characterized by lumbopelvic and hip pain associated with signs of systemic infection, such as fever, anorexia, and malaise. Individuals with this condition may present after a prolonged and varied course of antibiotics to address their symptoms.

Background Information

This condition is most common in immune-compromised individuals, such as patients in intensive care, patients receiving chemotherapy, patients with acquired immunodeficiency syndrome, and transplant recipients. This condition is most commonly due to *Candida* species infection, although *Aspergillus* also may be a culprit organism. The infection is transferred from health care worker to patient by way of hand contact. Serum pathology and molecular techniques confirm the diagnosis and direct appropriate pharmacologic management.[43]

■ Traumatic Spondylolisthesis

Chief Clinical Characteristics

This presentation can be characterized by low back pain following severe trauma with possible radiation to the thigh depending on affected level, neurological deficits, and cauda equina syndrome.[44]

Background Information

Local tenderness, swelling, and a palpable step-off between L5 and S1 are reported. Radiographic findings for diagnosis can include dislocated and locked facets with the inferior facets of L5 anterior to the S1 facets. Traumatic spondylolisthesis is considered rare and may occur following extreme hyperflexion, axial rotation, and compression forces. Surgical treatment may be warranted due to the frank instability of the injury.[44]

■ Tuberculosis of the Lumbar Spine (Pott's Disease)

Chief Clinical Characteristics

This presentation involves insidious onset of stiffness with pain over the involved vertebrae radiating into the buttock or lower extremity, low-grade fever, chills, weight loss, and nonspecific constitutional symptoms of varying duration.[45] Weakness, nerve root compression, and sensory involvement can be present to varying degrees.

Background Information

This condition usually results from the spread of a pulmonary or other primary infection involving *Mycobacterium tuberculosis*. If the disease affects one vertebral body, the intervertebral disk may be spared. However, collapse of the affected segment could occur due to impaired disk nutrition. Magnetic resonance imaging confirms the diagnosis. Treatment consists of antituberculosis medications, which are effective 90% of the time, or surgery in more advanced cases.[46]

■ Uterine Fibroids

Chief Clinical Characteristics

This presentation typically includes pelvic pain and pressure, with possible neurogenic pain in the thighs and lower legs due to impingement of the lumbosacral plexus. Symptoms and signs also may include abdominal distention, palpable evidence of a pelvic mass, heavy prolonged menstrual cycles, bladder pressure leading to constant urinary urgency, and constipation or bloating due to pressure on the bowels.[47]

Background Information

These are common benign tumors that develop in the muscular walls of the uterus. First detection usually occurs during routine gynecological examination since most are asymptomatic. Abdominal ultrasound confirms the diagnosis. If the fibroids are large enough to cause significant symptoms, treatment options will include surgical embolization or resection (myomectomy), as well as hysterectomy in severe cases.[47]

Local

■ Ankylosing Spondylitis

Chief Clinical Characteristics
This presentation may involve an insidious on-set of low back and symmetric posterior hip pain associated with a slowly progressive and significant loss of general spinal mobility.

Background Information
Symptoms may be worse in the morning and improve with light exercise. This condition is more common in males, as well as people of American indigenous descent, less than 40 years of age, or who carry the human leukocyte antigen B27.[51] It also may be associated with fever, malaise, and inflammatory bowel disease. The diagnosis is confirmed with plain radiographs of the sacroiliac joints and lumbar spine, which reveal characteristic findings of sacroiliitis and "bamboo spine." Blood panels including erythrocyte sedimentation rate are useful to track disease activity. Treatment typically includes a combination of steroidal, nonsteroidal, and biological anti-inflammatory medications combined with physical therapy to address postural and movement considerations associated with changing spinal position.

■ Avascular Necrosis of the Hip

Chief Clinical Characteristics
This presentation typically includes insidious onset of groin and anterolateral thigh pain.

Background Information
This condition may be associated with sickle cell anemia, femoral head or neck trauma, Gaucher's disease, alcoholism, Caisson disease, prolonged steroid use, irradiation, or pregnancy.[48] It is characterized by articular collapse of subchondral bone due to a lack of blood supply. The femoral head is most likely to be involved. Up to 20% of individuals with this condition have bilateral disease. Plain radiographs confirm the diagnosis, but early detection is difficult. Surgical decompression is typically performed to facilitate revascularization of the femoral head. Hemiarthroplasty may be considered if subchondral bone loss is extensive and the articular collapse is significant.

■ Brucellosis of the Hip

Chief Clinical Characteristics
This presentation can be characterized by a gradual onset of nonspecific myalgias, fever, malaise, and generalized hip or sacroiliac joint pain.

Background Information
This uncommon condition in the United States results from ingestion of bacteria that is found in nonpasteurized milk or other infected animal products. It is associated with sacroiliac joint effusions that produce some arthritic changes over time if left untreated. Treatment includes antibiotics.

BURSITIS

■ Ischiogluteal Bursitis

Chief Clinical Characteristics
This presentation typically includes traumatic or insidious onset of pain over the ischial tuberosity with possible radiation to the posterior thigh, worsened with palpation, active hip extension, and sitting. This uncommon condition may be worsened with hip motion, so the hip joint is sometimes erroneously implicated as the source of symptoms.

Background Information
Ischiogluteal bursitis can result from a direct injury to the bursa or from sitting for prolonged periods on hard surfaces. Inflammation of the bursa between the ischial tuberosity and proximal hamstrings causes this condition. Clinical examination confirms the diagnosis with additional certainty provided by magnetic resonance imaging. This condition is treated nonsurgically.

■ Trochanteric Bursitis

Chief Clinical Characteristics
This presentation typically involves an insidious onset of lateral hip, thigh, and buttock pain that is worsened with palpation, weight-bearing activities, laying on the involved side, and active/resisted hip abduction. Individuals with this condition may note improvement initially with walking, but return as they continue to walk. Symptoms from this condition may

radiate as far distally as the knee, and may be associated with crepitus over the greater trochanter with hip motion.

Background Information
Clinical examination confirms the diagnosis. This condition is treated nonsurgically.

■ Cellulitis

Chief Clinical Characteristics
This presentation typically includes lateral hip and thigh pain, associated with pain during activities involving compression of the superficial tissues, as well as redness and warmth of the affected region.

Background Information
Individuals with this condition may have a low-grade fever, and complete blood count may show an elevated white blood cell count. Individuals following hip surgery are at particular risk of developing this condition. Symptoms related to this condition may cause increasing difficulty with muscle activation about the hip, resulting in limited functional activities.[49] Clinical examination confirms the diagnosis. Treatment involves oral antibiotics and observation to ensure that the underlying infection does not spread to adjacent tissues.

■ Complex Regional Pain Syndrome

Chief Clinical Characteristics
This presentation may include a traumatic onset of severe chronic lower back pain accompanied by allodynia and hyperalgesia, as well as trophic, vasomotor, and sudomotor changes in later stages.

Background Information
This condition is characterized by disproportionate responses to painful stimuli. It is a regional neuropathic pain disorder that presents either without direct nerve trauma (Type I) or with direct nerve trauma (Type II) in any region of the body.[50] This condition may precipitate due to an event distant to the affected area. Thermography may confirm associated sympathetic dysfunction. Treatment may include physical therapy interventions to improve patient and client functioning, biofeedback, analgesic or anti-inflammatory medication, transcutaneous or spinal electrical nerve stimulation, and surgical or pharmacologic sympathectomy.

■ Fibromyalgia

Chief Clinical Characteristics
This presentation involves chronic widespread joint and muscle pain defined as bilateral upper body, lower body, and spine pain, associated with tenderness to palpating 11 of 18 specific muscle-tendon sites.

Background Information
Individuals with this condition will demonstrate lowered mechanical and thermal pain thresholds, high pain ratings for noxious stimuli, and altered temporal summation of pain stimuli.[51] The etiology of this condition is unclear; multiple body systems appear to be involved. Indistinct clinical boundaries between this condition and similar conditions (eg, chronic fatigue syndrome, irritable bowel syndrome, and chronic muscular headaches) pose a diagnostic challenge.[51] This condition is diagnosed by exclusion. Treatment will often include polypharmacy and elements to improve self-efficacy, physical training, and cognitive-behavioral techniques.[52]

FRACTURES (Fig. 19-2)

■ Acetabular Fracture

Chief Clinical Characteristics
This presentation can be characterized by constant pain in the groin and thigh region with an acute inability to weight bear through the pelvis or affected limb.

Background Information
This condition results from acute, high-energy trauma involving axial loading of the femur. The direction and magnitude of the force and position of the femoral head at impact determine the pattern of injury. Urethral, uterine, and vaginal ruptures should be considered, although bladder injury and clinically significant pelvic hemorrhage are not routinely observed in individuals with acetabular fracture unless a concomitant pelvic ring injury is present. Concomitant pelvic ring and extremity fractures are common. Plain radiographs confirm the diagnosis. The treatments for these fractures are initially directed at stabilization of fracture segments, eventually leading to restoration of normal movement.[53]

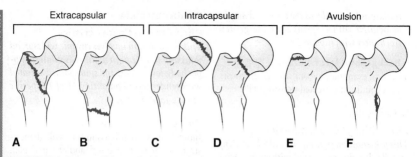

FIGURE 19-2 Fractures of the proximal femur and pelvis include (A) intertrochanteric fracture; (B) subtrochanteric fracture; (C) femoral head fracture; (D) femoral neck fracture; (E) avulsion of sartorius or rectis femoris off the anterior superior iliac spine; and (F) avulsion of hamstrings off the ischial tuberosity.

AVULSION FRACTURES

■ Hamstrings Off Ischial Tuberosity

Chief Clinical Characteristics
This presentation can involve a traumatic onset of pain in the buttock with possible radiation to the posterior thigh. Pain is worsened with sitting and resisted hip extension.

Background Information
This condition is more common in younger individuals, resulting from a sudden application of great muscular force to the ischial apophysis. The diagnosis is confirmed with plain radiographs that also are used to assess the displacement of fracture segments.

■ Rectus Femoris Off Anterior Inferior Iliac Spine

Chief Clinical Characteristics
This presentation involves groin and proximal medial thigh pain, swelling, and tenderness following acute trauma.

Background Information
These fractures are more common in younger individuals participating in high-speed activities due to the relative strength of tendons with respect to their attachment sites in this age group. Radiographs confirm the diagnosis, usually revealing minimal displacement of fracture fragments due to the strength of the surrounding periosteum. Stable injuries may be managed nonoperatively, although surgical treatment may be indicated to repair the avulsed segments if there is significant displacement.

■ Sartorius Off Anterior Superior Iliac Spine

Chief Clinical Characteristics
This presentation may include groin and proximal medial thigh pain, swelling, and tenderness following acute trauma.

Background Information
These fractures are more common in younger individuals participating in high-speed activities due to the relative strength of tendons with respect to their attachment sites in this age group. Radiographs confirm the diagnosis, usually revealing minimal displacement of fracture fragments due to the strength of the surrounding periosteum. Stable injuries may be managed nonoperatively, although surgical treatment may be indicated to repair the avulsed segments if there is significant displacement.

■ Extracapsular Femur Fracture

Chief Clinical Characteristics
This presentation can be characterized by a traumatic onset of constant anterior, anterior medial, or anterior lateral thigh region pain associated with an acute inability to bear weight or move the affected limb. Extracapsular fractures include intertrochanteric and femoral shaft fractures.

Background Information
This condition is often associated with bleeding into the soft tissues surrounding the fracture site. This blood accumulation is a potential source of infection.[54] Individuals suspected of having this condition should

receive a clinical neurovascular examination, because the associated swelling may cause compartment syndrome. Plain radiographs confirm the diagnosis. Surgical stabilization of fracture segments may be necessary.

■ Femoral Shaft Fracture

Chief Clinical Characteristics
This presentation typically includes a traumatic onset of severe circumferential pain and swelling about the femur over the fracture site. Characteristic symptoms include dull pain at rest, worsening with bearing weight, active motion, and passive motion. Hip and knee range of motion also may be limited as a protective response.

Background Information
Plain radiographs confirm the diagnosis. Immediate treatment for this condition includes immobilization of the extremity by a fracture brace or cast.

■ Intracapsular Femur Fracture

Chief Clinical Characteristics
This presentation may involve constant pain in the hip region following acute trauma. Pain is worsened with weight bearing or hip range of motion in any direction (see Fig. 19-2). The femur is often positioned in excessive internal or external rotation. There is also shortening of the limb.

Background Information
These fractures are usually associated with high-energy forces in normal bone (eg, a fall from height) or low-energy forces in pathological bone (eg, osteoporosis). Displaced fractures may disturb the nearby neurovascular bundle; patients suspected of this condition should be screened for distal neurological signs. Surgical treatment is aimed at anatomical reduction and ensuring stability of the fracture segment, as well as the decompression of the nerve if necessary.

■ Stress Fracture of the Femoral Neck

Chief Clinical Characteristics
This presentation typically includes an insidious onset of deep groin pain that may radiate to the knee. Symptoms are worsened with standing, walking, running, and at night; they usually are present over an extended period of time. Early stress fractures may cause only a minimal loss of hip range of motion and limping often is absent.

Background Information
Diagnostic delay may lead to fracture displacement. Therefore, individuals who report acute changes in training intensity and volume or pathology that weakens bone should be suspected of this condition. Bone scan and plain radiographs confirm the diagnosis. This condition is managed nonsurgically.

■ Gluteal Contusion

Chief Clinical Characteristics
This presentation includes a traumatic onset of ecchymosis and pain that is worsened with sitting, resisted hip extension, and activities that engage the gluteal musculature.

Background Information
Individuals competing in sports and working industrial jobs are at elevated risk. This condition occurs when capillaries in the affected musculature rupture due to blunt trauma. Clinical examination confirms the diagnosis. Treatment for this condition is usually nonsurgical, involving relative rest, protective padding or bracing, gentle exercise, and physical modalities.

■ Gout

Chief Clinical Characteristics
This presentation involves a sudden onset of deep stabbing pain in the hip joint. Pain is worsened with weight bearing and is associated with tenderness, warmth, and erythema of the superficial tissues.

Background Information
Increased prevalence is associated with advanced age, male sex, and alcohol consumption on a regular basis. This condition is less common in the hip. It is caused by a metabolic defect that results in overproduction of uric acid or a reduced ability to eliminate uric acid, allowing urate crystal deposition in affected joints. Blood tests or microscopic examination of aspirated synovial fluid confirms the diagnosis. Treatment usually involves anti-inflammatory medication and diet changes to address this condition's underlying metabolic dysfunction.

Greater Saphenous Vein Thrombophlebitis

Chief Clinical Characteristics

This presentation may be characterized by pain in the medial thigh along the course of the greater saphenous vein, which also may be associated with palpation of a tender cord-like band along its length. Generally, the range of motion of the hip joint or knee is not affected.

Background Information

The etiology of this condition is associated with Virchow's triad of intimal damage, stasis, or changes in blood composition.[55] Genetic predisposition also may cause elevated risk. Computed tomography, magnetic resonance angiography, and Doppler ultrasonography confirm the diagnosis. This condition is a medical emergency because the underlying thrombus may propagate proximally and cause pulmonary embolism.

HERNIAS

Femoral Hernia

Chief Clinical Characteristics

This presentation includes groin pain associated with a grape-sized lump, frequent constipation, and discomfort with rising to a standing position, coughing, and pushing heavy loads.

Background Information

This condition is more common in women than men. It is characterized by escape of the large bowel through a weakened portion of abdominal wall at the femoral canal. Discomfort also may be exacerbated with end range motion of the hip into full flexion or extension. For this reason, patients may relate their discomfort to a musculoskeletal problem. Treatment involves surgical repair of the contributing abdominal wall defect.

Inguinal Hernia

Chief Clinical Characteristics

This presentation typically may involve groin pain with a reducible lump, possibly worsened by activities that involve sprinting and direction change.

Background Information

Inguinal hernias are more common in men than women, and this herniation can also extend into the scrotum in males. This condition is a herniation of a portion of the intestines through a weakening in the abdominal wall at the site of the inguinal canal. Risk factors for developing this disorder include a parent or sibling with a hernia, chronic cough, and developmental dysplasia of the hip. Treatment involves surgical repair of the contributing abdominal wall defect.

Sports Hernia

Chief Clinical Characteristics

This presentation can involve an insidious onset of deep chronic groin pain that radiates along the inguinal ligament, perineum, rectus abdominis, and adductors. Symptoms are worsened with endurance running, kicking, coughing, sneezing, and the Valsalva maneuver.[56] *Physical findings include tenderness along the external ring and posterior wall of the inguinal canal, as well as spasm of the surrounding musculature. Testicular pain may be present in males, making testicular pathology an important differential diagnosis.*

Background Information

This condition is caused by weakness of the posterior inguinal wall. The diagnosis is confirmed with herniography due to the absence of classic palpation findings for hernia. Treatment involves surgical repair of the contributing abdominal wall defect.

Herpes Zoster

Chief Clinical Characteristics

This presentation typically includes an exquisitely painful rash or blisters along a specific dermatomal pattern accompanied by flu-like symptoms. Individuals with this condition also demonstrate a previous history of varicella exposure or infection. Pain associated with this condition may be disproportionate to the extent of skin irritation. The initial presentation of this condition may be confused with radiculopathy due to the distribution of symptoms. The presence of the rash, extreme pain, general malaise, and an unclear association with spinal movement aids in differential diagnosis.

Background Information

The virus remains dormant in the spinal ganglia until its reactivation during a period of stress, infection, or physical exhaustion.

Treatment includes the administration of antiviral agents as soon as the zoster eruption is noted, ideally within 48 to 72 hours. If timing is greater than 3 days, treatment is aimed at controlling pain and pruritus and minimizing the risk of secondary infection.[57]

■ Heterotopic Ossification

Chief Clinical Characteristics
This presentation can be characterized by groin and lateral hip pain with active and passive movement, associated with decreased hip range of motion, reduced flexibility of the associated musculature, and progressively firmer palpable mass.

Background Information
The palpable mass associated with this condition gradually becomes less tender and smaller, but its density increases. It develops as a result of direct soft tissue trauma (eg, blunt force or total hip arthroplasty) or in association with various central nervous system disorders (eg, traumatic brain injury, spinal cord injury, poliomyelitis, or Guillain-Barré syndrome). A previous history of this condition predisposes individuals to future occurrence. This condition involves abnormal bone formation within extraskeletal tissues.[58] Radiographs confirm the diagnosis. Surgical resection of heterotopic bone is associated with a high recurrence rate for this condition, but the surgery results in reestablishing joint range of motion and soft tissue flexibility.

■ Hip Dislocation

Chief Clinical Characteristics
This presentation typically includes extreme pain with weight bearing and range of motion of the affected hip, as well as shortening of the affected lower extremity following a traumatic event and extreme pain. Individuals with hip dislocation will present with an acute inability to walk or weight bear due to debilitating pain. They also may demonstrate external rotation of the affected lower extremity.

Background Information
This condition involves escape of the femoral head from the acetabulum, usually in a superior-posterior direction, due to a variety of acquired factors (eg, trauma) or congenital factors (eg, developmental dysplasia of the hip). The affected limb's shortened appearance is due to the proximal migration of the dislocated femoral head. Individuals suspected of this condition should be screened for neurovascular involvement, because the dislocated femoral head often compresses the sciatic nerve. This condition is a medical emergency.

■ Hip Osteoarthrosis/Osteoarthritis

Chief Clinical Characteristics
This presentation typically includes medial, anterior, or lateral hip pain that may refer to the anteromedial thigh, characterized by increased pain at end ranges of passive hip abduction and extension, and limping. This condition is the most common cause of hip pain in people older than 50 years of age.[59] It may be related to a prior injury or begin insidiously over the course of many months or years.

Background Information
This condition involves degeneration of the articular cartilage of the femoral head and acetabulum. Radiographs confirm the diagnosis, typically revealing a loss of joint space, osteophytes, and subchondral bone cysts. Treatment in mild to moderate stages involves lifestyle modification, exercises to maintain joint flexibility and strength, oral anti-inflammatory medication, and corticosteroid injections. In cases of severe pain and functional limitation, total joint arthroplasty is considered.

■ Iliac Artery Aneurysm

Chief Clinical Characteristics
This presentation typically includes lower back, abdominal, or groin pain with a pulsatile mass. Other symptoms may include lower extremity ischemia and erythema nodosum.

Background Information
This rare condition is more common in men than women.[60] It usually involves a defect in the wall of the common iliac artery. This condition occurs when the tunica intima, tunica media, or tunica adventitia becomes structurally compromised due to various acquired factors (eg, hypertension, cigarette smoking) or congenital factors (eg, Marfan's syndrome). Risk factors include arteriosclerosis, infection, lumbar or hip surgical trauma, and pregnancy. Computed tomography or magnetic resonance angiography confirm the

diagnosis. Elective open repair of the aneurysm is considered when the risk of rupture exceeds that of surgery.[2]

Iliac Crest Apophysitis

Chief Clinical Characteristics

This presentation typically includes pain over the lateral ilium with active movement and resisted abduction of the affected hip, as well as tenderness to palpation.

Background Information

This condition is more common in active, skeletally immature individuals.[61] It occurs after a sudden contraction of the abdominal muscles is opposed by simultaneous contraction of the gluteus medius and tensor fascia latae. Constant traction on the insertion site can lead to a chronic soreness of the lateral ilium. This condition is managed nonsurgically with relative rest, gentle exercise, and physical modalities.

Iliofemoral Venous Thrombosis

Chief Clinical Characteristics

This presentation typically includes an insidious onset of pain extending distal to the lesion, accompanied by diminished pulses and swelling in the affected lower extremity.

Background Information

Genetic predisposition may cause elevated risk. This condition also may manifest itself in pregnant women due to compression of the iliac vein. In addition, a history of malignancy or prior thrombosis increases the risk for this condition. The etiology of this condition is associated with Virchow's triad of intimal damage, stasis, and changes in blood composition.[55] Computed tomography, magnetic resonance angiography, and Doppler ultrasonography confirm the diagnosis. It is a medical emergency because of the risk for propagation of the thrombus to the lungs.

Iliopsoas Abscess

Chief Clinical Characteristics

This presentation typically includes hip, lateral lumbar, or abdominal pain with fever and limping.[25] Hip pain is present in approximately 29% of individuals with this condition.[62] Physical findings include an externally rotated hip, flank tenderness, and fullness in the lateral lumbar region. Other symptoms may include malaise, weight loss, or palpable mass.

Background Information

Primary iliopsoas abscesses mainly result from staphylococcal infections. Secondary abscesses may result from Crohn's disease, appendicitis, diverticulitis, ulcerative colitis, osteomyelitis, neoplasm, disk infection, renal infections, and trauma.[25,62] Abdominal computed tomography confirms the diagnosis. Treatment involves eliminating the underlying infection through medication or surgical debridement.

Iliopsoas Tendinitis

Chief Clinical Characteristics

This presentation includes deep groin or anteromedial thigh pain, worsened with resisted hip flexion, passive internal rotation during extension of the affected hip, and palpation of the iliopsoas muscle. The tenderness of the iliopsoas tendon may be palpated lateral to the femoral artery, inferior to the inguinal ligament in the femoral triangle.

Background Information

Both acute and repetitive trauma may contribute; overuse is the classic cause. Acute tendon inflammation may cause snapping or clicking during hip motion.[63] Clinical examination confirms the diagnosis. This condition is typically managed nonsurgically.

Iliopsoas Tendinosis

Chief Clinical Characteristics

This presentation includes deep groin or anteromedial thigh pain, worsened with resisted hip flexion, passive internal rotation during extension of the affected hip, and palpation of the iliopsoas muscle. The tenderness of the iliopsoas tendon may be palpated lateral to the femoral artery, inferior to the inguinal ligament in the femoral triangle.

Background Information

Both acute and repetitive trauma may contribute; overuse is the classic cause. Tendinosis involves disorganization of the intratendinous collagen matrix and angiofibroblastic hyperplasia.[64] Clinical examination confirms the diagnosis. This condition is typically managed nonsurgically.

■ Iliotibial Band Friction Syndrome

Chief Clinical Characteristics

This presentation may involve an insidious onset of sharp, burning lateral hip and thigh pain extending from the greater trochanter to the lateral femoral condyle.

Background Information

This condition may be associated with snapping during hip motion and significant tenderness to palpation of the iliotibial band. The etiology of this condition involves chronic overuse. It may be associated with a positive Ober test, although this finding itself is not pathognomic. Clinical examination confirms the diagnosis. This condition is typically managed nonsurgically.

■ Labral Tear

Chief Clinical Characteristics

This presentation involves either insidious or traumatic onset of stabbing hip and groin pain, worsened with weight bearing and associated with a global decrease in hip range of motion. This condition may be associated with a painful clunk or snapping with hip passive range of motion.

Background Information

Labral tears may lead to joint instability, leading some patients to report insecurity with their hip. Magnetic resonance imaging and therapeutic cortisone injections may confirm the diagnosis. Treatment includes both surgical[65] and nonoperative strategies, such as corticosteroid injections and physical therapy.

■ Metastases, Including From Primary Breast, Kidney, Lung, Prostate, and Thyroid Disease

Chief Clinical Characteristics

This presentation can be characterized by unremitting pain in individuals with these risk factors: previous history of cancer, age 50 years or older, failure to improve with conservative therapy, and unexplained weight change of more than 10 pounds in 6 months.[66]

Background Information

Cauda equina symptoms or nerve root compression of the spinal canal can be caused by vertebral collapse or infiltration of the tumor.[67] The skeletal system is the third most common site of metastatic disease; lumbar metastases account for 20% of cases.[68] Symptoms also may be related to pathological fracture in affected sites. Common primary sites causing metastases to bone include breast, prostate, lung, and kidney. Bone scan confirms the diagnosis. Common treatments for metastases include surgical resection, chemotherapy, radiation treatment, and palliation, depending on the tumor type and extent of metastasis.

MUSCLE STRAINS

■ Adductor Strain

Chief Clinical Characteristics

This presentation may include pain in the medial thigh and proximally to the area of the pubic symphysis. This condition is common among athletes who participate in sports requiring high-speed changes in direction. Adductor strains are characterized by pain with palpation of the affected muscle and pain with resisted adduction.

Background Information

Radiographs can exclude fractures or avulsions. The usual treatment for this condition is nonsurgical.

■ Hamstring Strain

Chief Clinical Characteristics

This presentation can include an acute onset of posterior thigh pain that is worsened with resisted action and stretch of the affected muscle.

Background Information

This condition is often associated with active overlengthening or eccentric contraction, as in acceleration and deceleration while sprinting. Palpation reproduces symptoms. Tissue edema may cause associated fullness and ecchymosis may be present in the posterior thigh. Radiographs may help exclude avulsion fractures. Usual treatment for this condition is nonsurgical.

■ Iliopsoas Strain

Chief Clinical Characteristics

This presentation may involve aching, throbbing groin pain with active movement and a preference toward passive positioning of the hip in flexion to slacken the iliopsoas. Deep palpation of the femoral triangle and passive hip extension stretching reproduce symptoms. A "snapping" sensation is associated with pain in 30% of cases.

Background Information
Iliopsoas strains may occur due to acute or repetitive trauma.[69] Usual treatment for this condition is nonsurgical.

■ Quadriceps Muscle Strain

Chief Clinical Characteristics
This presentation typically includes quadriceps muscle pain that is worsened with weight-bearing activities, palpation, acute stretch, and repeated eccentric muscular contractions. Symptoms are often reproduced with active knee extension and active or passive knee flexion.

Background Information
This condition is often associated with active overlengthening or eccentric contraction, as in acceleration and deceleration while sprinting. Tissue edema may cause associated fullness, and ecchymosis may be present. Clinical examination confirms the diagnosis. Usual treatment for this condition is nonsurgical.

■ Myositis Ossificans

Chief Clinical Characteristics
This presentation involves thigh or gluteal pain at the specific site of a prior trauma, associated with reduced hip flexibility and a tender, firm, somewhat mobile mass within the affected muscle belly.

Background Information
This condition results from abnormal bone growth within a hematoma in the soft tissues. Radiographs confirm the diagnosis 6 weeks after onset by showing centripetal ossification of a hematoma. Surgical resection of heterotopic bone is associated with a high recurrence rate for this condition, but the surgery results in reestablishing joint range of motion and soft tissue flexibility.

NERVE ENTRAPMENTS/ NEUROPATHY

■ Femoral Neuropathy

Chief Clinical Characteristics
This presentation typically includes a traumatic or insidious onset of anterior thigh or groin pain associated with quadriceps weakness, limited knee jerk, and intact sensation in the affected region.

Background Information
This condition may be associated with proximal compression of the femoral nerve due to contact with surgical instruments or development of a retroperitoneal hematoma due to intra-abdominal or lumbar surgery. Electromyographic studies may confirm the diagnosis. This condition is typically managed nonsurgically, and surgical intervention is reserved for cases in which the exact anatomical location of the entrapment has been identified.

■ Genitofemoral Nerve Entrapment

Chief Clinical Characteristics
This presentation typically involves burning medial thigh pain that radiates to the scrotum or labia majora and is worsened with hip extension and associated with tenderness over the inguinal canal. This condition most commonly presents after lower abdominal surgery. It is commonly mistaken for hernia, upper lumbar radiculopathy, or ilioinguinal nerve entrapment. The cremasteric reflex and perineal sensation may be absent.

Background Information
Selective nerve blocks confirm this diagnosis.[70] This condition is typically managed nonsurgically, and surgical intervention is reserved for cases in which the exact anatomical location of the entrapment has been identified.

■ Iliohypogastric Nerve Entrapment

Chief Clinical Characteristics
This presentation involves onset of burning inguinal and suprapubic pain with radiation to the genitals following lower abdominal surgery. Palpation of the surgical scar reproduces symptoms. Sensation loss is usually minimal.

Background Information
Selective nerve blocks confirm this diagnosis.[71] This condition is typically managed nonoperatively, and surgical intervention is reserved for cases in which the exact

anatomical location of the entrapment has been identified.

■ Ilioinguinal Nerve Entrapment

Chief Clinical Characteristics

This presentation may be characterized by an insidious onset of burning pain in the medial thigh that radiates to the scrotum or labia majora and is worsened with standing erect and hip motion. Abdominal surgery, pregnancy, and asphericity of the femoral head are risk factors for developing this condition. Palpation medial to the anterior superior iliac spine reproduces symptoms. Transversalis and internal oblique paralysis may be present, causing a small abdominal bulge that may be confused with a hernia. Perineal sensory loss also may be present.

Background Information

Selective nerve blocks confirm this diagnosis.[70] This condition is typically managed nonoperatively, and surgical intervention is reserved for cases in which the exact anatomical location of the entrapment has been identified.

■ Meralgia Paresthetica

Chief Clinical Characteristics

This presentation can involve unilateral proximal lateral thigh pain and numbness, which is relieved with sitting and worsened with standing and walking. Tapping over the inguinal ligament or moving the hip into extension may also provoke the symptoms.

Background Information

Focal compression of the lateral femoral cutaneous nerve as it passes beneath the inguinal ligament most commonly causes this condition. Pregnancy, obesity, diabetes, and tight-fitting clothes are among risk factors. Less frequently, this condition may be caused by blunt trauma, ischemia, or traction.[72] Clinical examination and electrodiagnostic studies confirm the diagnosis. Treatment for this condition includes removing the cause of the compression, which can include alteration of clothing as well as weight loss. In more severe cases, nerve blocks or surgical decompression may be warranted.

■ Obturator Nerve Entrapment

Chief Clinical Characteristics

This presentation may include unilateral medial thigh pain and paresthesias, worsened with hip abduction or extension, and is associated with hip adductor weakness. Individuals with this condition may walk with a wide-based gait. Sensory loss may extend from the midportion of the medial thigh to the region distal to the knee. Medial thigh wasting may be present, and the hip adductor tendon reflex may be absent.

Background Information

Electromyography confirms the diagnosis.[73] This condition is typically managed nonoperatively, and surgical intervention is reserved for cases in which the exact anatomical location of the entrapment has been identified.

■ Piriformis Syndrome

Chief Clinical Characteristics

This presentation can include traumatic or insidious onset of dull buttock pain with radiation to the posterior thigh. This condition may be associated with limping and painful weakness of hip musculature during resisted testing. Palpation over the muscle and sciatic notch usually results in symptom reproduction, as well as active and passive hip external rotation.

Background Information

Radiating pain is caused by compression of the sciatic nerve by the inflamed piriformis. Clinical examination confirms the diagnosis. This condition is typically managed nonsurgically, and surgical intervention is reserved for severe cases in which certainty regarding the role of the piriformis as a site of compression has been determined to be high.

■ Osteitis Pubis

Chief Clinical Characteristics

This presentation may involve a traumatic or insidious onset of lower abdominal and suprapubic pain that is worsened with walking and hip abduction.

Background Information

Individuals presenting with this condition may demonstrate a wide-based gait. This condition involves inflammation of the pubic symphysis following trauma, pelvic surgery, childbirth, or athletic overuse injuries. Its etiology is unclear. The diagnosis is confirmed with plain radiographs and technetium scan.[74] This condition is managed nonsurgically with activity modification and gentle exercise. Surgical intervention, including open reduction and internal fixation of the pubic symphysis, are typically reserved for more active individuals and individuals with recalcitrant symptoms that fail to respond to nonsurgical interventions.

■ Osteoblastoma of the Hip

Chief Clinical Characteristics

This presentation can involve an insidious onset of deep and aching pain, typically in males under 30 years of age. Pain associated with this condition is not usually worse at night. This condition may rarely affect the pelvic bones, and the proximal femoral epiphysis is even less commonly affected.

Background Information

This condition involves abnormal production of osteoid and primitive bone, although its specific etiology remains unclear. Biopsy and plain radiographs confirm the diagnosis. Computed tomography is necessary to define the tumor margins if surgical resection is considered.

■ Osteochondroma

Chief Clinical Characteristics

This presentation can be characterized by bone and joint pain that is usually only present when the lesion is mechanically stressed, typically in males less than 20 years of age.

Background Information

This condition is asymptomatic in most cases. It can arise in any bone that undergoes enchondral ossification, but is most common around the knee. Plain radiographs typically demonstrate bony projections from the areas adjacent to growth plates. Treatment includes surgical excision only with significant and persistent soft tissue irritation. If left untreated, lesions usually do not metastasize but can continue to grow.

■ Osteoid Osteoma

Chief Clinical Characteristics

This presentation may include focal bone pain at the site of the tumor that is associated with

tenderness and warmth to palpation, with significant increase in pain with activity and at night, and with substantial and immediate relief of pain with anti-inflammatory medication. This condition is more common in males than females, and it rarely presents in people younger than 5 or older than 40 years of age.

Background Information

The pathology of osteoid osteomas includes abnormal production of osteoid and primitive bone. The proximal femur is the most common site for this tumor. Pain associated with this condition is self-limiting and may resolve spontaneously over the course of 2 to 4 years.[75]

■ Osteomalacia

Chief Clinical Characteristics

This presentation can involve diffuse bone pain about the hip joint, associated with fatigue, malaise, generalized bone pain, fractures due to minor trauma, and possible joint deformity.

Background Information

This condition is analogous to rickets in children. It involves bone demineralization due to inadequate dietary intake of vitamin D, malabsorption of vitamin D by the intestines, inadequate exposure to the sunlight, renal deficiencies, and chronic use of anticonvulsant medications. Radiographs and laboratory tests help confirm the diagnosis, revealing decreased mineralization of bone and low phosphorous level, respectively. Treatment typically includes amelioration of contributing factors, including diet modification and vitamin D supplementation.

■ Pigmented Villonodular Synovitis

Chief Clinical Characteristics

This presentation can include an insidious onset of mild discomfort and stiffness of the affected hip that is relieved by positioning the hip in passive hip flexion and external rotation. This condition usually presents unilaterally.

Background Information

Pigmented villonodular synovitis is a rare, benign, idiopathic disorder of the synovium that results in villous (nodular) formation in joints, tendon sheaths, and bursae. This condition progresses slowly, although its long-term presence in the hip can result in femoral head erosions that lead to a degenerative condition.[76] Clinical imaging confirms the diagnosis. Treatment includes synovectomy and subsequent radiation therapy.

■ Polymyalgia Rheumatica

Chief Clinical Characteristics

This presentation typically includes the acute onset of proximal myalgias and stiffness involving the neck, shoulders, pelvic girdle, and hips that is worse at night and with movement and associated with fatigue, weight loss, fever, and sweats.

Background Information

Pelvic girdle involvement usually causes pain that radiates to the knee.[77] Diagnosis is confirmed with blood panels that demonstrate an elevated erythrocyte sedimentation rate.[77] This condition is associated with temporal arteritis, which can cause blindness if untreated, so urgent referral to a physician is necessary if this condition is suspected. Treatment of this condition mainly includes the use of low-dose oral prednisone in the morning.[77,78]

PRIMARY BONE TUMOR OF THE ACETABULUM OR PROXIMAL FEMUR

■ Ewing's Sarcoma

Chief Clinical Characteristics

This presentation includes anterior or lateral hip pain and swelling that persists for weeks or months, accompanied by intermittent fevers. Individuals with this condition may report resting and night pain, and their symptoms may be unchanged with activity.

Background Information

This condition is prevalent throughout the life span, and is most common during the first and second decades of life.[79] It affects Caucasian individuals more frequently than African American and/or Asian American individuals. Males are affected more often than females. Treatment includes surgical resection of the involved bone. Nonsurgical interventions usually fail to change symptoms in individuals with this condition.

■ Osteosarcoma

Chief Clinical Characteristics

This presentation may involve an insidious onset of pain that persists for weeks or months.

Pain due to this condition may be aggravated with activity, causing limping.

Background Information

This condition is frequently found in adolescents because of the active bone growth in this age group. African American individuals are affected slightly more often than Caucasian individuals. Plain films confirm the diagnosis, typically revealing tumors near metaphyseal growth plates of the femur. This condition can be especially fatal if metastasized to the lungs. Treatment for this condition involves extensive surgical resection of the involved bone along with orthopedic reconstruction.

■ Pseudogout

Chief Clinical Characteristics

This presentation includes a sudden onset of deep stabbing hip pain, worsened with weight bearing and hip passive range of motion, and is associated with tenderness, warmth, and redness of overlying soft tissues.

Background Information

This condition is more common in older males than females. It is less common in the hip joint. This condition's presentation mimics gout; however, calcium pyrophosphate dehydrate crystal deposits mediate its characteristic joint pain and articular cartilage destruction. Blood tests and microscopic examination of aspirated synovial fluid confirm the diagnosis. Treatment usually involves medication to address this condition's underlying metabolic dysfunction.

■ Reiter's Syndrome

Chief Clinical Characteristics

This presentation can involve pain and stiffness in the low back, sacroiliac, and posterior hip regions in the presence of conjunctivitis and urethritis.[26] These patients will have asymmetric distribution of pain between the hips and will most certainly have some form of spinal discomfort associated with this condition.

Background Information

This condition also has been called a reactive arthritis because it may present after other infections. Clinical examination confirms the diagnosis. Treatment includes anti-inflammatory medication to control inflammation, as well as antibiotics to prevent the development of chronic disease.

■ Rheumatoid Arthritis of the Hip

Chief Clinical Characteristics
This presentation may involve morning stiffness and generalized pain throughout multiple joints in a symmetric distribution, with possible tenderness and swelling of affected joints.

Background Information
Women are twice as likely to be affected as men. Symptoms associated with this progressive inflammatory joint disease are caused by synovial membrane thickening and cytokine production in synovial fluid. Articular cartilage erosion, synovial hypertrophy, and constant joint effusion[80] eventually cause bony erosions and joint deformities that have a significant impact on daily function. Younger age of onset is associated with a greater extent of disability later. Plain radiographs and blood tests confirm the diagnosis. Treatment typically includes a variety of steroidal, nonsteroidal, and biological anti-inflammatory medications.

RHEUMATOID ARTHRITIS–LIKE DISEASES

■ Inflammatory Muscle Diseases

Chief Clinical Characteristics
This presentation includes a gradual onset of mild muscle pain associated with proximal muscle weakness that causes difficulty with daily activities such as walking, ascending and descending stairs, and rising from chairs.

Background Information
This condition describes a group of pathologically, histologically, and clinically distinct disorders: polymyositis, dermatomyositis, and inclusion body myositis. They may be associated with other collagen, vascular, and immune disorders. Although proximal extremity weakness is a classic finding, up to 50% also demonstrate distal weakness that may be equally as severe.[32] Blood tests help confirm the diagnosis and track disease activity, revealing elevated serum levels of creatine phosphokinase. Treatment typically involves steroidal, nonsteroidal, and biological anti-inflammatory medications.

■ Psoriatic Arthritis

Chief Clinical Characteristics
This presentation involves an insidious onset of asymmetric posterior hip pain associated with psoriasis. Pitting nail lesions occur in 80% of individuals with this condition. Dactylitis, tenosynovitis, and peripheral arthritis also are common.

Background Information
The severity of arthritis is uncorrelated with the extent of skin involvement.[27] Radiographs of the distal phalanges may reveal a characteristic "pencil in cup" deformity. Blood tests including erythrocyte sedimentation rate are useful to track disease activity. Usual treatment includes a variety of steroidal, nonsteroidal, and biological anti-inflammatory medications.

■ Scleroderma

Chief Clinical Characteristics
This presentation typically includes myalgia, arthralgia, fatigue, weight loss, limited mobility, and hardened skin about the hands, knees, or elbows. This condition occurs in individuals between 25 and 55 years of age, and is four to five times more likely in women than men. Additional symptoms may include dry mouth and eyes, as well as Raynaud's phenomenon.

Background Information
This rare and progressive autoimmune disorder affects blood vessels and many internal organs, including the lungs and the gastrointestinal system. Overproduction of collagen in this condition eventually leads to poor blood flow in the extremities, which can cause ulcers in the fingers, changes in skin color, and a disappearance of creases in the skin. Continued damage to small-diameter vasculature leads to scar tissue production that impairs joint range of motion. Blood tests confirm the diagnosis. Treatment includes both steroidal and nonsteroidal anti-inflammatory medications and gentle exercise.

■ Systemic Lupus Erythematosus

Chief Clinical Characteristics
This presentation can be characterized by hip and groin pain associated with fatigue and

joint pain/swelling affecting the hands, feet, knees, and shoulders.

Background Information

This condition affects mostly women of childbearing age. It is a chronic autoimmune disorder that can affect any organ system, including skin, joints, kidneys, brain, heart, lungs, and blood. The diagnosis is confirmed by the presence of skin lesions; heart, lung, or kidney involvement; and laboratory abnormalities including low red or white cell counts, low platelet counts, or positive ANA and anti-DNA antibody tests.[33] Usual treatment includes a variety of steroidal, nonsteroidal, and biological anti-inflammatory medications.

■ Sacroiliac Joint Dysfunction

Chief Clinical Characteristics

This presentation typically includes either an acute or insidious onset of buttock pain with possible radiation to the groin, posterior thigh, and lower leg. Sacral sulcus tenderness shows high sensitivity but poor specificity for detecting individuals with this condition.[81]

Background Information

It is associated with articular and periarticular nociception due to pathological joint mechanics, although this theory remains contentious. A high index of suspicion for this condition is warranted for individuals with excessive ligamentous laxity (eg, pregnant women). Clinical examination and selective joint blockade confirm the diagnosis. Imaging usually is unhelpful to confirm the diagnosis. This condition is managed nonsurgically.

■ Septic Arthritis of the Hip

Chief Clinical Characteristics

This presentation involves an insidious onset of hip and groin pain with weight bearing and movement, accompanied by possible fever and malaise. Overlying tissue is usually swollen and inflamed, and this may extend to the anterior and lateral thigh.

Background Information

Septic arthritis of the hip occurs by way of bacterial, yeast, fungal, or viral infection of the hip joint. Sepsis also can damage articular cartilage, leading to osteoarthritis later in life. Culture of aspirated synovial fluid confirms

the diagnosis and directs medical management, which involves a regimen of antibiotic medication directed to the infective agent.

■ Sickle Cell Crisis

Chief Clinical Characteristics

This presentation may involve bone pain about the hip joint, worsened by cold weather, overexertion, dehydration, and being overly fatigued.

Background Information

This condition involves abnormal red blood cell morphology that causes them to become rigid and sticky, disrupting blood flow to bones, and resulting in painful bone infarcts. This condition may cause complications in multiple organ systems, including stroke, skin ulcers, and blindness. There is no cure for this condition; treatment is palliative and preventive.

■ Synovial Sarcoma

Chief Clinical Characteristics

This presentation can be characterized by pain and tenderness in a long-standing soft tissue nodule that has rapidly increased in size over a short period of time. This uncommon condition is typically found within 5 cm of the knee joints of people younger than 30 years of age.[82]

Background Information

Synovial sarcoma spreads along fascial planes, so the disease may be more widespread than apparent on initial evaluation. Biopsy confirms the diagnosis, and magnetic resonance imaging shows the extent of spread. This condition is slow growing and locally aggressive. Its recurrence rate within 5 years is significant. Surgical resection of the tumor and surrounding soft tissues is indicated.

■ Systemic Fungal Infection

Chief Clinical Characteristics

This presentation includes hip pain associated with signs of systemic infection, such as fever, anorexia, and malaise. Individuals with this condition may present after a prolonged and varied course of antibiotics to address their symptoms.

Background Information

This condition is most common in immune-compromised individuals, such as patients in intensive care, patients receiving chemotherapy, patients with acquired immunodeficiency syndrome, and transplant recipients. This condition is most commonly due to *Candida* species infection, although aspergillus also may be a culprit organism. The infection is transferred from health care worker to patient by way of hand contact. Scrum pathology and molecular techniques confirm the diagnosis and direct appropriate pharmacologic management.

■ Transient Osteoporosis of the Hip

Chief Clinical Characteristics
This presentation involves an acute or gradual onset of severe hip and groin pain that is worsened with bearing weight on the affected limb. This condition is associated with hip muscle tenderness, joint effusion, and nearly normal hip range of motion.[83]

Background Information
The etiology of this condition is unclear. Its pathology involves reversible bone demineralization. The diagnosis is confirmed with technetium scan and magnetic resonance imaging.[83] This condition's self-limiting course lasts approximately 9 months, with maximum symptoms at 2 months.[84]

■ Trochanteric Contusion (Hip Pointer)

Chief Clinical Characteristics
This presentation typically includes a traumatic onset of lateral hip pain that is worsened with weight-bearing activities, palpation of the affected tissues, and active/resisted hip abduction. This condition is particularly common in individuals playing contact sports due to a direct blow or fall on the greater trochanter. Individuals with this condition may demonstrate a Trendelenburg gait pattern, although this finding itself is not pathognomic.

Background Information
Clinical examination confirms the diagnosis. This condition is managed nonsurgically.

■ Tuberculosis of the Hip

Chief Clinical Characteristics
This presentation typically includes hip and low back pain with weight bearing that mimics osteoarthrosis/osteoarthritis, accompanied by fever, sweats, and fatigue. Individuals with this condition will demonstrate a slow loss of range of motion of affected joints due to articular cartilage erosion.

Background Information
This condition results from the hematogenous spread of a primary respiratory infection. Chest radiographs and culture of aspirated synovial fluid confirm the diagnosis. Magnetic resonance imaging confirms the diagnosis. Treatment consists of antituberculosis medications, which are effective 90% of the time, with surgery in more advanced cases.[46]

References

1. Magee DJ. *Orthopedic Physical Assessment.* 3rd ed. Philadelphia, PA: W. B. Saunders; 1997.
2. Anderson LA. Abdominal aortic aneurysm. *J Cardiovasc Nurs.* Jul 2001;15(4):1–14.
3. Kauppila LI, McAlindon T, Evans S, Wilson PW, Kiel D, Felson DT. Disk degeneration/back pain and calcification of the abdominal aorta. A 25-year follow-up study in Framingham. *Spine.* Aug 15, 1997;22(14):1642–1647; discussion 1648–1649.
4. Kurunlahti M, Tervonen O, Vanharanta H, Ilkko E, Suramo I. Association of atherosclerosis with low back pain and the degree of disk degeneration. *Spine.* Nov 15, 1999;24(20):2080–2084.
5. Gravereaux EC, Marin ML. Endovascular repair of diffuse atherosclerotic occlusive disease using stented grafts. *Mt Sinai J Med.* Dec 2003;70(6):410–417.
6. Shelton T, McKinlay R, Schwartz RW. Acute appendicitis: current diagnosis and treatment. *Curr Surg.* Sep–Oct 2003;60(5):502–505.
7. Berven S, Tay BB, Colman W, Hu SS. The lumbar zygapophyseal (facet) joints: a role in the pathogenesis of spinal pain syndromes and degenerative spondylolisthesis. *Semin Neurol.* Jun 2002;22(2):187–196.
8. Urban JP, Roberts S. Degeneration of the intervertebral disc. *Arthritis Res Ther.* 2003;5(3):120–130.
9. Biyani A, Andersson GB, Chaudhary H, An HS. Intradiscal electrothermal therapy: a treatment option in patients with internal disk disruption. *Spine.* 2003;28 (15 suppl):S8–14.
10. Wellbery C. Diagnosis and treatment of endometriosis [see comment]. *Am Fam Physician.* 1999;60(6):1753–1762. [Erratum appears in *Am Fam Physician.* May 1, 2000;61(9):2614.]
11. Stendel R, Danne M, Schulte T, Stoltenburg-Didinger G, Brock M. Chronic lumbar epidural haematoma presenting with acute paraparesis. *Acta Neurochir (Wien).* Nov 2003;145(11):1015–1018; discussion 1018.
12. Fukui S, Ohseto K, Shiotani M, Ohno K, Karasawa H, Naganuma Y. Distribution of referred pain from the lumbar zygapophyseal joints and dorsal rami. *Clin J Pain.* 1997;13(4):303–307.
13. Dreyfuss PH, Dreyer SJ, Nass. Lumbar zygapophysial (facet) joint injections. *Spine.* 2003;3(3 suppl):50S–59S.
14. Beckers R, Uyttebroeck A, Demaerel P. Acute lymphoblastic leukaemia presenting with low back pain. *Eur J Paediatr Neurol.* 2002;6(5):285–287.
15. Rubin DI, Schomberg PJ, Shepherd RF, Panneton JM. Arteritis and brachial plexus neuropathy as delayed

complications of radiation therapy. *Mayo Clin Proc.* Aug 2001;76(8):849–852.

16. Bradlow A, Barton C. Arthritic presentation of childhood leukaemia. *Postgrad Med J.* Jun 1991;67(788): 562–564.

17. Evans TI, Nercessian BM, Sanders KM. Leukemic arthritis. *Semin Arthritis Rheum.* Aug 1994;24(1):48–56.

18. Ostrov BE, Goldsmith DP, Athreya BH. Differentiation of systemic juvenile rheumatoid arthritis from acute leukemia near the onset of disease. *J Pediatr.* Apr 1993;122(4):595–598.

19. Garfin SR, Yuan HA, Reiley MA. New technologies in spine: kyphoplasty and vertebroplasty for the treatment of painful osteoporotic compression fractures. *Spine.* 2001;26(14):1511–1515.

20. Braunwald E, Harrison TR. *Harrison's Principles of Internal Medicine.* 11th ed. New York: McGraw-Hill; 1987.

21. anonymous. Case records of the Massachusetts General Hospital. Weekly clinicopathological exercises. Case 27-1996. A 31-year-old woman with lumbar and abdominal pain, hypertension, and a retroperitoneal mass. *New Engl J Med.* 1996;335(9):650–655.

22. Harwood-Nuss A, ed. *The Clinical Practice of Emergency Medicine.* Philadelphia, PA: Lippincott; 1991.

23. Igra V. Pelvic inflammatory disease in adolescents. *AIDS Patient Care & Stds.* 1998;12(2):109–124.

24. Mallick IH, Thoufeeq MH, Rajendran TP. Iliopsoas abscesses. *Postgrad Med J.* 2004;80(946):459–462.

25. Agrawal SN, Dwivedi AJ, Khan M. Primary psoas abscess. *Dig Dis Sci.* 2002;47(9):2103–2105.

26. Klippel JH, Weyand CM, Crofford LJ, Stone JH, Arthritis Foundation. *Primer on the Rheumatic Diseases.* 12th ed. Atlanta, GA: Arthritis Foundation; 2001.

27. Kataria RK, Brent LH. Spondyloarthropathies. *Am Fam Physician.* Jun 15 2004;69(12):2853–2860.

28. Vinen CS, Oliveira DB. Acute glomerulonephritis. *Postgrad Med J.* 2003;79(930):206–213; quiz 212–213.

29. Kawaguchi Y, Matsuno H, Kanamori M, Ishihara H, Ohmori K, Kimura T. Radiologic findings of the lumbar spine in patients with rheumatoid arthritis, and a review of pathologic mechanisms. *J Spinal Disord Tech.* 2003;16(1):38–43.

30. Knutson D, Greenberg G, Cronau H. Management of Crohn's disease—a practical approach. *Am Fam Physician.* Sep 15 2003;68(4):707–714.

31. Shapiro W. Inflammatory bowel disease. http://www.emedicine.com/emerg/topic106.htm. Accessed April 28, 2006.

32. Lotz BP, Engel AG, Nishino H, Stevens JC, Litchy WJ. Inclusion body myositis. Observations in 40 patients. *Brain.* Jun 1989;112(Pt 3):727–747.

33. Fauci AS, Haynes B, Katz P. The spectrum of vasculitis: clinical, pathologic, immunologic and therapeutic considerations. *Ann Intern Med.* Nov 1978;89(5 Pt 1): 660–676.

34. Honan M, White GW, Eisenberg GM. Spontaneous infectious discitis in adults. *Am J Med.* 1996;100(1):85–89.

35. Friedman JA, Maher CO, Quast LM, McClelland RL, Ebersold MJ. Spontaneous disk space infections in adults. *Surg Neurol.* 2002;57(2):81–86.

36. Koeller KK, Rosenblum RS, Morrison AL. Neoplasms of the spinal cord and filum terminale: radiologic-pathologic correlation. *Radiographics.* Nov–Dec 2000;20(6): 1721–1749.

37. Guerrero D. The management of primary spinal cord tumours. *Nurs Times.* Oct 21–27 2003;99(42):28–31.

38. Bagley CA, Gokaslan ZL. Cauda equina syndrome caused by primary and metastatic neoplasms. *Neurosurg Focus.* Jun 15, 2004;16(6):e3.

39. Arbit E, Pannullo S. Lumbar stenosis: a clinical review. *Clin Orthop.* Mar 2001(384):137–143.

40. Fritz JM, Delitto A, Welch WC, Erhard RE. Lumbar spinal stenosis: a review of current concepts in evaluation, management, and outcome measurements. *Arch Phys Med Rehabil.* Jun 1998;79(6):700–708.

41. Standaert CJ, Herring SA. Spondylolysis: a critical review. *Br J Sports Med.* Dec 2000;34(6):415–422.

42. Bono CM. Low-back pain in athletes. *J Bone Joint Surg Am.* Feb 2004;86A(2):382–396.

43. van Schalkwyk J. Systemic fungal infection. http://www.anaesthetist.com/icu/infect/fungi/serious.htm. Accessed April 28, 2006.

44. Roche PH, Dufour H, Graziani N, Jolivert J, Grisoli F. Anterior lumbosacral dislocation: case report and review of the literature. *Surg Neurol.* 1998;50(1):11–16.

45. Gorse GJ, Pais MJ, Kusske JA, Cesario TC. Tuberculous spondylitis. A report of six cases and a review of the literature. *Medicine.* 1983;62(3):178–193.

46. Dass B, Puet TA, Watanakunakorn C. Tuberculosis of the spine (Pott's disease) presenting as "compression fractures." *Spinal Cord.* 2002;40(11):604–608.

47. Umezurike C, Feyi-Waboso P. Successful myomectomy during pregnancy: a case report. *Reprod Health.* Aug 16 2005;2(1):6.

48. Steinberg ME, Larcom PG, Strafford B, et al. Core decompression with bone grafting for osteonecrosis of the femoral head. *Clin Orthop Relat Res.* May 2001(386): 71–78.

49. Rodriguez JA, Ranawat CS, Maniar RN, Umlas ME. Incisional cellulitis after total hip replacement. *J Bone Joint Surg Br.* Sep 1998;80(5):876–878.

50. Merskey H, Bogduk N. *Classification of Chronic Pain: Descriptions of Chronic Pain Syndromes and Definitions of Pain Terms.* Seattle, WA: IASP Press; 1994.

51. Goldenberg DL, Burckhardt C, Crofford L. Management of fibromyalgia syndrome [see comment]. *JAMA.* 2004;292(19):2388–2395.

52. Nampiaparampil DE, Shmerling RH. A review of fibromyalgia. *Am J Managed Care.* 2004;10(11 Pt 1):794–800.

53. Brandser E, Marsh JL. Acetabular fractures: easier classification with a systematic approach. *AJR Am J Roentgenol.* Nov 1998;171(5):1217–1228.

54. Brunner LC, Eshilian-Oates L, Kuo TY. Hip fractures in adults. *Am Fam Physician.* Feb 1, 2003;67(3):537–542.

55. Mammen EF. Pathogenesis of venous thrombosis. *Chest.* Dec 1992;102(6 suppl):640S–644S.

56. Lynch SA, Renstrom PA. Groin injuries in sport: treatment strategies. *Sports Med.* Aug 1999;28(2):137–144.

57. Chen TM, George S, Woodruff CA, Hsu S. Clinical manifestations of varicella-zoster virus infection. *Dermatol Clin.* Apr 2002;20(2):267–282.

58. Garland DE. A clinical perspective on common forms of acquired heterotopic ossification. *Clin Orthop Relat Res.* Feb 1991(263):13–29.

59. Recommendations for the medical management of osteoarthritis of the hip and knee: 2000 update. American College of Rheumatology Subcommittee on

Osteoarthritis Guidelines. *Arthritis Rheum.* Sep 2000; 43(9):1905–1915.

60. Lawrence PF, Lorenzo-Rivero S, Lyon JL. The incidence of iliac, femoral, and popliteal artery aneurysms in hospitalized patients. *J Vasc Surg.* Oct 1995;22(4):409–415; discussion 415–416.

61. Kujala UM, Orava S. Ischial apophysis injuries in athletes. *Sports Med.* Oct 1993;16(4):290–294.

62. Santaella RO, Fishman EK, Lipsett PA. Primary vs secondary iliopsoas abscess. Presentation, microbiology, and treatment. *Arch Surg.* Dec 1995;130(12):1309–1313.

63. O'Kane JW. Anterior hip pain. *Am Fam Physician.* Oct 15 1999;60(6):1687–1696.

64. Kraushaar BS, Nirschl RP. Tendinosis of the elbow (tennis elbow). Clinical features and findings of histological, immunohistochemical, and electron microscopy studies. *J Bone Joint Surg Am.* Feb 1999;81(2):259–278.

65. Czerny C, Hofmann S, Neuhold A, et al. Lesions of the acetabular labrum: accuracy of MR imaging and MR arthrography in detection and staging. *Radiology.* Jul 1996;200(1):225–230.

66. Joines JD, McNutt RA, Carey TS, Deyo RA, Rouhani R. Finding cancer in primary care outpatients with low back pain: a comparison of diagnostic strategies. *J Gen Intern Med.* 2001;16(1):14–23.

67. Hatrick NC, Lucas JD, Timothy AR, Smith MA. The surgical treatment of metastatic disease of the spine. *Radiother Oncol.* 2000;56(3):335–339.

68. Holman PJ, Suki D, McCutcheon I, Wolinsky JP, Rhines LD, Gokaslan ZL. Surgical management of metastatic disease of the lumbar spine: experience with 139 patients. *J Neurosurg Spine.* 2005;2(5):550–563.

69. Johnston CA, Wiley JP, Lindsay DM, Wiseman DA. Iliopsoas bursitis and tendinitis. A review. *Sports Med.* Apr 1998;25(4):271–283.

70. Reid V, Cros D. Proximal sensory neuropathies of the leg. *Neurol Clin.* Aug 1999;17(3):655–667, viii.

71. Stewart JD. *Focal Peripheral Neuropathies.* 3rd ed. Philadelphia, PA: Lippincott Williams & Wilkins; 2000.

72. Ivins GK. Meralgia paresthetica, the elusive diagnosis: clinical experience with 14 adult patients. *Ann Surg.* Aug 2000;232(2):281–286.

73. Busis NA. Femoral and obturator neuropathies. *Neurol Clin.* Aug 1999;17(3):633–653, vii.

74. Pauli S, Willemsen P, Declerck K, Chappel R, Vanderveken M. Osteomyelitis pubis versus osteitis pubis: a case presentation and review of the literature. *Br J Sports Med.* Feb 2002;36(1):71–73.

75. Crist BD, Lenke LG, Lewis S. Osteoid osteoma of the lumbar spine. A case report highlighting a novel reconstruction technique. *J Bone Joint Surg Am.* Feb 2005;87 (2):414–418.

76. Spanier D, Harrast M. Pigmented villonodular synovitis: an uncommon presentation of anterior hip pain. *Am J Phys Med Rehabil.* Feb 2005;84(2):131–135.

77. Salvarani C, Cantini F, Boiardi L, Hunder GG. Polymyalgia rheumatica and giant-cell arteritis. *N Engl J Med.* Jul 25, 2002;347(4):261–271.

78. Mandell BF. Polymyalgia rheumatica: clinical presentation is key to diagnosis and treatment. *Cleve Clin J Med.* Jun 2004;71(6):489–495.

79. Hillmann A, Hoffmann C, Gosheger G, Rodl R, Winkelmann W, Ozaki T. Tumors of the pelvis: complications after reconstruction. *Arch Orthop Trauma Surg.* Sep 2003;123(7):340–344.

80. Pincus T, Callahan LF. What is the natural history of rheumatoid arthritis? *Rheum Dis Clin North Am.* Feb 1993;19(1):123–151.

81. Dreyfuss P, Michaelsen M, Pauza K, McLarty J, Bogduk N. The value of medical history and physical examination in diagnosing sacroiliac joint pain. *Spine.* Nov 15, 1996;21(22):2594–2602.

82. Fisher C. Synovial sarcoma. *Ann Diagn Pathol.* Dec 1998; 2(6):401–421.

83. Toms AP, Marshall TJ, Becker E, Donell ST, Lobo-Mueller EM, Barker T. Regional migratory osteoporosis: a review illustrated by five cases. *Clin Radiol.* Apr 2005;60(4): 425–438.

84. Pantazopoulos T, Exarchou E, Hartofilakidis GA. Idiopathic transient osteoporosis of the hip. *J Bone Joint Surg Am.* Mar 1973;55(2):315–321.

CHAPTER 20

Case Demonstration: Hip Pain

▦ *Alison R. Scheid, PT, DPT, OCS, NCS* ▦ *Elizabeth M. Poppert, PT, DPT, MS, OCS*

NOTE: This case demonstration was developed using the diagnostic process described in Chapter 4 and demonstrated in Chapter 5. The reader is encouraged to use this diagnostic process in order to ensure thorough clinical reasoning. If additional elaboration is required on the information presented in this chapter, please consult Chapters 4 and 5.

THE DIAGNOSTIC PROCESS

Step 1 Identify the patient's chief concern.

Step 2 Identify *barriers to communication*.

Step 3 Identify *special concerns*.

Step 4 Create a symptom timeline and sketch the anatomy (if needed).

Step 5 Create a diagnostic hypothesis list considering all possible forms of *remote* and *local* pathology that could cause the patient's chief concern.

Step 6 Sort the diagnostic hypothesis list by epidemiology and specific case characteristics.

Step 7 Ask specific questions to rule specific conditions or pathological categories less likely.

Step 8 Re-sort the diagnostic hypothesis list based on the patient's responses to specific questioning.

Step 9 Perform tests to differentiate among the remaining diagnostic hypotheses.

Step 10 Re-sort the diagnostic hypothesis list based on the patient's responses to specific tests.

Step 11 Decide on a diagnostic impression.

Step 12 Determine the appropriate patient disposition.

Case Description

CD was a 43-year-old male who was referred to physical therapy by an orthopedic surgeon with a diagnosis of "right hip rectus femoris tendinosis." He presented with a 1-year history of hip pain that was originally diagnosed as avascular necrosis of the femoral head of unknown etiology with subsequent surgical replacement of the femoral head. Postsurgical therapy was discontinued after 1 month (patient self-discharged). However, the patient returned to therapy now due to his reports of an inability to return to prior level of function, discomfort with simple daily activities, and, although working, he was unable to resume full duties independently (climbing ladders and on his feet more than 8 hours per day).

He described the pain as feeling "stiff and achy," located mostly on the anterior and lateral area surrounding the right hip (not including groin) and denied any pain or pathology of the left lower extremity. He rated his minimum pain as 0/10 and his maximal pain during the last month at about 7/10 to 8/10. The morning and evenings were the worst because he felt stiffest at these times. Pain did not usually wake him up at night. His pain and stiffness started immediately upon moving and took about 3 to 4 minutes to decrease while weight bearing. However, if he sat or laid down, the pain immediately decreased. He reported Advil had a mild effect on pain relief. Walking (especially trying to take "longer/faster" steps and pain with the first several minutes of walking were the worst), squatting, using the elliptical, and going upstairs (more than down) all aggravated his pain.

Recent radiographs were taken 1 month prior to check placement of the femoral component and revealed mild degeneration at the acetabulum, with stable componentry. Due to a medical history of testicular cancer several years ago, he received a computed tomography scan of his abdomen and pelvis every 6 months. The most recent was 4 months ago and was clear for signs of cancerous changes. CD fractured his right tibial plateau 6 years ago, which was treated surgically, and he had arthroscopic surgery 3 to 4 years ago to clean out the knee after the original surgery. The only medication he took was Advil 3 to 4 times a day at the time of physical therapy evaluation.

STEP #1: Identify the patient's chief concern.

- Right hip pain

STEP #2: Identify *barriers to communication*.

- **Gender difference between patient and therapist.** When a male patient is evaluated by a female physical therapist, the type of information elicited from the history could be affected, both from the perspectives of the therapist's questions and the type of information the patient may be willing to share.
- **Negative tests and relatively young patient age.** Recent, negative imaging results and relatively young age could have led to

neglect of a pathology not appropriate for physical therapy intervention.

- **Report of limited physical therapy following hip replacement.** This report from the patient could have led to the therapist's assumption of unresolved mechanical factors for chronic pain. His pain did not appear to be "new" and his limited function brought him back to physical therapy.

STEP #3: Identify *special concerns*.

- Relatively recent history of cancer
- Avascular necrosis of unknown etiology

These factors raise the suspicion of cancer or other pathology that would require additional consultation with other health care providers.

STEP #4: Create a symptom timeline and sketch the anatomy (if needed).

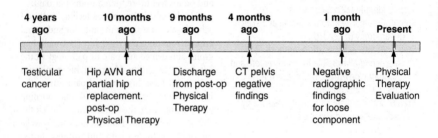

4 years ago	10 months ago	9 months ago	4 months ago	1 month ago	Present
Testicular cancer	Hip AVN and partial hip replacement. post-op Physical Therapy	Discharge from post-op Physical Therapy	CT pelvis negative findings	Negative radiographic findings for loose component	Physical Therapy Evaluation

STEP #5: Create a diagnostic hypothesis list considering all possible forms of *remote* and *local* pathology that could cause the patient's chief concern.

STEP #6: Sort the diagnostic hypothesis list by epidemiology and specific case characteristics.

Remote

T   Trauma

Acute lumbar sprain/strain

Disk disruption (with or without herniation)

Facet syndrome
Lumbar compression fracture

Remote

T   Trauma

~~Acute lumbar sprain/strain~~ (time course, presentation)

~~Disk disruption (with or without herniation)~~ (time course, presentation)

Facet syndrome
~~Lumbar compression fracture~~ (presentation, age, no mechanism of injury)

Lumbar radiculopathy
Traumatic spondylolisthesis

Lumbar radiculopathy
~~Traumatic spondylolisthesis~~ (presentation, no mechanism of injury)

I   Inflammation

Aseptic
Complex regional pain syndrome
Crohn's disease
Fibromyalgia
Reiter's syndrome of the lumbar spine
Rheumatoid arthritis of the lumbar spine

Septic
Appendicitis
Herpes zoster
Iliopsoas abscess

Pelvic inflammatory disease

Prostatitis
Renal or urinary tract infection

Retrocecal appendicitis

Retroperitoneal abscess

Septic discitis
Tuberculosis of the lumbar spine (Pott's disease)

I   Inflammation

Aseptic
Complex regional pain syndrome
Crohn's disease
Fibromyalgia
Reiter's syndrome of the lumbar spine
Rheumatoid arthritis of the lumbar spine

Septic
~~Appendicitis~~ (time course)
Herpes zoster
~~Iliopsoas abscess~~ (negative abdominal computed tomography scan)
~~Pelvic inflammatory disease~~ (uncommon in patient's sex)
~~Prostatitis~~ (time course)
~~Renal or urinary tract infection~~ (time course)
~~Retrocecal appendicitis~~ (negative abdominal computed tomography scan)
~~Retroperitoneal abscess~~ (negative abdominal computed tomography scan)
Septic discitis
Tuberculosis of the lumbar spine (Pott's disease)

M   Metabolic

Endometriosis

M   Metabolic

~~Endometriosis~~ (patient's sex)

Va   Vascular

Aortic arteriosclerosis
Aortic artery aneurysm
Epidural hematoma

Va   Vascular

Aortic arteriosclerosis
Aortic artery aneurysm
Epidural hematoma

De   Degenerative

Degenerative spondylolisthesis
Disk degeneration
Spinal stenosis
Spondylolysis

De   Degenerative

Degenerative spondylolisthesis
Disk degeneration
Spinal stenosis
Spondylolysis

Tu   Tumor

Malignant Primary, such as:
• Bone tumor of the lumbar spine
• Spinal cord tumor
Malignant Metastatic:
Not applicable
Benign, such as:
• Osteoblastoma
• Ovarian cysts
• Uterine fibroids

Tu   Tumor

Malignant Primary, such as:
• Bone tumor of the lumbar spine
• Spinal cord tumor
Malignant Metastatic:
Not applicable
Benign, such as:
• ~~Osteoblastoma~~ (patient age)
• ~~Ovarian cysts~~ (patient's sex)
• ~~Uterine fibroids~~ (patient's sex)

Co Congenital

Not applicable

Ne Neurogenic/Psychogenic

Anxiety
Depression
Malingering

Munchausen's syndrome

Secondary gain

Somatoform disorder

Local

T Trauma

Fractures:
- Extracapsular femur fracture

- Fracture of femoral shaft

Hip dislocation

Labral tear

Iliac crest apophysitis

Iliotibial band friction syndrome
Muscle strains:
- Iliopsoas strain
- Quadriceps muscle strain
Nerve entrapments/neuropathy:
- Femoral neuropathy
- Meralgia paresthetica
Sports hernia
Trochanteric contusion

I Inflammation

Aseptic
Complex regional pain syndrome
Fibromyalgia
Gout
Herpes zoster
Polymyalgia rheumatica
Pseudogout
Reiter's syndrome of the hip
Rheumatoid arthritis of the hip
Trochanteric bursitis

Co Congenital

Not applicable

Ne Neurogenic/Psychogenic

~~Anxiety~~ (time course)
Depression
~~Malingering~~ (presentation, no apparent external motives, return to work)
~~Munchausen's syndrome~~ (presentation of symptoms, medical attention not sought for months)
~~Secondary gain~~ (presentation, no external motives)
Somatoform disorder

Local

T Trauma

~~Fractures:~~
- ~~Extracapsular femur fracture~~ (no mechanism of injury; negative hip radiographs)
- ~~Fracture of femoral shaft~~ (no mechanism of injury; negative hip radiographs)

~~Hip dislocation~~ (no mechanism of injury; negative hip radiographs)

~~Labral tear~~ (presentation: lack of groin pain and clicking)

~~Iliac crest apophysitis~~ (location of symptoms, patient age)

Iliotibial band friction syndrome
Muscle strains:
- Iliopsoas strain
- Quadriceps muscle strain
Nerve entrapments/neuropathy:
- Femoral neuropathy
- Meralgia paresthetica
Sports hernia
~~Trochanteric contusion~~ (no mechanism of injury)

I Inflammation

Aseptic
Complex regional pain syndrome
Fibromyalgia
~~Gout~~ (time course)
Herpes zoster
~~Polymyalgia rheumatica~~ (age)
~~Pseudogout~~ (time course, age)
Reiter's syndrome of the hip
Rheumatoid arthritis of the hip
Trochanteric bursitis

Tendinitis:
* Iliopsoas
* Rectus femoris
* Sartorius
* Tensor fasciae latae

Septic
Cellulitis
Herpes zoster
Iliopsoas abscess

Sepsis
Tuberculosis of the hip

M   Metabolic

Transient osteoporosis of the hip

Va   Vascular

Iliac artery aneurysm

De   Degenerative

Failure of arthroplasty component

Hip osteoarthrosis (osteoarthritis)

Tendinoses:
* Iliopsoas
* Rectus femoris
* Sartorius
* Tensor fasciae latae

Tu   Tumor

Malignant Primary, such as:
* Bone tumor of the acetabulum or femur

Malignant Metastatic, such as:
* Metastases, including from primary breast, kidney, lung, prostate, thyroid disease, and testicular cancer
Benign, such as:
* Pigmented villonodular synovitis

Co   Congenital

Not applicable

Ne   Neurogenic/Psychogenic

Not applicable

~~Tendinitis:~~
* ~~Iliopsoas~~ (time course)
* ~~Rectus femoris~~ (time course)
* ~~Sartorius~~ (time course)
* ~~Tensor fasciae latae~~ (time course)

Septic
Cellulitis
Herpes zoster
~~Iliopsoas abscess~~ (negative abdominal computed tomographic scan)

Sepsis
Tuberculosis of the hip

M   Metabolic

~~Transient osteoporosis of the hip~~ (proximal femur replaced)

Va   Vascular

~~Iliac artery aneurysm~~ (negative pelvic computed tomography scan)

De   Degenerative

~~Failure of arthroplasty component~~ (negative radiographic findings)
~~Hip osteoarthrosis (osteoarthritis)~~ (mild radiographic changes)

Tendinoses:
* Iliopsoas
* Rectus femoris
* Sartorius
* Tensor fasciae latae

Tu   Tumor

Malignant Primary, such as:
* ~~Bone tumor of the acetabulum or femur~~ (negative radiographic findings)
Malignant Metastatic, such as:
* Metastases, including from primary breast, kidney, lung, prostate, thyroid disease, and testicular cancer
Benign, such as:
* ~~Pigmented villonodular synovitis~~ (negative radiographs; no femoral joint surface)

Co   Congenital

Not applicable

Ne   Neurogenic/Psychogenic

Not applicable

STEP #7: Ask specific questions to rule specific conditions or pathological categories less likely.

- **Have you been ill?** No, ruling less likely forms of septic inflammation.
- **Do you have pain in the pelvis or groin?** No, decreasing likelihood of referral from primary abdominal or pelvic pathology, including hernia.
- **Have you gained or lost weight that you didn't intend to gain or lose?** No, ruling less likely metastatic disease.
- **Do you have numbness, tingling, or weakness in your legs?** No, which makes pathology affecting the lumbar spine and peripheral nervous system of the lower extremities less likely.
- **Do you have pain in other joints?** No, decreasing the likelihood of lumbar involvement and rheumatic disease.

STEP #8: Re-sort the diagnostic hypothesis list based on the patient's responses to specific questioning.

> **Teaching Comment:** Despite CD's history of cancer, it appeared he did not present with cardinal signs or symptoms of metastatic cancer or other serious pathology. CD had regularly scheduled oncological follow-up appointments that included hip and pelvic imaging studies during the time symptoms were present, and his chronic symptoms remained consistent. Most lumbar and vascular pathologies were significantly less likely in the absence of low back pain during the months of hip pain. His chronic pain appeared to be consistent with local hip pathology.

Remote

T   Trauma

~~Facet syndrome~~ (no back pain)
Lumbar radiculopathy

I   Inflammation

Aseptic

~~Crohn's disease~~ (no abdominal pain)
Complex regional pain syndrome

~~Fibromyalgia~~ (no pain in multiple joints)
~~Reiter's syndrome of the lumbar spine~~ (no back pain)
~~Rheumatoid arthritis of the lumbar spine~~ (no back pain, patient sex, radiographic findings)

Septic

~~Herpes zoster~~ (no rash)
~~Septic discitis~~ (no back pain)
~~Tuberculosis of the lumbar spine (Pott's disease)~~ (no back pain)

M   Metabolic

Not applicable

Va   Vascular

~~Aortic arteriosclerosis~~ (no abdominal pain)
~~Aortic artery aneurysm~~ (no abdominal pain)
~~Epidural hematoma~~ (no back pain)

De   Degenerative

~~Degenerative spondylolisthesis~~ (no back pain, no lower extremity neurological symptoms)
~~Disk degeneration~~ (no back pain, no lower extremity neurological symptoms)
~~Spinal stenosis~~ (no back pain, patient age, no lower extremity neurological symptoms)
~~Spondylolysis~~ (no back pain)

Tu   Tumor

Malignant Primary, such as:
- ~~Bone tumor of the lumbar spine~~ (no back pain)
- ~~Spinal cord tumor~~ (no lower extremity neurological symptoms, no back pain)

Malignant Metastatic, such as:
- ~~Metastases, including from primary breast, kidney, lung, prostate, thyroid disease, and testicular cancer~~ (no weight change)

Benign:
Not applicable

Co   Congenital

Not applicable

Ne   Neurogenic/Psychogenic

~~Depression~~ (absence of generalized symptoms)
~~Somatoform disorder~~ (absence of generalized symptoms)

Local

T Trauma

Iliotibial band friction syndrome
Muscle strains:
- Iliopsoas strain
- Quadriceps muscle strain

Nerve entrapments/neuropathy:
- Femoral neuropathy
- ~~Meralgia paresthetica~~ (no lower extremity sensory symptoms)

Sports hernia

I Inflammation

Aseptic

Complex regional pain syndrome
~~Fibromyalgia~~ (no pain in multiple body regions)
Herpes zoster
~~Reiter's syndrome of the hip~~ (no illness, no pain in multiple joints)
~~Rheumatoid arthritis of the hip~~ (no pain in multiple joints, patient sex)
Trochanteric bursitis

Septic

Cellulitis
Herpes zoster
~~Sepsis~~ (no illness)
~~Tuberculosis of the hip~~ (no illness)

M Metabolic

Not applicable

Va Vascular

Not applicable

De Degenerative

Tendinoses:
- Iliopsoas
- Rectus femoris
- Sartorius
- Tensor fasciae latae

Tu Tumor

Malignant Primary:
Not applicable
Malignant Metastatic, such as:
- ~~Metastases, including from primary breast, kidney, lung, prostate, thyroid disease, and testicular cancer~~ (no weight change)

Benign:
Not applicable

Co Congenital

Not applicable

Teaching Comment: CD's young age, good overall health, and decreased likelihood of metastases from testicular cancer with recent negative imaging results all contributed to a continued search for other local causes of hip pain. The rate of metastases from testicular cancer to the hip/pelvic regions is small, with rates of inguinal metastases as low as 2%.[1]

Ne Neurogenic/Psychogenic

Not applicable

STEP #9: Perform tests to differentiate among the remaining diagnostic hypotheses.

- **Inspection.** No signs of rash.
- **Lower extremity reflexes.** 2+, decreasing likelihood of projected pain from lumbar spine pathology.
- **Prone knee bending.** Negative for reproduction of symptoms, but positive for limited muscle length.
- **Palpation.** Unremarkable for reproduction of symptoms (except for tenderness to palpation of hip flexor muscles).

STEP #10: Re-sort the diagnostic hypothesis list based on the patient's responses to specific tests.

Remote

T Trauma

~~Lumbar radiculopathy~~ (normal lower extremity deep tendon reflexes)

I Inflammation

Aseptic

~~Complex regional pain syndrome~~ (inspection unremarkable)

Septic

Not applicable

M Metabolic

Not applicable

Va Vascular

Not applicable

De Degenerative

Not applicable

Tu Tumor

Not applicable

Co Congenital

Not applicable

Ne Neurogenic/Psychogenic

Not applicable

Local

T Trauma

~~Iliotibial band friction syndrome~~ (negative palpation)

Muscle strains:

- ~~Iliopsoas strain~~ (negative palpation)
- ~~Quadriceps muscle strain~~ (negative palpation)

Nerve entrapments/neuropathy:

- ~~Femoral neuropathy~~ (negative prone knee bend)
- ~~Sports hernia~~ (negative palpation)

I Inflammation

Aseptic

~~Complex regional pain syndrome~~ (inspection unremarkable)

~~Trochanteric bursitis~~ (negative palpation)

Septic

~~Cellulitis~~ (inspection unremarkable)

~~Herpes zoster~~ (inspection unremarkable)

M Metabolic

Not applicable

Va Vascular

Not applicable

De Degenerative

Tendinoses:

- Iliopsoas
- Rectus femoris
- Sartorius
- Tensor fasciae latae

Tu Tumor

Not applicable

Co Congenital

Not applicable

Ne Neurogenic/Psychogenic

Not applicable

Teaching Comment: Many of the local pathologies specific to hip arthroplasty were difficult to rule out based on the initial exam, but their prevalence has been reported. In a study by Bhave and colleagues,[2] the rate of component malalignment was reported as 13%. Muscle contracture and weakness was much more common, 28% and 47% respectively.

STEP #11: Decide on a diagnostic impression.

- Tendinosis of the hip musculature vs. failure of arthroplasty component.

Teaching Comment: Upon objective examination, a 3-cm right leg length discrepancy was found, as was weakness of the proximal right lower extremity muscles, limited hip active and passive range of motion, right more than left, with pain only associated with the right passive flexion and rotation movements; some pain reproduction with palpation of hip flexor tendons; pain with quadriceps activation; gait and postural deviations. The local diagnoses remaining on the list most likely exist in combination and are not exclusive diagnoses.

STEP #12: Determine the appropriate patient disposition.

- Physical therapy was initiated with the caveat that failure of an arthroplasty component could not be completely excluded, but results of plain radiographs were encouraging. The patient would be monitored throughout intervention for signs of intolerance to treatment.

Case Outcome

CD was treated for the known impairments. Treatment included a shoe lift, strengthening exercises for hip/pelvic stabilization and lower extremity strength/endurance, and stretching exercises. He made measureable gains during the next 8 weeks for muscle strength, endurance, and flexibility. Upon resuming full work responsibilities, he developed increased anterior and lateral hip pain with distal symptoms into the knee. CD was referred to his physician. Follow-up radiographs and MRI confirmed loosening of the hip component. The hip joint was aspirated. CD had an allergic reaction to one of the metals contained in the femoral component and a revision of his arthroplasty was performed. Following revision surgery, CD quickly returned to full work responsibilities.

> **Teaching Comment:** In comparing outcomes in individuals with a primary diagnosis of avascular necrosis and osteoarthritis, a higher rate of mechanical failure and revision was reported in patients younger than 50 years old with avascular necrosis.[3]

References

1. Daugaard G, Karas V, Sommer P. Inguinal metastases from testicular cancer. *BJU Int.* Apr 2006;97(4): 724–726.
2. Bhave A, Marker DR, Seyler TM, Ulrich SD, Plate JF, Mont MA. Functional problems and treatment solutions after total hip arthroplasty. *J Arthroplasty.* Sep 2007;22(6 suppl 2):116–124.
3. Ortiguera CJ, Pulliam IT, Cabanela ME. Total hip arthroplasty for osteonecrosis: matched-pair analysis of 188 hips with long-term follow-up. *J Arthroplasty.* Jan 1999;14(1):21–28.

CHAPTER **21**

Knee Pain

■ *Della Lee, PT, DPT, OCS, ATC* ■ *Daniel Farwell, PT, DPT*

Description of the Symptom

This chapter describes pathology that may lead to knee pain, including general, anterior, lateral, medial, and posterior knee pain. **Local causes** of knee pain are defined as pathology occurring in the musculoskeletal, nervous, and vascular structures of the knee joint, between the midthigh and proximal one-third of the lower leg. **Remote causes** occur outside this area.

Special Concerns

- Decreased distal pulses
- Inability to bear weight
- Skin break and fever
- Warmth and swelling associated with a fever

CHAPTER PREVIEW: Conditions That May Lead to Knee Pain

T Trauma

REMOTE	LOCAL GENERALIZED	LOCAL ANTERIOR
COMMON		

Hip pathologies:
• Avascular necrosis 370
• Hip osteoarthrosis/
  osteoarthritis 370
	Acute patellar dislocation 372
	Patellofemoral pain
	  syndrome 380
		Not applicable

UNCOMMON		

Lumbar radiculopathies:
• L4 radiculopathy 370
• L5 radiculopathy 370
• S1 radiculopathy 371
	Fractures:
	• Intercondylar eminence fracture
	  of the tibia 375
	• Patellar fracture 376
	• Supracondylar fracture of the
	  femur 376
	Patellar instability 380
		Fractures:
		• Osteochondral fracture of the
		  patella 376
		• Patellar fracture 376

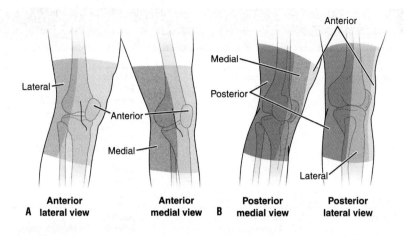

Anterior **A** **lateral view**	**Anterior** **medial view**	**Posterior** **B** **medial view**	**Posterior** **lateral view**

LOCAL LATERAL	LOCAL MEDIAL	LOCAL POSTERIOR
Iliotibial band friction syndrome 377 Muscle strains: • Biceps femoris muscle strain 378 Nerve entrapments: • Common peroneal nerve entrapment at the fibular head 379 Ruptures and tears: • Lateral collateral ligament sprain/rupture 382 • Lateral meniscus tear 382	Ruptures and tears: • Medial collateral ligament sprain/rupture 382 • Medial meniscus tear 383	Baker's cyst 372 Muscle strains: • Biceps femoris muscle strain 378 • Gastrocnemius muscle strain 378 Ruptures and tears: • Posterior cruciate ligament sprain/rupture 383
Not applicable	Muscle strains: • Semimembranosus muscle strain 379	Muscle strains: • Semimembranosus muscle strain 379

(continued)

KNEE PAIN

Trauma (*continued*)

REMOTE	LOCAL GENERALIZED	LOCAL ANTERIOR
RARE		
Not applicable	Not applicable	Ruptures and tears: • Quadriceps tendon rupture 384

I Inflammation

REMOTE	LOCAL GENERALIZED	LOCAL ANTERIOR
COMMON		
Not applicable	Not applicable	**Aseptic** Bursitis: • Infrapatellar bursitis 372 • Prepatellar bursitis 374 Tendinitis: • Patellar tendinitis 385 • Quadriceps tendinitis 385 **Septic** Not applicable
UNCOMMON		
Not applicable	**Aseptic** Fibromyalgia 375 Reiter's syndrome 381 Rheumatoid arthritis of the knee 382 **Septic** Osteomyelitis of the distal femur, proximal tibia, or proximal fibula 380 Septic arthritis 384	**Aseptic** Infrapatellar fat pad hypertrophy and inflammation (Hoffa's disease) 377 Plica syndrome 380 **Septic** Not applicable
RARE		
Not applicable	**Aseptic** Complex regional pain syndrome 374 **Septic** Not applicable	Not applicable

M Metabolic

REMOTE	LOCAL GENERALIZED	LOCAL ANTERIOR
COMMON		
Not applicable	Not applicable	Not applicable
UNCOMMON		
Not applicable	Gout 376 Pseudogout 381	Not applicable

LOCAL LATERAL	LOCAL MEDIAL	LOCAL POSTERIOR
Ruptures and tears: • Popliteus tendon rupture 383	Nerve entrapments: • Saphenous nerve entrapment 379	Ruptures and tears: • Plantaris muscle rupture 383 • Popliteus tendon rupture 383

LOCAL LATERAL	LOCAL MEDIAL	LOCAL POSTERIOR
Not applicable	**Aseptic** Bursitis: • Pes anserine bursitis 374 Tendinitis: • Pes anserine tendinitis 385 **Septic** Not applicable	**Aseptic** Tendonitis: • Hamstring tendinitis 385 **Septic** Not applicable
Aseptic Osteomyelitis of the distal femur, proximal tibia, or proximal fibula 380 **Septic** Not applicable	**Aseptic** Infrapatellar fat pad hypertrophy and inflammation (Hoffa's disease) 377 Plica syndrome 380 **Septic** Osteomyelitis of the distal femur, proximal tibia, or proximal fibula 380	**Aseptic** Tendinitis: • Popliteus tendinitis 385 **Septic** Not applicable
Not applicable	Not applicable	Not applicable

LOCAL LATERAL	LOCAL MEDIAL	LOCAL POSTERIOR
Not applicable	Not applicable	Not applicable
Not applicable	Not applicable	Not applicable

(continued)

Metabolic (continued)

REMOTE	LOCAL GENERALIZED	LOCAL ANTERIOR
RARE		
Not applicable	Not applicable	Not applicable

REMOTE	LOCAL GENERALIZED	LOCAL ANTERIOR
COMMON		
Not applicable	Not applicable	Not applicable
UNCOMMON		
Not applicable	Osteochondritis dissecans 379	Not applicable
RARE		
Not applicable	Arteriovenous malformation 372 Hemarthrosis 377 Sickle cell crisis 384	Deep venous thrombosis 374

De Degenerative

REMOTE	LOCAL GENERALIZED	LOCAL ANTERIOR
COMMON		
Not applicable	Primary osteoarthrosis/ osteoarthritis 381	Tendinoses: • Patellar tendinosis ("jumper's knee") 386 • Quadriceps tendinosis 387
UNCOMMON		
Not applicable	Not applicable	Not applicable
RARE		
Not applicable	Not applicable	Not applicable

Tu Tumor

REMOTE	LOCAL GENERALIZED	LOCAL ANTERIOR
COMMON		
Not applicable	Not applicable	Not applicable
UNCOMMON		
Not applicable	Not applicable	Not applicable
RARE		
Not applicable	*Malignant Primary, such as:* • Chondrosarcoma 387 • Osteosarcoma 388 • Parosteal osteosarcoma 388	Not applicable

LOCAL LATERAL	LOCAL MEDIAL	LOCAL POSTERIOR
Not applicable	Not applicable	Not applicable

LOCAL LATERAL	LOCAL MEDIAL	LOCAL POSTERIOR
Not applicable	Not applicable	Not applicable
Not applicable	Spontaneous avascular necrosis of the medial femoral condyle/proximal tibia 384	Deep venous thrombosis 374
Not applicable	Not applicable	Arteriovenous malformation 372 Popliteal artery occlusion 381

LOCAL LATERAL	LOCAL MEDIAL	LOCAL POSTERIOR
Lateral meniscus degeneration 377	Medial meniscus degeneration 378 Tendinoses: • Pes anserine tendinosis 386	Tendinoses: • Hamstring tendinosis 386
Not applicable	Not applicable	Tendinoses: • Popliteus tendinosis 386
Not applicable	Not applicable	Not applicable

LOCAL LATERAL	LOCAL MEDIAL	LOCAL SUPERIOR
Not applicable	Not applicable	Not applicable
Not applicable	Not applicable	Not applicable
Not applicable	Not applicable	*Malignant Primary, such as:* • Parosteal osteosarcoma 388 *Malignant Metastatic:* Not applicable

(continued)

Tumor *(continued)*

REMOTE	LOCAL GENERALIZED	LOCAL ANTERIOR
RARE		
	• Synovial sarcoma 389 *Malignant Metastatic, such as:* • Metastases to the knee, including from primary breast, kidney, lung, prostate, and thyroid disease 378 *Benign, such as:* • Chondroblastoma 387 • Ganglion cysts 387 • Giant cell tumor 387 • Osteochondroma 388 • Osteoid osteoma 388 • Pigmented villonodular synovitis 388 • Synovial chondromatosis 389	

Co Congenital

REMOTE	LOCAL GENERALIZED	LOCAL ANTERIOR
COMMON		
Not applicable	Not applicable	Not applicable
UNCOMMON		
Not applicable	Not applicable	Not applicable
RARE		
Not applicable	Not applicable	Not applicable

Ne Neurogenic/Psychogenic

REMOTE	LOCAL GENERALIZED	LOCAL ANTERIOR
COMMON		
Not applicable	Not applicable	Not applicable
UNCOMMON		
Not applicable	Not applicable	Not applicable
RARE		
Not applicable	Not applicable	Not applicable

Note: These are estimates of relative incidence because few data are available for the less common conditions.

Overview of Knee Pain

The intent of this chapter is to serve as a guide to differential diagnosis of knee pain based on the anatomical location of pain. However, because the knee joint itself has numerous structures that lie in proximity to each other and, in some cases, are physically connected, injury oftentimes results in pathology to multiple structures in multiple locations. Thus, during an examination of the knee, precise palpation in conjunction with the history of the pain will facilitate quickly ruling in or out common diagnoses. During a physical therapy evaluation of the knee, typically the most common causes of knee pain,

LOCAL LATERAL	LOCAL MEDIAL	LOCAL SUPERIOR
		Benign: Not applicable

LOCAL LATERAL	LOCAL MEDIAL	LOCAL SUPERIOR
Not applicable	Not applicable	Not applicable
Discoid meniscus 375	Not applicable	Not applicable
Not applicable	Not applicable	Not applicable

LOCAL LATERAL	LOCAL MEDIAL	LOCAL SUPERIOR
Not applicable	Not applicable	Not applicable
Not applicable	Not applicable	Not applicable
Not applicable	Not applicable	Not applicable

such as ligamentous sprains, meniscal lesions, and patellofemoral pain syndrome, are considered before the uncommon and rare causes of knee pain.

One of the primary purposes of this chapter is to introduce diagnoses that may not routinely be a part of the initial thought process during an evaluation of knee pain. Occasionally, remote causes of knee pain that commonly occur may also be initially overlooked by clinicians during an evaluation, such as pathologies arising from the lumbar spine and hip. Therefore, a secondary purpose of this chapter is to reinforce a clinician's knowledge of the common causes of knee pain and to serve as a reminder to be cognizant of diagnoses that may also originate from remote sources as well.

Description of Conditions That May Lead to Knee Pain

Remote

HIP PATHOLOGIES

■ Avascular Necrosis

Chief Clinical Characteristics
This presentation may involve insidious onset of groin and anterolateral thigh pain that radiates into the anteromedial aspect of the knee. An antalgic gait or a slight limp accompanied by hip pain may be observed. Unilateral, intermittent pain that radiates from the groin down the anterior thigh and knee typically indicates an intra-articular hip pathology.[1]

Background Information
This condition also may be associated with sickle cell anemia, femoral head or neck trauma, Gaucher's disease, alcoholism, Caisson disease, prolonged steroid use, irradiation, or pregnancy.[2] It is characterized by articular collapse of subchondral bone due to a lack of blood supply. The femoral head is most likely to be involved. Up to 20% of individuals with this condition have bilateral disease. Plain radiographs confirm the diagnosis, but early detection is difficult. Surgical decompression is typically performed to facilitate revascularization of the femoral head. Hemiarthroplasty may be considered if subchondral bone loss is extensive and the articular collapse is significant.

■ Hip Osteoarthrosis/ Osteoarthritis

Chief Clinical Characteristics
This presentation may include medial, anterior, or lateral hip pain that may refer to the anteromedial thigh, characterized by increased pain at the end ranges of passive hip abduction and extension and by limping (Fig. 21-1). This condition is the most common cause of hip pain in people older than 50 years of age.[3] It may be related to a prior injury or begin insidiously over the course of many months or years.

Background Information
This condition involves degeneration of the articular cartilage of the femoral head and acetabulum. Radiographs confirm the diagnosis, typically revealing a loss of joint space, osteophytes, and subchondral bone cysts. Treatment in mild to moderate stages involves lifestyle modification, exercises to maintain joint flexibility and strength, oral anti-inflammatory medication, and corticosteroid injections. In cases of severe pain and functional limitation, total joint arthroplasty is considered.

LUMBAR RADICULOPATHIES

■ L4 Radiculopathy

Chief Clinical Characteristics
This presentation can be characterized by pain in the lumbar spine and paresthesias radiating from the anterior aspect of the hip, thigh, and knee, sometimes ending anteromedially from the knee to the foot (see Fig. 21-1). Depending on the severity, the presentation may also include a decreased or absent patellar tendon reflex and motor loss in the muscles innervated by the L4 nerve. Prone knee bend may reproduce symptoms.

Background Information
A lumbar disk herniation is the most common cause of this condition. The diagnosis is confirmed with magnetic resonance imaging. Surgical intervention may be indicated in severe cases of lower extremity pain accompanied by neurological signs.

■ L5 Radiculopathy

Chief Clinical Characteristics
This presentation includes pain in the lumbar spine and paresthesias radiating from the lateral aspect of the hip and buttock to the lateral aspect of the knee, extending anterolaterally down to the foot (see Fig. 21-1). Depending on the severity, the presentation may also include motor loss in the muscles innervated by the L5 nerve root.

Background Information
A lumbar disk herniation is the most common cause for this condition. The diagnosis is confirmed with magnetic resonance imaging. Surgical intervention may be indicated

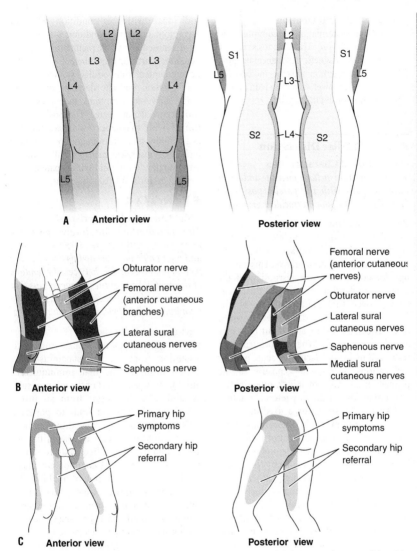

FIGURE 21-1 Referred and projected sources of knee pain, including (A) dermatomal patterns, (B) peripheral nerve patterns, and (C) hip joint referral patterns.

in severe cases of lower extremity pain accompanied by neurological signs.

■ S1 Radiculopathy

Chief Clinical Characteristics

This presentation typically includes pain in the lumbar spine and paresthesias radiating from *the buttock to the posterior aspect of the knee and extending posterolaterally from the knee to the foot (see Fig. 21-1). Depending on the severity, the presentation may also include a decreased or absent Achilles tendon reflex and motor loss in the muscles innervated by the S1 nerve.*

Background Information

A lumbar disk herniation is a common cause for this condition. The diagnosis is confirmed with magnetic resonance imaging. Surgical intervention may be indicated in severe cases of lower extremity pain accompanied by neurological signs.

Local

■ Acute Patellar Dislocation

Chief Clinical Characteristics

This presentation includes an acute and severe onset of pain with the patella positioned laterally over the femoral trochlear groove.

Background Information

The definition of a complete dislocation is the absence of contact between the patella and the trochlear groove. This pathology presents as a severe disruption of the extensor mechanism as a result of the patella sliding over the lateral portion of the trochlear groove. Acute dislocations are most often associated with trauma, but they may also be atraumatic. When associated with trauma, a major risk factor for acute patellar dislocations is frequent exposure to the primary mechanism of injury, oftentimes a noncontact lower extremity internal rotation and knee valgus stress on a fixed distal extremity. In nontraumatic dislocations, some form of patellar malalignment or abnormality such as patellar alta, ligamentous laxity, or increased Q angle is frequently observed. Rate of recurrence is high in children and preadolescents. Manual reduction is required, followed by conservative rehabilitation, emphasizing strengthening of the quadriceps and gluteal muscles, orthotic therapy, and flexibility of the lateral soft tissue structures of the knee. Surgical intervention is indicated when patellar instability continues after rehabilitation.

■ Arteriovenous Malformation

Chief Clinical Characteristics

This presentation may involve mild pain, edema, and disfigurement.

Background Information

This condition is a rare vascular anomaly that most frequently affects the knee joint. Individuals with this condition often are asymptomatic, so the condition is commonly misdiagnosed as juvenile rheumatoid arthritis, hemophilic arthropathy, tuberculous arthritis, or pigmented villonodular synovitis.[4] The malformation typically develops during infancy; however, symptoms may present in adolescence if not treated. Diagnosis is confirmed with magnetic resonance imaging, angiography, and ultrasonography. Treatment includes nonsurgical management in mildly symptomatic or asymptomatic patients, or surgical excision of localized lesions.

■ Baker's Cyst

Chief Clinical Characteristics

This presentation can involve posterior knee pain, stiffness, tenderness, edema, and a palpable mass located posterior to the medial femoral condyle between the tendons of the medial head of the gastrocnemius and semimembranosus muscles. The mass will be rounded, smooth, supple, and transilluminating.

Background Information

This condition typically results from fluid distention from the gastrocnemius-semimembranosus bursae that communicates with the posterior aspect of the joint capsule. In adults, it may result from an intraarticular pathology that leads to posterior effusion. Intra-articular knee disorders such as meniscal tears, primary osteoarthritis, and rheumatoid arthritis are frequently associated with this condition.[5,6] A common complication is rupture or dissection of fluid into the gastrocnemius muscle, which may mimic symptoms of a deep venous thrombosis. Diagnosis is confirmed by imaging studies including ultrasound and magnetic resonance imaging. Treatment typically consists of aspirating the knee effusion, although there is a high rate of recurrence when the underlying cause is unaddressed.

BURSITIS

■ Infrapatellar Bursitis

Chief Clinical Characteristics

This presentation includes localized edema over the inferior aspect of the patellofemoral joint and pain in the infrapatellar region with palpation (Fig. 21-2).

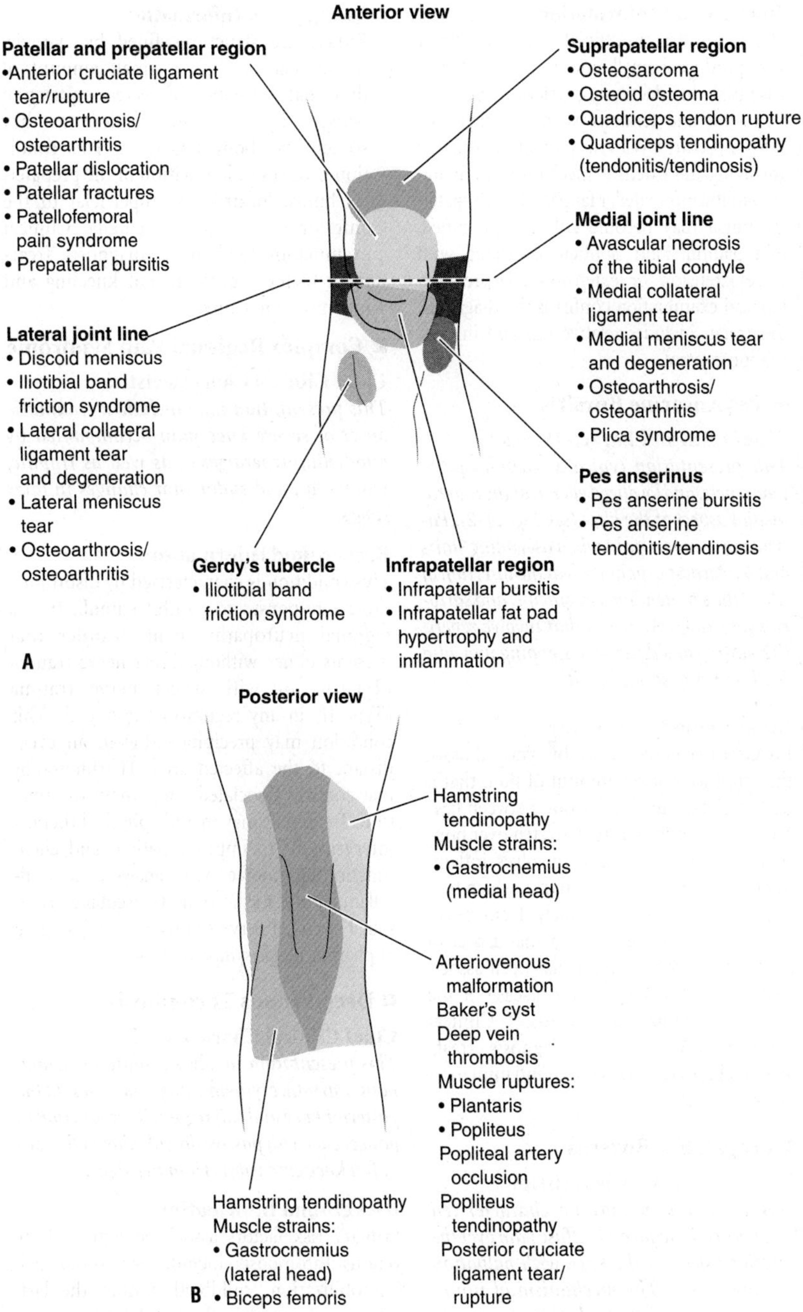

Anterior view

Patellar and prepatellar region
• Anterior cruciate ligament
  tear/rupture
• Osteoarthrosis/
  osteoarthritis
• Patellar dislocation
• Patellar fractures
• Patellofemoral
  pain syndrome
• Prepatellar bursitis

Suprapatellar region
• Osteosarcoma
• Osteoid osteoma
• Quadriceps tendon rupture
• Quadriceps tendinopathy
  (tendonitis/tendinosis)

Medial joint line
• Avascular necrosis
  of the tibial condyle
• Medial collateral
  ligament tear
• Medial meniscus tear
  and degeneration
• Osteoarthrosis/
  osteoarthritis
• Plica syndrome

Lateral joint line
• Discoid meniscus
• Iliotibial band
  friction syndrome
• Lateral collateral
  ligament tear
  and degeneration
• Lateral meniscus
  tear
• Osteoarthrosis/
  osteoarthritis

Pes anserinus
• Pes anserine bursitis
• Pes anserine
  tendonitis/tendinosis

Gerdy's tubercle
• Iliotibial band
  friction syndrome

Infrapatellar region
• Infrapatellar bursitis
• Infrapatellar fat pad
  hypertrophy and
  inflammation

A

Posterior view

Hamstring
  tendinopathy
Muscle strains:
• Gastrocnemius
  (medial head)

Arteriovenous
  malformation
Baker's cyst
Deep vein
  thrombosis
Muscle ruptures:
• Plantaris
• Popliteus
Popliteal artery
  occlusion
Popliteus
  tendinopathy
Posterior cruciate
  ligament tear/
  rupture

Hamstring tendinopathy
Muscle strains:
• Gastrocnemius
  (lateral head)
B • Biceps femoris

FIGURE 21-2 Surface anatomy of selected local sources of knee pain, causing either (A) anterior knee pain or (B) posterior knee pain.

Background Information

Bursae are structures lined by synovial tissue that produce a small amount of fluid that is essential in decreasing friction between ligaments and tendons as they stretch over bony structures. With movement dysfunction involving the extensor mechanism or irritation to the infrapatellar fat pad, the infrapatellar bursa may become enlarged, inflamed, and painful. Pain is often associated with hyperextension or extension overpressure. Clinical examination confirms the diagnosis. Treatment includes relative rest and inflammation control.

■ Pes Anserine Bursitis

Chief Clinical Characteristics

This presentation typically includes pain, tenderness, and localized edema at the anteromedial aspect of the knee (see Fig. 21-2). Patients may report pain when ascending stairs and tenderness to palpation at the insertion of site of the semitendinosus, gracilis, and sartorius insertions. Activities that involve repetitive cutting or side-to-side stepping may also result in pes anserine bursitis.

Background Information

Bursae are structures lined by synovial tissue that produce a small amount of fluid that is essential in decreasing friction between ligaments and tendons as they stretch over bony structures. This condition involves inflammation of the pes anserine bursa, which typically is located approximately 4 cm below the joint line at the anteromedial aspect of the knee.[7] Chronic bursitis has been associated with degenerative joint disease of the knee or rheumatoid arthritis.[8,9] Clinical examination confirms the diagnosis. Treatment includes relative rest and inflammation control.

■ Prepatellar Bursitis

Chief Clinical Characteristics

This presentation may be characterized by superficial edema and diffuse pain over the anterior aspect of the knee with palpation (see Fig. 21-2). The mechanism of injury typically involves repeated minor trauma or kneeling, inciting inflammation of the subcutaneous bursa over the patella.

Background Information

Bursae are structures lined by synovial tissue that produce a small amount of fluid that is essential in decreasing friction between ligaments and tendons as they stretch over bony structures. This condition involves inflammation of the prepatellar bursa, located just superficial to the anterior surface of the patella. Clinical examination confirms the diagnosis. Treatment includes avoidance of kneeling and inflammation control.

■ Complex Regional Pain Syndrome

Chief Clinical Characteristics

This presentation may include a traumatic onset of severe knee pain accompanied by allodynia, hyperalgesia, as well as trophic, vasomotor, and sudomotor changes in later stages.

Background Information

This condition is characterized by disproportionate responses to painful stimuli. It is a regional neuropathic pain disorder that presents either without direct nerve trauma (Type I) or with direct nerve trauma (Type II) in any region of the body.[10] This condition may precipitate due to an event distant to the affected area. Thermography may confirm associated sympathetic dysfunction. Treatment may include physical therapy interventions to improve patient and client functioning, biofeedback, analgesic or anti-inflammatory medication, transcutaneous or spinal electrical nerve stimulation, and surgical or pharmacologic sympathectomy.

■ Deep Venous Thrombosis

Chief Clinical Characteristics

This presentation involves unilateral edema, pain, warmth, erythema, and tenderness in the posterior knee and calf region. Reproduction of pain occurs with passive dorsiflexion of the foot in full knee extension (Homan's sign).

Background Information

Primary risk factors associated with a deep venous thrombosis include age, prolonged immobilization, childbirth within the last 6 months, surgery in the last 4 weeks, major trauma, cancer treatment, hormone replacement therapy, and long car or airplane travel in the last 4 weeks (Table 21-1). This condition involves a blood clot (thrombus) that develops in a deep vein, usually in the lower leg and thigh. A thrombus could interfere with circulation of the region, break off, and embolize to the brain, lungs, and heart. Doppler ultrasound confirms the diagnosis. Complications include severe tissue damage and death, making this condition a medical emergency.

TABLE 21-1

Does My Patient With Knee Pain Have Deep Venous Thrombosis? A Clinical Decision Rule for Diagnosis

CLINICAL FINDING	SCORE*
Activity cancer (treatment ongoing, within previous 6 months, or palliative)	1
Paralysis, paresis, or recent plaster immobilization of the lower extremities	1
Recently bedridden for > 3 days or major surgery within 4 weeks	1
Localized tenderness along the distribution of the deep venous system[†]	1
Entire leg swelling	1
Calf swelling by > 3 cm when compared with the asymptomatic leg[‡]	1
Pitting edema (greater in the symptomatic leg)	1
Collateral superficial veins (nonvaricose)	1
Alternative diagnosis as likely or greater than that of PDVT[§]	-2

*A score is obtained by summing all items that are judged to be present; score of ≤ 0 = low probability of PDVT; score of 1 or 2 = moderate probability of PDVT; score of ≥ 3 = high probability of PDVT.

[†]Tenderness along the deep venous system is assessed by firm palpation in the center of the posterior calf, the popliteal space, and along the area of the femoral vein in the anterior thigh and groin.

[‡]Measured with a tape measure 10 cm below tibial tuberosity.

[§]More common alternative diagnoses are cellulitis, calf strain, Baker's cyst, or postoperative swelling.

Reprinted with permission from Wells PS, Anderson DR, Bormanis J, et al. Value of assessment of pretest probability of deep-vein thrombosis in clinical management. *Lancet.* 1997;350[9094]:1795–1798.

■ Discoid Meniscus

Chief Clinical Characteristics
This presentation typically includes pain, edema, locking, and catching. This condition may involve a "snapping knee" or an audible, palpable, or visible pop near terminal knee extension that most commonly presents in children.

Background Information
A discoid meniscus is an anatomical variant with a propensity for tearing and is most commonly present in the lateral meniscus.[11,12] Magnetic resonance imaging confirms the diagnosis. Surgical intervention usually is required. The type of surgical intervention depends on the nature of this condition. Treatment options include partial or total meniscectomies, meniscal stabilization, and saucerization.

■ Fibromyalgia

Chief Clinical Characteristics
This presentation typically includes chronic widespread joint and muscle pain defined as bilateral upper body, lower body, and spine pain, associated with tenderness to palpation at 11 of 18 specific muscle-tendon sites. Individuals with this condition will demonstrate lowered mechanical and thermal pain thresholds, high pain ratings for noxious stimuli, and altered temporal summation of pain stimuli.[13]

Background Information
The etiology of this condition is unclear; multiple body systems appear to be involved. Indistinct clinical boundaries between this condition and similar conditions (eg, chronic fatigue syndrome, irritable bowel syndrome, and chronic muscular headaches) pose a diagnostic challenge.[13] This condition is diagnosed by exclusion. Treatment will often include polypharmacy and elements to improve self-efficacy, physical training, and cognitive-behavioral techniques.[14]

FRACTURES

■ Intercondylar Eminence Fracture of the Tibia

Chief Clinical Characteristics
This presentation typically includes pain, joint effusion, and the inability to bear weight.

Background Information

Fracture has been reported to occur most commonly after a fall from a bicycle and the mechanism of injury is usually a hyperextension force with or without a valgus or rotational moment about the knee.[15] This condition often is observed in patients prior to skeletal maturity, resulting from injuries that would ordinarily cause anterior cruciate ligament tears in adults. When the tibia is forcefully anteriorly displaced on the femur, the incompletely ossified tibial eminence will fail before the anterior cruciate ligament. The diagnosis is confirmed with plain radiographs. Depending on the extent of the fracture, treatment typically includes immobilization with protected weight bearing, surgical fixation, or reduction.

■ Osteochondral Fracture of the Patella

Chief Clinical Characteristics

This presentation includes patellar tenderness, edema, and a history of direct or indirect injury. Injuries that damage articular cartilage and adversely affect the subchondral bone are often referred to as osteochondral fractures.

Background Information

This condition most commonly occurs as a result of a direct or indirect blow and from patellar dislocations. Compared to adults, children are more susceptible to this type of fracture because they have greater patellar mobility. Diagnosis may be confirmed by plain radiographs. The fracture occurs at the point of contact, with the separate fracture fragment containing articular cartilage, subchondral bone, and supporting trabecular bone. These fragments may be displaced intra-articularly and become loose bodies, or they may be in place and heal. Surgical intervention for the removal of loose bodies may be indicated if pain persists.

■ Patellar Fracture

Chief Clinical Characteristics

This presentation ranges from mild concerns of instability in the knee, to severe pain and complete inability to actively flex or extend the knee. Bearing weight on the affected limb (especially in any angle of knee flexion) is often significantly painful.

Background Information

Patellar fractures most commonly occur in relatively young patients due to a direct force to the knee.[16] In young patients, patellar fractures are most often transverse due to the mechanism of injury being from a distraction or "pulling apart" of the patella by a forceful active contraction of the quadriceps.[17] Comminuted fractures result from a direct force to the patella while the quadriceps is under tension. Differential diagnosis includes patellar bursitis, dislocation, and bipartite patella (typically asymptomatic). The diagnosis is confirmed with plain radiographs. Usual treatment involves immobilization, although surgical fixation of fracture segments may be indicated if the fracture is displaced.

■ Supracondylar Fracture of the Femur

Chief Clinical Characteristics

This presentation includes pain, edema, limb deformity, and an inability to bear weight. In the absence of osteoporosis, the patient will often have some history of trauma.

Background Information

Supracondylar femur fractures typically result from low-energy trauma to osteoporotic bone in elderly persons or high-energy trauma in young patients. These fractures are most commonly observed in elderly patients with multiple medical comorbidities and osteoporosis. Surgical treatment almost always is indicated, involving reduction followed by external or internal fixation to maintain alignment.

■ Gout

Chief Clinical Characteristics

This presentation includes severe pain, edema, warmth, erythema, and localized tenderness. Systemic findings may include fever, chills, malaise, and sweating. Patients typically report an acute onset of symptoms within several hours. Pain may be triggered by low alcohol abuse, dehydration, trauma, surgery, septic arthritis, protein fasting, excessive purine ingestion, and allopurinol or uricosuric agents.

Background Information

This condition is a peripheral arthritis that results from the deposition of sodium urate crystals in one or more joints. A variety of conditions, including renal disease, have been implicated as contributory, but most cases are idiopathic. Gout most commonly affects the feet, ankles, hands, wrists, elbows, and knees. This diagnosis is confirmed with microscopic study of synovial fluid aspirated from affected joints. Treatment involves medication to ameliorate the underlying metabolic dysfunction.

■ Hemarthrosis

Chief Clinical Characteristics

This presentation may involve joint effusion, pain with motion and weight bearing, and a fixed flexion deformity. The knee, ankle, and elbow are most susceptible to this condition.[18]

Background Information

Hemarthrosis is commonly associated with hemophilia, an X-linked hematologic disorder characterized by a propensity to hemorrhage due to the inability to produce clotting factors VIII and IX. Acute bleeding increases the pressure in the synovial cavity and bone marrow, which leads to severe pain and possible avascular necrosis or pseudotumoral mass. Intra-articular hemorrhage may occur spontaneously or result from insignificant trauma. Diagnosis is confirmed with ultrasound, plain radiographs, and magnetic resonance imaging. Treatment involves a combination of factor replacement, joint aspiration, rest (with or without splinting), joint injections of radioactive substances to control hemorrhage, and surgical joint replacements for end-stage disease.

■ Iliotibial Band Friction Syndrome

Chief Clinical Characteristics

This presentation typically includes a gradual and progressive onset of pain and localized tenderness over the lateral aspect of the knee that increases with activities involving repetitive knee flexion (see Fig. 21-2).

Background Information

This condition is an inflammatory injury that results from friction between the iliotibial band and the lateral femoral condyle. It is commonly observed among long-distance runners, cyclists, downhill skiers, and military recruits. In runners, the pain often begins at a predictable distance, is relieved when the knee is maintained in full extension, and is aggravated by repetitive knee flexion, specifically at 30 degrees of knee flexion.[19] Factors that may contribute to the development of this syndrome include sudden changes in training volume, genu varus, decreased flexibility of the iliotibial band, hip abduction weakness, rearfoot varus, and pes cavus.[19] Clinical examination confirms the diagnosis. Treatment involves nonsurgical interventions, such as relative rest, exercise, and physical modalities for symptom and inflammation control.

■ Infrapatellar Fat Pad Hypertrophy and Inflammation (Hoffa's Disease)

Chief Clinical Characteristics

This presentation includes pain, edema, and tenderness over the anterior or medial aspect of the knee in the region of the patellar tendon. Patients will report pain with end-range knee extension. Palpation may reveal local tenderness and a hypertrophied infrapatellar fat pad.

Background Information

Inflammation of the infrapatellar fat pad may result from the impingement of the fat pad in the tibiofemoral joint during knee extension or from direct trauma.[20] This diagnosis may present as an acute or chronic condition. Clinical examination confirms the diagnosis. Acute management includes rest and inflammation control. In chronic conditions, restoration of extension range of motion, strength, and quadriceps muscle flexibility should be emphasized.

■ Lateral Meniscus Degeneration

Chief Clinical Characteristics

This presentation can involve localized pain in the region of the lateral joint line. Pain is worsened with squatting activities and ascending/descending stairs (see Fig. 21-2). Reports of locking and catching are less common with degenerative tears as opposed to acute traumatic tears.

Background Information

This condition occurs when the collagen fibers within the meniscus start to break down and lend less support to the structure of the meniscus. Age is a risk factor; 60% of individuals over the age of 65 present with this condition.[21] Degenerative tears may result from repetitive activities over time such as squatting and kneeling, but may also occur over time secondary to trauma or previous history of surgery. Magnetic resonance imaging confirms the diagnosis. Nonsurgical intervention is commonly attempted first, and severe cases may require partial or total knee replacements.

■ Medial Meniscus Degeneration

Chief Clinical Characteristics
This presentation may include localized pain in the region of the medial joint line. Patient reports pain with squatting activities and ascending/descending stairs (see Fig. 21-2).

Background Information
Degenerative meniscal tears occur as part of the aging process when the collagen fibers within the meniscus start to break down and lend less support to the structure of the meniscus. Age is a risk factor; 60% of individuals over the age of 65 have degenerative meniscal tears.[21] Degenerative tears may result from repetitive activities over time such as squatting and kneeling, but may also occur over time secondary to trauma or previous history of surgery. Patients are less likely to report locking and catching with degenerative tears as opposed to acute traumatic tears. Diagnosis is confirmed with magnetic resonance imaging. Degenerative tears are typically associated with articular cartilage degeneration; therefore, arthroscopic surgical outcomes may not be as successful as those for acute traumatic tears. Nonsurgical intervention is commonly attempted first. Severe cases may require partial or total knee replacements.

■ Metastases to the Knee, Including From Primary Breast, Kidney, Lung, Prostate, and Thyroid Disease

Chief Clinical Characteristics
This presentation typically includes unremitting pain in individuals with these risk factors: previous history of cancer, age 50 years or older, failure to improve with conservative therapy, and unexplained weight change of more than 10 pounds in 6 months.[22]

Background Information
The skeletal system is the third most common site of metastatic disease.[23] Symptoms also may be related to pathological fracture in affected sites. Common primary sites causing metastases to bone include breast, prostate, lung, and kidney. Bone scan confirms the diagnosis. Common treatments for metastases include surgical resection, chemotherapy, radiation treatment, and palliation, depending on the tumor type and extent of metastasis.

MUSCLE STRAINS

■ Biceps Femoris Muscle Strain

Chief Clinical Characteristics
This presentation can involve pain and tenderness over the posterolateral thigh and knee, with a history of sudden onset during activity. Symptoms include pain with resisted knee flexion and passive knee extension. The biceps femoris muscle is the most commonly injured muscle of the hamstring complex,[24–26] often occurring in athletes who run, kick, and jump.

Background Information
Injury is most likely to occur while the musculotendinous junction undergoes maximum strain during an eccentric contraction of the hamstrings. A hamstring strain can occur during an isolated event or result from persistent repetitive stress. Ecchymosis and edema are typically present in second- and third-degree strains. The diagnosis is confirmed on the basis of clinical examination. Treatment includes inflammation control and strength and flexibility exercises. Caution should be taken to avoid early aggressive stretching. Surgical intervention is required only in the case of complete rupture of the proximal or distal attachment.

■ Gastrocnemius Muscle Strain

Chief Clinical Characteristics
This presentation may involve pain and tenderness to palpation at the origin of the gastrocnemius muscle and posterior calf. Depending on the severity of the injury, pain may radiate into the ankle. Symptoms are aggravated by passive ankle dorsiflexion and active ankle plantarflexion.

Background Information
This condition results from a forceful push-off with the foot. Tennis, jumping, hill

running, and sprinting are commonly associated with this injury. The medial head of the gastrocnemius is most frequently involved. Clinical examination confirms the diagnosis. Treatment includes rest, inflammation control, gentle, pain-free ankle range of motion, use of a heel lift, and strength and flexibility exercises. Caution should be taken to avoid early, aggressive stretching.

■ Semimembranosus Muscle Strain

Chief Clinical Characteristics
This presentation includes a sudden onset of pain and tenderness over the posteromedial thigh and knee. Ecchymosis and edema are more commonly present in second- and third-degree strains. Symptoms include pain with resisted knee flexion and passive knee extension. Strains most commonly occur in athletes who run, kick, and jump.

Background Information
Injury is most likely to occur while the musculotendinous junction undergoes maximum strain during eccentric contraction of the hamstrings. This condition can occur following an isolated event or persistent repetitive stress. Clinical examination confirms the diagnosis. Treatment usually includes inflammation control, strength, and flexibility. Caution should be taken to avoid early, aggressive stretching. Surgical intervention is required only in the case of complete rupture of the proximal or distal attachment.

NERVE ENTRAPMENTS

■ Common Peroneal Nerve Entrapment at the Fibular Head

Chief Clinical Characteristics
This presentation may be characterized by a partial or total loss of sensation in the distribution of the peroneal nerve. Weakness with ankle dorsiflexion and extension of the toes and a positive Tinel's sign at the fibular head may also be present.

Background Information
Pain is an uncommon feature unless it is related to the specific cause of the nerve entrapment, such as entrapment secondary to soft tissue swelling and inflammation from direct trauma. Causes include sitting

crossed-legged, prolonged immobility in bed against bedrails or firm mattresses, trauma, squatting, crouching, kneeling, and idiopathic origins. Dynamic entrapments also may occur during activities such as running. The common peroneal nerve may be injured at any location along the nerve; however, entrapment most frequently occurs at the fibular head. The nerve may become compressed under the fibrous arch in the region where the bifurcation of the nerve into its deep and superficial branches occurs.[27,28] An electrodiagnostic evaluation, including a nerve conduction velocity test and needle electromyography, may confirm the diagnosis. Treatment is generally conservative; however, surgical decompression may be indicated in recalcitrant cases in which the anatomical site of entrapment is well characterized.

■ Saphenous Nerve Entrapment

Chief Clinical Characteristics
This presentation involves pain and/or paresthesias in the medial thigh and knee, tenderness to palpation over the adductor canal, and normal motor function of the affected extremity. Symptoms include a deep ache that may radiate into the foot along the saphenous nerve distribution. Symptoms are exacerbated by prolonged walking or standing.

Background Information
Entrapment typically occurs where the saphenous nerve pierces the fascia of the adductor canal, resulting in inflammation. Mechanisms for saphenous nerve entrapment may be traumatic, nontraumatic, or iatrogenic (eg, following knee surgery or saphenous vein harvest). Diagnosis may be confirmed with injection of local anesthetic. Symptoms typically improve following an injection with a local anesthetic and steroids and avoiding aggravating activities. Neurolysis or neurectomy may be performed if nonsurgical treatment fails in recalcitrant cases in which the anatomical site of entrapment is well characterized.[29]

■ Osteochondritis Dissecans

Chief Clinical Characteristics
This presentation typically includes vague knee pain and effusion without a history of recent

trauma. Pain increases with activity and patient may report a history of locking or catching if a loose body is present.

Background Information

This condition is a partial or total separation of intra-articular bone fragment and/or articular cartilage without a history of specific trauma. It is associated with acute bone necrosis. In adults and adolescents, these lesions are classically located on the lateral aspect of the medial femoral condyle.[30] This diagnosis is confirmed with plain radiographs, computed tomography, or magnetic resonance imaging. Treatment includes immobilization and rest; however, surgical treatment may be indicated if no progression toward healing is seen on radiographs or if the lesion becomes unstable.

■ Osteomyelitis of the Distal Femur, Proximal Tibia, or Proximal Fibula

Chief Clinical Characteristics

This presentation involves local pain, edema, and erythema with associated systemic findings such as malaise, chills, night sweats, and an abrupt onset of fever.

Background Information

This condition is an acute or chronic infection of bone secondary to infection with pyogenic organisms. The two primary types of acute osteomyelitis are direct inoculation and hematogenous. Direct inoculation osteomyelitis primarily occurs in adults and is the result of direct contact of tissue and bacteria during trauma or surgery. Hematogenous osteomyelitis is an infection caused by bacterial seeding from the blood and most commonly occurs in children. The diagnosis is confirmed with blood panels demonstrating elevated white blood cell count and plain radiographs. Treatment involves intravenous antibiotic therapy and surgical treatment of the lesion.

■ Patellar Instability

Chief Clinical Characteristics

This presentation includes vague anterior knee pain and swelling with a history of patellar subluxations or reports of the knee "giving way." A positive patellar apprehension test and palpable tenderness over the lateral condyle, medial soft tissue, or the anterior aspect of the

knee may be present. Symptoms occur with jumping, running, or quick changes in direction.

Background Information

The most common mechanism of patellar dislocation is lower extremity internal rotation with combined knee valgus on a planted foot (noncontact). Younger children and adolescents are at greater risk for instability. A number of risk factors are associated with patellar instability, including ligament laxity, decreased strength and muscle mass, patella alta, increased Q angle, increased femoral anteversion, iliotibial band tightness, and excessive midfoot pronation. Treatment typically involves rehabilitation, although surgical intervention is indicated if patellar instability continues after rehabilitation, with concomitant osteochondral lesions, if palpable disruption of the medial patellofemoral ligament-vastus medialis obliquus-adductor mechanism occurs, or if participation in high-level athletics is required.

■ Patellofemoral Pain Syndrome

Chief Clinical Characteristics

This presentation involves pain in the anterior aspect or deep inside the knee joint (see Fig. 21-2). Symptoms may begin insidiously or following trauma. Patients report pain with squatting, prolonged sitting, and ascending or descending stairs.

Background Information

In the absence of trauma or acute inflammation, minimal effusion will be present and pain with palpation is often absent. The mechanism of injury can present acutely following an episode of trauma to the knee joint (falling or any compressive force directly on the knee) or symptoms may develop over a prolonged period of time (overuse from repeated running or squatting activities). Treatment involves relative rest, proximal lower extremity muscle strengthening and flexibility exercises, and physical modalities for symptom control.

■ Plica Syndrome

Chief Clinical Characteristics

This presentation typically includes an acute onset of pain and tenderness just anterior and medial to the joint line. Localized tenderness over the medial femoral condyle and medial patella may be present. Patient may report snapping between 50 and 70 degrees of knee flexion.[20] *Symptoms may mimic loose bodies, a meniscal lesion, or patellofemoral pain syndrome.*

Background Information

Plicae are redundant folds of synovium, located in the knee, that may become inflamed and symptomatic as a result of direct trauma or overuse. There are three major types of plica: the infrapatellar, suprapatellar, and mediopatellar plicae. The mediopatellar plica is most often implicated. Arthroscopy is the gold standard for diagnosis of plica syndrome.[31] Nonsurgical intervention is typically initiated first, which includes patellar mobilization, stretching, and anti-inflammatory medication. Surgical intervention to excise the pathological plica is rare, but may be successful.

■ Popliteal Artery Occlusion

Chief Clinical Characteristics

This presentation includes an acute onset of severe claudication, dependent rubor, absent ankle pulses, and decreased temperature to palpation distally.

Background Information

In severe chronic conditions, pain at rest, cyanosis, or a nonhealing ischemic ulcer may be present. This condition is caused by trauma, atherosclerosis, emboli, popliteal artery aneurysm, cystic adventitial disease, and popliteal entrapment syndrome. Patients at risk include elderly patients and patients with diabetes mellitus and cardiovascular disease. Diagnosis is confirmed with angiography, ultrasonography, and the ankle brachial index. Surgical and nonsurgical treatment of an arterial occlusion depends on the cause of the occlusion, with interventions ranging from drug therapy to bypass surgery.

■ Primary Osteoarthrosis/ Osteoarthritis

Chief Clinical Characteristics

This presentation typically includes joint pain, stiffness, and radiographic evidence of articular cartilage degeneration. Other signs and symptoms may include limited range of motion, intermittent aching associated with activity, or constant deep pain. This condition

is the most common joint disease for middle-aged and older individuals.[32]

Background Information

Primary osteoarthrosis/osteoarthritis involves a progressive loss of articular cartilage, remodeling and sclerosis of subchondral bone, and osteophyte formation. Risk factors include age, joint injury, excessive repetitive joint loading, and joint dysplasia.[32] Plain radiographs confirm the diagnosis. Nonoperative treatment may include inflammation control, patient education for weight control, exercise (avoiding high-impact activities), and foot orthoses. In severe cases, osteotomy, arthroscopy, chondroplasty, or joint replacement may be indicated.

■ Pseudogout

Chief Clinical Characteristics

This presentation includes warmth and erythematous, tender, and asymmetrical edema of the knee. This condition is characterized by an insidious onset of symptoms over several days. The most commonly affected joints are the knees, wrists, and shoulders.

Background Information

Many cases are idiopathic; however, pseudogout also has been associated with aging, trauma, and metabolic abnormalities such as hyperparathyroidism and hemochromatosis. This condition involves joint inflammation caused by calcium pyrophosphate crystals and is often referred to as calcium pyrophosphate disease. This diagnosis is confirmed with microscopic study of synovial fluid aspirated from affected joints. Treatment involves medication to ameliorate the underlying metabolic dysfunction.

■ Reiter's Syndrome

Chief Clinical Characteristics

This presentation may be characterized by joint pain and stiffness, involved with a classic triad of arthritis, urethritis, and conjunctivitis. Disease incidence peaks during the third decade of life, with a male-to-female ratio of 5:1.[33]

Background Information

This condition is typically preceded by either an episode of dysentery or infectious arthritis, and individuals with the HLA-B27 genetic makeup are at greater risk. Asymmetric arthropathy involving the knee, ankle, foot, and sacroiliac joint is common. It is generally a self-limiting disease that typically resolves in 3 to 4 months. However, it is common for approximately half of all patients to have recurring symptoms. Medications are used in the treatment of the disease and physical therapy intervention should be targeted toward restoration of range of motion, flexibility, and strength.

■ Rheumatoid Arthritis of the Knee

Chief Clinical Characteristics
This presentation includes morning stiffness and generalized pain throughout multiple joints in a symmetric distribution, with possible tenderness and swelling of affected joints. Women are twice as likely to be affected as men.

Background Information
Symptoms associated with this progressive inflammatory joint disease are caused by synovial membrane thickening and cytokine production in synovial fluid. Articular cartilage erosion, synovial hypertrophy, and constant joint effusion eventually cause bony erosions and joint deformities that have a significant impact on daily function.[50] Younger age of onset is associated with a greater extent of disability later. Plain radiographs and blood tests confirm the diagnosis. Treatment typically includes a variety of steroidal, nonsteroidal, and biological anti-inflammatory medications.

RUPTURES AND TEARS

■ Lateral Collateral Ligament Sprain/Rupture

Chief Clinical Characteristics
This presentation involves pain, localized edema along the lateral aspect of the knee, and lateral joint line tenderness (see Fig. 21-2). Pain and/or laxity is present with varus stress testing at 30 degrees of knee flexion. This injury generally results in minimal effusion and pain with walking; however, the patient may report difficulty with running and cutting activities.

Background Information
Mechanism of injury is typically from a varus stress applied to the knee, such as a direct blow to the medial aspect of the knee.

During varus stress testing, pain with no joint laxity is a Grade I (stretch) injury. Laxity with a firm end-feel is a Grade II (partial tear) injury and no firm end-feel is a Grade III (complete tear) injury.[34] Clinical examination and magnetic resonance imaging confirm the diagnosis. Grade I, II, and III injuries are managed nonsurgically.[34,35] Surgical repair may be necessary to address associated meniscal or combined ligament tears.

■ Lateral Meniscus Tear

Chief Clinical Characteristics
This presentation may involve pain, lateral joint line tenderness, and reports of catching, clicking, and locking (see Fig. 21-2). Mild joint line effusion is present and pain or a palpable click may be provoked with McMurray's and Apley's compression tests.

Background Information
Mechanism of injury involves an acute, non-contact rotatory force with the knee flexed and the foot planted. Meniscal compromise leads to increased stress on the articular cartilage and early degenerative changes. Magnetic resonance imaging confirms this diagnosis.[36–38] Tears located in the peripheral one-third of the meniscus respond well to surgical intervention. Some researchers advocate that tears in the middle one-third zone also be repaired.[39,40]

■ Medial Collateral Ligament Sprain/Rupture

Chief Clinical Characteristics
This presentation includes pain, localized edema along the medial aspect of the knee, and medial joint line tenderness (see Fig. 21-2). Pain and/or laxity is present with valgus stress testing at 30 degrees of knee flexion. This injury generally results in minimal effusion and pain with walking; however, it also may cause difficulty with running and cutting.

Background Information
Mechanism of injury involves a valgus stress applied to the knee, such as a direct blow to the lateral aspect of the knee. The incidence of medial meniscus tears increases with increased severity of the sprain because of its attachment to the medial collateral ligament.

With valgus stress testing, pain with no joint laxity is a Grade I injury (stretch). Laxity with a firm end-feel is a Grade II injury (partial tear) and no firm end-feel is a Grade III injury (complete tear).[34] Clinical examination and magnetic resonance imaging confirm the diagnosis. Tears located in the peripheral one-third of the meniscus respond well to surgical intervention. Some researchers advocate that tears in the middle one-third zone also be repaired.[39,40]

■ Medial Meniscus Tear

Chief Clinical Characteristics
This presentation can be characterized by pain, medial joint line tenderness, and reports of catching, clicking, and locking (see Fig. 21-2). Mild joint line effusion is present and pain or a palpable click may be provoked with McMurray's and Apley's compression tests. Mechanism of injury involves an acute, noncontact rotatory force with the knee flexed and the foot planted.

Background Information
The medial meniscus is more commonly injured than the lateral meniscus because it is less mobile.[39] This condition often is associated with medial collateral ligament injuries because of its rigid attachment to the ligament and the joint capsule. Meniscal compromise leads to increased stress on the articular cartilage and early degenerative changes. Magnetic resonance imaging confirms the diagnosis.[36–38] Typically, tears located in the peripheral one-third of the meniscus respond well with surgical intervention. Some researchers advocate that tears in the middle one-third zone also be repaired.[39,40]

■ Plantaris Muscle Rupture

Chief Clinical Characteristics
This presentation may include pain, tenderness, the presence of a hematoma, and retraction of the muscle over the proximal, posteromedial aspect of the calf. A "pop" in the calf is commonly experienced. This condition results from a forceful push-off with the foot.

Background Information
Tennis, jumping, hill running, and sprinting are commonly associated with this injury.

Rupture of the plantaris muscle rarely occurs in isolation and is most commonly associated with strain of the medial head of the gastrocnemius.[41,42] The diagnosis is confirmed by magnetic resonance imaging. This condition is typically treated nonsurgically. When surgical intervention is indicated, the retracted muscle is resected.[41]

■ Popliteus Tendon Rupture

Chief Clinical Characteristics
This presentation involves acute, lateral joint line and posterolateral knee pain and decreased range of motion. Acute symptoms may be associated with a crack or pop at the time of the injury and difficulty bearing weight on the affected limb.

Background Information
Mechanism of injury involves a rapid external rotation of the tibia with the knee in a flexed and fixed position; however, rupture may also occur without a history of trauma.[43] Isolated ruptures of the popliteus tendon are rare. This condition occurs more frequently with posterolateral corner injuries in which there is concomitant disruption of the arcuate ligament complex, the lateral collateral ligament, the anterior/posterior cruciate ligaments, or the menisci.[44] The diagnosis is confirmed with magnetic resonance imaging. Intervention requires surgical reattachment of the ruptured tendon.

■ Posterior Cruciate Ligament Sprain/Rupture

Chief Clinical Characteristics
This presentation typically includes pain, edema, and tenderness in the region of the popliteal fossa. Positive posterior sag sign of the tibia with the hip and knee flexed to 90 degrees and a positive posterior drawer test may be present.

Background Information
Mechanism of injury is typically from a hyperextension force or a direct anterior blow to the knee in a flexed position. This condition occurs with falls onto a flexed knee with the foot in plantarflexion, causing the tibial tubercle to contact the ground first, and in motor vehicle accidents resulting from contact with the dashboard. Magnetic

resonance imaging confirms the diagnosis. Even complete ruptures are not usually repaired surgically.

■ Quadriceps Tendon Rupture

Chief Clinical Characteristics

This presentation typically involves acute, severe pain over the anterior aspect of the knee and the inability to actively extend the knee. Superior dislocation of the patella and hemarthrosis often result immediately. A palpable gap in the suprapatellar region may be present, although this is often masked by hemarthrosis. This condition is frequently observed in patients older than 40 years of age and in patients with comorbid medical conditions, such as metabolic disease, obesity, and long-term steroid use.[45]

Background Information

Mechanism of injury is often associated with a strong concentric contraction of the quadriceps in association with forced flexion of the knee. Diagnosis is confirmed with magnetic resonance imaging. Incomplete ruptures are typically managed nonsurgically with the knee immobilized in full extension for 6 weeks followed by protected range of motion and strengthening once the patient is able to exhibit good quadriceps control and perform a straight leg raise with minimal discomfort. Surgical repair is indicated for complete ruptures.

■ Septic Arthritis

Chief Clinical Characteristics

This presentation may involve severe aching pain, edema, erythema, stiffness, general malaise, and fever. The fever may be low grade and there also may be a restriction to active and passive range of motion.

Background Information

Common risk factors include rheumatoid arthritis, immunodeficiency, intravenous drug use, and joint replacement. This condition involves inflammation of the synovial membrane with purulent effusion into the joint capsule, usually due to bacterial infection. In adults, septic arthritis most commonly affects the knee. The diagnosis is confirmed by elevated white blood cell count and erythrocyte sedimentation rate and needle aspiration.

Treatment includes antibiotic therapy and aspiration. Surgical intervention may be necessary in cases that do not respond to aspiration.

■ Sickle Cell Crisis

Chief Clinical Characteristics

This presentation includes an acute, severe onset of pain and limited range of motion that may be associated with fever, cold weather, dehydration, infection, and physical/psychological stress in individuals with sickle cell anemia.[46]

Background Information

An acute exacerbation of the signs and symptoms associated with sickle cell disease is known as a crisis. There are four patterns of an acute crisis based on their location: bone crisis, acute chest syndrome, abdominal crisis, and joint crisis. During a bone crisis, the tibia, femur, and humerus are commonly involved and single or multiple joints may be affected. This condition is a group of inherited disorders with abnormalities caused by hemoglobin S. This condition typically is associated with pain due to tissue infarction and/or worsening anemia. Diagnosis of a crisis is confirmed with plain radiographs and magnetic resonance imaging. This condition is a medical emergency.

■ Spontaneous Avascular Necrosis of the Medial Femoral Condyle/Proximal Tibia

Chief Clinical Characteristics

This presentation can be characterized by a sudden onset of severe medial knee pain that is exacerbated by weight-bearing activities and frequently present at rest and worst at night. This condition most commonly occurs after the sixth decade of life, and women are affected three times more frequently than men.[47–51]

Background Information

This condition is the result of circulatory impairments to an area of bone that result in infarct due to either primary vascular insufficiency, minor trauma, or repetitive insults, leading to microfractures in the subchondral bone. Unilateral involvement dominates and lesions most frequently are observed at either the medial femoral condyle or the medial tibial plateau.[47–49,51,52] The diagnosis is confirmed with magnetic resonance imaging. This diagnosis may be managed nonsurgically with protective weight bearing, inflammation control, and strengthening of the quadriceps and hamstring muscles. When surgical intervention is required, treatment options are arthroscopy, tibial osteotomy, osteochondral grafts, core decompression, unicondylar knee arthroplasty, and total knee arthroplasty.

TENDINITIS

■ Hamstring Tendinitis

Chief Clinical Characteristics
This presentation involves acute, localized pain, tenderness, and edema over the involved tendon. Symptoms include pain with resisted knee flexion and passive knee extension. History is usually significant for repetitive hamstring muscle strains.

Background Information
This condition most commonly occurs in athletes who run, kick, and jump. Clinical examination and magnetic resonance imaging confirm an acute inflammation of the hamstring tendon. Treatment includes rest, inflammation control, and improving muscle flexibility of the quadriceps and hamstring muscles.

■ Patellar Tendinitis

Chief Clinical Characteristics
This presentation may be characterized by acute, localized pain and edema at the inferior pole of the patella (origin), the tibial tubercle (insertion), or the patellar tendon itself (see Fig. 21-2). Pain is most often localized at the insertion of the patellar tendon and onset is typically insidious; however, most patients may relate a period of onset with increased activity or sport. Patient reports pain with squatting and jumping activities.

Background Information
Mechanism of injury is most often from repetitive eccentric overload of the knee in flexion ranges, resulting in microscopic destruction of the patellar tendon. Magnetic resonance imaging confirms the diagnosis. Treatment includes rest, inflammation control, and improving muscle flexibility of the quadriceps and hamstring muscles.

■ Pes Anserine Tendinitis

Chief Clinical Characteristics
This presentation typically includes acute pain, tenderness, and edema localized anteromedially (see Fig. 21-2). Patient reports pain with ascending stairs and tenderness to palpation at the insertion of site of the three tendons that comprise the pes anserine group (semitendinosus, gracilis, and sartorius).

Background Information
Pain is typically located approximately 4 cm below the joint line at the anteromedial aspect of the knee.[7] This diagnosis is often observed in long-distance runners.[53] Symptoms may mimic or be associated with pes anserine bursitis. Treatment includes rest, control of inflammation, orthotic therapy, and strengthening to reduce stress on the medial structures of the knee.

■ Popliteus Tendinitis

Chief Clinical Characteristics
This presentation involves acute pain, tenderness, and edema over the posterolateral aspect of the knee and along the proximal course of the popliteal tendon. Activities that require frequent deceleration, such as downhill running or hiking, may produce and exacerbate symptoms. Reproduction of symptoms occurs with resisted tibial external rotation at 90 degrees of knee flexion.

Background Information
Overuse or fatigue of the quadriceps may lead to inflammation of the popliteus musculotendinous unit, causing overuse of the popliteus musculotendinous unit.[54] Magnetic resonance imaging confirms the diagnosis. Treatment includes rest and control of inflammation.

■ Quadriceps Tendinitis

Chief Clinical Characteristics
This presentation may involve acute pain, tenderness, and edema on the anterior aspect of the thigh, just along the superior border of the patella (see Fig. 21-2). Patient reports pain with eccentric or concentric quadriceps contractions.

Background Information
This condition typically results from repetitive hyperextension of the hip or a combination of

hip extension and knee flexion. Injury is most often associated with athletic activity, such as running and jumping. Diagnosis is confirmed with magnetic resonance imaging. Treatment includes rest, inflammation control, and improving muscle flexibility of the quadriceps and hamstring muscles.

TENDINOSES

■ Hamstring Tendinosis

Chief Clinical Characteristics
This presentation includes a history of chronic pain and tenderness over the involved tendon with the absence of inflammation. Symptoms include pain with resisted knee flexion and passive knee extension. History is usually significant for repetitive hamstring muscle strains.

Background Information
This condition most commonly occurs in athletes who run, kick, and jump. Tendinosis is characterized as noninflammatory intratendinous collagen degeneration and the disordered, haphazard healing of collagen with vascular ingrowth.[55] Clinical examination, ultrasonography, and magnetic resonance imaging confirm this diagnosis. A combination of patient/client education, unloading the affected musculotendinous unit, controlled mechanical reloading, and preventive measures appear effective to manage this condition.[56]

■ Patellar Tendinosis ("Jumper's Knee")

Chief Clinical Characteristics
This presentation may include a history of chronic pain at the inferior pole of the patella (origin), the tibial tubercle (insertion), or the patellar tendon itself (see Fig. 21-2). Pain is most often localized at the insertion of the patellar tendon and onset is typically insidious; however, most patients may relate a period of onset with increased activity or sport. Patient reports pain with squatting and jumping activities.

Background Information
Mechanism of injury is most often from repetitive eccentric overload of the knee in flexion ranges. Tendinosis is characterized as noninflammatory intratendinous collagen

degeneration and the disordered, haphazard healing of collagen with vascular ingrowth.[55] Clinical examination, ultrasonography, and magnetic resonance imaging confirm this diagnosis. Present research supports the use of eccentric exercise to reduce pain and facilitate return to sport in chronic cases.[57,58]

■ Pes Anserine Tendinosis

Chief Clinical Characteristics
This presentation typically includes a history of chronic pain and tenderness localized anteromedially (see Fig. 21-2). Patient reports pain when ascending stairs and tenderness to palpation at the insertion of site of the three tendons that comprise the pes anserine group (semitendinosus, gracilis, and sartorius). Pain is typically located approximately 4 cm below the joint line at the anteromedial aspect of the knee.[7] This diagnosis is often observed in long-distance runners.[53]

Background Information
Tendinosis is characterized as noninflammatory intratendinous collagen degeneration and the disordered, haphazard healing of collagen with vascular ingrowth.[55] Clinical examination, ultrasonography, and magnetic resonance imaging confirm this diagnosis. Treatment includes rest, control of inflammation, orthotic therapy, and strengthening to reduce stress on the medial structures of the knee.

■ Popliteus Tendinosis

Chief Clinical Characteristics
This presentation can be characterized by a chronic history of pain over the posterolateral aspect of the knee and tenderness along the proximal course of the popliteal tendon. Reproduction of symptoms occurs with resisted tibial external rotation at 90 degrees of knee flexion.

Background Information
Overuse or fatigue of the quadriceps may lead to inflammation of the popliteus muscle, causing overuse of the popliteus musculotendinous unit.[54] Thus, activities that require frequent deceleration, such as downhill running or hiking, may produce and exacerbate symptoms. Tendinosis is characterized as noninflammatory intratendinous collagen degeneration and the disordered,

haphazard healing of collagen with vascular ingrowth.[55] Clinical examination, ultrasonography, and magnetic resonance imaging confirm this diagnosis. A combination of patient/client education, unloading the affected musculotendinous unit, controlled mechanical reloading, and preventive measures appears to be effective for managing this condition.[56]

■ Quadriceps Tendinosis

Chief Clinical Characteristics
This presentation includes a history of chronic pain on the anterior aspect of the thigh, just along the superior border of the patella, without signs of inflammation (see Fig. 21-2). Patient reports pain with eccentric or concentric quadriceps contractions.

Background Information
Quadriceps tendinosis typically results from repetitive hyperextension of the hip or a combination of hip extension and knee flexion. Injury is most often associated with athletic activity, such as running and jumping. Tendinosis is characterized as noninflammatory intratendinous collagen degeneration and the disordered, haphazard healing of collagen with vascular ingrowth.[55] Clinical examination, ultrasonography, and magnetic resonance imaging confirm this diagnosis. A combination of patient/client education, unloading the affected musculotendinous unit, controlled mechanical reloading, and preventive measures appears to be effective for managing this condition.[56]

TUMORS

■ Chondroblastoma

Chief Clinical Characteristics
This presentation typically includes nonspecific pain, edema, local tenderness to palpation, decreased range of motion, and joint stiffness. This condition most commonly presents between the ages of 10 and 20 years, with a male-to-female ratio of 2:1.[59]

Background Information
This condition arises from the development of a benign neoplasm of cartilaginous origin. It is typically found in the epiphysis or apophysis of long bones in younger individuals. Diagnosis is confirmed with biopsy and imaging studies including plain radiographs, bone scan, and magnetic resonance imaging. Treatment consists of curettage, en bloc resection, and radiation therapy.[60]

■ Chondrosarcoma

Chief Clinical Characteristics
This presentation includes pain that is dull in character, has been present for months, and may be worst at night. When the tumor is located near a joint, effusion and limited range of motion may be present.

Background Information
This condition is a malignant tumor of cartilaginous origin, in which the tumor matrix formation is entirely chondroid in nature and may arise within the medullary canal or in the periphery as either a primary or secondary lesion. Tumors are most commonly found in the pelvis, femur, humerus, ribs, scapula, sternum, and spine. The proximal metaphysis is more frequently involved than the distal end of the bone. This type of tumor is generally unresponsive to chemotherapy, thus treatment involves surgical resection.

■ Ganglion Cysts

Chief Clinical Characteristics
This presentation involves a nonpainful or minimally painful soft tissue mass. Pain, clicking and locking, decreased range of motion, and effusion are commonly present with intra-articular cysts.

Background Information
This condition frequently is found at the insertion sites of ligaments, near the region of the epiphysis, and may result from minor trauma or be congenital in origin. Intra-articular cysts typically present with greater losses of range of motion compared to intraosseous cysts.[61] Diagnosis is confirmed by plain radiographs and magnetic resonance imaging. Aspiration or surgical excision may be necessary in some cases; however, most cysts do not require surgical intervention.

■ Giant Cell Tumor

Chief Clinical Characteristics
This presentation can be characterized by pain and tenderness but the tumor is typically asymptomatic.

Background Information

If pain is present, it may be the result of an associated inflammatory response. This condition involves benign, locally aggressive bone tumors that occur between the ages of 20 and 40 years and affects females more often than males.[62] They are frequently found in the epiphysis of long bones, with the majority located at the distal femur and proximal tibia. Giant cell tumors are characterized by their locally aggressive behavior. Diagnosis is confirmed by plain radiographs and computed tomography. Treatment may include radiation therapy, intralesional curettage with and without bone graft or insertion of polymethylmethacrylate, cryotherapy, and surgical resection.

■ Osteochondroma

Chief Clinical Characteristics

This presentation involves a palpable mass that is typically painless. This condition is typically asymptomatic, but a decrease in range of motion may present depending on the location of the lesion.

Background Information

This condition is the most common benign tumor of bone that originates near the ends of long bones and typically grows away from the joint. They generally occur as single lesions, with most occurring at the knee.[63,64] Plain radiographs confirm the diagnosis; this condition often is incidentally detected while examining films obtained for another reason. Treatment generally involves surgical resection of the lesion.

■ Osteoid Osteoma

Chief Clinical Characteristics

This presentation may include localized pain, often greatest at night, and adjacent soft tissue edema. Classically, pain is readily relieved by aspirin.

Background Information

This condition is a benign skeletal neoplasm of unknown etiology that is composed of osteoid and woven bone and is most frequently found in young children and adolescents.[65] It is usually found in the long bones of the lower extremity, particularly the proximal femur. The diagnosis is confirmed with

plain radiographs. Pain associated with this condition is self-limiting and may resolve spontaneously over the course of 2 to 4 years, but surgical excision also may be effective.[66]

■ Osteosarcoma

Chief Clinical Characteristics

This presentation may involve localized pain, soft tissue swelling or mass, muscle atrophy, and decreased knee range of motion.

Background Information

This condition is the most common bone malignancy. It is more common in males than females, with a peak incidence in the second decade of life.[67] The most commonly affected sites are the distal femur, proximal tibia, and proximal humerus. Diagnosis is confirmed with a biopsy. This type of tumor is generally unresponsive to chemotherapy, thus treatment involves surgical resection.

■ Parosteal Osteosarcoma

Chief Clinical Characteristics

This presentation can be characterized by an insidious onset of pain, edema, decreased range of motion, and a palpable mass.

Background Information

This condition is a variant of osteosarcoma and is often found in the metaphysis of long bones; it is present on the posterior aspect of the distal femur in 75% of cases.[68] The lesion arises from the surface of the bone and has a tendency to encircle the bone. Radiographically, parosteal osteosarcoma is characterized by a large, dense, lobulated mass broadly attached to the underlying bone without involvement of the medullary canal. Diagnosis is confirmed with biopsy and imaging studies, including plain radiographs, magnetic resonance imaging, and computed tomography. Wide excision of the lesion is the preferred treatment and there is normally no role for chemotherapy.

■ Pigmented Villonodular Synovitis

Chief Clinical Characteristics

This presentation may involve diffuse, recurrent edema that is initially pain free, repeated hemarthrosis in the absence of trauma, progressive and insidious onset of pain, palpable nodules, and decreased range of motion. Symptoms may include locking and catching.

Background Information
This condition is a benign, proliferative pathology of unknown etiology that affects synovial tissue. It results in various degrees of villous and/or nodular changes in the joint, with the knee being the most commonly involved.[69-72] The two forms of the disorder are diffuse and focal. The diffuse form involves large joints and the entire synovial lining, resulting in destructive changes to the joint. The focal form involves small joints, such as the hands and feet, and results in mechanical symptoms such as locking and catching. Diagnosis is confirmed with plain radiographs and magnetic resonance imaging. Treatment includes synovectomy and subsequent radiation therapy.

■ Synovial Chondromatosis
Chief Clinical Characteristics
This presentation involves a chronic history of pain, edema, stiffness, progressive loss of range of motion, and joint locking. Palpable nodules may also present. This condition commonly presents between 30 and 50 years of age,[73] is observed more often in males than females, and frequently occurs on the right side of the body (4:1 ratio).[74]

Background Information
This condition is a benign disorder of unknown etiology that is characterized by synovial membrane proliferation and metaplasia. Nodular proliferation of synovial lining occurs and fragments may break off into the joint to calcify and grow, resulting in gradual joint degeneration and secondary osteoarthritis. Almost any joint can be affected; however, the knee is involved in more than half of cases. Diagnosis is confirmed with imaging studies, including plain radiographs, computed tomography and computed tomographic arthrograms, and magnetic resonance imaging. Treatment requires surgical excision of the proliferating synovium. Total synovectomy minimizes the risk of recurrence.

■ Synovial Sarcoma
Chief Clinical Characteristics
This presentation may include a dull, deep pain that is accompanied by a slowly enlarging mass. Vague pain may occur for months without a mass being appreciated. Tumors located near the joint may also result in decreased range of motion.

Background Information
This condition is a malignant mesenchymal neoplasm that arises from soft tissue, representing 10% of all soft tissue sarcomas and most commonly affecting the lower extremities of young adults.[75] Diagnosis is confirmed with biopsy and imaging studies including plain radiographs, computed tomography scan, and magnetic resonance imaging. Treatment includes a combination of chemotherapy and surgical resection.

References
1. Troum OM, Crues JV 3rd. The young adult with hip pain: diagnosis and medical treatment, circa 2004. *Clin Orthop Relat Res.* Jan 2004(418):9–17.
2. Steinberg ME, Larcom PG, Strafford B, et al. Core decompression with bone grafting for osteonecrosis of the femoral head. *Clin Orthop Relat Res.* May 2001(386): 71–78.
3. Recommendations for the medical management of osteoarthritis of the hip and knee: 2000 update. American College of Rheumatology Subcommittee on Osteoarthritis Guidelines. *Arthritis Rheum.* Sep 2000;43(9): 1905–1915.
4. Bennett GE, Cobey MC. Hemangioma of joints: report of five cases. *Arch Surg.* 1939;38:487–500.
5. Handy JR. Popliteal cysts in adults: a review. *Semin Arthritis Rheum.* Oct 2001;31(2):108–118.
6. Sansone V, De Ponti A. Arthroscopic treatment of popliteal cyst and associated intra-articular knee disorders in adults. *Arthroscopy.* May 1999;15(4): 368–372.
7. Marquis AM. Pes anserine bursitis. *Ona J.* Oct 1979;6(10):418–419.
8. Larsson LG, Baum J. The syndrome of anserine bursitis: an overlooked diagnosis. *Arthritis Rheum.* 1985;28: 1062–1065.
9. Zeiss J, Coombs RJ, Booth RL Jr, Saddemi SR. Chronic bursitis presenting as a mass in the pes anserine bursa: MR diagnosis. *J Comput Assist Tomogr.* Jan–Feb 1993;17(1):137–140.
10. Merskey H, Bogduk N. *Classification of Chronic Pain: Descriptions of Chronic Pain Syndromes and Definitions of Pain Terms.* Seattle, WA: IASP Press; 1994.
11. Dickhaut SC, DeLee JC. The discoid lateral meniscus syndrome. *J Bone Joint Surg Am.* 1982;64:1068–1073.
12. Kocher MS, Klingele K, Rassman SO. Meniscal disorders: normal, discoid, and cysts. *Orthop Clin North Am.* Jul 2003;34(3):329–340.

KNEE PAIN

13. Goldenberg DL, Burckhardt C, Crofford L. Management of fibromyalgia syndrome [see comment]. *JAMA.* 2004;292(19):2388–2395.

14. Nampiaparampil DE, Shmerling RH. A review of fibromyalgia. *Am J Managed Care.* 2004;10(11 Pt 1):794–800.

15. Accousti WK, Willis RB. Tibial eminence fractures. *Orthop Clin North Am.* Jul 2003;34(3):365–375.

16. Bostrom A. Fracture of the patella. A study of 422 patellar fractures. *Acta Orthop Scand Suppl.* 1972;143:1–80.

17. Sanders R. Patella fractures and extensor mechanism injuries. In: Brownder BD, Jupitter JB, Levine AM, eds. *Skeletal Trauma: Fractures, Dislocations, Ligamentous Injuries.* Philadelphia, PA: W. B. Saunders; 1992: 1685–1716.

18. Mann HA, Goddard NJ, Lee CA, Brown SA. Periarticular aneurysm following total knee replacement in hemophilic arthropathy. A case report. *J Bone Joint Surg Am.* Dec 2003;85A(12):2437–2440.

19. Gunter P, Schwellnus MP. Local corticosteroid injection in iliotibial band friction syndrome in runners: a randomised controlled trial. *Br J Sports Med.* Jun 2004;38(3):269–272; discussion 272.

20. Shea KG, Pfeiffer R, Curtin M. Idiopathic anterior knee pain in adolescents. *Orthop Clin North Am.* Jul 2003;34(3):377–383, vi.

21. Mackenzie R, Dixon AK, Keene GS, Hollingworth W, Lomas DJ, Villar RN. Magnetic resonance imaging of the knee: assessment of effectiveness. *Clin Radiol.* Apr 1996;51(4):245–250.

22. Joines JD, McNutt RA, Carey TS, Deyo RA, Rouhani R. Finding cancer in primary care outpatients with low back pain: a comparison of diagnostic strategies. *J Gen Intern Med.* 2001;16(1):14–23.

23. Holman PJ, Suki D, McCutcheon I, Wolinsky JP, Rhines LD, Gokaslan ZL. Surgical management of metastatic disease of the lumbar spine: experience with 139 patients. *J Neurosurg Spine.* 2005;2(5):550–563.

24. Verrall GM, Slavotinek JP, Barnes PG, Fon GT. Diagnostic and prognostic value of clinical findings in 83 athletes with posterior thigh injury: comparison of clinical findings with magnetic resonance imaging documentation of hamstring muscle strain. *Am J Sports Med.* Nov—Dec 2003;31(6):969–973.

25. Koulouris G, Connell D. Evaluation of the hamstring muscle complex following acute injury. *Skeletal Radiol.* Oct 2003;32(10):582–589.

26. DeSmet AA, Best TM. MR imaging of the distribution and location of acute hamstring injuries in athletes. *AJR.* 2000;174:393–399.

27. Kopell HP, Thompson WAL. Peripheral entrapment neuropathies. Baltimore, MD: Williams and Wilkins; 1963:34–47.

28. Maudsley RH. Fibular tunnel syndrome. In proceedings of the North-West Metropolitan Orthopaedic Club. *J Bone Joint Surg.* 1967;49B:384.

29. Deese MJ, Baxter DE. Compressive neuropathies of the lower extremity. *J Musculoskelet Med.* 1988;5(11):68–91.

30. Wall E, Von Stein D. Juvenile osteochondritis dissecans. *Orthop Clin North Am.* Jul 2003;34(3):341–353.

31. Tindel NL, Nisonson B. The plica syndrome. *Orthop Clin North Am.* Oct 1992;23(4):613–618.

32. Buckwalter JA, Saltzman C, Brown T. The impact of osteoarthritis: implications for research. *Clin Orthop Relat Res.* Oct 2004(427 suppl):S6–15.

33. Wollschlaeger B. Epileptic seizures as a neurological complication of Reiter disease. *J Am Board Fam Pract.* May–Jun 1995;8(3):233–236.

34. Kruse RW. Evaluation of Knee Injuries. In: Lilliegard WA, Rucker KS, eds. *Handbook of Sports Medicine. A Symptom-Oriented Approach.* Newton, MA: Andover Medical Publishers; 1993:135–149.

35. Indelicato PA. Nonoperative treatment of complete tears of the medial collateral ligament of the knee. *J Bone Joint Surg Am.* Mar 1983;65(3):323–329.

36. Ekstrom JE. Arthrography. Where does it fit in? *Clin Sports Med.* Jul 1990;9(3):561–566.

37. Mink JH, Levy T, Crues JV 3rd. Tears of the anterior cruciate ligament and menisci of the knee: MR imaging evaluation. *Radiology.* Jun 1988;167(3):769–774.

38. Reicher MA, Hartzman S, Duckwiler GR, Bassett LW, Anderson LJ, Gold RH. Meniscal injuries: detection using MR imaging. *Radiology.* Jun 1986;159(3):753–757.

39. McCarty EC, Marx RG, DeHaven KE. Meniscus repair: considerations in treatment and update of clinical results. *Clin Orthop Relat Res.* Sep 2002(402):122–134.

40. van Trommel MF, Simonian PT, Potter HG, Wickiewicz TL. Arthroscopic meniscal repair with fibrin clot of complete radial tears of the lateral meniscus in the avascular zone. *Arthroscopy.* May–Jun 1998;14(4): 360–365.

41. Hamilton W, Klostermeier T, Lim E, J.S. M. Surgically documented rupture of the plantaris muscle: A case report and literature review. *Foot Ankle Int.* 1997; 18(8):522–523.

42. Helms CA, Fritz RC, Garvin GJ. Plantaris muscle injury: evaluation with MR imaging. *Radiology.* Apr 1995;195(1):201–203.

43. Murray JR, Grundy JR, Collins IE, Mundil N, Pongratz R, Woods DA. Spontaneous rupture of the popliteus tendon in a 74-year-old woman and review of the literature. *Arthroscopy.* Oct 2004;20(8):860–864.

44. Westrich GH, Hannafin JA, Potter HG. Isolated rupture and repair of the popliteus tendon. *Arthroscopy.* Oct 1995;11(5):628–632.

45. Ilan DI, Tejwani N, Keschner M, Leibman M. Quadriceps tendon rupture. *J Am Acad Orthop Surg.* May–Jun 2003;11(3):192–200.

46. Okpala I. The management of crisis in sickle cell disease. *Eur J Haematol.* Jan 1998;60(1):1–6.

47. Aglietti P, Insall JN, Buzzi R, Deschamps G. Idiopathic osteonecrosis of the knee. Aetiology, prognosis and treatment. *J Bone Joint Surg Br.* Nov 1983;65(5): 588–597.

48. Ahlback S, Bauer GC, Bohne WH. Spontaneous osteonecrosis of the knee. *Arthritis Rheum.* Dec 1968;11(6):705–733.

49. Al-Rowaih A, Lindstrand A, Bjorkengren AG, Wingstrand H, Thorngren KG. Osteonecrosis of the knee. Diagnosis and outcome in 40 patients. *Acta Orthop Scand.* 1991;62:19–23.

50. Rozing PM, Insall J, Bohne WH. Spontaneous osteonecrosis of the knee. *J Bone Joint Surg Am.* Jan 1980;62(1):2–7.

51. Narvaez J, Narvaez JA, Rodriguez-Moreno J, Roig-Escofet D. Osteonecrosis of the knee: differences among idiopathic and secondary types. *Rheumatology (Oxford).* Sep 2000;39(9):982–989.

52. Houpt JB, Pritzker KP, Alpert B, Greyson ND, Gross AE. Natural history of spontaneous osteonecrosis of the

knee (SONK): a review. *Semin Arthritis Rheum.* Nov 1983;13(2):212–227.

53. Safran MR, Fu FH. Uncommon causes of knee pain in the athlete. *Orthop Clin North Am.* Jul 1995;26(3): 547–559.

54. Nyland J, Lachman N, Kocabey Y, Brosky J, Altun R, Caborn D. Anatomy, function, and rehabilitation of the popliteus musculotendinous complex. *J Orthop Sports Phys Ther.* Mar 2005;35(3):165–179.

55. Sharma P, Maffulli N. Tendon injury and tendinopathy: healing and repair. *J Bone Joint Surg Am.* Jan 2005;87(1):187–202.

56. Davenport TE, Kulig K, Matharu Y, Blanco CE. The EdUReP model for nonsurgical management of tendinopathy. *Phys Ther.* Oct 2005;85(10):1093–1103.

57. Jensen K, Di Fabio RP. Evaluation of eccentric exercise in treatment of patellar tendinitis. *Phys Ther.* Mar 1989;69(3):211–216.

58. Cannell LJ, Taunton JE, Clement DB, Smith C, Khan KM. A randomised clinical trial of the efficacy of drop squats or leg extension/leg curl exercises to treat clinically diagnosed jumper's knee in athletes: pilot study. *Br J Sports Med.* Feb 2001;35(1):60–64.

59. Endo H, Kawai A, Naito N, Sugihara S, Inoue H. Knee pain in a 16-year-old girl. *Clin Orthop Relat Res.* Dec 2001(393):345–349.

60. Nishihara RM, Helmstedter CS. Chondroblastoma: an unusual cause of knee pain in the adolescent. *J Adolesc Health.* Jan 2000;26(1):49–52.

61. Ellen MI, Gilhool JJ, Rogers DP. Nonoperative treatment of an interosseous ganglion cyst. *Am J Phys Med Rehabil.* Jul 2001;80(7):536–539.

62. Turcotte RE, Wunder JS, Isler MH, et al. Giant cell tumor of long bone: a Canadian Sarcoma Group study. *Clin Orthop Relat Res.* Apr 2002(397):248–258.

63. Reith JD, Bauer TW, Joyce MJ. Paraarticular osteochondroma of the knee: report of 2 cases and review of the literature. *Clin Orthop Relat Res.* Jan 1997(334): 225–232.

64. Vasseur MA, Fabre O. Vascular complications of osteochondromas. *J Vasc Surg.* Mar 2000;31(3):532–538.

65. Bhat I, Zerin JM, Bloom DA, Mooney JF 3rd. Unusual presentation of osteoid osteoma mimicking osteomyelitis in a 27-month-old infant. *Pediatr Radiol.* Jun 2003;33 (6):425–428.

66. Crist BD, Lenke LG, Lewis S. Osteoid osteoma of the lumbar spine. A case report highlighting a novel reconstruction technique. *J Bone Joint Surg Am.* Feb 2005;87(2):414–418.

67. Paluska SA. Persistent knee pain in a recreational runner. *J Am Board Fam Pract.* Sep–Oct 2003;16(5): 435–442.

68. Ahuja SC, Villacin AB, Smith J. Juxtacortical (parosteal) osteogenic sarcoma. *J Bone Joint Surg.* 1977;59: 632–647.

69. Flandry F, Hughston JC. Pigmented villonodular synovitis. *J Bone Joint Surg Am.* Jul 1987;69(6):942–949.

70. Hamlin BR, Duffy GP, Trousdale RT, Morrey BF. Total knee arthroplasty in patients who have pigmented villonodular synovitis. *J Bone Joint Surg Am.* Jan 1998;80(1):76–82.

71. Johansson JE, Ajjoub S, Coughlin LP, Wener JA, Cruess RL. Pigmented villonodular synovitis of joints. *Clin Orthop Relat Res.* Mar 1982(163):159–166.

72. Myers BW, Masi AT. Pigmented villonodular synovitis and tenosynovitis: a clinical epidemiologic study of 166 cases and literature review. *Medicine (Baltimore).* May 1980;59(3):223–238.

73. Langguth DM, Klestov A, Denaro C. Synovial osteochondromatosis. *Intern Med J.* Aug 2002;32(8): 419–420.

74. Lucas JH, Quinn P, Foote J, Baker S, Bruno J. Recurrent synovial chondromatosis treated with meniscectomy and synovectomy. *Oral Surg Oral Med Oral Pathol Oral Radiol Endod.* Sep 1997;84(3):253–258.

75. Kartha SS, Bumpous JM. Synovial cell sarcoma: diagnosis, treatment, and outcomes. *Laryngoscope.* Nov 2002;112(11):1979–1982.

CHAPTER 22

Lower Leg Pain

■ *Jason R. Cozby, PT, DPT, OCS*

Description of the Symptom

This chapter describes pathology that may lead to lower leg pain, including generalized, anteromedial, anterolateral, and posterior lower leg pain. **Local causes** of lower leg pain are defined as pathology occurring between the proximal one-third of the tibia and the area just proximal to the medial and lateral malleoli of the tibia. **Remote causes** are defined as occurring outside this region.

Special Concerns
■ Decreased sensation
■ Diminished femoral, popliteal, tibial, or dorsalis pedis pulses
■ Fever or signs of systemic disease
■ Inability to bear weight on the affected lower extremity
■ Pain increased at night and/or rest
■ Palpable warmth and swelling
■ Skin breakdown

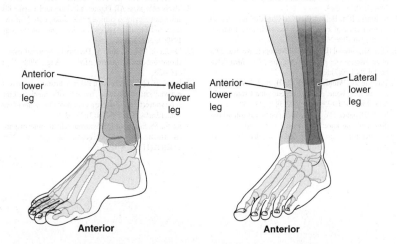

Anterior lower leg — Medial lower leg

Anterior

Anterior lower leg — Lateral lower leg

Anterior

CHAPTER PREVIEW: Conditions That May Lead to Lower Leg Pain

T **Trauma**		
REMOTE	**LOCAL GENERALIZED**	**LOCAL ANTEROMEDIAL**
COMMON		
Lumbar radiculopathies: • L4 radiculopathy 400 • L5 radiculopathy 400 • S1 radiculopathy 400	Not applicable	Fractures: • Stress fracture of the tibia 405 • Tibia 405 Shin splints: • Posteromedial shin splints 411

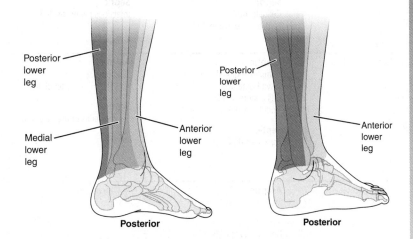

Posterior
lower
leg

Medial
lower
leg

Anterior
lower
leg

Posterior

Posterior
lower
leg

Anterior
lower
leg

Posterior

LOCAL ANTEROLATERAL

LOCAL POSTERIOR

Muscle strains:
• Anterior compartment muscle strain 407
• Lateral compartment muscle strain 407
Shin splints:
• Anterolateral shin splints 411

Muscle strains:
• Gastrocnemius muscle strain 407
• Soleus muscle strain 407
Rupture of the Achilles tendon 411

(continued)

Trauma *(continued)*

REMOTE	LOCAL GENERALIZED	LOCAL ANTEROMEDIAL
UNCOMMON		
Not applicable	Not applicable	Nerve entrapments: • Saphenous nerve 408
RARE		
Not applicable	Not applicable	Not applicable

I Inflammation

REMOTE	LOCAL GENERALIZED	LOCAL ANTEROMEDIAL
COMMON		
Not applicable	**Aseptic** Delayed onset muscle soreness secondary to exercise 403 **Septic** Cellulitis 402 Erythema nodosum 404	**Aseptic** Tendinitis: • Tibialis posterior tendinitis 413 **Septic** Infectious periostitis 406
UNCOMMON		
Not applicable	**Aseptic** Complex regional pain syndrome 403 Gas gangrene 405 Nodular panniculitis 409 **Septic** Erysipelas 404	**Aseptic** Tendinitis: • Tibialis anterior tendinitis 413 **Septic** Osteomyelitis of the tibia 410
RARE		
Not applicable	**Aseptic** Erythema induratum 404 **Septic** Necrotizing fasciitis 408 Nonclostridial myositis 409	Not applicable

M Metabolic

REMOTE	LOCAL GENERALIZED	LOCAL ANTEROMEDIAL
COMMON		
Not applicable	Distal symmetric polyneuropathy, including from acquired immunodeficiency syndrome, alcohol/drug abuse, carcinoma, diabetes mellitus, and kidney failure 404	Not applicable

LOCAL ANTEROLATERAL	LOCAL POSTERIOR
Fractures: • Fibula 405 Nerve entrapments: • Superficial peroneal nerve 408	Hematoma of the calf 406 Nerve entrapments: • Sciatic nerve 408 • Sural nerve 408 • Tibial nerve 409
Not applicable	Not applicable

LOCAL ANTEROLATERAL	LOCAL POSTERIOR
Aseptic Tendinitis: • Peroneal tendinitis 413 **Septic** Not applicable	**Aseptic** Tendinitis: • Achilles tendinitis 412 **Septic** Not applicable
Aseptic Paratenonitis of the extensor tendons of the foot and toes 410 Tendinitis: • Extensor digitorum longus tendinitis 412 • Extensor hallucis longus tendinitis 413 **Septic** Not applicable	**Aseptic** Achilles paratenonitis 401 **Septic** Not applicable
Aseptic Not applicable **Septic** Pyomyositis 410	**Aseptic** Inflammatory muscle disease 406 **Septic** Pyomyositis 410

LOCAL ANTEROLATERAL	LOCAL POSTERIOR
Not applicable	Benign muscle cramps 402

(continued)

Metabolic *(continued)*

REMOTE	LOCAL GENERALIZED	LOCAL ANTEROMEDIAL
UNCOMMON		
Not applicable	Not applicable	Not applicable
RARE		
Not applicable	Malnutrition 406	Not applicable

Va Vascular

REMOTE	LOCAL GENERALIZED	LOCAL ANTEROMEDIAL
COMMON		
Not applicable	Not applicable	Not applicable
UNCOMMON		
Not applicable	Acute femoropopliteal arterial occlusion 401 Sickle cell crisis 411 Skin ulcers: • Arterial or hypertensive ulcers 412 • Systemic vasculitis with ulceration 412	Compartment syndromes: • Distal deep posterior compartment syndrome 402 Greater saphenous vein thrombophlebitis 405
RARE		
Not applicable	Not applicable	Not applicable

De Degenerative

REMOTE	LOCAL GENERALIZED	LOCAL ANTEROMEDIAL
COMMON		
Baker's cyst 399	Not applicable	Tendinoses: • Tibialis posterior tendinosis 415
UNCOMMON		
Not applicable	Not applicable	Tendinoses: • Tibialis anterior tendinosis 415
RARE		
Not applicable	Not applicable	Not applicable

Tu Tumor

REMOTE	LOCAL GENERALIZED	LOCAL ANTEROMEDIAL
COMMON		
Not applicable	Not applicable	Not applicable
UNCOMMON		
Not applicable	Not applicable	Not applicable

LOCAL ANTEROLATERAL	LOCAL POSTERIOR
Not applicable	Not applicable
Not applicable	Acute rhabdomyolysis 401

LOCAL ANTEROLATERAL	LOCAL POSTERIOR
Not applicable	Posterior tibial vein thrombosis 410
Anterior tibial vein thrombosis 401 Compartment syndromes: • Anterior compartment syndrome 402	Compartment syndromes: • Posterior compartment syndrome 403
Compartment syndromes: • Lateral compartment syndrome 403	Arteriovenous malformation 402

LOCAL ANTEROLATERAL	LOCAL POSTERIOR
Tendinoses: • Peroneal tendinosis 414	Tendinoses: • Achilles tendinosis 413
Tendinoses: • Extensor digitorum longus tendinosis 414 • Extensor hallucis longus tendinosis 414	Not applicable
Not applicable	Not applicable

LOCAL ANTEROLATERAL	LOCAL POSTERIOR
Not applicable	Not applicable
Not applicable	Not applicable

(continued)

Tumor *(continued)*

REMOTE	LOCAL GENERALIZED	LOCAL ANTEROMEDIAL
RARE		
Not applicable	*Malignant Primary, such as:* • Osteosarcoma 410 *Malignant Metastatic, such as:* • Metastases to the lower leg, including from primary breast, kidney, lung, prostate, and thyroid disease 406 • Multiple myeloma 407 *Benign, such as:* • Osteoid osteoma 409	*Malignant Primary:* Not applicable *Malignant Metastatic:* Not applicable *Benign, such as:* • Osteoid osteoma 409

Co **Congenital**

REMOTE	LOCAL GENERALIZED	LOCAL ANTEROMEDIAL
COMMON		
Not applicable	Not applicable	Not applicable
UNCOMMON		
Not applicable	Not applicable	Not applicable
RARE		
Not applicable	Not applicable	Not applicable

Ne **Neurogenic/Psychogenic**

REMOTE	LOCAL GENERALIZED	LOCAL ANTEROMEDIAL
COMMON		
Not applicable	Not applicable	Not applicable
UNCOMMON		
Fear and avoidance 400	Not applicable	Not applicable
RARE		
Psychological effect of complex regional pain syndrome 400	Not applicable	Not applicable

Note: These are estimates of relative incidence because few data are available for the less common conditions.

Overview of Lower Leg Pain

The lower leg is subject to internal trauma as a result of ground reaction forces, stress from the powerful muscle attachments in the region, or forces that may occur to correct deficiencies at the foot, ankle, or hip. These deficiencies may be weakness, congenital anomalies, limitations in flexibility, or decreased range of motion, to name a few. Although trauma accounts for many of the potential diagnoses, multiple peripheral nerves and blood vessels traverse the region and therefore diagnoses may also be related to vascular compromise, a peripheral nerve compression, or systemic disease. The lower leg is often an end target site for multiple disease processes, so even if mechanical trauma is associated with the presentation, diagnosis should consider all potential possibilities.

LOCAL ANTEROLATERAL	LOCAL POSTERIOR
Malignant Primary:	*Malignant Primary:*
Not applicable	Not applicable
Malignant Metastatic:	*Malignant Metastatic:*
Not applicable	Not applicable
Benign, such as:	*Benign, such as:*
• Osteoid osteoma 409	• Osteoid osteoma 409

LOCAL ANTEROLATERAL	LOCAL POSTERIOR
Not applicable	Not applicable
Not applicable	Not applicable
Not applicable	Not applicable

LOCAL ANTEROLATERAL	LOCAL POSTERIOR
Not applicable	Not applicable
Not applicable	Not applicable
Not applicable	Not applicable

Description of Conditions That May Lead to Lower Leg Pain

Remote

■ Baker's Cyst

Chief Clinical Characteristics

This presentation involves posterior knee pain, stiffness, tenderness, edema, and a palpable mass located posterior to the medial femoral condyle between the tendons of the medial head of the gastrocnemius and semimembranosus muscles. The mass will be rounded, smooth, supple, and transilluminating.

Background Information

This condition typically results from fluid distention from the gastrocnemius-semimembranosus bursae that communicates with the posterior aspect of the joint capsule. In adults, it also may result from an intra-articular pathology that leads to posterior effusion. Intra-articular knee disorders such as meniscal tears, primary osteoarthritis, and rheumatoid arthritis are frequently associated with this condition.[1,2] A common complication is rupture or dissection of fluid into the gastrocnemius muscle, which may mimic symptoms of a deep venous thrombosis. Diagnosis is confirmed by imaging studies including ultrasound and magnetic resonance imaging. Treatment typically consists of aspirating the knee effusion, although there is a high rate of recurrence when the underlying cause is unaddressed.

■ Fear and Avoidance

Chief Clinical Characteristics

This presentation may include avoiding the use of an extremity as a result of apprehension about onset of pain.

Background Information

Injury to the foot and ankle may contribute to the disuse of the lower extremity even with minimal injury. Fear of reinjury, pain, or other factors will need to be explored. In all cases the basis of pathology must be thoroughly explored before this presentation is considered. If this condition is present, a team approach ensures optimal treatment.

LUMBAR RADICULOPATHIES

■ L4 Radiculopathy

Chief Clinical Characteristics

This presentation can be characterized by pain in the lumbar spine and paresthesias radiating from the anterior aspect of the hip, thigh, and knee, sometimes extending anteromedially from the knee to the foot. Depending on the severity, the presentation may also include a decreased or absent patellar tendon reflex and motor loss in the muscles innervated by the L4 nerve. Prone knee bend may reproduce symptoms.

Background Information

A lumbar disk herniation is the most common cause for this condition. The diagnosis is confirmed with magnetic resonance imaging. Surgical intervention may be indicated in severe cases of lower extremity pain accompanied by neurological signs.

■ L5 Radiculopathy

Chief Clinical Characteristics

This presentation includes pain in the lumbar spine and paresthesias radiating from the lateral aspect of the hip and buttock to the lateral aspect of the knee, extending anterolaterally down to the foot. Depending on the severity, the presentation may also include motor loss in the muscles innervated by the L5 nerve root.

Background Information

A lumbar disk herniation is the most common cause for this condition. The diagnosis is confirmed with magnetic resonance imaging. Surgical intervention may be indicated in severe cases of lower extremity pain accompanied by neurological signs.

■ S1 Radiculopathy

Chief Clinical Characteristics

This presentation typically includes pain in the lumbar spine and paresthesias radiating from the buttock to the posterior aspect of the knee and extending posterolaterally from the knee to the foot. Depending on the severity, the presentation may also include a decreased or absent Achilles tendon reflex and motor loss in the muscles innervated by the S1 nerve.

Background Information

A lumbar disk herniation is a common cause for this condition. The diagnosis is confirmed with magnetic resonance imaging. Surgical intervention may be indicated in severe cases of lower extremity pain accompanied by neurological signs.

■ Psychological Effect of Complex Regional Pain Syndrome

Chief Clinical Characteristics

This presentation typically includes a traumatic onset of severe chronic ankle and foot pain accompanied by allodynia, hyperalgesia, and, in later stages, trophic, vasomotor, and sudomotor changes. This condition is characterized by disproportionate responses to painful stimuli.

Background Information

This regional neuropathic pain disorder presents either without direct nerve trauma (Type I) or with direct nerve trauma (Type II) in any region of the body.[3] This condition may precipitate due to an event distant to the affected area. Thermography may confirm associated sympathetic dysfunction. This condition has been shown to have a psychological component and may be influenced by cortical mechanisms.[4] Treatment may include physical therapy interventions to improve patient/client functioning, biofeedback, analgesic or anti-inflammatory medication, transcutaneous or spinal electrical nerve stimulation, and surgical or pharmacologic sympathectomy. However, a team approach ensures optimal treatment for individuals with this condition.

Local

■ Achilles Paratenonitis

Chief Clinical Characteristics
This presentation typically includes diffuse pain, tenderness, and thickening and swelling along the Achilles tendon, especially 2 to 6 cm from the calcaneal insertion. However, the painful palpable thickening does not move with dorsiflexion or plantarflexion because the tendon moves with this action but the paratenon does not. Pain is greatest in the mornings or at the start of a physical activity, but the pain will often decrease with continued walking or activity as the tendon begins to move more freely inside the paratenon.

Background Information
The paratenon is usually the site of inflammatory injury related to overuse, but it may also be damaged from direct traumatic pressure. The diagnosis is determined clinically, but magnetic resonance or ultrasound imaging may be necessary for confirmation if the clinical diagnosis is unclear. Treatment includes rest, inflammation control, improving flexibility of the calf muscle group, and improving strength of the antipronator (supinator) muscle groups.

■ Acute Femoropopliteal Arterial Occlusion

Chief Clinical Characteristics
This presentation usually involves diffuse lower leg pain, coldness, pallor, paresthesias, muscle weakness, and diminished or absent distal pulses. The onset may be abrupt with deep achy and/or burning pain as a result of an occlusion at the bifurcation just distal to the last detectable pulse.

Background Information
Common causes include trauma, embolus, or thrombus.[5] Symptoms often will reverse if the occlusion is treated and relieved within 6 hours; otherwise, complications include gangrene and residual weakness or sensory impairment. Diagnosis is most often confirmed with Doppler ultrasonography; however, angiography, assessment of systolic blood pressure, and magnetic resonance angiography also may be utilized. This condition is a medical emergency in its acute form due to the risk for compromise of the distal tissues. Treatment usually involves pharmacologic or surgical thrombolysis.

■ Acute Rhabdomyolysis

Chief Clinical Characteristics
This presentation includes calf pain, generalized tenderness, swelling, darkened urine, and aggravation of symptoms with bearing weight on the affected lower extremity and muscle contraction.

Background Information
Toxic syndrome from alcoholic binge drinking is the most common etiology, followed by trauma and infection.[6] Urine darkening associated with this condition is caused by the excretion of myoglobin. The diagnosis is confirmed with histopathological testing that reveals muscle fiber necrosis and myophagocytosis. This condition requires urgent referral for evaluation by a physician.

■ Anterior Tibial Vein Thrombosis

Chief Clinical Characteristics
This presentation can be characterized by anterolateral lower leg pain, tenderness, lower extremity swelling, cramping, erythema, palpable warmth, engorged veins, and potentially a low-grade fever and pain along the course of the vein. Individuals with this condition usually demonstrate thromboses at other sites within the lower leg. This condition may be effort induced or spontaneous.

Background Information
The etiology of this condition is associated with Virchow's triad of intimal damage, stasis,

or changes in blood composition.[7] Computed tomography, magnetic resonance angiography, and Doppler ultrasonography confirm the diagnosis. It is a medical emergency because of the risk for propagation of the thrombus to the lungs.

■ Arteriovenous Malformation

Chief Clinical Characteristics
This presentation includes lower leg pain and fatigue in the presence of possible limb hypertrophy, hypotrophy, or length discrepancy. Numerous clinical constellations of skin, muscle, and skeletal complications are common, including skin ulceration secondary to impaired peripheral circulation.[8] These changes are usually present in early childhood, although they may remain unaddressed until they cause disability in adulthood.

Background Information
Arteriovenous malformations include vascular tumors (eg, hemangiomas) and vascular malformations. Vascular malformations may include capillary, lymphatic, venous, and arterial deformities. The specific etiology of arteriovenous malformation is suggested by magnetic resonance imaging. Treatment may involve surgical resection and thrombosis treatment techniques.

■ Benign Muscle Cramps

Chief Clinical Characteristics
This presentation involves painful muscle cramps, palpable tightness, and induration that is often correlated with a sustained contraction of the affected muscle.[9] This condition may last several minutes to approximately one-half hour, with tenderness for several hours following an acute episode.

Background Information
This condition is associated with an insidious onset following muscle overuse. Other potential causes include dehydration, hyponatremia, hypomagnesemia, geriatric nocturnal leg cramps, or association with pregnancy.[9] Treatment typically involves addressing the underlying cause of muscle cramps. Quinine sulfate is an established pharmacologic treatment that also has potential adverse cardiac side effects.

■ Cellulitis

Chief Clinical Characteristics
This presentation may involve pain, erythema, edema, warmth, and tenderness spreading from the region of the initial infection. Vesicles, bullae, and necrosis may be present with occasional petechiae and ecchymosis. Fever, chills, headaches, malaise, hypotension, tachycardia, and delirium are common signs of systemic involvement.

Background Information
This condition usually results from a wound infection by staphylococcal and streptococcal species. Edema is a significant risk factor. Laboratory tests help determine the causative pathogen. Most cases are self-limiting. Severe cases involve necrosis and may require surgical debridement and antibiotic therapy.

COMPARTMENT SYNDROMES

■ Anterior Compartment Syndrome

Chief Clinical Characteristics
This presentation typically includes early signs of paresthesia and hypesthesia in the anterior lower leg and dorsal foot, followed by significant pain, massive edema, ecchymoses, soft tissue tenderness, erythema, palpable warmth, and weakness of the foot and toe dorsiflexor muscle group. Pulses and capillary refill often remain normal until the pressure increases to the level of severe injury.

Background Information
This condition can occur spontaneously in patients with diabetes mellitus.[10] Altered vessel perfusion and edema result in increased intercompartmental pressure that disrupts the oxygen diffusion and results in ischemia.[11] This condition often is the result of trauma. Clinical presentation and intercompartmental pressure measurements confirm the diagnosis.[12] This condition is a medical emergency and requires urgent surgical decompression.

■ Distal Deep Posterior Compartment Syndrome

Chief Clinical Characteristics
This presentation may be characterized by early signs of paresthesia and hypesthesia in

the lower leg and foot, followed by significant pain, massive edema, ecchymosis, soft tissue tenderness, erythema, palpable warmth, and weakness of the foot plantarflexor-invertors and toe flexor muscle groups. Pulses and capillary refill often remain normal until the pressure increases to the level of severe injury.

Background Information
This condition can occur spontaneously in patients with diabetes mellitus.[10] Altered vessel perfusion and edema result in increased intercompartmental pressure that disrupts the oxygen diffusion and results in ischemia.[11] This condition often is the result of trauma. Clinical presentation and intercompartmental pressure measurements confirm the diagnosis.[12] This condition is a medical emergency and requires urgent surgical decompression.

■ Lateral Compartment Syndrome
Chief Clinical Characteristics
This presentation can involve early signs of paresthesia and hypesthesia, followed by significant pain, massive edema, ecchymosis, soft tissue tenderness, erythema, palpable warmth, and weakness of the foot plantarflexor-evertor muscle group. Pulses and capillary refill often remain normal until the pressure increases to the level of severe injury.

Background Information
This condition can occur spontaneously in patients with diabetes mellitus.[10] Altered vessel perfusion and edema result in increased intercompartmental pressure that disrupts the oxygen diffusion and results in ischemia.[11] This condition often is the result of trauma. Clinical presentation and intercompartmental pressure measurements confirm the diagnosis.[12] This condition is a medical emergency and requires urgent surgical decompression.

■ Posterior Compartment Syndrome
Chief Clinical Characteristics
This presentation typically includes early signs of paresthesia and hypesthesia in the

lower leg and foot, followed by significant pain, massive edema, ecchymosis, soft tissue tenderness, erythema, palpable warmth, and weakness of the plantarflexors or toe flexors. Pulses and capillary refill often remain normal until the pressure increases to the level of severe injury.

Background Information
This condition can occur spontaneously in patients with diabetes mellitus.[10] Altered vessel perfusion and edema result in increased intercompartmental pressure that disrupts the oxygen diffusion and results in ischemia.[11] This condition often is the result of trauma. Clinical presentation and intercompartmental pressure measurements confirm the diagnosis.[12] This condition is a medical emergency and requires urgent surgical decompression.

■ Complex Regional Pain Syndrome
Chief Clinical Characteristics
This presentation may include a traumatic onset of severe chronic ankle and foot pain accompanied by allodynia, hyperalgesia, and, in later stages, trophic, vasomotor, and sudomotor changes. This condition is characterized by disproportionate responses to painful stimuli.

Background Information
This regional neuropathic pain disorder presents either without direct nerve trauma (Type I) or with direct nerve trauma (Type II) in any region of the body.[3] This condition may precipitate due to an event distant to the affected area. Thermography may confirm associated sympathetic dysfunction. Treatment may include physical therapy interventions to improve patient/client functioning, biofeedback, analgesic or anti-inflammatory medication, transcutaneous or spinal electrical nerve stimulation, and surgical or pharmacologic sympathectomy.

■ Delayed Onset Muscle Soreness Secondary to Exercise
Chief Clinical Characteristics
This presentation may be characterized by pain, soreness, swelling, restricted range of motion, and tenderness to palpation and stretching. Self-limiting symptoms are usually aggravated with

bearing weight on the affected lower extremity or muscle contraction, but also may be present at rest.

Background Information

This condition is caused by muscle damage and immune response following exercise at an unaccustomed intensity and duration. Clinical examination confirms the diagnosis. Blood panels may reveal increased serum creatine kinase levels, which usually begin to increase 24 to 48 hours following exercise. Rare complications may include rhabdomyolysis or myoglobinuria. This condition is usually self-limiting, but can respond favorably to gentle flexibility exercises.

■ Distal Symmetric Polyneuropathy, Including From Acquired Immunodeficiency Syndrome, Alcohol/Drug Abuse, Carcinoma, Diabetes Mellitus, and Kidney Failure

Chief Clinical Characteristics

This presentation may be characterized by decreased distal deep tendon reflexes, as well as pain, dysesthesia, or paresthesia in the feet and toes.

Background Information

Peripheral neuropathy is one of the more common complications in patients presenting with acquired immunodeficiency syndrome, diabetes, renal failure, hypothyroidism, toxins, malignancy, and malnutrition. It is characterized by retrograde axonal degeneration, so this condition commonly progresses from distal to proximal. Electromyographic studies and biopsy confirm the diagnosis. Vibration and light touch sensation (10-g Semmes Weinstein monofilament) tests are useful to assess protective sensation. Curative treatment of this condition remains controversial, so the focus of intervention typically includes patient education to maintain blood glucose control and care for the insensate regions to prevent progression and complications secondary to this condition.

■ Erysipelas

Chief Clinical Characteristics

This presentation may include tenderness, shiny and red erythema, induration, vesicles, bullae, and possibly lymphadenopathy. Fever, chills, and malaise are common signs of systemic involvement.

The lower legs and feet are primarily affected, but involvement of the arms and face also is common.[13]

Background Information

This condition results from a superficial interdigital fungal infection with lymphatic involvement. Blood tests and pathological staining techniques confirm the diagnosis and guide medical management. Antibiotic medications directed toward the underlying infective agent comprise the typical treatment for this condition.

■ Erythema Induratum

Chief Clinical Characteristics

This presentation can involve brown or blue subcutaneous nodules on the lower leg that may be accompanied by painful ulcerations that are present for a significant length of time. Necrosis or plaques also may be present.

Background Information

This condition is a dermatological disorder that is most common to the calf. Diagnosis is confirmed with biopsy of the nodules or ulcerations. This condition may be treated with rest in combination with a polypharmaceutical antibiotic approach. Intralesional corticosteroids to address inflammation also may be necessary.

■ Erythema Nodosum

Chief Clinical Characteristics

This presentation can include pretibial pain, edema, and arthralgia that may be associated with knee or ankle pain. Characteristic findings include bilateral red subcutaneous nodules that may resemble bruises in the early stages, later changing to a darker brown. Systemic signs of infection often include fever and malaise.

Background Information

This condition most commonly appears in individuals ranging from 20 to 40 years of age. Upper respiratory infections are the common source of infection in children, while streptococcal and sarcoidal infections are the common causes in adults. Diagnosis is often one of exclusion. Diagnosis may be assisted with determination of the causative agent. Also, many individuals presenting with this condition often have an elevated erythrocyte sedimentation rate. This condition often resolves spontaneously along with treatment of the underlying infection, although anti-inflammatory and antibiotic medications also may be used.

FRACTURES

■ Fibula

Chief Clinical Characteristics
This presentation typically includes pain, poor tolerance to bearing weight on the affected lower extremity, tenderness to palpation, swelling, and ecchymosis, with possible crepitus and pain with vibration.

Background Information
This condition has either traumatic or pathological etiology. It is more commonly traumatic and may be associated with fractures of the tibia. Isolated fibula fractures are more commonly associated with ankle injuries. Pathological fractures may have an unknown etiology, but are often associated with comorbidities of metastases, leukemia, bone lesions, or osteoporosis. The diagnosis is confirmed with plain radiographs. Depending on fracture stability, treatment options range from immobilization to reduction and fixation.

■ Stress Fracture of the Tibia

Chief Clinical Characteristics
This presentation includes pain and palpable tenderness over the posteromedial border of the tibia. Pain is aggravated with bearing weight on the affected lower extremity, such as with running; it is alleviated with rest.

Background Information
This condition usually occurs in runners and is associated with an abrupt increase in training. The clinical examination, plain radiographs, and bone scan confirm the diagnosis. The fracture usually heals in approximately 6 to 8 weeks as a result of no weight bearing or weight-bearing restrictions. In the meantime, continued activity in a reduced-impact environment may be considered to maintain general strength and conditioning.

■ Tibia

Chief Clinical Characteristics
This presentation may involve pain, poor tolerance to bearing weight on the affected lower extremity, tenderness to palpation, swelling, ecchymosis, crepitus, and pain with vibration through the tibia.

Background Information
The pain is usually severe when the fracture is located in the tibial shaft. Limb shortening may be seen in the involved extremity. Fractures of the tibia tend to be of either traumatic or pathological etiology. Traumatic fractures are more common and related to direct trauma. Pathological fractures are associated with comorbidities such as metastases, leukemia, bone lesions, or osteoporosis. Plain radiographs confirm the diagnosis and guide medical management. Depending on fracture stability, treatment options range from immobilization to reduction and fixation.

■ Gas Gangrene

Chief Clinical Characteristics
This presentation may involve severe local wound pain, edema, tenderness to palpation, pallor, a malodorous brown and serous discharge, and, in the later stages, gas crepitation. Skin may appear pale at the early stages and later turn a red or bronze color. Systemic signs of infection may include pallor, diaphoresis, fever, hypotension, apathy, drowsiness, agitation, stupor, or coma.

Background Information
This condition is caused by a clostridial infection that usually follows trauma to deep tissues or infection of postoperative wounds. This condition can progress within several hours to several days. It is a medical emergency. Diagnosis is confirmed with Gram staining. Surgical exploration may be necessary to reveal the extent of myonecrosis.[14]

■ Greater Saphenous Vein Thrombophlebitis

Chief Clinical Characteristics
This presentation includes anteromedial lower leg pain, tenderness, edema, erythema, palpable warmth, engorged veins, and possibly a low-grade fever and pain along the course of the vein. An indurated cord may be palpated along the course of the vein.

Background Information
This condition involves thrombosis and inflammation of the involved vein. The etiology

of this condition is associated with Virchow's triad of intimal damage, stasis, and changes in blood composition[7]; it usually occurs due to trauma to the vein or surrounding tissue, but also may present spontaneously. Saphenous venous thrombosis is correlated with hypercoagulability.[15] Computed tomography, magnetic resonance angiography, and Doppler ultrasonography confirm the diagnosis. It is a medical emergency because of the risk for propagation of the thrombus to the lungs.

■ Hematoma of the Calf

Chief Clinical Characteristics
This presentation can involve pain, swelling, tenderness to palpation, and occasional ecchymosis with symptoms very similar to thrombophlebitis. Pain is aggravated with bearing weight on the affected lower extremity, muscle contraction, and passive ankle dorsiflexion. Symptoms may have an abrupt or gradual onset, depending on the nature of the bleed.

Background Information
Intercompartmental pressure may elevate to the level of a compartment syndrome, causing neuralgia or ischemia. This condition is caused by muscle tear, fracture, direct blunt trauma, or rupture of the lower extremity vasculature. The clinical examination in combination with magnetic resonance or ultrasound imaging confirms the diagnosis. This condition may be managed with evacuation of the hematoma and rest.

■ Infectious Periostitis

Chief Clinical Characteristics
This presentation may be characterized by aching to severe pain with tenderness and edema of the infected bone. Suppuration may be present and an individual with this condition will often exhibit systemic signs of infection, such as fever, chills, and fatigue.

Background Information
This condition involves a chronic infection of the periosteum from a hematogenous source or trauma to the affected region. Not all cases of periostitis are the result of an infection; therefore, the diagnosis is confirmed by radiographic imaging revealing necrosis of the affected bone and bone scan revealing increased uptake. This condition is usually managed with antibiotic medication appropriately directed to the infective agent.

■ Inflammatory Muscle Disease

Chief Clinical Characteristics
This presentation includes a gradual onset of mild muscle pain associated with proximal muscle weakness that causes difficulty with daily activities such as walking, ascending and descending stairs, and rising from chairs.

Background Information
This condition describes a group of pathologically, histologically, and clinically distinct disorders: polymyositis, dermatomyositis, and inclusion body myositis. They may be associated with other collagen, vascular, and immune disorders. Although proximal extremity weakness is a classic finding, up to 50% also demonstrate distal weakness that may be equally as severe.[16] Blood panels help confirm the diagnosis and track disease activity, revealing elevated serum levels of creatine phosphokinase. Treatment typically involves steroidal, nonsteroidal, and biological anti-inflammatory medications.

■ Malnutrition

Chief Clinical Characteristics
This presentation typically includes muscle cramps and muscular pain that more often affect the calf musculature. Systemic signs may include lethargy, mental and physical fatigue, apathy, impaired learning ability, diminished immune system function, and delayed healing response.

Background Information
Morphological changes are observed in the later stages. Etiology includes starvation, alcoholic malnutrition, inadequate diet, eating disorders, or imbalanced diet. Hypomagnesemia and hyponatremia are common causes of the muscular symptoms. Clinical and biochemical tests confirm the diagnosis. Treatment includes amelioration of diet.

■ Metastases to the Lower Leg, Including From Primary Breast, Kidney, Lung, Prostate, and Thyroid Disease

Chief Clinical Characteristics
This presentation typically includes unremitting pain in individuals with these risk factors:

previous history of cancer, age 50 years or older, failure to improve with conservative therapy, and unexplained weight change of more than 10 pounds in 6 months.[17]

Background Information
The skeletal system is the third most common site of metastatic disease.[18] Symptoms also may be related to pathological fracture in affected sites. Common primary sites causing metastases to bone include breast, prostate, lung, and kidney. Bone scan confirms the diagnosis. Common treatments for metastases include surgical resection, chemotherapy, radiation treatment, and palliation, depending on the tumor type and extent of metastasis.

■ Multiple Myeloma
Chief Clinical Characteristics
This presentation involves unexplained skeletal pain in the feet, lower legs, arms, hands, back, and thorax. This may be associated with renal failure, recurrent bacterial infections, pathological fractures, and anemia.

Background Information
This condition is an insidious plasma cell cancer that originates in the bone marrow and can affect multiple areas with multiple lytic and osteosclerotic affects. Pain results from either neuropathy or bone pain. Radiographically, the bones will have lesions of a punched-out appearance with generalized osteoporosis. Diagnosis may be confirmed with blood tests, urinalysis, serum protein electrophoresis, bone scan, magnetic resonance imaging, and bone marrow aspiration and biopsy. Depending on the aggressiveness of this condition, treatment may range from "watchful waiting" to chemotherapy and bone marrow transplantation.

MUSCLE STRAINS
■ Anterior Compartment Muscle Strain
Chief Clinical Characteristics
This presentation typically includes pain and tenderness, difficulty bearing weight on the affected lower extremity, and possible edema and ecchymosis in the anterolateral lower leg. Symptoms may be reproduced with either muscle action or stretching.

Background Information
The three dorsiflexor muscles in the anterolateral compartment may be injured individually or in combination. This condition often occurs during activities that place excessive eccentric demand on the anterior compartment muscles.[19] The diagnosis is confirmed by magnetic resonance imaging or computed tomography. Usual treatment is nonsurgical.

■ Gastrocnemius Muscle Strain
Chief Clinical Characteristics
This presentation may involve pain, tenderness, pain with contraction, difficulty weight bearing and sometimes swelling or ecchymoses in the region of the gastrocnemius muscle.

Background Information
Injury to the muscle often occurs during activities that place excessive eccentric demand on the gastrocnemius, usually on an extended knee.[19] Diagnosis may be aided by magnetic resonance imaging. Treatment is often nonsurgical and healing usually takes 6 to 10 weeks.

■ Lateral Compartment Muscle Strain
Chief Clinical Characteristics
This presentation includes pain, tenderness, difficulty bearing weight on the affected extremity and walking, and possible edema or ecchymosis in the region of the peroneal muscles. Symptoms may be reproduced by either muscle action or stretching.

Background Information
Injury to the muscle often occurs during activities that place excessive eccentric demand on the peroneal muscles.[19] The diagnosis is confirmed by magnetic resonance imaging or computed tomography. Usual treatment is nonsurgical.

■ Soleus Muscle Strain
Chief Clinical Characteristics
This presentation may involve pain, tenderness, pain with contraction, difficulty bearing weight on the affected lower extremity, and possibly edema or ecchymosis over the soleus muscle.

Background Information
The injured area is often more distal and deep to the gastrocnemius; this may be

assessed through an individual's history and palpation. This condition often occurs during activities that place excessive eccentric demand on the soleus, more often with a flexed knee.[19] Magnetic resonance imaging confirms the diagnosis. Usual treatment is nonsurgical.

■ Necrotizing Fasciitis

Chief Clinical Characteristics
This presentation involves pain with erythema, warmth, swelling, possible skin discoloration, blisters, gangrene, and joint crepitus. Systemic signs of an infection may include fever, tachycardia, hypotension, diaphoresis, chills, malaise, and altered mental status. The wound may be odorous and sometimes subcutaneous gas is observed.

Background Information
The underlying infection often is caused by a bacterium following trauma or infection of an open wound or ulcer. This condition often is mistaken for cellulitis in its early stages. Diagnosis may be confirmed with radiographs, abnormal blood serum tests, and a Gram stain of the infected tissue. This condition is a medical emergency. Treatment includes debridement of necrotic tissue and an aggressive regimen of antibiotic medication.

NERVE ENTRAPMENTS

■ Saphenous Nerve

Chief Clinical Characteristics
This presentation involves pain, paresthesias, dysesthesias, or numbness on the medial aspect of the lower leg and distal to the medial ankle and foot. This condition also may be associated with medial knee pain.[20]

Background Information
The saphenous nerve is a cutaneous afferent, so entrapment produces no motor deficits. Potential entrapment sites include the adductor hiatus and the distal sartorius muscle. Knee surgery, surgical excision of the saphenous vein, femoral neuropathy, or knee trauma may cause this condition.[21] The diagnosis is confirmed with the clinical examination, with additional studies potentially useful to detect contributory conditions. Typical treatment is nonsurgical, with surgical exploration and release of entrapment

sites reserved for cases in which the site of entrapment is well characterized.

■ Sciatic Nerve

Chief Clinical Characteristics
This presentation may include diminished Achilles deep tendon reflex, weakness of the hamstrings or ankle plantarflexors and dorsiflexors, pain, and buttock, posterior thigh, posterior lower leg, and foot paresthesias or hypesthesias.

Background Information
Common etiologies include entrapment at the sciatic notch or the hamstrings. This condition is a diagnosis of exclusion after lumbar radiculopathy is ruled less likely. The clinical examination, including the straight leg raise test and a standard neurological examination, and electrodiagnostic tests confirm the diagnosis. Typical treatment is nonsurgical, with surgical exploration and release of entrapment sites reserved for cases in which the site of entrapment is well-characterized.

■ Superficial Peroneal Nerve

Chief Clinical Characteristics
This presentation can involve pain, paresthesias, dysesthesias, or numbness on the anterolateral lower leg and dorsum of the foot. Plantarflexion and foot inversion are often aggravating factors, and Tinel's sign over the superficial peroneal nerve also may reproduce pain. Associated motor deficits may include weakness of foot eversion.

Background Information
Etiology includes compression due to trauma or idiopathic entrapment.[22] This condition is a diagnosis of exclusion after lumbar radiculopathy is ruled out. The clinical examination, including the straight leg raise test and a standard neurological examination, and electrodiagnostic tests confirm the diagnosis. Typical treatment is nonsurgical, with surgical exploration and release of entrapment sites reserved for cases in which the site of entrapment is well characterized.

■ Sural Nerve

Chief Clinical Characteristics
This presentation can be characterized by hypesthesias or paresthesias and pain along

the posterior calf, posterolateral ankle, or the dorsolateral foot. Tinel's sign also may reproduce pain. This condition does not include motor involvement because the sural nerve is a sensory afferent.

Background Information

Common etiologies include ankle sprains, stretch injury, Achilles injury, trauma, nerve compression due to ganglion cyst, or calcaneal fracture. This condition is a diagnosis of exclusion after lumbar radiculopathy has been ruled out. The clinical examination, including the straight leg raise test and a standard neurological examination, and electrodiagnostic tests confirm the diagnosis. Typical treatment is nonsurgical, with surgical exploration and release of entrapment sites reserved for cases in which the site of entrapment is well characterized.

■ Tibial Nerve

Chief Clinical Characteristics

This presentation may involve hypesthesias or paresthesias and pain along the posterior calf, medial ankle, and plantar surface of the foot. Motor symptoms are less common. Pain may be aggravated with bearing weight on the affected lower extremity and walking, manual compression over the nerve, or Tinel's sign.

Background Information

Common etiologies include space-occupying lesions, fractures, calluses, arthritis and osteophytes, edema, bursitis, tendonitis or tenosynovitis, accessory bones, or other prolonged pressure. This condition is a diagnosis of exclusion after lumbar radiculopathy has been ruled out. The clinical examination, including the straight leg raise test and a standard neurological examination, and electrodiagnostic tests confirm the diagnosis. Typical treatment is nonsurgical, with surgical exploration and release of entrapment sites reserved for cases in which the site of entrapment is well characterized.

■ Nodular Panniculitis

Chief Clinical Characteristics

This presentation may be characterized by painfully tender plaques and nodules that are often reddish in color on the lower extremities. The nodules may necrose with a "pus-like"

drainage that can be stained as free fat. Skin lesions are the primary sign; fever, leukocytosis, ecchymoses, pulmonary lesions, and elevated serum amylase and lipase levels also may be present.

Background Information

This condition often has a systemic cause such as connective tissue disorders, lymphoproliferative disorders, alpha$_1$-antitrypsin deficiency, or lipodystrophy. Histological examination of the affected tissue confirms the diagnosis. Intralesional corticosteroids to address inflammation also may be necessary.

■ Nonclostridial Myositis

Chief Clinical Characteristics

This presentation involves pain, erythema, edema, malodorous discharge, and possibly tissue crepitus. Symptoms may vary depending on the nature of the infection. In advanced cases, dark areas of gangrene are present.

Background Information

This condition usually results from penetrating trauma, complications of diabetes mellitus, ischemia, or direct infection from an outside source. Laboratory tests determine the pathogen, plain radiographs confirm tissue gas, and surgical exploration may confirm the myonecrosis or myositis as well as guide medical management. Typical treatment involves an aggressive regimen of antibiotic medication and surgical drainage.

■ Osteoid Osteoma

Chief Clinical Characteristics

This presentation may involve focal bone pain at the site of the tumor that is associated with tenderness and warmth to palpation, with significant increase in pain with activity and at night, as well as substantial and immediate relief of pain with anti-inflammatory medication.

Background Information

This condition is more common in males than females, and it rarely presents in people younger than age 5 or older than 40 years of age. Its pathology includes abnormal production of osteoid and primitive bone. The proximal femur is the most common site for this tumor. Pain associated with this condition is self-limiting and may resolve spontaneously over the course of

2 to 4 years.[23] Pain relief also may be achieved by surgical removal of the tumor.

■ Osteomyelitis of the Tibia

Chief Clinical Characteristics

This presentation typically involves localized tenderness, warmth, erythema, swelling, and systemic signs of infection such as weight loss and fatigue. The toes may present with a "sausage toe" deformity.

Background Information

This condition is an inflammation and necrosis of bone as a result of an infection. The calcaneus is the most common site of infection in the foot, followed by the metatarsals, tarsals, and then the phalangeal bones. Biopsy, magnetic resonance imaging, and histology confirm the diagnosis and guide medical intervention.[24] Treatment may involve an aggressive regimen of antibiotic medications, with surgical resection of affected areas potentially necessary.

■ Osteosarcoma

Chief Clinical Characteristics

This presentation may be characterized by an insidious onset of pain that persists for weeks or months. Pain due to this condition may be aggravated with activity, causing limping.

Background Information

This condition is frequently found in adolescents because of the active bone growth in this age group. African American individuals are affected slightly more often than Caucasian individuals. This condition can be especially fatal if metastasized to the lungs. Plain films confirm the diagnosis. Treatment includes chemotherapy and surgery to remove the cancerous cells or tumors.

■ Paratenonitis of Extensor Tendons of the Foot and Toes

Chief Clinical Characteristics

This presentation includes pain, possible swelling, erythema, and tenderness to palpation over the anterior ankle and may include crepitus with active or passive movements if the tendon sheaths are inflamed.

Background Information

This condition usually occurs with a sudden onset following increases in walking intensity or distance, change of shoe, tightness in the shoe laces over the tendons, midtarsal joint hyperostosis, or tightness of the posterior calf muscles. Differentiation among extensor tendons can be achieved by passive stretching and active contraction of the specific muscles. Clinical examination confirms the diagnosis. Usual treatment is nonsurgical.

■ Posterior Tibial Vein Thrombosis

Chief Clinical Characteristics

This presentation may include calf pain, tenderness, lower extremity swelling, cramping, erythema, palpable warmth, engorged veins, sometimes a low-grade fever, and pain potentially along the course of the vein. The thrombosis can affect superficial or deep veins, but the popliteal and calf veins are more commonly affected.

Background Information

Venous thrombosis may be effort induced or spontaneous. This condition involves thrombosis and inflammation of the involved vein. The etiology of this condition is associated with Virchow's triad of intimal damage, stasis, and changes in blood composition[7]; it usually occurs due to trauma to the vein or surrounding tissue, but also may present spontaneously. Homan's sign, D-dimer assay measurement, computed tomography, magnetic resonance angiography, and Doppler ultrasonography confirm the diagnosis.[25,26] This condition is a medical emergency because of the risk for propagation of the thrombus to the lungs.

■ Pyomyositis

Chief Clinical Characteristics

This presentation often involves cramping pain and edema with early-stage induration, followed by increased pain and edema in the later stages. Systemic signs of infection may include fever, chills, and sometimes diaphoresis. Leukocytosis is common. Abscess formation due to Staphylococcus aureus infection often follows muscle tissue trauma.

Background Information

Risk factors include poorly controlled diabetes mellitus, presence of a contiguous bone or soft tissue infection, malnutrition, or a compromised immune system. Diagnosis is confirmed by the clinical examination, computed tomography or magnetic resonance imaging, and Gram-stained culture of the aspirated pus.[27] Treatment is directed at the underlying infection.

■ Rupture of the Achilles Tendon

Chief Clinical Characteristics

This presentation may include a sudden onset of pain, palpable tenderness, significant weakness, and sometimes a palpable sulcus, usually 2 to 6 cm proximal to the distal insertion of the Achilles tendon (Fig. 22-1).

Background Information

This condition often occurs spontaneously during an activity that places loading on the plantarflexors. It is associated with age over 40 years and a history of Achilles tendinopathy. The Thompson test and magnetic resonance or ultrasound imaging confirm the diagnosis. This condition is treated with surgical repair of the affected tendon.

SHIN SPLINTS

■ Anterolateral Shin Splints

Chief Clinical Characteristics

This presentation includes pain and palpable tenderness along the involved anterior tibial muscles immediately adjacent to the

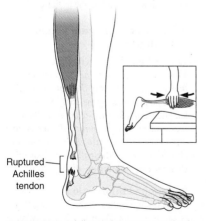

Ruptured Achilles tendon

FIGURE 22-1 Achilles tendon rupture may be detected by the Thompson test (inset), in which manual circumferential pressure is exerted against the calf. A normal response includes passive ankle plantarflexion. A positive test is absence of ankle movement.

tibia. The pain usually lessens following warm-up exercises of the involved muscles, but is often present during activity with soreness following the activity. Pain usually is absent at night.

Background Information

Shin splints are the result of eccentric overuse, leading to an inflammatory musculotendinous injury along the lateral aspect of the tibia, with potential muscular avulsion from the tibia.[28] Diagnosis is usually based on the clinical presentation. Imaging is usually unhelpful, although fat-suppressed magnetic resonance imaging may allow differentiation between stress fractures and shin splints.[29] Usual treatment is nonsurgical.

■ Posteromedial Shin Splints

Chief Clinical Characteristics

This presentation involves pain and palpable tenderness along the muscles attached to the posteromedial aspect of the tibia within the deep posterior compartment. Pain is usually less often located directly over the tibia. Pain is aggravated with stretching into foot dorsiflexion and eversion, and with active contraction of the involved muscles. Pain usually lessens following warm-up of the muscles, there is usually pain during activity with soreness following the activity, and there is usually no pain during the night.

Background Information

Shin splints are due to an eccentric overuse, leading to musculotendinous injury along the posteromedial attachment of the tibia, resulting in a periostitis.[30,31] Diagnosis is based on the clinical presentation. Imaging is usually unhelpful, although fat-suppressed magnetic resonance imaging may help differentiate between stress fractures and shin splints.[29] Typical treatment is nonsurgical.

■ Sickle Cell Crisis

Chief Clinical Characteristics

This presentation may be characterized by bone pain about the hip joint, worsened by cold weather, overexertion, dehydration, and being overly fatigued.

Background Information
Sickle cell crisis involves abnormal red blood cell morphology that causes the cells to become rigid and sticky, disrupting blood flow to bones and resulting in painful bone infarcts. This condition is a group of inherited disorders with abnormalities caused by hemoglobin S. This condition typically is associated with pain due to tissue infarction and/or worsening anemia. Diagnosis of a crisis is confirmed with plain radiographs and magnetic resonance imaging. This condition is a medical emergency.

SKIN ULCERS

■ Arterial or Hypertensive Ulcers

Chief Clinical Characteristics
This presentation involves small, painful, and tender ulcers measuring from several millimeters to a few centimeters in size. They are more commonly found in the pretibial region. Associated symptoms may include palpable coolness and trophic changes such as hair loss.

Background Information
This condition commonly is associated with hypertension or peripheral vascular disease with ulcerations at the ends of the arterial branches.[32] Wound management in combination with endovascular or bypass surgical interventions may be necessary as treatments.

■ Systemic Vasculitis With Ulceration

Chief Clinical Characteristics
This presentation may include subcutaneous erythematous nodules on the lower leg that are usually painful and may develop into purulent ulcerations.

Background Information
This condition results from inflammation of the blood vessels that may result from systemic lupus erythematosus, polyarteritis nodosa, rheumatoid arthritis, Wegener's granulomatosis, or sickle cell anemia. Diagnosis may be focused toward determining the tissue involved via histological analysis or angiography. Typical treatment involves wound management in combination with treatment for the underlying pathology.

TENDINITIS

■ Achilles Tendinitis

Chief Clinical Characteristics
This presentation can involve a sharp, aching, or burning pain with point tenderness 2 to 6 cm proximal to the calcaneal insertion. Insertional tendinopathy may be located at the distal insertion at the calcaneus. Symptoms are reproduced with palpation of the tendon, passive dorsiflexion, and active resisted plantarflexion. Palpable crepitus may be present with movement, and an increased thickening of the tendon that moves with tendon excursion may be palpable in comparison to the asymptomatic side. Calf atrophy may be observed, the patient may have limitations in ankle dorsiflexion, and the patient may report increased stiffness in the morning.

Background Information
Achilles tendinitis is associated with overuse from repetitive loading of the involved tendon. This injury is most common in 15- to 45-year-old active individuals, most commonly runners. Diagnosis is often made clinically. If the diagnosis is difficult, then confirmation may be made with magnetic resonance imaging. Usual treatment is nonsurgical, consisting of anti-inflammatory medication, rest, and gentle exercise.

■ Extensor Digitorum Longus Tendinitis

Chief Clinical Characteristics
This presentation can be characterized by pain over the dorsum of the foot and tenderness to palpation along the extensor digitorum longus tendons. Resisted extension of the lesser toes and passive flexion of the lesser toes often increase the pain. Pain may also be elicited with resisted dorsiflexion of the ankle. Walking and running are often painful.

Background Information
The pathology of this tendinitis is usually the result of overuse. Diagnosis is usually made clinically, but may be confirmed with magnetic resonance or ultrasound imaging. Nonsurgical treatments may be indicated, such as anti-inflammatory medication, rest, and gentle exercise.

■ Extensor Hallucis Longus Tendinitis

Chief Clinical Characteristics
This presentation may include pain and palpable tenderness along the extensor hallucis tendon. Resisted extension of the hallux and passive flexion of the hallux often increase the pain. Pain may also be elicited with resisted dorsiflexion of the ankle. Walking and running are often painful.

Background Information
The pathology of this tendinitis is usually the result of overuse.[33] Diagnosis is usually made clinically, but may be confirmed with magnetic resonance or ultrasound imaging. Treatment usually involves nonsurgical interventions, such as anti-inflammatory medication, rest, and gentle exercise.

■ Peroneal Tendinitis

Chief Clinical Characteristics
This presentation can involve pain anywhere along the lateral lower leg to the posterior lateral malleolus and along the lateral foot at the location of the cuboid or at the plantar aspect of the foot where the peroneus longus tendon inserts at the base of the first metatarsal. The pain may also be present at the base of the fifth metatarsal where the peroneus brevis tendon inserts. The pain is often aggravated with a stretch into foot and ankle dorsiflexion and inversion or a muscle contraction into foot and ankle plantarflexion and/or eversion.

Background Information
Common causes of peroneal tendon injury include overuse and inversion injury mechanisms. Diagnosis is usually made clinically, but may be confirmed with magnetic resonance or ultrasound imaging. Nonsurgical treatments may be indicated, such as anti-inflammatory medication, rest, and gentle exercise.

■ Tibialis Anterior Tendinitis

Chief Clinical Characteristics
This presentation typically includes pain and tenderness to palpation of the tibialis anterior tendon.

Background Information
Pain is often present at initial contact and during the loading response of gait, due to the eccentric loading of the tendon and muscle. Pain is often increased with passive stretch into plantarflexion or resisted dorsiflexion of the ankle. The pathology of tibialis anterior tendinitis is usually overuse.[33] Diagnosis is usually made clinically, but may be confirmed with magnetic resonance or ultrasound imaging. Usual treatment is nonsurgical, consisting of anti-inflammatory medication, rest, and gentle exercise.

■ Tibialis Posterior Tendinitis

Chief Clinical Characteristics
This presentation may involve pain and swelling with palpable tenderness along the medial aspect of the midfoot and sometimes posterior to the medial malleolus. Pain is often worsened with weight bearing, walking, performing a heel rise, or stretching the tendon. Attenuation of this tendon is sometimes seen and can lead to a flat foot deformity. Palpation may be assisted with muscle contraction of the tibialis posterior muscle.

Background Information
Injury to this tendon is often the result of overuse that is caused by a hypermobile midfoot and excessive foot pronation. The tibialis posterior is the most significant active stabilizer of the arch.[34] Diagnosis is usually made clinically, but may be confirmed with magnetic resonance or ultrasound imaging. Nonsurgical treatments may be indicated, such as anti-inflammatory medication, rest, and gentle exercise.

TENDINOSES

■ Achilles Tendinosis

Chief Clinical Characteristics
This presentation typically includes sharp, aching, or burning pain with point tenderness usually along the medial aspect of the middle one-third of the Achilles tendon. Some of these patients are pain free. Symptoms, if present, may be reproduced with palpation of the Achilles tendon, passive dorsiflexion, or active resisted plantarflexion. Palpable increased thickening of the tendon may be present in comparison to the uninvolved tendon. Calf atrophy, limitations in ankle dorsiflexion, and reports of increased stiffness

in the morning may be observed. Pain is often worse with weight bearing and walking, and these patients often have difficulty performing a heel rise.

Background Information

Tendinosis is a state of increased tenocyte and cellular activity that leads to disorganized collagen and vascular hyperplasia.[35,36] Tendinosis is usually a chronic degenerative process that is initiated by an injury to the tendon. Diagnosis is usually based on the clinical presentation. If pathology is severe or the clinical diagnosis is unclear, then magnetic resonance or ultrasound imaging may confirm the diagnosis and allow for prognosis and staging of the tendinosis. A combination of patient/client education, unloading the affected musculotendinous unit, controlled mechanical reloading, and preventive measures appears to be effective for managing this condition.[37]

■ **Extensor Digitorum Longus Tendinosis**

Chief Clinical Characteristics

This presentation typically includes pain over the dorsum of the foot and tenderness to palpation along the extensor digitorum longus tendons. Walking and running often are painful. Resisted extension of the lesser toes and passive flexion of the lesser toes often increase the pain. Pain also may be elicited with resisted dorsiflexion of the ankle.

Background Information

Tendinosis is a state of increased tenocyte and cellular activity that leads to disorganized collagen and vascular hyperplasia.[35,36] Tendinosis is usually a chronic degenerative process that is initiated by an injury to the tendon. Clinical examination confirms the diagnosis. If pathology is severe or the clinical diagnosis is unclear, then magnetic resonance or ultrasound imaging may confirm the diagnosis and allow for prognosis and staging of the tendinosis. A combination of patient/client education, unloading the affected musculotendinous unit, controlled mechanical reloading, and preventive measures appears to be effective for managing this condition.[37]

■ **Extensor Hallucis Longus Tendinosis**

Chief Clinical Characteristics

This presentation typically includes pain and palpable tenderness along the extensor hallucis tendon. Walking and running are often painful. Resisted extension of the hallux and passive flexion of the hallux often increase the pain. Pain may also be elicited with resisted dorsiflexion of the ankle.

Background Information

Extensor hallucis longus tendinosis is a state of increased tenocyte and cellular activity that leads to disorganized collagen and vascular hyperplasia.[35,36] Tendinosis is usually a chronic degenerative process that is initiated by an injury to the tendon. Clinical examination confirms the diagnosis. If pathology is severe or the clinical diagnosis is unclear, then magnetic resonance or ultrasound imaging may confirm the diagnosis and allow for prognosis and staging of the tendinosis. A combination of patient/client education, unloading the affected musculotendinous unit, controlled mechanical reloading, and preventive measures appears to be effective for managing this condition.[37]

■ **Peroneal Tendinosis**

Chief Clinical Characteristics

This presentation typically includes pain anywhere along the lateral lower leg to the posterior lateral malleolus and along the lateral foot at the location of the cuboid or at the plantar aspect of the foot where the peroneus longus tendon inserts at the base of the first metatarsal. The pain may also be present at the base of the fifth metatarsal where the peroneus brevis tendon inserts. The pain is often aggravated with a stretch into dorsiflexion and inversion or a muscle contraction into plantarflexion and/or eversion. Weakness may be noted into plantarflexion and/or eversion due to degenerative thickening, lengthening, and tearing of the tendon.

Background Information

Common causes of peroneal tendon injury include overuse and inversion injury mechanisms that may lead to the chronic degenerative process of tendinosis. Tendinosis is a state of increased tenocyte and cellular activity that leads to disorganized collagen and vascular hyperplasia.[35,36] Final diagnosis is confirmed with magnetic resonance or ultrasound imaging. A combination of patient/client education, unloading the affected musculotendinous unit, controlled mechanical reloading, and preventive measures appears to be effective for managing this condition.[37]

■ Tibialis Anterior Tendinosis

Chief Clinical Characteristics
This presentation typically includes pain and tenderness to palpation of the tibialis anterior tendon.

Background Information
Pain is often present at initial contact and during the loading response of gait, due to the eccentric loading of the tendon and muscle. Pain is often increased with passive stretch into plantarflexion or resisted dorsiflexion of the ankle. Tendinosis is a state of increased tenocyte and cellular activity that leads to disorganized collagen and vascular hyperplasia.[35,36] Tendinosis is usually a chronic degenerative process that is initiated by an injury to the tendon. Diagnosis is usually made clinically, but may be confirmed with magnetic resonance or ultrasound imaging. Usual treatment is nonsurgical, consisting of anti-inflammatory medication, rest, and gentle exercise.

■ Tibialis Posterior Tendinosis

Chief Clinical Characteristics
The patient presentation typically includes pain and swelling with palpable tenderness along the medial aspect of the midfoot and posterior to the medial malleolus. Pain is often worse with weight bearing and walking, and these patients often have difficulty performing a heel rise. Attenuation of this tendon is sometimes seen as a result of tendinosis, and the development of posterior tibialis tendon dysfunction may lead to a flat foot deformity and a caudal drop of the navicular. These patients have a very difficult time contracting the tibialis posterior muscle, even during a manual muscle test.

Background Information
Injury to this tendon is often the result of overuse with a hypermobile midfoot. The tibialis posterior is the most significant active stabilizer of the arch.[34] Tendinosis is a state of increased tenocyte and cellular activity that leads to disorganized collagen and vascular hyperplasia. Tendinosis is usually a chronic degenerative process that is initiated by injury to the tendon. Diagnosis is usually based on the clinical presentation; however, magnetic resonance imaging may confirm the diagnosis and allow for prognosis and staging of the tendinosis. A combination of patient/client education, unloading the affected musculotendinous unit, controlled mechanical reloading, and preventive measures appears to be effective for managing this condition.[37]

References
1. Handy JR. Popliteal cysts in adults: a review. *Semin Arthritis Rheum.* Oct 2001;31(2):108–118.
2. Sansone V, De Ponti A. Arthroscopic treatment of popliteal cyst and associated intra-articular knee disorders in adults. *Arthroscopy.* May 1999;15(4):368–372.
3. Merskey H, Bogduk N. *Classification of Chronic Pain: Descriptions of Chronic Pain Syndromes and Definitions of Pain Terms.* Seattle, WA: IASP Press; 1994.
4. Moseley GL. Imagined movements cause pain and swelling in a patient with complex regional pain syndrome. *Neurology.* May 11, 2004;62(9):1644.
5. Mosley JG. Arterial problems in athletes. *Br J Surg.* Dec 2003;90(12):1461–1469.
6. Joshi MK, Liu HH. Acute rhabdomyolysis and renal failure in HIV-infected patients: risk factors, presentation, and pathophysiology. *AIDS Patient Care Stds.* Oct 2000;14(10):541–548.
7. Mammen EF. Pathogenesis of venous thrombosis. *Chest.* Dec 1992;102(6 suppl):640S–644S.
8. Breugem CC, Maas M, Breugem SJ, Schaap GR, van der Horst CM. Vascular malformations of the lower limb with osseous involvement. *J Bone Joint Surg Br.* Apr 2003;85(3):399–405.
9. Parisi L, Pierelli F, Amabile G, et al. Muscular cramps: proposals for a new classification. *Acta Neurol Scand.* Mar 2003;107(3):176–186.
10. Jose RM, Viswanathan N, Aldlyami E, Wilson Y, Moiemen N, Thomas R. A spontaneous compartment syndrome in a patient with diabetes. *J Bone Joint Surg Br.* Sep 2004;86(7):1068–1070.
11. Mubarak SJ, Hargens AR. Acute compartment syndromes. *Surg Clin North Am.* Jun 1983;63(3):539–565.
12. Tiwari A, Haq AI, Myint F, Hamilton G. Acute compartment syndromes. *Br J Surg.* Apr 2002;89(4):397–412.
13. Bonnetblanc JM, Bedane C. Erysipelas: recognition and management. *Am J Clin Dermatol.* 2003;4(3):157–163.
14. Stephens MB. Gas gangrene: potential for hyperbaric oxygen therapy. *J Postgrad Med.* Apr 1996;99(4):217–220, 224.

15. Hanson JN, Ascher E, DePippo P, et al. Saphenous vein thrombophlebitis (SVT): a deceptively benign disease. *J Vasc Surg.* Apr 1998;27(4):677–680.

16. Lotz BP, Engel AG, Nishino H, Stevens JC, Litchy WJ. Inclusion body myositis. Observations in 40 patients. *Brain.* Jun 1989;112(Pt 3):727–747.

17. Joines JD, McNutt RA, Carey TS, Deyo RA, Rouhani R. Finding cancer in primary care outpatients with low back pain: a comparison of diagnostic strategies. *J Gen Intern Med.* 2001;16(1):14–23.

18. Holman PJ, Suki D, McCutcheon I, Wolinsky JP, Rhines LD, Gokaslan ZL. Surgical management of metastatic disease of the lumbar spine: experience with 139 patients. *J Neurosurg Spine.* 2005;2(5):550–563.

19. Kirkendall DT, Garrett WE Jr. Clinical perspectives regarding eccentric muscle injury. *Clin Orthop.* Oct 2002(403 suppl):S81–89.

20. Morganti CM, McFarland EG, Cosgarea AJ. Saphenous neuritis: a poorly understood cause of medial knee pain. *J Am Acad Orthop Surg.* Mar–Apr 2002;10(2):130–137.

21. Pyne D, Jawad AS, Padhiar N. Saphenous nerve injury after fasciotomy for compartment syndrome. *Br J Sports Med.* Dec 2003;37(6):541–542.

22. Lundborg G, Dahlin LB. Anatomy, function, and pathophysiology of peripheral nerves and nerve compression. *Hand Clin.* May 1996;12(2):185–193.

23. Crist BD, Lenke LG, Lewis S. Osteoid osteoma of the lumbar spine. A case report highlighting a novel reconstruction technique. *J Bone Joint Surg Am.* Feb 2005;87(2):414–418.

24. Lipman BT, Collier BD, Carrera GF, et al. Detection of osteomyelitis in the neuropathic foot: nuclear medicine, MRI and conventional radiography. *Clin Nucl Med.* Feb 1998;23(2):77–82.

25. Tamariz LJ, Eng J, Segal JB, et al. Usefulness of clinical prediction rules for the diagnosis of venous thromboembolism: a systematic review. *Am J Med.* Nov 1, 2004;117(9):676–684.

26. Wells PS, Hirsh J, Anderson DR, et al. Accuracy of clinical assessment of deep-vein thrombosis. *Lancet.* May 27, 1995;345(8961):1326–1330.

27. King RJ, Laugharne D, Kerslake RW, Holdsworth BJ. Primary obturator pyomyositis: a diagnostic challenge. *J Bone Joint Surg Br.* Aug 2003;85(6):895–898.

28. Slocum DB. The shin splint syndrome. Medical aspects and differential diagnosis. *Am J Surg.* Dec 1967;114(6):875–881.

29. Aoki Y, Yasuda K, Tohyama H, Ito H, Minami A. Magnetic resonance imaging in stress fractures and shin splints. *Clin Orthop.* Apr 2004(421):260–267.

30. Michael RH, Holder LE. The soleus syndrome. A cause of medial tibial stress (shin splints). *Am J Sports Med.* Mar–Apr 1985;13(2):87–94.

31. Beck BR, Osternig LR. Medial tibial stress syndrome. The location of muscles in the leg in relation to symptoms. *J Bone Joint Surg Am.* Jul 1994;76(7):1057–1061.

32. Sieggreen MY, Kline RA. Arterial insufficiency and ulceration: diagnosis and treatment options. *Nurse Pract.* Sep 2004;29(9):46–52.

33. Karlsson J, Lundin O, Lossing IW, Peterson L. Partial rupture of the patellar ligament. Results after operative treatment. *Am J Sports Med.* Jul–Aug 1991;19(4):403–408.

34. Thordarson DB, Schmotzer H, Chon J, Peters J. Dynamic support of the human longitudinal arch. A biomechanical evaluation. *Clin Orthop.* Jul 1995(316):165–172.

35. Mafi N, Lorentzon R, Alfredson H. Superior short-term results with eccentric calf muscle training compared to concentric training in a randomized prospective multicenter study on patients with chronic Achilles tendinosis. *Knee Surg Sports Traumatol Arthrosc.* 2001;9(1):42–47.

36. Kraushaar BS, Nirschl RP. Tendinosis of the elbow (tennis elbow). Clinical features and findings of histological, immunohistochemical, and electron microscopy studies. *J Bone Joint Surg Am.* Feb 1999;81(2):259–278.

37. Davenport TE, Kulig K, Matharu Y, Blanco CE. The EdUReP model for nonsurgical management of tendinopathy. Oct 2005;85(10):1093–1103.

CHAPTER 23

Ankle Pain

■ *Jason R. Cozby, PT, DPT, OCS* ■ *Lisa Meyer, PT, DPT, OCS*
■ *Stephen F. Reischl, PT, DPT, OCS*

Description of the Symptom

This chapter describes pathology that may lead to ankle pain, including generalized, lateral, medial, anterior, and posterior ankle pain. Local causes of ankle pain are defined as pathology occurring between the distal one-third of the tibia and the ankle joint, inclusive of musculoskeletal and neurovascular structures that cross the ankle joint. Remote causes are defined as occurring outside this area.

Special Concerns

■ Ankle symptoms associated with fever
■ Decreased sensation
■ Diminished popliteal, dorsalis pedis, or tibial arterial pulses
■ Inability to bear weight
■ Pain that increases at night and/or with rest
■ Skin breakdown
■ Warmth and swelling

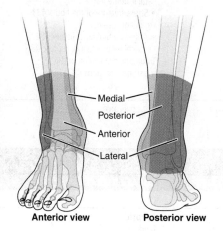

Anterior view   Posterior view

CHAPTER PREVIEW: Conditions That May Lead to Ankle Pain

T Trauma

REMOTE	LOCAL GENERALIZED	LOCAL LATERAL
COMMON		
Lumbar radiculopathies:	Fractures:	Anterolateral shin splints 427
• L4 radiculopathy 425	• Lateral malleolus 429	Fractures:
• L5 radiculopathy 425	• Medial malleolus 430	• Lateral malleolus 429
• S1 radiculopathy 426	Ligament sprains:	Ligament sprains:
	• Anterior talofibular	• Anterior talofibular ligament 432
	ligament 432	• Subtalar joint 434
	• Calcaneofibular ligament	Peroneal tendon tear or rupture 436
	(isolated) 433	Traumatic dislocation of the
	• Deltoid ligament 434	peroneal tendons 442
UNCOMMON		
Not applicable	Ankle dislocation 427	Fractures:
	Fractures:	• Lateral process of the talus 429
	• Anterior or posterior lip of the	• Lateral tubercle of the posterior
	tibial articular surface 429	process of the talus 430
	• Talus, neck or body 431	• Osteochondral fracture of the
		talar dome 430
		• Stress fracture of the fibula 431
		Ligament sprains:
		• Anterior tibiofibular ligament 432
		Peroneal tendon tear or rupture 436
		Traumatic dislocation of the
		peroneal tendons 442
RARE		
Not applicable	Ankle dislocation 427	Not applicable

I Inflammation

REMOTE	LOCAL GENERALIZED	LOCAL LATERAL
COMMON		
Not applicable	**Aseptic**	**Aseptic**
	Reiter's syndrome 437	Tendinitis:
	Rheumatoid arthritis 437	• Peroneal tendinitis 440
	Rubella and rubella	
	vaccine–associated	**Septic**
	arthritis 437	Not applicable
	Septic	
	Not applicable	

LOCAL MEDIAL	LOCAL ANTERIOR	LOCAL POSTERIOR
Fractures: • Medial malleolus 430 • Stress fracture of the tibia 431 Ligament sprains: • Deltoid ligament 434 Posteromedial shin splints 436 Tarsal tunnel syndrome 438	Anterior ankle impingement 427 Tibiofibular synostosis 441	Not applicable
Fractures: • Medial tuberosity of the posterior process of the talus 430 • Osteochondral fracture of the talar dome 430 • Sustentaculum tali 431	Fractures: • Anterior lip of the distal tibial articular surface 429 Ligament sprains: • Anterior tibiofibular ligament 432 • Cruciate crural ligament 434	Rupture of the Achilles tendon 438 Talar compression syndrome/impingement 438
Not applicable	Not applicable	Fractures: • Posterosuperior calcaneal tuberosity 430

LOCAL MEDIAL	LOCAL ANTERIOR	LOCAL POSTERIOR
Aseptic Tendinitis: • Tibialis posterior tendinitis 440 **Septic** Infectious periostitis 432	**Aseptic** Paratenonitis of extensor tendons of the foot and toes 436 **Septic** Not applicable	**Aseptic** Tendinitis: • Achilles tendinitis 439 **Septic** Not applicable

(continued)

Inflammation *(continued)*

REMOTE	LOCAL GENERALIZED	LOCAL LATERAL
UNCOMMON		
Not applicable	**Aseptic** Acute rheumatic fever 427 Arthritis associated with inflammatory bowel disease 427 Complex regional pain syndrome 428 Hepatitis B–associated arthritis 432 Reiter's syndrome 437 **Septic** Lyme arthritis 434 Septic arthritis 438	Not applicable
RARE		
Not applicable	**Aseptic** Rubella and rubella vaccine–associated arthritis 437 **Septic** Osteomyelitis 436	Not applicable

M Metabolic

REMOTE	LOCAL GENERALIZED	LOCAL LATERAL
COMMON		
Not applicable	Distal symmetric polyneuropathy, including from acquired immunodeficiency syndrome, alcohol/drug abuse, carcinoma, diabetes mellitus, and kidney failure 428 Gout 432	Not applicable
UNCOMMON		
Not applicable	Pseudogout 437	Distal symmetric polyneuropathy, including from acquired immunodeficiency syndrome, alcohol/drug abuse, carcinoma, diabetes mellitus, and kidney failure 428
RARE		
Not applicable	Transient migratory osteoporosis 442	Not applicable

LOCAL MEDIAL	LOCAL ANTERIOR	LOCAL POSTERIOR
Aseptic Tendinitis: • Flexor digitorum longus tendinitis 439 • Flexor hallucis longus tendinitis 440 • Tibialis anterior tendinitis 440 **Septic** Not applicable	**Aseptic** Tendinitis: • Extensor digitorum longus tendinitis 439 • Extensor hallucis longus tendinitis 439 **Septic** Not applicable	**Aseptic** Achilles paratenonitis 426 Bursitis: • Retrocalcaneal bursitis 428 • Subcutaneous Achilles bursitis 428 **Septic** Not applicable
Not applicable	Not applicable	Not applicable

LOCAL MEDIAL	LOCAL ANTERIOR	LOCAL POSTERIOR
Not applicable	Not applicable	Not applicable
Distal symmetric polyneuropathy, including from acquired immunodeficiency syndrome, alcohol/drug abuse, carcinoma, diabetes mellitus, and kidney failure 428	Distal symmetric polyneuropathy, including from acquired immunodeficiency syndrome, alcohol/drug abuse, carcinoma, diabetes mellitus, and kidney failure 428	Distal symmetric polyneuropathy, including from acquired immunodeficiency syndrome, alcohol/drug abuse, carcinoma, diabetes mellitus, and kidney failure 428
Not applicable	Not applicable	Not applicable

(continued)

Va Vascular

REMOTE	LOCAL GENERALIZED	LOCAL LATERAL
COMMON		
Not applicable	Not applicable	Not applicable
UNCOMMON		
Not applicable	Hemophilic arthropathy 432 Osteochondritis dissecans 435	Not applicable
RARE		
Not applicable	Acute hemarthrosis 426	Not applicable

De Degenerative

REMOTE	LOCAL GENERALIZED	LOCAL LATERAL
COMMON		
Not applicable	Osteoarthrosis/osteoarthritis of the ankle joint 435	Tendinosis: • Peroneal tendinosis 441
UNCOMMON		
Not applicable	Not applicable	Not applicable
RARE		
Not applicable	Not applicable	Not applicable

REMOTE	LOCAL GENERALIZED	LOCAL LATERAL
COMMON		
Not applicable	Not applicable	Not applicable
UNCOMMON		
Not applicable	*Malignant Primary:* Not applicable *Malignant Metastatic:* Not applicable *Benign, such as:* • Dysplasia epiphysealis hemimelica (Trevor's disease) 429 • Osteoid osteoma 435	Not applicable
RARE		

Not applicable	*Malignant Primary, such as:*
	• Osteosarcoma 436
	Malignant Metastatic, such as:
	• Metastases to the ankle,
	  including from primary breast,
	  kidney, lung, prostate, and
	  thyroid disease 434
	• Multiple myeloma 435
	Benign:
	Not applicable
		Not applicable

LOCAL MEDIAL	LOCAL ANTERIOR	LOCAL POSTERIOR
Not applicable	Not applicable	Not applicable
Not applicable	Not applicable	Not applicable
Not applicable	Not applicable	Not applicable

LOCAL MEDIAL	LOCAL ANTERIOR	LOCAL POSTERIOR
Tendinosis: • Tibialis posterior tendinosis 441	Tendinitis: • Tibialis anterior tendinitis 440	Tendinosis: • Achilles tendinosis 440
Not applicable	Not applicable	Not applicable
Not applicable	Not applicable	Not applicable

LOCAL MEDIAL	LOCAL ANTERIOR	LOCAL POSTERIOR
Not applicable	Not applicable	Not applicable
Not applicable	Not applicable	Not applicable
Not applicable	Not applicable	Not applicable

(continued)

Co Congenital

REMOTE	LOCAL GENERALIZED	LOCAL LATERAL
COMMON		
Not applicable	Not applicable	Not applicable
UNCOMMON		
Not applicable	Not applicable	Not applicable
RARE		
Not applicable	Not applicable	Not applicable

Ne Neurogenic/Psychogenic

REMOTE	LOCAL GENERALIZED	LOCAL LATERAL
COMMON		
Not applicable	Not applicable	Not applicable
UNCOMMON		
Fear and avoidance 424	Not applicable	Ganglion cyst 431
RARE		
Psychological effect of complex regional pain syndrome 426	Not applicable	Not applicable

Note: These are estimates of relative incidence because few data are available for the less common conditions.

Overview of Ankle Pain

Pain that is experienced in the ankle region is often due to injury or mechanical disorders affecting the underlying structures, especially because the ankle experiences very high forces from the ground reaction forces, forces originating from functional activities, and forces that arise during attempts to control body weight and momentum. However, pain also may be associated with vascular compromise, a proximal nerve compression, or systemic disease. The lower leg, ankle, and foot are end target sites for multiple disease processes, so all potential diagnoses should be considered even if mechanical trauma is associated with the presentation.

Description of Conditions That May Lead to Ankle Pain

Remote

■ Fear and Avoidance

Chief Clinical Characteristics
This presentation may include avoiding the use of an extremity as a result of apprehension of onset of pain.

Background Information
Injury to the foot and ankle may contribute to the disuse of the lower extremity even with minimal injury. Fear of reinjury, pain, or other factors will need to be explored. In all cases the basis of pathology must be thoroughly explored before this presentation

LOCAL MEDIAL	LOCAL ANTERIOR	LOCAL POSTERIOR
Not applicable	Not applicable	Not applicable
Not applicable	Not applicable	Not applicable
Not applicable	Not applicable	Not applicable

LOCAL MEDIAL	LOCAL ANTERIOR	LOCAL POSTERIOR
Not applicable	Not applicable	Not applicable
Not applicable	Not applicable	Not applicable
Not applicable	Not applicable	Not applicable

is to be considered. If this condition is present, a team approach ensures optimal treatment.

LUMBAR RADICULOPATHIES

■ L4 Radiculopathy

Chief Clinical Characteristics
This presentation can be characterized by pain in the lumbar spine and paresthesias radiating from the anterior aspect of the hip, thigh, and knee, sometimes extending anteromedially from the knee to the foot. Depending on the severity, the presentation may also include a decreased or absent patellar tendon reflex and motor loss in the muscles innervated by the L4 nerve. Prone knee bend may reproduce symptoms.

Background Information
A lumbar disk herniation is the most common cause for this condition. The diagnosis is confirmed with magnetic resonance imaging. Surgical intervention may be indicated in severe cases of lower extremity pain accompanied by neurological signs.

■ L5 Radiculopathy

Chief Clinical Characteristics
This presentation includes pain in the lumbar spine and paresthesias radiating from the lateral aspect of the hip and buttock to the lateral aspect of the knee, extending anterolaterally down to the foot. Depending on the severity, the presentation may also include motor loss in the muscles innervated by the L5 nerve root.

Background Information

A lumbar disk herniation is the most common cause for this condition. The diagnosis is confirmed with magnetic resonance imaging. Surgical intervention may be indicated in severe cases of lower extremity pain accompanied by neurological signs.

■ S1 Radiculopathy

Chief Clinical Characteristics

This presentation typically includes pain in the lumbar spine and paresthesias radiating from the buttock to the posterior aspect of the knee and extending posterolaterally from the knee to the foot. Depending on the severity, the presentation may also include a decreased or absent Achilles tendon reflex and motor loss in the muscles innervated by the S1 nerve.

Background Information

A lumbar disk herniation is a common cause for this condition. The diagnosis is confirmed with magnetic resonance imaging. Surgical intervention may be indicated in severe cases of lower extremity pain accompanied by neurological signs.

■ Psychological Effect of Complex Regional Pain Syndrome

Chief Clinical Characteristics

This presentation typically includes a traumatic onset of severe chronic ankle and foot pain accompanied by allodynia, hyperalgesia, and trophic, vasomotor, and sudomotor changes in later stages. This condition is characterized by disproportionate responses to painful stimuli.

Background Information

This regional neuropathic pain disorder presents either without direct nerve trauma (Type I) or with direct nerve trauma (Type II) in any region of the body.[1] This condition may precipitate due to an event distant to the affected area. Thermography may confirm associated sympathetic dysfunction. This condition has been shown to have a psychological component and may be influenced by cortical mechanisms.[2] Treatment may include physical therapy interventions to improve patient/client functioning, biofeedback, analgesic or anti-inflammatory medication, transcutaneous or

spinal electrical nerve stimulation, and surgical or pharmacologic sympathectomy. However, a team approach ensures optimal treatment for individuals with this condition.

Local

■ Achilles Paratenonitis

Chief Clinical Characteristics

This presentation involves diffuse pain, tenderness, and thickening and swelling along the Achilles tendon, especially 2 to 6 cm from the calcaneal insertion. However, the painful palpable thickening does not move with dorsiflexion or plantarflexion because the tendon moves with this action but the paratenon does not. Pain is greatest in the mornings or at the start of a physical activity, but the pain will often decrease with continued walking or activity as the tendon begins to move more freely inside the paratenon.

Background Information

The paratenon is usually the site of inflammatory injury related to overuse, but it may also be damaged from direct traumatic pressure. The diagnosis is determined clinically, but magnetic resonance or ultrasound imaging may be necessary for confirmation if the clinical diagnosis is unclear. Treatment includes rest, inflammation control, improving flexibility of the calf muscle group, and improving strength of the antipronator muscle groups.

■ Acute Hemarthrosis

Chief Clinical Characteristics

This presentation typically includes pain, swelling, tenderness to palpation, decreased range of motion with a possible soft end feel, difficulty bearing weight, and pain with squatting. Individuals with hemophilia are more at risk to develop a hemarthrosis.[3]

Background Information

This condition is rare in the ankle; however, injury to the joint capsule can lead to a hemarthrosis. The presence of blood in aspirated synovial fluid aspirated from affected joints confirms the diagnosis. Complications include risks associated with acute bleeding, as well as the arthropathy that may result from chronic bleeding.[4] The patient should seek medical attention to treat the acute bleeding and prevent arthropathy.[4]

■ Acute Rheumatic Fever

Chief Clinical Characteristics

This presentation may involve warm, red, swollen, and tender joints with systemic signs of infection including fever, abdominal pain, anorexia, lethargy, malaise, and fatigue. Rheumatic fever usually has five major manifestations that include migratory polyarthritis, carditis, chorea, subcutaneous nodules, and erythema marginatum (flat to slightly indurated lesions on the skin of the extensor surfaces of the extremities or trunk).

Background Information

This condition is an acute inflammation as a result of group A streptococcal infection.[5] The pain is usually the result of an aseptic inflammation of the joints. Diagnosis is made with confirmation of a group A streptococcal infection in association with two of the five major manifestations. Monoarthritis and low-grade fever are important considerations to avoid underdiagnosis.[5] Usual treatment consists of antibiotic, anti-inflammatory, and antipyretic medications.

■ Ankle Dislocation

Chief Clinical Characteristics

This presentation can involve severe pain with gross deformity, usually with an inability to weight bear through the involved extremity.

Background Information

Trauma is usually severe and directed to the tibia on a fixed foot. Most cases result in either complete rupture of the ankle ligaments, fracture of the ankle, or various combinations of the two. Standard radiographs of the ankle usually visualize these fractures and confirm the diagnosis of the dislocation. Treatment consists of surgical reduction and stabilization. Acute dislocations are a medical emergency secondary to potential compromise of neurovascular structures.

■ Anterior Ankle Impingement

Chief Clinical Characteristics

This presentation includes pain at the anterior ankle during dorsiflexion activities. The ankle may be tender to palpation if osteophytes are present on the talus or tibia.

Background Information

The impingement is caused by compression of osseous or soft tissue structures, possibly including a meniscoid lesion of organized scar tissue that may be present due to thickening of the anterior capsule after multiple sprains and decreased talar gliding. Usual treatment is nonsurgical with possible arthroscopic debridement in cases of recalcitrant symptoms and disability.

■ Anterolateral Shin Splints

Chief Clinical Characteristics

This presentation may involve pain and palpable tenderness along the involved anterior tibial muscles immediately adjacent to the tibia. The pain usually lessens following warm-up exercises of the involved muscles, but is often present during activity with soreness following the activity. Pain usually is absent at night.

Background Information

Shin splints are the result of eccentric overuse, leading to an inflammatory musculotendinous injury along the lateral aspect of the tibia, with potential muscular avulsion from the tibia.[6] Diagnosis is usually based on the clinical presentation. Imaging is usually unhelpful, although fat-suppressed magnetic resonance imaging may allow differentiation between stress fractures and shin splints.[7] Usual treatment is nonsurgical.

■ Arthritis Associated with Inflammatory Bowel Disease

Chief Clinical Characteristics

This presentation typically includes migratory polyarthritic pain with abdominal pain, diarrhea, abdominal cramping, and other gastrointestinal symptoms. Commonly affected joints include the metatarsophalangeal joints, ankle, knee, elbow, wrist, and hand. Other extraintestinal manifestations include episcleritis, ankylosing spondylitis, sacroiliitis, anterior uveitis, aphthous stomatitis, erythema nodosum, pyoderma gangrenosum, or growth and development retardation.

Background Information

One-third of patients with inflammatory bowel disease have at least one musculoskeletal

ANKLE PAIN

manifestation, and in children the extraintestinal manifestations may dominate.[8] Colonoscopy with mucosal biopsy confirms the diagnosis. Treatment typically involves aminosalicylates, corticosteroids, anti–tumor necrosis factor medications, diet changes, and surgical resection of the involved portion of bowel.

BURSITIS

■ Retrocalcaneal Bursitis

Chief Clinical Characteristics
This presentation can involve pain, palpable warmth, tenderness to palpation, and some swelling at the medial and lateral aspects of the Achilles tendon. Pain is reproduced with firm palpation of the tissue anterior to the tendon, as well as with dorsiflexion of the ankle.

Background Information
This condition is the result of inflammation within the bursa that lies between the Achilles tendon and the calcaneus. Predisposing factors include trauma, systemic disease, and biomechanical or structural factors such as prominent posterosuperior calcaneal tuberosity (Haglund's deformity) and rearfoot varus. Clinical examination confirms the diagnosis. Treatment is nonsurgical, and typically involves footwear modification.

■ Subcutaneous Achilles Bursitis

Chief Clinical Characteristics
This presentation includes local pain, tenderness to palpation, and swelling just posterior to the Achilles tendon insertion at the calcaneal tuberosity. Palpable warmth and observable redness may be present in the same area.

Background Information
Subcutaneous Achilles bursitis is a result of inflammation and swelling of the bursa between the Achilles tendon and the skin. This may occur from mechanical trauma to the tendon or it may be associated with insertional Achilles tendinopathy (tendinitis/tendinosis) or retrocalcaneal bursitis. Continued irritation of the inflamed and swollen bursa may lead to thickening of the bursal walls and fibrosis. Clinical examination confirms the diagnosis.

Treatment is nonsurgical, and typically involves footwear modification.

■ Complex Regional Pain Syndrome

Chief Clinical Characteristics
This presentation may include a traumatic onset of severe chronic ankle and foot pain accompanied by allodynia, hyperalgesia, and trophic, vasomotor, and sudomotor changes in later stages. This condition is characterized by disproportionate responses to painful stimuli.

Background Information
This regional neuropathic pain disorder presents either without direct nerve trauma (Type I) or with nerve trauma (Type II) in any region of the body.[1] This condition may precipitate due to an event distant to the affected area. Thermography may confirm associated sympathetic dysfunction. Treatment may include physical therapy interventions to improve patient and client functioning, biofeedback, analgesic or anti-inflammatory medication, transcutaneous or spinal electrical nerve stimulation, and surgical or pharmacologic sympathectomy.

■ Distal Symmetric Polyneuropathy, Including From Acquired Immunodeficiency Syndrome, Alcohol/Drug Abuse, Carcinoma, Diabetes Mellitus, and Kidney Failure

Chief Clinical Characteristics
This presentation may be characterized by decreased distal deep tendon reflexes, as well as pain, dysesthesia, or paresthesia in the feet and toes.

Background Information
Peripheral neuropathy is one of the more common complications in patients presenting with acquired immunodeficiency syndrome, diabetes, renal failure, hypothyroidism, toxins, malignancy, and malnutrition. It is characterized by retrograde axonal degeneration, so this condition commonly progresses from distal to proximal. Electromyographic studies and biopsy confirm the diagnosis. Vibration and light touch sensation (10-g Semmes Weinstein monofilament) tests are useful to assess protective sensation. Curative treatment of this

condition remains controversial, so the focus of intervention typically includes patient education to maintain blood glucose control and care for the insensate regions to prevent progression and complications secondary to this condition.

■ Dysplasia Epiphysealis Hemimelica (Trevor's Disease)

Chief Clinical Characteristics
This presentation can include a limp that may be accompanied by joint swelling, restricted joint movement, or muscle wasting. Males are more likely to be affected than females.

Background Information
This condition is a congenital bone development disorder that is the result of an intra-articular osteochondromatosis (localized overgrowth of the cartilage) that is present in the epiphyses of the joint. This affects both sides of the epiphyses and joint deformity is often the result. This condition is most common at the medial ankle, but it also may be seen in the femur, the wrist, or the foot. Radiographs often reveal the structural changes to the joint. Treatment usually consists of surgical excision of the mass, as well as correction of any angular deformity that may have resulted. Nonsurgical intervention includes immobilization.

FRACTURES

■ Anterior Lip of the Distal Tibial Articular Surface

Chief Clinical Characteristics
This presentation typically includes limited weight bearing on the affected leg as well as pain, tenderness, and swelling around the location of the fracture.

Background Information
These fractures usually do not traverse into the articular cartilage of the talocrural joint, but may be associated with ligamentous injuries. The fracture to the anterior lip of the tibia more often occurs with an injury with the foot pronated and the ankle in dorsiflexion. Standard radiograph views of the ankle confirm the diagnosis. Surgery may be required if the fracture is unstable.

■ Anterior or Posterior Lip of the Tibial Articular Surface

Chief Clinical Characteristics
This presentation may involve limited weight bearing on the affected leg as well as pain, tenderness, and swelling around the location of the fracture.

Background Information
These fractures usually do not traverse into the articular cartilage of the talocrural joint, but may be associated with ligamentous injuries. The fracture to the anterior lip of the tibia more often occurs with an injury with the foot pronated and the ankle in dorsiflexion. The fracture to the posterior lip of the tibia may occur with the foot and ankle in various positions; however, it is more commonly associated with talar eversion and posterior displacement. Standard radiograph views of the ankle confirm the diagnosis. If the fracture is unstable, surgical fixation may be necessary.

■ Lateral Malleolus

Chief Clinical Characteristics
This presentation can include significant pain at the lateral malleolus, swelling, and possible ecchymosis with pain increasing with inversion, eversion, plantarflexion, and dorsiflexion motions.

Background Information
The fracture usually results during a forceful inversion sprain of the lateral ligaments, but may also occur during eversion sprains, direct trauma, or torsional injuries. Associated injuries include medial malleolar lesions, ligamentous injury, talar dome and body lesions, or peroneal tendon injury. Diagnosis may be made clinically, assisted by the Ottawa ankle rules, and radiographs are necessary for confirmation of a fracture.[9] Surgery is indicated for displaced fractures; nondisplaced fractures typically are treated with immobilization.

■ Lateral Process of the Talus

Chief Clinical Characteristics
This presentation may be characterized by pain, swelling, and tenderness along the anterior and inferior lateral ankle located

ANKLE PAIN

directly over the lateral process of the talus. Pain increases with weight bearing, talocrural plantarflexion and dorsiflexion, and subtalar joint movement. The mechanism of injury is usually a dorsiflexion and inversion motion common in motor vehicle accidents, direct trauma, or snowboarding accidents.

Background Information
Chronic pain may be indicative of avascular necrosis. Bone scans, computed tomography, and magnetic resonance imaging often assist in the diagnosis, staging, and prognosis of the injury. Surgical treatment is indicated for large or displaced fractures; otherwise, nonsurgical treatment is indicated.[10]

■ Lateral Tubercle of the Posterior Process of the Talus

Chief Clinical Characteristics
This presentation can involve posterolateral ankle pain, swelling, and tenderness over the lateral tubercle. Pain increases while walking downhill or downstairs, as well as with ankle and subtalar movement, active first toe flexion, or forced first toe dorsiflexion.

Background Information
This condition results from talocalcaneal ligament avulsion, posterior talofibular ligament avulsion, or a compressive force. It is associated with lateral ankle sprains, lateral malleolus avulsion fractures, and osteochondral defects on the talar dome. Clinical examination findings and radiographs confirm the diagnosis.[10] Surgical treatment is necessary for nonunion or displaced fractures.[10]

■ Medial Malleolus

Chief Clinical Characteristics
This presentation typically involves local pain, swelling, and point tenderness present over the fracture site. Pain is most severe within the first 24 hours of the injury. The fracture usually is the result of an abduction or external rotation force on a pronated foot, but also can result from a high-force inversion sprain that may lead to a compression fracture.

Background Information
Associated findings may include a deltoid ligament rupture, syndesmosis tear, lateral ankle sprain, lateral malleolus fracture, or subtalar dislocation. Diagnosis is confirmed with the clinical examination, and the fracture can be confirmed with plain radiographs. Surgical treatment is necessary for nonunion or displaced fractures.

■ Medial Tuberosity of the Posterior Process of the Talus

Chief Clinical Characteristics
This presentation typically includes ankle pain that is posterior to the medial malleolus and anterior to the Achilles tendon. The injury often results from dorsiflexion-pronation ankle injuries, ankle dislocation, or possibly an avulsion fracture from a posterior tibiotalar injury.

Background Information
Bone scan, computed tomography scan, or magnetic resonance imaging may assist in the diagnosis, staging, and prognosis. In the event of unstable fractures or nonunion, surgical fixation may be necessary.

■ Osteochondral Fracture of the Talar Dome

Chief Clinical Characteristics
This presentation includes variable symptoms based on the site of the osteochondral lesion. Lateral dome lesions commonly present with localized pain at the central and lateral ankle anterior to the lateral malleolus. Medial dome lesions present with tenderness posterior to the medial malleolus and at the posterior talus.

Background Information
Osteochondral defects may loosen and cause joint pain, locking, and swelling. Lateral dome injuries are frequently associated with trauma, usually the result of an inversion-dorsiflexion mechanism. Medial dome injuries may either be the result of inversion-plantarflexion trauma or present insidiously. Radiographs, magnetic resonance imaging, and arthroscopy confirm the diagnosis. Patients should be monitored because joint degeneration is common following these injuries.[11]

■ Posterosuperior Calcaneal Tuberosity

Chief Clinical Characteristics
This presentation can include pain, swelling, and possible ecchymosis located at the calcaneal insertion of the Achilles tendon, the

posterior heel, and the posterior ankle. The patient will often have a functional loss of plantarflexion, such as with a single-leg heel raise, due to the avulsion fracture. This condition is most common in older individuals with advanced age, diabetes mellitus, or osteoporosis.

Background Information

The mechanism of injury is a rapid pull of the Achilles tendon. A positive Thompson test and a palpable sulcus may be present if the tendon is avulsed. Associated findings may include an Achilles tendon tear or other extra-articular calcaneal fractures. Plain radiographs confirm the diagnosis. Surgical fixation under traction may be necessary for displaced fractures.

■ **Stress Fracture of the Fibula**

Chief Clinical Characteristics

This presentation may involve focused, localized, superficial aching or sharp pain directly at the site of the fracture (usually within 15 cm [6 in.] of the distal fibula). Pain is worse with prolonged standing and weight-bearing activities that require dorsiflexion and rotation. Pain is rarely present at rest unless the fracture is severe.

Background Information

This condition occurs as a result of abnormal loading from a sudden increase in or change in training, improper footwear, or ankle and foot dysfunction that may lead to excessive loading of the fibula. Clinical presentation and bone scan confirm the diagnosis. This condition typically is treated with relative rest, including general conditioning in an environment that is characterized by low-impact training.

■ **Stress Fracture of the Tibia**

Chief Clinical Characteristics

This presentation can be characterized by pain and palpable tenderness over the posteromedial border of the tibia, more commonly at the middle to proximal one-third of the tibia. Pain also may be present at the distal tibia, leading to ankle pain. Pain usually is aggravated with weight bearing and running and alleviated with rest in a non–weight-bearing position.

Background Information

This condition occurs in runners and is associated with an increase in training. A clinical examination and bone scan confirm the diagnosis. This condition typically is treated with relative rest, including general conditioning in an environment that is characterized by low-impact training.

■ **Sustentaculum Tali**

Chief Clinical Characteristics

This presentation may involve pain, swelling, and tenderness over the medial heel and ankle, inferior to the medial malleolus. Pain is increased with passive rearfoot inversion and passive hyperextension of the first phalanx.

Background Information

This fracture may result from a fall onto the heel with an inverted foot, but it is uncommon to have this condition as an isolated injury. Plain radiographs confirm the diagnosis. Complications may include nonunion, nerve irritation, and toe flexor injury. Surgery is indicated if the fracture is unstable.

■ **Talus, Neck or Body**

Chief Clinical Characteristics

This presentation includes pain, swelling, and tenderness at the sinus tarsi or just distal to the lateral malleolus, following extreme compression or shear loading of the foot. Pain usually is present with active or passive subtalar motion. This injury is commonly associated with spasm of the peroneal muscles, resulting in palpable tenderness. A valgus deformity of the hindfoot may be present.

Background Information

The diagnosis is confirmed with imaging that may include plain radiographs, magnetic resonance imaging, and bone scan. This condition includes fractures of the talar neck and body, as well as osteochondral lesions of the trochlear surface that often require surgical treatment.[12]

■ **Ganglion Cyst**

Chief Clinical Characteristics

This presentation often involves the presence of a mildly painful or painless cystic lesion over the posterior, inferolateral aspect of the ankle usually detected following an inversion ankle sprain. *Rest will sometimes decrease the pressure and alleviate some of the pain.*

Background Information

Cysts are often tender to palpation; they may arise from a joint or tendon sheath, increasing in size and pressure during ambulation as the associated motion increases the pressure. Clinical examination confirms the diagnosis. If the pain causes dysfunction or is recalcitrant, then aspiration and steroid treatment may help. If nonsurgical treatment is unsuccessful, surgical excision of the ganglion is required. Recurrence is possible if excision is incomplete.

■ Gout

Chief Clinical Characteristics

This presentation includes severe pain, edema, warmth, erythema, and very localized tenderness. Systemic findings may include fever, chills, malaise, and sweating. The areas typically involved are the first metatarsophalangeal joint, the talocrural joint, the calcaneal region, and the tarsals of the instep. Pain is usually provoked by hard movements, or may follow alcohol abuse, dehydration, trauma, surgery, septic arthritis, protein fasting, excessive purine ingestion, and allopurinol or uricosuric agents.

Background Information

Sustained hyperuricemia levels lead to deposition of monosodium urate crystals in and around the tendons and joints. Men are eight times more likely to be affected than women.[13] Needle aspiration is required to confirm the diagnosis. Treatment commonly involves a combination of anti-inflammatory medication and colchicine in individuals with normal liver function. Preventive treatment should be undertaken to control uric acid levels by way of diet and medication in individuals with chronic gout.

■ Hemophilic Arthropathy

Chief Clinical Characteristics

This presentation can involve a painful, swollen, and tender joint culminating in range-of-motion limitation and difficulty bearing weight through the affected limb.

Background Information

Recurrent hemarthroses lead to inflammation of the joint and result in joint degeneration.[3] This condition commonly affects the knees, elbows, and ankles. The diagnosis is confirmed by the presence of blood in aspirated synovial fluid from affected joints and joint deterioration apparent on plain radiographs. Immediate medical treatment of acute hemarthrosis is necessary to minimize the extent of arthropathy. This may include immobilization of the affected joint and systemic infusion of the deficient blood factor.

■ Hepatitis B–Associated Arthritis

Chief Clinical Characteristics

This presentation typically includes a symmetrical polyarthralgia that can affect the toes and, more commonly, the fingers. The common symptoms include anorexia, malaise, nausea, vomiting, and fever. Jaundice usually develops in approximately 1 to 2 weeks.

Background Information

Hepatitis is an inflammation of the liver as a result of viral infection with necrosis of the liver. The arthralgia is usually the result of an aseptic inflammation of the joints. Blood tests confirm the diagnosis.

■ Infectious Periostitis

Chief Clinical Characteristics

This presentation may be characterized by aching to severe pain with tenderness and edema of the infected bone. Suppuration may be present and an individual with this condition will often experience systemic signs of infection, such as fever, chills, and fatigue.

Background Information

This condition involves a chronic infection of the periosteum from a hematogenous source or trauma to the affected region. Not all cases of periostitis are the result of an infection; therefore, the diagnosis is confirmed by radiographic imaging revealing necrosis of the affected bone and bone scan revealing increased uptake. This condition is usually managed with antibiotic medication appropriately directed to the infective agent.

LIGAMENT SPRAINS

■ Anterior Talofibular Ligament

Chief Clinical Characteristics

This presentation can include pain, swelling, tenderness to palpation, and possible ecchymosis just anterior and inferior to the lateral malleolus, directly over the ligament (Fig. 23-1). Weight bearing and combined inversion/plantarflexion motions of the foot will be painful and may be limited by pain. If the ligament is completely torn, then pain may or may not be present with excessive inversion.

Background Information

Injury to the ligament is usually caused by an inversion and plantarflexion mechanism to the ankle. Associated injuries may include calcaneofibular ligament sprain, syndesmotic ligament sprain, sinus tarsi syndrome with a subtalar sprain, superficial peroneal nerve injury, fifth metatarsal fracture, medial ankle impingement, a medial or lateral malleolar fracture, talar or osteochondral fractures, or peroneal tendon injury. Diagnosis is usually based on the clinical presentation,

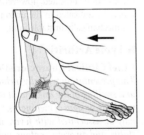

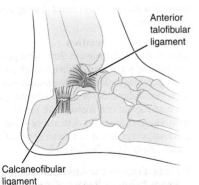

Anterior
talofibular
ligament

Calcaneofibular
ligament

FIGURE 23-1 Lateral ankle sprain, including tear of the anterior talofibular ligament, calcaneofibular ligament, and posterior talofibular ligament. The anterior drawer test (*inset*) is one method used to grade lateral ankle sprains.

mechanism of injury, and a positive anterior translation test of the talus. If pain or instability persists, then radiographs are helpful to rule out fractures, osteochondral defects, or structural instability with stress. Nonsurgical intervention is commonly indicated; however, surgical stabilization may be indicated in the event of a mechanically unstable joint.

■ Anterior Tibiofibular Ligament

Chief Clinical Characteristics

This presentation may involve tenderness and pain at the superomedial aspect of the lateral malleolus and the anterior aspect of the syndesmosis. Pain is present with weight bearing, forced dorsiflexion of the ankle, and extreme eversion or external rotation of the ankle, and is often reproduced with the squeeze test or external rotation of the foot while the knee is flexed to 90 degrees.[14,15]

Background Information

This injury (commonly referred to as a high ankle sprain) usually occurs with abduction or abduction-external rotation injuries directly to the foot and ankle, or with forced internal rotation of the body over a planted foot. Associated injuries include lateral ankle ligament sprains, interosseous membrane injury, deltoid ligament rupture, fibular fracture, bone bruising or osteochondral defects, and avascular necrosis. Diagnosis is based on patient presentation, mechanism of injury, and external rotation stress radiographs. Nonsurgical intervention is commonly indicated; however, surgical stabilization may be indicated in the event of a mechanically unstable joint.

■ Calcaneofibular Ligament (Isolated)

Chief Clinical Characteristics

This presentation can be characterized by swelling and tenderness along the lateral ankle, inferior to the lateral malleolus, along the ligament (see Fig. 23-1). Pain increases with foot inversion.

Background Information

Injury to the ligament occurs during an inversion mechanism of the ankle, with the ankle in neutral or even sometimes dorsiflexion.

This injury rarely occurs independently, and is commonly associated with anterior talofibular ligament sprains, lateral malleolus fractures, and syndesmotic injuries. Diagnosis is based on the clinical presentation, and the use of radiographs may be useful to rule out any additional injuries or complications. Nonsurgical intervention is commonly indicated; however, surgical stabilization may be indicated in the event of a mechanically unstable joint.

■ Cruciate Crural Ligament

Chief Clinical Characteristics

This presentation may include pain and tenderness to palpation along the ligament on the dorsum of the ankle and foot. Pain is intensified with plantarflexion of the toes, but is present even at rest. Paresthesias or weakness may be present if the injury causes increased intracompartmental pressure.

Background Information

Injury to this ligament may be due to either direct or indirect trauma. Complications may include injury to the blood vessels or nerves on the surface of the foot. Palpation for pedal pulses, neurological examination, and possibly a Doppler should be used to determine the extent of the injury to the nerves or vasculature. Treatment will often consist of rest to allow for healing, provided that nerve and vascular injuries are absent.

■ Deltoid Ligament

Chief Clinical Characteristics

This presentation involves medial ankle pain, swelling, ecchymosis, tenderness along the ligaments, pain with weight bearing, and pain with eversion of the ankle.

Background Information

Injury results from an abduction and/or external rotation force on the ankle with severe eversion of the calcaneus, or when the body moves over a fixed foot. The injury can occur independently or may be associated with lateral malleolus fractures, fracture of the anterior distal tip of the tibial articular surface, or distal tibiofibular syndesmosis injuries. Diagnosis is made based on the clinical presentation and magnetic resonance imaging. Nonsurgical intervention is

commonly indicated; however, surgical stabilization may be indicated in the event of a mechanically unstable joint.

■ Subtalar Joint

Chief Clinical Characteristics

This presentation often includes pain at the lateral ankle with tenderness in the sinus tarsi and pain aggravated with excessive inversion or subtalar motion.

Background Information

This condition may be associated with an inversion ankle injury followed by persistent difficulty with walking on uneven surfaces. The injury also may be associated with grade II calcaneofibular ligament injuries occurring in a neutral or plantarflexed position, and synovitis of the subtalar joint if excessive motion occurs. If the clinical examination is not definitive, then magnetic resonance imaging may be necessary. Nonsurgical intervention is commonly indicated; however, surgical fusion may be indicated in the uncommon event of a mechanically unstable joint.

■ Lyme Arthritis

Chief Clinical Characteristics

This presentation typically includes arthralgia and swelling of the ankle joint or other joints, myalgias, or signs of meningitis. Symptoms also may be associated with fever, altered mental status, and an erythematous and pruritic skin lesion that demonstrates central clearing and satellite rings.

Background Information

This condition results when the *Borrelia burgdorferi* infection is transferred through a tick bite. Serologic testing confirms the diagnosis. In most cases, this condition can be treated with prompt administration of oral antibiotics or parenteral agent. However, musculoskeletal and neurological consequences appear in a minority of individuals despite the medication used.

■ Metastases to the Ankle, Including From Primary Breast, Kidney, Lung, Prostate, and Thyroid Disease

Chief Clinical Characteristics

This presentation typically includes unremitting pain in individuals with these risk factors: previous history of cancer, age 50 years or older, failure to improve with conservative therapy, and unexplained weight change of more than 10 pounds in 6 months.[16]

Background Information

The skeletal system is the third most common site of metastatic disease.[17] Symptoms also may be related to pathological fracture in affected sites. Common primary sites causing metastases to bone include breast, prostate, lung, and kidney. Bone scan confirms the diagnosis. Common treatments for metastases include surgical resection, chemotherapy, radiation treatment, and palliation, depending on the tumor type and extent of metastasis.

■ Multiple Myeloma

Chief Clinical Characteristics

This presentation involves unexplained skeletal pain in the feet, lower legs, arms, hands, back, and thorax. This may be associated with renal failure, recurrent bacterial infections, pathological fractures, and anemia.

Background Information

This condition is an insidious plasma cell cancer that originates in the bone marrow and can affect multiple areas with multiple lytic and osteosclerotic effects. Pain results from either neuropathic or bone pain. Radiographically, the bones will have lesions of a punched-out appearance with generalized osteoporosis. Diagnosis may be confirmed with blood tests, urinalysis, serum protein electrophoresis, bone scan, magnetic resonance imaging, and bone marrow aspiration and biopsy. Depending on the aggressiveness of this condition, treatment may range from "watchful waiting" to chemotherapy and bone marrow transplantation.

■ Osteoarthrosis/Osteoarthritis of the Ankle Joint

Chief Clinical Characteristics

This presentation includes pain with localized tenderness at the involved joint, range-of-motion limitations, a hard end feel, and crepitus, depending on the extent of the joint damage. Onset of pain is usually gradual, symptoms are worsened by exercise and weight-bearing activities, and patients usually report increased pain and stiffness in the morning and following prolonged static postures.

Background Information

The etiology of osteoarthritis is either idiopathic or secondary to conditions that affect the intra-articular environment (such as infection, inflammation, genetic defects, instability, or trauma). The clinical presentation will lead to a preliminary diagnosis with radiographs confirming the diagnosis and revealing the extent of joint damage. Treatment for this condition ranges from nonsurgical options, such as physical therapy intervention and intra-articular corticosteroid injections, to total joint arthroplasty.

■ Osteochondritis Dissecans

Chief Clinical Characteristics

This presentation involves pain, swelling, and tenderness at the sinus tarsi, just distal to the lateral malleolus or around the peroneal tendons as a result of muscle spasm. Symptoms increase with subtalar motion and a valgus deformity of the hindfoot may be present.

Background Information

This condition, also called osteochondral lesion of the talus, occurs on both the medial and lateral trochlea and has been linked to injuries related to movement of the talus inside the mortise of the ankle following ligamentous disruption. The medial lesions are seen most often in bilateral lower extremities, indicating some genetic or predisposition to these injuries. This condition can occur secondary to abnormal blood flow, resulting in a poor prognosis.[18] Bone scan, computed tomography, and magnetic resonance imaging assist in the diagnosis, staging, and prognosis of this pathology. This condition is often staged based on magnetic resonance imaging findings. Four stages are used to describe the extent of articular damage as well as the stability of the joint. Intervention may include immobilization during early-stage disease or arthroscopic debridement and drilling for advanced lesions.

■ Osteoid Osteoma

Chief Clinical Characteristics

This presentation typically includes focal bone pain at the site of the tumor that is associated with tenderness and warmth to palpation, with a significant increase in pain with activity and at night, and with substantial and immediate relief of pain with use of anti-inflammatory medication. This condition is more common in males than females, and it rarely presents in people younger than 5 or older than 40 years of age.

Background Information

The pathology of this condition includes abnormal production of osteoid and primitive bone. The proximal femur is the most common site for this tumor. Pain associated with this condition is self-limiting and may resolve spontaneously over the course of 2 to 4 years.[19] Relief also may be obtained by surgical removal of the tumor.

■ Osteomyelitis

Chief Clinical Characteristics

This presentation typically includes localized tenderness, warmth, erythema, swelling, and systemic signs of infection such as weight loss and fatigue. The toes may present with a "sausage toe" deformity.

Background Information

This condition is an inflammation and necrosis of bone as a result of an infection. The calcaneus is the most common site of infection in the foot, followed by the metatarsals, tarsals, and then the phalangeal bones. Biopsy, magnetic resonance imaging, and histology confirm the diagnosis.[20] Treatment may involve an aggressive regimen of antibiotic medications, with surgical resection of the affected areas potentially necessary.

■ Osteosarcoma

Chief Clinical Characteristics

This presentation may be characterized by an insidious onset of pain that persists for weeks or months. Pain due to this condition may be aggravated with activity, causing limping.

Background Information

This condition is frequently found in adolescents because of the active bone growth in this age group. African American individuals are affected slightly more often than Caucasian individuals. This condition can be especially fatal if metastasized to the lungs. Plain films confirm the diagnosis. Treatment includes chemotherapy and surgery to remove the cancerous cells or tumors.

■ Paratenonitis of Extensor Tendons of the Foot and Toes

Chief Clinical Characteristics

This presentation often involves pain, possible swelling, erythema, and tenderness to palpation over the anterior ankle and may include crepitus with active or passive movements if the tendon sheaths are inflamed.

Background Information

This condition usually occurs with a sudden onset following increases in walking intensity or distance, change of shoe, tightness in the shoelaces over the tendons, midtarsal joint hyperostosis, or tightness of the posterior calf muscles. Differentiation among extensor tendons can be achieved by passive stretching and active contraction of the specific muscles. Clinical examination confirms the diagnosis. Typical intervention is nonsurgical, involving gentle exercise, physical modalities, and footwear modification.

■ Peroneal Tendon Tear or Rupture

Chief Clinical Characteristics

This presentation can include lateral ankle pain, edema, weakness, and tenderness between the tip of the fibula and the fifth metatarsal. Painful weakness is present with resistance into plantarflexion and eversion, and ankle instability is common.

Background Information

The presentation of this condition differs from peroneal tendinopathy (tendinitis/tendinosis) because symptoms often will persist even with treatment. If there is a complete rupture, which is more common with the peroneus longus tendon, an audible pop may have been observed. This injury often is associated with ankle fractures, severe lateral ankle sprains, peroneal tenosynovitis, or a previous history of peroneal tendon injuries. Magnetic resonance imaging confirms the diagnosis. Treatment ranges from nonsurgical options, such as physical therapy intervention, to surgical options, such as debridement of partial tears and repair of complete tears.

■ Posteromedial Shin Splints

Chief Clinical Characteristics

This presentation often is characterized by pain and palpable tenderness along the muscles attached to the posteromedial aspect of the tibia within the deep posterior compartment. Pain is usually less often located directly over the tibia. Pain is aggravated with stretching into foot dorsiflexion and eversion, and with active contraction of the involved muscles. Pain usually lessens following warm-up of the muscles. Pain is usually present during activity with soreness following the activity, but pain does not usually occur during the night.

Background Information

Shin splints are due to an eccentric overuse, leading to musculotendinous injury along the posteromedial attachment of the tibia, resulting in a periostitis.[21,22] Diagnosis is based on the clinical presentation. Imaging is usually unhelpful, although fat-suppressed magnetic resonance imaging may help differentiate between stress fractures and shin splints.[7] Usual intervention is nonsurgical.

■ Pseudogout

Chief Clinical Characteristics

This presentation may include pain, edema, warmth, erythema, and tenderness of the involved joint or joints. The arthritis may mimic other types of arthritis, but attacks usually are less severe than those experienced with gout. The first metatarsophalangeal joint, ankle, dorsum of the foot, knees, wrists, or shoulders may be affected. This condition is prevalent in individuals over 60 years of age.

Background Information

Causes for the contributory calcium pyrophosphate crystal deposition in synovial joints are unknown. Diagnosis is based on the clinical presentation, the pattern of joints involved, radiographic intra-articular and periarticular involvement, and aspiration of calcium pyrophosphate crystals in the joint fluid.[23] Anti-inflammatory medication comprises the usual treatment for this condition. Unlike with gout, uric acid–lowering medications are not used.

■ Reiter's Syndrome

Chief Clinical Characteristics

This presentation typically includes asymmetric and varying severity of joint pain and stiffness of the subtalar joint, the metatarsophalangeal joints, interphalangeal joints, tarsal joints, calcaneal abnormalities, and knees.

Other symptoms can include tendon synovitis, fasciitis, back pain, mucocutaneous lesions, skin lesions, or cardiac involvement. Joint pain accompanies urethritis and conjunctivitis.

Background Information

This disease typically follows either an episode of dysentery or infectious arthritis, and persons with the HLA-B27 genetic makeup are at greater risk.[24] Diagnosis is usually based on the patient's history, radiographs, and blood tests to rule out other forms of arthritis or potentially associated infections. This is usually a self-limiting condition and resolves in 3 to 4 months. When provided, treatment involves a combination of antibiotic medications directed toward the infective agent that is responsible for the autoimmune response that characterizes this condition, in combination with anti-inflammatory medication.

■ Rheumatoid Arthritis

Chief Clinical Characteristics

This presentation can involve symmetric foot pain with localized tenderness, swelling, and early morning stiffness. The feet may be the first region affected by the arthritis; however, multiple joints are often affected. After the initial stages, subcutaneous rheumatoid nodules and joint deformities may present, most commonly flexion deformities. The metatarsophalangeal joints are the joints most commonly affected by rheumatoid arthritis.[25]

Background Information

This is a progressive systemic condition with unknown etiology. Diagnosis, according to the American Rheumatism Association, includes at least a 6-week presentation with any four of the seven following manifestations: morning stiffness for more than 1 hour, arthritis of three or more joints, arthritis of the hand joints, symmetric arthritis, rheumatoid nodules, serum rheumatoid factor, or radiographic changes. Treatment typically includes a variety of steroidal, nonsteroidal, and biological anti-inflammatory medications.

■ Rubella and Rubella Vaccine–Associated Arthritis

Chief Clinical Characteristics

This presentation includes symmetric polyarthralgia that is often correlated with joint stiffness and preceded by a prodromal stage of malaise, low-grade fever, and lymphadenopathy and by skin rash. The rash is similar in appearance to the measles. Arthralgias are more common in children, whereas the joint stiffness is more common in adults.

Background Information
This condition is caused by a ribonucleic acid viral infection and diagnosis is usually confirmed with laboratory tests (serology) and clinical examination. It is usually self-limiting and the symptoms usually alleviate in several weeks.

■ Rupture of the Achilles Tendon

Chief Clinical Characteristics
This presentation may be characterized by a sudden onset of pain, palpable tenderness, significant weakness, and sometimes a palpable sulcus, usually 2 to 6 cm proximal to the distal insertion of the Achilles tendon.

Background Information
This condition often occurs spontaneously during an activity that places loading on the plantarflexors. It is associated with age over 40 years and a history of Achilles tendinitis/tendinosis. The Thompson test and magnetic resonance or ultrasound imaging confirm the diagnosis. Surgical intervention is indicated for repair of the Achilles tendon in most individuals.

■ Septic Arthritis

Chief Clinical Characteristics
This presentation includes achy to throbbing pain, erythema, edema, and palpable warmth. Systemic signs of infection may include fever or malaise. This condition more often is monarticular and can have a sudden onset.

Background Information
Septic arthritis can result from a fungal, bacterial, or viral pathogen infecting the periarticular or synovial tissues; Staphylococcus aureus is the most common cause in all ages. Computed tomography and magnetic resonance imaging combined with culture and staining of aspirated joint fluid commonly confirm the diagnosis. Treatment usually involves a combination of an aggressive antibiotic medication and joint drainage, perhaps by way of open drainage and/or surgical lavage.

■ Talar Compression Syndrome/Impingement

Chief Clinical Characteristics
This presentation can involve pain, swelling, and tenderness to palpation over the posterior aspect of the lateral ankle, between the Achilles tendon and peroneals, and that pain is increased with forced plantarflexion.

Background Information
The mechanism of injury is a compression of the posterior structures, between the posterior tibia and the talar process, or an os trigonum (accessory center of ossification), if present. This injury is common in ballet dancers, gymnasts, and ice skaters. Associated injuries include flexor hallucis longus stenosing tenosynovitis, hypertrophic posterior capsulitis, and calcific debris. Diagnosis is based on the clinical examination, and imaging for confirmation if a clinical diagnosis is unclear. Relative rest with progressive reloading comprises the typical treatment for this condition, although arthroscopic debridement may be necessary in cases of recalcitrant disability.

■ Tarsal Tunnel Syndrome

Chief Clinical Characteristics
This presentation may include hypesthesias, pain, and paresthesias due to compression of the tibial nerve at the ankle, located around the medial aspect of the ankle and the plantar surface of the foot. Symptoms often are worse with walking, with compression, and with a dorsiflexion-eversion test. They present with a positive Tinel's sign. Rest alleviates symptoms. Weakness of the flexor hallucis and flexor digitorum brevis muscles is rarely present.

Background Information
Common etiologies are space-occupying lesions, fractures, edema, tendinitis or tenosynovitis, accessory bones, or prolonged direct and indirect pressures from inflammation and fluid retention as a result of systemic diseases (rheumatoid arthritis, ankylosing spondylitis) or significant hindfoot pronation that causes tibial nerve stretch. Diagnosis is confirmed with the clinical examination and nerve conduction studies. Nonsurgical treatment—such as physical therapy intervention, orthoses, and corticosteroid injections—may be used to address this condition. Surgical intervention

may be considered for individuals with persistent disability.

TENDINITIS
■ Achilles Tendinitis
Chief Clinical Characteristics
This presentation can involve a sharp, aching, or burning pain with point tenderness 2 to 6 cm proximal to the calcaneal insertion. Insertional tendinopathy may be located at the distal insertion at the calcaneus. Symptoms are reproduced with palpation of the tendon, passive dorsiflexion, and active resisted plantarflexion. Palpable crepitus may be present with movement, and an increased thickening of the tendon that moves with tendon excursion may be palpable in comparison to the asymptomatic side. Calf atrophy may be observed, the patient may have limitations in ankle dorsiflexion, and the patient may report increased stiffness in the morning.

Background Information
Achilles tendinitis is associated with overuse from repetitive loading of the involved tendon. This injury is most common in 15- to 45-year-old active individuals, most commonly runners. Diagnosis is often made clinically. If the diagnosis is difficult, then confirmation may be made with magnetic resonance imaging. Usual treatment is nonsurgical, consisting of anti-inflammatory medication, rest, and gentle exercise.

■ Extensor Digitorum Longus Tendinitis
Chief Clinical Characteristics
This presentation can be characterized by pain over the dorsum of the foot and tenderness to palpation along the extensor digitorum longus tendons. Resisted extension of the lesser toes and passive flexion of the lesser toes often increases the pain. Pain may also be elicited with resisted dorsiflexion of the ankle. Walking and running are often painful.

Background Information
The pathology of this tendinitis is usually the result of overuse. Diagnosis is usually made clinically, but may be confirmed with magnetic resonance or ultrasound imaging. Nonsurgical treatments may be indicated, such as anti-inflammatory medication, rest, and gentle exercise.

■ Extensor Hallucis Longus Tendinitis
Chief Clinical Characteristics
This presentation may include pain and palpable tenderness along the extensor hallucis tendon. Walking and running are often painful. Resisted extension of the hallux and passive flexion of the hallux often increase the pain. Pain may also be elicited with resisted dorsiflexion of the ankle.

Background Information
This pathology is usually the result of overuse of the affected musculotendinous unit.[26] Diagnosis is usually made clinically, but may be confirmed with magnetic resonance or ultrasound imaging. Treatment usually involves nonsurgical interventions, such as anti-inflammatory medication, rest, and gentle exercise.

■ Flexor Digitorum Longus Tendinitis
Chief Clinical Characteristics
This presentation can be characterized by pain, tenderness, and swelling along the plantar hindfoot and midfoot with tenderness along the tendon of the flexor digitorum longus. Pain is aggravated with walking and weight bearing.

Background Information
A common site of irritation is deep to the flexor retinaculum at the posteromedial ankle. Palpation can be aided with the use of muscle contraction or active movement of the toes. If the tendons are inflamed, then pain is often reproduced with stretching of the toes into extension or contraction into flexion. The pathology is often related to trauma or overuse of the affected musculotendinous unit. Diagnosis is often determined clinically and may be confirmed with magnetic resonance or ultrasound imaging. Treatment usually involves nonsurgical interventions, such as anti-inflammatory medication, rest, and gentle exercise.

■ Flexor Hallucis Longus Tendinitis

Chief Clinical Characteristics

This presentation typically includes pain and tenderness to the flexor hallucis longus tendon. Pain is aggravated with walking, weight bearing, or stretching of the tendon. Swelling is often noted in the region of the pathology.

Background Information

The location of the pathology is often at the medial aspect of the midfoot and can usually be isolated along the tendon with palpation. A common site of irritation is under the flexor retinaculum at the posteromedial ankle. Palpation can be aided with the use of muscle contraction or movement of the hallux. The pathology is often related to overuse of the affected musculotendinous unit. Diagnosis is usually made clinically, but may be confirmed with magnetic resonance or ultrasound imaging. Management typically involves a combination of anti-inflammatory medication, rest, and gentle exercise.

■ Peroneal Tendinitis

Chief Clinical Characteristics

This presentation can involve pain anywhere along the lateral lower leg to the posterior lateral malleolus and along the lateral foot at the location of the cuboid or at the plantar aspect of the foot where the peroneus longus tendon inserts at the base of the first metatarsal. The pain may also be present at the base of the fifth metatarsal where the peroneus brevis tendon inserts. The pain is often aggravated with a stretch into foot and ankle dorsiflexion and inversion or a muscle contraction into foot and ankle plantarflexion and/or eversion.

Background Information

Common causes of peroneal tendon injury include overuse and inversion injury mechanisms. Diagnosis is usually made clinically, but may be confirmed with magnetic resonance or ultrasound imaging. Nonsurgical treatments may be indicated, such as anti-inflammatory medication, rest, and gentle exercise.

■ Tibialis Anterior Tendinitis

Chief Clinical Characteristics

This presentation typically includes pain and tenderness to palpation of the tibialis anterior tendon.

Background Information

Pain is often present at initial contact and during the loading response of gait, due to the eccentric loading of the tendon and muscle. Pain is often increased with passive stretch into plantarflexion or resisted dorsiflexion of the ankle. Tibialis anterior tendinitis is usually caused by overuse.[26] Diagnosis is usually made clinically, but may be confirmed with magnetic resonance or ultrasound imaging. Usual treatment is nonsurgical, consisting of anti-inflammatory medication, rest, and gentle exercise.

■ Tibialis Posterior Tendinitis

Chief Clinical Characteristics

This presentation may involve pain and swelling with palpable tenderness along the medial aspect of the midfoot and sometimes posterior to the medial malleolus. Pain is often worsened with weight bearing, walking, performing a heel rise, or stretching the tendon. Attenuation of this tendon is sometimes seen and can lead to a flat-foot deformity. Palpation may be assisted with muscle contraction of the tibialis posterior muscle.

Background Information

Injury to this tendon is often the result of overuse that is caused by a hypermobile midfoot and excessive foot pronation. The tibialis posterior is the most significant active stabilizer of the arch.[27] Diagnosis is usually made clinically, but may be confirmed with magnetic resonance or ultrasound imaging. Nonsurgical treatments may be indicated, such as anti-inflammatory medication, rest, and gentle exercise.

TENDINOSIS

■ Achilles Tendinosis

Chief Clinical Characteristics

This presentation typically includes sharp, aching, or burning pain with point tenderness usually along the medial aspect of the middle one-third of the Achilles tendon. Some patients with Achilles tendinosis are pain free. Symptoms, if present, may be reproduced with palpation of the Achilles tendon, passive dorsiflexion, or active resisted plantarflexion. Palpable increased thickening of the tendon may be present in comparison to the uninvolved tendon. Calf atrophy, limitations in ankle dorsiflexion, and reports of increased stiffness in the morning may be observed. Pain is often worse with weight bearing and walking, and these patients often have difficulty performing a heel rise.

Background Information

Tendinosis is a state of increased tenocyte and cellular activity that leads to disorganized collagen and vascular hyperplasia.[28,29] Tendinosis is usually a chronic degenerative process that is initiated by an injury to the tendon. Diagnosis is usually based on the clinical presentation. If pathology is severe or the clinical diagnosis is unclear, then magnetic resonance or ultrasound imaging may confirm the diagnosis and allow for prognosis and staging of the tendinosis. A combination of patient/client education, unloading of the affected musculotendinous unit, controlled mechanical reloading, and preventive measures appears to be effective to manage this condition.[30]

■ Peroneal Tendinosis

Chief Clinical Characteristics

This presentation typically includes pain anywhere along the lateral lower leg to the posterior lateral malleolus and along the lateral foot at the location of the cuboid or at the plantar aspect of the foot where the peroneus longus tendon inserts at the base of the first metatarsal. The pain may also be present at the base of the fifth metatarsal where the peroneus brevis tendon inserts. The pain is often aggravated with a stretch into dorsiflexion and inversion or a muscle contraction into plantarflexion and/or eversion. Weakness may be noted into plantarflexion and/or eversion due to degenerative thickening, lengthening, and tearing of the tendon.

Background Information

Common causes of peroneal tendon injury include overuse and inversion injury mechanisms that may lead to the chronic degenerative process of tendinosis. Tendinosis is a

state of increased tenocyte and cellular activity that leads to disorganized collagen and vascular hyperplasia.[28,29] Final diagnosis is confirmed with magnetic resonance or ultrasound imaging. A combination of patient/client education, unloading of the affected musculotendinous unit, controlled mechanical reloading, and preventive measures appears to be effective to manage this condition.[30]

■ Tibialis Posterior Tendinosis

Chief Clinical Characteristics

This presentation typically includes pain and swelling with palpable tenderness along the medial aspect of the midfoot and posterior to the medial malleolus. Pain is often worse with weight bearing and walking, and these patients often have difficulty performing a heel rise. Attenuation of this tendon is sometimes seen as a result of tendinosis and the development of posterior tibialis tendon dysfunction may lead to a flat-foot deformity and a caudal drop of the navicular. These patients have a very difficult time contracting the tibialis posterior muscle, even during a manual muscle test.

Background Information

Injury to this tendon is often the result of overuse with a hypermobile midfoot. The tibialis posterior is the most significant active stabilizer of the arch.[27] Tendinosis is a state of increased tenocyte and cellular activity that leads to disorganized collagen and vascular hyperplasia. Tendinosis is usually a chronic degenerative process that is initiated by injury to the tendon. Diagnosis is usually based on the clinical presentation; however, magnetic resonance imaging may confirm the diagnosis and allow for prognosis and staging of the tendinosis. A combination of patient/client education, unloading of the affected musculotendinous unit, controlled mechanical reloading, and preventive measures appears to be effective to manage this condition.[30]

■ Tibiofibular Synostosis

Chief Clinical Characteristics

This presentation typically includes pain at the anterior ankle and lower leg and instability with activities such as cutting, pivoting, running, or performing agility activities.

ANKLE PAIN

Background Information

This condition is associated with a history of recurrent inversion ankle sprains that remain symptomatic due to widening of the inferior tibiofibular joint and bone formation in the interosseous membrane. The mechanism of injury for the fracture is the same as the original injury. With a synostosis present in the absence of a fracture, pain may be present with dorsiflexion and pushing off. Injuries to associated structures could include the anterior and posterior inferior tibiofibular ligaments, the interosseous membrane, the lateral ankle ligaments, and possibly the talar dome lesions. A clinical impingement test and radiographs confirm the diagnosis. Typical intervention is nonsurgical.

■ Transient Migratory Osteoporosis

Chief Clinical Characteristics

This presentation typically includes pain and swelling at the ankle joint, progressing over time to adjacent joints with symptoms usually lasting 6 months to a year. Pitting edema, palpable warmth, erythema, or trophic changes are unlikely.

Background Information

The etiology of this condition is unknown. Transient migratory osteoporosis differs from senile osteoporosis in the presentation of pain and edema, in addition to multiple joints affected in the same individual. Radiographic evidence of osteoporosis in the presence of normal laboratory tests confirms the diagnosis.[31] It is sometimes difficult to differentiate from avascular necrosis. This condition is usually self-limiting and resolves within 1 year.

■ Traumatic Dislocation of the Peroneal Tendons

Chief Clinical Characteristics

This presentation typically includes sudden onset of posterolateral ankle pain and swelling, with possible snapping posterior to and over the lateral malleolus and tenderness over the peroneal tendons. Resisted dorsiflexion on a plantarflexed and everted foot will often reproduce pain and may reproduce the tendon dislocation.

Background Information

This injury results from dorsiflexion force on an inverted ankle during muscle contraction of the peroneals, and commonly occurs during skiing, ice skating, running, basketball, and football. Associated injuries include lateral ankle retinaculum tear, avulsion fracture of the inferior tip of the lateral malleolus, and posterior talofibular ligament injury. Diagnosis is based on the clinical examination. Treatment ranges from nonsurgical reduction and immobilization to surgical fixation of the dislocated tendons.

References

1. Merskey H, Bogduk N. *Classification of Chronic Pain: Descriptions of Chronic Pain Syndromes and Definitions of Pain Terms.* Seattle, WA: IASP Press; 1994.
2. Moseley GL. Imagined movements cause pain and swelling in a patient with complex regional pain syndrome. *Neurology.* May 11, 2004;62(9):1644.
3. Abshire T. An approach to target joint bleeding in hemophilia: prophylaxis for all or individualized treatment? *J Pediatr.* Nov 2004;145(5):581–583.
4. Rodriguez-Merchan EC. Management of musculoskeletal complications of hemophilia. *Semin Thromb Hemost.* Feb 2003;29(1):87–96.
5. Carapetis JR, Currie BJ. Rheumatic fever in a high incidence population: the importance of monoarthritis and low grade fever. *Arch Dis Child.* Sep 2001;85(3):223–227.
6. Slocum DB. The shin splint syndrome. Medical aspects and differential diagnosis. *Am J Surg.* Dec 1967;114(6):875–881.
7. Aoki Y, Yasuda K, Tohyama H, Ito H, Minami A. Magnetic resonance imaging in stress fractures and shin splints. *Clin Orthop.* Apr 2004;(421):260–267.
8. Salvarani C, Vlachonikolis IG, van der Heijde DM, et al. Musculoskeletal manifestations in a population-based cohort of inflammatory bowel disease patients. *Scand J Gastroenterol.* Dec 2001;36(12):1307–1313.
9. Springer BL, Clarkson PM. Two cases of exertional rhabdomyolysis precipitated by personal trainers. *Med Sci Sports Exerc.* Sep 2003;35(9):1499–1502.
10. Judd DB, Kim DH. Foot fractures frequently misdiagnosed as ankle sprains. *Am Fam Physician.* Sep 1, 2002;66(5):785–794.
11. Canale ST, Belding RH. Osteochondral lesions of the talus. *J Bone Joint Surg Am.* Jan 1980;62(1):97–102.
12. Loomer R, Fisher C, Lloyd-Smith R, Sisler J, Cooney T. Osteochondral lesions of the talus. *Am J Sports Med.* Jan–Feb 1993;21(1):13–19.
13. Kramer HM, Curhan G. The association between gout and nephrolithiasis: the National Health and Nutrition Examination Survey III, 1988–1994. *Am J Kidney Dis.* Jul 2002;40(1):37–42.
14. Xenos JS, Hopkinson WJ, Mulligan ME, Olson EJ, Popovic NA. The tibiofibular syndesmosis. Evaluation of the ligamentous structures, methods of fixation, and radiographic assessment. *J Bone Joint Surg Am.* Jun 1995;77(6):847–856.
15. Sangeorzan BJ. Painful disorders of the ankle and heel. In Loeser JD, eds. *Bonica's Management of Pain.* 3rd ed. Philadelphia, PA: Lippincott Williams & Wilkins; 2001:1637–1646.

16. Joines JD, McNutt RA, Carey TS, Deyo RA, Rouhani R. Finding cancer in primary care outpatients with low back pain: a comparison of diagnostic strategies. *J Gen Intern Med*. 2001;16(1):14–23.

17. Holman PJ, Suki D, McCutcheon I, Wolinsky JP, Rhines LD, Gokaslan ZL. Surgical management of metastatic disease of the lumbar spine: experience with 139 patients. *J Neurosurg Spine*. 2005;2(5):550–563.

18. Kelberine F, Frank A. Arthroscopic treatment of osteochondral lesions of the talar dome: a retrospective study of 48 cases. *Arthroscopy*. Jan–Feb 1999;15(1):77–84.

19. Crist BD, Lenke LG, Lewis S. Osteoid osteoma of the lumbar spine. A case report highlighting a novel reconstruction technique. *J Bone Joint Surg Am*. Feb 2005;87(2):414–418.

20. Lipman BT, Collier BD, Carrera GF, et al. Detection of osteomyelitis in the neuropathic foot: nuclear medicine, MRI and conventional radiography. *Clin Nucl Med*. Feb 1998;23(2):77–82.

21. Michael RH, Holder LE. The soleus syndrome. A cause of medial tibial stress (shin splints). *Am J Sports Med*. Mar–Apr 1985;13(2):87–94.

22. Beck BR, Osternig LR. Medial tibial stress syndrome. The location of muscles in the leg in relation to symptoms. *J Bone Joint Surg Am*. Jul 1994;76(7):1057–1061.

23. Cassetta M, Gorevic PD. Crystal arthritis. Gout and pseudogout in the geriatric patient. *Geriatrics*. Sep 2004; 59(9):25–30; quiz 31.

24. Eapen BR. A new insight into the pathogenesis of Reiter's syndrome using bioinformatics tools. *Int J Dermatol*. Mar 2003;42(3):242–243.

25. Smyth CJ, Janson RW. Rheumatologic view of the rheumatoid foot. *Clin Orthop*. Jul 1997(340):7–17.

26. Karlsson J, Lundin O, Lossing IW, Peterson L. Partial rupture of the patellar ligament. Results after operative treatment. *Am J Sports Med*. Jul–Aug 1991;19(4): 403–408.

27. Thordarson DB, Schmotzer H, Chon J, Peters J. Dynamic support of the human longitudinal arch. A biomechanical evaluation. *Clin Orthop*. Jul 1995(316): 165–172.

28. Mafi N, Lorentzon R, Alfredson H. Superior short-term results with eccentric calf muscle training compared to concentric training in a randomized prospective multicenter study on patients with chronic Achilles tendinosis. *Knee Surg Sports Traumatol Arthrosc*. 2001;9(1): 42–47.

29. Kraushaar BS, Nirschl RP. Tendinosis of the elbow (tennis elbow). Clinical features and findings of histological, immunohistochemical, and electron microscopy studies. *J Bone Joint Surg Am*. Feb 1999;81(2):259–278.

30. Davenport TE, Kulig K, Matharu Y, Blanco CE. The EdUReP model for nonsurgical management of tendinopathy. *Phys Ther*. Oct 2005;85(10):1093–1103.

31. McCarthy EF. The pathology of transient regional osteoporosis. *Iowa Orthop J*. 1998;18:35–42.

CHAPTER 24

Foot Pain

■ *Jason R. Cozby, PT, DPT, OCS* ■ *Lisa Meyer, PT, DPT, OCS*
■ *Stephen F. Reischl, PT, DPT, OCS*

Description of the Symptom

This chapter describes pathology that may lead to foot pain, including generalized, dorsal foot, forefoot and toe, hindfoot, and midfoot. **Local causes** of foot pain are defined as pathology that occurs within the foot, either deep to or distal to the medial and lateral malleoli of the tibia. **Remote causes** are defined as occurring outside this region.

Special Concerns

- Decreased sensation
- Diminished dorsalis pedis or tibial pulses
- Pain that increases at night or with rest
- Skin breakdown
- Warmth and edema

CHAPTER PREVIEW: Conditions That May Lead to Foot Pain

T Trauma

REMOTE	LOCAL GENERALIZED	LOCAL DORSAL
COMMON		
Lumbar radiculopathies: • L5 radiculopathy 455 • S1 radiculopathy 456	Nerve entrapments: • Tarsal tunnel syndrome 475	Bite injuries 459 Fractures: • Metatarsal 466

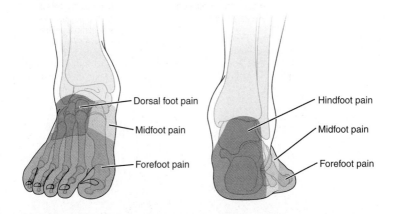

Dorsal foot pain
Midfoot pain
Forefoot pain

Hindfoot pain
Midfoot pain
Forefoot pain

LOCAL FOREFOOT AND TOE	LOCAL HINDFOOT	LOCAL MIDFOOT

Calluses 460
Corns 461
Crush injury 461
Fractures:
• Hallucal sesamoid disorders 465
• Metatarsal 466
• Toe 468
Hammer toe deformity 469
Ligament sprains:
• Forefoot 472
Metatarsalgia 473
Shoe vamp ulcer and bursitis 480
	Fractures:
	• Calcaneus 464
	Ligament sprains:
	• Anterior talofibular
	  ligament 471
	• Calcaneofibular ligament
	  (isolated) 472
	Nerve entrapments:
	• Tarsal tunnel syndrome 475
	Plantar fasciitis 477
	Strain of the peroneal
	  muscles 481
		Longitudinal arch
		  strain 472
		Plantar fasciitis 477
		Positional faults:
		• Calcaneocuboid joint 477
		• Talonavicular joint 478

(continued)

Trauma *(continued)*

REMOTE	LOCAL GENERALIZED	LOCAL DORSAL
UNCOMMON		
Lumbar radiculopathies: • L4 radiculopathy 455	Bite injuries 459 Cold injuries 460 Crush injury 461 Nerve entrapments: • Deep peroneal nerve 475 • Superficial peroneal nerve 475 • Sural nerve 475	Fractures: • Osteochondral fracture of the subtalar joint 466 Ligament sprains: • Cruciate crural ligament 472 Nerve entrapments: • Deep peroneal nerve 475 • Superficial peroneal nerve 475
RARE		
Not applicable	Not applicable	Not applicable

I Inflammation

REMOTE	LOCAL GENERALIZED	LOCAL DORSAL
COMMON		
Not applicable	**Aseptic** Dermatitis 462 Reiter's syndrome 479 Rheumatoid arthritis 479	**Aseptic** Tendinitis: • Extensor digitorum longus tendinitis 481 • Extensor hallucis longus tendinitis 482 • Tibialis anterior tendinitis 482

LOCAL FOREFOOT AND TOE	LOCAL HINDFOOT	LOCAL MIDFOOT
Dislocations: • Interphalangeal joint 462 Ligament sprains: • Metatarsophalangeal joint 472 Mallet toe deformity 473 Morton's neuroma 474	Calcaneal apophysitis (Sever's disease) 459 Fat pad syndrome 464 Fractures: • Lateral process of the talus 465 • Lateral tubercle of the posterior process of the talus 465 • Medial process of the sustentaculum tali of the calcaneus 465 • Medial tuberosity of the posterior process of the talus 466 • Osteochondral fracture of the talar dome 466 • Posterosuperior calcaneal tuberosity 467 • Stress fracture of the calcaneus 467 • Stress fracture of the lateral malleolus 467 Nerve entrapments: • First branch of the lateral plantar nerve 475 • Sural nerve 475 Ruptures: • Achilles tendon 480 • Plantar fascia 480	Fractures: • Fifth metatarsal 464 • Navicular 466 Interosseous myositis 470
Dislocations: • Metatarsophalangeal joint 462 Joplin's neuroma 471	Nerve entrapments: • Calcaneal branch neurodynia 474	Fractures: • Osteochondral fracture of the subtalar joint 466 • Tarsometatarsal joint (Lisfranc's) fracture or dislocation 467

LOCAL FOREFOOT AND TOE	LOCAL HINDFOOT	LOCAL MIDFOOT
Aseptic Not applicable **Septic** Paronychia 477 Tinea pedis (athlete's foot) 485 Warts 486	**Aseptic** Achilles paratenonitis 456 Bursitis: • Retrocalcaneal bursitis 459 • Subcutaneous Achilles bursitis 459	Not applicable

(continued)

FOOT PAIN

Inflammation *(continued)*

REMOTE	LOCAL GENERALIZED	LOCAL DORSAL
COMMON		
	Septic Bite injuries 459 Cellulitis 460 Tinea pedis (athlete's foot) 485	**Septic** Cellulitis 460
UNCOMMON		
Not applicable	**Aseptic** Acute rheumatic fever 457 Ankylosing spondylitis 457 Arthritis associated with inflammatory bowel disease 458 Complex regional pain syndrome 461 Hepatitis B–associated arthritis 469 Herpes zoster 469 Hypersensitivity vasculitis 470 Polyarteritis nodosa 477 Rheumatoid arthritis–like diseases of the foot: • Psoriatic arthritis 479 • Systemic lupus erythematosus 479 Rubella and rubella vaccine– associated arthritis 480 **Septic** Abscess 456 Hand-foot-and-mouth disease 469 Osteomyelitis 476	**Aseptic** Interosseous myositis 470 **Septic** Not applicable
RARE		
Not applicable	**Aseptic** Allergic angiitis and granulomatosis (Churg-Strauss disease) 457 Erosive lichen planus 463 Fixed drug eruption 464 **Septic** Necrotizing fasciitis 474	**Aseptic** Herpes zoster 469 **Septic** Abscess 456 Osteomyelitis 476 Septic arthritis 480

LOCAL FOREFOOT AND TOE	LOCAL HINDFOOT	LOCAL MIDFOOT
	Tendinitis: • Achilles tendinitis 481 • Peroneal tendinitis 482 • Tibialis posterior tendinitis 483 **Septic** Not applicable	
Aseptic Idiopathic metatarsophalangeal synovitis 470 **Septic** Candidiasis 460 Infected blister 470	**Aseptic** Haglund's syndrome 468 Tendinitis: • Flexor digitorum longus tendinitis 482 • Flexor hallucis longus tendinitis 482 **Septic** Not applicable	**Aseptic** Tendinitis: • Flexor hallucis longus tendinitis 482 • Peroneal tendinitis 482 • Tibialis posterior tendinitis 483 **Septic** Abscess 456 Osteomyelitis 476
Aseptic Not applicable **Septic** Osler's nodules 476 Pulp-space infection 478 Septic arthritis 480	**Aseptic** Not applicable **Septic** Osteomyelitis 476	Not applicable

M Metabolic

REMOTE	LOCAL GENERALIZED	LOCAL DORSAL
COMMON		
Not applicable	Benign muscle cramps 459 Distal symmetric polyneuropathy, including from acquired immunodeficiency syndrome, alcohol/drug abuse, carcinoma, diabetes mellitus, and kidney failure 462 Envenomation 463 Gout 468	Envenomation 463 Gout 468
UNCOMMON		
Not applicable	Pseudogout 478	Pseudogout 478
RARE		
Not applicable	Fabry's disease 463 Intermittent acute porphyria 470 Primary amyloidosis 478 Vitamin B deficiency 485	Not applicable

Va Vascular

REMOTE	LOCAL GENERALIZED	LOCAL DORSAL
COMMON		
Not applicable	Arterial insufficiency 457 Sickle cell crisis 480	Not applicable
UNCOMMON		
Not applicable	Arterial occlusion 457 Cholesterol embolism 460	Not applicable
RARE		
Not applicable	Arteriosclerosis obliterans 458 Compartment syndrome 461 Cryoglobulinemia 461 Erythromelalgia 463 Thromboangiitis (Buerger's disease) 485 Waldenstrom's macroglobulinemia 486	Avascular necrosis of the navicular 458

LOCAL FOREFOOT AND TOE	LOCAL HINDFOOT	LOCAL MIDFOOT
Gout 468	Not applicable	Not applicable
Distal symmetric polyneuropathy, including from acquired immunodeficiency syndrome, alcohol/drug abuse, carcinoma, diabetes mellitus, and kidney failure 462 Pseudogout 478	Not applicable	Not applicable
Not applicable	Not applicable	Not applicable

LOCAL FOREFOOT AND TOE	LOCAL HINDFOOT	LOCAL MIDFOOT
Ischemic ulceration of the toes 471 Subungual hematoma 481	Not applicable	Not applicable
Arterial insufficiency 457 Freiberg's disease 468 Raynaud's disease 478	Not applicable	Not applicable
Not applicable	Not applicable	Avascular necrosis of the navicular 458

De Degenerative

REMOTE	LOCAL GENERALIZED	LOCAL DORSAL
COMMON		
Not applicable	Not applicable	Osteoarthrosis/osteoarthritis: • Midfoot (tarsometatarsal joints) 476 Tendinosis: • Extensor digitorum longus tendinosis 483 • Extensor hallucis longus tendinosis 483 • Tibialis anterior tendinosis 484
UNCOMMON		
Not applicable	Not applicable	Not applicable
RARE		
Not applicable	Not applicable	Not applicable

Tu Tumor

REMOTE	LOCAL GENERALIZED	LOCAL DORSAL
COMMON		
Not applicable	Not applicable	Not applicable
UNCOMMON		
Not applicable	Not applicable	Not applicable
RARE		
Not applicable	*Malignant Primary, such as:* • Leukemia 471 • Lymphoma 473 • Multiple myeloma 474 *Malignant Metastatic, such as:* • Metastases to the foot, including from primary breast, kidney, lung, prostate, and thyroid disease 473 *Benign:* Not applicable	Not applicable

LOCAL FOREFOOT AND TOE	LOCAL HINDFOOT	LOCAL MIDFOOT

Hallux rigidus 469
Hallux valgus 469
Osteoarthrosis/osteoarthritis:
• Interphalangeal joint 476
• Small toes 476
	Tendinosis:
	• Achilles tendinosis 483
	• Peroneal tendinosis 484
	• Tibialis posterior
	  tendinosis 485
		Osteoarthrosis/osteoarthritis:
		• Midfoot (tarsometatarsal
		  joints) 476

Not applicable	Atrophic fat pad disorder 458
	Tendinosis:
	• Flexor digitorum longus
	  tendinosis 484
	• Flexor hallucis longus
	  tendinosis 484
		Tendinosis:
		• Flexor hallucis longus
		  tendinosis 484
		• Peroneal tendinosis 484
		• Tibialis posterior
		  tendinosis 485

Calcific tendinitis of the flexor hallucis longus or brevis 460	Not applicable	Not applicable

LOCAL FOREFOOT AND TOE	LOCAL HINDFOOT	LOCAL MIDFOOT
Not applicable	Not applicable	Not applicable
Malignant Primary: Not applicable *Malignant Metastatic:* Not applicable *Benign, such as:* • Submetatarsal cyst 481	*Malignant Primary:* Not applicable *Malignant Metastatic:* Not applicable *Benign, such as:* • Fat pad separation secondary to a cyst 463 • Piezogenic papules 477	Not applicable
Not applicable	*Malignant Primary:* Not applicable *Malignant Metastatic:* Not applicable *Benign, such as:* • Glomus tumor 468	Not applicable

Co Congenital

REMOTE	LOCAL GENERALIZED	LOCAL DORSAL
COMMON		
Not applicable	Not applicable	Not applicable
UNCOMMON		
Not applicable	Dysplasia epiphysealis hemimelica (Trevor's disease) 462	Not applicable
RARE		
Not applicable	Not applicable	Not applicable

Ne Neurogenic/Psychogenic

REMOTE	LOCAL GENERALIZED	LOCAL DORSAL
COMMON		
Not applicable	Not applicable	Not applicable
UNCOMMON		
Fear and avoidance 454	Not applicable	Not applicable
RARE		
Psychological effect of complex regional pain syndrome 456	Not applicable	Not applicable

Note: These are estimates of relative incidence because few data are available for the less common conditions.

Overview of Foot Pain

Pain that is experienced in the foot is commonly the result of traumatic injury or mechanical disorders that affect the underlying structures. The foot is the structure of the lower extremity that comes in direct contact with the ground and therefore experiences very high forces due to ground reaction forces, forces originating from functional activities, and forces that arise during attempts to control body weight and momentum. Injury to the foot may lead to alignment issues as well as damage to multiple joints or tissues. Furthermore, damage to multiple structures may lead to a more generalized pain. Nevertheless, the foot also may experience pain as a result of vascular compromise, proximal nerve compression, or systemic disease. The foot often is an end target site for multiple disease processes, so all potential diagnoses should be considered even if mechanical trauma is associated with the presentation.

Description of Conditions That May Lead to Foot Pain

Remote

■ Fear and Avoidance

Chief Clinical Characteristics
This presentation may include avoiding the use of an extremity as a result of apprehension of onset of pain.

Background Information
Injury to the foot and ankle may contribute to the disuse of the lower extremity even with minimal injury. Fear of reinjury, pain, or other

LOCAL FOREFOOT AND TOE	LOCAL HINDFOOT	LOCAL MIDFOOT
Not applicable	Not applicable	Not applicable
Not applicable	Not applicable	Not applicable
Not applicable	Not applicable	Not applicable

LOCAL FOREFOOT AND TOE	LOCAL HINDFOOT	LOCAL MIDFOOT
Not applicable	Not applicable	Not applicable
Not applicable	Not applicable	Not applicable
Not applicable	Not applicable	Not applicable

factors will need to be explored. In all cases the basis of pathology must be thoroughly explored before this presentation is to be considered. If this condition is present, a team approach ensures optimal treatment.

LUMBAR RADICULOPATHIES

■ L4 Radiculopathy

Chief Clinical Characteristics

This presentation can be characterized by pain in the lumbar spine and paresthesias radiating from the anterolateral thigh, the anteromedial lower leg, the medial malleolus, and distally into the medial aspect of the foot. The patient may have weakness of the tibialis anterior muscle. Depending on the severity, the presentation may also include a decreased or absent patellar tendon reflex and motor loss in the muscles innervated by
the L4 nerve. Prone knee bend may reproduce symptoms.

Background Information

A lumbar disk herniation is the most common cause for this condition. The diagnosis is confirmed with magnetic resonance imaging. Surgical intervention may be indicated in severe cases of lower extremity pain accompanied by neurological signs.

■ L5 Radiculopathy

Chief Clinical Characteristics

This presentation includes pain in the lumbar spine and paresthesias radiating from the lateral aspect of the hip and buttock to the lateral aspect of the knee, extending from the anterolateral lower leg down into the dorsum of the foot. Depending on the severity, the presentation may also include motor loss in the muscles innervated by the L5 nerve root, including extensor hallucis longus and extensor digitorum longus.

Background Information
A lumbar disk herniation is the most common cause for this condition. The diagnosis is confirmed with magnetic resonance imaging. Surgical intervention may be indicated in severe cases of lower extremity pain accompanied by neurological signs.

■ S1 Radiculopathy

Chief Clinical Characteristics
This presentation typically includes pain in the lumbar spine and paresthesias radiating from the buttock to the posterior aspect of the knee and extending posterolaterally along the lower leg, the lateral heel, and the lateral plantar foot. Depending on the severity, the presentation may also include a decreased or absent Achilles tendon reflex and motor loss in the muscles innervated by the S1 nerve, including the peroneal muscles, gastrocnemius, and soleus.

Background Information
A lumbar disk herniation is a common cause for this condition. The diagnosis is confirmed with magnetic resonance imaging. Surgical intervention may be indicated in severe cases of lower extremity pain accompanied by neurological signs.

■ Psychological Effect of Complex Regional Pain Syndrome

Chief Clinical Characteristics
This presentation typically includes a traumatic onset of severe chronic ankle and foot pain accompanied by allodynia, hyperalgesia, and trophic, vasomotor, and sudomotor changes in later stages. This condition is characterized by disproportionate responses to painful stimuli.

Background Information
This regional neuropathic pain disorder presents either without direct nerve trauma (Type I) or with direct nerve trauma (Type II) in any region of the body.[1] This condition may precipitate due to an event distant to the affected area. Thermography may confirm associated sympathetic dysfunction. This condition has been shown to have a psychological component

and may be influenced by cortical mechanisms.[2] Treatment may include physical therapy interventions to improve patient/client functioning, biofeedback, analgesic or anti-inflammatory medication, transcutaneous or spinal electrical nerve stimulation, and surgical or pharmacologic sympathectomy. However, a team approach ensures optimal treatment for individuals with this condition.

Local

■ Abscess

Chief Clinical Characteristics
This presentation often includes a severe, deep, and throbbing pain, with pus surrounded by a region of erythema, edema, and warmth, as well as systemic signs of infection that may include fever, chills, malaise, anorexia, and delirium.

Background Information
This condition most commonly affects the central plantar compartment. It often follows minor skin trauma. Localized cellulitis may accompany the abscess. Magnetic resonance imaging with contrast confirms the diagnosis.[3] Treatment may involve options ranging from rest and antibiotic medications to surgical drainage.

■ Achilles Paratenonitis

Chief Clinical Characteristics
This presentation involves diffuse pain, tenderness, and thickening and swelling along the Achilles tendon, especially 2 to 6 cm from the calcaneal insertion. However, the painful palpable thickening does not move with dorsiflexion or plantarflexion because the tendon moves with this action but the paratenon does not. Pain is greatest in the mornings or at the start of a physical activity, but the pain will often decrease with continued walking or activity as the tendon begins to move more freely inside the paratenon.

Background Information
The paratenon is usually the site of inflammatory injury related to overuse, but it may also be damaged from direct traumatic pressure. The diagnosis is determined clinically, but magnetic resonance or ultrasound imaging may be necessary for confirmation if the clinical diagnosis is unclear. Treatment includes

rest, inflammation control, improving flexibility of the calf muscle group, and improving strength of the antipronator muscle groups.

■ Acute Rheumatic Fever

Chief Clinical Characteristics
This presentation may involve warm, red, swollen, and tender joints with systemic signs of infection including fever, abdominal pain, anorexia, lethargy, malaise, and fatigue. Rheumatic fever usually has five major manifestations that include migratory polyarthritis, carditis, chorea, subcutaneous nodules, and erythema marginatum (flat to slightly indurated lesions on the skin of the extensor surfaces of the extremities or trunk).

Background Information
This condition is an acute inflammation as a result of group A streptococcal infection.[4] The pain is usually the result of an aseptic inflammation of the joints. Diagnosis is made with confirmation of a group A streptococcal infection in association with two of the five major manifestations. Monoarthritis and low-grade fever are important considerations to avoid underdiagnosis.[4] Usual treatment consists of antibiotic, anti-inflammatory, and antipyretic medications.

■ Allergic Angiitis and Granulomatosis (Churg-Strauss Disease)

Chief Clinical Characteristics
This presentation can be characterized by fever, abdominal pain, peripheral neuropathy, mononeuritis multiplex, weakness, weight loss, hypertension, edema, oliguria, and uremia in association with pulmonary symptoms. This disorder is always associated with bronchial asthma.

Background Information
Other signs and symptoms include skin nodules, eosinophilia, mononeuropathy or polyneuropathy, and small blood vessel occlusion that may result in toe and foot gangrene. Drug allergies or infection are theoretical causes. Clinical examination confirms the diagnosis in the presence of rhinitis, sinusitis, or asthma. Usual treatment includes corticosteroids. Because of the multisystem nature of this condition, other supportive interventions also may be necessary.

■ Ankylosing Spondylitis

Chief Clinical Characteristics
This presentation may include an insidious onset of low back and symmetric posterior hip pain associated with a slowly progressive and significant loss of general spinal mobility. Some individuals with late-stage disease also will develop characteristic syndesmophytes in the foot region.

Background Information
Symptoms may be worse in the morning and improve with light exercise. This condition is more common in males, as well as people of American indigenous descent, less than 40 years of age, or who carry the human leukocyte antigen B27. It also may be associated with fever, malaise, and inflammatory bowel disease. The diagnosis is confirmed with plain radiographs of the sacroiliac joints and lumbar spine, which reveal characteristic findings of sacroiliitis and "bamboo spine." Blood panels including erythrocyte sedimentation rate are useful to track disease activity. Treatment typically includes a combination of steroidal, nonsteroidal, and biological anti-inflammatory medications combined with physical therapy to address postural and movement considerations associated with changing spinal position.

■ Arterial Insufficiency

Chief Clinical Characteristics
This presentation may involve pain in the foot and lower leg that is worst at night, possibly causing awakening from sleep. Symptoms often decrease when the leg is placed in a dependent position or after walking.

Background Information
More severe cases of arterial insufficiency may be associated with skin ulceration. This condition is a result of decreased mean arterial pressure while sleeping; ischemia causes foot pain. Doppler ultrasonography confirms the diagnosis. The goal of treatment is to prevent the progression of this condition to acute arterial occlusion.[5] Treatment may involve exercise, risk factor modification, stenting, balloon angioplasty, bypass grafting, or amputation.

■ Arterial Occlusion

Chief Clinical Characteristics
This presentation includes an abrupt onset of deep achy and/or burning pain, often on the

plantar surface of the foot. Diminished sensation, weakness, pallor, coldness, and cyanotic mottling also may be present. The pulses in the feet, and often the entire lower extremity, may be absent.

Background Information

Common causes of this condition include trauma, embolus, or a thrombus.[6] It is located at the bifurcation just distal to the last detectable pulse. If the occlusion is present for longer than 6 hours, the patient is likely to contract gangrene and/or have residual symptoms of weakness or sensory impairment. Diagnosis is most often confirmed with Doppler ultrasonography; however, angiography, assessment of systolic blood pressure, and magnetic resonance angiography may be utilized. This condition is a medical emergency in its acute form due to the risk for compromise of the distal tissues. Treatment usually involves pharmacologic or surgical thrombolysis.

■ Arteriosclerosis Obliterans

Chief Clinical Characteristics

This presentation typically includes painful toes or feet in association with symptoms of palpable coolness, and trophic changes such as hair loss or nail changes. Affected toes may be blue or black in color. Pulses are diminished or absent in the lower leg and foot.

Background Information

This condition is a vascular disease in which the arteries become thickened and lose elasticity, resulting in vessel occlusion.[7,8] It can lead to ulceration or gangrene of the foot or toes. The kidneys, brain, and heart also may be affected. The diagnosis is confirmed with Doppler ultrasonography or angiography. Treatment may involve exercise, risk factor modification, stenting, balloon angioplasty, bypass grafting, or amputation.

■ Arthritis Associated with Inflammatory Bowel Disease

Chief Clinical Characteristics

This presentation may be characterized by migratory polyarthritic pain with abdominal pain, diarrhea, abdominal cramping, and other gastrointestinal symptoms. Commonly affected joints include the metatarsophalangeal joints, ankle, knee, elbow, wrist, and hand. Other

extraintestinal manifestations include episcleritis, ankylosing spondylitis, sacroiliitis, anterior uveitis, aphthous stomatitis, erythema nodosum, pyoderma gangrenosum, or growth and development delay.

Background Information

One-third of patients with inflammatory bowel disease have at least one musculoskeletal manifestation, and in children the extraintestinal manifestations may dominate.[9] Colonoscopy with mucosal biopsy confirms the diagnosis. Treatment typically involves aminosalicylates, corticosteroids, anti–tumor necrosis factor medications, diet changes, and surgical resection of the involved portion of bowel.

■ Atrophic Fat Pad Disorder

Chief Clinical Characteristics

This presentation can involve pain on the plantar surface of the heel with tenderness to palpation. Pain increases with barefoot walking, especially in the morning.

Background Information

This condition results from thinning or spreading of the fat pad that occurs more often in the elderly, long-distance runners, individuals who train on hard surfaces, and individuals who wear open-heeled or unsupportive shoes. Clinical examination confirms the diagnosis. Treatment usually involves nonsurgical interventions, such as orthoses and footwear modification, relative rest, and strengthening and flexibility exercises for the lower quarter.

■ Avascular Necrosis of the Navicular

Chief Clinical Characteristics

This presentation includes severe medial midfoot pain accompanied by edema and erythema. This condition is more common in individuals with a severe pes planus foot posture.

Background Information

This condition results from an alteration in blood supply that does not allow for proper healing after initial trauma to the bone, most commonly as a dorsal avulsion fracture or direct trauma (such as a blow to the bone). The diagnosis is confirmed with plain radiographs. Intervention may include immobilization in early-stage disease or arthroscopic debridement and drilling for advanced lesions.

■ Benign Muscle Cramps

Chief Clinical Characteristics

This presentation involves painful muscle cramps, palpable tightness, and induration that is often correlated with a sustained contraction of the affected muscle.[10] *This condition may last several minutes to approximately one-half hour, with tenderness for several hours following an acute episode.*

Background Information

This condition is associated with an insidious onset following muscle overuse. Other potential causes include dehydration, hyponatremia, hypomagnesemia, geriatric nocturnal leg cramps, or association with pregnancy.[10] Treatment typically involves addressing the underlying cause of muscle cramps. Quinine sulfate is an established pharmacologic treatment that also has potential adverse cardiac side effects.

■ Bite Injuries

Chief Clinical Characteristics

This presentation may involve pain with ecchymosis, edema, abrasion, and lesions or puncture wounds at the location of the bite.

Background Information

Common bites include those by humans, dogs, and cats. Potential complications include nerve damage, blood vessel damage, or crush injury resulting in tissue damage or a fracture. Any bite injury may develop septicemia and its associated signs of systemic infection. The history will reveal the cause and circumstances of the bite. This condition is treated prophylactically with antibiotics due to the risk for septicemia.[11,12]

BURSITIS

■ Retrocalcaneal Bursitis

Chief Clinical Characteristics

This presentation typically includes pain, palpable warmth, tenderness to palpation, and some edema at the medial and lateral aspects of the Achilles tendon. Pain is reproduced with compressing the tissue anterior to the tendon, as well as with dorsiflexion of the ankle.

Background Information

This condition is the result of inflammation within the bursa that lies between the Achilles tendon and the calcaneus. Biomechanical or structural factors, such as Haglund's deformity or rearfoot varus, may lead to increased stress on this region. Systemic inflammatory diseases or direct trauma also may lead to this disorder. Clinical examination confirms the diagnosis. Usual intervention includes activity and footwear modification.

■ Subcutaneous Achilles Bursitis

Chief Clinical Characteristics

This presentation can include local pain, tenderness to palpation, and edema just posterior to the Achilles tendon insertion at the calcaneal tuberosity. Warmth and redness may be present.

Background Information

This condition results from inflammation and edema of the bursa located between the Achilles tendon insertion and the skin. Continued irritation of the inflamed and swollen bursa may lead to thickening of the bursal walls and fibrosis. Clinical examination confirms the diagnosis. Treatment is typically nonsurgical, including physical therapy intervention, orthoses, and footwear and activity modification.

■ Calcaneal Apophysitis (Sever's Disease)

Chief Clinical Characteristics

This presentation may include pain along the medial and lateral heel or distal Achilles insertion. Edema and warmth may be present. Pain increases with higher level weight-bearing activities and decreases with rest. This condition is common in young athletes.

Background Information

Calcaneal apophysitis occurs when the open calcaneal physis of adolescents is disrupted by direct trauma, excessive shearing forces, or traction injury from tight calf musculature. This condition resolves with maturity and the closing of the epiphysis. The diagnosis is confirmed with the clinical examination. This condition is typically treated nonsurgically with rehabilitative interventions, including physical modalities and gentle flexibility and strengthening exercises for the lower quarter.

■ Calcific Tendinitis of the Flexor Hallucis Longus or Brevis

Chief Clinical Characteristics

This presentation may involve pain, edema, redness, and palpable tenderness on the plantar aspect of the first ray along the tendon. Pain is aggravated with bearing weight on the affected limb, walking, and passive stretching or action of the hallux flexors.

Background Information

The etiology of this condition is unclear. It is self-limiting. The diagnosis is confirmed with plain radiographs and biopsy. This condition is usually treated nonsurgically; however, surgical debridement of the affected tendon may be necessary in cases of recalcitrant disability.

■ Calluses

Chief Clinical Characteristics

This presentation includes tenderness located at a broad and diffuse hyperkeratotic lesion.

Background Information

This condition usually is the result of excessive friction or pressure, and usually is located under the first metatarsal head. Clinical examination confirms the diagnosis. Treatment usually includes mitigation of the callus with an abrasive block. In the case of recurring disease, analysis of plantar foot pressures should be undertaken in order to determine the optimal preventive footwear modification of orthoses.

■ Candidiasis

Chief Clinical Characteristics

This presentation can include burning pain, maceration, weeping lesions, and itching between the toes. Individuals with poor general health or immunosuppression are at particular risk for this condition.

Background Information

This condition results from a fungal infection from the *Candida* species. Microscopic laboratory culture confirms the diagnosis. Topical antifungal medication is the usual treatment of choice for this condition.

■ Cellulitis

Chief Clinical Characteristics

This presentation may involve pain, erythema, edema, warmth, and tenderness spreading from the region of the initial infection. Vesicles, bullae, necrosis, petechiae, and ecchymosis may be present. Fever, chills, headaches, malaise, hypotension, tachycardia, and delirium are the common signs of systemic involvement.

Background Information

This condition often results from a wound complication. Edema is a significant risk factor. There are multiple causative pathogens, of which *Staphylococcus* and *Streptococcus* species are the most common. Laboratory tests confirm the causative pathogen. Most cases are self-limiting. However, severe cases involve necrosis and may require surgical debridement and antibiotic therapy.

■ Cholesterol Embolism

Chief Clinical Characteristics

This presentation can be characterized by unilateral or bilateral foot pain associated with toes of a blue-black color, foot and toe gangrene, foot ulceration, and ischemia. Diminished or absent pulse is common in the affected artery.

Background Information

The embolism may develop as an atherosclerotic plaque is dislodged, resulting in complete or partial arterial occlusion. It is a rare but potentially fatal complication of cardiac catheterization, particularly using the descending thoracic aorta as a route.[13] Complications include renal embolism, penile gangrene, bowel infarction, or spinal cord infarction. The diagnosis is confirmed with Doppler ultrasonography, abnormal laboratory blood tests, histological conformation of involved tissues, or angiography. Treatment is symptomatic.

■ Cold Injuries

Chief Clinical Characteristics

This presentation often involves pain, paresthesias, and numbness followed by hyperemia and hypesthesias for at least several weeks following the injury. Frostnip is a reversible epithelial injury presenting as firm, cold white areas on the affected skin, changing to burning sensation with redness during rewarming, followed by peeling and blistering 24 to 72 hours after the presentation. Frostbite results in more serious tissue damage as a result of cells freezing. It presents as cold, white, hard, and anesthetic skin. Frostbitten skin may develop blistering with dry or wet gangrene of the deeper tissue.

Background Information

Clinical examination confirms the diagnosis. Treatment typically includes progressive rewarming of affected tissue. Tissues injured by cold tend toward additional damage during rewarming as a result of inflammation.[14]

■ Compartment Syndrome

Chief Clinical Characteristics

This presentation includes paresthesia and hypesthesia, followed by significant pain, massive edema, ecchymosis, soft tissue tenderness, erythema, palpable warmth, and weakness of the plantarflexors or toe flexors. Pulses and capillary refill often remain normal until the pressure increases to the level of severe injury.

Background Information

Compartment syndrome often is the result of trauma; however, it can occur spontaneously in patients with diabetes mellitus.[15] Altered vessel perfusion and edema result in increased intercompartmental pressure that disrupts the oxygen diffusion and results in ischemia. Clinical examination and intercompartmental pressure measurements confirm the diagnosis. This condition is a medical emergency and requires urgent surgical decompression.

■ Complex Regional Pain Syndrome

Chief Clinical Characteristics

This presentation may include a traumatic onset of severe chronic ankle and foot pain accompanied by allodynia, hyperalgesia, and trophic, vasomotor, and sudomotor changes in later stages. This condition is characterized by disproportionate responses to painful stimuli.

Background Information

This regional neuropathic pain disorder presents either without direct nerve trauma (Type I) or with direct nerve trauma (Type II) in any region of the body.[1] This condition may precipitate due to an event distant to the affected area. Thermography may confirm associated sympathetic dysfunction. Treatment may include physical therapy interventions to improve patient and client functioning, biofeedback, analgesic or anti-inflammatory medication, transcutaneous or spinal electrical nerve stimulation, and surgical or pharmacologic sympathectomy.

■ Corns

Chief Clinical Characteristics

This presentation includes painful and tender hyperkeratotic lesions that are small and conical. Pain often is localized to the site of the lesion with increased pain during weight bearing.

Background Information

This condition develops at the site of excessive or repetitive mechanical trauma or friction. The most common type is a hard corn. Soft corns result from the absorption of a considerable amount of perspiration, so they are usually more painful than hard corns. Clinical examination confirms the diagnosis. Treatment usually includes mitigation of the corn. In the case of recurring disease, analysis of plantar foot pressures should be undertaken to determine the optimal preventive footwear modification or orthoses.

■ Crush Injury

Chief Clinical Characteristics

This presentation can be characterized by pain with possible inability to bear weight on the affected limb following a crush injury.

Background Information

Clinical examination should determine if the source of pain is related to epithelial injury, soft tissue injury, or fracture. The nature and extent of the injury depends on the weight and composition of the object as well as the duration of time that it is applied to the foot. Even if the injury seems insignificant, the diagnosis may require clinical imaging to confirm the specific structures that are affected. Treatment depends on the extent and type of tissue involvement.

■ Cryoglobulinemia

Chief Clinical Characteristics

This presentation typically includes pain, weakness, paresthesia, sensory loss, Raynaud's phenomenon, toe gangrene, ulceration of the feet or toes, purpura, signs of glomerulonephritis, or gastrointestinal bleeding. Tissues and skin of the extremities are commonly affected.

Background Information

This condition is the result of macroglobulins that precipitate when plasma cools, leading to small-vessel damage in the tissues. Blood tests confirm the diagnosis. Usual treatments involve a combination of anti-inflammatory, interferon, and monoclonal antibody medications with plasmapheresis.

■ Dermatitis

Chief Clinical Characteristics
This presentation may involve superficial skin irritation characterized by epidermal edema, vesicles, erythema, oozing, crusting, scaling, usually pruritus, and lichenification. Sweating may be normal, diminished, or excessive.

Background Information
The three major types of dermatitis in the feet include contact dermatitis, atopic dermatitis, and dyshidrosis (pompholyx). Most cases of contact or atopic dermatitis are related to exposure of the skin to an irritating agent. Atopic dermatitis has a genetic susceptibility and exacerbations may be related to environmental irritants, emotional stress, temperature changes, bacterial skin infections, certain fabric softeners, nutritional deficiencies, and wool. Most cases of dyshidrosis are chronic forms of dermatitis and are idiopathic. Clinical examination confirms the diagnosis. Treatment typically involves a combination of risk factor modification with topical medication appropriately directed at the source of dermatitis if it can be identified.

DISLOCATIONS
■ Interphalangeal Joint

Chief Clinical Characteristics
This presentation can include pain, edema, difficulty weight bearing, tenderness to palpation, and gross deformity of the hallux interphalangeal joint.

Background Information
The interphalangeal joint of the hallux is the most common to dislocate, usually caused by axial loading of the hallux. The dislocation occurs in a dorsal direction. The sesamoid bone may become lodged between the distal phalanx and proximal phalanx as a possible complication. Plain radiographs confirm the diagnosis. Reduction of the dislocated joint is a usual treatment, and immobilization or surgical fixation may be necessary.

■ Metatarsophalangeal Joint

Chief Clinical Characteristics
This presentation may be characterized by pain, edema, tenderness, and gross deformity of the metatarsophalangeal joint. Hallux dislocation is the most common of all metatarsophalangeal dislocations.

Background Information
This condition may be complicated with injury to the sesamoid complex of the hallux. This dislocation usually is related to high-impact trauma and often involves injury to the joints of the midfoot. Plain radiographs confirm the diagnosis. Reduction of the dislocated joint is a usual treatment, and immobilization or surgical fixation may be necessary.

■ Distal Symmetric Polyneuropathy, Including From Acquired Immunodeficiency Syndrome, Alcohol/Drug Abuse, Carcinoma, Diabetes Mellitus, and Kidney Failure

Chief Clinical Characteristics
This presentation may be characterized by decreased distal deep tendon reflexes, as well as pain, dysesthesia, or paresthesia in the feet and toes.

Background Information
Peripheral neuropathy is one of the more common complications in patients presenting with acquired immunodeficiency syndrome, diabetes, renal failure, hypothyroidism, toxins, malignancy, and malnutrition. It is characterized by retrograde axonal degeneration, so this condition commonly progresses from distal to proximal. Electromyographic studies and biopsy confirm the diagnosis. Vibration and light touch sensation (10-g Semmes Weinstein monofilament) tests are useful to assess protective sensation. Curative treatment of this condition remains controversial, so the focus of intervention typically includes patient education to maintain blood glucose control and care for the insensate regions to prevent progression and complications secondary to this condition.

■ Dysplasia Epiphysealis Hemimelica (Trevor's Disease)

Chief Clinical Characteristics
This presentation can include a limp that may be accompanied by joint swelling, restricted

joint movement, or muscle wasting. Males are more likely to be affected than females.

Background Information
This condition is a congenital bone development disorder that is the result of an intra-articular osteochondromatosis (localized overgrowth of the cartilage) that is present in the epiphyses of the joint. This affects both sides of the epiphyses and joint deformity is often the result. This condition is most common at the medial ankle, but it also may be seen in the femur, the wrist, or the foot. Radiographs often reveal the structural changes to the joint. Treatment usually consists of surgical excision of the mass, as well as correction of any angular deformity that may have resulted. Nonsurgical intervention includes immobilization.

■ **Envenomation**
Chief Clinical Characteristics
This presentation may include immediate pain and redness at the location of the sting or venomous bite. Depending on the nature of the sting, the patient may have ecchymosis, edema, bullae, necrosis, ulceration, or gangrene.

Background Information
The extent of the injury will be determined by the nature of the bite or sting and the type of venom. Most stings are from sea urchins, fish, insects, or arthropods. Most common venomous bites are from snakes and spiders. Snake venom may be neurotoxic, hemotoxic, or cardiotoxic. Spider venom may be neurotoxic or necrotizing. Clinical examination confirms the diagnosis. This condition can be a medical emergency.

■ **Erosive Lichen Planus**
Chief Clinical Characteristics
This presentation typically includes cutaneous lesions that involve itchy and violaceous polygonal papules. Characteristic lesions are marked by Wickham's striae (itchy, violaceous, flat papules that are highlighted by white dots or lines). Papules often unite to form rough, scaly patches.

Background Information
Skin degeneration may occur with ulceration on the plantar, medial, or lateral surfaces of the foot. Several drug interactions and infections are suspected causes. Clinical examination confirms the diagnosis. These lesions are self-limiting and may take months or years to resolve.[16]

■ **Erythromelalgia**
Chief Clinical Characteristics
This presentation involves symmetric burning pain in the hands and feet of mild to disabling intensity with observable redness. Pain usually presents as attacks that are often aggravated by vasodilation, such as exposure to warmth or exercise. Alleviating factors include rest, elevation, and cryotherapy. The lower extremities are more often involved than the upper extremities.

Background Information
This disease is a result of paroxysmal vasodilation of unknown etiology. Doppler ultrasonography, transcutaneous oximetry, and nerve conduction studies confirm the diagnosis. Treatment may include anti-inflammatory medications.

■ **Fabry's Disease**
Chief Clinical Characteristics
This presentation often includes males with symmetrical skin lesions on the lower trunk (angiokeratomas), with common symptoms of burning pain in the lower extremities and feet. Pain in the hands or more proximal extremities, corneal opacities, cardiac involvement, and renal disease are other associated symptoms.

Background Information
This condition is a rare X-linked genetic disorder that leads to abnormal lipid metabolism. Heterozygous females are usually asymptomatic, but may display an attenuated version of this disease that is characterized by corneal opacities. Blood test or prenatal assay confirms the diagnosis. Treatment includes supportive intervention for the multisystem effects of this condition, as well as enzyme replacement therapy.

■ **Fat Pad Separation Secondary to a Cyst**
Chief Clinical Characteristics
This presentation may involve pain at the plantar heel, edema, and tenderness to palpation and pressure.

Background Information
This condition is caused by a fluid-filled bursa or cyst. The cyst or bursa may be palpable and

aid in the diagnosis. Treatment requires drainage of the cyst and rest to allow the fat pad to adhere to the calcaneus.

■ Fat Pad Syndrome

Chief Clinical Characteristics
This presentation includes pain and palpable tenderness on the plantar surface of the heel. Pain often increases with bearing weight on the affected limb, especially with barefoot walking and in the morning.

Background Information
Atrophy or inflammation of the heel fat pad may cause this condition, often as the result of repetitive traumatic compression of the fat pad secondary to repetitive overuse, overtraining, weak or fatigued lower extremity muscles, or training on hard surfaces. Clinical examination confirms the diagnosis. Usual treatment involves footwear modification, orthoses, activity modification, and strengthening weak muscles that may contribute to this condition.

■ Fixed Drug Eruption

Chief Clinical Characteristics
This presentation can often involve either immediate or delayed eruptions of the skin or mucous membranes as a result of administration of a drug. Redness, edema, pain, and tenderness of the affected skin often are observed. Responses can vary from a mild rash to epidermal necrolysis.

Background Information
In the feet, this condition often is secondary to oral drug administration (such as Antabuse, isoniazid, and other drugs that may cause sensory or sensorimotor neuropathy). Clinical examination confirms the diagnosis. Treatment typically includes ceasing the medication responsible for this condition. Individuals suspected of having this condition should be referred to a physician for further investigation and to supervise changes in an individual's medication regimen.

FRACTURES

■ Calcaneus

Chief Clinical Characteristics
This presentation includes severe heel pain associated with significant plantar edema, ecchymosis, tenderness, and occasional widening of the heel or development of a valgus deformity. Pain may be described as diffuse or sharp. Pain and edema presenting inferior to the medial malleolus and increased with inversion of the calcaneus or hyperextension of the great toe may indicate sustentaculum tali involvement. Pain inferior to the medial malleolus and reproduction of symptoms with forced dorsiflexion of the foot or toes may indicate possible medial calcaneal process involvement.

Background Information
This condition is caused by a fall or jump from height. Associated conditions may include diabetes mellitus, spinal and ankle fractures, severe ankle sprains, bilateral calcaneal fractures, peroneal injuries, flexor hallucis longus injury, and compartment syndrome. Complications may include loss of sensation and paresthesias of the distal foot, excruciating pain with toe movements, compartment syndrome, or subtalar arthritis. Plain radiographs confirm the diagnosis. Treatment ranges from immobilization and protected weight-bearing status in the event of a stable fracture, to surgical fixation for unstable or nonunion fractures.

■ Fifth Metatarsal

Chief Clinical Characteristics
This presentation involves pain and tenderness at the lateral aspect of the foot around the base of the fifth metatarsal.

Background Information
Typical fractures are either avulsion fractures or diaphyseal fractures. Avulsion fractures result from an inversion motion that is correlated with reflexive contraction of the peroneus brevis. Diaphyseal fractures are caused by loading through a foot that is in a plantarflexed and inverted position. Pain at the base of the fifth metatarsal or inability to bear weight on the affected limb may lead the clinician to utilize radiographs, which largely confirm the diagnosis.[17] Usual treatment ranges from immobilization and protected weight-bearing status in the event of a stable fracture, to surgical fixation for unstable or nonunion fractures.

■ Hallucal Sesamoid Disorders

Chief Clinical Characteristics
This presentation often involves pain and tenderness with palpation of the involved sesamoid, as well as dorsiflexion of the first metatarsophalangeal joint (Fig. 24-1).

Background Information
Fracture of either the medial (tibial) or lateral (fibular) sesamoid can occur with direct trauma, an avulsion injury, or from repetitive trauma. Bone scan, magnetic resonance imaging, or computed tomography confirms the diagnosis. Typically, treatment involves immobilization and protected weight-bearing status. In the event of recalcitrant pain and disability, however, surgical excision of the affected sesamoid(s) may be considered.

■ Lateral Process of the Talus

Chief Clinical Characteristics
This presentation may be characterized by pain, swelling, and tenderness along the anterior and inferior lateral ankle located directly over the lateral process of the talus. Pain increases with weight bearing, talocrural plantarflexion and dorsiflexion, and subtalar joint movement. The mechanism of injury is usually a dorsiflexion and inversion motion common in motor vehicle accidents, direct trauma, or snowboarding accidents.

Background Information
Chronic pain may be indicative of avascular necrosis. Bone scans, computed tomography,

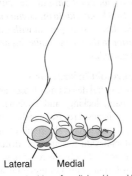

Lateral   Medial

FIGURE 24-1 Position of medial and lateral hallucal sesamoids.

and magnetic resonance imaging often assist in the diagnosis, staging, and prognosis of the injury. Surgical treatment is indicated for large or displaced fractures; otherwise, nonsurgical treatment is indicated.[18]

■ Lateral Tubercle of the Posterior Process of the Talus

Chief Clinical Characteristics
This presentation can involve posterolateral ankle pain, swelling, and tenderness over the lateral tubercle. Pain increases while walking downhill or downstairs, as well as with ankle and subtalar movement, active first toe flexion, or forced first toe dorsiflexion.

Background Information
This condition results from talocalcaneal ligament avulsion, posterior talofibular ligament avulsion, or a compressive force. It is associated with lateral ankle sprains, lateral malleolus avulsion fractures, and osteochondral defects on the talar dome. Clinical examination findings and radiographs confirm the diagnosis.[18] Surgical treatment is necessary for nonunion or displaced fractures.[18]

■ Medial Process of the Sustentaculum Tali of the Calcaneus

Chief Clinical Characteristics
This presentation typically includes pain, edema, and tenderness over the medial ankle, just inferior to the medial malleolus and along the heel. Pain increases with passive rearfoot inversion. Passive hyperextension of the first phalanx may increase pain due to the position of the flexor hallucis longus, just inferior to this structure.

Background Information
This condition may result from a fall onto the heel with an inverted foot; it is uncommon in isolation. Complications may include nonunion, nerve irritation, and toe flexor injury. Bone scan, computed tomography, or magnetic resonance imaging confirms the diagnosis. Surgical fixation may be necessary in the event of an unstable or nonunion fracture.

■ Medial Tuberosity of the Posterior Process of the Talus

Chief Clinical Characteristics

This presentation typically includes ankle pain that is posterior to the medial malleolus and anterior to the Achilles tendon. The injury often results from dorsiflexion-pronation ankle injuries, ankle dislocation, or possibly an avulsion fracture from a posterior tibiotalar injury.

Background Information

Bone scan, computed tomography scan, or magnetic resonance imaging may assist in the diagnosis, staging, and prognosis. In the event of unstable fractures or nonunion, surgical fixation may be necessary.

■ Metatarsal

Chief Clinical Characteristics

This presentation may be characterized by pain, tenderness, and sometimes edema around the location of the injury. Pain is aggravated when bearing weight on the affected limb and alleviated with rest in a non–weight-bearing position.

Background Information

Most commonly, this condition involves a fracture along one or more of the metatarsal shafts. Repetitive overuse commonly causes this condition, although it also could result from acute trauma. Common fractures may include an avulsion, diaphyseal fracture, or stress fracture, which may share a common clinical presentation. Clinical examination confirms the diagnosis. Additional certainty may be obtained with plain radiographs.[19] Treatment depends on severity and ranges from nonsurgical to surgical interventions.

■ Navicular

Chief Clinical Characteristics

This presentation includes pain and tenderness that is located at the medial and dorsal aspect of the midfoot. Pain is provoked with weight-bearing activities and running.

Background Information

Stress fractures are more common in the athletic population due to repetitive high-impact trauma. They may present without significant edema, while traumatic or avulsion fractures typically present with edema. Traumatic fractures are due to avulsion of the distal insertion of the posterior tibialis tendon; less commonly, trauma to the navicular or the calcaneus may lead to a direct fracture or dislocation. Diagnosis is confirmed with plain radiographs, magnetic resonance imaging, or computed tomography. Usually, treatment depends on severity and ranges from nonsurgical to surgical interventions.

■ Osteochondral Fracture of the Subtalar Joint

Chief Clinical Characteristics

This presentation typically includes pain, edema, and tenderness at the sinus tarsi or just distal to the lateral malleolus. Pain is worsened with subtalar passive motion. Peroneal muscle spasm and tenderness may be present.

Background Information

Often, osteochondral lesions of the subtalar joint are idiopathic. The diagnosis is confirmed with magnetic resonance imaging. Treatment is usually nonsurgical, with arthrodesis considered for individuals with recalcitrant pain and disability.[20]

■ Osteochondral Fracture of the Talar Dome

Chief Clinical Characteristics

This presentation includes variable symptoms based on the site of the osteochondral lesion. Lateral dome lesions commonly present with localized pain at the central and lateral ankle anterior to the lateral malleolus. Medial dome lesions present with tenderness posterior to the medial malleolus and at the posterior talus.

Background Information

Osteochondral defects may loosen and cause joint pain, locking, and swelling. Lateral dome injuries are frequently associated with trauma, usually the result of an inversion-dorsiflexion mechanism. Medial dome injuries may either be the result of inversion-plantarflexion trauma or present insidiously. Radiographs, magnetic resonance imaging, and arthroscopy confirm the diagnosis. Patients should be monitored because joint degeneration is common following these injuries.[21]

■ Posterosuperior Calcaneal Tuberosity

Chief Clinical Characteristics
This presentation may be characterized by pain, swelling, and possible ecchymosis located at the calcaneal insertion of the Achilles tendon, the posterior heel, and the posterior ankle. The patient will often have a functional loss of plantarflexion, such as with a single-leg heel raise, due to the avulsion fracture. This condition is most common in older individuals with advanced age, diabetes mellitus, or osteoporosis.

Background Information
The mechanism of injury is a rapid pull of the Achilles tendon. A positive Thompson test and a palpable sulcus may be present if the tendon is avulsed. Associated findings may include an Achilles tendon tear or other extra-articular calcaneal fractures. Plain radiographs confirm the diagnosis. Treatment may range from nonsurgical interventions, such as protected weight bearing and immobilization, to surgical fixation of unstable or nonunion fractures.

■ Stress Fracture of the Calcaneus

Chief Clinical Characteristics
This presentation can include diffuse pain, edema, and possible erythema in the heel. Pain increases with bearing weight on the affected limb and decreases with rest.

Background Information
This condition develops through repetitive overuse, overtraining, weak or fatigued lower extremity muscles, or training on hard surfaces. This presentation may be associated with low to flat arch height and weak intrinsic foot musculature. Clinical examination, including the squeeze test, confirms the diagnosis. Additional certainty may be obtained with bone scan. Usual treatment involves protected weight bearing in combination with activity modification, footwear

modification, orthoses, and strengthening and flexibility exercises for weak or tight lower quarter muscles that may be responsible for contributory pathomechanics.

■ Stress Fracture of the Lateral Malleolus

Chief Clinical Characteristics
This presentation may involve focused, localized, superficial aching or sharp pain directly on the lateral malleolus at the site of the fracture (usually within 15 cm [6 in.] of the distal fibula). Mild edema may be present but is not required for the diagnosis. Tenderness usually is present with direct palpation, and pain may be provoked with vibration testing. Pain rarely is present at rest unless the fracture is severe.

Background Information
This condition occurs as a result of abnormal loading from a sudden increase in training, repetitive forces, training on hard surfaces, improper footwear, or ankle and foot dysfunction (such as a valgus deformity or severe flat-foot deformity). Bone scan confirms the diagnosis. Treatment typically involves protected weight bearing in combination with activity modification, footwear modification, orthoses, and strengthening and flexibility exercises for weak or tight lower quarter muscles that may be responsible for contributory pathomechanics.

■ Tarsometatarsal Joint (Lisfranc's) Fracture or Dislocation

Chief Clinical Characteristics
This presentation can include pain, tenderness, and edema at the location of the involved joint or joints. Pain may be reproduced with active supination, pronation, or weight bearing, and deformity may be present.

Background Information
This condition is caused by axial loading through a plantarflexed foot. Even seemingly mild injuries may lead to degeneration at the tarsometatarsal joints, which lead to future complications and pain.[22] This injury is commonly associated with tarsometatarsal ligament sprain. The diagnosis

is confirmed with plain radiographs. Treatment commonly involves surgical reduction and fixation.

■ Toe

Chief Clinical Characteristics
This presentation involves pain, edema, tenderness to palpation, ecchymosis, and often a subungual hematoma. This condition is associated with difficulty bearing weight on the affected lower extremity, with terminal stance gait abnormalities to reduce loading on the forefoot and toes.

Background Information
This condition usually occurs as a result of direct trauma to a toe. Ligament damage is a potential complication. Plain radiographs confirm the diagnosis. Usual treatment includes immobilization and protected weight bearing; however, reduction and fixation may be considered for unstable or nonunion fractures.

■ Freiberg's Disease

Chief Clinical Characteristics
This presentation often involves pain, tenderness, and edema over the second and third metatarsal heads. The second metatarsal head is involved 75% of the time and females are more commonly affected.

Background Information
This condition is a form of osteochondrosis with avascular necrosis that follows repetitive trauma. Radiography, radionuclide bone scan, and magnetic resonance imaging confirm the diagnosis. Immobilization is a primary treatment, with surgical debridement reserved for cases of advanced disease.

■ Glomus Tumor

Chief Clinical Characteristics
This presentation typically includes localized pain and tenderness on the plantar heel. A palpable nodule may be present. Pain will not increase with dorsiflexion of the toes, although cold often aggravates the symptoms.

Background Information
This condition results from an organized arteriovenous anastomosis. Diagnosis may be confirmed with imaging, including ultrasound or

magnetic resonance imaging. Surgical excision is a common treatment.

■ Gout

Chief Clinical Characteristics
This presentation includes severe pain, edema, warmth, erythema, and very localized tenderness. Systemic findings may include fever, chills, malaise, and sweating. The areas typically involved are the first metatarsophalangeal joint, the talocrural joint, the calcaneal region, and the tarsals of the instep. Pain is usually provoked by hard movements, or may follow alcohol abuse, dehydration, trauma, surgery, septic arthritis, protein fasting, excessive purine ingestion, and allopurinol or uricosuric agents.

Background Information
Sustained hyperuricemia levels lead to deposition of monosodium urate crystals in and around the tendons and joints. Men are eight times more likely to be affected than women.[23] Needle aspiration is required to confirm the diagnosis. Treatment commonly involves a combination of anti-inflammatory medication and colchicine in individuals with normal liver function. Preventive treatment should be undertaken to control uric acid levels by way of diet and medication in individuals with chronic gout.

■ Haglund's Syndrome

Chief Clinical Characteristics
This presentation can be characterized by pain and edema along the posterior heel and Achilles tendon, near the distal insertion at the calcaneus. Symptoms are reproduced with direct palpation, passive or forceful dorsiflexion, and resisted plantarflexion. Walking and running are very painful during late stance phase, and high shoe heel counters also will aggravate symptoms.

Background Information
This condition is a prominent superior calcaneal tuberosity. Haglund's syndrome is the combination of retrocalcaneal bursitis, superficial Achilles bursitis, Achilles tendinopathy, and Haglund's deformity—a prominent posterior superior tuberosity of the calcaneus.[24] The diagnosis is confirmed with the combination of plain radiographs and clinical examination. Treatment is typically nonsurgical, with surgical reshaping of the superior calcaneal tuberosity combined with debridement

of the Achilles tendon insertion reserved for cases of recalcitrant symptoms and disability.

■ Hallux Rigidus

Chief Clinical Characteristics

This presentation can include pain, decreased range of motion, edema, possible bony prominence with redness, and tenderness at the first metatarsophalangeal joint. Common gait abnormalities include a decreased terminal stance phase and rolling the foot into supination. Pain may be present with metatarsophalangeal extension.

Background Information

Hallux rigidus or limitus results from degenerative changes to the first metatarsophalangeal joint. Clinical examination confirms the diagnosis. Usual nonsurgical treatments involve physical therapy intervention, footwear modification, and orthoses. Surgical treatments include wedge osteotomy.

■ Hallux Valgus

Chief Clinical Characteristics

This presentation may involve medial pain, edema, redness, metatarsalgia pain, and tenderness as a result of the prominence of the great toe. This condition may progress to the point that deviation develops in other toes. An adventitious bursa may develop, and patients also may have difficulty wearing desired footwear.

Background Information

This condition is truly an abductus deformity, better termed *hallux abductovalgus*. It is associated with cartilage damage within the first metatarsophalangeal joint; the degree of cartilage damage and angle of deformity are directly related. Clinical examination confirms the diagnosis. Usual nonsurgical treatments involve physical therapy intervention, footwear modification, and orthoses. Surgical treatments include a variety of techniques to correct the deformity.

■ Hammer Toe Deformity

Chief Clinical Characteristics

This presentation typically includes pain, redness, tenderness, blister formation, or the presence of a corn or callus formation. Some of these patients will present with a history of subungual hematomas as a result of the repetitive trauma.

Background Information

A hammer toe deformity is a position of proximal interphalangeal joint flexion with distal interphalangeal joint extension. The injuries to the toes are a result of this deformity, whether flexible or rigid, that leads to altered mechanical pressure and friction. Typical treatments for clinically significant forms of this condition that cause intolerable pain and disability involve surgical procedures to straighten the toes.

■ Hand-Foot-and-Mouth Disease

Chief Clinical Characteristics

This presentation can include vesicular eruption around the buccal mucosa or the tongue, as well as similar lesions on the palms of the hands and the soles of the feet. Skin lesions are painful to palpation and pressure.

Background Information

The disease is a result of a viral infection, most often by Coxsackie virus A 16.[25] This condition is more common in young children than adults. Molecular assay confirms the diagnosis.[26] Typically, treatment is supportive pending resolution of the underlying viral infection.

■ Hepatitis B–Associated Arthritis

Chief Clinical Characteristics

This presentation involves a symmetric polyarthralgia that can affect the toes, and more commonly, the fingers. The common symptoms include anorexia, malaise, nausea, vomiting, and fever. Jaundice usually develops in approximately 1 to 2 weeks.

Background Information

Hepatitis is an inflammation of the liver as a result of viral infection with necrosis of the liver. Arthralgia usually is the result of an aseptic inflammation of the joints. Blood tests confirm the diagnosis.

■ Herpes Zoster

Chief Clinical Characteristics

This presentation typically includes an exquisitely painful rash or blisters along a specific dermatomal pattern accompanied by flu-like symptoms. Individuals with this condition also demonstrate a previous history of varicella exposure or infection. Pain associated with this condition may be disproportionate to the extent of skin irritation. The initial presentation of this condition may be confused with radiculopathy due to the distribution of symptoms. The presence of the rash, extreme pain, general malaise, and unclear association with spinal movement aids in differential diagnosis.

Background Information

The virus remains dormant in the spinal ganglia until its reactivation during a period of stress, infection, or physical exhaustion. Treatment includes the administration of antiviral agents as soon as the zoster eruption is noted, ideally within 48 to 72 hours. If timing is greater than 3 days, treatment is aimed at controlling pain and pruritus and minimizing the risk of secondary infection.[27]

■ Hypersensitivity Vasculitis

Chief Clinical Characteristics

This presentation often includes pruritic skin lesions, necrosis, and painful ulcerations of the feet and toes. Associated conditions may include joint pain, hepatosplenomegaly, lymphadenopathy, or glomerulonephritis.

Background Information

This condition is an inflammation of the postcapillary venule that is caused by a drug interaction or immune complex interaction, resulting in leukocytoclastic angiitis.[28] Biopsy and subsequent histological investigation confirm the diagnosis. This condition is often self-limiting and resolves without specific treatment. Topical or oral anti-inflammatory medication may be necessary for individuals with persistent symptoms.

■ Idiopathic Metatarsophalangeal Synovitis

Chief Clinical Characteristics

This presentation may involve tenderness, pain, and edema of the involved joints. Pain is aggravated with forced flexion of the metatarsophalangeal joint. Monoarticular metatarsophalangeal joint synovitis is more common than multiple joint involvement. Commonly, the second ray is more affected.

Background Information

A history of trauma or injury is not frequently reported. Clinical examination confirms the diagnosis, and plain radiographs often will be unremarkable. Nonsurgical interventions are often preferred, including footwear modification, orthoses, taping, and rehabilitative exercises. Synovectomy may be required in individuals with persistent symptoms and disability.

■ Infected Blister

Chief Clinical Characteristics

This presentation can be characterized by burning and pain at the site of a blister. Purulence of the blister fluid with redness and edema around the blister are associated signs. Signs of systemic involvement may include fever, chills, malaise, or myalgia.

Background Information

Blisters of the feet may result from friction between the skin and a sock or shoe.[29] Clinical examination confirms the diagnosis. Treatment for this condition usually includes risk factor mitigation, wound dressing, and oral antibiotic medication.

■ Intermittent Acute Porphyria

Chief Clinical Characteristics

This presentation includes neurovisceral symptoms with abdominal pain attacks and associated symptoms of nausea, vomiting, constipation, or diarrhea. Exacerbating factors include drugs, hormones, or dietary restrictions (eg, low-calorie or low-carbohydrate diets).

Background Information

Neuropathy can lead to burning pain in the feet and/or hands, paresthesias, numbness, dysesthesias, myalgias, and symmetrical or asymmetrical weakness. Associated symptoms also may include bladder and urinary symptoms, behavioral changes, hypertension, tachycardia, and cardiac or respiratory failure. Reflexes may be diminished or absent. This condition is an autosomal dominant disorder that results from porphobilinogen deaminase deficiency.[30] Urine, blood, and deoxyribonucleic acid tests confirm the diagnosis. Treatment involves medications to reduce heme synthesis, as well as supportive interventions for the multisystem effects of this condition.

■ Interosseous Myositis

Chief Clinical Characteristics

This presentation involves pain and palpable tenderness in between the metatarsal bones with pain aggravated by weight-bearing and frontal plane movements. Pain usually is worst in the morning.

Background Information

Midfoot and forefoot support often alleviate the pain associated with this condition, such as when wearing shoes. Overuse injury of the interosseous muscles may cause this condition. Magnetic resonance imaging confirms the diagnosis. The usual treatment for this condition is nonsurgical, including footwear and activity modification, orthoses, and oral nonsteroidal anti-inflammatory medication.

■ Ischemic Ulceration of the Toes

Chief Clinical Characteristics

This presentation can involve pain, tenderness, ulceration, and blackening of the great toe. The foot or toe may be cold, pulseless, and pale.

Background Information

This condition results from tissue ischemia, and the nature of vascular compromise determines the affected distribution of foot and toes. This condition is caused by thrombus, embolism, vasculitis, or small artery occlusion. Doppler ultrasonography confirms the diagnosis. Treatment includes wound management strategies combined with interventions to improve tissue perfusion. Interventions to improve tissue perfusion are appropriately directed to the cause of ischemia.

■ Joplin's Neuroma

Chief Clinical Characteristics

This presentation can include pain and paresthesia at the medial plantar surface of the foot, just distal to the first metatarsophalangeal joint and into the first digit. Pain may be worsened during weight bearing on the affected limb or when wearing certain shoes.

Background Information

Entrapment of the medial plantar nerve near the hallux causes this condition. Clinical examination, including Tinel's or compression sign along the involved nerve, confirms the diagnosis. Usual treatment is nonsurgical, with surgical intervention reserved for cases in which the site of entrapment is well characterized.

■ Leukemia

Chief Clinical Characteristics

This presentation typically includes a variety of symptoms including bony foot pain, malaise, fatigue, excessive bruising or bleeding, night sweats, and weight loss. Acute disorders have a more rapid onset with illness.[31]

Background Information

Leukemic cells will accumulate in the bone marrow and replace the normal hematopoietic cells, which may then infiltrate any other organ. Acute myelogenous leukemias constitute 85% of adult acute leukemias. Chronic lymphocytic leukemia is responsible for 30% of all leukemias in the Western countries and the median age of onset is the seventh decade; whereas acute lymphoblastic leukemia is responsible for 80% of childhood cases.[32] Foot pain may result from either an arthritis or symmetrical peripheral polyneuropathy. The diagnosis is confirmed with the presence of disabling bone pain, night pain, hematologic findings in the blood tests, leucopenia, or positive findings in a bone marrow biopsy.[33–35] Typical treatments for this condition involve chemotherapy, radiation, monoclonal antibody medication, and stem cell transplantation.

LIGAMENT SPRAINS

■ Anterior Talofibular Ligament

Chief Clinical Characteristics

This presentation can include pain, swelling, tenderness to palpation, and possible ecchymosis just anterior and inferior to the lateral malleolus, directly over the ligament. Weight bearing and combined inversion/plantarflexion motions of the foot will be painful and may be limited by pain. If the ligament is completely torn, then pain may or may not be present with excessive inversion.

Background Information

Injury to the ligament is usually caused by an inversion and plantarflexion mechanism to the ankle. Associated injuries may include calcaneofibular ligament sprain, syndesmotic ligament sprain, sinus tarsi syndrome with a subtalar sprain, superficial peroneal nerve injury, fifth metatarsal fracture, medial ankle impingement, a medial or lateral malleolar fracture, talar or osteochondral fractures, or peroneal tendon injury. Diagnosis is usually based on the clinical presentation, mechanism of injury, and a positive anterior translation test of the talus. If pain or instability persists, then radiographs are helpful to rule out fractures, osteochondral defects, or structural instability with stress. Nonsurgical intervention is commonly indicated; however, surgical stabilization may be indicated in the event of a mechanically unstable joint.

■ Calcaneofibular Ligament (Isolated)

Chief Clinical Characteristics

This presentation can be characterized by swelling and tenderness along the lateral ankle, inferior to the lateral malleolus, along the ligament. Pain increases with foot inversion.

Background Information

Injury to the ligament occurs during an inversion mechanism of the ankle, with the ankle in neutral or even sometimes dorsiflexion. This injury rarely occurs independently, and is commonly associated with anterior talofibular ligament sprains, lateral malleolus fractures, and syndesmotic injuries. Diagnosis is based on the clinical presentation and the use of radiographs may be useful to rule out any additional injuries or complications. Nonsurgical intervention is commonly indicated; however surgical stabilization may be indicated in the event of a mechanically unstable joint.

■ Cruciate Crural Ligament

Chief Clinical Characteristics

This presentation may include pain and tenderness to palpation along the ligament on the dorsum of the ankle and foot. Pain is intensified with plantarflexion of the toes, but is present even at rest. Paresthesias or weakness may be present if the injury causes increased intracompartmental pressure.

Background Information

Injury to this ligament may be due to either direct or indirect trauma. Complications may include injury to the blood vessels or nerves on the surface of the foot. Palpation for pedal pulses, neurological examination, and possibly a Doppler should be used to determine the extent of the injury to the nerves or vasculature. Treatment will often consist of rest to allow for healing, provided that nerve and vascular injuries are absent.

■ Forefoot

Chief Clinical Characteristics

This presentation may be characterized by pain, edema, and tenderness to palpation. Symptoms are aggravated with range of motion or weight bearing through a dorsiflexed or extended joint. Deformity may result if there is significant damage to the ligamentous and other passive stabilizing structures.

Background Information

This condition results from movement beyond the normal range of the joint in any of the planes of movement, usually through a hyperextension injury of the metatarsophalangeal joints. Clinical examination confirms the diagnosis, and plain radiographs may be useful to rule out fracture. Treatment usually consists of activity and footwear modification along with anti-inflammatory medications, with arthrodesis necessary in the presence of symptoms and disability related to gross mechanical instability.

■ Metatarsophalangeal Joint

Chief Clinical Characteristics

This presentation typically includes pain, edema, and tenderness to palpation. Pain is aggravated with range of motion or bearing weight on the affected limb through the affected joint while it is dorsiflexed.

Background Information

This condition is commonly caused by a hyperextension injury of the metatarsophalangeal joint. Clinical examination confirms the diagnosis. Plain radiographs may be helpful to exclude avulsion fractures and disruptions of the sesamoid and flexor hallucis longus complex. Typical treatment involves rest and footwear modification along with anti-inflammatory medications.

■ Longitudinal Arch Strain

Chief Clinical Characteristics

This presentation involves pain on the plantar aspect of the foot, primarily along the medial aspect of the foot. Pain is aggravated by weight bearing or dorsiflexion of the foot, and alleviated by rest or plantarflexion of the foot.

Background Information
Prolonged weight bearing that results in ligament sprain or muscle fatigue causes this condition. Individuals with excessive foot pronation, pes cavus, pes planus, or excessive ligament laxity are usually more prone to this condition. Clinical examination confirms the diagnosis. Typical treatment involves rest and footwear modification along with anti-inflammatory medications, as well as stretching and strengthening of muscle length and strength deficits that may contribute to this condition.

■ **Lymphoma**
Chief Clinical Characteristics
This presentation may include foot pain, tingling, paresthesias, or weakness that results from a sometimes present polyneuropathy.[36] Some of the most common symptoms include fever, night sweats, or weight loss.

Background Information
Congestion and edema of the face and neck as well as ureteral compression are common in individuals with non-Hodgkin's lymphoma. Hodgkin's lymphoma is caused by malignant proliferation of tumor cells in the lymphoreticular system, while non-Hodgkin's lymphoma is proliferation of lymphoid cells within the immune system. Diagnosis may be confirmed with histological study of a biopsy or excised tissue. Treatment will vary based on the type of lymphoma. Common treatments include chemotherapy, radiation, and bone marrow transplantation.

■ **Mallet Toe Deformity**
Chief Clinical Characteristics
This presentation can involve pain, redness, tenderness, blister formation, or the presence of a corn or callus formation. Some of these patients will present with a history of subungual hematomas as a result of the repetitive trauma.

Background Information
A mallet toe deformity is a position of distal and proximal interphalangeal joint flexion. This condition is often termed "claw toe" deformity. The injuries to the toes are a result of this deformity, whether flexible or rigid, that leads to altered mechanical pressure and friction. Typical treatments for clinically significant forms of this condition that cause intolerable pain and disability involve surgical procedures to straighten the toes.

■ **Metastases to the Foot, Including From Primary Breast, Kidney, Lung, Prostate, and Thyroid Disease**
Chief Clinical Characteristics
This presentation can be characterized by unremitting pain in individuals with these risk factors: previous history of cancer, age 50 years or older, failure to improve with conservative therapy, and unexplained weight change of more than 10 pounds in 6 months.[37]

Background Information
The skeletal system is the third most common site of metastatic disease.[38] Symptoms also may be related to pathological fracture in affected sites. Common primary sites causing metastases to bone include breast, prostate, lung, and kidney. Bone scan confirms the diagnosis. Common treatments for metastases include surgical resection, chemotherapy, radiation treatment, and palliation, depending on the tumor type and extent of metastasis.

■ **Metatarsalgia**
Chief Clinical Characteristics
This presentation can include pain and palpable tenderness on the plantar aspect of the metatarsal heads. Pain is aggravated with weight bearing, especially with a heel rise or during the terminal stance in gait.

Background Information
This condition is the result of imbalanced weight distribution across the metatarsal heads, leading to overuse trauma to the bones, joints, and surrounding tissues. Clinical examination confirms the diagnosis. Additional certainty may be obtained by plantar pressure measurement during walking. Typical treatment involves rest and footwear modification, anti-inflammatory medications, and gentle exercise for lower quarter muscle length and strength deficits that may lead to this condition.

■ Morton's Neuroma

Chief Clinical Characteristics

This presentation involves sharp or burning forefoot pain or numbness that may be generalized or in the distribution of a specific digital nerve (Fig. 24-2). Pain may be particularly present while wearing shoes, with additional increases while bearing weight on the metatarsal heads, and during walking, standing, or active ankle dorsiflexion.

Background Information

This condition is caused by thickening and fibrosis of the interdigital nerve; it is most common in the third intermetatarsal space. Clinical examination, including palpation and Mulder's test, and response to local corticosteroid injections confirm the diagnosis.[39] Corticosteroid injection is a diagnostic test as well as a form of treatment. Other usual treatments include footwear and activity modification, orthoses, anti-inflammatory medications, and gentle exercise for lower quarter muscle length and strength deficits that may lead to this condition.

■ Multiple Myeloma

Chief Clinical Characteristics

This presentation may involve unexplained skeletal pain in the feet, lower legs, arms, hands, back, and thorax. This may be associated with renal failure, recurrent bacterial infections, pathological fractures, and anemia.

Background Information

This condition is an insidious plasma cell cancer that originates in the bone marrow and can affect multiple areas with multiple lytic and osteosclerotic effects. Pain results from either

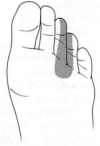

FIGURE 24-2 Distribution of symptoms in Morton's neuroma.

neuropathy or bone pain. Radiographically, the bones will have lesions of a punched-out appearance with generalized osteoporosis. Diagnosis may be confirmed with blood tests, urinalysis, serum protein electrophoresis, bone scan, magnetic resonance imaging, and bone marrow aspiration and biopsy. Depending on the aggressiveness of this condition, treatment may range from "watchful waiting" to chemotherapy and bone marrow transplantation.

■ Necrotizing Fasciitis

Chief Clinical Characteristics

This presentation often is characterized by pain with erythema, warmth, swelling, possible skin discoloration, blisters, gangrene, and joint crepitus. Systemic signs of an infection may include fever, tachycardia, hypotension, diaphoresis, chills, malaise and altered mental status. The wound may be odorous and sometimes subcutaneous gas is observed.

Background Information

The underlying infection often is caused by a bacterium following trauma or infection of an open wound or ulcer. This condition often is mistaken for cellulitis in its early stages. Diagnosis may be confirmed with radiographs or abnormal blood serum tests, and a Gram stain of the infected tissue will often provide the best diagnostic information. This condition is a medical emergency. Treatment includes debridement of necrotic tissue and an aggressive regimen of antibiotic medication.

NERVE ENTRAPMENTS

■ Calcaneal Branch Neurodynia

Chief Clinical Characteristics

This presentation includes local medial heel pain, located inferior and posterior to the tarsal tunnel. Pain often is increased with weight bearing, direct palpation, or neural tension testing with the ankle in dorsiflexion and foot eversion. A valgus hindfoot posture is common.

Background Information

This condition results from compression or tension on the calcaneal branch of the tibial nerve. It may be caused by space-occupying lesions, fractures, calluses, arthritis and osteophytes, edema, bursitis, tendinitis or tenosynovitis, accessory bones, or prolonged direct and indirect pressures. The clinical examination, including neurodynamic testing, confirms the diagnosis. Usual treatment is nonsurgical, with surgical release of entrapment sites reserved for cases in which the site of entrapment is well characterized.

■ Deep Peroneal Nerve

Chief Clinical Characteristics
This presentation involves pain, numbness, dysesthesias, and/or paresthesias at the first dorsal web space of the foot. Ankle plantarflexion or foot inversion may aggravate symptoms. This condition may present as anterolateral ankle pain or weakness of ankle dorsiflexion.

Background Information
The extensor retinaculum is the most common site of entrapment. However, other sources of compression may include tight shoelaces, anterior compartment syndrome, ankle fracture, ganglion, and other forms of trauma. Electromyographic tests confirm the diagnosis. Treatment is typically nonsurgical, with surgical exploration and release of entrapment sites reserved for cases in which the site of entrapment is well characterized.

■ First Branch of the Lateral Plantar Nerve

Chief Clinical Characteristics
This presentation may involve pain and tenderness present over the plantar aspect of the heel, just slightly anterior and medial to the plantar fascia insertion on the calcaneal tuberosity. Pain also may be palpable at the distal tibial nerve, along the medial plantar foot.

Background Information
The most common entrapment site is distal to the tarsal tunnel. Clinical examination, including neurodynamic testing, confirms the diagnosis. Treatment is typically nonsurgical, with surgical exploration and release of entrapment sites reserved for cases in which the site of entrapment is well characterized.

■ Superficial Peroneal Nerve

Chief Clinical Characteristics
This presentation can include pain, paresthesia, dysesthesia, or numbness on the anterolateral lower leg and dorsum of the foot. Plantarflexion and foot inversion are often aggravating factors, and Tinel's sign over the superficial peroneal nerve also may reproduce pain. Associated motor deficits may include weakness or foot eversion.

Background Information
Etiology includes compression due to trauma or idiopathic entrapment.[40] This condition is a diagnosis of exclusion after lumbar radiculopathy has been ruled out. The clinical examination, including the straight leg raise test and a standard neurological examination, and electrodiagnostic tests confirm the diagnosis. Treatment is typically nonsurgical, with surgical release of entrapment sites reserved for cases in which the site of entrapment is well characterized.

■ Sural Nerve

Chief Clinical Characteristics
This presentation may often include hypesthesia or paresthesia and pain along the posterior calf, posterolateral ankle, or dorsolateral foot. Tinel's sign also may reproduce pain. This condition does not include motor involvement because the sural nerve is a sensory afferent.

Background Information
Common etiologies include ankle sprains, stretch injury, Achilles injury, trauma, nerve compression due to ganglion cyst, or a calcaneal fracture. This condition is a diagnosis of exclusion after lumbar radiculopathy is ruled out. The clinical examination, including the straight leg raise test and a standard neurological examination, and electrodiagnostic tests confirm the diagnosis. Typically, treatment is nonsurgical, with surgical exploration and release of entrapment sites reserved for cases in which the site of entrapment is well characterized.

■ Tarsal Tunnel Syndrome

Chief Clinical Characteristics
This presentation involves hypesthesia, pain, and paresthesia due to compression of the tibial nerve at the ankle, located around the medial aspect of the ankle and the plantar surface of the foot. Symptoms often are worse with walking, with compression, and with a dorsiflexion-eversion test. They present with

a positive Tinel's sign. Rest alleviates symptoms. Weakness of the flexor hallucis and flexor digitorum brevis muscles is rarely present.

Background Information

Common etiologies are space-occupying lesions, fractures, edema, tendinitis or tenosynovitis, accessory bones, or prolonged direct and indirect pressures from inflammation and fluid retention as a result of systemic diseases (rheumatoid arthritis, ankylosing spondylitis) or significant hindfoot pronation that causes tibial nerve stretch. Diagnosis is confirmed with the clinical examination and nerve conduction studies. Usual treatment is nonsurgical, with surgical release of entrapment sites reserved for cases in which the site of entrapment is well characterized.

■ Osler's Nodules

Chief Clinical Characteristics

This presentation may be characterized by painfully tender, small, red lesions with a central elevation on the tips of the toes. Systemic signs of infection may include fever, myalgia, pallor, anorexia, a heart murmur, and encephalopathy.

Background Information

This condition involves small microabscesses that are associated with bacterial endocarditis. Blood cultures and echocardiography confirm the diagnosis. Treatment involves antibiotic intervention directed toward the underlying organism, which is Staphylococcus aureus.

OSTEOARTHROSIS/ OSTEOARTHRITIS

■ Interphalangeal Joint

Chief Clinical Characteristics

This presentation typically includes pain, tenderness, and edema. Pain is worsened with active and passive range of motion to the joint.

Background Information

The pain and arthritis usually are initiated by either acute trauma or cumulative stress that results from changes in anatomical and functional alignment. Plain radiographs that indicate spurring or joint space narrowing confirm the diagnosis. Treatment is typically nonsurgical, except in cases of intractable symptoms and disability in which arthrodesis may be considered.

■ Midfoot (Tarsometatarsal Joints)

Chief Clinical Characteristics

This presentation typically includes pain, localized tenderness, crepitus, and joint noise located at the involved joint. Patients usually report increased pain and stiffness in the morning and after prolonged static postures. Onset of pain is usually gradual and symptoms are often worsened by exercise.

Background Information

In the midfoot, some of the more common sites of osteoarthrosis include the first metatarsocuneiform joint and the cuboid-metatarsal joint. Osteoarthrosis is a progressive disorder that usually starts in the second or third decade of life. The cause of osteoarthrosis is often thought of as either idiopathic or secondary to conditions that affect the environment of the joint (such as infection, inflammation, genetic defects, or trauma). Radiographs will often confirm the diagnosis and reveal damage to the involved joint, such as narrowing of the joint space, formation of osteophytes, and formation of pseudocysts in the subchondral bone. Usual treatment is nonsurgical, with arthrodesis considered for cases of recalcitrant symptoms and disability.

■ Small Toes

Chief Clinical Characteristics

This presentation typically includes pain, tenderness, and edema of the involved joint or joints. Active and passive range of motion may reproduce symptoms.

Background Information

This condition usually is initiated by trauma or increased stress that results from changes in lower extremity alignment. Plain radiographs that demonstrate joint space narrowing and bone spurs confirm the diagnosis. Typically, treatment is nonsurgical, except in cases of intractable symptoms and disability in which arthrodesis may be considered.

■ Osteomyelitis

Chief Clinical Characteristics

This presentation typically includes localized tenderness, warmth, erythema, edema, and systemic signs of infection such as weight loss and fatigue. The toes may present with a "sausage toe" deformity.

Background Information

This condition is an inflammation and necrosis of bone as a result of an infection. The calcaneus is the most common site of infection in the foot, followed by the metatarsals, tarsals, and then the phalangeal bones. Biopsy, magnetic resonance imaging, and histology confirm the diagnosis and guide medical intervention.[41] Treatment may involve an aggressive regimen of antibiotic medications, with surgical resection of affected areas potentially necessary.

■ Paronychia

Chief Clinical Characteristics

This presentation typically includes pain and tenderness with possible redness to the paronychium around the nail. Purulent drainage is common in the region of the infection.

Background Information

Chronic cases tend to be nonsuppurative. This condition involves infection to the epidermis surrounding the nail, which usually is caused by some puncture or laceration to the tissue. The diagnosis is confirmed by clinical examination. Treatment typically involves drainage and oral antibiotic medications.

■ Piezogenic Papules

Chief Clinical Characteristics

This presentation typically includes pain and tenderness at the plantar heel. Symptoms are worsened when bearing weight on the affected limb, especially in a rigid shoe or when barefoot on a hard floor.

Background Information

Oversized fat nodules may cause compressive pain on the fat pad. These nodules are often observable clinically. Pain may result from subcutaneous fat herniations. Diagnosis is made clinically. Footwear modifications, orthoses, and activity modification may be considered as common treatments.

■ Plantar Fasciitis

Chief Clinical Characteristics

This presentation typically includes pain and tenderness at the calcaneal insertion of the

plantar fascia, as well the plantar aspect of the midfoot. Pain is more intense with the first few steps in the morning and activities that involve bearing weight on the affected limb, such as walking, running, and ankle dorsiflexion with extension of the toes.

Background Information

Overuse and overloading of the plantar fascia cause this condition. Plain radiographs may reveal a calcaneal heel spur. However, these have been shown as the source of pain in only a minority of cases. Clinical examination confirms the diagnosis. Treatment commonly consists of nonsurgical interventions, such as footwear modification, orthoses, and gentle exercise to improve ankle dorsiflexion and plantar fascial mobility. In individuals with recalcitrant symptoms and disability, surgical debridement also may be considered.

■ Polyarteritis Nodosa

Chief Clinical Characteristics

This presentation typically includes fever, abdominal pain, peripheral neuropathy, mononeuritis multiplex, weakness, weight loss, hypertension, edema, oliguria, and uremia (in order of commonness). This condition is most common in males between 40 and 50 years of age.

Background Information

Neuropathy can result in sensory loss, hypesthesia, or weakness. Pain associated with this condition results from peripheral neuropathy, myalgia, or arthralgia. This condition involves inflammation and necrosis of the medium-sized arteries that result in ischemia, and it may occur as an effect of hepatitis B.[42] The diagnosis is confirmed with angiography, tissue biopsy, or magnetic resonance imaging.[43,44] Corticosteroid medication combined with cyclophosphamide comprises a common treatment.

POSITIONAL FAULTS

■ Calcaneocuboid Joint

Chief Clinical Characteristics

This presentation typically includes pain at the plantar aspect of the calcaneocuboid joint or lateral to the joint line. Pain usually is increased with impact activities, when performing a heel raise, or with a manual muscle test of the peroneus longus. Localized edema and peroneus longus weakness may be present.

Background Information

Theoretical causes include lateral ankle sprains, calcaneocuboid joint abnormalities, or torque from the peroneus longus tendon. Diagnosis is usually made by clinical presentation, weakness of the peroneus longus, and localized palpable pain. The diagnosis is confirmed with the clinical examination, and radiographs usually are unhelpful. Common treatment is nonsurgical, involving mobilization or manipulation of the cuboid.

■ Talonavicular Joint

Chief Clinical Characteristics

This presentation typically includes pain at the plantar and medial aspect of the foot, around the navicular. Pain is aggravated with weight bearing on the affected limb, impact activities, and manual muscle testing of the posterior tibialis muscle. Weakness of the posterior tibialis muscle, mild edema, and hypomobility of the talonavicular joint usually are present.

Background Information

Torsion of the medial forefoot is thought to medially displace the navicular, causing this condition. Clinical examination confirms the diagnosis, and radiographs usually are unhelpful. Common treatment is nonsurgical, involving mobilization or manipulation of the navicular.

■ Primary Amyloidosis

Chief Clinical Characteristics

This presentation typically includes pain, paresthesia, hypesthesia, and loss of light touch and temperature sensation in the feet and toes.

Background Information

This condition occurs when amyloid, a protein-like substance, is deposited in between cells in many tissues of the body. Renal failure with proteinemia and uremia are the most common complications; however, the patient also may have cardiac and gastrointestinal involvement. Diagnosis of primary amyloidosis neuropathy must correlate the neuropathy with other comorbidities that may result from amyloidosis. If organ involvement is suspected, then a tissue biopsy may confirm this diagnosis. Prognosis may range from mild changes to death. Typical goals of treatment include addressing contributory conditions and organ failure.

■ Pseudogout

Chief Clinical Characteristics

This presentation may include pain, edema, warmth, erythema, and tenderness of the involved joint or joints. The arthritis may mimic other types of arthritis but attacks usually are less severe than those experienced with gout. The first metatarsophalangeal joint, ankle, dorsum of the foot, knees, wrists, or shoulders may be affected. This condition is prevalent in individuals over 60 years of age.

Background Information

Causes for the contributory calcium pyrophosphate crystal deposition in synovial joints are unknown. Diagnosis is based on the clinical presentation, the pattern of joints involved, radiographic intra-articular and periarticular involvement, and aspiration of calcium pyrophosphate crystals in the joint fluid.[45] Anti-inflammatory medication comprises the usual treatment for this condition. Unlike with gout, uric acid–lowering medications are not used.

■ Pulp-Space Infection

Chief Clinical Characteristics

This presentation typically includes pain, redness, edema, tenderness, and sometimes palpable warmth at the plantar aspect of the first toe. Signs of systemic involvement include fever, malaise, weight loss, or fatigue.

Background Information

The cause of this rare condition is a puncture wound. Clinical examination confirms the diagnosis. Treatment typically involves oral antibiotic medications.

■ Raynaud's Disease

Chief Clinical Characteristics

This presentation typically includes a period of pallor and cyanosis followed by skin rubor and pain. Symptoms are often aggravated with cold or emotional stress. It is most common in the fingers, although toes also may be affected. Paresthesia tends to occur during the later stages.

Background Information
This phenomenon may be idiopathic, or related to vascular disease or a drug reaction. Clinical examination confirms the diagnosis. Typical treatment of this condition involves prevention of future episodes.

■ **Reiter's Syndrome**

Chief Clinical Characteristics
This presentation typically includes asymmetric and varying severity of joint pain and stiffness of the subtalar joint, metatarsophalangeal joints, interphalangeal joints, tarsal joints, calcaneal abnormalities, and knees. Other symptoms can include tendon synovitis, fasciitis, back pain, mucocutaneous lesions, skin lesions, and cardiac involvement. Joint pain accompanies urethritis and conjunctivitis.

Background Information
This disease typically follows either an episode of dysentery or infectious arthritis, and persons with the HLA-B27 genetic makeup are at greater risk.[46] Diagnosis is usually based on the patient's history, radiographs, and blood tests to rule out other forms of arthritis or potentially associated infections. This usually is a self-limiting condition and resolves in 3 to 4 months. When provided, treatment involves a combination of antibiotic medications directed toward the infective agent that is responsible for the autoimmune response that characterizes this condition, in combination with anti-inflammatory medication.

■ **Rheumatoid Arthritis**

Chief Clinical Characteristics
This presentation can involve symmetric foot pain with localized tenderness, swelling, and early morning stiffness. The feet may be the first region affected by the arthritis; however, multiple joints are often affected. After the initial stages, subcutaneous rheumatoid nodules and joint deformities may present, most commonly flexion deformities. The metatarsophalangeal joints are the joints most commonly affected by rheumatoid arthritis.[47]

Background Information
This is a progressive systemic condition with unknown etiology. Diagnosis, according to the American Rheumatism Association, includes at least a 6-week presentation with any four of the seven following manifestations: morning stiffness for more than 1 hour, arthritis of three or more joints, arthritis of the hand joints, symmetric arthritis, rheumatoid nodules, serum rheumatoid factor, or radiographic changes. Treatment typically includes a variety of steroidal, nonsteroidal, and biological anti-inflammatory medications.

RHEUMATOID ARTHRITIS–LIKE DISEASES OF THE FOOT

■ **Psoriatic Arthritis**

Chief Clinical Characteristics
This presentation can be characterized by an insidious onset of lumbopelvic and hip pain associated with psoriasis. The severity of arthritis is uncorrelated with the extent of skin involvement.[48] Pitting nail lesions occur in 80% of individuals with this condition. Dactylitis, tenosynovitis, and peripheral arthritis also are common.

Background Information
Radiographs of the distal phalanges may reveal a characteristic "pencil in cup" deformity. Blood panels including erythrocyte sedimentation rate are useful to track disease activity. Management usually includes use of salicylates, corticosteroids, antibiotics, and immunosuppressants depending on the severity of the pathology.[49]

■ **Systemic Lupus Erythematosus**

Chief Clinical Characteristics
This presentation can involve fatigue and joint pain/swelling affecting the hands, feet, knees, and shoulders. This condition affects mostly women of childbearing age, but men also may be affected.

Background Information
This condition is a chronic autoimmune disorder that can affect virtually any organ system of the body, including skin, joints, kidneys, brain, heart, lungs, and blood. There may be some ankle tendon involvement, more often in the Achilles tendon. The diagnosis is confirmed by the presence of skin lesions; heart, lung, or kidney involvement; and laboratory abnormalities including low red or white cell counts, low platelet counts, or positive ANA and anti-DNA antibody tests.[42]

Rubella and Rubella Vaccine–Associated Arthritis

Chief Clinical Characteristics

This presentation typically includes symmetric polyarthralgia that often is correlated with joint stiffness and preceded by a prodromal stage of malaise, low-grade fever, and lymphadenopathy and by skin rash. The rash is similar in appearance to the measles. Arthralgias are more common in children, whereas the joint stiffness is more common in adults.

Background Information

This condition is caused by a ribonucleic acid viral infection and diagnosis usually is confirmed with laboratory tests (serology) and clinical examination. It usually is self-limiting and the symptoms usually alleviate in several weeks.

RUPTURES

Achilles Tendon

Chief Clinical Characteristics

This presentation may involve a sudden onset of pain, palpable tenderness, significant weakness, and sometimes a palpable sulcus, usually 2 to 6 cm proximal to the distal insertion of the Achilles tendon.

Background Information

This condition often occurs spontaneously during an activity that places loading on the plantarflexors. It is associated with age over 40 years and a history of Achilles tendinopathy. The Thompson test and magnetic resonance or ultrasound imaging confirm the diagnosis. This condition is treated with surgical repair of the affected tendon.

Plantar Fascia

Chief Clinical Characteristics

This presentation can include sudden onset of severe pain during walking, running, jumping, or climbing stairs. Pain is described as a "tearing" or "ripping" pain in the heel and midfoot that prevents activities that involve bearing weight on the affected limb. Ecchymosis along the plantar fascia may appear 24 to 48 hours following the injury. Pain may be reproduced with weight bearing, palpation, or with dorsiflexion of the ankle and extension of the toes.

Background Information

A history of plantar fasciitis with one or more corticosteroid injections may predispose individuals to this condition. It may be caused by degeneration of the plantar fascia, chronic microtrauma, or a single acute trauma. Clinical examination confirms the diagnosis. Surgical repair may be indicated.

Septic Arthritis

Chief Clinical Characteristics

This presentation includes achy to throbbing pain, erythema, edema, and palpable warmth. Systemic signs of infection may include fever or malaise. This condition more often is monoarticular and can have a sudden onset.

Background Information

Septic arthritis can result from a fungal, bacterial, or viral pathogen infecting the periarticular or synovial tissues; *Staphylococcus aureus* is the most common cause in all ages. Computed tomography and magnetic resonance imaging combined with culture and staining of aspirated joint fluid commonly confirms the diagnosis. Treatment usually involves a combination of an aggressive antibiotic medication and joint drainage, perhaps by way of open drainage potentially combined with surgical lavage.

Shoe Vamp Ulcer and Bursitis

Chief Clinical Characteristics

This presentation may involve erythema, tenderness, pain, and superficial ulceration to the dorsal aspect of the hallux.

Background Information

Ulceration of skin, bursitis, and blistering occur from friction with the shoe vamp. Ulcers in patients with vascular or neuropathic deficits are of concern because healing may be compromised. Clinical examination confirms the diagnosis. Treatment usually includes footwear modification to reduce friction between the shoe vamp and foot.

Sickle Cell Crisis

Chief Clinical Characteristics

This presentation includes bone pain about the hip joint that is worsened by cold weather, overexertion, dehydration, and being overly fatigued.

Background Information

This condition involves abnormal red blood cell morphology that causes the cells to become rigid and sticky, disrupting blood flow to bones, and resulting in painful bone infarcts. This condition may cause complications in multiple organ systems, including stroke, skin ulcers, and blindness. Diagnosis may be confirmed with a blood test, the most common being hemoglobin electrophoresis. This condition is a medical emergency.

■ Strain of the Peroneal Muscles

Chief Clinical Characteristics

This presentation involves pain, tenderness, and possible edema or ecchymosis at the lateral lower leg and ankle, in the region of the peroneal muscles. Pain may be aggravated with passive dorsiflexion and inversion of the foot, or with contraction of the muscle with active plantarflexion and eversion of the foot. Bearing weight on the affected limb may be difficult, such as with walking and running. Focal tenderness may be present.

Background Information

This condition occurs as a result of rapid eccentric muscle contractions involved with activities like acceleration and deceleration. Clinical examination confirms the diagnosis. Additional certainty may be obtained with magnetic resonance imaging or computed tomography. Usual treatment is nonsurgical, including physical therapy intervention, orthoses, and footwear and activity modification.

■ Submetatarsal Cyst

Chief Clinical Characteristics

This presentation can involve a tender cyst just plantar to the metatarsal heads.

Background Information

This condition is a dermal plantar mass that is benign and usually is residing in the dermal layer. As opposed to a submetatarsal bursa, the cyst is palpable and adhered to the dermis. Sebaceous material may discharge through a small pore. Treatment may include drainage.

■ Subungual Hematoma

Chief Clinical Characteristics

This presentation involves a painful toenail that is very tender to pressure.

Background Information

Trauma or repetitive use, a medication reaction, systemic pathology, and aging may initiate the characteristic hematoma under the nail. Clinical examination confirms the diagnosis with the appearance of a blackened toenail. Usual treatment involves drainage.

TENDINITIS

■ Achilles Tendinitis

Chief Clinical Characteristics

This presentation can involve a sharp, aching, or burning pain with point tenderness 2 to 6 cm proximal to the calcaneal insertion. Insertional tendinopathy may be located at the distal insertion at the calcaneus. Symptoms are reproduced with palpation of the tendon, passive dorsiflexion, and active resisted plantarflexion. Palpable crepitus may be present with movement, and an increased thickening of the tendon that moves with tendon excursion may be palpable in comparison to the asymptomatic side. Calf atrophy may be observed, the patient may have limitations in ankle dorsiflexion, and the patient may report increased stiffness in the morning.

Background Information

Achilles tendinitis is associated with overuse from repetitive loading of the involved tendon. This injury is most common in 15- to 45-year-old active individuals, most commonly runners. Diagnosis is often made clinically. If the diagnosis is difficult then confirmation may be made with magnetic resonance imaging. Usual treatment is nonsurgical, consisting of anti-inflammatory medication, rest, and gentle exercise.

■ Extensor Digitorum Longus Tendinitis

Chief Clinical Characteristics

This presentation can be characterized by pain over the dorsum of the foot and tenderness to palpation along the extensor digitorum longus tendons. Resisted extension of the lesser toes and passive flexion of the lesser toes often increases the pain. Pain may also be elicited with resisted dorsiflexion of the ankle. Walking and running are often painful.

Background Information
The pathology of this tendinitis is usually the result of overuse. Diagnosis is usually made clinically, but may be confirmed with magnetic resonance or ultrasound imaging. Nonsurgical treatments may be indicated, such as anti-inflammatory medication, rest, and gentle exercise.

■ Extensor Hallucis Longus Tendinitis

Chief Clinical Characteristics
This presentation may include pain and palpable tenderness along the extensor hallucis tendon. Walking and running are often painful. Resisted extension of the hallux and passive flexion of the hallux often increase the pain. Pain may also be elicited with resisted dorsiflexion of the ankle.

Background Information
The pathology of this tendinitis is usually the result of overuse.[50] Diagnosis is usually made clinically, but may be confirmed with magnetic resonance or ultrasound imaging. Treatment usually involves nonsurgical interventions, such as anti-inflammatory medication, rest, and gentle exercise.

■ Flexor Digitorum Longus Tendinitis

Chief Clinical Characteristics
This presentation typically includes pain, tenderness, and swelling along the plantar hindfoot and midfoot with tenderness along the tendon of the flexor digitorum longus. Pain is aggravated with walking and weight bearing.

Background Information
A common site of irritation is deep to the flexor retinaculum at the posteromedial ankle. Palpation can be aided with the use of muscle contraction or active movement of the toes. If the tendons are inflamed, then pain is often reproduced with stretching of the toes into extension or contraction into flexion. The pathology is often related to trauma or overuse of the affected musculotendinous unit. Diagnosis is often determined clinically and may be confirmed with magnetic resonance or ultrasound imaging. Treatment usually involves nonsurgical interventions, such as anti-inflammatory medication, rest, and gentle exercise.

■ Flexor Hallucis Longus Tendinitis

Chief Clinical Characteristics
This presentation typically includes pain and tenderness to the flexor hallucis longus tendon. Pain is aggravated with walking, weight bearing, or stretching of the tendon. Swelling is often noted in the region of the pathology.

Background Information
The location of the pathology is often at the medial aspect of the midfoot and can usually be isolated along the tendon with palpation. A common site of irritation is under the flexor retinaculum at the posteromedial ankle. Palpation can be aided with the use of muscle contraction or movement of the hallux. The pathology is often related to overuse of the affected musculotendinous unit. Diagnosis is usually made clinically, but may be confirmed with magnetic resonance or ultrasound imaging. Management typically involves a combination of anti-inflammatory medication, rest, and gentle exercise.

■ Peroneal Tendinitis

Chief Clinical Characteristics
This presentation can involve pain anywhere along the lateral lower leg to the posterior lateral malleolus and along the lateral foot at the location of the cuboid or at the plantar aspect of the foot where the peroneus longus tendon inserts at the base of the first metatarsal. The pain may also be present at the base of the fifth metatarsal where the peroneus brevis tendon inserts. The pain is often aggravated with a stretch into foot and ankle dorsiflexion and inversion or a muscle contraction into foot and ankle plantarflexion and/or eversion.

Background Information
Common causes of peroneal tendon injury include overuse and inversion injury mechanisms. Diagnosis is usually made clinically, but may be confirmed with magnetic resonance or ultrasound imaging. Nonsurgical treatments may be indicated, such as anti-inflammatory medication, rest, and gentle exercise.

■ Tibialis Anterior Tendinitis

Chief Clinical Characteristics
This presentation typically includes pain and tenderness to palpation of the tibialis anterior tendon.

Background Information

Pain is often present at initial contact and during the loading response of gait, due to the eccentric loading of the tendon and muscle. Pain is often increased with passive stretch into plantarflexion or resisted dorsiflexion of the ankle. Tibialis anterior tendinitis is usually caused by overuse.[50] Diagnosis is usually made clinically, but may be confirmed with magnetic resonance or ultrasound imaging. Usual treatment is nonsurgical, consisting of anti-inflammatory medication, rest, and gentle exercise.

■ Tibialis Posterior Tendinitis

Chief Clinical Characteristics

This presentation may involve pain and swelling with palpable tenderness along the medial aspect of the midfoot and sometimes posterior to the medial malleolus. Pain is often worsened with weight bearing, walking, performing a heel rise, or stretching the tendon. Attenuation of this tendon is sometimes seen and can lead to a flat-foot deformity. Palpation may be assisted with muscle contraction of the tibialis posterior muscle.

Background Information

Injury to this tendon is often the result of overuse that is caused by a hypermobile midfoot and excessive foot pronation. The tibialis posterior is the most significant active stabilizer of the arch.[51] Diagnosis is usually made clinically, but may be confirmed with magnetic resonance or ultrasound imaging. Nonsurgical treatments may be indicated, such as anti-inflammatory medication, rest, and gentle exercise.

TENDINOSIS

■ Achilles Tendinosis

Chief Clinical Characteristics

This presentation typically includes sharp, aching, or burning pain with point tenderness usually along the medial aspect of the middle one-third of the Achilles tendon. Some patients with Achilles tendinosis are pain free. Symptoms, if present, may be reproduced with palpation of the Achilles tendon, passive dorsiflexion, or active resisted plantarflexion. Palpable increased thickening of the tendon may be present in comparison to the uninvolved tendon. Calf atrophy, limitations in

ankle dorsiflexion, and reports of increased stiffness in the morning may be observed. Pain is often worse with weight bearing and walking, and these patients often have difficulty performing a heel rise.

Background Information

Tendinosis is a state of increased tenocyte and cellular activity that leads to disorganized collagen and vascular hyperplasia.[52,53] Tendinosis is usually a chronic degenerative process that is initiated by an injury to the tendon. Diagnosis is usually based on the clinical presentation. If pathology is severe or the clinical diagnosis is unclear, then magnetic resonance or ultrasound imaging may confirm the diagnosis and allow for prognosis and staging of the tendinosis. A combination of patient/client education, unloading of the affected musculotendinous unit, controlled mechanical reloading, and preventive measures appears to be effective to manage this condition.[54]

■ Extensor Digitorum Longus Tendinosis

Chief Clinical Characteristics

This presentation is characterized by pain over the dorsum of the foot and tenderness to palpation along the extensor digitorum longus tendons. Resisted extension of the lesser toes or passive flexion of the lesser toes often increases the pain. Pain may also be elicited with resisted dorsiflexion of the ankle. Walking and running are often painful.

Background Information

The pathology of this tendinosis is usually the result of sustained overuse. Diagnosis is usually made clinically, but may be confirmed with magnetic resonance or ultrasound imaging. Nonsurgical treatments may be indicated, such as anti-inflammatory medication, rest, and gentle exercise.

■ Extensor Hallucis Longus Tendinosis

Chief Clinical Characteristics

This presentation may include pain and palpable tenderness along the extensor hallucis tendon. Walking and running are often painful. Resisted extension of the hallux or passive flexion of the hallux often increases the pain. Pain may also be elicited with resisted dorsiflexion of the ankle. Walking and running are often painful.

Background Information

The pathology of this tendinosis is usually the result of sustained overuse.[50] Diagnosis is usually made clinically, but may be confirmed with magnetic resonance or ultrasound imaging. Treatment usually involves nonsurgical interventions, such as anti-inflammatory medication, rest, and gentle exercise.

■ Flexor Digitorum Longus Tendinosis

Chief Clinical Characteristics

This presentation typically includes pain, tenderness, and swelling along the plantar hindfoot and midfoot with tenderness along the tendon of the flexor digitorum longus. Pain is aggravated with walking and weight bearing.

Background Information

A common site of irritation is deep to the flexor retinaculum at the posteromedial ankle. Palpation can be aided with the use of muscle contraction or active movement of the toes. If the tendons are chronically inflamed, then pain is often reproduced with stretching of the toes into extension or contraction into flexion. The pathology is often related to sustained trauma or overuse of the affected musculotendinous unit. Diagnosis is often determined clinically and may be confirmed with magnetic resonance or ultrasound imaging. Treatment usually involves nonsurgical interventions, such as anti-inflammatory medication, rest, and gentle exercise.

■ Flexor Hallucis Longus Tendinosis

Chief Clinical Characteristics

This presentation typically includes pain and tenderness to the flexor hallucis longus tendon. Pain is aggravated with walking, weight bearing, or stretching of the tendon. Swelling is often noted in the region of the pathology.

Background Information

The location of the pathology is often at the medial aspect of the midfoot and can usually be isolated along the tendon with palpation. A common site of irritation is under the

flexor retinaculum at the posteromedial ankle. Palpation can be aided with the use of muscle contraction or movement of the hallux. The pathology is often related to chronic overuse of the affected musculotendinous unit. Diagnosis is usually made clinically, but may be confirmed with magnetic resonance or ultrasound imaging. Management typically involves a combination of anti-inflammatory medication, rest, and gentle exercise.

■ Peroneal Tendinosis

Chief Clinical Characteristics

This presentation typically includes pain anywhere along the lateral lower leg to the posterior lateral malleolus and along the lateral foot at the location of the cuboid or at the plantar aspect of the foot where the peroneus longus tendon inserts at the base of the first metatarsal. The pain may also be present at the base of the fifth metatarsal where the peroneus brevis tendon inserts. The pain is often aggravated with a stretch into dorsiflexion and inversion or a muscle contraction into plantarflexion and/or eversion. Weakness may be noted into plantarflexion and/or eversion due to degenerative thickening, lengthening, and tearing of the tendon.

Background Information

Common causes of peroneal tendon injury include overuse and inversion injury mechanisms that may lead to the chronic degenerative process of tendinosis. Tendinosis is a state of increased tenocyte and cellular activity that leads to disorganized collagen and vascular hyperplasia.[52,53] Final diagnosis is confirmed with magnetic resonance or ultrasound imaging. A combination of patient/client education, unloading of the affected musculotendinous unit, controlled mechanical reloading, and preventive measures appears to be effective to manage this condition.[54]

■ Tibialis Anterior Tendinosis

Chief Clinical Characteristics

This presentation typically includes pain and tenderness to palpation of the tibialis anterior tendon.

Background Information

Pain is often present at initial contact and during the loading response of gait, due to the eccentric loading of the tendon and muscle. Pain is often increased with passive stretch into plantarflexion or resisted dorsiflexion of the ankle. The pathology of tibialis anterior tendinosis is usually caused by sustained overuse.[50] Diagnosis is usually made clinically, but may be confirmed with magnetic resonance or ultrasound imaging. Usual treatment is nonsurgical, consisting of anti-inflammatory medication, rest, and gentle exercise.

■ Tibialis Posterior Tendinosis

Chief Clinical Characteristics

This presentation typically includes pain and swelling with palpable tenderness along the medial aspect of the midfoot and posterior to the medial malleolus. Pain is often worse with weight bearing and walking, and these patients often have difficulty performing a heel rise. Attenuation of this tendon is sometimes seen as a result of tendinosis and the development of posterior tibialis tendon dysfunction may lead to a flat-foot deformity and a caudal drop of the navicular. These patients have a very difficult time contracting the tibialis posterior muscle, even during a manual muscle test.

Background Information

Injury to this tendon is often the result of overuse with a hypermobile midfoot. The tibialis posterior is the most significant active stabilizer of the arch.[51] Tendinosis is a state of increased tenocyte and cellular activity that leads to disorganized collagen and vascular hyperplasia. Tendinosis is usually a chronic degenerative process that is initiated by injury to the tendon. Diagnosis is usually based on the clinical presentation; however, magnetic resonance imaging may confirm the diagnosis and allow for prognosis and staging of the tendinosis. A combination of patient/client education, unloading of the affected musculotendinous unit, controlled mechanical reloading, and preventive measures appears to be effective to manage this condition.[54]

■ Thromboangiitis (Buerger's Disease)

Chief Clinical Characteristics

This presentation typically includes pain that is worse in early stages, as well as coldness, numbness, tingling, paresthesia, ulcerations, and gangrene. Signs of intermittent claudication are common in the calf or the arch of the foot. Distal pulses of the lower and upper extremities are often decreased or absent with a proximal progression. This condition is prevalent in males ages 20 to 40 years with a history of smoking.

Background Information

This condition is characterized by an obliteration of the small and medium arteries and veins through autoimmunity triggered by smoking nicotine.[55,56] Angiography confirms the diagnosis. The only known effective intervention is nicotine smoking cessation.

■ Tinea Pedis (Athlete's Foot)

Chief Clinical Characteristics

This presentation typically includes itching, pain, inflammation, vesiculation, and maceration of affected web spaces, as well as thickening and distortion of infected toenails. Symptoms range from mild to severe.

Background Information

This condition usually starts in the third web space, and may spread to the plantar surface of the feet. The common infecting organism is the *Trichophyton rubrum* fungus, which is transmitted from person to person or animal to person. Fungal culture confirms the diagnosis. Topical antifungal agents form the most common treatment for this condition.

■ Vitamin B Deficiency

Chief Clinical Characteristics

This presentation typically includes burning pain on the soles of the feet with erythematous mottling and systemic symptoms include anorexia, weakness, and weight loss.

Background Information

This condition can result in damage to peripheral nerves, the heart, and the central nervous system. In developed countries, this deficiency is more likely in individuals with a history of chronic alcohol abuse, debilitating illness, long-term unsupplemented parenteral nutrition, and pernicious vomiting. Blood tests confirm the diagnosis. Vitamin B supplementation is a common treatment for this condition, as well as addressing underlying diseases that may contribute to this condition.

■ Waldenstrom's Macroglobulinemia

Chief Clinical Characteristics
This presentation typically includes bleeding and peripheral neuropathy. Neuropathy associated with this condition may present as lower extremity and foot pain, sensation loss, or weakness.

Background Information
Common associated findings include fatigue, weakness, visual disturbances, headaches, and skin and mucosal bleeding. Cardiovascular impairment, recurrent infections, sensitivity to cold, lymphadenopathy, hepatosplenomegaly, or engorgement of retinal veins also may be present. This disease is a result of bone marrow infiltration that leads to increased amounts of macroglobulin circulating in the plasma. The survival rate usually is in the range of 5 to 10 years.[57] Laboratory tests that reveal altered immunoglobulin M monoclonal proteins and neoplastic infiltration of tissues confirm the diagnosis. Treatments for this condition may include nucleoside analogs, alkylators, combination chemotherapy, and stem cell transplantation.[58]

■ Warts

Chief Clinical Characteristics
This presentation typically includes pain and tenderness to palpation or weight bearing on the lesion.

Background Information
Warts result from human papillomavirus infection; plantar warts are commonly present beneath points that bear high pressures. This condition involves skin lesions that have a rough keratotic surface with an outer rim of thickened skin and punctate black dots, which are thrombosed capillaries. Clinical examination confirms the diagnosis.

References
1. Merskey H, Bogduk N. *Classification of Chronic Pain: Descriptions of Chronic Pain Syndromes and Definitions of Pain Terms.* Seattle, WA: IASP Press; 1994.
2. Moseley GL. Imagined movements cause pain and swelling in a patient with complex regional pain syndrome. *Neurology.* May 11, 2004;62(9):1644.
3. Ledermann HP, Schweitzer ME, Morrison WB. Nonenhancing tissue on MR imaging of pedal infection: characterization of necrotic tissue and associated limitations for diagnosis of osteomyelitis and abscess. *Am J Roentgenol.* Jan 2002;178(1):215–222.
4. Carapetis JR, Currie BJ. Rheumatic fever in a high incidence population: the importance of monoarthritis and low grade fever. *Arch Dis Child.* Sep 2001;85(3): 223–227.
5. Weitz JI, Byrne J, Clagett GP, et al. Diagnosis and treatment of chronic arterial insufficiency of the lower extremities: a critical review. *Circulation.* Dec 1, 1996;94(11):3026–3049.
6. Mosley JG. Arterial problems in athletes. *Br J Surg.* Dec 2003;90(12):1461–1469.
7. Williams KJ, Tabas I. The response-to-retention hypothesis of early atherogenesis. *Arterioscler Thromb Vasc Biol.* May 1995;15(5):551–561.
8. Schwartz SM, deBlois D, O'Brien ER. The intima. Soil for atherosclerosis and restenosis. *Circ Res.* Sep 1995;77 (3):445–465.
9. Salvarani C, Vlachonikolis IG, van der Heijde DM, et al. Musculoskeletal manifestations in a population-based cohort of inflammatory bowel disease patients. *Scand J Gastroenterol.* Dec 2001;36(12):1307–1313.
10. Parisi L, Pierelli F, Amabile G, et al. Muscular cramps: proposals for a new classification. *Acta Neurol Scand.* Mar 2003;107(3):176–186.
11. Morgan MS. Prophylaxis should be considered even for trivial animal bites. *BMJ.* May 10, 1997;314(7091): 1413.
12. Toolan BC, Sangeorzan BJ, Hansen ST, Jr. Complex reconstruction for the treatment of dorsolateral peritalar subluxation of the foot. Early results after distraction arthrodesis of the calcaneocuboid joint in conjunction with stabilization of, and transfer of the flexor digitorum longus tendon to, the midfoot to treat acquired pes planovalgus in adults. *J Bone Joint Surg Am.* Nov 1999;81 (11):1545–1560.
13. Fukumoto Y, Tsutsui H, Tsuchihashi M, Masumoto A, Takeshita A. The incidence and risk factors of cholesterol embolization syndrome, a complication of cardiac catheterization: a prospective study. *J Am Coll Cardiol.* Jul 16, 2003;42(2):211–216.
14. Murphy JV, Banwell PE, Roberts AH, McGrouther DA. Frostbite: pathogenesis and treatment. *J Trauma.* Jan 2000;48(1):171–178.
15. Jose RM, Viswanathan N, Aldlyami E, Wilson Y, Moiemen N, Thomas R. A spontaneous compartment syndrome in a patient with diabetes. *J Bone Joint Surg Br.* Sep 2004;86(7):1068–1070.
16. Handa S, Sahoo B. Childhood lichen planus: a study of 87 cases. *Int J Dermatol.* Jul 2002;41(7):423–427.
17. Pao DG, Keats TE, Dussault RG. Avulsion fracture of the base of the fifth metatarsal not seen on conventional radiography of the foot: the need for an additional projection. *Am J Roentgenol.* Aug 2000;175(2):549–552.
18. Judd DB, Kim DH. Foot fractures frequently misdiagnosed as ankle sprains. *Am Fam Physician.* Sep 1, 2002;66(5):785–794.
19. Fanciullo JJ, Bell CL. Stress fractures of the sacrum and lower extremity. *Curr Opin Rheumatol.* Mar 1996;8(2): 158–162.

20. Choi CH, Ogilvie-Harris DJ. Occult osteochondral fractures of the subtalar joint: a review of 10 patients. *J Foot Ankle Surg*. Jan–Feb 2002;41(1):40–43.

21. Canale ST, Belding RH. Osteochondral lesions of the talus. *J Bone Joint Surg Am*. Jan 1980;62(1):97–102.

22. Buoncristiani AM, Manos RE, Mills WJ. Plantar-flexion tarsometatarsal joint injuries in children. *J Pediatr Orthop*. May–Jun 2001;21(3):324–327.

23. Kramer HM, Curhan G. The association between gout and nephrolithiasis: the National Health and Nutrition Examination Survey III, 1988–1994. *Am J Kidney Dis*. Jul 2002;40(1):37–42.

24. Sella EJ, Caminear DS, McLarney EA. Haglund's syndrome. *J Foot Ankle Surg*. Mar–Apr 1998;37(2):110–114; discussion 173.

25. Haamann P, Kessel L, Larsen M. Monofocal outer retinitis associated with hand, foot, and mouth disease caused by coxsackievirus. *Am J Ophthalmol*. Apr 2000;129 (4):552–553.

26. Tsao KC, Chang PY, Ning HC, et al. Use of molecular assay in diagnosis of hand, foot and mouth disease caused by enterovirus 71 or coxsackievirus A 16. *J Virol Methods*. Apr 2002;102(1–2):9–14.

27. Chen TM, George S, Woodruff CA, Hsu S. Clinical manifestations of varicella-zoster virus infection. *Dermatol Clin*. Apr 2002;20(2):267–282.

28. Younger DS. Vasculitis of the nervous system. *Curr Opin Neurol*. Jun 2004;17(3):317–336.

29. Knapik JJ, Hamlet MP, Thompson KJ, Jones BH. Influence of boot-sock systems on frequency and severity of foot blisters. *Mil Med*. Oct 1996;161(10):594–598.

30. Periasamy V, al Shubaili A, Girsh Y. Diagnostic dilemmas in acute intermittent porphyria. A case report. *Med Princ Pract*. Apr–Jun 2002;11(2):108–111.

31. Beckers R, Uyttebroeck A, Demaerel P. Acute lymphoblastic leukaemia presenting with low back pain. *Eur J Paediatr Neurol*. 2002;6(5):285–287.

32. Rubin DI, Schomberg PJ, Shepherd RF, Panneton JM. Arteritis and brachial plexus neuropathy as delayed complications of radiation therapy. *Mayo Clin Proc*. Aug 2001;76(8):849–852.

33. Bradlow A, Barton C. Arthritic presentation of childhood leukaemia. *Postgrad Med J*. Jun 1991;67(788): 562–564.

34. Evans TI, Nercessian BM, Sanders KM. Leukemic arthritis. *Semin Arthritis Rheum*. Aug 1994;24(1):48–56.

35. Ostrov BE, Goldsmith DP, Athreya BH. Differentiation of systemic juvenile rheumatoid arthritis from acute leukemia near the onset of disease. *J Pediatr*. Apr 1993; 122(4):595–598.

36. Wada M, Kurita K, Tajima K, Kawanami T, Kato T. A case of inflammatory demyelinating polyradiculoneuropathy associated with T-cell lymphoma. *Acta Neurol Scand*. Jan 2003;107(1):62–66.

37. Joines JD, McNutt RA, Carey TS, Deyo RA, Rouhani R. Finding cancer in primary care outpatients with low back pain: a comparison of diagnostic strategies. *J Gen Intern Med*. 2001;16(1):14–23.

38. Holman PJ, Suki D, McCutcheon I, Wolinsky JP, Rhines LD, Gokaslan ZL. Surgical management of metastatic disease of the lumbar spine: experience with 139 patients. *J Neurosurg Spine*. 2005;2(5):550–563.

39. Sharp RJ, Wade CM, Hennessy MS, Saxby TS. The role of MRI and ultrasound imaging in Morton's neuroma and the effect of size of lesion on symptoms. *J Bone Joint Surg Br*. Sep 2003;85(7):999–1005.

40. Lundborg G, Dahlin LB. Anatomy, function, and pathophysiology of peripheral nerves and nerve compression. *Hand Clin*. May 1996;12(2):185–193.

41. Lipman BT, Collier BD, Carrera GF, et al. Detection of osteomyelitis in the neuropathic foot: nuclear medicine, MRI and conventional radiography. *Clin Nucl Med*. Feb 1998;23(2):77–82.

42. Fauci AS, Haynes B, Katz P. The spectrum of vasculitis: clinical, pathologic, immunologic and therapeutic considerations. *Ann Intern Med*. Nov 1978;89(5 pt 1): 660–676.

43. Henderson J, Cohen J, Jackson J, Wiselka M. Polyarteritis nodosa presenting as a pyrexia of unknown origin. *Postgrad Med J*. Nov 2002;78(925):685–686.

44. Gallien S, Mahr A, Rety F, et al. Magnetic resonance imaging of skeletal muscle involvement in limb restricted vasculitis. *Ann Rheum Dis*. Dec 2002;61(12):1107–1109.

45. Cassetta M, Gorevic PD. Crystal arthritis. Gout and pseudogout in the geriatric patient. *Geriatrics*. Sep 2004;59 (9):25–30; quiz 31.

46. Eapen BR. A new insight into the pathogenesis of Reiter's syndrome using bioinformatics tools. *Int J Dermatol*. Mar 2003;42(3):242–243.

47. Smyth CJ, Janson RW. Rheumatologic view of the rheumatoid foot. *Clin Orthop*. Jul 1997(340):7–17.

48. Kataria RK, Brent LH. Spondyloarthropathies. *Am Fam Physician*. Jun 15, 2004;69(12):2853–2860.

49. Knutson D, Greenberg G, Cronau H. Management of Crohn's disease—a practical approach. *Am Fam Physician*. Sep 15, 2003;68(4):707–714.

50. Karlsson J, Lundin O, Lossing IW, Peterson L. Partial rupture of the patellar ligament. Results after operative treatment. *Am J Sports Med*. Jul–Aug 1991;19(4):403–408.

51. Thordarson DB, Schmotzer H, Chon J, Peters J. Dynamic support of the human longitudinal arch. A biomechanical evaluation. *Clin Orthop*. Jul 1995(316): 165–172.

52. Mafi N, Lorentzon R, Alfredson H. Superior short-term results with eccentric calf muscle training compared to concentric training in a randomized prospective multicenter study on patients with chronic Achilles tendinosis. *Knee Surg Sports Traumatol Arthrosc*. 2001;9(1): 42–47.

53. Kraushaar BS, Nirschl RP. Tendinosis of the elbow (tennis elbow). Clinical features and findings of histological, immunohistochemical, and electron microscopy studies. *J Bone Joint Surg Am*. Feb 1999;81(2):259–278.

54. Davenport TE, Kulig K, Matharu Y, Blanco CE. The EdUReP model for nonsurgical management of tendinopathy. *Phys Ther*. Oct 2005;85(10):1093–1103.

55. Sulzberger MB. Hypersensitivity to tobacco glycoprotein in human peripheral vascular disease. *Ann Allergy*. Dec 1981;47(6):476.

56. Adar R, Papa MZ, Halpern Z, et al. Cellular sensitivity to collagen in thromboangiitis obliterans. *N Engl J Med*. May 12 1983;308(19):1113–1116.

57. Garcia-Sanz R, Montoto S, Torrequebrada A, et al. Waldenstrom macroglobulinaemia: presenting features and outcome in a series with 217 cases. *Br J Haematol*. Dec 2001;115(3):575–582.

58. Chen CI. Treatment for Waldenstrom's macroglobulinemia. *Ann Oncol*. Apr 2004;15(4):550–558.

FOOT PAIN

CHAPTER **25**

Foundations of Neurological Differential Diagnosis

■ *Bernadette M. Currier, PT, DPT, MS, NCS* ■ *Beth E. Fisher, PT, PhD*

IN THIS CHAPTER:

■ Rationale for considering nervous system pathology in diagnosis
■ Summary of relevant clinical neuroanatomy
■ Relationship between neuroanatomy and clinical syndromes

Introduction

Numbness, tingling, weakness, and dizziness are just a few symptoms commonly encountered in physical therapist practice that may indicate pathology of the neurological system. Resultant difficulty in mobility and function is what frequently drives an individual to seek physical therapy services. As specialists in the diagnosis and treatment of movement dysfunction, physical therapists must have the knowledge base and clinical skills to confirm that impairments are consistent with a given medical diagnosis. As Gordon and Watts discuss in Chapter 1, physical therapists must engage in the *diagnostic process* as part of their overall evaluation. The process must lead to a decision regarding the probable pathological or pathophysiological cause of an individual's problem, followed by a determination of whether physical therapy intervention is the most appropriate to address the pathology underlying the condition. We advocate that the use of this process should extend to physical therapists working with individuals who display symptoms and signs consistent with nervous system pathology.

Nervous System Pathology is Important to Consider in Diagnostic Reasoning

We believe it is imperative for physical therapists to be as skilled in the process of diagnosis for individuals reporting concerns of activity restrictions for reasons other than pain, as it is when diagnosing individuals reporting concerns of pain. As Landel describes in Chapter 2, it is the responsibility of the physical therapist to encourage individuals to describe what activities are limited as a result of their chief concern. Unlike individuals with pain, however, individuals with neurological diagnoses rarely report problems at the level of body structures and functions as a chief concern. Individuals are not likely to state that they are experiencing ataxia, spasticity, or problems with force production. Rather, these problems manifest as limitations specific to *activity* or participation in a social context, and these limitations are frequently the chief concern. Regardless of whether activity restrictions are the result of pain or impairments resulting from nervous system pathology, the physical therapist is encouraged to conduct the examination to establish causative pathology and the appropriate plan of care. Determining appropriateness for physical therapy and identifying the primary problems influencing the movement dysfunction are the primary goals of the physical therapy evaluation.

To illustrate the importance of considering nervous system pathology during the process of differential diagnosis, throughout the chapter we will use the example of a 34-year-old Caucasian female schoolteacher whose chief concern involves not being able to reach high enough to effectively write on the chalkboard. Patient interview reveals the individual has experienced this difficulty reaching for the past 3 weeks. Past medical history is unremarkable with the exception of nearsightedness for which the individual wears corrective lenses. The individual states that she has experienced intermittent problems with her vision for the past several months, and attributes this to missing her eye exam this year with the need for a new eyeglass prescription.

As Davenport introduces in Chapter 3 and Watts elaborates on in Chapter 4, a process of backward reasoning should be used to create and test clinical hypotheses related to the cause of this individual's symptoms and signs. A physical therapist who incorporates a *backward reasoning pattern* will start with a list of all the possible pathologies that may cause the patient's disablement in order to guide additional history and physical examination. Further questioning of this individual reveals she has been experiencing difficulty tying her students' shoes during the past few weeks, and attributes this to work-related stress. She also admits to an episode of visual changes a few years prior to this visit. Because those changes resolved spontaneously within just a few days, the individual did not feel the need to seek medical consultation. Upon hearing these concerns, the physical

therapist applying a backward reasoning thought process to establish differential diagnoses would further investigate the possible reasons for difficulty tying shoes along with multiple episodes of "visual changes."

Given that the patient history in this case includes the possible presence of *special concerns* related to the nervous system, the physical therapist should immediately consider causative pathologies beyond an isolated musculoskeletal system disorder such as shoulder impingement. Watts discusses common special concerns in Chapter 4. In addition, Box 25-1 provides a list of signs and symptoms caused by neurological pathology that should alert the physical therapist as to the appropriate course of action—emergent or nonemergent referral to a medical provider. Optic neuritis, tumor, and multiple sclerosis are additional examples of pathologies that should be included in the list of hypotheses.

Neurological testing should include mental status, cranial nerve function, force production, deep tendon and pathological reflexes, coordination, gait, and sensory integrity.[1] For the example in this chapter, an abnormal Babinski reflex and upper limb ataxia are found. As described by Landel in Chapter 2, when determining if managing the causative pathology is within the scope of physical therapy practice, the decision-making process involves three possible outcomes:

- Physical therapy is not indicated;
- Physical therapy is indicated but a consultation to another health care provider is required; or
- Physical therapy can proceed independent of additional consultation.

The constellation of findings from the history and physical examination in the case of the 34-year-old schoolteacher should indicate that physical therapy is not indicated. The physical therapist should refer this individual to a neurologist promptly for further medical workup.

Summary of Neurological Differential Diagnosis

How did the physical therapist in the above scenario determine that the individual was not only inappropriate for physical therapy services, but also in need of referral to a

---

BOX 25-1 Special Concerns Specific to Nervous System Pathology[2]

Emergency Situations (Immediate Medical Assistance Required)

- Loss of consciousness or difficult to arouse
- Extreme confusion not consistent with premorbid status
- Uncontrolled seizure activity (status epilepticus)
- Acute infection with other associated neurological signs such as nuchal rigidity or intense, localized back pain
- Rapid onset of focal neurological deficits (suggesting stroke in progress):
  - Weakness, numbness or tingling of face, arm, or leg, especially on one side of body
  - Blurred or decreased vision in one or both eyes or double vision
  - Loss of speech or trouble understanding speech
  - Headache that is sudden, severe, and unusual
  - Dizziness, loss of balance or coordination with any of other signs.
- Evidence of spinal column instability (eg, decrement in motor and sensory status with position change from supine to sit or sit to stand, bilateral upper extremity paresthesias with neck flexion)
- Nonresponsive autonomic dysreflexia

Nonemergency Situations (Outside Referral Required)

- Acute onset of neurological signs such as incontinence, saddle paresthesia, abnormal reflexes
- Progressive neurological signs in a known neurological diagnosis that is not degenerative (ie, decrement in motor, sensory, or cognitive status)

- Evidence of motor neuron disease (fasciculation, atrophy, weakness in limbs or trunk) not previously diagnosed
- New onset of involuntary movements or tremor
- Change in autonomic status (RR, HR, HP, body temperature, autonomic dysreflexia, orthostatic hypotension)
- Bulbar and other cranial nerve signs/symptoms, progressive change in swallowing, dysarthria, voice hoarseness, visual changes such as gaze palsies or report of diplopia, nystagmus, ptosis, impaired papillary responses, facial weakness or sensory changes, hearing loss, dizziness, vertigo (*Note:* Acute onset or changes in any of these signs or symptoms would require immediate medical assistance.)
- Constant headache that worsens over time
- Patient report of transient ischemic attack symptoms (stroke-in-progress symptoms from above that resolve within 24 hours)
- Vertebral artery insufficiency (neck motions discontinued immediately)
- Neurological signs inconsistent with diagnosis
- Signs or symptoms of systemic illness (fever, diaphoretic, poor exercise tolerance)
- Significant changes in personality or cognitive status (memory loss, impaired language ability, visuospatial deficits)

---

neurologist for further medical evaluation? How is the symptom-based diagnostic process described in the previous chapters applied to individuals with neurological diagnoses? Consistent with pathology of other body systems, we encourage the use of a hypothesis-driven reasoning strategy to formulate a list of possible diagnoses and establish an appropriate course of action when physical therapists suspect that pathology related to the nervous system is the probable cause for an individual's chief concern.

Sullivan and colleagues[2] adapted an existing process of neurological differential diagnosis[3] to provide physical therapists with a framework for establishing a hypothesized lesion location within the neuraxis. In this model, information from the chart review, subjective examination, and objective testing are combined to create a hypothesized anatomical lesion location. The hypothesized lesion location can assist physical therapists with determining which among the list of hypothesized forms of pathology can be ruled less likely. In turn, forms of pathology that can be excluded will assist in the decision to treat the individual, refer him or her to another health care provider for additional evaluation, or both.

Chart Review

When available in physical therapy settings, the medical record can be a primary source of information for obtaining the individual's temporal features such as age, history of present illness, past medical history, past surgical history, lab and radiology reports, family history, and medications. It is the responsibility of the physical therapist to confirm that the information gathered from the medical record is consistent with the individual's chief concern and clinical presentation. To determine this, the physical therapist must extract pertinent information from the subjective examination and combine it with information obtained from the objective examination. In some settings, however, medical records are inaccessible and the physical therapist must use solely his or her interaction with the individual to gain this information.

History/Subjective Examination

The patient interview should include a skilled set of questions posed by the physical therapist with the goal of distinguishing among hypothetical causes of the patient's disablement. If the individual is unable to fully participate in the subjective interview due to cognitive or language barriers, a caregiver or interpreter, respectively, may be a necessary participant in the interview. Key pieces of information should include the individual's goals for physical therapy, the family's goals for physical therapy if the individual is unable to express these, current and prior levels of function, perceived limitations to the individual's participation in societal roles and relevant activities, social history, and temporal features.

The physical therapist should then determine, based on the information gathered from the subjective interview, whether or not it is appropriate to continue with the physical therapy examination of the individual. If the information from the subjective history reveals information consistent with the referred medical diagnosis, the physical therapist is encouraged to proceed with the exam. In the event that the individual's history either does not appear consistent with the given diagnosis or suggests the presence of *special concerns*, the physical therapist is encouraged to continue by performing a neurological screen and utilizing those results to determine the appropriate course of action (see Box 25-1).

Objective Examination

Following the subjective interview, an objective examination should be performed (1) to determine if the individual's clinical presentation is consistent with pathology that is potentially amenable to physical therapy and then (2) to establish causes for movement dysfunction including the identification of direct impairments and compensations. Given that the individual's chief concern is often a limitation at the functional level, observation and analysis of task performance is the next step in the objective examination. Comparison of what the physical therapist considers to be "ideal" with the actual demonstration of the task gives the clinician valuable insight into what impairments and compensations might be influencing the production of movement.[4] The physical therapist can then test those impairments to confirm or negate working hypotheses as to the cause(s) of the present movement dysfunction.

Clinical Neurological Tests

In addition to testing hypothesized impairments, clinical neurological tests should be performed for any individual whose given medical diagnosis, subjective history, or clinical presentation suggests underlying pathology of the nervous system. These tests include examination of mental status, cranial nerve function, force production, deep tendon and pathological reflexes, coordination, gait, and sensory integrity.[1] The following examples of presentations should cue the clinician to perform additional neurological testing:

- *Mental status:* Confusion, inability to follow simple directions, no recall of events from the recent past, or emotional lability.
- *Cranial nerve function:* Eyes that are offset from one another, facial asymmetry or weakness, slurred speech, drooling, poor hearing, or balance problems.
- *Force production:* Slowness in movement or signs of weakness. Often these signs are noticed during observation of functional tasks such as moving from a sitting position to standing, walking, and reaching.

- *Deep tendon and pathological reflexes:* Neck or low back pain with radiating pain or sensory disturbances down an extremity. Pathological reflex testing should be performed to help determine the presence of an upper motor neuron lesion, which is described in a later section of this chapter.
- *Coordination:* Uncoordinated trunk or extremity movement, indicated by tremors or inability to accurately reach targets. Gait may appear unsteady and individuals may lose their balance while walking.
- *Gait:* Stagger, limp, maintain a wide base of support, or require an assistive device in order to be able to walk.
- *Sensory integrity:* Inconsistent foot placement or the need to look down at the floor while walking, or report of sensory disturbances such as numbness or tingling.

Diagnostic Impression

The results of clinical neurological testing in combination with other information gleaned through movement analysis and specific impairment testing should enable the physical therapist to hypothesize lesion location(s). Based on the lesion location, this hypothesis will aid in the decision to proceed with physical therapy and/or refer the individual to a neurologist. Box 25-1 lists signs and symptoms that may warrant referral to a medical provider. In addition to the signs and symptoms listed in Box 25-1, if involvement of specific neuroanatomical structures is suspected in an individual with an otherwise unknown pathology, referral to a neurologist should take place.

To provide an example of how going through this process will generate a diagnostic impression, let's consider the 34-year-old female who reports difficulty reaching, tying shoes, and seeing clearly. Because impairment testing revealed an abnormal Babinski sign and upper limb ataxia, involvement of neuroanatomical structures should be suspected. Specifically, the abnormal Babinski reflex suggests the presence of a disorder that affects the upper motor neurons, and the presence of the ataxia suggests a disorder that involves the cerebellum. The process of linking examination findings to neuroanatomy is elaborated on next.

Linking Examination Findings to Neuroanatomy

We suggest that the decision to refer the patient to a medical care provider in the case of suspected nervous system pathology is facilitated by the physical therapist's ability to interpret examination findings and concisely communicate the most important findings. To be able to accurately associate impairments with neuroanatomical locations, a physical therapist must have a sound background in neuroanatomy with the ability to efficiently utilize neuroanatomy resources to supplement his or her knowledge as needed. In this section, the anatomy and function of the nervous system, and pathological processes associated with specific brain regions, spinal cord regions, and peripheral nerves, are reviewed in order to assist the reader in determining possible lesion locations as a part of the differential diagnosis process.

Anatomy and Functions of the Nervous System

The nervous system is divided into two main parts, the central nervous system (CNS) and the peripheral nervous system (PNS). The CNS is comprised of the brain and spinal cord. It is made up of white matter (myelinated axons) and gray matter (cell bodies; Fig. 25-1). The PNS is comprised of the cranial, spinal, sympathetic and parasympathetic nerves, and ganglia. Neuroanatomical structures work individually and together to perform specific functions. We discuss the anatomy and common functions of the neuroanatomical structures in this section.

The ultrastructure of the brain is characterized by two cerebral hemispheres, each of which has frontal, parietal, temporal, and occipital lobes (Fig. 25-2). The interhemispheric fissure separates the two hemispheres, while the corpus callosum connects the paired lobes of each hemisphere. The central sulcus divides the brain into anterior (precentral) and posterior (postcentral) regions. Cortices made up of gray matter cover the surfaces of the cerebral hemispheres and serve important functions. The primary motor cortex is located in the precentral gyrus of the frontal lobe. The primary somatosensory cortex is within the

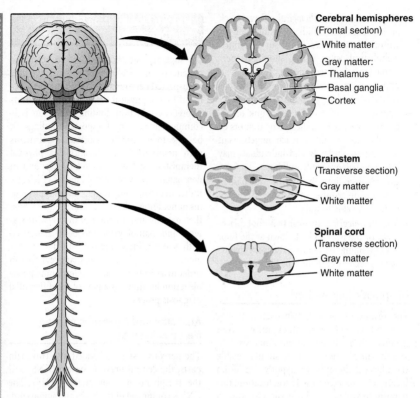

FIGURE 25-1 Relative position of gray matter and white matter in the neuraxis. In the brain, the gray matter is primarily located in the periphery, the thalamus, and the basal ganglia. By contrast, the gray matter is located centrally within the spinal cord.

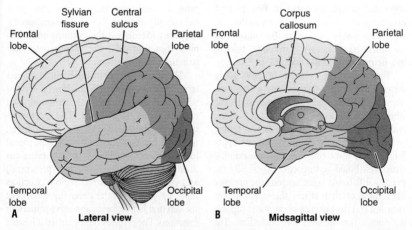

FIGURE 25-2 Ultrastructure of the brain, including (A) lateral view and (B) midsagittal view of the cerebrum and its component lobes.

postcentral gyrus of the parietal lobe. The primary visual cortex is in the occipital lobe. The primary auditory cortex is in the temporal lobe.

The cerebral cortex is topographically organized. The somatotopic map is characterized by the motor and sensory homunculi, by which motor and sensory regions of the body are represented by regions of the brain. The motor homunculus represents the areas within the motor cortex that control movement of respective parts of the body, and the sensory homunculus within the sensory cortex receives sensory input from respective parts of the body.

Several brain structures are involved in the production of movement. These include the cerebral cortex (Table 25-1), brainstem, thalamus, basal ganglia, and cerebellum. Movement information is transferred between these structures via motor pathways. The lateral corticospinal tract is the primary motor pathway. The cell bodies, or upper motor neurons, are located within the primary motor cortex. Axons then travel down as white matter through the brainstem to cross over at the level of the medulla to reach the spinal cord, specifically to project to lower motor neurons within the anterior horn. The cerebellum, basal ganglia, and thalamus are subcortical structures located within both the right and left sides of the brain. Table 25-1 reviews the primary functions of the main regions within the cerebral hemispheres. The functions of other structures involved in motor pathways are as follows:

- *Basal ganglia:* Regulates the descending motor pathway, eye movements, emotion, and cognition.
- *Brainstem:* Cardiorespiratory function; provides sensory and motor innervation to face and neck, passageway for ascending sensory tracts and descending motor pathways, regulation of consciousness and sleep/wake cycle.
- *Cerebellum:* Integrates information to produce smooth movement, motor planning, and learning.
- *Lateral motor pathways (lateral corticospinal and rubrospinal tracts):* Control movement of the extremities.
- *Lower motor neurons:* Provide the connection between upper motor neurons and the periphery.
- *Medial motor pathways (anterior corticospinal, vestibulospinal, reticulospinal, and tectospinal tracts):* Control movements of the trunk and its relationship to postural stability and balance, head and neck orientation, and automaticity of gait.
- *Thalamus:* Conveys sensory, motor, and limbic information to the cerebral cortex.
- *Upper motor neurons:* Involved in movement and tone of the trunk and extremities.

TABLE 25-1 ■ Functions of Selected Brain Structures

BRAIN STRUCTURE	FUNCTION(S)

Frontal lobe
   Broca's area (left hemisphere)
	Initiation, judgment, memory, impulse control, sequencing, social behavior
	   Expressive language

Parietal lobe	Sensory integration, awareness of body image and environment

Temporal lobe
   Wernicke's area (left hemisphere)
	Long-term memory, auditory processing
	   Processing of speech

Occipital lobe	Visual field, color discrimination

Cerebral cortex
   Motor cortex (motor homunculus)
   Somatosensory cortex (sensory homunculus)
   Visual cortex
   Auditory cortex
	
	Contralateral control of movement
	Contralateral perception of sensation
	Contralateral perception of vision
	Bilateral reception of auditory input

Corpus callosum	Facilitates communication between the right and left hemispheres of the brain

Each motor pathway described above originates at the primary motor cortex. The axons come together to form the corona radiata and internal capsule prior to traversing through the brainstem to reach the spinal cord and finally synapse with alpha motor neurons in the ventral horns. The interrelationships among structures that form specific motor pathways are depicted in Figure 25-3.

A common way of describing pathology to the CNS or PNS is by using the terms *upper motor neuron (UMN) disorder* or *lower motor neuron (LMN) disorder*. The term UMN disorder signifies that there is a lesion within the CNS, specifically involving the descending motor pathways, whereas the term LMN disorder signifies that there is a lesion within the PNS. Certain classic signs, summarized in Table 25-2, suggest the presence of a lesion.

Somatic sensation travels through the ascending pathways of the somatosensory system, the dorsal column/medial lemniscus pathways, and the anterolateral pathways. The axons traveling through the dorsal column cross at the level of the medulla prior to ascending to the contralateral thalamus in order to reach the somatosensory cortex. Axons of the anterolateral pathway cross within the gray matter of the spinal cord and ascend through the thalamus to terminate at the somatosensory cortex.

Somatosensory pathways convey information from the periphery to the brain:

- *Anterolateral pathways:* Convey pain and temperature sensations.
- *Medulla:* Area where the dorsal column/medial lemniscal pathways cross over.
- *Dorsal column:* Conveys proprioception, vibration, and light touch.
- *Somatosensory cortex:* Receives and integrates sensory information.
- *Thalamus:* Conveys sensory, motor, and limbic information to the cerebral cortex.

To summarize, the dorsal column carries the sensory modalities of proprioception, vibration, and light touch. Peripheral sensory receptors initially receive the stimuli, and information is carried from ascending peripheral nerves through spinal nerves to reach the dorsal column of the spinal cord. The medial lemniscal pathways carry this information ipsilaterally up the spinal cord, where it crosses over at the level of the medulla to then ascend through the rest of the brainstem and thalamus to eventually be received and integrated within the somatosensory cortex.

The spinothalamic tracts carry the sensory modalities of pain and temperature. As is the case with the pathways of proprioception, vibration, and light touch, peripheral sensory receptors initially receive the stimuli, and information is then carried from ascending peripheral nerves through spinal nerves to reach the spinal cord. Pain and temperature modalities are transmitted in the anterolateral rather than dorsal column of the spinal cord. Rather than ascending ipsilaterally as the dorsal column does, pathways carrying pain and temperature cross over through Lissauer's tract to the opposite side of the spinal cord within a few levels of entry to then ascend the anterolateral tract contralaterally. The spinothalamic tracts ascend through the brainstem and thalamus to also be received and integrated within the somatosensory cortex. Figure 25-4 depicts the structures responsible for somatosensory processing, which are generally organized into the dorsal column–medial lemniscal pathway and the anterolateral system.

The brainstem houses the reticular formation and cranial nerves. It is comprised of the midbrain, pons, and medulla. The brainstem has many important functions, especially those responsible for maintaining vital life functions:

- *Midbrain:* Controls consciousness, maintenance of open eyelids, pupil dilation; acts as the pathway for ascending and descending long tracts.
- *Pons:* Controls facial sensation, muscles of mastication, eye movements, facial expression, vestibular and hearing sense; acts as the pathway for ascending and descending long tracts.
- *Medulla:* Relays signals between the brain and spinal cord; controls autonomic functions including respiration, blood pressure, vomiting, and reflexes.

The paired internal carotid arteries (ICAs) and vertebral arteries provide the blood supply to the brain. Anterior circulation is provided by the ICAs, which give rise to the anterior and middle cerebral arteries. The anterior cerebral

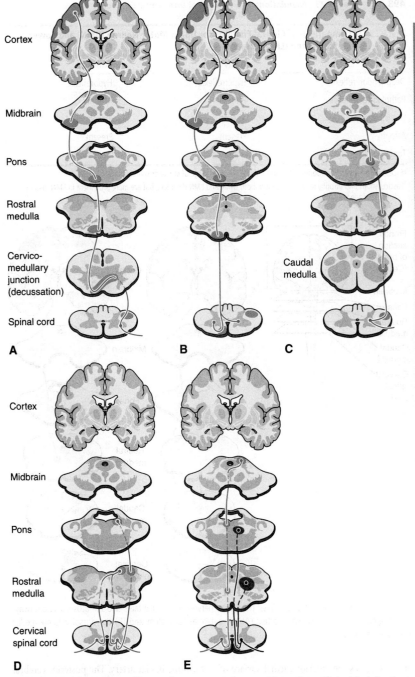

FIGURE 25-3 Motor pathways. The central nervous system has two motor pathways that originate in primary motor cortex: (A) the lateral corticospinal tract and (B) the anterior corticospinal tract. Additionally, motor pathways originate in the midbrain: (C) rubrospinal tract and pons and rostral medulla; (D) vestibulospinal tracts and midbrain and pons; (E) tectospinal tract and reticulospinal tract.

TABLE 25-2 ■ **Comparison of Clinical Findings for Upper Motor Neuron (UMN) and Lower Motor Neuron (LMN) Disease**

	UMN	LMN
Deep tendon reflexes	Hyperreflexic[a]	Hyporeflexic
Pathological reflexes	Present	Absent[a]
Fasciculations[b]	Absent	Present
Atrophy[b]	Present	Present
Tone	Increased[a]	Decreased

[a]Except in the case of newborns and individuals in the acute stage of stroke or spinal injury.

[b]Fasciculations and atrophy may be present in both UMN and LMN disorders, but are more prominent in LMN disorders due to profound weakness.

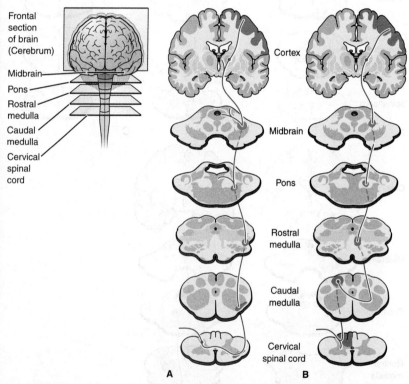

Frontal section of brain (Cerebrum)

Midbrain
Pons
Rostral medulla
Caudal medulla
Cervical spinal cord

Cortex
Midbrain
Pons
Rostral medulla
Caudal medulla
Cervical spinal cord

A   B

FIGURE 25-4 Somatosensory pathways. The central nervous system contains two somatosensory pathways that originate in primary sensory cortex: (A) the anterolateral system and (B) the dorsal column–medial lemniscal pathway.

artery supplies the anterior medial surface of the cortex, and the middle cerebral artery supplies the lateral frontal, temporal, and parietal lobes. Posterior circulation is provided by the vertebral arteries, which come together to form the basilar artery. The posterior cerebral artery arises from the basilar artery. The basilar artery supplies the brainstem and cerebellum, while the posterior cerebral artery supplies the brainstem, cerebellum, inferior and medial temporal lobes, and medial occipital cortex.

The ICAs and basilar artery meet to form the circle of Willis, which is an anastomotic ring that gives rise to additional arteries that supply the cerebral hemispheres. This structure allows brain vasculature to be somewhat redundant, so that if one vessel is damaged and cannot provide blood supply to a certain region of the brain, another will provide some degree of circulation.

The spinal cord is housed within the bony vertebral canal (Fig. 25-5). The vertebral canal is made up of 7 cervical, 12 thoracic, and 5 lumbar vertebrae, along with a fused sacrum. The spinal cord ends at the level of the first or second lumbar vertebrae. Both gray and white matter are located within the cord, with the gray matter housing cell bodies and myelinated axons that travel within the posterior column and anterolateral ascending pathways. The single anterior and two posterior spinal arteries provide the blood supply to the spinal cord.

The spinal cord is a central component of the pathways that transmit information to and from the brain and periphery. Structures within the spinal cord have many functions that serve this purpose. The posterior column receives ipsilateral axons to convey information of proprioception, vibration, and light touch sensation to the brain. Within the posterior column, the gracile fasciculus transmits information from the lower trunk and legs, and the cuneate fasciculus transmits information from the upper trunk, arms, and neck. The anterolateral pathways receive contralateral axons two to three spinal segments superior to convey information of pain and temperature sensation to the brain

The PNS is comprised of lower motor neurons (LMNs), peripheral nerves (including cranial nerves), spinal nerve roots, and the autonomic nervous system. LMNs have cell bodies located within the brainstem and anterior horns of the spinal cord.

There are 12 pairs of cranial nerves (CNs) (Table 25-3). CN I, the olfactory tract, traverses the surface of the frontal lobes (Fig. 25-6). CN II, the optic nerve, comes together at the optic chiasm, forming the optic tracts that enter the thalamus. The remainder of the cranial nerves are located within and exit from the brainstem. CNs III and IV exit the midbrain,

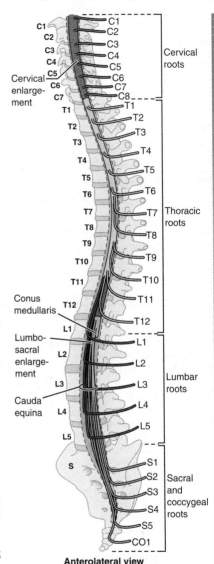

Anterolateral view

FIGURE 25-5 The spinal cord, composed of the cervical, thoracic, lumbar, and sacral cord. The spinal cord terminates at the conus medullaris (T12–L1 level). Traversing lumbosacral roots continue within the spinal canal in the cauda equina.

CN V exits the pons, CN VI the ponto-medullary junction, and CNs VII tkhrough X the pontomedullary junction and medulla, inferiorly in that respective order. The cerebellopontine angle is the exit point for CNs VII, VIII,

TABLE 25-3 ▪ **Cranial Nerves and Functions**

NUMBER	NAME	FUNCTION
I	Olfactory nerve	Sense of smell
II	Optic nerve	Visual acuity, color vision, visual fields, papillary responses
III	Oculomotor nerve	Smooth pursuit, convergence
IV	Trochlear nerve	Smooth pursuit, convergence
V	Trigeminal nerve	Facial sensation, muscles of mastication
VI	Abducens nerve	Smooth pursuit, convergence
VII	Facial nerve	Facial expression, taste
VIII	Vestibulocochlear nerve	Vestibular and hearing sensation, vestibulo-ocular reflex
IX	Glossopharyngeal nerve	Palate elevation and gag reflex
X	Vagus nerve	Palate elevation and gag reflex, visceral innervation
XI	Spinal accessory nerve	Cervical rotation, side-bending, flexion, and shoulder elevation
XII	Hypoglossal nerve	Tongue movements

and IX. CN XI is located within the cervical spinal cord, and CN XII exits the medulla.

The spinal cord gives rise to nerve roots at each level bilaterally (see Fig. 25-6). There are 8 cervical (C1–C8), 12 thoracic (T1–T12), 5 lumbar (L1–L5), 5 sacral (S1–S5) and 1 coccygeal (Co1) pairs of nerve roots. Nerve roots exit each segment of the spinal cord through the intervertebral foramina to then merge into peripheral nerves that traverse the upper extremities, trunk, and lower extremities. Two major plexuses are formed by the nerve roots and peripheral nerves: the brachial plexus, which supplies the upper extremities, and the lumbosacral plexus, which supplies the lower extremities.

The spinal cord terminates as the conus medullaris at the level of L1 or L2. At or around this level, nerve roots converge to become the cauda equina. Both the conus medullaris and cauda equina are considered parts of the PNS. The *conus medullaris* is the caudal end of the spinal cord where lumbar, sacral, and coccygeal nerve roots begin to form. The *cauda equina* is a collection of L1–S2 nerve roots that receive sensory information and provide motor innervation to the legs; they also control bowel and bladder function.

The brachial plexus receives sensory information from and provides a conduit for motor innervation to the upper extremities. The brachial plexus forms from the roots of C5–T1 spinal levels to then merge to become the superior, middle, and inferior trunks. Each trunk then divides in two to form anterior and posterior divisions. These six divisions then merge to become the posterior, lateral, and medial cords. Branches of these cords (in addition to a few exceptions of branches from previous structures within the plexus) make up the peripheral nerves, which are the dorsal scapular, long thoracic, subclavius, suprascapular, lateral pectoral, musculocutaneous, median, upper subscapular, thoracodorsal, lower subscapular, axillary, radial, medial pectoral, medial cutaneous of the arm, medial cutaneous of the forearm, and ulnar nerves. An analogy to this structure is found in the lower extremities in the *lumbosacral plexus*, which receives sensory information from and provides motor innervation to the legs. The lumbosacral plexus forms from the 12 thoracic, 5 lumbar, 5 sacral, and 1 coccygeal spinal nerves. The branches of these spinal nerves form the peripheral nerves, which include the iliohypogastric, ilioinguinal, genitofemoral, lateral femoral cutaneous, obturator, femoral, superior gluteal,

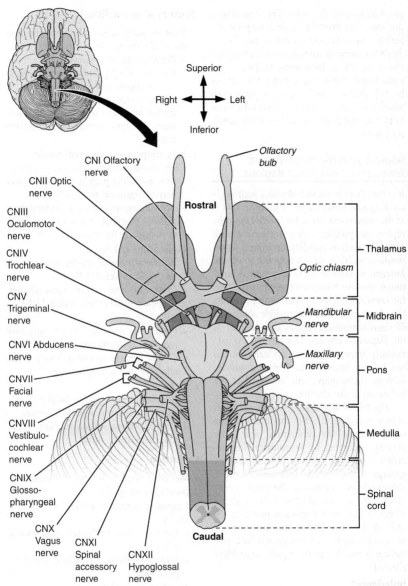

Superior

Right ◄───► Left

Inferior

CNI Olfactory nerve

Olfactory bulb

CNII Optic nerve

Rostral

CNIII Oculomotor nerve

Thalamus

CNIV Trochlear nerve

Optic chiasm

CNV Trigeminal nerve

Mandibular nerve

Midbrain

CNVI Abducens nerve

Maxillary nerve

Pons

CNVII Facial nerve

CNVIII Vestibulo-cochlear nerve

Medulla

CNIX Glosso-pharyngeal nerve

CNX Vagus nerve

CNXI Spinal accessory nerve

CNXII Hypoglossal nerve

Spinal cord

Caudal

FIGURE 25-6 Twelve cranial nerves exit from the midbrain, pons, and brainstem.

inferior gluteal, posterior cutaneous femoral, sciatic, common fibular, tibial, pudendal, and coccygeal nerves.

Dermatomes are an area of skin that is primarily supplied by a single spinal nerve. *Myotomes* are a group of muscles innervated

by the same spinal nerve. Dysfunction in dermatomal distributions, myotomal distributions, or both indicates pathology that causes a spinal nerve root lesion.

The autonomic nervous system (ANS) is comprised of the sympathetic and parasympathetic divisions. The sympathetic division arises from T1–L2, and the parasympathetic from the cranial nerves and S2–S4. The ANS primarily controls consciousness and visceral functions. Its *sympathetic division* elevates blood pressure and heart rate, causes bronchodilation, and increases pupil size, whereas its *parasympathetic division* decreases heart rate and pupil size and increases gastric secretions.

Neurological Impairments and Associated Anatomical Regions

It is rare that an individual with a neurological diagnosis would report a problem that is at the impairment level. Individuals typically report the problems they are having with activities, such as standing up from a seated position, walking, or reaching for an object. Movement analysis of these identified functional activities points to the appropriate tests for impairments. Once specific impairments have been identified, the possible source list of neuroanatomical regions becomes key in the diagnostic process. This approach is particularly important for individuals who do not have a known neurological diagnosis, such as those individuals described at the beginning of this chapter.

The following section provides examples of how neurological health conditions may be considered in the differential diagnostic process, organized by neurological impairments commonly seen in physical therapy settings. These include imbalance, sensory abnormalities, cognition, abnormal movement, stiffness, and weakness. A thorough list of neuroanatomical regions is provided for each of the impairments, and the clinician must follow up by narrowing down the hypothetical source list to the regions *most likely* affected.

Imbalance[5]

- **Peripheral nervous system:** inner ear (membranous and bony labyrinths, hair cells), sensory receptors, ascending peripheral nerves, spinal nerves, vestibulocochlear nerve (CN VIII)
- **Central nervous system:** spinal cord, brainstem, cerebellum, thalamus, basal ganglia

Sensory Abnormalities[1]

- Joint position sense, vibration, and fine, discriminative touch:
  - *Peripheral nervous system:* sensory receptors, ascending peripheral nerves, spinal nerves, trigeminal nerve
  - *Central nervous system:* dorsal column, medial lemniscus of spinal cord, brainstem, thalamus, primary somatosensory cortex
- Pain, temperature, and crude touch:
  - *Peripheral nervous system:* sensory receptors, ascending peripheral nerves, spinal nerves, trigeminal nerve (CN V)
  - *Central nervous system:* anterolateral pathway of spinal cord, brainstem, thalamus, primary somatosensory cortex
- Visual acuity and fields:
  - *Peripheral nervous system:* visual receptors, optic nerves (CN II)
  - *Central nervous system:* optic chiasm, thalamus, visual cortex, occipital lobe
- Smell:
  - *Peripheral nervous system:* olfactory receptors, olfactory nerves (CN I)
  - *Central nervous system:* olfactory tracts, olfactory cortex, temporal lobe
- Taste:
  - *Peripheral nervous system:* facial (CN VII) and glossopharyngeal (CN IX) nerves
  - *Central nervous system:* medulla, thalamus, taste cortex, insula

Cognition[1]

- **Memory:** medial temporal lobes, hippocampus, amygdala
- **Language:** dominant hemisphere (usually the left)
  - *Expressive aphasia:* Broca's area (frontal lobe)
  - *Receptive aphasia:* Wernicke's area (temporal lobe)
- **Attention:** frontal lobe
- **Perseveration:** frontal lobe
- **Impulsivity:** frontal lobe

Abnormal Movement

- **Tremor:** cerebellum, basal ganglia
- **Incoordination:** spinocerebellar pathways, cerebellum, basal ganglia

Stiffness[1]

- **Spasticity:** descending motor pathways at the cortical, brainstem, or spinal cord levels
- **Rigidity:** basal ganglia
- **Hypertonicity:** descending motor pathways, especially the reticulospinal and corticospinal
- **Hypotonicity:** cerebellum, descending motor pathways, and spinal cord in the acute stage of injury

Weakness

- **Upper extremity:**
  - *Peripheral nervous system:* spinal nerves, brachial plexus, peripheral nerves
  - *Central nervous system:* upper extremity region of motor homunculus, primary motor cortex, descending motor pathways, brainstem, cervical spinal cord
- **Lower extremity:**
  - *Peripheral nervous system:* spinal nerves, lumbosacral plexus, cauda equina, conus medullaris, peripheral nerves
  - *Central nervous system:* lower extremity region of motor homunculus, primary motor cortex, descending motor pathways, brainstem
- **Trunk:**
  - *Peripheral nervous system:* spinal nerves, peripheral nerves
  - *Central nervous system:* trunk region of motor homunculus, primary motor cortex, descending motor pathways, brainstem, thoracic spinal cord
- **Face:**
  - *Peripheral nervous system:* facial nerve (CN VII)
  - *Central nervous system:* face region of motor homunculus, primary motor cortex, corticobulbar pathways.

Conclusion

The purpose of this chapter was to outline the foundations of neurological differential diagnosis. To review, the process of neurological differential diagnosis entails formation of a "database" of hypothetical causes for disablement; chart review; focused subjective examination to determine the chief concern and help to discern the type of pathology that may be responsible for causing the chief concern; objective examination, including focused testing that can rule more or less likely involvement of pathology affecting various neuroanatomical structures; identification of neurological impairments and associated neuroanatomical regions; and synthesis of information to determine the appropriate disposition.

References

1. Blumenfeld H. *Neuroanatomy Through Clinical Cases.* Sunderland, MA: Sinauer Associates; 2002.
2. Sullivan KJ, Hershberg J, Howard R, Fisher BE. Neurologic differential diagnosis for physical therapy. *J Neurol Phys Ther.* 2004;28:162–168.
3. Victor M, Ropper A. *Adams and Victor's Principles of Neurology.* 7th ed. New York, NY: McGraw-Hill; 2001.
4. Fisher B, Yakura J. Movement analysis: A different perspective. *Orthop Phys Ther Clin North Am.* 1993;2:1–24.
5. Herdman SJ. *Vestibular Rehabilitation.* 3rd ed. Philadelphia, PA: F. A. Davis; 2007.

FOUNDATIONS OF NEUROLOGICAL DIFFERENTIAL DIAGNOSIS

CHAPTER 26

Cardiovascular and Pulmonary Clues from Examination

■ *Jesus F. Dominguez, PT, PhD*

IN THIS CHAPTER:

■ Rationale for diagnosis of cardiac and pulmonary pathologies by physical therapists
■ Diagnostic relevance of the clinical examination for cardiac and pulmonary pathologies
■ Interpretation of common examination findings with respect to pathology affecting the cardiovascular and pulmonary systems

OUTLINE

Introduction

Physical therapy is becoming a more common route of first entry into the health care delivery system. This development necessitates that physical therapists quickly and accurately recognize the pathology underlying patients' clinical presentations, especially those pathologies that require referral to other health care providers. Of particular importance is the appreciation of cardiovascular and pulmonary disorders that may present in patients who are being seen for unrelated musculoskeletal or neuromuscular dysfunction.

Most patients who experience acute cardiovascular or pulmonary symptoms do not initially seek the services of a physical therapist. Patients may mention these symptoms to a physical therapist or manifest signs of compromised cardiovascular or pulmonary function during the course of treatment for another disorder. In such situations, the physical therapist should establish the patient's cardiovascular and pulmonary status quickly by means of a thorough line of questioning, evaluation of current signs and symptoms, and application of appropriate definitive assessment tools.

During this process, the physical therapist must decide on the appropriate course of action to ensure the health and safety of the patient in a timely manner. Depending on the patient's medical stability, this can include expeditious referral to the patient's primary care physician, direct contact with the primary care provider while the patient is still in the presence of the physical therapist, administration of basic cardiopulmonary life support techniques, or activation of the emergency medical services system.

This chapter is not intended to present a comprehensive cardiovascular and pulmonary examination sequence; rather, it provides an overview of how observation and fundamental evaluation tools contribute to the diagnostic process with respect to cardiovascular and pulmonary pathology.

General Observation is an Important Initial Basis for Diagnosing Cardiovascular and Pulmonary Pathologies

Patients with various cardiovascular and pulmonary diseases commonly adopt recognizable body positions that should prompt the therapist to examine further the pathological reasons behind these preferences. Individuals with chronic obstructive pulmonary disease often assume the "professional position," which consists of leaning forward with hands or elbows resting on knees or another stationary object. This strategy helps to stabilize the shoulder girdle so that the accessory muscles of ventilation can function more optimally in elevating the clavicle and upper ribs. Patients with

chronic obstructive pulmonary disease may also avoid tasks that require the arms to be held at or above shoulder level because of the altered ventilatory mechanics and increased energy cost associated with overhead activities.[1]

The effects of gravity on the distribution of pulmonary edema secondary to chronic congestive heart failure may lead some patients to assume a **semi-Fowler's position** (the head of the bed is elevated and the knees may be slightly elevated) during bedtime and they will state that they require one or several pillows under their head and shoulders to prevent the shortness of breath associated with lying flat on their back. Once in this position, the pulmonary edema is preferentially distributed to the lung bases and the patient is afforded some relief from dyspnea. This condition is called **orthopnea**. The therapist may rate the degree of cardiopulmonary compromise by the number of pillows used by the patient. For example, "two-pillow orthopnea" occurs when the patient uses two pillows to achieve relief.

The patient's general appearance can often suggest the presence of latent or undiagnosed cardiopulmonary disorders.[2] The following physical characteristics represent clues to primary disorders that have secondary cardiopulmonary implications. Anasarca, which is edema or general accumulation of serous fluid in various tissues of the body, may result from congestive heart failure, cirrhosis of the liver, renal failure, or hypoalbuminemia. A tall and thin frame with long extremities, pes cavus, genu valgum, pectus excavatum or carinatum, and flushed cheeks suggest a patient with homocystinuria and a corresponding predisposition toward increased thrombus formation and embolic incidents. Patients with large neck circumferences who are morbidly obese and appear somnolent may have obstructive sleep apnea and associated sequelae that include systemic hypertension and cor pulmonale.

Individuals with Duchenne muscular dystrophy present with accentuated lumbar lordosis, a waddling gait, and pseudohypertrophy of the calves. Duchenne muscular dystrophy is associated with hypertrophic cardiomyopathy and respiratory failure as the disease progresses. Young children who present with cyanosis, fatigue easily, and exhibit a preferential squatting posture are likely to have tetralogy of Fallot. This posture serves as a compensatory strategy by increasing peripheral and aortic pressure so that the right-to-left shunt through the ventricular septal defect is lessened and more blood enters the pulmonary circulation to be oxygenated.

Adiposity in the abdomen and upper torso, peripheral muscle atrophy and weakness, alopecia in women, the presence of a round, plump face, and a fat deposit in the back of the neck and upper shoulders are highly suggestive of Cushing's syndrome. Associated findings include hypertension and elevated blood sugar levels in the diabetic range. Acromegaly leads to enlargement of the hands, feet, and nasal bone with protrusion of the lower jaw and brow. Patients with this condition typically develop systemic hypertension and cardiomyopathy, and often succumb to lethal dysrhythmias. Women with Turner's syndrome present with a webbed neck, short stature, low nuchal hairline, and edema of the lower extremities. This condition may be associated with hypertension or coarctation of the aorta.

Careful inspection and palpation of the head and neck areas during the course of the initial interview and subsequent physical exam also can reveal important clues regarding underlying cardiac or pulmonary pathology. For example, patients with myxedema (cutaneous and dermal edema secondary to deposition of connective tissues often associated with severe hypothyroidism) present with a dull and puffy facies, significant periorbital edema, course hair, and dry skin. In contrast, patients with hyperthyroidism exhibit exophthalmos, palpitations, excessive sweating, and enlargement of the thyroid gland (goiter), which is noted by both visual inspection and palpation. Hypertrophy of the accessory muscles of ventilation (ie, the scalenes and sternocleidomastoids), excessive upper rib cage and clavicular movement, and nasal flaring suggest the presence of chronic obstructive pulmonary disease as the patient attempts to expand an already hyperinflated thoracic cage. These same patients may exhibit pursed-lip breathing and prolonged expiratory time in attempts to maintain airway patency and maximize expired air volume.

Deviation of the trachea from the midline may indicate the presence of a tumor, mediastinal shift, or pneumothorax (deviation toward a simple pneumothorax and away from a tension

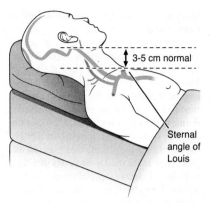

FIGURE 26-1 Assessment of jugular venous distension.

pneumothorax). A corneal arcus (thin, grayish white or yellowish arc around the outer edges of the cornea) in young people suggests, but does not confirm, hyperlipoproteinemia, and individuals with dental caries and advanced gingivitis are at risk for bacterial endocarditis and cardiac valvular lesions. Jugular venous distention (JVD) is a manifestation of heart failure, cardiac tamponade, or constrictive pericarditis. JVD is measured while the patient is semirecumbent with the upper torso at a 45-degree angle (Fig. 26-1). A ruler is used to measure the vertical distance between the sternal angle (angle of Louis) and the highest point of jugular venous pulsation. A value greater than 3 to 5 cm above the sternal angle is considered the criteria for elevated jugular venous pressure.

Assessment of Skin Provides Clues Regarding the Status of Cardiac and Pulmonary Function

Observation of the patient's skin also provides important clues regarding potential underlying cardiovascular or pulmonary pathology. When assessing the patient's skin for signs of cardiovascular and/or pulmonary involvement, the physical therapist should evaluate color, temperature, mobility, and turgor and also identify the presence of lesions or marks.

Color May Indicate the Presence of Impaired Blood Oxygenation

Changes in skin color can be evaluated by examining the lips, the mucous membranes including the oral mucosa, and the peripheral extremities including the nailbeds. **Cyanosis** is a bluish or purplish discoloration of the skin and mucous membranes and may be better appreciated in the perioral area and nailbeds. Cyanosis can result from desaturating disorders that include congestive heart failure with pulmonary edema and chronic obstructive pulmonary disease. Cyanosis is also caused by impaired blood flow associated with peripheral arterial disease. These conditions lead to oxygen desaturation, which causes the bluish appearance characteristic of cyanotic tissue. In the case of impaired flow, an excess amount of oxygen is removed from the circulation and the venous blood is further desaturated. Hypoxemia that is associated with cyanosis may suggest the presence of various congenital heart defects producing right-to-left shunts, such as tetralogy of Fallot, ventricular septal defect, and patent ductus arteriosus, or abnormalities in hemoglobin structure, including methemoglobinemia and sulfhemoglobinemia.[3]

Cyanosis can be classified as central or peripheral, depending on the etiology. Peripheral cyanosis is localized only to the extremities and nailbeds, suggesting compromised blood flow through the arterial tree. Anxiety or cold weather–induced arterial vasoconstriction can also present as transient peripheral cyanosis. Central cyanosis is best appreciated in the lips, oral mucosa, and tongue. It suggests a primary cardiovascular or pulmonary etiology. It is generally accepted that central cyanosis associated with hypoxemia becomes evident only when there are 5 g/dL of unsaturated hemoglobin in the capillaries, and that patients with normal hemoglobin levels manifest cyanosis at higher partial pressures of oxygen and higher hemoglobin saturation levels than patients with lower hemoglobin values.[4] It is likely that patients with low hemoglobin levels will demonstrate signs of acute hypoxemia well before cyanosis becomes evident.

In addition to cyanosis, patients who are chronically hypoxemic often present with digital clubbing (a condition in which the distal segments of the fingers and toes become enlarged) and the nailbeds take on a more convex appearance (similar to the beak of a parrot). A cardinal feature of digital clubbing is a positive Schamroth sign and it is often used to confirm the observation. The sign is observed by having the patient place the dorsal surfaces of two opposing fingers (usually the thumbs) together. Normally, a diamond-shaped window is formed between the distal interphalangeal (DIP) joints and the tips of the nails. A positive Schamroth sign is associated with obliteration of the window as the distal fingertips approximate one another (Fig. 26-2). Digital clubbing is usually associated with such cardiovascular and pulmonary diseases as congenital cyanotic heart disease, endocarditis, atrial myxoma, idiopathic pulmonary fibrosis, chronic lung infections, malignancy, and interstitial pulmonary diseases.

Once cyanosis is identified and hypoxemia is suspected, further evaluation is warranted by means of pulse oximetry to assess hemoglobin oxygen saturation. Cyanosis with associated rapid heart and respiratory rates and altered

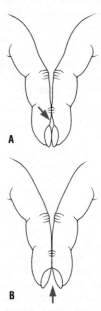

FIGURE 26-2 Schamroth sign: (A) normal appearance of diamond-shaped window between DIP joints and tips of nails (negative Schamroth sign); (B) positive Schamroth sign (obliteration of diamond-shaped window).

mental status are signs that emergency medical intervention is required.

Surface Temperature Reflects the Rate of Underlying Tissue Metabolism

Physical therapists can make a general assessment of skin temperature using the dorsum of the hand and fingers. Warmth noted over an area of localized tenderness, erythema, and swelling may indicate the presence of venous obstruction such as deep venous thrombosis or cellulitis, whereas extremities that appear cold to the touch are often associated with arterial insufficiency. This latter finding can be associated with the presence of diminished pulses. On auscultation, a harsh, vibratory noise secondary to interruption of normal laminar flow through a vessel may be appreciated. This noise is called a **bruit**. If the arterial obstruction or occlusion is severe, a palpable vibration or **thrill** that may also be felt with the palmar aspect of the hand. Generalized warmth is often associated with fever or hyperthyroidism, whereas patients with hypothyroidism exhibit generalized skin coolness.

Mobility and Turgor Suggest the Status of Nutrition, Hydration, and Vascular Competence

Evaluation of skin mobility and turgor can be accomplished by gently lifting up a fold of skin in the distal extremities and observing how quickly it returns to its place. Persistence of elevated skinfolds after they are released indicates decreased turgor. This finding usually occurs in patients with dehydration or malnutrition. Edema is characterized by reduced tissue mobility secondary to extravascular congestion. It can be classified as nonpitting or pitting, with the anterior tibia being a useful site for distinguishing between the two forms. The therapist presses on the skin over a bony area for 10 seconds using three or four fingers and looks or feels for *hills and valleys* (depressions and ridges) after the pressure is released. If the depressions made by the fingers resolve immediately, the edema is nonpitting. If however, the depressions persist, the edema is considered to be pitting. Resolution of the pitting within 30 to 40 seconds is typically associated with low plasma albumin levels, and the persistence of pitting beyond 1 minute favors increased vascular hydrostatic pressure as the contributing source. The latter is termed congestive pitting edema and may be due to such conditions as congestive heart failure, hypertension, medication-induced vasodilation, or venous obstruction. In cases where edema is accompanied by rapid and significant weight gain, such as an increase of 2 to 3 pounds overnight, the patient should be referred to his or her medical practitioner for further workup, because this finding is suggestive of acute fluid retention and heart failure.

The severity of edema has traditionally been assessed on a 0 to 4+ scale, although considerable variation in opinion exists between the precise depth of tissue depression for each value.[5] Alternative methods include taking circumferential or figure-8 girth measurements at several sites along the limb or recording volumetric water displacement by immersing the involved limb in a container filled with water.[6] When utilizing these methods, the therapist should remember to record the precise landmarks used for measurements so that subsequent assessments will more accurately track true changes in limb girths and volumes.

Lesions and Marks can Provide Clues to the Presence of Important Medical Comorbidities

The presence of certain skin lesions or marks may at times alert the physical therapist to the possibility of underlying cardiovascular and pulmonary disorders in their patients. For example, *xanthomas*, which are raised, yellowish, waxy-appearing skin lesions due to deposits of fatty material under the surface of the skin, are often associated with an increase in blood lipid levels. These lesions appear most frequently on the elbows, knees, hands, feet, or buttocks. Underlying metabolic disorders often linked with the presence of xanthomas include diabetes, biliary cirrhosis, and familial hypercholesterolemia. Xanthomas can also appear on the eyelids and are termed xanthelasma palpebra. A butterfly-shaped rash that covers both cheeks and often crosses the bridge of the nose, or **malar rash**, is often observed in patients with systemic lupus erythematosus. Patients with this condition can develop pericarditis or pleurisy some time during the progression of the disease. **Vitiligo**, which refers to white patches of skin appearing on different parts of the body secondary to destruction of melanocytes, may present in patients with hyperthyroidism.

Examination of the Thorax Provides Diagnostic Information Regarding the Cardiovascular and Pulmonary Systems

Examination of the chest yields useful information about the function and integrity of the cardiopulmonary system and provides clues to the presence of pathology. When evaluating the chest wall, the therapist should routinely observe the general contours of the thoracic cage from an anteroposterior (AP) and lateral perspective and assess for obvious asymmetries between the left and right sides. Examination of chest wall excursion, together with breathing rate, rhythm, and depth, should be noted in order to assess ventilatory pump function and identify potential impairments in oxygenation capacity. Palpation, percussion, and auscultation may often be required to appreciate the origin of identified impairments more fully. Examination of the thorax should include assessment of the chest wall configuration and excursion, chest palpation, auscultation, and performance of mediate percussion.

Configuration of the Chest Wall May Indicate the Presence of Chronic Pulmonary Pathology

The normal circumferential pattern of the chest wall is elliptical with an AP-to-lateral diameter ratio of 1:2. Additionally, the ribs typically form an angle of 45 degrees below horizontal where they articulate with the vertebral bodies. AP-to-lateral diameter ratios greater than 1:2 and rib angles that approach the horizontal result in the thoracic cage taking on a more rounded contour that adversely affects chest wall dynamics. The term **barrel chest** is used to describe this observation and is usually associated with pulmonary hyperinflation secondary to chronic obstructive pulmonary disease.

A patient with traumatic flail chest secondary to rib fractures will present with depression of the involved area during inhalation and protrusion during expiration, which is an example of a **paradoxical breathing** pattern. Severe deformities of the chest wall and thoracic spine may impair ventilatory mechanics. For example, patients with moderate to severe scoliosis or kyphoscoliosis may manifest symptoms of hypoinflation, restrictive lung disease, or **cor pulmonale** secondary to excessive pulmonary vascular resistance if chest wall mechanics are significantly compromised. In patients who are morbidly obese (especially those with central adiposity), the increased abdominal mass may impair the descent of the diaphragm and lead to restrictive lung dysfunction. Visible pulsations of the tissue overlying the thorax or abdomen in symptomatic patients are often suggestive of large vessel pathology (ie, aneurysm or dissection) and constitute a medical emergency. In most cases, there is a palpable mass beneath the area of pulsation and a bruit is commonly heard upon auscultation with a stethoscope.

Chest Wall Excursion Reflects the Status of Ventilatory Mechanics

During the initiation of inspiration, the diaphragm descends and the rib cage expands by way of contraction of the parasternals and scalenes to generate the negative intrapleural pressure necessary for lung expansion. The descent of the diaphragm also compresses the abdominal contents, causing the abdominal wall to protrude slightly. Normally, the chest and abdominal walls rise to a similar extent during inspiration, although thoracic excursion is less obvious when the patient is in the supine position. The therapist may choose to evaluate chest wall expansion in any patient who presents with symptoms of potential cardiac or pulmonary pathology, but overt abnormalities in chest wall configuration warrant special attention to thoracic mobility.

Several techniques are available for evaluating the extent and quality of chest wall expansion. One method is to place the thumbs on the posterior aspect of the patient's thorax at the midline and the fingers in parallel orientation to the rib cage approximately at the level of the 10th rib. The thumbs are then brought close together so that a fold of skin is formed at the midline of the patient's back. As the patient is instructed to breathe in deeply, the hands are allowed to travel with the movement of the rib cage (Fig. 26-3). The same procedure can be utilized to evaluate motion in the midthorax, with thumbs placed at the level of the xiphoid process and fingers parallel with the rib cage, and upper thorax, with thumbs placed at the level of the suprasternal notch and fingers perpendicular to the clavicles.

An alternate method is to place a measuring tape around the upper, middle, and lower thorax and evaluate excursion as the patient breathes deeply. The tape should be held loosely so that chest movement is not restricted. In general, the typical excursion in most areas of the thoracic cage ranges from 3 to 10 cm.[7] The therapist is reminded to measure chest wall excursion both during quiet breathing and with deep breathing to evaluate possible restrictions in range of motion. Although excursion deficits should be noted in all cases, the measurements obtained are best suited for purposes of tracking changes within a particular patient.

The magnitude of chest expansion and symmetry of movement can provide the therapist with clues as to the presence of cardiopulmonary dysfunction. For example, a patient with lobar pneumonia, hemi-diaphragm paralysis secondary to phrenic nerve injury during cardiac bypass surgery, or a thoracic surgical incision may present with diminished excursion on the involved side, whereas a patient with chronic obstructive pulmonary disease may demonstrate a symmetric decrease in chest wall motion.

Globally diminished chest wall excursion may be observed in patients with ankylosing spondylitis as the disease progresses. Unilateral lag usually indicates pathology of the underlying lung or pleura. Paradoxical breathing patterns may be noted in individuals with spinal cord injury and severe chronic obstructive pulmonary disease. In individuals with spinal cord injury, the limited abdominal and intercostal muscle control causes exaggerated abdominal protrusion and intercostal retraction during inspiration. This is characterized as an upper chest paradox with pronounced abdominal rise. Individuals with chronic obstructive pulmonary disease typically present with abdominal and lower rib cage retraction during inspiration, while expansion of the upper chest is accentuated because of accessory muscle overuse. This pattern is characterized as an abdominal paradox with pronounced upper chest rise. Retraction of the intercostal spaces during inspiratory effort suggests the presence of severe airway obstruction, which is typically accompanied by a loud, clearly audible, high-pitched wheezing sound called **stridor**. These signs indicate that the patient is rapidly decompensating and in need of immediate medical attention.

Palpation of the Thorax Provides Information Regarding the Physical Composition and Orientation of Thoracic Organs

Tactile fremitus is a normal phenomenon resulting from transmission of vocal sounds via the bronchopulmonary tree to the surface of the thorax. The vibration of tactile fremitus is best appreciated with the palmar

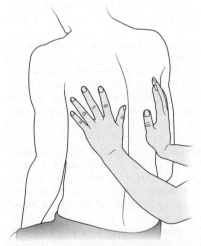

FIGURE 26-3 Evaluation of chest wall excursion.

surface of the metacarpal heads or the hypothenar eminence. The therapist instructs the patient to repeat the words "one–two–three" or "ninety-nine" as both sides of the posterior thorax are palpated simultaneously to compare intensity and symmetry of the vibration. Because of the location of the scapulae and heart, as well as the natural decay in transmission volume, tactile fremitus is most prominent in the interscapular regions, while the left side and posterior lung bases are associated with decreased vibration.

With experience, the novice therapist will be able to discern normal from abnormal patterns. Because of the physical properties of different media, sound volume is transmitted more effectively through fluid as compared to air. Consolidation of the underlying lung tissue secondary to fluid accumulation and pneumonia enhances the intensity of tactile fremitus. Conversely, other conditions that cause impedance of sound transmission are associated with diminished tactile fremitus, such as bronchial obstruction, hyperinflation associated with chronic obstructive pulmonary disease, pneumothorax, and obesity. The therapist should auscultate with a stethoscope over areas of altered vibration to assess further for the presence of underlying pulmonary involvement.

Palpation over the precordium can yield valuable information about the patient's cardiac status as well. The *apical impulse* refers to the point at which the apex of the heart strikes the thoracic wall during ventricular systole, whereas the *point of maximal impulse* is a term used to identify the specific location where the heart strikes the thoracic wall with the greatest force. The apical impulse and the point of maximal impulse can be grossly identified by palpation using the palmar aspect of the phalanges; finer localization can then be accomplished using one finger. Normally, both occur at the fifth intercostal space along the midclavicular line. At times, the apical impulse and the point of maximal impulse are not coincident and the point of maximal impulse may be displaced medially or laterally from the fifth intercostal space. This may occur in individuals with ventricular hypertrophy or dilation, aortic dilation or aneurysm, pulmonary artery enlargement, pneumothorax, or a space-occupying tumor. An extreme rightward deviation of the apical impulse is associated with the rare condition of **dextrocardia** in which the heart is rotated 180 degrees and is anatomically located in the right margin of the mediastinum. Additional investigation of these palpatory findings should include cardiac auscultation.

Masses observed on the abdominal or thoracic walls should be palpated to identify the presence of thrills as the result of vascular obstruction or dilation. Some of the most common conditions associated with palpable thrills are aortic aneurysms, aortic dissections, atherosclerosis, arteriovenous malformations, or arteriovenous fistulas. The therapist will often appreciate a bruit when auscultating over the area where the thrill is identified. This finding further supports the presence of vascular pathology and warrants timely consultation with the patient's physician.

Tonal Quality of Sound Transmitted Through the Thorax Provides Information Regarding the Composition of the Lungs

The ability to appreciate the subtle, yet distinct, sounds produced by percussion of the chest wall and discriminate sound quality that suggests the presence of air, fluid, or consolidation within the underlying tissues is vital to the emerging trend of autonomous practice in physical therapy. The technique of mediate percussion begins with hyperextension of the middle finger (referred to as the **pleximeter**) of the nondominant hand and placement of its distal interphalangeal joint on the surface to be percussed. Care should be taken to keep the other four fingers raised away from the patient's skin so as not to dampen the transmission of sound. The tip of the middle finger of the dominant hand (referred to as the **plexor**) is used to strike the distal interphalangeal joint of the pleximeter sharply by allowing the wrist to flex freely (Fig. 26-4). After the strike, the plexor is quickly withdrawn.

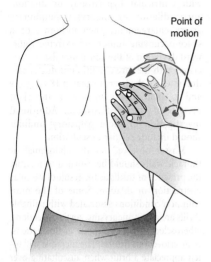

Point of motion

FIGURE 26-4 The technique of mediate percussion.

The resulting sound is categorized according to its quality and should prompt the therapist to evaluate the area in question more thoroughly by employing more directed auscultatory techniques (discussed later in this chapter). From a physical therapy perspective, the most likely candidates for the application of mediate percussion techniques are those patients who present with pulmonary symptoms and in whom auscultatory findings warrant further evaluation. The

nature of pulmonary pathology is related to the tonal quality that results from mediate percussion (Table 26-1).[8]

Vital Signs Provide Direct Information Regarding Various Aspects of Cardiovascular and Pulmonary Functioning

The arterial pulse is produced when the left ventricle contracts and ejects blood through the aorta and out to the peripheral arterial tree. Thus, the pulse is coincident with the period of ventricular systole. The pulse is measured at the wrist by palpating the radial artery and counting the number of beats felt in 10, 15, or 30 seconds and multiplying by 6, 4, or 2, respectively, to arrive at an average heart rate (HR) in beats per minute (bpm). If the pulse is noted to be irregular, as discussed later in this section, then the length of assessment should be increased to 60 seconds in order to minimize error in estimation.

The therapist should routinely assess the pulse quality bilaterally to rule out asymmetries between limbs, which is suggestive of peripheral vascular compromise. It is also wise practice to assess all peripheral arteries in order to compare pulse characteristics of the neck (carotid), upper extremities (ie, brachial and radial arteries), and lower extremities (femoral, popliteal, posterior tibial, and dorsalis pedis arteries). For

TABLE 26-1 ■ **Characteristics of Percussion Notes and Associated Pathologies**

PERCUSSION NOTE	RELATIVE INTENSITY OR LOUDNESS	RELATIVE PITCH OR FREQUENCY	RELATIVE DURATION	EXAMPLE OF LOCATION FOR COMPARISON	EXAMPLE OF ASSOCIATED CONDITION
Flatness	Soft	High	Short	Thigh	Large pleural effusion
Dullness	Medium	Medium	Medium	Liver	Lobar pneumonia
Resonance	Loud	Low	Long	Normal lung	Normal, chronic bronchitis
Hyperresonance	Very loud	Lower	Longer	None normally	Emphysema, pneumothorax
Tympany	Loud	High[a]	[a]	Gastric air bubble or puffed-out cheek	Large pneumothorax

[a]Distinguished mainly by its musical timbre.

example, diminished strength or absence of pulses in the left vs. right upper extremity or the lower vs. upper extremity is associated with coarctation of the aorta or advanced peripheral vascular disease. Evaluation of the rate, rhythm, and quality of the patient's pulse can provide the therapist with information regarding the status of the cardiac pump.

Heart Rate Indicates the Cardiovascular System's Response to Different Levels of Activity

The normal resting heart rate lies within the range of 60 to 100 bpm. This is referred to as a *normal sinus rhythm*. Patients may present with a resting pulse that is less than 60 bpm (bradycardia) or greater than 100 bpm (tachycardia) which may manifest symptoms of underperfusion, including dizziness, lightheadedness, diaphoresis, visual disturbance, cognitive impairment, shortness of breath/chest discomfort, or syncope. However, resting heart rates that deviate from the normal range do not always indicate the presence of pathology. Because of the potential for deficits in cardiac output, bradycardia or tachycardia must be evaluated within the context of the patient's entire clinical picture.

The therapist can further evaluate the cardiac rate response to various perturbations, including ventilatory maneuvers and positional changes (Box 26-1). For example, some individuals exhibit a variation in heart rate that is influenced by the ventilatory cycle and is mediated by the respiratory centers in the medulla. The heart rate is felt to increase as the patient inhales and to decrease as the patient exhales. This phenomenon is called *respiratory sinus dysrhythmia* and is considered to be a normal variant in children and young adults, as well as highly conditioned athletes. Additionally, asking an individual to move from the supine to sitting or standing position renders the cardiovascular system more susceptible to the influence of gravity. This maneuver induces temporary venous pooling in the lower extremities and would lead to a reduction in venous return and cardiac output if it were not for the normal reflexive response of increasing the heart rate in addition to vascular adjustments

---

BOX 26-1 How is the Appropriateness of Heart Rate Determined for a Given Functional Activity?

The chronotropic index (ratio of heart rate reserve to metabolic reserve) is often used in the clinic to assess the appropriateness of the heart rate response to a particular workload. For a given workload, the percentage of heart rate (HR) reserve used is represented by the following equation:

$$\% \text{ HR reserve} = [(HR_{stage} - HR_{rest}) / (220 - \text{age in years} - HR_{rest})] \times 100.$$

Similarly, the percentage of metabolic reserve used is represented by the following equation:

$$\% \text{ Metabolic reserve} = [(MET_{stage} - MET_{rest}) / (MET_{peak} - MET_{rest})] \times 100,$$

where MET refers to the metabolic equivalent (ie, 1 MET = 3.5 mL O_2/kg/min consumed at rest) and MET_{peak} refers to the peak oxygen consumption during a maximal symptom-limited exercise test.

The chronotropic index is expressed as the ratio between the % HR reserve and the % metabolic reserve. A ratio of <0.8 is considered to be a low chronotropic index and suggestive of *chronotropic incompetence*. An alternative determination is that heart rate should increase by approximately 10 to 15 bpm from resting values during *normal* walking speeds (ie, 2.0 to 3.0 mph). Chronotropic incompetence is highly suggestive of sympathetic autonomic nervous system dysfunction and warrants referral to the appropriate health care practitioner.

---

to maintain left ventricular output. It has been suggested that no change or a decrease in heart rate when assuming a more vertical position is indicative of a compromised cardiovascular system.[9]

Pulse Rhythm Suggests the Status of Electrical Conduction and Cardiac Output

Heartbeat rhythm is described by one of the following three terms:

1. Regular,
2. Regularly irregular, or
3. Irregularly irregular.

A *regular* rhythm implies that the cadence of the palpated pulse does not vary appreciably from beat to beat and usually, although not always, identifies normal sinus rhythm. A rhythm that is *regularly irregular* refers to an irregularity in the palpated pulse that occurs in a regular, repeating pattern. Examples of this include normal sinus rhythm with premature atrial contractions, premature junctional contractions, premature ventricular contractions, and supraventricular tachycardias with a fixed atrial/ventricular block.

Atrial fibrillation is perhaps the best example of an *irregularly irregular* rhythm, and it is characterized by erratic variations in the time between successive beats. The pulse rhythm varies from beat to beat and can alternate between fast and slow rates. An irregular rhythm should prompt the therapist to auscultate the heart with a stethoscope while palpating the pulse to correlate cardiac contraction with the peripheral pulse. In some instances, premature beats do not generate a peripheral pulse because cardiac diastolic filling time is compromised. This is referred to as a *pulse deficit*. Irregular rhythms may affect cardiac output and should therefore be a consideration for referral to the appropriate health care practitioner.

Pulse Quality Provides Information Regarding the Status of Contractile Force and Cardiac Output

In general terms, the quality of the pulse refers to its strength when palpated and to the presence of associated findings such as palpable thrills. Physical therapists should consider examining the brachial and carotid pulses in the event of abnormal findings on radial artery examination. The pulse can be characterized based on its strength (Table 26-2). The

characteristics discussed next may also be identified. They are typically appreciated best at the carotid artery but can, on occasion, be felt in other peripheral arteries.

COLLAPSING PULSE
The pulse is noted to be strong initially and then disappears quickly. This finding is also common in patients with severe aortic regurgitation and is caused by a larger than normal stroke volume yielding a forceful contraction followed by rapid collapse of the pulse strength as blood regurgitates back into the left ventricle. For this reason, the difference between systolic and diastolic blood pressures will be wide.

PULSUS BISFERIENS
In *pulsus bisferiens* (*bis* = two and *feriere* = to beat), the pulse is noted to have two distinct systolic peaks separated by a slight drop during midsystole. The dip is primarily due to regurgitation of blood back into the left ventricle during midsystole. This finding is common in patients with significant aortic regurgitation and hypertrophic cardiomyopathy. In the latter, the mechanism involves rapid ejection of blood in early systole, followed by a trough, culminating in a second ventricular ejection wave (the second peak). Pulsus bisferiens is also commonly associated with a wide pulse pressure.

PULSUS ALTERNANS
In an otherwise healthy individual, the pulse strength may decrease slightly during inspiration as the result of pulmonary vascular engorgement associated with decreased intrapleural pressures. This, in turn, diminishes return to the left heart and the pulse is noted to be softer because of the slightly lower stroke volume. Although not commonly

TABLE 26-2 ■ **Classification of Peripheral Pulses**

GRADE	PHYSICAL FINDING	EXAMPLE OF ASSOCIATED CONDITION
0	Absent	Arterial obstruction or cardiovascular collapse
1+	Weak and thready	Hypovolemic or hypotensive
2+	Normal force	Normal
3+	Full	Elevated temperature (fever), anxiety, or exercise
4+	Bounding	Hypervolemic or hypertensive

observed, this is considered to be a normal phenomenon. However, significant variations in pulse strength timed with the breathing cycle typically indicate the presence of a pathological condition. The appreciation of a strong pulse alternating with a weak pulse in a cyclic pattern is referred to as *pulsus alternans*.

If pulsus alternans is suspected, the patient is asked to hold his or her breath during mid-inspiration to avoid ventilatory cycle influence. The physical therapist should then assess the pulse strength for alternating weak and strong beats. The systolic pressure is noted to alternate between higher and lower values as well. It is thought that the variation in pulse strength is a manifestation of decreased myocardial contractility secondary to failure of certain myocytes to contract on alternate cardiac cycles. The decreased myocardial contractility leads to decreased stroke volume (weaker pulse). This results in increased end-diastolic volume prior to the next systole. Via the Frank-Starling mechanism, the next systole produces a more forceful contraction (stronger pulse). The cycle then repeats itself. Pulsus alternans is almost always associated with severe left ventricular systolic dysfunction. In some individuals, **electrical alternans** (visible as fluctuations in QRS amplitude or electrical axis on ECG) is also present. This is often observed in patients with severe pericardial effusion and cardiac temponade. It is thought to result from the heart "wobbling" back and forth within the fluid-filled pericardial sac.[10]

PULSUS PARADOXUS

The term *pulsus paradoxus* was coined by Adolph Kussmaul in 1873 to describe an absence of the palpated pulse and auscultated contraction correlated to the ventilatory cycle.[11] The pulse strength diminishes slightly during inspiration and returns again during expiration. More appropriately, the term is used to describe an exaggerated fall ($\geq$10 mm Hg) in systolic blood pressure during inspiration. During inspiration, venous return to the right heart is enhanced and this causes a bowing of the interventricular septum toward the left ventricle, reducing the left ventricle's dimensions during diastole and limiting end-diastolic volume. In addition, the reduction in intrapleural pressure during inspiration favors pooling in the pulmonary vasculature and further reduces left ventricular end-diastolic volume. Both factors

combine to cause the diminished pulse strength and systolic blood pressure during this maneuver and the magnitude of the drop is exaggerated by disease states. Pulsus paradoxus is associated with cardiopulmonary pathologies that include cardiac tamponade, constrictive pericarditis, acute myocardial infarction, pulmonary embolus, and severe asthma.

BIGEMINAL PULSE

The term used to describe a pulse in which the beats seem to occur in pairs with a slight pause between coupled beats is referred to as *pulsus bigeminus*. The most likely cause of this finding is premature contraction of the ventricles, which may be of ventricular or supraventricular origin. Typically, the second beat is noted to be weaker than the first, suggesting that the beat occurred prematurely and limited ventricular diastolic filling. Although the distinction is typically made on the basis of ECG criteria, longer pauses between paired beats suggests an ectopic focus of ventricular origin.

PALPABLE VIBRATION (THRILL)

Normally, blood flowing through vessels does so in a streamlined fashion, a phenomenon referred to as laminar flow. In peripheral arteries, when there is an obstruction to flow or when flow velocities are enhanced, the resulting turbulence is appreciated as a *palpable thrill*, often described as a vibration best felt with the palmar aspect of the metacarpals or hypothenar eminence. The thrill is almost always associated with a bruit when the vessel is auscultated with a stethoscope. Bruits in the peripheral vessels are thus analogous to cardiac murmurs. As mentioned previously, palpable thrills are observed in patients with various conditions, including peripheral vascular disease, cardiac valvular stenosis or regurgitation, arteriovenous malformations, or arteriovenous fistulas.

Blood Pressure Responds to Changes in Position and Activity in a Predictable Fashion and Provides Important Clues to Organ Perfusion

Measurement of arterial pressure is a skill that every physical therapist can master with experience and diligence. This often requires little more effort than routinely measuring blood pressure (BP) in all patients coming into the clinic or being seen at the bedside. With the patient seated quietly and his or her arm supported by the therapist, a cuff is placed around the patient's arm and inflated until the pressure in the cuff exceeds the systolic blood pressure. The degree to which the cuff should be inflated is easily estimated by palpating the patient's radial or brachial pulse as the pressure in the cuff increases. The therapist should note the point at which the pulse becomes absent; this is a general approximation of the systolic blood pressure. The cuff is deflated and the patient is allowed to rest for 1 minute. The therapist then inflates the cuff 20 to 30 mm Hg higher than the point where the pulse became absent and begins listening to the Korotkoff sounds with a stethoscope as the bladder is deflated.[12]

To ensure inter- and intra-tester reliability and accurately monitor patient status, the therapist should be familiar with the American Heart Association (AHA) standardization guidelines for the measurement of blood pressure.[12] According to these guidelines, the systolic blood pressure is recorded when the therapist first hears discernable tapping sounds as the pressure in the cuff is released (coincident with the first Korotkoff sound). The cuff is allowed to continue deflating and the diastolic pressure is recorded when the sounds disappear altogether (or at the point when they are last heard). Diastolic blood pressure corresponds to this fifth Korotkoff sound. In some cases (eg, in infants and small children), the tapping sounds may be heard all the way down to the 0 mm Hg mark on the dial. When this occurs, the diastolic pressure should be recorded when the therapist hears the tapping sound muffle distinctly (corresponding to the fourth Korotkoff sound). Most experts feel that the fifth Korotkoff sound (disappearance) more closely approximates true adult diastolic pressure, whereas the fourth Korotkoff sound (muffling)

is a better estimate of diastolic pressure in infants and children. Table 26-3 represents the most recent AHA recommendations for resting BP values in adults and their classification.[12]

Blood pressure measurements should be routinely taken in both arms when seeing the patient for the first time. It is common for BP to differ between right and left arms on the order of ≤10 mm Hg (although greater differences have been recorded) with the higher reading frequently measured in the right arm. Clinical evidence suggests that the mortality hazard (risk of all-cause death) increases significantly for every 10 mm Hg difference in systolic BP between arms.[13] As a matter of convention, the arm with the higher reading is used to monitor blood pressure and determine the presence of hypertension. A difference of >10 mm Hg usually necessitates further investigation, including assessment of lower extremity pressures. Depending on location, coarctation of the aorta and aortic dissection are associated with higher pressures in the right vs. left arm, or higher pressures in the upper vs. lower extremities.

The therapist can gather important information about a patient's cardiovascular health by measuring blood pressure while the patient assumes different body positions. Blood pressure is measured in the supine position after the patient has been lying quietly for 5 to 10 minutes and then immediately after the patient stands up. In most cases, diastolic pressure is lower in the supine compared to the standing position. The increase in diastolic BP with standing reflects the effects of gravity on venous pooling that are offset by an increase in peripheral vascular tone. In contrast, systolic BP changes very little during the transition from supine to standing in otherwise healthy individuals (a finding that is consistent with maintenance of

TABLE 26-3 ■ American Heart Association Classification for Adult Blood Pressure Values

CLASSIFICATION	SYSTOLIC BP (mm HG)	DIASTOLIC BP (mm HG)
Normal	<120	<80
Prehypertension	120–139	80–89
Stage 1 hypertension	140–159	90–99
Stage 2 hypertension	≥160	≥100

venous return supported by increased diastolic pressure). A diastolic blood pressure that drops when the patient stands likely indicates vascular incompetence or a dysfunctional autonomic nervous system (especially if there is no compensatory increase in heart rate). By definition, *orthostatic hypotension* refers to a drop in systolic and/or diastolic BP when going from the supine position to sitting or standing. The accepted criteria is a drop of ≥20 mm Hg in systolic pressure and/or a drop of ≥10 mm Hg in diastolic pressure within 3 minutes of standing up.[14] Associated symptoms can include dizziness, light-headedness, shortness of breath, chest discomfort, urinary incontinence, and syncope.

In some patients, an exaggerated reflex tachycardia (usually an increase in heart rate of 30 bpm) is noted as the sympathetic nervous system attempts to compensate for the drop in arterial pressure.[15] The condition is termed **positional orthostatic tachycardia syndrome**. Absence of a blood pressure increase in the presence of hypotension may imply a neurological component to the disorder.

Other factors to consider in the diagnosis of orthostatic hypotension include the patient's neurological status, use of vasoactive medications, prolonged bed rest, and hemorrhagic or hypovolemic states. Furthermore, maintenance of (or an increase in) systolic blood pressure in the face of a lower diastolic blood pressure in the standing position may be an early sign of cardiac pump failure. In this example, the left ventricle operates more efficiently when the patient stands because of the reduced venous return.[9]

As mentioned during the discussion of pulse assessment, blood pressure also demonstrates variations timed with the ventilatory cycle. Specifically, systolic blood pressure is lower during inspiration because of the associated pulmonary vascular engorgement and decreased left ventricular end-diastolic volume. The typical difference in systolic pressure between inspiration and expiration is on the order of ≤10 mm Hg. Certain pathologies exaggerate the inspiratory drop in systolic blood pressure, including cardiac tamponade and constrictive pericarditis. When these conditions are suspected, the therapist should check for the presence of pulsus paradoxus. First, the therapist takes the patient's blood pressure as usual. The therapist then asks the patient to inspire and hold their breath. Blood pressure is now taken while the patient continues to hold his or her breath and systolic pressure is noted. A drop of >10 mm Hg in systolic BP with inspiration confirms pulsus paradoxus.[16] An alternate approach is to have the patient breathe normally as the therapist takes the blood pressure by deflating the cuff at a slightly slower rate. This will allow the therapist to note when the systolic blood pressure is heard only during expiration and then when it is heard during both inspiration and expiration.

Systolic BP demonstrates typical responses to increasing physical workload, which can be altered in various disease states (Table 26-4).[17,18] Because systolic BP is a function of cardiac output and total peripheral resistance, the

TABLE 26-4 ■ **Criteria for Normal and Abnormal Blood Pressure (BP) Responses to Graded Exercise**

DESCRIPTION	CRITERIA	EXAMPLE OF ASSOCIATED CONDITION
Normal	*Systolic BP:* 7–12 mm Hg increase per MET *Diastolic BP:* ± 10 mm Hg from resting values throughout test	Normal BP response
Hypertensive	*Systolic BP:* ≥15–20 mm Hg increase per MET *Diastolic BP:* ≥90 mm Hg	Systemic hypertension, coronary artery disease, arteriosclerosis
Blunted or flat	*Systolic BP:* <5–7 mm Hg increase per MET	Overmedication, ventricular failure, coronary artery disease
Hypoadaptive	*Systolic BP:* ≥20 mm Hg drop after an initial rise	Severe ventricular failure, multivessel coronary artery disease, significant overmedication

relationship can be expressed in terms of the following equation: systolic BP ≈ CO × TPR. Recalling also that cardiac output is the product of heart rate and left ventricular stroke volume, increasing workload leads to an increase in cardiac output (because of its direct effects on heart rate and stroke volume). To support this increase in cardiac output, systemic vascular tone is adjusted such that total peripheral resistance actually decreases as the intensity of exercise progresses.

In response to graded exercise, systolic BP increases in a fairly linear fashion, such that for every 1 metabolic equivalent (MET) increase in workload, the systolic BP increases 7 to 12 mm Hg from resting values.[17] The conclusion drawn from this observation is that cardiac output increases to a greater degree than total peripheral resistance decreases, and the net result is an increase in systolic BP. In contrast, diastolic blood pressure is more directly influenced by total peripheral resistance and changes very little from resting values in response to exertion (on the order of ±10 mm Hg).

Respiratory Rate Suggests the Status of Ventilatory Mechanics and Blood Oxygenation

Measurement of respiratory rate provides important basic diagnostic information regarding pulmonary function. At rest, the typical respiratory rate in adults is 10 to 20 breaths per minute; in infants it may be 20 to 40 breaths per minute. In newborns, the respiratory rate may be as high as 40 to 50 breaths per minute. Because most individuals alter their

respiratory rate subconsciously if they know they are being watched, the therapist should adopt a strategy that minimizes this confounding factor. One strategy is to assess the patient's pulse for 30 seconds and continue to palpate the pulse for another 30 seconds while inconspicuously counting breaths. The respiratory rate is then calculated by multiplying the breaths counted in 30 seconds by 2.

Breathing rhythm is important to observe, because various forms of pathology may affect it (Table 26-5). Normally, the inspiratory phase is half as long as the expiratory phase. Patients with small airway obstruction often present with prolonged expiratory times (and may exhibit pursed-lip breathing), whereas patients with restrictive lung disease may shorten both the inspiratory and expiratory phases leading to a reduced tidal volume. In the latter case, respiratory rate is usually elevated and represents a pattern termed **tachypnea**. Patients with restrictive lung disease often adopt this pattern of breathing because of the relatively high metabolic cost associated with maintaining normal tidal volume.

Other diagnoses associated with tachypnea include pleuritic or incisional chest pain, elevated or hemi-diaphragm, and partial upper airway obstruction. Although hyperventilation has been used historically in reference to either rapid or deep breathing, the term **hyperpnea** is probably more appropriate and indicates that the breathing pattern is rapid and deep. Hyperpnea may be caused by relatively benign factors that include exercise and anxiety, but can also be associated with more serious conditions such as metabolic acidosis. Patients with

---

TABLE 26-5 ■ **Characteristics of Abnormal Breathing Patterns**

BREATHING PATTERN	CHARACTERISTICS	EXAMPLE OF ASSOCIATED CONDITION
Cheyne-Stokes breathing	Periods of hyperpnea followed by periods of apnea (no breathing)	Uncompensated congestive heart failure, drug-induced respiratory depression, brain injury, uremia secondary to kidney failure
Biot's (ataxic) breathing	Periods of hyperpnea, tachypnea, or apnea with no predictable regularity	Meningitis, brain injury
Apneustic breathing	Deep inspiration followed by a pause, ending in rapid exhalation	Brain injury (pontine lesion)

diabetes mellitus and severe ketoacidosis may demonstrate a characteristic deep, labored, and gasping breathing pattern called **Kussmaul breathing**. Likewise, **bradypnea**, which is slow breathing in which the respiratory rate is <10 breaths per minute, may be a manifestation of an exercise-trained pulmonary system or concentration on a specific task, but can also result from drug-induced respiratory depression, diabetic coma, or traumatic brain injury with elevation of intracranial pressure.

With respect to graded exercise, the first adjustment made by the ventilatory system is usually an increase in tidal volume. As exercise intensity progresses, the respiratory rate increases in order to support the metabolic demands of the exercising muscles. Anxiety can often lead to a rapid increase in respiratory rate at the start of an exercise bout and should not be interpreted as an abnormal finding.

Heart and Lung Sounds Reveal Clues About Cardiac and Pulmonary Pathology

Although a comprehensive tutorial on cardiac and pulmonary auscultation is beyond the scope of this chapter, all physical therapists should be able to identify more obvious abnormal heart sounds that can be readily distinguished from normal heart sounds. We advocate that any stethoscope that will be used for auscultating heart and lung sounds must have a diaphragm (the flat head that is pressed firmly against the skin and used for listening to high-frequency sounds) and a bell (the cup-shaped head that is placed softly against the skin and is useful for hearing low-frequency sounds). Using a stethoscope that only has a diaphragm will result in failure to appreciate some abnormal cardiac sounds.

Cardiac Auscultation

To perform a competent auscultatory examination of the heart, the therapist should adopt a systematic approach which includes:

1. Proper positioning of the patient,
2. Listening to the major auscultatory areas on the chest wall with the diaphragm, and
3. Listening to those same areas again with the bell of the stethoscope.

Sounds produced by the aortic valve are usually heard best in the aortic area (second intercostal space along the right sternal border), whereas the pulmonic valve sounds are appreciated best in the pulmonic area (second intercostal space along the left sternal border). The tricuspid area (fourth or fifth intercostal space along the left sternal border) and mitral area (fifth intercostal space at the midclavicular line) represent the remaining landmarks for auscultation (Fig. 26-5). These sites are typically auscultated with the patient supine, but having the patient assume the left lateral decubitus position or sitting up and leaning forward while holding the breath can be useful to accentuate heart sounds that are otherwise faint or inaudible.

Normal heart sounds are thought to originate from the closure of specific heart valves (or the reverberating sound made by blood colliding with a valve as it is closing). The first normal heart sound (the *lub* in *lub-dub*) is called S_1 and is associated with closure of the mitral (M_1 component of S_1) and tricuspid (T_1 component of S_1) valves. The second normal heart sound (the *dub* in *lub-dub*) is called S_2 and is associated with closure of the aortic (A_2 component of S_2) and pulmonic (P_2 component of S_2) valves. Ventricular systole, then, is represented by the period between S_1 and S_2, whereas diastole occurs between S_2 and the next S_1. Although S_1 and S_2 are high frequency in nature and usually appreciated as single

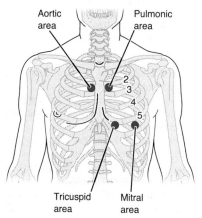

FIGURE 26-5 Primary sites for cardiac auscultation of the anterior chest wall.

sounds when using the diaphragm, individual components of each sound are sometimes distinguishable. In this case, the sound is said to be **split**. This occurs because cardiac mechanical events on the left slightly precede those on the right. That is to say, the mitral valve closes slightly before the tricuspid valve and the aortic valve closes slightly before the pulmonic valve.

A useful maneuver to aid the therapist in distinguishing between the S_1 and S_2 sounds (and especially difficult task with faster pulse rates) is to palpate the carotid artery while auscultating the heart. The carotid pulse is coincident with the beginning of ventricular systole, and so it is timed with S_1. Because S_1 is associated with closure of the mitral and tricuspid valves, S_1 is louder than S_2 in the mitral and tricuspid areas. Conversely, S_2 is louder than S_1 in the aortic and pulmonic areas. The tricuspid area is the best place to listen for a normal splitting of S_1, whereas the pulmonic area is best for appreciating a splitting of S_2 (the pulmonic valve closes slightly later than the aortic valve). While a split S_1 is not affected by the ventilatory cycle, a split S_2 can be further evaluated on the basis of changes related to inspiration or expiration. A **physiological** split S_2 (a normal phenomenon) exhibits a widening of the A_2 and P_2 sounds upon inspiration and a fusion of the two sounds upon expiration. The drop in intrathoracic pressure during inspiration leads to increased venous return and prolongs right ventricular ejection, causing the pulmonic valve to close later than usual.

Several abnormal heart sounds can be auscultated:

- A split S_2 that either:
  1. is not affected by the ventilatory cycle (fixed split S_2)
  2. widens with inspiration and approximates, but does not fuse, with expiration (persistent split S_2); or
  3. widens with expiration and fuses with inspiration (paradoxical split S_2); these are associated with various cardiac anatomical and conduction abnormalities.
- A third heart sound (S_3) can be heard with the bell of the stethoscope in patients with congestive heart failure and occurs as a low-frequency sound immediately after S_2. An S_3

is thought to result from the reverberating sound produced by blood as it enters the ventricle during the early part of diastole and collides against a stiff myocardium that has lost normal compliance.[19] Another name for an S_3 is a **ventricular gallop**. In addition to congestive heart failure, an S_3 can be heard in patients with thyrotoxicosis, significant anemia, and conditions characterized by large left-to-right shunts such as ventricular septal defect and patent ductus arteriosus. The sound can be of right or left ventricular origin and is heard best at the cardiac apex. When an S_3 is heard in children, pregnant females, or young, well-conditioned individuals, it is considered to be a normal variant (possibly secondary to hyperdynamic ventricular function) and is called a physiological S_3. All other patients exhibiting an S_3 should be referred to the appropriate health care provider for further evaluation.

- An S_4 (the fourth heart sound) is also heard with the bell of the stethoscope in patients with cardiovascular syndromes that include chronic systemic hypertension, hypertensive heart disease, myocardial infarction, and acute mitral regurgitation secondary to chordae tendineae rupture. The mechanism of sound production is similar to that of an S_3, with the exception that the sound occurs immediately after atrial contraction forces blood into the ventricle during late ventricular diastole (the sound occurs immediately before S_1). Because of its atrial component, an S_4 is also referred to as an **atrial gallop**.

When the novice first hears any of these abnormal heart sounds, a question may arise as to how they can be distinguished from a split S_2. To make the distinction consistently, the therapist can rely on a physical property of the stethoscope itself. As discussed, high-frequency sounds are best heard by pressing the diaphragm firmly against the patient's skin so as to leave a slight impression when it is removed. The bell, on the other hand, should be held gently with little more than its own weight resting on the patient's skin so that it can transmit low-frequency sounds through its cone. If firm pressure is applied to the bell, the patient's own skin acts as a diaphragm (like the skin of a drum) and the bell is less able to transmit lower frequencies. The therapist need only adjust the pressure applied to the bell in order to differentiate between the normal variant and the abnormal sounds. For example, a sound that is heard with the stethoscope's bell held gently on the skin and not when the bell is pressed firmly favors an S_3 or S_4 (the latter two are then distinguished on the basis of proximity to S_1 or S_2).

Cardiac murmurs may be appreciated during auscultation of the heart. Cardiac murmurs are usually the result of:

1. High-velocity flow through normal or abnormal heart valves,
2. Forward flow through a restricted (stenotic) valve, past an area of obstruction, or into a dilated vessel/chamber,
3. Backward flow through an incompetent (regurgitant) valve, or
4. High-velocity flow through nonvalvular communications between cardiac chambers or large vessels.

An entry-level practitioner can acquire a level of aptitude in auscultating cardiac murmurs by remembering a few key concepts.[20] First, the timing of the murmur will indicate if it is systolic (heard between S_1 and S_2) or diastolic (heard between S_2 and S_1). Once the timing is noted, the auscultatory area where the murmur is heard loudest provides further clues to its origin. Finally, remembering the state of the valve during the particular phase of the cardiac cycle will usually implicate the specific valvular dysfunction. For example, a murmur that is heard between S_1 and S_2 and is loudest at the second intercostal space along the left sternal border would suggest pulmonic stenosis, since the pulmonary valve should be open at that time.

Murmurs are also graded in terms of their relative loudness and associated physical findings. Some murmurs merit special consideration in the clinical setting:

- **Aortic stenosis** is a pathological narrowing of the aortic valve that can impede left ventricular outflow during systole. Calcification of the stenotic leaflets can further impair left ventricular outflow. The murmur of aortic stenosis is usually a harsh, medium- to high-pitched sound with a crescendo–decrescendo quality, which rises to a peak in midsystole

and decays in late systole. It is heard best at the aortic area with the diaphragm of the stethoscope. When severe, the sound may radiate to the carotid arteries. Symptoms associated with aortic stenosis include dyspnea, chest pain, and near or frank syncope. The patient may occasionally present with palpitations, fatigue, and a narrowed pulse pressure.

- **Hypertrophic obstructive cardiomyopathy** is a result of abnormal blood flow through the left ventricular outflow tract. The obstruction is below the level of the aortic valve and involves thickening of the interventricular septum and left ventricular free wall. When the ventricle contracts, the thickened septum and free wall approximate below the aortic valve and the anterior mitral leaflet is sometimes pulled into the outflow path.[21] The obstruction is less severe if the end-diastolic volume (and thus, the left ventricular dimensions) is increased. This murmur is a harsh and rough murmur whose intensity is usually maintained throughout all of systole (*holosystolic*). It is heard loudest along the left sternal border with the diaphragm of the stethoscope and often radiates to the apex rather than the aortic area. Patients with significant hypertrophic obstructive cardiomyopathy present with symptoms similar to aortic stenosis.

- **Aortic regurgitation** is characterized by a high-pitched, blowing murmur heard during diastole that has a decrescendo pattern that decreases in intensity with time. It is usually loudest along the left sternal border and heard best with the diaphragm of the stethoscope. It may radiate to the cardiac apex. Aortic regurgitation can be the result of such pathologies as rheumatic fever, chronic systemic hypertension (leading to dilation of the aortic root and aortic annulus), and congenital bicuspid valve. Patients with Marfan's syndrome and ankylosing spondylitis are at higher risk for developing this condition. The typical symptoms include signs and symptoms of left heart failure, worsening fatigue, hypotension, pallor, tachycardia, palpitations, and chest pain. Associated findings often include a widened pulse pressure and pulsus bisferiens.

- **Mitral stenosis** exhibits a low-frequency, rumbling diastolic murmur that is heard best with the bell of the diaphragm at the cardiac apex. The etiology is almost always rheumatic valvular disease. The typical presentation includes exertional dyspnea, fatigue, pulmonary edema, and hemoptysis secondary to elevated pulmonary vascular pressure.

- **Mitral regurgitation** can be due to any factor that interferes with the normal function of the mitral complex, including papillary muscle dysfunction, rupture of the chordae tendineae, and rheumatic valvular disease. The holosystolic murmur is high pitched and has a blowing quality. It is heard best with the diaphragm of the stethoscope at the cardiac apex and often radiates to the left axilla. Patients with mitral regurgitation can present with pulmonary edema, fatigue, dyspnea, edema, and tachycardia. Associated findings can include *mitral valve prolapse* in which one of the leaflets bulges back into the left atrium during systole (possibly due to elongation of the chordae tendineae). Mitral valve prolapse occurs more often in females than males and exhibits a high-pitched click occurring in mid- to late systole that is heard best with the diaphragm of the stethoscope. Quite often, the disorder is benign and patients remain asymptomatic.[22] Patients with clinically significant mitral valve prolapse may present with symptoms of dizziness, weakness, chest pain, awareness of the heartbeat, fatigue, anxiety, and palpitations.

- **Pericardial friction rubs** are often described as squeaking or scratching sounds heard best with the diaphragm of the stethoscope and are likened to the rubbing of sandpaper or dry leather. Friction rubs indicate the presence of pericarditis that is more severe in nature, often involving both the visceral and parietal layers. Pericarditis may result from such conditions as myocardial infarction or infection or may occur post-pericardiotomy or as a result of trauma. Patients often report chest pain and may present with tachycardia, tachypnea, hypotension, and fever. A simple maneuver to help the therapist distinguish between a pericardial friction rub and a rub of pulmonary origin is to ask the patient to hold his or her breath during auscultation. If the sound persists, then it is pericardial in nature.

Pulmonary Auscultation

As with cardiac auscultation, pulmonary auscultation begins with proper positioning of the patient. The lung fields are best auscultated with the patient sitting at the edge of the bed or plinth so that the therapist can assess both the anterior and posterior chest wall. Because the majority of lung sounds are of medium to high frequency, the diaphragm of the stethoscope should be used for auscultation. Posteriorly, the therapist should begin by listening to the apices and then move down along either side of the vertebral column (asking the patient to protract the shoulders prevents scapular interference), finally terminating in the basal-lateral aspects of the rib cage. The anterior chest should be auscultated in a similar fashion while avoiding direct auscultation over the sternum (Fig. 26-6).

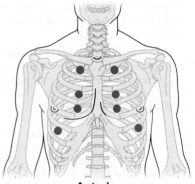

Anterior

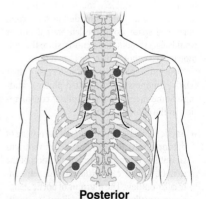

Posterior

FIGURE 26-6 Primary sites for pulmonary auscultation of the chest wall.

Most therapists find it efficient to alternate from right to left at each level so as to better compare discrepancies between sides. Auscultation through clothes dampens sound transmission and may simulate pathological sounds, so the therapist should auscultate over bare skin while maintaining proper draping techniques. The patient should be asked to breathe deeply through the mouth to maximize airflow and enhance sound fidelity.

Normal breath sounds can be classified into three main groups:

1. Bronchial,
2. Bronchovesicular, and
3. Vesicular.

Bronchial breath sounds are loud, high-pitched sounds that have an almost equal inspiratory and expiratory phase separated by a discernable pause. They are heard primarily over the trachea and mainstem bronchi. Bronchovesicular sounds share similar characteristics with bronchial sounds, but they are much softer and lack a discernable pause between phases (the inspiratory component fuses with the expiratory component). They are heard over the junctions of the mainstem bronchi and the various segmental bronchi (in the interscapular region). Vesicular sounds are very soft, low-pitched sounds having an expiratory phase that is approximately one-third of the inspiratory phase (at times, the expiratory phase may actually be inaudible). They also lack a discernable pause between phases and are heard over most of the peripheral lung fields.

Generally speaking, the absence of a normal breath sound when one would be expected or appreciation of a normal breath sound over an area in which it is not usually heard should prompt further examination. For example, a patient with pneumonia may have an area of consolidation in the peripheral lung fields secondary to accumulation of secretions in the alveoli. In this case, fluid has displaced the air in the peripheral lung tissue, increasing its relative density. The increased density causes the sounds from the larger airways to be transmitted more readily to the surface of the chest. As a result, bronchial breath sounds may be heard in an area where vesicular sounds are normally heard. Conversely, a patient with severe emphysema may have such a degree of pulmonary hyperinflation that breath sounds are poorly transmitted to the surface of the chest. In this case, significantly diminished breath sounds may be appreciated during auscultation. Finally, a patient with a pneumothorax will present with absent breath sounds over the involved area.

When sound transmission is altered, the therapist can apply several techniques to further characterize the degree or severity of pulmonary involvement. **Egophony** (also called the *E to A change*) is observed when the patient is asked to say "E" and the auscultated sound is "A." The second abnormal sound characteristic is called **bronchophony** and is demonstrated by asking the patient to repeat "ninety-nine" or "one–two–three." The therapist will hear the words with greater intensity and higher pitch during auscultation (normally, the words are muffled and hard to decipher). Egophony and bronchophony usually occur together in patients with diffuse pulmonary consolidation, pleural effusion, or compression atelectasis.

The last abnormal characteristic is referred to as **whispered pectoriloquy**, and is elicited by asking the patient to whisper the words "ninety-nine" or "one–two–three" and the words are clearly heard through the stethoscope (normally, the words are unintelligible). Whispered pectoriloquy may be appreciated even in the absence of egophony and bronchophony, and allows for the identification of more subtle consolidation or hyperinflation. As a general rule, louder and more pronounced words are heard in the presence of consolidation, whereas hyperinflation states are associated with softer and less intelligible sound transmission.

Adventitious breath sounds refer to abnormal extrinsic breath sounds that can be heard throughout the bronchopulmonary tree. According to the American Thoracic Society, they are classified as being either continuous or discontinuous:

- **Wheezes** are continuous, high- or low-pitched sounds of varying duration auscultated during expiration (although they may also be heard during inspiration). High-pitched expiratory wheezes are associated with intrathoracic airway obstruction as can occur with bronchospasm secondary to asthma or obstruction by secretions secondary to chronic bronchitis. Although some clinicians still label low-pitched, continuous sounds as **rhonchi**, they are more correctly referred to as *low-pitched wheezes*. Inspiratory wheezes usually indicate a more severe airway obstruction and may coexist with expiratory wheezes. A laryngeal or tracheal obstruction produces a loud, high-pitched sound that is readily audible without a stethoscope. Examples of large airway obstruction include foreign body aspiration, epiglottitis, croup, and tumors. This sound is referred to as *stridor* and is usually heard during inspiration, but may be heard during both phases of the ventilatory cycle. The presence of stridor necessitates expeditious evaluation and treatment (especially when associated with cyanosis) because it represents a potentially life-threatening condition.

- **Crackles** are discontinuous, low-pitched sounds similar in quality to the carbonation of a soft drink or Velcro ripping and can be associated with either restrictive or obstructive lung diseases. The therapist can simulate the sound by rubbing hair between the fingertips next to the ear. Crackles are heard primarily during inspiration (but can also be heard during expiration) and are further described as *fine* or *coarse*. The mechanism of sound production usually involves the sudden opening of previously closed airways (including alveoli) or the movement of air through secretions that have accumulated in the air spaces. Early inspiratory crackles are consistent with chronic obstructive pulmonary disease, whereas late inspiratory crackles suggest the presence of restrictive lung diseases, such as congestive heart failure, pneumonia, atelectasis, and interstitial pulmonary fibrosis.

- Inflammation of the pleural membranes typically produces another adventitious lung sound referred to as a **pleural friction rub**. The sound made by a pleural rub is likened to that of two pieces of dry leather or sandpaper being rubbed together. It is almost always heard during inspiration and expiration. Patients often will report chest pain with a pleuritic component in that the pain worsens with deep inspiration and is aggravated by coughing or sneezing. As mentioned previously, pleural friction rubs are distinguished from pericardial friction rubs on the basis of the effect breath-holding has on the sound, where disappearance of the sound indicates a pleural friction rub while persistence of the sound favors a pericardial friction rub.

Conclusion

This chapter provided an overview of the physical clues suggestive of cardiovascular and/or pulmonary dysfunction and reviewed specific clinical evaluation tools that are available to the physical therapist to further assess its presence and severity. Understanding the clues given by cardiovascular and pulmonary pathologies will provide physical therapists with the tools necessary to suspect and determine the presence of cardiovascular and/or pulmonary involvement in their patients who may be receiving physical therapy intervention for seemingly unrelated disorders. Awareness of the possibility of cardiovascular and pulmonary comorbidities in patients will also allow the physical therapist to design appropriate treatment plans, accurately interpret the patient's physiological responses to exertion, modify assessment and treatment approaches as needed, and initiate a referral to an appropriate health care provider when the patient's needs fall outside the scope of physical therapist practice.

References

1. Panka GFL, Oliveira MM, Franca DC, et al. Ventilatory and muscular assessment in healthy subjects during an activity of daily living with unsupported arm elevation. *Rev Bras Fisioter*. Jul/Aug 2010;14(4);337–344.
2. Mangione S. The skin, the neck, the cardiovascular system, and chest inspection, palpation, and percussion. In: Mangione S, ed. *Physical Diagnosis Secrets*. Philadelphia, PA; Elsevier Health Sciences; 2008.
3. Stack AM. Etiology and evaluation of cyanosis in children. In: UpToDate, Basow DS (Ed), UpToDate, Waltham, MA, 2009.
4. Martin L, Khalil H. How much reduced hemoglobin is necessary to generate central cyanosis? *Chest*. Jan 1990;97(1):182–185.
5. Welsh JR, Arzouman JM, Holm K. Nurses' assessment and documentation of peripheral edema. *Clin Nurse Spec*. Jan 1996;10(1):7–10.
6. Brodovicz KG, McNaughton K, Uemura N, et al. Reliability and feasibility of methods to quantitatively assess peripheral edema. *C M & R*. 2009;7(1/2):21–31
7. Plathow C, Ley S, Fink C, et al. Evaluation of chest motion and volumetry during the breathing cycle by dynamic MRI in healthy subjects: comparison with pulmonary function tests. *Invest Radiol*. Apr 2004;39(4):202–209.

8. Bickley LS, Szilagyi PG. *Bates' Guide to Physical Examination and History Taking*. Philadelphia, PA: Lippincott Williams & Wilkins; 2003.

9. Cahalin LP. Cardiovascular evaluation. In: DeTurk WE, Cahalin LP, eds. *Cardiovascular and Pulmonary Physical Therapy: An Evidence–Based Approach*. New York, NY: McGraw Hill Medical; 2011.

10. Kodama M, Kato K, Hirono S. Linkage between mechanical and electrical alternans in patients with chronic heart failure. *J Cardiovasc Electrophysiol*. 2004;15(3):295–299.

11. Wagner HR. Paradoxical pulse: 100 years later. *Am J Cardiol*. Jul 1973;32(1):91–92.

12. Pickering TG, Hall JE, Appel LJ, et al. Recommendations for blood pressure measurement in humans and experimental animals: part 1: blood pressure measurement in humans: a statement for professionals from the Subcommittee of Professional and Public Education of the American Heart Association Council on High Blood Pressure Research. *Circulation*. Feb 8, 2005;111(5):697–716.

13. Agarwal R, Bunaye Z, Bekele DM. Prognostic significance of between-arm blood pressure differences. *Hypertension*. 2008;51:657–662.

14. Bradley JG, Davis KA. Orthostatic hypotension. *Am Fam Physician*. Dec 15, 2003;68(12):2393–2398.

15. Stewart JM. Chronic orthostatic intolerance and the postural tachycardia syndrome (POTS). *J Pediatr*. Dec 2004;145(6):725–730.

16. Khasnis A, Lokhandwala Y. Clinical signs in medicine: pulsus paradoxus. *J Postgrad Med*. Jan–Mar 2002; 48(1):46–49.

17. Le V-V, Mitiku T, Sungar G, et al. The blood pressure response to dynamic exercise testing: a systematic review. *Prog Cardiovasc Dis*. Sept/Oct 2008;51(2):135–160.

18. Watchie J. Cardiopulmonary implications of specific diseases. In: Hillegass E, ed. *Essentials of Cardiopulmonary Physical Therapy*. St. Louis, MO: Elsevier Saunders; 2011.

19. Richardson TR, Moody JM, Jr. Bedside cardiac examination: constancy in a sea of change. *Curr Probl Cardiol*. Nov 2000;25(11):783–825.

20. Chizner MA. Cardiac auscultation: rediscovering the lost art. *Curr Prob Cardiol*. July 2008;33:326–408.

21. Lee CT, Dec GW, Lilly LS. The cardiomyopathies. In: Lilly LS, ed. *Pathophysiology of Heart Disease: A Collaborative Project of Medical Students and Faculty*. 5th ed. Baltimore, MD: Lippincott Williams & Wilkins; 2011.

22. Freed LA, Benjamin EJ, Levy D, et al. Mitral valve prolapse in the general population: the benign nature of echocardiographic features in the Framingham Heart Study. *J Am Coll Cardiol*. Oct 2, 2002;40(7):1298–1304.

CHAPTER 27

Dizziness

■ *Rob Landel, PT, DPT, OCS, CSCS, FAPTA*

Description of the Symptom

This chapter describes pathology that may lead to dizziness. Dizziness is described as a sensation of movement of self or surroundings (vertigo), light-headedness (presyncope), or imbalance (disequilibrium).

Special Concerns

Dizziness in the presence of any of the following symptoms and signs:

■ Chest pain
■ Irregular heartbeat
■ A new onset of, or a change in, neurological status, including:
 ■ Weakness or paralysis in the face, arm, or leg, especially on one side of the body
 ■ Tremor
 ■ Change in mental status, such as confusion, memory loss, hallucinations
 ■ Difficulty talking
 ■ Difficulty understanding speech
 ■ Trouble seeing with one or both eyes
 ■ Loss of coordination
 ■ Loss of balance
 ■ Nystagmus that is spontaneous (resting), direction changing, or gaze evoked
 ■ Oculomotor abnormalities including abnormal smooth pursuit and saccades.
 ■ Loss of sensation

■ History of head or neck trauma and concerns of:
 ■ Changes in neurological status, as noted above
 ■ Long tract signs elicited by head or neck movements
 ■ Dizziness with sustained head or neck positions
 ■ Unwillingness to move the neck
 ■ Facial numbness or paresthesias
■ Palpitations that are:
 ■ Followed by loss of consciousness
 ■ Associated with significant shortness of breath, chest discomfort, light-headedness, or presyncopal symptoms
 ■ Associated with marked hypertension (ie, >220/110) or hypotension (ie, <90/60 in an individual who is typically normotensive)
 ■ Of sudden onset and last longer than 15 to 20 minutes
 ■ Occurring in an individual with a family history of sudden death.
■ Fever, chills, accompanied by a very stiff neck or other signs of infection
■ Unrelenting headache
■ Hyperpnea or dyspnea
■ Anxiety
■ Sudden hearing loss
■ Ear pain

CHAPTER PREVIEW: Conditions That May Lead to Dizziness

T Trauma

COMMON

Benign paroxysmal positional vertigo 532
Cervicogenic dizziness (cervical vertigo) 533
Whiplash injury (whiplash-associated disorder) 546

UNCOMMON

Brainstem–eighth nerve complex injury 533
Labyrinthine concussion 537
Traumatic brain injury 544

Trauma *(continued)*

RARE

Perilymph fistula 542
Superior canal dehiscence syndrome 544

I   Inflammation

COMMON

Aseptic
Not applicable

Septic
Labyrinthitis and neuronitis 537

UNCOMMON

Aseptic
Multiple sclerosis 540

Septic
Not applicable

RARE

Aseptic
Autoimmune inner ear disease 532
Paraneoplastic syndromes 542

Septic
Herpes zoster oticus (Ramsey Hunt syndrome) 535
Otosyphilis 541

M   Metabolic

COMMON

Adverse effect or side effect of medications 530
Dehydration/hypovolemia 534
Hypoglycemia 536
Pregnancy 543

UNCOMMON

Exposure to toxic chemicals 535
Hyperthyroidism/thyrotoxicosis 535
Hypothyroidism 536

RARE

Vestibular ototoxicity 546

Va   Vascular

COMMON

Anemia 530
Orthostatic hypotension 541

UNCOMMON

Dysrhythmias/arrhythmias 535
Mitral valve prolapse 539
Transient ischemic attack 544

(continued)

DIZZINESS

Vascular *(continued)*

RARE

Arteriovenous malformation 532
Idiopathic intracranial hypertension 537
Lateral medullary infarction (Wallenberg's syndrome) 537
Postural tachycardia syndrome 543
Vertebrobasilar artery insufficiency 545

De Degenerative

COMMON

Not applicable

UNCOMMON

Not applicable

RARE

Multiple system atrophy with orthostatic hypotension (striatonigral degeneration, olivopontocerebellar atrophy, Shy-Drager syndrome) 540

Tu Tumor

COMMON

Not applicable

UNCOMMON

Malignant Primary, such as:
• Brain primary tumors 533
Malignant Metastatic, such as:
• Brain metastases 532
Benign:
Not applicable

RARE

Malignant Primary, such as:
• Brain primary tumors 533
• Spinal primary tumors 544
Malignant Metastatic, such as:
• Brain metastases 532
• Spinal metastases 543
Benign, such as:
• Acoustic neuroma (vestibular schwannoma) 530
• Angiomatosis (Von Hippel-Lindau disease) 531
• Neurosarcoidosis 541

Co Congenital

COMMON

Not applicable

UNCOMMON

Not applicable

Congenital *(continued)*

RARE
Cholesteatoma 534
Hereditary neuropathies 535

Ne Neurogenic/Psychogenic

COMMON
Anxiety disorder/panic attacks 531
Vasovagal syncope 545

UNCOMMON
Ménière's disease 538
Migraine-related dizziness:
• Basilar migraines 539
• Benign recurrent vertigo 539
• Vestibular migraine 539

RARE
Mal de débarquement 538
Vestibular epilepsy (vestibular seizures) 545

Note: These are estimates of relative incidence because few data are available for the less common conditions.

Overview of Dizziness

Dizziness manifests itself in many forms and includes vertigo, defined as a whirling or tilting sensation with a tendency to fall[1,2]; disequilibrium or imbalance; and light-headedness or presyncope. Individuals may use the term *dizziness* to describe any of the preceding symptoms. Individuals may report dizziness but upon further questioning may describe a feeling of being off-balance, unsteady, lightheaded, spacey, or feeling as if they are rocking or floating. It is important to distinguish between the sensations and determine as well as possible what the individual is experiencing, because the description will help narrow down the diagnostic possibilities.[1,3,4] Disequilibrium or imbalance can be due to multiple factors including sensory deficits, motor deficits, and impairment in the central nervous system processing of the two. Causes of falling and limited balance are covered in Chapter 28. Light-headedness such as that felt with orthostatic hypotension is typically a sign of presyncope or near syncope and suggests impaired central nervous system perfusion. Checking the change in blood pressure between supine and standing positions will help rule in orthostatic hypotension; a drop of 20 mm Hg or more in systolic blood pressure is significant. This chapter focuses on vertigo or the illusion of movement, typically spinning, either of the individual or of the surrounding environment.

There are many causes of dizziness, and while most are benign, serious pathologies must be identified. One study suggests that vertigo or vomiting combined with a positive Dix-Hallpike test has an 85% positive predictive value (PPV) for being benign. In addition, the presence of vertigo in an individual 69 years old or younger, with no neurological deficits, has an 88% negative predictive value for serious pathology. Over the age of 69, vertigo combined with neurological deficits has a 40% PPV for serious pathology. This suggests that performing a neurological exam on the person presenting with vertigo is essential.[5]

Once the individual's concerns have been narrowed to vertigo, differentiation must be made between central causes (lesions in the central nervous system) and peripheral causes (lesions in the vestibular labyrinth or nerve or both).[1,4] The presence of other neurological symptoms such as generalized weakness, difficulty with speech, problems with walking, tremor, and so on in addition to vertigo suggests central involvement. The location of the lesion will determine the symptoms of most central vertigo syndromes, but the etiology of a particular lesion may vary. For example, traumatic, inflammatory, vascular, or neoplastic lesions will produce the same symptoms if they affect the same location. The presence of other otologic symptoms, such as hearing loss, tinnitus, and aural fullness, suggests a peripheral cause. The intensity of the vertigo in central conditions is typically more moderate and persistent than in peripheral conditions.

The duration of symptoms can be helpful in making the diagnosis. Short episodes of vertigo suggest a peripheral cause such as benign paroxysmal positional vertigo, the most common cause of vertigo. Vertigo lasting 20 to 30 minutes is suggestive of transient ischemic attacks or migrainous vertigo. Vertigo lasting hours is typical of Ménière's disease, and vestibular neuronitis resolves after days or weeks. Peripheral vertigo other than benign paroxysmal positional vertigo will resolve gradually due to central compensation, whereas central vertigo will persist for a long time and fluctuates little if at all in intensity.

Associated symptoms may assist in making the diagnosis. The presence of headaches suggests migrainous vertigo; panic attacks, anxiety, hyperventilation, and agoraphobia suggest psychogenic causes. The medical history should include questions about drug use; metabolic, cardiovascular, or immunologic conditions; impaired vision; symptoms of infection; or generalized neuropathies.

Description of Conditions That May Lead to Dizziness

■ Acoustic Neuroma (Vestibular Schwannoma)

Chief Clinical Characteristics

This presentation may include hearing loss, tinnitus, vertigo, or disequilibrium in the early stages.[5-11] Vestibular nerve function may be gradually lost without much balance disturbance. Symptoms worsen as the tumor grows, and the individual may also report having a

headache. If untreated, brainstem compression can occur, with concerns of generalized headache, facial twitch and weakness, visual loss, diplopia, lower cranial nerve dysfunction causing aspiration, hoarseness, dysphagia, shoulder weakness, tongue weakness, and long tract signs.[6]

Background Information

Acoustic neuromas arise from the Schwann cells of the eighth cranial nerve within the internal auditory canal, eventually growing out into and compressing the brainstem. Audiometry, electronystagmography, auditory brainstem response, computed tomography, and magnetic resonance imaging with gadolinium contrast confirm the diagnosis, with the latter providing the most specificity.[6] Treatment is surgical removal of the tumor, with risk of permanent changes in hearing, balance and facial sensation, and motion. Loss of a preoperatively functioning vestibular nerve will result in disequilibrium for which vestibular adaptation exercises and balance rehabilitation are appropriate.[11]

■ Adverse Effect or Side Effect of Medications

Chief Clinical Characteristics

This presentation commonly includes onset of dizziness with use of certain prescription and over-the-counter medications, as well as illicit drugs.

Background Information

The medications, both prescribed and over the counter, that have dizziness or lightheadedness as a side effect are too numerous to describe here. The prudent clinician will obtain from the individual a complete list of prescription and nonprescription drugs the individual is taking and determine if any of them induce dizziness or light-headedness. Consultation with a pharmacist may be advisable in order to determine drug interactions. Recreational drugs should not be overlooked.

■ Anemia

Chief Clinical Characteristics

This presentation can be characterized by lightheadedness, associated with lethargy, cold skin, depression, easy fatigability, shortness of breath, and cognitive impairment.[12]

DIZZINESS

Background Information

Comorbid conditions that render the individual susceptible to anemia include recent major surgery (ie, orthopedic and cardiopulmonary surgeries), pregnancy, lesions of the gastrointestinal tract, sickle cell trait, and cancer.[13] Anemia is defined as a decrease in the oxygen-carrying capacity of blood secondary to a decrease in the erythrocyte (red blood cell) content of blood, a diminished content of hemoglobin per erythrocyte, or a combination of both.[14] It can arise from failed synthesis, premature destruction, hemorrhage, or deficiencies in iron, B_{12}, or folic acid. The resultant reduction in the blood's oxygen-carrying capacity initiates a reflex sinus tachycardia in attempts to maintain adequate tissue oxygenation while blood pressure is usually within the normal resting range.[15] The pulse is felt to be rapid and regular upon palpation, supporting the presence of sinus tachycardia. If anemia is suspected, the individual should be referred to his or her primary care practitioner for further evaluation. The diagnosis is confirmed by routine blood testing, including complete blood count.

■ Angiomatosis (Von Hippel-Lindau Disease)

Chief Clinical Characteristics

This presentation commonly includes headaches, problems with balance and walking, dizziness, weakness of the limbs, vision problems, and high blood pressure.

Background Information

This condition is a rare, genetic multisystem condition characterized by the abnormal growth of tumors in certain parts of the body (angiomatosis). The tumors of the central nervous system are benign and are comprised of a nest of blood vessels and are called hemangioblastomas (or angiomas in the eye). Hemangioblastomas may develop in the brain, the retina of the eyes, and other areas of the nervous system. Other types of tumors develop in the adrenal glands, the kidneys, or the pancreas. Cysts (fluid-filled sacs) and/or tumors (benign or cancerous) may develop around the hemangioblastomas and cause the symptoms listed above. Specific symptoms vary among individuals and depend on the size and location of the tumors. Individuals with this condition are also at a higher risk than normal for certain types of cancer, especially kidney cancer. Treatment varies according to the location and size of the tumor and its associated cyst. In general, the objective is to treat the tumors when they are causing symptoms but are still small. Treatment of most cases usually involves surgical resection. Certain tumors can be treated with focused high-dose irradiation. Individuals with this condition need careful monitoring by a physician and/or medical team familiar with the condition.

■ Anxiety Disorder/Panic Attacks

Chief Clinical Characteristics

This presentation typically includes repeated panic or anxiety attacks. Symptoms include increased heart rate and respiratory rate, pupil dilation, and trembling and sweating with feelings of fear and dread. The symptoms usually subside in 15 to 30 minutes.

Background Information

This condition is a nonspecific syndrome and can be due to a variety of medical or psychiatric syndromes or observed as part of a drug withdrawal or drug intoxication effect. The diagnosis of an anxiety condition is based on criteria from the DSM-IV-TR.[16] Anxiety conditions are classified into specific categories. One category, panic condition, has dizziness as one of its features. Panic condition is defined by recurrent attacks with at least four of the following features: increased heart rate, sweating, trembling or shaking, dyspnea, sensation of choking, chest pain or discomfort, nausea or abdominal distress, feelings of dizziness, fear of losing control, fear of dying, paresthesias, and chills or hot flashes. The etiology of anxiety conditions includes genetic factors, social and psychological factors, and physiological and biochemical abnormalities.[17] Treatment includes cognitive-behavioral therapy, relaxation exercises, and pharmacologic treatment.[17] The course of this condition is variable; most individuals maintain normal social lives. Clinicians are encouraged to consider referral of individuals suspected of having this condition to a mental health specialist for evaluation and treatment.

■ Arteriovenous Malformation

Chief Clinical Characteristics

This presentation may be characterized by seizures and severe headache. Hemorrhage may result in paresis, ataxia, dyspraxia, dizziness, visual disturbances, aphasia, paresthesias, and cognitive deficits.[18]

Background Information

This condition is caused by a tangle of arteries and veins that cause abnormal communication within the vasculature. Approximately 12% of the 300,000 individuals in the United States with this condition are symptomatic. This condition is caused by a developmental abnormality that likely arises during embryonic or fetal development. Neurological damage occurs due to reduction of oxygen delivery, hemorrhage, or compression upon nearby structures of the brain or spinal cord. Computed tomography, magnetic resonance imaging, and arteriography confirm the diagnosis. Ligation and embolization may be used to reduce the size of the lesion prior to surgical excision, which is the preferred method of treatment. Stereotactic radiation and proton beam therapy are alternative approaches to invasive methods of intervention. Up to 90% of individuals who experience a hemorrhagic arteriovenous malformation survive.[18]

■ Autoimmune Inner Ear Disease

Chief Clinical Characteristics

This presentation involves progressive bilateral sensorineural hearing loss often accompanied by bilateral loss of vestibular function.[19]

Background Information

The symptoms may occur as a direct assault by the immune system on the inner ear, or may be related to the deposition of antibody–antigen complex in the inner ear structures. This condition may occur as a result of a concomitant autoimmune condition, such as rheumatoid arthritis, psoriasis, ulcerative colitis, or Cogan's syndrome (iritis accompanied by vertigo and sensorineural hearing loss). Treatment is primarily pharmacologic, because this condition represents bilateral involvement of the vestibular system. Controlled physical exercises to promote substitution for the lost peripheral vestibular input may promote some clinical benefit.

■ Benign Paroxysmal Positional Vertigo

Chief Clinical Characteristics

This presentation commonly involves dizziness or vertigo (typically described as a spinning sensation), light-headedness, imbalance, and nausea. Symptoms are precipitated by a position change of the head relative to gravity, such as getting out of bed, rolling over in bed, or looking up.[20,21]

Background Information

This condition is thought to occur when free-floating debris becomes trapped in the semicircular canal (canalithiasis) or becomes adhered to the cupula (cupulolithiasis), rendering the semicircular canal sensitive to gravity and thus changes in head position rather than head motion. The etiology of benign paroxysmal positional vertigo is unknown in most cases, but it is associated with head trauma, vestibular neuritis, and vertebrobasilar ischemia and can occur after ear surgery or prolonged bed rest.[22] This condition occurs more often in the elderly, and tends to recur in up to 15% of cases within 1 year and 50% of cases within 40 months.[23] The diagnosis is confirmed with the Hallpike maneuver, in which the head is rotated 45 degrees and tilted back while hanging off the end of the table. This position will elicit torsional and vertical nystagmus when the vertical semicircular canals are involved. Duration of vertigo while in the Hallpike position will determine if the individual has *canalithiasis* (short duration, <1 minute) or *cupulolithiasis* (long duration, >1 minute). When the horizontal (lateral) semicircular canals are involved, turning the head while the patient is supine will elicit horizontal nystagmus and vertigo. A nonsurgical treatment consisting of a series of positional changes to move the debris out of the canals, known as the canalith repositioning maneuver, can be very successful.[22–28] In recalcitrant cases, the offending canal can be plugged surgically.[29]

■ Brain Metastases

Chief Clinical Characteristics

This presentation may include headaches, seizures, dysphagia, weakness, cognitive changes, behavioral changes, dizziness, vomiting, alterations in the level of consciousness, ataxia, aphasia, nystagmus, visual disturbances, dysarthria, balance deficits, falls, lethargy, and incoordination.[18,30]

Background Information

The majority of individuals with brain metastases have been previously diagnosed with a primary tumor; however, a small percentage of individuals are diagnosed concomitantly with brain metastases and the primary tumor. The most common cancers resulting in subsequent brain metastases include lung, breast, melanoma, colorectal, and genitourinary tract. The new onset of neurological symptoms after a primary tumor warrants imaging such as magnetic resonance imaging or computed tomography to confirm the diagnosis. Treatment may include corticosteroids, brain irradiation, surgery, chemotherapy, radiotherapy, and rehabilitative therapies. The prognosis is poor with death typically occurring within 6 months.

■ Brain Primary Tumors

Chief Clinical Characteristics

This presentation may include headaches, seizures, dysphagia, weakness, cognitive changes, behavioral changes, dizziness, vomiting, alterations in the level of consciousness, ataxia, aphasia, nystagmus, visual disturbances, dysarthria, balance deficits, falls, lethargy, and incoordination.[18]

Background Information

With the excessive proliferation of cells, a tumor mass eventually results in compression of the brain. This compression may displace cerebrospinal fluid, thereby increasing intracranial pressure and resulting in ischemia to the same tissues. Glioblastoma multiforme, astrocytoma, oligodendroglioma, metastatic tumors, primary central nervous system lymphomas, ganglioglioma, neuroblastoma, meningioma, arachnoid cysts, hemangioblastoma, medulloblastoma, and acoustic neuroma/schwannoma are some of the more common brain tumors. The first test to diagnose brain and spinal column tumors is a neurological examination. Specific diagnoses for brain tumors may be confirmed with imaging and biopsy. Treatment is variable depending on the type, size, and location of the tumor and may include surgical resection, chemotherapy, radiation, corticosteroids, and rehabilitative therapies. Prognosis is

also variable and depends on the type and grade of tumor, severity of compression, and duration of compression.

■ Brainstem–Eighth Nerve Complex Injury[20]

Chief Clinical Characteristics

This presentation can be characterized by acute signs of vertigo, leading to constant unsteadiness, which worsens in darkness and during fatigue and contributes to motion intolerance. The symptoms are generally chronic, as the vestibular disturbance remains uncompensated. Symptoms and signs for this condition are similar to those for labyrinthine concussion.

Background Information

A reduced vestibular response is apparent on caloric testing, and rotary chair tests show gain asymmetry and an increased phase lag. Posturography is typically abnormal. Experimental and autopsy reports have described a shearing effect on the root entry zone of cranial nerves with head trauma. Even mild trauma leads to hemorrhages often in the brainstem and especially in the area of the vestibular nuclei. Magnetic resonance imaging confirms the diagnosis when it reveals this anatomical finding. Treatment involves vestibular habituation exercises.

■ Cervicogenic Dizziness (Cervical Vertigo)

Chief Clinical Characteristics

This presentation typically involves a non-specific form of dizziness that is related to neck pain and impairments such as decreased cervical spine range of motion. It can include unsteady gait, postural disturbances, ataxia, or headaches. Individuals with this condition often will report a history of cervical trauma such as whiplash.

Background Information

Cervicogenic dizziness is defined as a nonspecific sensation of altered orientation in space and dysequilibrium originating from abnormal afferent activity from the neck,[31] and vertigo induced by changes of position of the neck or vertigo originating from the cervical region.[32] The vestibular system is not involved in true cervicogenic dizziness. This condition is thought to result from malfunction or disturbance in the afferent flow of impulses from deep cervical tissues and cervical proprioceptors.[33,34] The diagnosis of this condition is by exclusion. When the onset is related to trauma, upper cervical hypermobility and cervical fractures must be ruled out as both can produce symptoms of dizziness. Physical examination will reveal soft tissue tenderness of the cervical spine, limited neck motion, and abnormal intervertebral mobility. The neck torsion nystagmus test, where dizziness and nystagmus are produced when the head remains fixed while the neck and body are rotated, is thought to be a sign of cervicogenic dizziness,[20] but it is non-specific for the condition.[31] The smooth pursuit neck torsion test may be used, which reveals smooth pursuit abnormalities when the head is held rotated in individuals with whiplash-associated conditions who report dizziness, as well as posturography that is conducted while inducing postural perturbations using head and neck vibration.[35] Disturbances in balance may be present[36] although not likely enough to produce falls unless other comorbidities exist. Interventions such as cervical and thoracic mobilization and manipulation, traction, exercise including activities to improve cervical joint position error and head control, physical modalities, postural re-education, active range of motion, soft tissue mobilization, balance retraining, trigger point injections, muscle relaxants, and soft collars are typical treatments.[31-34,36-39]

Cholesteatoma

Chief Clinical Characteristics
This presentation typically includes gradual onset, persistent intermittent discharge from the ear, and, rarely, dizziness and facial palsy.[40,41] While not often painful, infection can occasionally occur, causing pain and swelling behind the ear.

Background Information
This is a rare condition caused by a skin cyst behind the eardrum, which grows into the middle ear and mastoid. The cyst gradually expands, generally causing destruction of the eardrum and ossicles, and can erode the surrounding bone; if it progresses to the point of eroding the bony labyrinth, dizziness will occur. Most cases are congenital, and some are acquired due to metaplastic tissue, or overgrowth of tympanic membrane epithelial cells after a

perforation, or the formation of a pocket that accumulates keratin debris. The diagnosis is made primarily from the history and physical examination. Computed tomography can be used preoperatively to plan surgery. Treatment consists of periodic ear cleaning but in almost all cases surgery is necessary to remove the lesion. Hearing loss, dizziness, facial paralysis, tinnitus, and taste abnormalities are possible postoperative complications.

Dehydration/Hypovolemia

Chief Clinical Characteristics
This presentation can be characterized by palpitations, lethargy, poor concentration, tremors, light-headedness, constipation, dry mouth, and syncope. If this condition is severe, cyanosis of the lips, sunken eyes, cold extremities, failure of skin to bounce back when it is lightly pinched and released, confusion, and lethargy may be noted.

Background Information
Dehydration due to sweat loss and/or inadequate fluid replacement during physical exertion can lead to a significant decrease in central blood volume. Mild to moderate dehydration and/or hypovolemia initiates a sympathetic nervous system reflex manifested by an increase in heart rate and contractile force in order to sustain mean arterial pressure. In addition, the tachycardic response is highly correlated with the degree of hypovolemia. The individual may sense this increase in heart rate and contractility as palpitations. In most cases, the rhythm is sinus tachycardia and the therapist will note a rapid but regular pulse that may be slightly diminished. Dehydration can be avoided by reminding the individual to drink fluids during exercise sessions in the clinic, especially if the exercise is aerobic and will be maintained for greater than 20 to 30 minutes. Mild hypovolemia necessitates fluid replacement, which may be accomplished by having the individual lie semirecumbent and drink water as the therapist monitors signs and symptoms. More severe cases of hypovolemia usually require activation of the emergency medical system and administration of intravenous fluids by appropriate health care personnel.

■ Dysrhythmias/Arrhythmias

Chief Clinical Characteristics

This presentation involves light-headedness, and associated symptoms of palpitations, shortness of breath, chest discomfort, headache, slurred speech, fatigue, lethargy, and anxiety.

Background Information

A variety of pathologies result in this condition, including myocardial infarction, sick sinus syndrome, pacemaker failure, electrolyte imbalance, pregnancy, dehydration/hypovolemia, Wolff-Parkinson-White syndrome, and congestive heart failure. If palpable, the pulse is abnormal. Pulse may be either more rapid or slower than expected, and either regular or irregular in beat. Blood pressure may be abnormal. Cardiac auscultation may be abnormal. Referral to a physician or activating the emergency medical system is warranted, particularly for individuals with a new onset or changing signs and symptoms.

■ Exposure to Toxic Chemicals

Chief Clinical Characteristics

This presentation includes acute onset of dizziness associated with exposure to chemical irritants.

Background Information

Any individual who reports dizziness or light-headedness should be asked about potential exposure to toxic chemicals. There should be a temporal association between the exposure and the onset of symptoms. Common chemicals include household cleaners, insect sprays, fertilizers, and paints. The most common toxic cause of acute vertigo is ethyl alcohol. Position changes during a hangover exacerbate vertigo, possibly due to the production of a density gradient from the different diffusion rates of alcohol into the endolymph and the cupula, rendering the cupula gravity sensitive. Other toxic agents include organic compounds of heavy metals. Referral to a physician for evaluation and treatment is warranted.

■ Hereditary Neuropathies

Chief Clinical Characteristics

This presentation includes distal sensory abnormalities, such as numbness and tingling of the feet, and muscle weakness of distal musculature. Individuals affected with this condition may also report sweating and dizziness upon standing.

Background Information

This condition includes hereditary motor and sensory neuropathy, hereditary sensory neuropathy, hereditary motor neuropathy, and hereditary sensory and autonomic neuropathy. The majority of neuropathies composing this condition are Charcot-Marie-Tooth neuropathy. This condition is caused by genetic abnormalities. Diagnosis is made by nerve conduction and electromyographic studies. Prognosis for hereditary sensory neuropathies is poor due to intractable pain.[42] Prognosis for hereditary motor and sensory neuropathies has also been found to be unfavorable due to slowing of conduction velocity with age.[43] Intervention is typically directed at the underlying cause when possible.

■ Herpes Zoster Oticus (Ramsay Hunt Syndrome)

Chief Clinical Characteristics

This presentation commonly includes intense ear pain; a rash around the ear, mouth, face, neck, and scalp; and paralysis of facial nerves. Other symptoms may include hearing loss, vertigo, and tinnitus. Taste loss in the tongue and dry mouth and eyes may also occur. Sensory losses precede facial paralysis. Vestibular deficits are more frequent than hearing loss (80% vs. 26%, respectively), although hearing loss may go unnoticed.[44]

Background Information

This condition is a common complication of herpes zoster. This condition is an infection caused by the spread of varicella-zoster virus, which is the virus that causes chickenpox, to facial nerves. This condition occurs in people who have had chickenpox and represents a reactivation of the dormant varicella-zoster virus. When treatment is needed, medications such as antiviral drugs or corticosteroids may be prescribed. Vertigo also may be treated with the drug diazepam.

■ Hyperthyroidism/Thyrotoxicosis

Chief Clinical Characteristics

This presentation involves high cardiac output, hypertension, dyspnea (orthopnea, exertional dyspnea, and paroxysmal nocturnal dyspnea), and dysrhythmias associated with palpitations that may lead to feelings of dizziness or light-headedness.[45–47] Associated signs and symptoms include nervousness, heat intolerance, fatigue, weight loss despite increased appetite, sweating, tremors, and exophthalmos.

Background Information

A supportive clinical finding is a minimal decrease in resting heart rate during the individual's sleeping hours, which may be confirmed by nocturnal heart rate monitoring. Palpitations in these individuals are typically chronic, felt during resting states, and exaggerated with activity. This condition results from overactivity of the thyroid gland and primarily results in elevated levels of thyroid hormones in the bloodstream, while thyrotoxicosis refers to the clinical syndrome resulting from hyperthyroidism. Typical etiologies of hyperthyroidism include Graves' disease, excessive thyroid hormone replacement therapy, toxic adenoma, thyroiditis, goiter, and hyperthyroidism due to amiodarone and iodine-containing radiographic contrast agents. Thyroid hormones are known to enhance myocardial contractility and elevate the body's metabolic rate, leading to arterial vasodilation and possible hypotension. A reflex tachycardia may ensue to counteract the hypotension. The most common dysrhythmia associated with hyperthyroidism is sinus tachycardia, although supraventricular dysrhythmias (particularly atrial fibrillation) can occur and may pose a serious health risk for individuals with known coronary artery disease or history of stroke. Often, diagnosis is made by blood test on the basis of elevated thyroid hormone levels. If the therapist suspects hyperthyroidism in a previously undiagnosed individual, the individual should be referred to a physician for definitive assessment.

■ Hypoglycemia

Chief Clinical Characteristics

This presentation commonly involves headache, slurred speech, dizziness, feelings of "vagueness," palpitations, impaired motor function, anxiety, sweating, hypotension, and sinus tachycardia.[48]

Background Information

The sensation of palpitations is quite often a reflex sinus tachycardia in response to the hypoglycemic insult and resolves quickly after the condition is corrected. This condition in individuals with diabetes mellitus may result from excess ingestion of insulin/oral hypoglycemic agents or insufficient food intake in relation to insulin/oral hypoglycemic dose. In individuals without diabetes mellitus, hypoglycemia may result from insufficient caloric intake or an abnormal increase in physical activity or exercise in the absence of proper nutrition. The onset of signs and symptoms typically occurs when blood sugar falls below 50 mg/dL and findings can be divided into two categories: those related to the activation of the autonomic nervous system and those caused by altered cerebral function. The diagnosis is confirmed by blood glucose testing. Having the individual immediately ingest a source of concentrated carbohydrate such as sugar, honey, candy, or orange juice can readily reverse the condition. The practitioner should monitor vital signs until they return to normal values. The therapist should be prepared to administer supportive care or activate the emergency medical services should the individual lapse into a diabetic coma (typically preceded by convulsions and unresponsiveness). Individuals with diabetes mellitus should be reminded to check blood glucose levels periodically and to avoid exercising in combination with the peak insulin effect to avoid episodes of hypoglycemia.

■ Hypothyroidism

Chief Clinical Characteristics

This presentation may be characterized by dizziness in combination with edema of the eyelids, face, and dorsum of the hand. Myxedema also may be present.

Background Information

This condition develops as a result of decreased production or levels of T_4 and T_3 hormones.[3,28] This condition may be suspected if an individual presents with pretibial edema and unusual fatigue that does not improve with rest.[28,29] Lab values for thyroid-stimulating hormone are elevated and can be detected before abnormal plasma levels of T_3 and T_4 hormones are observed. Blood values for serum T_3 and free T_4 are elevated, while serum TSH is decreased and radioactive iodine uptake is increased. Thyroid hormone replacement therapy is given for individuals with this condition. In many cases, the thyroid gland is surgically removed and hormone replacement therapy is required.

DIZZINESS

■ Idiopathic Intracranial Hypertension

Chief Clinical Characteristics

This presentation includes headaches, visual disturbances, dizziness, or tinnitus.[49]

Background Information

Diagnostic criteria include the presence of symptoms that reflect generalized intracranial hypertension or papilledema, elevated intracranial pressure (>250 mm H_2O per lumbar puncture), normal cerebrospinal fluid composition, absence of lesions on magnetic resonance imaging or computed tomography, and no other cause identified.[50] Also known as pseudotumor cerebri or benign intracranial hypertension, this condition is characterized by increased intracranial pressure without associated space-occupying lesions or hydrocephalus. Approximately one-third of individuals with idiopathic intracranial hypertension recover within 6 months following repeated lumbar punctures and drainage of cerebrospinal fluid to maintain the pressure at near normal or normal levels. Weight reduction and surgical gastric placation are effective forms of treatment.[18]

■ Labyrinthine Concussion

Chief Clinical Characteristics

This presentation commonly involves acute signs of vertigo, leading to constant unsteadiness, which worsens in darkness and during fatigue, and results in motion intolerance.[20] The symptoms are generally chronic, because the vestibular disturbance remains uncompensated. There is significant overlap in clinical presentation between this condition and brainstem–eighth nerve complex injury.

Background Information

A reduced vestibular response is apparent on caloric testing and rotary chair tests show gain asymmetry and an increased phase lag. Posturography is typically abnormal. The exact etiology is unknown but damage to the semicircular canal epithelium is an accepted cause. Magnetic resonance imaging will reveal hemorrhage in the semicircular canals, differentiating this condition from a brainstem–eighth nerve complex injury. Treatment is labyrinthectomy or selective vestibular nerve section. Vestibular rehabilitation in the form of vestibular habituation exercises is warranted postsurgically.

■ Labyrinthitis and Neuronitis

Chief Clinical Characteristics

This presentation may be characterized by a relatively sudden onset of severe, constant rotary vertigo (made worse by head movement) that resolves after days or weeks.[1,51] This condition is associated with spontaneous nystagmus, postural imbalance, and nausea without accompanying cochlear or neurological symptoms.[51] The specific presentation varies depending on the site of the infection. If the vestibular system is affected, the symptoms will include dizziness and difficulty with vision and/or balance. If the inflammation affects the cochlea, this condition will produce disturbances in hearing, such as tinnitus or hearing loss. The symptoms can be mild or severe, temporary or permanent, depending on the severity of the infection.

Background Information

The etiology is a bacterial or viral infection causing inflammation of the vestibular nerve (neuronitis) or the labyrinth (labyrinthitis). The terms are often used interchangeably because it is difficult to distinguish neuronitis from labyrinthitis.[1] The diagnostic hallmark is unilateral hyporesponsiveness with caloric testing.[51] Regardless of the type of infection, the treatment consists of destroying the bacteria by means of antibiotics. If the labyrinthitis is caused by a break in the membranes separating the middle and inner ears, surgery may also be required to repair the membranes to prevent a recurrence of the disease. Residual vertigo can be reduced with vestibular habituation exercises.[52]

■ Lateral Medullary Infarction (Wallenberg's Syndrome)

Chief Clinical Characteristics

This presentation can include nystagmus, oscillopsia, vertigo, nausea, vomiting, impairment of pain and thermal sense over half of the body, ipsilateral Horner syndrome including miosis, ptosis, anhidrosis, hoarseness, dysphagia, ipsilateral paralysis of palate and vocal cord with a diminished gag reflex, vertical diplopia or sensation of tilting vision, ipsilateral ataxia of limbs, loss of balance to ipsilateral side, and

DIZZINESS

impaired sensation of ipsilateral half of the face.[18,53,54]

Background Information
In 75% of cases, onset was sudden. Main etiologic factors associated with this condition include large-vessel infarction, arterial dissection, small-vessel infarction, cardiac embolism, tumor, hemorrhage, and other unknown factors. The most typical cause is occlusion of the vertebral artery, with the posterior inferior cerebellar artery being involved to a lesser degree. A thorough history, clinical examination, and magnetic resonance imaging may confirm the diagnosis. An emergency response is required for individuals experiencing new onset of symptoms. Residual symptoms include balance deficits (most common), dysphagia, dizziness, and numbness, which may be addressed with physical, occupational, and speech therapy.

■ Mal de Débarquement

Chief Clinical Characteristics
This presentation may involve vague concerns of unsteadiness and disequilibrium, as well as the illusion of movement such as rocking or swaying. Tilting, nausea, headache, and jumping or blurred vision are also associated concerns.[55]

Background Information
Symptoms generally ease during actual movement. Rotational vertigo is not a concern, but other otologic symptoms such as fullness, tinnitus, hyperacusis, otalgia, and decreased hearing may be reported. The symptoms typically follow travel by sea, air, or train, space flight, or experience within a slowly rotating room. Duration of symptoms is important to making the differential diagnosis; although postmotion vertigo lasting up to 48 hours is not uncommon (referred to as "landsickness"), this condition persists for longer periods. Although the cause is unknown, the strong predominance of this condition in women of postmenarchal and premenopausal ages suggests that female hormones may play a role. Another theory is persistent central nervous system adaptation to the moving environment. Medications such as benzodiazepines, amitriptyline hydrochloride, methazolamide, Fioricet, Percocet, and morphine have had some success at reducing symptoms. Meclizine and scopolamine, typically given to individuals

with dizziness, appear to be ineffective. Two-thirds of individuals find small benefit from vestibular rehabilitation.

■ Ménière's Disease

Chief Clinical Characteristics
This presentation is characterized by recurrent episodic spontaneous attacks of vertigo (exacerbated by head movements and accompanied by nausea and vomiting), fluctuating sensorineural hearing loss, aural fullness, and tinnitus.[51,56–63] In the late stages the symptoms are more severe, hearing loss is less likely to fluctuate, and tinnitus and aural fullness may be more constant. Sudden unexplained falls without loss of consciousness or vertigo (drop attacks) may occur. Attacks can be preceded by an aura consisting of a sense of fullness in the ear, increasing tinnitus, and a decrease in hearing,[61] but can also occur without warning. The typical duration of an attack is 2 to 3 hours, ranging from minutes to hours in length. Attacks can be single or multiple, with short or long intervening periods of remission during which the individual may be asymptomatic.

Background Information
The cause of this condition is thought to be overproduction or underabsorption of endolymph (endolymphatic hydrops), resulting in distortion of the membranous labyrinth. Ruptures of the membranous labyrinth, autoimmune disease processes, and viral infection are among other proposed causes.[61] Appropriate tests include caloric testing to determine amount of vestibular asymmetry; audiometry, which often shows a low-frequency loss more often than high frequencies; and exclusion of other causes (typically with gadolinium-enhanced magnetic resonance imaging). The head thrust test can be negative despite caloric asymmetry. Restricting salt intake and using diuretics may be useful in over half of individuals with this condition. Approximately 10% of individuals with this condition will have persistent vertigo and require other forms of treatment. These include surgery to decompress or drain the endolymphatic sac, selective vestibular neurectomy or labyrinthectomy, and intratympanic injections of aminoglycosides such as gentamicin[58] to reduce or abolish vestibular function on the affected side.

MIGRAINE-RELATED DIZZINESS

■ Basilar Migraines

Chief Clinical Characteristics

This presentation consists of two or more neurological problems (vertigo, tinnitus, decreased hearing, ataxia, dysarthria, visual symptoms in both hemifields of both eyes, diplopia, bilateral paresthesia or paresis, decreased level of consciousness) followed by a throbbing headache. It occurs in individuals primarily before age 20 years, and the duration of symptoms is 5 to 60 minutes.

Background Information

This condition is a form of migraine with aura. Audiograms are often normal. Diagnostic clues include having been diagnosed with migraine headaches or having a family history of migraines, but the diagnosis is one of exclusion. The diagnosis can be substantiated by medical efficacy in treating (ergotamines) and preventing (metoprolol, flunarizine) attacks, and exclusion of similar diagnoses, such as posterior fossa tumors, transient ischemic attacks (shorter duration, lasting only a few minutes), Ménière's disease, and vestibular paroxysmia. In addition to pharmacotherapy, vestibular rehabilitation may help, as may education regarding avoiding migraine triggers such as stress, nicotine, estrogen, and foods known to exacerbate migraines.

■ Benign Recurrent Vertigo

Chief Clinical Characteristics

This presentation can be characterized by vertigo spells, occasionally with tinnitus but without hearing loss, with or without headaches, that last minutes to hours.[64]

Background Information

If there is no headache, this may be referred to as migraine aura without headache. These spells occur between 20 and 60 years of age. Diagnostic clues include having been diagnosed with migraine headaches or having a family history of migraines, but the diagnosis is one of exclusion. The diagnosis can be substantiated by medical efficacy in treating (ergotamines) and preventing (metoprolol, flunarizine) attacks, and exclusion of similar diagnoses, such as

posterior fossa tumors, transient ischemic attacks (shorter duration, lasting only a few minutes), Ménière's disease, and vestibular paroxysmia. In addition to pharmacotherapy, vestibular rehabilitation may help, as may education regarding avoiding migraine triggers such as stress, nicotine, estrogen, and foods known to exacerbate migraines.

■ Vestibular Migraine

Chief Clinical Characteristics

This presentation may include episodic vertigo, primarily rotational but also of the rocking type.[65–67] *The vertigo often occurs before or with a headache but not always (32% to 36%). Associated symptoms are phonophobia, photophobia, visual disturbances, imbalance, nausea, and vomiting. The duration is most often a few minutes to several hours but can be quite variable.*

Background Information

When symptom free, ocular motor signs (saccadic pursuit, gaze-evoked nystagmus, positional nystagmus, and spontaneous nystagmus) can still be found. Diagnostic clues include having been diagnosed with migraine headaches or having a family history of migraines, but the diagnosis is one of exclusion. The diagnosis can be substantiated by medical efficacy in treating (ergotamines) and preventing (metoprolol, flunarizine) attacks, and exclusion of similar diagnoses, such as posterior fossa tumors, transient ischemic attacks (shorter duration, lasting only a few minutes), Ménière's disease, and vestibular paroxysmia. In addition to pharmacotherapy, vestibular rehabilitation may help, as may education regarding avoiding migraine triggers such as stress, nicotine, estrogen, and foods known to exacerbate migraines.

■ Mitral Valve Prolapse

Chief Clinical Characteristics

This presentation may include palpitations, chest pain, shortness of breath, fatigue, and light-headedness, and the individual may experience periodic syncopal episodes.[68] *The great majority of individuals with this condition are asymptomatic and the condition may go undiagnosed for years.*

Background Information

The palpitations are usually supraventricular in origin and occur paroxysmally. If palpable, the pulse is typically rapid and regular. The palpitation episodes commonly are self-limiting and last several minutes (less often, for hours), during which the individual may experience the other associated symptoms. Typically, the associated symptoms follow a benign course. Upon cardiac auscultation, a midsystolic click is often appreciated best over the fifth intercostal space left of the sternum. This may be followed by a late systolic murmur. This condition occurs when one or both valve leaflets exhibit exaggerated systolic bowing beyond the mitral annulus. This diagnosis is confirmed with echocardiography or angiography. Individuals diagnosed with this condition may be instructed by their physician to cough forcefully or perform a Valsalva maneuver (bearing down against a closed glottis) during episodes of palpitations in an effort to break the abnormal rhythm through vagal mediation. Quite often, these individuals are also prescribed calcium channel blockers or beta blockers to suppress the occurrence of palpitations. Occasionally, the tachycardia may be prolonged and immediate medical intervention is usually warranted, especially if the individual has underlying coronary artery disease and becomes hemodynamically unstable.

■ Multiple Sclerosis

Chief Clinical Characteristics

This presentation may include paresthesias, weakness, spasticity, hypertonicity, hyperreflexia, positive Babinski, incoordination, optic neuritis, ataxia, vertigo, dysarthria, diplopia, bladder incontinence, tremor, balance deficits, falls, and cognitive deficits.[18]

Background Information

This condition may present as relapsing-remitting, primary progressive, or secondary progressive. The disease occurs most frequently in women between the ages of 20 and 40 years. Only a small number of children or individuals between 50 and 60 years are diagnosed with this condition.[18] This condition was originally thought to be secondary to environmental and genetic factors, but evidence suggests an autoimmune response to a viral infection, which subsequently targets myelin.[18] The diagnosis may be confirmed by a thorough history, physical examination, magnetic resonance imaging, analysis of cerebrospinal fluid, and evoked potentials.[18,69,70] Life expectancy and cause of mortality are similar for all types of this condition.[18] Clinical characteristics that are associated with a longer time interval for progression of disability include female sex, younger age of onset, relapsing-remitting type, complete recovery after the first relapse, and longer time interval between first and second exacerbation.[71] Medical management may include the use of methylprednisolone, prednisone, cyclophosphamide, immunosuppressant treatment, and beta interferon.[18] Physical, occupational, and speech therapy may be indicated to prevent secondary sequelae and to optimize functional activity and mobility. Some individuals may benefit from psychological/psychiatric and social support as the disease progresses.

■ Multiple System Atrophy with Orthostatic Hypotension (Striatonigral Degeneration, Olivopontocerebellar Atrophy, Shy-Drager Syndrome)

Chief Clinical Characteristics

This presentation involves tremor, rigidity, akinesia, and/or postural imbalance along with signs of cerebellar, pyramidal, and autonomic dysfunction. Autonomic symptoms such as orthostatic hypotension, dry mouth, loss of sweating, impotence, and urinary incontinence or retention are the initial feature in 41% of individuals, with 74% to 97% of individuals developing some degree of autonomic dysfunction during the course of the disease.[72] *This condition is a combination of parkinsonian and non-parkinsonian symptoms and signs.*

Background Information

Diagnostic criteria are based on the clinical presentation, which includes poor response to levodopa, presence of autonomic features, presence of speech or bulbar problems, absence of dementia, absence of toxic confusion, and presence of falls.[73] The disease course ranges between 0.5 and 24 years after diagnosis with a mean survival time of 6.2 years.[74] This condition is a progressive condition of the central and autonomic nervous systems that rarely occurs without orthostatic hypotension. There are three types of this condition. The parkinsonian-type includes symptoms of Parkinson's disease such as slow movement, stiff muscles, and tremor. The cerebellar type causes problems with coordination and speech. The combined type includes symptoms of both parkinsonism and cerebellar failure. Older age at onset is associated with a shorter survival time.[74] Average age of onset is 54 years, with mean age at death being 60.3 years.[72] Most individuals with this condition receive a trial of levodopa although only a minority respond.[72] Additional treatment addresses symptoms and involves physical and occupational therapy to maintain mobility and address safety issues related to the progression of imbalance.

■ Neurosarcoidosis

Chief Clinical Characteristics
This presentation may be characterized by facial palsy, impaired taste, sight, smell, or swallowing, vertigo, loss of sensation in a stocking/glove pattern, and weakness in a distal greater than proximal distribution.[18]

Background Information
This condition is a manifestation of sarcoidosis with central and/or peripheral nervous system involvement. It is characterized by formation of granulomas in the central nervous system. The lesion consists of lymphocytes and mononuclear phagocytes surrounding a noncaseating epithelioid cell granuloma. These granulomas represent an autoimmune response to central nervous system tissues. This condition includes 5% of individuals with sarcoidosis. The diagnosis is established by the presence of clinical features, along with clinical and biopsy evidence of sarcoid granulomas in tissues outside the nervous system. Approximately two-thirds of individuals experience this illness only once, whereas the remainder experience chronic relapses. Primary treatment for neurosarcoidosis is the administration of corticosteroids.

■ Orthostatic Hypotension

Chief Clinical Characteristics
This presentation commonly involves dizziness, light-headedness, and blurred vision that generally occur after sudden standing. In more severe forms of this condition, individuals may experience seizures, transient ischemic attacks, or syncope.

Background Information
This condition is caused by a sudden decrease of greater than 20 mm Hg in systolic blood pressure or greater than 10 mm Hg in diastolic blood pressure that occurs when a person assumes a standing position. It may be caused by hypovolemia resulting from the excessive use of diuretics, vasodilators, or other types of vasoactive medications (eg, calcium channel blockers and beta blockers), dehydration, or prolonged bed rest. Other factors to consider include the individual's neurological status and hemorrhagic/hypovolemic states. The condition may be associated with Addison's disease, atherosclerosis, diabetes, and certain neurological conditions including Shy-Drager syndrome and other dysautonomias. Hypovolemia due to medications is reversed by adjusting the dosage or by discontinuing the medication. If prolonged bed rest is the cause, improvement may occur by sitting up with increasing frequency each day. In some cases, physical counterpressure such as elastic hose or whole-body inflatable suits may be required. Dehydration is treated with salt and fluids. Individuals with this condition can be instructed to rise slowly from bed in the mornings or when moving from a sitting/squatting to standing position. Symptoms usually dissipate when the individual is placed in a semirecumbent or supine position, although some individuals may progress to frank syncope. In this case, the clinician should be prepared to activate the emergency medical system if the individual fails to regain consciousness with basic life support measures.

■ Otosyphilis

Chief Clinical Characteristics
This presentation may involve severe episodic vertigo, fluctuating hearing loss, low-frequency hearing loss in the early stages of the disease, and flat audiometric patterns in the later stages of the disease.[75,76] The hearing loss is usually bilateral in most individuals; the loss in speech discrimination is usually out of proportion to the speech reception threshold. Vestibular disturbances could be present in

as many as 80% of individuals with this condition. This condition's presentation is similar to that of Ménière's disease.

Background Information

Otosyphilis is caused by the spirochete *Treponema pallidum*. Both congenital and acquired forms of syphilis infection can lead to this condition with subsequent degeneration of the audiovestibular system. Histopathological findings are identical for both the congenital and acquired forms. The underlying syphilis infection causes meningoneurolabyrinthitis in the early congenital form and in the acute period of the secondary and tertiary acquired forms. It causes temporal bone osteitis with secondary involvement of the membranous labyrinth in the late congenital, late latent, and tertiary syphilis stages. Endolymphatic hydrops and degenerative changes in the sensory and neural structures are seen in both the congenital and acquired forms. Poor prognosis is indicated by endolymphatic sac obstruction by microgummata. The goal of treatment is to halt the progression of the disease. Treatment includes antibiotic and steroidal anti-inflammatory medication, and the medication of choice differs with the clinical stage of the disease.

■ Paraneoplastic Syndromes

Chief Clinical Characteristics

This presentation commonly includes dizziness in combination with a variety of different neurological symptoms and signs in an individual with cancer. Specific neurological symptoms and signs depend on the location of involvement of the central or peripheral nervous system.

Background Information

Paraneoplastic encephalomyelitis and focal encephalitis may present with ataxia, vertigo, balance deficits, nystagmus, nausea, vomiting, cranial nerve palsies, seizures, sensory neuropathy, anxiety, depression, cognitive changes, and hallucinations. For individuals presenting with ataxia, dysarthria, dysphagia, and diplopia, paraneoplastic cerebellar degeneration may be suspected. Paraneoplastic opsoclonus/myoclonus tends to affect both children and adults with signs and symptoms

including hypotonia, ataxia, irritability, truncal ataxia, gait difficulty, balance deficits, and frequent falls. Stiff-man syndrome presents with spasms and fluctuating rigidity of axial musculature, legs, and possibly shoulders, upper extremities, and neck. Paraneoplastic sensory neuropathy presents with asymmetric, progressive sensory alterations involving the limbs, trunk, and face, sensorineural hearing loss, autonomic dysfunction, and pain. Other conditions in this category include vasculitis, Lambert-Eaton myasthenia syndrome, myasthenia gravis, dermatomyositis, neuromyotonia, and various neuropathies.[18,77] These conditions result from an immune-mediated response to the presence of tumor or metastases. Antibodies or T cells respond to the presence of the tumor, but also attack normal cells of the nervous system.[78,79] Over 60% of individuals present with this condition prior to the discovery of the cancer.[77] The underlying tumor is treated according to the type of cancer. Additional treatment is dependent on this condition's type and may include steroids, plasmapheresis, immunotherapy, chemotherapy, radiation, or cyclophosphamide.[77] Physical, occupational, and speech therapy may be indicated to address functional limitations.

■ Perilymph Fistula

Chief Clinical Characteristics

This presentation may involve dizziness, vertigo, imbalance, nausea, and vomiting.[51] Some individuals with this condition experience ringing or fullness in the ears, and many notice a hearing loss. Most people with fistulas find that their symptoms get worse with changes in altitude (elevators, airplanes, travel over mountain passes) or air pressure (weather changes), as well as with exertion and activity.

Background Information

The cause of this condition is a tear or defect in the oval or round window in one or both ears, allowing pressure changes in the middle ear to stimulate the inner ear and cause symptoms. Head trauma via a direct blow and whiplash injury, barotrauma sustained during diving, weightlifting, and childbirth are among common causes. This condition also may be present from birth or may result from chronic, severe ear infections. Clinical tests suggestive of a fistula include reproduction of symptoms during a Valsalva maneuver or when applying pressure to the external auditory canal. The definitive diagnosis is made by direct visualization during tympanotomy. Surgical repair with grafting is indicated if symptoms persist despite nonsurgical care consisting of activity restriction aimed at avoiding lifting, straining (Valsalva maneuver), bending over, and changes in pressure.

■ Postural Tachycardia Syndrome

Chief Clinical Characteristics

This presentation includes rapid heartbeat, light-headedness or dizziness with prolonged standing, headache, chronic fatigue, exercise intolerance, weakness, hyperpnea or dyspnea, tremulousness, nausea/abdominal pain, sweating, anxiety/palpitations, chest pain, and other nonspecific concerns.

Background Information

This condition is characterized by orthostatic intolerance associated with a pulse rate that increases 30 beats per minute or greater when the individual moves from a supine to standing position.[80] Causes usually are not identified but symptoms are related to reduced cerebral blood flow associated with inadequate systemic venous return to the right heart. Reversible causes such as low blood volume should be ruled out. Treatment depends on the severity of the symptoms. This condition is self-limiting, but individuals are usually advised to increase their fluid and salt intake. Body stockings may provide some relief. Drug therapy, with fludrocortisone, beta blockers, midodrine, or clonidine, can be beneficial. Physical exercise, such as walking and gluteal and calf muscle resistance training, also may help.[80] Some individuals may require and benefit from insertion of a cardiac pacemaker. Individuals with this condition can be instructed to rise slowly from bed in the mornings (eg, sitting at the edge of the bed and performing ankle/calf exercises) or when going from a sitting/squatting to standing position. Symptoms usually dissipate when the individual is placed in a semirecumbent or supine position, although some individuals may progress to frank syncope. In this case, the therapist should be prepared to activate the emergency medical system if the individual fails to regain consciousness with basic life support measures.

■ Pregnancy

Chief Clinical Characteristics

This condition is commonly characterized by reports of palpitations associated with shortness of breath, dizziness, presyncope, or syncope in a pregnant woman.

Background Information

During pregnancy, significant changes occur in hormonal and hemodynamic function that predispose women to the development of dysrhythmias. Changes in hormone levels during pregnancy (particularly progesterone) have been associated with enhanced sympathetic activity and the precipitation of dysrhythmias.[81] The enhanced maternal blood volume and associated increase in stroke volume may lead to the sensation of a forceful, bounding pulse in some individuals. The type of dysrhythmia often associated with palpitations is often sinus tachycardia or supraventricular tachycardia. Very rarely is atrial fibrillation or ventricular tachycardia the source of the dysrhythmia.[82] The episodes are usually benign and self-limiting, can often be associated with shortness of breath, and there may be an increased occurrence of symptoms to term.[83] At times, the palpitations may also be associated with dizziness, presyncope, or frank syncope. If palpitations are associated with these latter symptoms, the individual should be referred back to her primary care physician for evaluation. In the event of cardiovascular compromise, the therapist should be prepared to provide supportive interventions and activate the emergency medical system if warranted.

■ Spinal Metastases

Chief Clinical Characteristics

This presentation can involve spasticity, weakness, sensory alterations, bowel and bladder incontinence, neck pain, back pain, radicular pain, atrophy, cerebellar signs, balance deficits, falls, and cranial nerve involvement.[18,84,85]

Background Information

This condition is the most frequent neoplasm involving the spine.[85] The most common types and locations of primary tumors that result in spinal metastases include breast, lung, lymphoma, prostate, kidney, gastrointestinal tract, and thyroid.[18,86] The diagnosis is confirmed with gadolinium-enhanced magnetic resonance imaging and computed tomography.[18,85] Treatment is variable depending on the tumor and may include surgical resection, chemotherapy, radiation, corticosteroids, and rehabilitative therapies.[18] Although the long-term prognosis is poor, individuals without paresis or pain and who are still ambulatory have longer survival rates.[86]

■ Spinal Primary Tumors

Chief Clinical Characteristics
This presentation may include spasticity, weakness, sensory alterations, bowel/bladder incontinence, back pain, radicular pain, atrophy, cerebellar signs, balance deficits, falls, and cranial nerve involvement.[18]

Background Information
Types of this condition include myeloma, neurofibroma, lymphoma, metastasis, meningioma, schwannoma, and astrocytoma. The first test to diagnose brain and spinal column tumors is a neurological examination. Special imaging techniques (computed tomography, magnetic resonance imaging, and positron emission tomography) are also employed. Specific diagnoses may be confirmed with imaging and biopsy. Treatment is variable depending on the type, size, and location of the tumor and may include surgical resection, chemotherapy, radiation, corticosteroids, and rehabilitative therapies. Prognosis is variable and depends on the type and grade of tumor, severity of compression, and duration of compression.

■ Superior Canal Dehiscence Syndrome

Chief Clinical Characteristics
This presentation typically involves recurrent attacks of vertigo and oscillopsia (movement of the visual field) induced by changes in intracranial or middle ear pressure or by loud noises.

Background Information
This condition is a variant of perilymph fistula. It is caused by a dehiscence of the bone overlying the superior (anterior) semicircular canal, which allows pressure changes to be transmitted to the canal. Clinical tests suggestive of superior canal dehiscence are reproduction of symptoms with coughing, tragal pressure, or Valsalva maneuver. Computed tomography and click-evoked myogenic potentials are important diagnostic tools. Treatment involves plugging the dehiscence surgically.

■ Transient Ischemic Attack

Chief Clinical Characteristics
This presentation can include numbness or weakness in the face, arm, or leg, especially on one side of the body; confusion or difficulty in talking or understanding speech; trouble seeing with one or both eyes; and difficulty with walking, dizziness, or loss of balance and coordination.

Background Information
This condition is a transient stroke that lasts only a few minutes. It occurs when the blood supply to part of the brain is briefly interrupted. Symptoms of this condition, which usually occur suddenly, are similar to those of stroke but do not last as long. Most symptoms disappear within an hour, although they may persist for up to 24 hours. Because it is impossible to differentiate between symptoms from this condition and acute stroke, individuals should assume that all stroke-like symptoms signal a medical emergency. A prompt evaluation (within 60 minutes) is necessary to identify the cause of this condition and determine appropriate therapy. Depending on the individual's medical history and the results of a medical examination, the doctor may recommend drug therapy or surgery to reduce the risk of stroke. Antiplatelet medications, particularly aspirin, are a standard treatment for individuals suspected of having this condition and who also are at risk for stroke, including individuals with atrial fibrillation.

■ Traumatic Brain Injury

Chief Clinical Characteristics
This presentation typically includes disequilibrium in the presence of cognitive changes, altered level of consciousness, seizures, nausea, vomiting, coma, dizziness, headache, pupillary changes, tinnitus, weakness, incoordination, behavioral changes, spasticity, hypertonicity, cranial nerve lesions, sensory, and motor deficits.[18,87]

Background Information

This condition can be classified as mild, moderate, or severe based on the Glasgow Coma Scale, length of coma, and duration of post-traumatic amnesia.[87] Magnetic resonance imaging may be used to confirm the diagnosis.[84] Treatment initiated at the scene of the accident and during the acute phase is focused on medical stabilization. It should be initiated during the acute phase in order to minimize complications.[88] Low Glasgow Coma Scale, longer length of coma, longer duration of post-traumatic amnesia, and older age tend to be associated with poor outcomes.[89] Optimal rehabilitation is interdisciplinary and customized to address each specific individual's disablement.

■ Vasovagal Syncope

Chief Clinical Characteristics

This presentation commonly includes dizziness, as well as prodromal symptoms of nausea, headache, paresthesias, light-headedness, dizziness, palpitations, shortness of breath, diaphoresis, and chest pain.[90] The therapist will usually note the individual's pulse to be rapid and regular, and blood pressure may be hypotensive.

Background Information

Individuals susceptible to vasovagal syncope usually have difficulty standing for prolonged periods of time and exhibit delayed or diminished neurocardiovascular responses when assuming an upright posture. The precise mechanism responsible for this condition is not well understood. Predisposing factors include hypovolemia, anemia, and sympathetic blocking/antihypertensive medications. The tilt-table test is the diagnostic procedure of choice for confirming vasovagal syncope, and the individual should be referred to his or her primary care physician for definitive assessment. Treatment involves the individual assuming a more recumbent position and administering fluids. These treatments will often cause the symptoms to abate.

■ Vertebrobasilar Artery Insufficiency

Chief Clinical Characteristics

This presentation commonly involves symptoms consistent with a cerebrovascular accident involving the vertebrobasilar artery

system, usually the anterior inferior cerebellar artery.[91] Headache or neck pain was found to be the prominent feature in 88% of 26 individuals presenting with vertebral artery dissection. The most common focal neurological symptom was vertigo (57%).[92] In cases of stroke following cervical spine manipulation purported to be due to vertebral artery dissection, the presenting neurological symptoms were loss of coordination (52%), dizziness/vertigo/nausea/vomiting (50%), speech/swallowing dysfunction, visual disturbances, and numbness, nystagmus, loss of consciousness, hearing deficits/tinnitus, and death.[93]

Background Information

Less severe but similar symptoms may be expected in lesser degrees of vertebrobasilar insufficiency. The circulation to the inner ear arises from the vertebrobasilar artery system, which leads to dizziness when this circulation is impaired.[91,94] If the insufficiency is great enough to progress to stroke there are generally other associated neurological symptoms typical of central nervous system lesions but these can be absent.[91,94] A classic sequela of stroke related to this condition is lateral medullary (Wallenberg's) syndrome. Proposed causes of vascular compromise include trauma (including participation in sports or manipulation of the cervical spine), cervical spine rotation and/or extension, and complications due to risk factors such as age, gender, migraine headaches, hypertension, diabetes, birth control pills, cervical spondylosis, and smoking.[93,95,96] However, systematic reviews of the literature suggest there is no definitive way to identify who is at risk for vertebrobasilar insufficiency, either by history, clinical examination, or special tests.[93,95,97,98] Individuals suspected of having this condition should be referred for medical evaluation urgently.

■ Vestibular Epilepsy (Vestibular Seizures)

Chief Clinical Characteristics

This presentation can be characterized by sensations of horizontal or vertical rotation, or of falling and rising. Individuals may describe vertigo and light-headedness as part of the epileptic aura in complex partial seizures with temporal or extratemporal foci.[99]

Background Information

Associated symptoms may be typical of simple partial seizures (no loss of consciousness) or of complex partial seizures (loss of consciousness) or of generalized tonic-clonic seizures (loss of consciousness and movements of the extremities). There may be associated eye, head, and body deviations or epileptic nystagmus. This condition is caused by focal discharge in the thalamus, temporal lobe, or parietal association cortex. Treatment commonly includes antiepileptic medications.

■ Vestibular Ototoxicity

Chief Clinical Characteristics

This presentation includes fluctuating or constant tinnitus and hearing loss ranging from mild to complete deafness if the cochlea is involved; vertigo, vomiting, nystagmus, and imbalance if the vestibular system is involved unilaterally; and headache, ear fullness, oscillopsia, an inability to tolerate head movement, a wide-based gait, difficulty walking in the dark, a feeling of unsteadiness and actual unsteadiness while moving, imbalance to the point of being unable to walk, light-headedness, and severe fatigue in bilateral involvement. Any combination of the above is possible since either the cochlea or the vestibular system individually, or both in combination, can be affected, either unilaterally or bilaterally.

Background Information

The severity, type, and particular combination of symptoms are variable, depending on the medication exposure, whether it is unilateral or bilateral, the speed of onset, and the individual. A slow unilateral loss may produce few symptoms since the brain can compensate through other mechanisms, whereas a fast bilateral loss can produce significant disability. Because these symptoms are similar to many other conditions, the key diagnostic feature is a history of drug or chemical exposure. Medications that are known to be vestibulotoxic include aspirin and quinine, loop diuretics (bumetanide [Bumex], ethacrynic acid [Edecrin], furosemide [Lasix], torsemide [Demadex]), aminoglycoside antibiotics (amikacin, dihydrostreptomycin, gentamicin, kanamycin, Neomycin, netilmicin, ribostamycin, streptomycin, tobramycin), and anticancer medications such as carboplatin and cisplatin. Some medications produce a temporary dysfunction, while others produce permanent loss. Treatment involves removing exposure to the medication if possible and post-exposure compensatory vestibular habituation and balance exercises.

■ Whiplash Injury (Whiplash-Associated Disorder)

Chief Clinical Characteristics

This presentation is characterized by a collection of symptoms that occur following damage to the neck, usually because of sudden extension and flexion such as might happen in an automobile accident. Symptoms commonly include nonspecific dizziness in combination with neck pain, stiffness, headache, abnormal sensations such as burning or prickling, or shoulder or back pain.[21] There may also be complaints of unsteadiness and visual disturbances, as well as signs of altered postural stability, cervical proprioception, and head and eye movement control.[34]

Background Information

Damage to the cervical spine, especially the upper cervical region, leads to disruption of cervicocephalic kinesthesia that may be responsible for this condition.[31,34,100,101] Sensorimotor deficits are common. In addition, some people experience cognitive, somatic, or psychological conditions such as memory loss, concentration impairment, nervousness/irritability, sleep disturbances, fatigue, or depression. Symptoms such as neck pain may be present directly after the injury or may be delayed for several days. The condition may include injury to intervertebral joints, disks, and ligaments, cervical muscles, and nerve roots. The trauma may dislodge otoconia in the inner ear, leading to benign paroxysmal positional vertigo, and complaints of dizziness upon change of position.[25] The need for radiographs can be determined through a careful history; they are not always necessary.[102] Otolaryngologic evaluation may reveal abnormal findings suggestive of central and/or peripheral vestibular involvement.[103,104] Treatment for individuals with an acute whiplash may include pain medications, physical therapy modalities, nonsteroidal anti-inflammatory drugs, antidepressants, muscle relaxants, and use of a cervical collar. Range of motion and strengthening exercises are key aspects of long-term management. Treatment for decreased kinesthetic awareness involves eye–head–neck–trunk coordination exercises.[39]

References

1. Froehling DA, Silverstein MD, Mohr DN, Beatty CW. Does this dizzy patient have a serious form of vertigo? *JAMA.* 1994;271(5):385–388.
2. Venes D, ed. *Taber's Cyclopedic Medical Dictionary.* 20th ed. Philadelphia, PA: F. A. Davis; 2001.
3. Baloh RW. Dizziness: neurological emergencies. *Neurol Clin.* May 1998;16(2):305–321.
4. Baloh RW. Differentiating between peripheral and central causes of vertigo. *Otolaryngol Head Neck Surg.* 1998;119:55–59.
5. Lee DJ, Westra WH, Staecker H, Long D, Niparko JK, Slattery WH 3rd. Clinical and histopathologic features of recurrent vestibular schwannoma (acoustic neuroma) after stereotactic radiosurgery. *Otol Neurotol.* Jul 2003;24(4):650–660; discussion 660.
6. Murphy MR, Selesnick SH. Cost-effective diagnosis of acoustic neuromas: a philosophical, macroeconomic, and technological decision. *Otolaryngol Head Neck Surg.* Oct 2002;127(4):253–259.
7. Ho SY, Kveton JF. Acoustic neuroma. Assessment and management. *Otolaryngol Clin North Am.* Apr 2002; 35(2):393–404.
8. Rosenberg SI. Natural history of acoustic neuromas. *Laryngoscope.* Apr 2000;110(4):497–508.
9. Ramina R, Maniglia JJ, Meneses MS, et al. Acoustic neurinomas. Diagnosis and treatment. *Arquivos de Neuro-Psiquiatria.* Sep 1997;55(3A):393–402.
10. Kartush JM, Brackmann DE. Acoustic neuroma update. *Otolaryngol Clin North Am.* Jun 1996;29(3):377–392.
11. Herdman SJ, Clendaniel RA, Mattox DE, Holliday MJ, Niparko JK. Vestibular adaptation exercises and recovery: acute stage after acoustic neuroma resection. *Otolaryngol Head Neck Surg.* 1995;113(1):77–87.
12. Ludwig H, Strasser K. Symptomatology of anemia. *Semin Oncol.* 2001;28(2 suppl 8):7–14.
13. Pujade-Lauraine E, Gascon P. The burden of anaemia in patients with cancer. *Oncology.* 2004;67(suppl 1):1–4.
14. Widmaier EP, Raff H, Strang KT. *Vander, Sherman, and Luciano's Human Physiology: The Mechanisms of Body Function.* New York, NY: McGraw-Hill; 2004.
15. Toy P, Feiner J, Viele MK. Fatigue during acute isovolemic anemia in healthy, resting humans. *Transfusion.* 2000;40:457–460.
16. *Diagnostic and Statistical Manual of Mental Disorders, Text Revision.* 4th ed. Washington, DC: American Psychiatric Association; 2000.
17. Halgin RP, Whitbourne SK. *Abnormal Psychology. The Human Experience of Psychological Disorders.* 2nd ed. Madison, WI: Brown and Benchmark; 1997.
18. Victor M, Ropper AH. *Adams and Victor's Principles of Neurology.* 7th ed. New York, NY: McGraw-Hill; 2001.
19. Fetter M. Vestibular system disorders. In: Herdman S, ed. *Vestibular Rehabilitation.* 2nd ed. Philadelphia, PA: F. A. Davis; 2000:91–102.
20. Fitzgerald DC. Head trauma: hearing loss and dizziness.[see comment]. *J Trauma-Injury Infect Crit Care.* 1996;40(3):488–496.
21. Herdman S, ed. *Vestibular Rehabilitation.* 2nd ed. Philadelphia, PA: F. A. Davis; 2000.
22. Hilton M, Pinder D. The Epley (canalith repositioning) manoeuvre for benign paroxysmal positional vertigo [update of Cochrane Database Syst Rev. 2002;(1): CD003162; PMID: 11869655]. *Cochrane Database Syst Rev.* 2004(2):CD003162.
23. Nunez RA, Cass SP, Furman JM. Short- and long-term outcomes of canalith repositioning for benign paroxysmal positional vertigo. *Otolaryngol Head Neck Surg.* 2000;122:647–652.
24. Froehling DA, Bowen JM, Mohr DN, et al. The canalith repositioning procedure for the treatment of benign paroxysmal positional vertigo: a randomized controlled trial. *Mayo Clin Proc.* Jul 2000;75(7):695–700.
25. Parnes LS, Agrawal SK, Atlas J. Diagnosis and management of benign paroxysmal positional vertigo (BPPV). *CMAJ.* Sep 30 2003;169(7):681–693.
26. Tusa RJ. Benign paroxysmal positional vertigo. *Curr Neurol Neurosci Rep.* Sep 2001;1(5):478–485.
27. Dornhoffer JL, Colvin GB. Benign paroxysmal positional vertigo and canalith repositioning: clinical correlations. *Am J Otol.* Mar 2000;21(2):230–233.
28. Cohen HS, Jerabek J. Efficacy of treatments for posterior canal benign paroxysmal positional vertigo. *Laryngoscope.* Apr 1999;109(4):584–590.
29. Agrawal SK, Parnes LS. Human experience with canal plugging. *Ann NY Acad Sci.* Oct 2001;942:300–305.
30. Tosoni A, Ermani M, Brandes AA. The pathogenesis and treatment of brain metastases: a comprehensive review. *Crit Rev Oncol Hematol.* 2004;52:199–215.
31. Wrisley DM, Sparto PJ, Whitney SL, Furman JM. Cervicogenic dizziness: a review of diagnosis and treatment. *J Orthop Sports Phys Ther.* 2000;30(12):755–766.
32. Reid S, Rivett DA. Manual therapy treatment of cervicogenic dizziness: a systematic review. *Man Ther.* 2005; 10:4–13.
33. Brandt T, Bronstein AM. Cervical vertigo. *J Neurol Neurosurg Psychiatry.* 2001;71(1):8–12.
34. Kristjansson E, Treleaven J. Sensorimotor function and dizziness in neck pain: Implications for assessment and management. *J Orthop Sports Phys Ther.* 2009; 39(5):364–377.
35. Tjell C, Rosenhall U. Smooth pursuit neck torsion test: a specific test for cervical dizziness. *Am J Otol.* Jan 1998;19(1):76–81.
36. Stapley PJ, Beretta MV, Dalla Toffola E, Schieppati M. Neck muscle fatigue and postural control in patients with whiplash injury. *Clin Neurophysiol.* 2006;117;610–622.
37. Bracher ES, Almeida CI, Almeida RR, Duprat AC, Bracher CB. A combined approach for the treatment of cervical vertigo. *J Manipulative Physiol Ther.* Feb 2000;23(2):96–100.
38. Clendaniel RA. Cervical vertigo. In: Herdman S, ed. *Vestibular Rehabilitation.* 2nd ed. Philadelphia, PA: F. A. Davis; 2000:494–509.
39. Revel M, Minguet M, Gregoy P, Vaillant J, Manuel JL. Changes in cervicocephalic kinesthesia after a proprioceptive rehabilitation program in patients with neck pain: a randomized controlled study. *Arch Phys Med Rehabil.* 1994;75(8):895–899.
40. Holt JJ. Cholesteatoma and otosclerosis: two slowly progressive causes of hearing loss treatable through corrective surgery. *Clin Med Res.* Apr 2003;1(2):151–154.

41. Shohet JA, de Jong AL. The management of pediatric cholesteatoma. *Otolaryngol Clin North Am.* Aug 2002;35(4):841–851.

42. Mitsumoto H, Wilbourn AJ. Causes and diagnosis of sensory neuropathies: a review. *J Clin Neurophysiol.* Nov 1994;11(6):553–567.

43. Rossi LN, Lutschg J, Meier C, Vassella F. Hereditary motor sensory neuropathies in childhood. *Dev Med Child Neurol.* 1983;25(1):19–31.

44. Boemo RL, Navarrete ML, García-Arumí AM, et al. Ramsay Hunt syndrome. Our experience. *Acta Otorrinolaringol Esp.* 2010; 61(6):418–421.

45. Aronow WS. The heart and thyroid disease. *Clin Geriatr Med.* 1995;11(2):219–229.

46. Chohan ND, Cray JV. *Professional Guide to Signs and Symptoms.* Springhouse, PA: Springhouse; 2003.

47. Rosana GMC, Leonardo F, Dicandia C. Acute electrophysiologic effects of estradiol 17 in menopausal women. *Am J Cardiol.* 2000;86:1385–1387.

48. Cryer PE. Symptoms of hypoglycemia, thresholds for their occurrence, and hypoglycemia unawareness. *Endocrinol Metab Clin North Am.* 1991;28(3):495–500.

49. Galvin JA, Van Stavern GP. Clinical characterization of idiopathic intracranial hypertension at the Detroit Medical Center. *J Neurol Sci.* 2004;30(223(2)):157–160.

50. Friedman DI, Jacobson DM. Diagnostic criteria for idiopathic intracranial hypertension. *Neurology.* 2002;59: 1492–1495.

51. Strupp M, Arbusow V. Acute Vestibulopathy. *Curr Opin Neurol.* 2001;14(1):11–20.

52. Yardley L, Beech S, Zander L, Evans T, Weinman J. A randomized controlled trial of exercise therapy for dizziness and vertigo in primary care [see comments]. *Br J Genl Pract.* 1998;48(429):1136–1140.

53. Kim JS. Pure lateral medullary infarction: clinical-radiological correlation of 130 acute, consecutive patients. *Brain.* 2003;126:1864–1872.

54. Nelles G, Contois KA, Valente SL, Jacobs DH, Kaplan JD, Pessin MS. Recovery following lateral medullary infarction. *Neurology.* 1998;50(5):1418–1422.

55. Hain TC, Hanna PA, Rheinberger MA. Mal de debarquement. *Acta Otolaryngol Head Neck Surg.* 1999;125:615–620.

56. Thorp MA, Shehab ZP, Bance ML, Rutka JA. The AAO-HNS Committee on Hearing and Equilibrium guidelines for the diagnosis and evaluation of therapy in Meniere's disease: have they been applied in the published literature of the last decade? *Clin Otolaryngol Allied Sci.* Jun 2003;28(3):173–176.

57. Carey J. Intratympanic gentamicin for the treatment of Meniere's disease and other forms of peripheral vertigo. *Otolaryngol Clin North Am.* Oct 2004;37(5):1075–1090.

58. Cohen-Kerem R, Kisilevsky V, Einarson TR, Kozer E, Koren G, Rutka JA. Intratympanic gentamicin for Meniere's disease: a meta-analysis. *Laryngoscope.* Dec 2004;114(12):2085–2091.

59. Ervin SE. Meniere's disease: identifying classic symptoms and current treatments. *AAOHN J.* Apr 2004; 52(4):156–158.

60. James A, Thorp M. Meniere's disease [update of *Clin Evid.* 2003 Jun;(9):565–73; PMID: 12967379]. *Clin Evid.* Jun 2004(11):664–672.

61. Minor LB, Schessel DA, Carey JP. Meniere's disease. *Curr Opin Neurol.* Feb 2004;17(1):9–16.

62. Neuhauser H, Lempert T. Vertigo and dizziness related to migraine: a diagnostic challenge [see comment]. *Cephalalgia.* Feb 2004;24(2):83–91.

63. Boyev KP. Meniere's disease or migraine? The clinical significance of fluctuating hearing loss with vertigo [see comment]. *Arch Otolaryngol Head Neck Surg.* May 2005;131(5):457–459.

64. Tusa RJ. Diagnosis and management of neuro-otological disorders due to migraine. In: Herdman S, ed. *Vestibular Rehabilitation.* 2nd ed. Philadelphia, PA: F. A. Davis; 2001:298–315.

65. Dieterich M, Brandt T. Episodic vertigo related to migraine (90 cases): vestibular migraine? *J Neurol.* Oct 1999;246(10):883–892.

66. Furman JM, Marcus DA, Balaban CD. Migrainous vertigo: development of a pathogenetic model and structured diagnostic interview. *Curr Opin Neurol.* Feb 2003;16(1):5–13.

67. Furman JM, Whitney SL. Central causes of dizziness. *Phys Ther.* Feb 2000;80(2):179–187.

68. Bouknight DP, O'Rourke RA. Current management of mitral valve prolapse. *Am Fam Physician.* 2000;61: 3343–3350, 3353–3354.

69. McDonald WI, Compston A, Edan G, et al. Recommended diagnostic criteria for multiple sclerosis: guidelines from the International Panel on the diagnosis of multiple sclerosis. *Ann Neurol.* Jul 2001;50(1): 121–127.

70. Thompson AJ, Montalban X, Barkhof F, et al. Diagnostic criteria for primary progressive multiple sclerosis: a position paper. *Ann Neurol.* Jun 2000;47(6):831–835.

71. Confavreux C, Vukusic S, Adeleine P. Early clinical predictors and progression of irreversible disability in multiple sclerosis: an amnesic process. *Brain.* Apr 2003;126(Pt 4):770–782.

72. Wenning GK, Tison F, Ben Shlomo Y, Daniel SE, Quinn NP. Multiple system atrophy: a review of 203 pathologically proven cases. *Mov Disord.* Mar 1997;12(2): 133–147.

73. Wenning GK, Ben-Shlomo Y, Hughes A, Daniel SE, Lees A, Quinn NP. What clinical features are most useful to distinguish definite multiple system atrophy from Parkinson's disease? *J Neurol Neurosurg Psychiatry.* Apr 2000;68(4):434–440.

74. Ben-Shlomo Y, Wenning GK, Tison F, Quinn NP. Survival of patients with pathologically proven multiple system atrophy: a meta-analysis. *Neurology.* Feb 1997;48(2): 384–393.

75. Fayad JN, Linthicum FH, Jr. Temporal bone histopathology case of the month: otosyphilis. *Am J Otology.* Mar 1999;20(2):259–260.

76. Klemm E, Wollina U. Otosyphilis: report on six cases. *J Eur Acad Dermatol Venereol.* Jul 2004;18(4):429–434.

77. Bataller L, Dalmau J. Paraneoplastic neurologic syndromes: approaches to diagnosis and treatment. *Semin Neurol.* Jun 2003;23(2):215–224.

78. Darnell RB, Posner JB. Paraneoplastic syndromes involving the nervous system. *N Engl J Med.* Oct 16 2003;349(16):1543–1554.

79. Dalmau JO, Posner JB. Paraneoplastic syndromes. *Arch Neurol.* Apr 1999;56(4):405–408.

80. Stewart JM. Chronic orthostatic intolerance and the postural tachycardia syndrome (POTS). *J Pediatr.* 2004;45:725–730.

81. Rosano GM, Rillo M, Leonardo F. Palpitations: what is the mechanism, and when should we treat them? *Int J Fertil Women's Med.* 1997 42(2):94–100.

82. Wolbrette D. Treatment of arrhythmias during pregnancy. *Curr Women's Health Rep.* 2003;3(2):135–139.

83. Choi HS, Han SS, Choi HA. Dyspnea and palpitation during pregnancy. *Korean J Intern Med.* 2001; 16(4):247–249.

84. Lindsay KW, Bone I, Callander, R. *Neurology and Neurosurgery Illustrated.* 3rd ed. New York, NY: Churchill Livingstone; 1997.

85. Perrin RG, Laxton AW. Metastatic spine disease: epidemiology, pathophysiology, and evaluation of patients. *Neurosurg Clin N Am.* Oct 2004;15(4):365–373.

86. Hosono N, Ueda T, Tamura D, Aoki Y, Yoshikawa H. Prognostic relevance of clinical symptoms in patients with spinal metastases. *Clin Orthop Relat Res.* Jul 2005(436):196–201.

87. Bruns J, Hauser WA. The epidemiology of traumatic brain injury: a review. *Epilepsia.* 2003;44(suppl 10):2–10.

88. Das-Gupta R, Turner-Stokes L. Traumatic brain injury. *Disabil Rehabil.* 2002;24(13):654–665.

89. Hukkelhoven CWPM, Steyerberg EW, Rampen AJJ, et al. Patient age and outcome following severe traumatic brain injury: an analysis of 5600 patients. *J Neurosurg.* 2003;99:666–673.

90. Nair N, Padder FA, Kantharia BK. Pathophysiology and management of neurocardiogenic syncope. *Am J Managed Care.* 2003;9(4):327–334, 335–336.

91. Baloh RW, Honrubia V. *Clinical Neurophysiology of the Vestibular System.* 3rd ed. New York, NY: Oxford University Press; 2001.

92. Saeed AB, Shuaib A, Al-Sulaiti G, Emery D. Vertebral artery dissection: warning symptoms, clinical features and prognosis in 26 patients. *Can J Neurol Sci.* 2000;27:292–296.

93. Haldeman S, Kohlbeck FJ, McGregor M. Unpredictability of cerebrovascular ischemia associated with cervical spine manipulation therapy: a review of sixty-four cases after cervical spine manipulation [comment]. *Spine.* 2002;27(1):49–55.

94. Baloh RW. Episodic vertigo: central nervous system causes. *Curr Opin Neurobiol.* 2002;15:17–21.

95. Haldeman S, Kohlbeck FJ, McGregor M. Risk factors and precipitating neck movements causing vertebrobasilar artery dissection after cervical trauma and spinal manipulation. *Spine.* 1999;24(8):785–794.

96. Hurwitz EL, Aker PD, Adams AH, Meeker WC, Shekelle PG. Manipulation and mobilization of the cervical spine. A systematic review of the literature [see comment]. *Spine.* Aug 1 1996;21(15):1746–1759; discussion 1759–1760.

97. Cote P, Kreitz BG, Cassidy JD, Thiel H. The validity of the extension-rotation test as a clinical screening procedure before neck manipulation: a secondary analysis [see comments]. *J Manipulative Physiol Ther.* 1996;19(3):159–164.

98. Childs JD, Flynn TW, Fritz J, et al. Screening for vertebrobasilar insufficiency in patients with neck pain: manual therapy decision-making in the presence of uncertainty. *J Orthop Sports Phys Ther.* 2005;35:300–306.

99. Brandt T, Dieterich M. Assessment and management of central vestibular disorders. In: Herdman S, ed. *Vestibular Rehabilitation.* 2nd ed. Philadelphia, PA: F.A. Davis; 2000:264–297.

100. Revel M, Andre-Deshays C, Minguet M. Cervicocephalic kinesthetic sensibility in patients with cervical pain. *Arch Phys Med Rehabil.* 1991;72(5):288–291.

101. Treleaven J, Jull G, Sterling M. Dizziness and unsteadiness following whiplash injury: characteristic features and relationship with cervical joint position error. *J Rehabil Med.* 2003;35(1):36–43.

102. Stiell IG, Wells GA, Vandemheen KL, et al. The Canadian C-spine rule for radiography in alert and stable trauma patients [comment]. *JAMA.* 2001;286(15):1841–1848.

103. Oosterveld WJ, Kortschot HW, Kingma GG, de Jong HA, Saatci MR. Electronystagmographic findings following cervical whiplash injuries. *Acta Otolaryngol.* 1991;111:201–205.

104. Toglia JU. Acute flexion-extension injury of the neck: electronystagmographic study of 309 patients. *Neurology.* 1976;26:808–814.

CHAPTER 28

Loss of Balance and Falls

■ *Robbin Howard, PT, DPT, NCS* ■ *Didi Matthews, PT, DPT, NCS*

Description of the Symptom

This chapter describes pathology that may lead to a loss of balance and falls. A loss of balance can be defined as unsteadiness when sitting, standing, or walking that may result in a stumble, trip, and/or fall. A fall is an unintentional event that results in an individual coming to rest at a lower surface.[1]

Special Concerns

■ Sudden onset of balance problems or falls
■ Balance problems that occur after trauma that have not yet been discussed with a physician

CHAPTER PREVIEW: Conditions That May Lead to a Loss of Balance and Falls

T Trauma

COMMON

Benign paroxysmal positional vertigo 554
Traumatic brain injury 566

UNCOMMON

Not applicable

RARE

Not applicable

I Inflammation

COMMON

Not applicable

UNCOMMON

Aseptic
Labyrinthitis and neuronitis 558
Multiple sclerosis 560

Septic
Encephalitis 556
Meningitis:
• Bacterial meningitis 559
• Viral meningitis 559

RARE

Aseptic
Behçet's disease 554
Creutzfeldt-Jakob disease 556
Inflammatory muscle disease 557
Lyme disease (tick paralysis) 558

Inflammation *(continued)*

RARE

Paraneoplastic syndromes 563
Vasculitis (giant cell arteritis, temporal arteritis, cranial arteritis) 566

Septic

Neurosyphilis (tabes dorsalis, syphilitic spinal sclerosis, progressive locomotor ataxia) 562

M Metabolic

COMMON

Neuropathy secondary to diabetes mellitus 561

UNCOMMON

Not applicable

RARE

Vestibular ototoxicity 567

Va Vascular

COMMON

Orthostatic hypotension 562
Stroke (cerebrovascular accident) 565

UNCOMMON

Cerebral aneurysm 555
Transient ischemic attack 565

RARE

Lateral medullary infarction (Wallenberg's syndrome) 558
Vasculitis (giant cell arteritis, temporal arteritis, cranial arteritis) 566
Vertebrobasilar artery insufficiency 566

De Degenerative

COMMON

Parkinson's disease 563

UNCOMMON

Dementia with Lewy bodies 556

RARE

Corticobasal degeneration 555
Fahr's syndrome (familial idiopathic basal ganglia calcification, bilateral striopallidodentate calcinosis) 557
Multiple system atrophy with orthostatic hypotension (striatonigral degeneration, olivopontocerebellar atrophy, Shy-Drager syndrome) 560
Progressive supranuclear palsy (Richardson-Steele-Olszewski syndrome) 564
Spinocerebellar ataxia (spinocerebellar atrophy, spinocerebellar degeneration) 565

Tu Tumor

COMMON

Not applicable

(continued)

Tumor *(continued)*

UNCOMMON

Malignant Primary, such as:
• Brain primary tumors 554
Malignant Metastatic, such as:
• Brain metastases 554
Benign:
Not applicable

RARE

Malignant Primary, such as:
• Spinal primary tumors 565
Malignant Metastatic, such as:
• Spinal metastases 564
Benign, such as:
• Acoustic neuroma (vestibular schwannoma) 553
• Angiomatosis (Von Hippel-Lindau disease) 553
• Neurofibromatosis 560

Co Congenital

COMMON

Hydrocephalus 557

UNCOMMON

Not applicable

RARE

Not applicable

Ne Neurogenic/Psychogenic

COMMON

Peripheral neuropathy 564

UNCOMMON

Ménière's disease 559
Neurological complications of acquired immunodeficiency syndrome 561

RARE

Not applicable

Note: These are estimates of relative incidence because few data are available for the less common conditions.

Overview of Loss of Balance and Falls

Any disease affecting cognition, alertness, motivation, or planning also may affect balance.[2] It is common for a patient or family members to report a history of falls or loss of balance. Sixty-five percent of the population over the age of 60 may experience dizziness or loss of balance on a daily basis.[2] In addition, approximately one-third to one-fourth of the population over the age of 65 has experienced a fall in the past 12 months.[1] The etiology of imbalance and falls may be associated with a single risk factor or may be multifactorial in nature. These risk factors are commonly categorized as being either intrinsic (related to the patient) or extrinsic (related to the environment).[1,3]

Intrinsic risk factors may include:

- Older age and female sex[1,3]
- Gait deviations[1,4]
- Balance deficits[1,4]
- Weakness[4,5]
- Medications (eg, antidepressants, sedatives, benzodiazepines, diuretics, analgesics, antihypertensives, anticoagulants, and anticonvulsants)[1,3,4]
- Diagnosis and possible comorbidities (eg, orthostatic hypotension, dizziness, syncope, Parkinson's disease, polyneuropathy, motor neuron disease, epilepsy, transient ischemic attacks, hydrocephalus, bilateral vascular white matter disease, vestibular and brainstem disease, and emotional conditions)[1,4,5]
- Visual impairments (eg, glaucoma, cataracts, macular degeneration, and impaired visual acuity and depth perception)[3,6]
- Altered mental status[7]
- Alcohol use.[3]

Extrinsic factors may include:

- Obstacles[1,3]
- Inadequate lighting[1,3]
- Slippery surfaces[1,3]
- Inadequate/inappropriate assistive device[1]
- Poorly fitting shoes or no shoes.[1]

Description of Conditions That May Lead to Loss of Balance and Falls

■ Acoustic Neuroma (Vestibular Schwannoma)

Chief Clinical Characteristics
This presentation may include hearing loss, tinnitus, vertigo, or dysequilibrium in the early stages.[8–14] Vestibular nerve function may be gradually lost without much balance disturbance. Symptoms worsen as the tumor grows, and the individual may also report having a headache. If untreated, brainstem compression can occur, with concerns of generalized headache, facial twitch and weakness, visual loss, diplopia, lower cranial nerve dysfunction causing aspiration, hoarseness, dysphagia, shoulder weakness, tongue weakness, and long tract signs.[9]

Background Information
Acoustic neuromas arise from the Schwann cells of the eighth cranial nerve within the

internal auditory canal, eventually growing out into and compressing the brainstem. Audiometry, electronystagmography, auditory brainstem response, computed tomography, and magnetic resonance imaging with gadolinium contrast confirm the diagnosis, with the latter providing the most specificity.[9] Treatment is surgical removal of the tumor, with risk of permanent changes in hearing, balance, and facial sensation and motion. Loss of a preoperatively functioning vestibular nerve will result in dysequilibrium for which vestibular adaptation exercises and balance rehabilitation are appropriate.[14]

■ Angiomatosis (Von Hippel-Lindau Disease)

Chief Clinical Characteristics
This presentation commonly includes headaches, problems with balance and walking, dizziness, weakness of the limbs, vision problems, and high blood pressure.

Background Information
This condition is a rare, genetic multisystem condition characterized by the abnormal growth of tumors in certain parts of the body (angiomatosis). Tumors of the central nervous system are benign, are comprised of a nest of blood vessels, and are called hemangioblastomas (or angiomas in the eye). Hemangioblastomas may develop in the brain, the retina of the eye, and other areas of the nervous system. Other types of tumors develop in the adrenal glands, the kidneys, or the pancreas. Cysts (fluid-filled sacs) and/or tumors (benign or cancerous) may develop around the hemangioblastomas and cause the symptoms listed above. Specific symptoms vary among individuals and depend on the size and location of the tumors. Individuals with this condition are also at a higher risk than normal for certain types of cancer, especially kidney cancer. Treatment varies according to the location and size of the tumor and its associated cyst. In general, the objective is to treat them when they are causing symptoms but are still small. Treatment of most cases usually involves surgical resection. Certain tumors can be treated with focused high-dose irradiation. Individuals with this condition need careful monitoring by a physician and/or medical team familiar with the condition.

■ Behçet's Disease

Chief Clinical Characteristics

This presentation may include bilateral pyramidal signs, headache, memory loss, hemiparesis, cerebellar ataxia, balance deficits, sphincter dysfunction, or cranial nerve palsies. In addition to these neurological signs, individuals with this condition also may present with arthritis; renal, gastrointestinal, vascular, and cardiac diseases; and genital, oral, and cutaneous ulcerations.[15]

Background Information

Mean age of onset is in the third decade of life. Diagnostic criteria according to an international study group include presence of recurrent oral ulceration, recurrent genital ulceration, eye lesions, skin lesions, papulopustular lesions, and/or a positive pathergy test.[15,16] Medical treatment typically consists of corticosteroids and immunosuppressants. Neurological symptoms tend to clear within weeks, but can sometimes recur or result in permanent deficits.[16] Onset before the age of 25 and male sex indicate a poorer prognosis.

■ Benign Paroxysmal Positional Vertigo

Chief Clinical Characteristics

This presentation commonly involves dizziness or vertigo (typically described as a spinning sensation), light-headedness, imbalance, and nausea. Symptoms are precipitated by a position change of the head relative to gravity, such as getting out of bed, rolling over in bed, or looking up.[17,18]

Background Information

This condition is thought to occur when free-floating debris becomes trapped in the semicircular canal (canalithiasis) or becomes adhered to the cupula (cupulolithiasis), rendering the semicircular canal sensitive to gravity and thus changes in head position rather than head motion. The etiology of benign paroxysmal positional vertigo is unknown in most cases, but is associated with head trauma, vestibular neuritis, and vertebrobasilar ischemia, and can occur after ear surgery or prolonged bed rest.[19] This condition occurs more often in the elderly, and tends to recur in up to 15% of cases within 1 year and 50% of cases within 40 months.[20] The diagnosis is confirmed with the Hallpike maneuver, in which the head is rotated 45 degrees and tilted back while hanging off the end of the table. This position will elicit torsional and vertical nystagmus when the vertical semicircular canals are involved. Duration of vertigo while in the Hallpike position will determine if the individual has *canalithiasis* (short duration, <1 minute) or *cupulolithiasis* (long duration, >1 minute). Turning the head while supine will elicit horizontal nystagmus and vertigo when the horizontal (lateral) semicircular canals are involved. Nonsurgical treatment consisting of a series of positional changes to move the debris out of the canals, known as the canalith repositioning maneuver, can be very successful.[19,21–25] In recalcitrant cases, the offending canal can be plugged surgically.[26]

BRAIN TUMORS

■ Brain Metastases

Chief Clinical Characteristics

This presentation may include headaches, seizures, dysphagia, weakness, cognitive changes, behavioral changes, dizziness, vomiting, alterations in the level of consciousness, ataxia, aphasia, nystagmus, visual disturbances, dysarthria, balance deficits, falls, lethargy, and incoordination.[16,27]

Background Information

The majority of individuals with brain metastases have been previously diagnosed with a primary tumor; however, a small percentage of individuals are diagnosed concomitantly with brain metastases and the primary tumor. The most common cancers resulting in subsequent brain metastases include lung, breast, melanoma, colorectal, and genitourinary tract. The new onset of neurological symptoms after a primary tumor warrants the use of imaging such as magnetic resonance imaging or computed tomography to confirm the diagnosis. Treatment may include corticosteroids, brain irradiation, surgery, chemotherapy, radiotherapy, and rehabilitative therapies. The prognosis is poor with death typically occurring within 6 months.

■ Brain Primary Tumors

Chief Clinical Characteristics

This presentation may include headaches, seizures, dysphagia, weakness, cognitive changes, behavioral changes, dizziness, vomiting, alterations in the level of consciousness, ataxia, aphasia, nystagmus, visual disturbances, dysarthria, balance deficits, falls, lethargy, and incoordination.[16]

Background Information
With the excessive proliferation of cells, a tumor mass eventually results in compression of the brain. This compression may displace cerebrospinal fluid, thereby increasing intracranial pressure and resulting in ischemia to the same tissues. Glioblastoma multiforme, astrocytoma, oligodendroglioma, metastatic tumors, primary central nervous system lymphomas, ganglioglioma, neuroblastoma, meningioma, arachnoid cysts, hemangioblastoma, medulloblastoma, and acoustic neuroma/schwannoma are some of the more common brain tumors. The first test to diagnose brain and spinal column tumors is a neurological examination. Specific diagnoses for brain tumors may be confirmed with imaging and biopsy. Treatment is variable depending on the type, size, and location of the tumor and may include surgical resection, chemotherapy, radiation, corticosteroids, and rehabilitative therapies. Prognosis is also variable and depends on the type and grade of tumor, severity of compression, and duration of compression.

■ Cerebral Aneurysm
Chief Clinical Characteristics
This presentation may involve loss of balance in combination with a whole host of other neurological symptoms and signs that depend on the affected cerebral tissue. Any associated signs or symptoms may not be reported due to the fact that this condition is typically asymptomatic prior to rupture. However, if the aneurysm results in a mass effect, ischemia, or hemorrhage, then neurological signs and symptoms are dependent on the affected location.[16,28,29]

Background Information
There has been some description of genetic factors in this condition.[28] Cigarette smoking, hypertension, and heavy alcohol use have all been found to be correlated with increased risk of aneurysm development.[28,29] Factors associated with increased risk of rupture include size of aneurysm, location in the posterior circulation, and a previous history of aneurismal

subarachnoid hemorrhage.[30,31] Definitive diagnosis is based on catheter angiography; however, magnetic resonance angiography, magnetic resonance imaging, and computed tomography may aid in the diagnosis. Unruptured aneurysms are sometimes surgically treated. Aneurysm size, location, and prior history of a subarachnoid hemorrhage help to determine if the risk of surgical treatment is worth the potential benefits. Most aneurysms that have hemorrhaged must be treated surgically. Patients with a previous rupture are at an 11 times greater risk of having a second intracranial aneurysm rupture. When aneurysms do rupture, many patients die within 1 month of the rupture, and those who survive often have residual neurological deficits.[28]

■ Corticobasal Degeneration
Chief Clinical Characteristics
This presentation typically includes limb ideomotor apraxia and unilateral parkinsonism that is unresponsive to levodopa, gait disturbances, tremor, postural instability, and dementia.[32,33]

Background Information
A proposed set of criteria for the diagnosis of this condition includes core features of:

1. Insidious onset and progressive course
2. No identifiable cause
3. Cortical dysfunction (ideomotor apraxia, alien-limb phenomenon, cortical sensory loss, visual or sensory hemineglect, constructional apraxia, focal or asymmetric myoclonus, apraxia of speech, or nonfluent aphasia)
4. Extrapyramidal dysfunction (rigidity that does not respond to levodopa therapy and dystonia).[34]

This condition is a sporadic disease with an average age of onset of 63 years.[33] There have been reports of familial cases; however, for most cases there is no known cause.[32] Diagnosis is made based on clinical presentation. A definitive diagnosis can only be made postmortem. Medical treatment is not typically successful; it has been found that only about 24% of these patients will respond to levodopa therapy aimed at addressing the extrapyramidal features of the disease.[35] Physical and occupational therapy are used to maintain mobility and address safety issues related to the progression of imbalance. Mean survival is 7.9 years with a range of 2.5 to 12.5 years.[33] Early presence of bilateral parkinsonism or frontal lobe signs indicates a less favorable prognosis.[33]

■ Creutzfeldt-Jakob Disease

Chief Clinical Characteristics
This presentation may involve rapidly progressive dementia, cerebellar ataxia, balance deficits, myoclonus, cortical blindness, pyramidal signs, extrapyramidal signs, and akinetic mutism.[36]

Background Information
Different forms of this condition have been described including sporadic, iatrogenic, and variant. Sporadic and iatrogenic forms of this condition typically affect older individuals, whereas the variant form affects younger individuals.[37] The early stages of the variant form are characterized by psychiatric symptoms, including depression and anxiety.[37] The condition is rare and affects only one to two people per million worldwide per year.[36,37] It is caused by a conformational change of the normal prion protein, which is encoded by human chromosome 20 to a disease-related prion protein. Diagnosis is suggested by a thorough history and physical examination, electroencephalography, and cerebrospinal fluid analysis.[37] Computed tomography and magnetic resonance imaging are typically normal in sporadic and iatrogenic forms and help to exclude other diagnoses.[36,38] Diagnosis for all forms of this condition is only confirmed postmortem.[38] There is no proven treatment.[37,38] Death in sporadic and iatrogenic forms occurs in a matter of months with death occurring at a mean age of 66 years.[39] Mean duration of illness in the variant form is 14 months.[37]

■ Dementia With Lewy Bodies

Chief Clinical Characteristics
This presentation can be characterized by fluctuating cognitive dysfunction, particularly visuospatial problems and executive dysfunction, visual hallucinations, and parkinsonism features such as masked facies, autonomic dysfunction, rigidity, and bradykinesia. Other signs and symptoms may include postural instability, falls, sleep disturbances, memory problems, syncope, transient loss of consciousness, and sensitivity to antipsychotic and anti-Parkinson medications.[39]

Background Information
This progressive condition is the second most common dementia after Alzheimer's disease.[39] The specific etiology of this condition is unknown. The characteristic Lewy bodies are eosinophilic inclusion bodies found within the cytoplasm of neurons in the cerebral cortex and limbic system.[39] A thorough clinical examination, laboratory screen, and imaging are important to rule out other causes of dementia. The definitive diagnosis for this condition is made postmortem; however, it appears that the use of single-photon emission computed tomography and positron emission tomography may be useful in the identification of occipital hypoperfusion, which may be associated with the visual hallucinations.[39,40] Management includes caregiver education to assist in minimizing factors that may contribute to problematic behaviors. Medication therapy may be indicated, but should be monitored closely due to potential exacerbation of symptoms.[39] Life expectancy for individuals with this condition is similar to that of Alzheimer's disease. The average survival time is between 6 and 8 years from the onset of dementia.[39,41]

■ Encephalitis

Chief Clinical Characteristics
This presentation includes confusion, delirium, convulsions, problems with speech or hearing, memory loss, hallucinations, drowsiness, and coma. Loss of balance and/or falls may be present.

Background Information
This condition is an inflammation of nerve cells in the brain. It usually refers to the viral form, although bacterial, parasitic, and fungal agents also can cause this condition. Up to 20,000 new cases of viral forms of this condition are reported annually in the United States. Diagnosis is established by clinical presentation suggesting dysfunction of the cerebrum, brainstem, or cerebellum, cellular reaction and elevated protein in spinal fluid, and possible demonstration of diffuse edema or enhancement of the brain on magnetic resonance imaging or computed tomography. Treatment is primarily pharmacologic, with drugs such

as corticosteroids, antiviral agents, and anticonvulsants. The majority of individuals with encephalitis do recover, but irreversible brain damage and death can result.[16]

■ Fahr's Syndrome (Familial Idiopathic Basal Ganglia Calcification, Bilateral Striopallidodentate Calcinosis)

Chief Clinical Characteristics
This presentation may involve features of parkinsonism, such as chorea, athetosis, rigidity, dystonia, and tremor in addition to cognitive impairments, cerebellar impairments, gait and balance disorder, psychiatric features, pain, pyramidal signs (such as weakness, hyperreflexia in the deep tendon reflexes, hypertonia, clonus, and/or a positive Babinski sign), sensory changes, and speech disorder.[42]

Background Information
This condition occurs due to bilateral symmetric calcification of the basal ganglia with or without calcification of the dentate nucleus. The disease has been described as both familial and nonfamilial.[16] Diagnosis is established using computed tomography or magnetic resonance imaging of the brain; however, computed tomography has been found to be more sensitive for identifying calcium deposits.[43] Treatment aimed at minimizing calcium deposits has been unsuccessful.[44] Individuals with this condition may be responsive to levodopa for treatment of their parkinsonian features.[16]

■ Hydrocephalus

Chief Clinical Characteristics
This presentation commonly includes frontal lobe signs such as slowness of mental response, inattentiveness, distractibility, perseveration, inability to sustain complex cognitive function, and incontinence. Other symptoms include gait deterioration, frequent falls, occipital or frontal headaches, nausea and vomiting, diplopia, and lethargy. Advanced stages are associated with coma and extensor posturing.

Background Information
Intracranial pressure can be increased due to many mechanisms including a cerebral or extracerebral mass, generalized brain swelling, increased venous pressure, obstruction to the flow and absorption of cerebrospinal fluid, or

volume expansion of cerebrospinal fluid.[16] Magnetic resonance imaging and the presence of papilledema are commonly used to establish the diagnosis of hydrocephalus. Medical treatment may include restriction of fluid intake and drugs with an osmotic effect, or the addition of diuretics.[45] Surgical treatment depends on the chronicity of the hydrocephalus. The acute form of this condition is considered fatal and is emergently treated via lumbar puncture or ventricular catheter.[45] The chronic form of this condition is treated with placement of a ventricular shunt or with surgical removal of a mass if that is the cause of the hydrocephalus. Although surgical procedures for hydrocephalus have a high success rate and a good prognosis, it is common to have shunt complications such as infection, occlusion, and over- or underdrainage. Thus, patients who have been treated for this condition must continue to be medically managed and educated regarding the indications of shunt compromise.

■ Inflammatory Muscle Disease

Chief Clinical Characteristics
This presentation involves asymmetric weakness of the quadriceps, wrist, and finger flexors. Individuals with this condition can present with proximal muscle weakness as well, which may lead to balance deficits and falls. This condition eventually will cause dysphagia in 40% to 60% of individuals with this condition.[46]

Background Information
A set of diagnostic criteria has been proposed, including duration of illness greater than 6 months, age over 30 years, and muscle weakness that must affect proximal and distal muscles of arms and legs with at least one of the following groups:

1. Finger flexor weakness
2. Wrist flexor greater than wrist extensor weakness
3. Quadriceps muscle weakness.[47]

Progression is slow such that patients may have symptoms for up to 10 years before diagnosis. The disease is more common in men over the age of 50 years.[46,48] Effective treatment for this condition has not been found. Individuals with this condition are generally unresponsive to steroid treatment[49] and controlled studies have found no benefit with intravenous immunoglobulin or immuno-suppressive treatments.[46,49] In individuals over the age of 60 years, disease progression is accelerated, resulting in an early need for an assistive device.[48]

■ Labyrinthitis and Neuronitis

Chief Clinical Characteristics

This presentation may be characterized by a relatively sudden onset of severe, constant rotary vertigo (made worse by head movement) that resolves after days or weeks.[50,51] This condition is associated with spontaneous nystagmus, postural imbalance, and nausea without accompanying cochlear or neurological symptoms.[51] The specific presentation varies depending on the site of the infection. If the vestibular system is affected, the symptoms will include dizziness and difficulty with vision and/or balance. If the inflammation affects the cochlea, this condition will produce disturbances in hearing, such as tinnitus or hearing loss. The symptoms can be mild or severe, temporary or permanent, depending on the severity of the infection.

Background Information

The etiology of this condition is a bacterial or viral infection causing inflammation of the vestibular nerve (neuronitis) or the labyrinth (labyrinthitis). The terms are often used interchangeably because it is difficult to distinguish neuronitis from labyrinthitis.[50] The diagnostic hallmark is unilateral hyporesponsiveness with caloric testing.[51] Regardless of the type of infection, the treatment consists of destroying the bacteria by means of antibiotics. If the labyrinthitis is caused by a break in the membranes separating the middle and inner ears, surgery may also be required to repair the membranes to prevent a recurrence of the disease. Residual vertigo can be reduced with vestibular habituation exercises.[52]

■ Lateral Medullary Infarction (Wallenberg's Syndrome)

Chief Clinical Characteristics

This presentation can include nystagmus, oscillopsia, vertigo, nausea, vomiting, impairment of pain and thermal sense over half of the body, ipsilateral Horner syndrome including miosis, ptosis, anhidrosis, hoarseness, dysphagia, ipsilateral paralysis of palate and vocal cord with a diminished gag reflex, vertical diplopia or sensation of tilting vision, ipsilateral ataxia of limbs, loss of balance to ipsilateral side, and impaired sensation of ipsilateral half of the face.[16,53,54]

Background Information

In 75% of cases, onset of this condition was sudden. Main etiologic factors associated with this condition include large-vessel infarction, arterial dissection, small-vessel infarction, cardiac embolism, tumor, hemorrhage, and other unknown factors. The most typical cause is occlusion of the vertebral artery, with the posterior inferior cerebellar artery being involved to a lesser degree. A thorough history, clinical examination, and magnetic resonance imaging may confirm the diagnosis. An emergency response is required for individuals experiencing the new onset of symptoms. Residual symptoms include balance deficits (most common), dysphagia, dizziness, and numbness, which may be addressed with physical, occupational, and speech therapy.

■ Lyme Disease (Tick Paralysis)

Chief Clinical Characteristics

This presentation can include fluctuating signs or symptoms such as headache, neck stiffness, nausea, vomiting, malaise, fever, pain, fatigue, and presence of a "bull's-eye" rash.[16] Over time, additional symptoms may include sensory changes, irritability, cognitive changes, depression, behavioral changes, seizures, ataxia, chorea movements, pain, weakness, balance deficits, arthritis, and cranial nerve involvement.[16,38]

Background Information

Borrelia burgdorferi, an organism that infects ticks, is responsible for the transmission of this condition to a human host.[16] The diagnosis is confirmed with a thorough history, clinical assessment, enzyme-linked immunosorbent assay, and Western blot or immunoblot analysis. In addition, magnetic resonance imaging or computed tomography may reveal multifocal or periventricular cerebral lesions.[16] Medical management includes treatment with oral tetracycline, penicillin, or intravenous ceftriaxone.[16] Many individuals experience full recovery with treatment; however, residual deficits may persist for individuals with chronic Lyme disease.[16]

■ Ménière's Disease

Chief Clinical Characteristics

This presentation is characterized by recurrent episodic spontaneous attacks of vertigo (exacerbated by head movements and accompanied by nausea and vomiting), fluctuating sensorineural hearing loss, aural fullness, and tinnitus.[51,55–62] In the late stages the symptoms are more severe, hearing loss is less likely to fluctuate, and tinnitus and aural fullness may be more constant. Sudden unexplained falls without loss of consciousness or vertigo (drop attacks) may occur. Attacks can be preceded by an aura consisting of a sense of fullness in the ear, increasing tinnitus, and a decrease in hearing,[60] but can also occur without warning. The typical duration of an attack is 2 to 3 hours, ranging from minutes to hours in length. Attacks can be single or multiple, with short or long intervening periods of remission during which the individual may be asymptomatic.

Background Information

The cause of this condition is thought to be overproduction or underabsorption of endolymph (endolymphatic hydrops), resulting in distortion of the membranous labyrinth. Ruptures of the membranous labyrinth, autoimmune disease processes, and viral infection are among other proposed causes.[60] Appropriate tests include caloric testing to determine amount of vestibular asymmetry; audiometry, which often shows a low-frequency loss rather than a high-frequency one; and exclusion of other causes (typically with gadolinium-enhanced magnetic resonance imaging). The head thrust test can be negative despite caloric asymmetry. Restricting salt intake and using diuretics may be useful in over half of individuals with this condition. Approximately 10% of individuals with this condition will have persistent vertigo and require other forms of treatment. These include surgery to decompress or drain the endolymphatic sac, selective vestibular neurectomy or labyrinthectomy, and intratympanic injections of aminoglycosides such as gentamicin[57] to reduce or abolish vestibular function on the affected side.

MENINGITIS

■ Bacterial Meningitis

Chief Clinical Characteristics

This presentation includes acute symptoms such as fever, severe headache, neck stiffness, seizures, changes in consciousness, facial and ocular palsies, positive Kernig and Brudzinski signs, and possible hemiparesis, which may lead to falls. Chronic symptoms include hydrocephalus, vomiting, immobility, impaired alertness, hemiplegia, decorticate or decerebrate posturing, cortical blindness, stupor, or coma.[63]

Background Information

This condition results from an infection and inflammation of the meninges surrounding the brain and spinal cord. Lumbar puncture for spinal fluid pressure and cerebrospinal fluid culture, blood cultures, and radiologic studies confirm the diagnosis.[63] This condition is considered a medical emergency. Medical management includes maintenance of blood pressure, treatment for septic shock, and administration of intravenous antibiotics for 10 to 14 days.[63] Prognosis depends on the strain of bacteria; approximately 5% to 15% of patients with bacterial meningitis do not survive.[63] Residual effects after the infection resolves are variable and patients with pneumococcal and *H. influenzae* bacterial meningitis are more likely to have lasting neurological deficits.[63]

■ Viral Meningitis

Chief Clinical Characteristics

This presentation can be characterized by an acute onset of fever, headache, and neck stiffness. Drowsiness, lethargy, and irritability may occur, but overall symptoms tend to be relatively mild.[63] Although not a common presenting sign, falls or imbalance may occur due to drowsiness and lethargy.

Background Information

This condition is an infection and inflammation of the meninges surrounding the brain and spinal cord. Also known as aseptic meningitis, this condition is most commonly caused by the echovirus or coxsackie virus.[63] Cerebrospinal fluid analysis and blood work are used to determine the diagnosis.[63,64] There is no specific treatment, although supportive care may include administration of analgesics. This condition is rarely fatal and most patients demonstrate a full recovery.[63]

Multiple Sclerosis

Chief Clinical Characteristics

This presentation may include paresthesias, weakness, spasticity, hypertonicity, hyperreflexia, positive Babinski sign, incoordination, optic neuritis, ataxia, vertigo, dysarthria, diplopia, bladder incontinence, tremor, balance deficits, falls, and cognitive deficits.[16]

Background Information

This condition may present as relapsing-remitting, primary progressive, or secondary progressive. The disease occurs most frequently in women between the ages of 20 and 40 years. Only a small number of children or individuals between 50 and 60 years of age are diagnosed with this condition.[16] This condition was originally thought to be secondary to environmental and genetic factors, but evidence suggests an autoimmune response to a viral infection, which subsequently targets myelin.[16] The diagnosis may be confirmed by a thorough history, physical examination, magnetic resonance imaging, analysis of cerebrospinal fluid, and evoked potentials.[16,65,66] Life expectancy and cause of mortality are similar for all types of this condition.[16] Clinical characteristics that are associated with a longer time interval for progression of disability include female sex, younger age of onset, relapsing-remitting type, complete recovery after the first relapse, and longer time interval between first and second exacerbation.[67] Medical management may include the use of methylprednisolone, prednisone, cyclophosphamide, immunosuppressant treatment, and beta-interferon.[16] Physical, occupational, and speech therapy may be indicated to prevent secondary sequelae and to optimize functional activity and mobility. Some individuals may benefit from psychology/psychiatry and social support as the disease progresses.

Multiple System Atrophy With Orthostatic Hypotension (Striatonigral Degeneration, Olivopontocerebellar Atrophy, Shy-Drager Syndrome)

Chief Clinical Characteristics

This presentation involves tremor, rigidity, akinesia, and/or postural imbalance along with signs of cerebellar, pyramidal, and autonomic dysfunction. Autonomic symptoms such as orthostatic hypotension, dry mouth, loss of sweating, impotence, and urinary incontinence or retention are the initial feature in 41% of individuals, with 74% to 97% of individuals developing some degree of autonomic dysfunction during the course of the disease.[68] This condition is a combination of parkinsonian and non-parkinsonian symptoms and signs.

Background Information

Diagnostic criteria are based on the clinical presentation, which includes poor response to levodopa, presence of autonomic features, presence of speech or bulbar problems, absence of dementia, absence of toxic confusion, and presence of falls.[69] The disease course ranges between 0.5 and 24 years after diagnosis with a mean survival time of 6.2 years.[70] This condition is a progressive condition of the central and autonomic nervous systems that rarely occurs without orthostatic hypotension. There are three types of this condition. The parkinsonian-type includes symptoms of Parkinson's disease such as slow movement, stiff muscles, and tremor. The cerebellar type causes problems with coordination and speech. The combined type includes symptoms of both parkinsonism and cerebellar failure. Older age at onset is associated with a shorter survival time.[70] Average age of onset is 54 years, with mean age at death being 60.3 years.[68] Most individuals with this condition receive a trial of levodopa although only a minority respond.[68] Additional treatment addresses symptoms and involves physical and occupational therapy to maintain mobility and address safety issues related to the progression of imbalance.

Neurofibromatosis

Chief Clinical Characteristics

This presentation depends on the type of neurofibromatosis. Neurofibromatosis type 1 (NF1,

Von Recklinghausen's disease) may include café au lait spots, neurofibromas, pathological fractures, syringomyelia, scoliosis, stroke, neoplasms, learning difficulties, and hyperactivity. Neurofibromatosis type 2 (NF2) is characterized by bilateral vestibular schwannomas, progressive hearing loss, and possible intracranial or intraspinal neoplasms.[16,38]

Background Information

This condition is an autosomal dominant disorder on chromosome 17 for NF1 and on chromosome 22 for NF2. The tumors in NF1 occur due to the excessive proliferation of cells within the meninges, vascular system, skin, viscera, peripheral, and central nervous systems.[16,38] The tumors in NF2 arise from the posterior nerve roots. Depending on the type of this condition, the diagnosis may be confirmed by a thorough family history, the presence of six or more café au lait spots, imaging, and genetic testing. If indicated, the tumors that result from this condition may be surgically removed.[38] Both forms of this condition are progressive and the prognosis varies depending on the severity of lesions.[16]

■ **Neurological Complications of Acquired Immunodeficiency Syndrome**

Chief Clinical Characteristics

This presentation is variable and dependent on the affected neuroanatomical structures in an individual with acquired immunodeficiency syndrome.[71]

Background Information

This condition may be categorized by:

1. Meningitic symptoms including headache, malaise, and fever (such as secondary to meningitis, cryptococcal meningitis, tuberculous meningitis, and human immunodeficiency virus headache)
2. Focal cerebral symptoms including hemiparesis, aphasia, apraxia, sensory deficits, homonymous hemianopia, cranial nerve involvement, balance deficits, incoordination, and/or ataxia (such as secondary to cerebral toxoplasmosis, primary central nervous system lymphoma, and progressive multifocal leukoencephalopathy)

3. Diffuse cerebral symptoms that involve cognitive deficits, altered level of consciousness, hyperreflexia, Babinski sign, presence of primitive reflexes (such as secondary to postinfectious encephalomyelitis, acquired immunodeficiency dementia complex, cytomegalovirus encephalitis)
4. Myelopathy associated with gait difficulties, spasticity, ataxia, balance deficits, and hyperreflexia (such as secondary to herpes zoster myelitis, vacuolar myelopathy that occurs with acquired immunodeficiency syndrome dementia complex)
5. Peripheral involvement associated with sensory changes, weakness, balance deficits, and pain (such as secondary to peripheral neuropathy, acute and chronic inflammatory demyelinating polyneuropathies).[16,71]

Abnormal neurological findings are observed during a clinical examination in approximately one-third of patients with acquired immunodeficiency syndrome; however, on autopsy, most individuals with this condition have abnormalities within the nervous system.[16] Diagnosis of the variable neurological complications associated with this condition may be confirmed with laboratory tests, cerebrospinal fluid cultures, imaging, nerve conduction studies, and physical examination.[16,38,71] Treatment appears to be limited primarily to the use of antiviral medications.[71] Physical and occupational therapy may be indicated to address equipment needs and caregiver/patient training related to functional mobility.

■ **Neuropathy Secondary to Diabetes Mellitus**

Chief Clinical Characteristics

This presentation is variable, including manifestations such as acute diabetic mononeuropathies, which may include involvement of cranial nerves (eg, oculomotor or abducens nerve involvement) or peripheral nerves[16]; multiple mononeuropathies and radiculopathies, which may include unilateral or asymmetric pain, low back pain with or without symptoms in leg, weakness, atrophy, diminished or absent deep tendon reflexes, and sensory deficits[16]; distal polyneuropathy, the most common diabetic neuropathy, which consists of chronic, symmetric, distal sensory deficits (eg, numbness and tingling), diminished or absent deep tendon reflexes, balance deficits, and weakness[16]; and autonomic neuropathy, which may involve resting tachycardia, orthostatic hypotension, sexual impotence, exercise intolerance, abnormal sweating, pupil abnormalities, weakness, sensory deficits, and gastroparesis.[16,38,72,73]

Background Information
Approximately 15% to 20% of people with diabetes may present with the signs and symptoms of this condition.[16,72] However, approximately 50% will have neuropathic symptoms and may have abnormalities in nerve conduction testing.[16] Commonly considered a metabolic disorder, this condition may be a result of vascular complications disrupting the supply of nutrients to the nerves.[38,74] A thorough history, physical examination (specifically including the assessment of deep tendon reflexes and sensory examination), electromyography/nerve conduction testing, and laboratory screen helps to differentiate other causes of neuropathy.[72,73] Treatment consists of maintaining a normal range of blood glucose levels.[16,72,73] In addition, individuals with this condition may prevent complications by completing visual inspection of the skin and routine podiatry care.[73] Medications may help to control symptoms such as paresthesias or pain.[16,38] Additional management may include consultations with an orthotist to ensure proper fitting of footwear and physical therapy to minimize disability by addressing impairments associated with limitations in functional mobility.[74]

■ Neurosyphilis (Tabes Dorsalis, Syphilitic Spinal Sclerosis, Progressive Locomotor Ataxia)

Chief Clinical Characteristics
This presentation can be characterized by hemiparesis, ataxia, aphasia, gait instability, falls, neuropathy, personality and cognitive changes, seizures, diplopia, visual impairments, hearing loss, psychotic disorders, loss of bowel/bladder function, pain, hyporeflexia, and hypotonia.[75,76]

Background Information
Treponema pallidum infects the human host by way of contact with contaminated body fluids or lesions.[75] This spirochete is responsible for the diagnosis of syphilis; however, when *T. pallidum* is present within the central nervous system the individual is diagnosed with neurosyphilis.[76] This condition occurs in approximately 10% of individuals with untreated syphilis, and in 81% of these cases it presents as meningovascular, meningeal, and general paresis. Treatment includes use of various forms of penicillin or alternative choices for those allergic to penicillin[75] and may involve rehabilitative therapies depending on the individual's activity limitations or participation restrictions. A better prognosis has been observed for individuals treated during early neurosyphilis.[76]

■ Orthostatic Hypotension

Chief Clinical Characteristics
This presentation commonly involves dizziness, light-headedness, and blurred vision that generally occur after sudden standing. In more severe forms of this condition, individuals may experience seizures, transient ischemic attacks, or syncope.

Background Information
This condition is caused by a sudden decrease of greater than 20 mm Hg in systolic blood pressure or greater than 10 mm Hg in diastolic blood pressure, which occurs when a person assumes a standing position. It may be caused by hypovolemia resulting from the excessive use of diuretics, vasodilators, or other types of vasoactive medications (eg, calcium channel blockers and beta blockers), dehydration, or prolonged bed rest. Other factors to consider include the individual's neurological status and hemorrhagic/hypovolemic states. The condition may be associated with Addison's disease, atherosclerosis, diabetes, and certain neurological conditions including Shy-Drager syndrome and other dysautonomias. Hypovolemia due to medications is reversed by adjusting the dosage or by discontinuing the medication. If prolonged bed rest is the cause, improvement may occur by sitting up with increasing frequency each day. In some cases, physical counterpressure such as elastic hose or whole-body inflatable suits may be required. Dehydration is treated with salt and fluids. Individuals with this condition can be instructed to rise slowly from bed in the mornings or when moving from a sitting/squatting to standing position. Symptoms

usually dissipate when the individual is placed in a semirecumbent or supine position, although some individuals may progress to frank syncope. In this case, the clinician should be prepared to activate the emergency medical system if the individual fails to regain consciousness with basic life support measures.

■ Paraneoplastic Syndromes

Chief Clinical Characteristics
This presentation includes dizziness in combination with a variety of different neurological symptoms and signs in an individual with cancer. Specific neurological symptoms and signs depend on the location of involvement of the central or peripheral nervous system.

Background Information
Paraneoplastic encephalomyelitis and focal encephalitis may present with ataxia, vertigo, balance deficits, nystagmus, nausea, vomiting, cranial nerve palsies, seizures, sensory neuropathy, anxiety, depression, cognitive changes, and hallucinations. For individuals presenting with ataxia, dysarthria, dysphagia, and diplopia, paraneoplastic cerebellar degeneration may be suspected. Paraneoplastic opsoclonus/myoclonus tends to affect both children and adults with signs and symptoms including hypotonia, ataxia, irritability, truncal ataxia, gait difficulty, balance deficits, and frequent falls. Stiff-man syndrome presents with spasms and fluctuating rigidity of axial musculature, legs and possibly shoulders, upper extremities, and neck. Paraneoplastic sensory neuropathy presents with asymmetric, progressive sensory alterations involving the limbs, trunk, and face, sensorineural hearing loss, autonomic dysfunction, and pain. Other conditions in this category include vasculitis, Lambert-Eaton myasthenia syndrome, myasthenia gravis, dermatomyositis, neuromyotonia, and various neuropathies.[16,77] These conditions result from an immune-mediated response to the presence of tumor or metastases. Antibodies or T-cells respond to the presence of the tumor, but also attack normal cells of the nervous system.[78,79] Over 60% of individuals present with this condition prior to the discovery of the cancer.[77] The underlying tumor is treated according to the type of cancer. Additional treatment is dependent on this condition's type and may include steroids, plasmapheresis, immunotherapy, chemotherapy, radiation, or cyclophosphamide.[77] Physical, occupational, and speech therapy may be indicated to address functional limitations.

■ Parkinson's Disease

Chief Clinical Characteristics
This presentation commonly involves resting tremor, bradykinesia, rigidity, and postural instability. Falls are a common problem in individuals with this condition, with up to 68% falling within a 1-year period and approximately 50% of these individuals falling multiple times within that same year.[80] Other common signs and symptoms include festination, freezing, micrographia, hypophonia (hypokinetic dysarthria), akinesia, masked facies, drooling, difficulty turning over in bed, dystonia, dyskinesia, falls, dementia, and depression.[16]

Background Information
This condition occurs due to the depletion or injury of dopamine-producing cells in substantia nigra pars compacta. Clinical signs and symptoms are not typically present until after approximately 80% of dopamine-producing cells are lost. The definitive diagnosis is made postmortem. However, a clinically definitive diagnosis may be made with the presence of at least two of three criteria—asymmetric resting tremor, bradykinesia, or rigidity—and a positive response to anti-Parkinson medications.[16,81] Imaging may be useful to exclude vascular involvement. Medical management may include use of dopamine agonists, levodopa, and other medications to address nonmotor symptoms, such as depression, constipation, autonomic symptoms, and sexual dysfunction. Surgical management also may be considered, including deep brain stimulation or pallidotomy.[81] Forced use or higher intensity, challenging activities may provide a neuroprotective benefit for individuals with early forms of this condition.[82] With the high incidence of depression, consultation with a psychologist or psychiatrist may be warranted. Individuals with a late onset tend to progress more rapidly.[83,84] Poor prognostic indicators for disability include initial presentation without tremor, early dependence, dementia, balance impairments, older age, and the

postural instability/gait difficulty dominant type.[83,84]

■ Peripheral Neuropathy

Chief Clinical Characteristics
This presentation may be characterized by falls, loss of balance, weakness, and sensory alterations, as well as diminished or absent deep tendon reflexes, fasciculations, syncope, abnormal sweating, orthostatic hypotension, resting tachycardia, and trophic changes.[16,85]

Background Information
The patterns of peripheral neuropathies are variable and may present as polyneuropathy, polyradiculopathy, neuronopathy, mononeuropathy, mononeuropathy multiplex, and plexopathy.[16] Some of the etiologies associated with peripheral neuropathies include trauma, inflammation (eg, herpes zoster, Lyme disease, human immunodeficiency virus, Guillain-Barré syndrome), metabolic causes (eg, diabetes mellitus, uremia), nutritional causes (eg, vitamin B deficiencies commonly associated with alcohol abuse, eating disorders, and individuals with malabsorption syndromes), congenital and idiopathic causes (eg, aging or unknown causes), and toxic etiology (eg, exposure to lead, arsenic, thallium; chemotherapeutic drugs such as vincristine, cisplatin).[85] Twenty percent of individuals over the age of 60 are affected by a type of peripheral neuropathy.[86] The diagnosis of the specific disorder may be differentiated by the pattern of peripheral neuropathy and temporal features. The diagnosis may be confirmed after completing a thorough history, physical examination, gait assessment, balance assessment, laboratory testing, and electromyography/nerve conduction testing.[16,87] Treatment and prognosis will vary depending on the etiology and severity of this condition.

■ Progressive Supranuclear Palsy (Richardson-Steele-Olszewski Syndrome)

Chief Clinical Characteristics
This presentation classically includes vertical gaze palsy, prominent instability, and falls within the first year of disease onset.[88] Other characteristics may include rigidity, akinesia, dysarthria, dysphagia, and mild dementia. Falls were found to be the most commonly reported

symptom with the majority of falls being backward falls.[89] Difficulty with voluntary vertical eye movements (usually downward) and involuntary saccades are relatively early features. The disease progresses to the point at which all voluntary eye movements are lost.

Background Information
Some patients may not demonstrate difficulties with ocular movements for 1 to 3 years after disease onset. Most cases are sporadic; however, a pattern of inheritance compatible with autosomal dominant transmission has been described.[16] Diagnosis is based on clinical presentation, which includes a gradually progressive disorder with age of onset at 40 years or older, vertical supranuclear palsy, and postural instability with falls within the first year of disease onset.[90] Medical treatment is typically unsuccessful, because the majority of these patients are not responsive to levodopa therapy aimed at addressing the extrapyramidal features of the disease.[35] Physical and occupational therapy are used to maintain mobility and address safety issues related to the progression of imbalance. The disease course is progressive with a mean survival time of 5.6 years.[89] Older age at disease onset, early onset of falls, incontinence, dysarthria, dysphagia, insertion of a percutaneous gastrostomy, and diplopia have all been described as being predictive of shorter survival time.[89]

■ Spinal Metastases

Chief Clinical Characteristics
This presentation can involve spasticity, weakness, sensory alterations, bowel and bladder incontinence, neck pain, back pain, radicular pain, atrophy, cerebellar signs, balance deficits, falls, and cranial nerve involvement.[16,38,91]

Background Information
This condition is the most frequent neoplasm involving the spine.[91] The most common types and locations of primary tumors that result in spinal metastases include breast, lung, lymphoma, prostate, kidney, gastrointestinal tract, and thyroid.[16,92] The diagnosis is confirmed with gadolinium-enhanced magnetic resonance imaging and computed tomography.[16,91] Treatment is variable depending on the tumor and may include surgical resection, chemotherapy, radiation, corticosteroids, and rehabilitative therapies.[16] Although the long-term prognosis

is poor, individuals without paresis or pain and who are still ambulatory have longer survival rates.[92]

■ Spinal Primary Tumors

Chief Clinical Characteristics
This presentation may include spasticity, weakness, sensory alterations, bowel/bladder incontinence, back pain, radicular pain, atrophy, cerebellar signs, balance deficits, falls, and cranial nerve involvement.[16]

Background Information
Types of this condition include myeloma, neurofibroma, lymphoma, metastasis, meningioma, schwannoma, and astrocytoma. The first test to diagnose brain and spinal column tumors is a neurological examination. Special imaging techniques (computed tomography, magnetic resonance imaging, and positron emission tomography) are also employed. Specific diagnoses may be confirmed with imaging and biopsy. Treatment is variable depending on the type, size, and location of the tumor and may include surgical resection, chemotherapy, radiation, corticosteroids, and rehabilitative therapies. Prognosis is variable and depends on the type and grade of tumor, severity of compression, and duration of compression.

■ Spinocerebellar Ataxia (Spinocerebellar Atrophy, Spinocerebellar Degeneration)

Chief Clinical Characteristics
This presentation can involve ataxia, incoordination, supranuclear ophthalmoplegia, slow saccades, optic atrophy, dysarthria, balance deficits, falls, tremor, myoclonus, chorea, nystagmus, dementia, amyotrophy, and peripheral neuropathy.[93,94]

Background Information
This condition refers to a group of progressive, neurodegenerative, autosomal dominant disorders affecting the cerebellum, brainstem, and spinal cord. Twelve variants have been identified: SCA 1, 2, 3, 6, 7, 8, 10, 12, 14, 17, FGF10-SCA, and dentatorubral-pallidoluysian atrophy.[94] The disorders occur due to expansions of CAG triplet repeats that are subsequently transcribed into long polyglutamine tracts. Diagnosis is confirmed by deoxyribonucleic acid testing. There is no current medical treatment for the various forms of this condition.[93,94] Individuals with this condition may benefit from physical, occupational, and speech therapy to address activity limitations and participation restrictions.

■ Stroke (Cerebrovascular Accident)

Chief Clinical Characteristics
This presentation may include a wide range of symptoms that correspond to specific areas of the brain that are affected, potentially including balance deficits or falls. The initial symptoms can include numbness or weakness, especially on one side of the body or face; confusion or aphasia; visual disturbances; or sudden severe headache with no known cause.

Background Information
This condition occurs when blood flow to the brain is interrupted either by blockage (ischemia or infarction) or from hemorrhagic disruption. A thrombosis or embolic occlusion of an artery causes an ischemic type of this condition. A hemorrhagic type of this condition can be caused by arteriovenous malformation, hypertension, aneurysm, neoplasm, drug abuse, and trauma. This condition is the most common and disabling neurological disorder in adults and occurs in 114 of every 100,000 people.[95] This condition is diagnosed using clinical presentation and positive findings on computed tomography and magnetic resonance imaging. Medication, surgery, and interdisciplinary therapy are the most common treatments for this condition. The prognosis for recovery is predicted by the magnitude of initial deficit. Factors that are associated with poor outcomes include coma, poor cognition, severe aphasia, severe hemiparesis with little return within 1 month, visual perceptual disorders, depression, and incontinence after 2 weeks.[96,97]

■ Transient Ischemic Attack

Chief Clinical Characteristics
This presentation can include numbness or weakness in the face, arm, or leg, especially on one side of the body; confusion or difficulty in talking or understanding speech; trouble seeing in one or both eyes; and difficulty with walking, dizziness, or loss of balance and coordination.

Background Information

This condition is a transient stroke that lasts only a few minutes. It occurs when the blood supply to part of the brain is briefly interrupted. Symptoms of this condition, which usually occur suddenly, are similar to those of stroke but do not last as long. Most symptoms disappear within an hour, although they may persist for up to 24 hours. Because it is impossible to differentiate between symptoms from this condition and acute stroke, individuals should assume that all stroke-like symptoms signal a medical emergency. A prompt evaluation (within 60 minutes) is necessary to identify the cause of this condition and determine appropriate therapy. Depending on the individual's medical history and the results of a medical examination, the doctor may recommend drug therapy or surgery to reduce the risk of stroke. Antiplatelet medications, particularly aspirin, are a standard treatment for individuals suspected of this condition and who also are at risk for stroke, including individuals with atrial fibrillation.

■ Traumatic Brain Injury

Chief Clinical Characteristics

This presentation typically includes dysequilibrium in the presence of cognitive changes, altered level of consciousness, seizures, nausea, vomiting, coma, dizziness, headache, pupillary changes, tinnitus, weakness, incoordination, behavioral changes, spasticity, hypertonicity, cranial nerve lesions, and sensory and motor deficits.[16,98]

Background Information

This condition can be classified as mild, moderate, or severe based on Glasgow Coma Scale, length of coma, and duration of post-traumatic amnesia.[98] Magnetic resonance imaging may be used to confirm the diagnosis.[38] Treatment initiated at the scene of the accident and during the acute phase is focused on medical stabilization. It should be initiated during the acute phase in order to minimize complications.[99] Low Glasgow Coma Scale, longer length of coma, longer duration of post-traumatic amnesia, and older age tend to be associated with poor outcomes.[100] Optimal rehabilitation is interdisciplinary and customized to address the specific individuals' disablement.

■ Vasculitis (Giant Cell Arteritis, Temporal Arteritis, Cranial Arteritis)

Chief Clinical Characteristics

This presentation can be characterized by headaches, psychiatric syndromes, dementia, peripheral or cranial nerve involvement, pain, seizures, hypertension, hemiparesis, balance deficits, neuropathies, myopathies, organ involvement, fever, and weight loss.[16,38,101]

Background Information

This condition is the result of an immune-mediated response resulting in the inflammation of vascular structures.[16,101] It includes a variety of disorders such as giant cell/temporal arteritis (which is the most common form), primary angiitis of the central nervous system, Takayasu's disease, periarteritis nodosa, Kawasaki disease, Churg-Strauss syndrome, Wegener's granulomatosis, and secondary vasculitis associated with systemic lupus erythematous, rheumatoid arthritis, and scleroderma.[101] The diagnosis is confirmed through history, physical examination, laboratory testing, angiography, biopsy, and imaging.[16,38,101] Corticosteroids, cytotoxic agents, intravenous immunoglobulin, and plasmapheresis may be used in the treatment of vasculitis.[38,101] Prognosis is variable and depends on the specific underlying disorder. For example, giant cell arteritis is typically self-limiting within 1 to 2 years; however, death usually occurs within 1 year for individuals with primary angiitis of the central nervous system.[101]

■ Vertebrobasilar Artery Insufficiency

Chief Clinical Characteristics

This presentation commonly involves symptoms consistent with a cerebrovascular accident involving the vertebrobasilar artery system, usually the anterior inferior cerebellar artery.[102] Headache or neck pain was found to be the prominent feature in 88% of 26 individuals presenting with vertebral artery dissection. The most common focal neurological symptom was vertigo (57%).[103] In cases of stroke following cervical spine manipulation purported to be due to vertebral artery dissection, the presenting neurological symptoms were loss of coordination

(52%), dizziness/vertigo/nausea/vomiting (50%), speech/swallowing dysfunction, visual disturbances, and numbness, nystagmus, loss of consciousness, hearing deficits/tinnitus, and death.[104]

Background Information

Less severe but similar symptoms may be expected in lesser degrees of vertebrobasilar insufficiency. The circulation to the inner ear arises from the vertebrobasilar artery system, which leads to dizziness when this circulation is impaired.[102,105] If the insufficiency is great enough to progress to stroke, generally other associated neurological symptoms typical of central nervous system lesions are present, but these can be absent.[102,105] A classic sequel of stroke related to this condition is lateral medullary (Wallenberg's) syndrome. Proposed causes of vascular compromise include trauma resulting from participation in sports or manipulation of the cervical spine, cervical spine rotation and/or extension, and complications due to risk factors such as age, gender, migraine headaches, hypertension, diabetes, use of birth control pills, cervical spondylosis, and smoking.[104,106,107] However, systematic reviews of the literature suggest there is no definitive way to identify who is at risk for vertebrobasilar insufficiency, either by history, clinical examination, or special tests.[104,106,108,109] Individuals suspected of having this condition should be referred for medical evaluation urgently.

■ **Vestibular Ototoxicity**

Chief Clinical Characteristics

This presentation includes fluctuating or constant tinnitus and hearing loss ranging from mild to complete deafness if the cochlea is involved; vertigo, vomiting, nystagmus, and imbalance if the vestibular system is involved unilaterally; and headache, ear fullness, oscillopsia, an inability to tolerate head movement, a wide-based gait, difficulty walking in the dark, a feeling of unsteadiness and actual unsteadiness while moving, imbalance to the point of being unable to walk, light-headedness, and severe fatigue in bilateral involvement. Any combination of the above is possible because either the cochlea or the vestibular system individually, or both in combination, can be affected, either unilaterally or bilaterally.

Background Information

The severity, type, and particular combination of symptoms are variable, depending on the medication exposure, whether it is unilateral or bilateral, the speed of onset, and the individual. A slow unilateral loss may produce few symptoms since the brain can compensate through other mechanisms, whereas a fast bilateral loss can produce significant disability. Because these symptoms are similar to many other conditions, the key diagnostic feature is a history of drug or chemical exposure. Medications that are known to be vestibulotoxic include aspirin and quinine, loop diuretics (bumetanide [Bumex], ethacrynic acid [Edecrin], furosemide [Lasix] torsemide [Demadex]), aminoglycoside antibiotics (amikacin, dihydrostreptomycin, gentamicin, kanamycin, Neomycin, netilmicin, ribostamycin, streptomycin, tobramycin), and anticancer medications such as carboplatin and cisplatin. Some medications produce a temporary dysfunction, while others produce permanent loss. Treatment involves removing exposure to the medication if possible, and vestibular habituation and balance exercises.

References

1. Stolze H, Klebe S, Zechlin C, Baecker C, Friege L, Deuschl G. Falls in frequent neurological diseases—prevalence, risk factors and aetiology. *J Neurol.* Jan 2004;251(1):79–84.
2. Hobeika CP. Equilibrium and balance in the elderly. *Ear Nose Throat J.* Aug 1999;78(8):558–562, 565–566.
3. Sattin RW. Falls among older persons: a public health perspective. *Annu Rev Public Health.* 1992;13:489–508.
4. Tinetti ME, Williams TF, Mayewski R. Fall risk index for elderly patients based on number of chronic disabilities. *Am J Med.* Mar 1986;80(3):429–434.
5. Dominguez RO, Bronstein AM. Assessment of unexplained falls and gait unsteadiness: the impact of age. *Otolaryngol Clin North Am.* Jun 2000;33(3):637–657.
6. Tinetti ME, Speechley M. Risk factors for falls among elderly persons living in the community. *N Engl J Med* 1998;319:1701–1707.
7. Stalenhoef PA, Diederiks JP, Knottnerus JA, Kester AD, Crebolder HF. A risk model for the prediction of recurrent falls in community-dwelling elderly: a prospective cohort study. *J Clin Epidemiol.* Nov 2002;55(11):1088–1094.
8. Lee DJ, Westra WH, Staecker H, Long D, Niparko JK, Slattery WH 3rd. Clinical and histopathologic features of recurrent vestibular schwannoma (acoustic neuroma) after stereotactic radiosurgery. *Otol Neurotol.* Jul 2003;24(4):650–660; discussion 660.
9. Murphy MR, Selesnick SH. Cost-effective diagnosis of acoustic neuromas: a philosophical, macroeconomic, and technological decision. *Otolaryngol Head Neck Surg.* Oct 2002;127(4):253–259.

10. Ho SY, Kveton JF. Acoustic neuroma. Assessment and management. *Otolaryngol Clin North Am.* Apr 2002; 35(2):393–404.

11. Rosenberg SI. Natural history of acoustic neuromas. *Laryngoscope.* Apr 2000;110(4):497–508.

12. Ramina R, Maniglia JJ, Meneses MS, et al. Acoustic neurinomas. Diagnosis and treatment. *Arquivos de Neuro-Psiquiatria.* Sep 1997;55(3A):393–402.

13. Kartush JM, Brackmann DE. Acoustic neuroma update. *Otolaryngol Clin North Am.* Jun 1996;29(3):377–392.

14. Herdman SJ, Clendaniel RA, Mattox DE, Holliday MJ, Niparko JK. Vestibular adaptation exercises and recovery: acute stage after acoustic neuroma resection. *Otolaryngol Head Neck Surg.* 1995;113(1):77–87.

15. Al-Otaibi LM, Porter SR, Poate TW. Behcet's disease: a review. *J Dent Res.* Mar 2005;84(3):209–222.

16. Victor M, Ropper AH. *Adams and Victor's Principles of Neurology.* 7th ed. New York, NY: McGraw-Hill; 2001.

17. Fitzgerald DC. Head trauma: hearing loss and dizziness [see comment]. *J Trauma-Injury Infect Crit Care.* 1996;40(3):488–496.

18. Herdman S, ed. *Vestibular Rehabilitation.* 2nd ed. Philadelphia, PA: F. A. Davis; 2000.

19. Hilton M, Pinder D. The Epley (canalith repositioning) manoeuvre for benign paroxysmal positional vertigo. [update of *Cochrane Database Syst Rev.* 2002;(1):CD003162; PMID: 11869655]. *Cochrane Database Syst Rev.* 2004;(2):CD003162.

20. Nunez RA, Cass SP, Furman JM. Short- and long-term outcomes of canalith repositioning for benign paroxysmal positional vertigo. *Otolaryngol Head Neck Surg.* 2000;122:647–652.

21. Froehling DA, Bowen JM, Mohr DN, et al. The canalith repositioning procedure for the treatment of benign paroxysmal positional vertigo: a randomized controlled trial. *Mayo Clin Proc.* Jul 2000;75(7):695–700.

22. Parnes LS, Agrawal SK, Atlas J. Diagnosis and management of benign paroxysmal positional vertigo (BPPV). *CMAJ.* Sep 30 2003;169(7):681–693.

23. Tusa RJ. Benign paroxysmal positional vertigo. *Curr Neurol Neurosci Rep.* Sep 2001;1(5):478–485.

24. Dornhoffer JL, Colvin GB. Benign paroxysmal positional vertigo and canalith repositioning: clinical correlations. *Am J Otol.* Mar 2000;21(2):230–233.

25. Cohen HS, Jerabek J. Efficacy of treatments for posterior canal benign paroxysmal positional vertigo. *Laryngoscope.* Apr 1999;109(4):584–590.

26. Agrawal SK, Parnes LS. Human experience with canal plugging. *Ann NY Acad Sci.* Oct 2001;942:300–305.

27. Tosoni A, Ermani M, Brandes AA. The pathogenesis and treatment of brain metastases: a comprehensive review. *Crit Rev Oncol Hematol.* 2004;52:199–215.

28. Schievink WI. Intracranial aneurysms. *N Engl J Med.* Jan 2 1997;336(1):28–40.

29. Vogel T, Verreault R, Turcotte JF, Kiesmann M, Berthel M. Intracerebral aneurysms: a review with special attention to geriatric aspects. *J Gerontol A Biol Sci Med Sci.* Jun 2003;58(6):520–524.

30. Consensus statement on the definition of orthostatic hypotension, pure autonomic failure, and multiple system atrophy. The Consensus Committee of the American Autonomic Society and the American Academy of Neurology. *Neurology.* May 1996;46(5):1470.

31. Unruptured intracranial aneurysms—risk of rupture and risks of surgical intervention. International Study of Unruptured Intracranial Aneurysms Investigators. *N Engl J Med.* Dec 10 1998;339(24):1725–1733.

32. Mahapatra RK, Edwards MJ, Schott JM, Bhatia KP. Corticobasal degeneration. *Lancet Neurol.* Dec 2004;3(12):736–743.

33. Wenning GK, Litvan I, Jankovic J, et al. Natural history and survival of 14 patients with corticobasal degeneration confirmed at postmortem examination. *J Neurol Neurosurg Psychiatry.* Feb 1998;64(2):184–189.

34. Boeve BF, Lang AE, Litvan I. Corticobasal degeneration and its relationship to progressive supranuclear palsy and frontotemporal dementia. *Ann Neurol.* 2003;54(suppl 5):S15–19.

35. Kompoliti K, Goetz CG, Boeve BF, et al. Clinical presentation and pharmacological therapy in corticobasal degeneration. *Arch Neurol.* Jul 1998;55(7):957–961.

36. Collinge J. Molecular neurology of prion disease. *J Neurol Neurosurg Psychiatry.* Jul 2005;76(7):906–919.

37. Knight RS, Will RG. Prion diseases. *J Neurol Neurosurg Psychiatry.* Mar 2004;75(suppl 1):36–42.

38. Lindsay KW, Bone I, Callander R. *Neurology and Neurosurgery Illustrated.* 3rd ed. New York, NY: Churchill Livingstone; 1997.

39. Geldmacher DS. Dementia with Lewy bodies: diagnosis and clinical approach. *Cleve Clin J Med.* Oct 2004;71(10):789–790, 792–794, 797–798 passim.

40. Small GW. Neuroimaging as a diagnostic tool in dementia with Lewy bodies. *Dement Geriatr Cogn Disord.* 2004;17(suppl 1):25–31.

41. Walker Z, Allen RL, Shergill S, Mullan E, Katona CL. Three years survival in patients with a clinical diagnosis of dementia with Lewy bodies. *Int J Geriatr Psychiatry.* Mar 2000;15(3):267–273.

42. Manyam BV, Walters AS, Narla KR. Bilateral striopallidodentate calcinosis: clinical characteristics of patients seen in a registry. *Mov Disord.* Mar 2001;16(2):258–264.

43. Manyam BV, Bhatt MH, Moore WD, Devleschoward AB, Anderson DR, Calne DB. Bilateral striopallidodentate calcinosis: cerebrospinal fluid, imaging, and electrophysiological studies. *Ann Neurol.* Apr 1992;31(4):379–384.

44. Manyam BV. What is and what is not 'Fahr's disease.' *Parkinsonism Relat Disord.* Mar 2005;11(2):73–80.

45. Arriada N, Sotelo J. Review: treatment of hydrocephalus in adults. *Surg Neurol.* Dec 2002;58(6):377–384; discussion 384.

46. Kissel JT. Misunderstandings, misperceptions, and mistakes in the management of the inflammatory myopathies. *Semin Neurol.* Mar 2002;22(1):41–51.

47. Griggs RC, Askanas V, DiMauro S, et al. Inclusion body myositis and myopathies. *Ann Neurol.* Nov 1995;38(5):705–713.

48. Peng A, Koffman BM, Malley JD, Dalakas MC. Disease progression in sporadic inclusion body myositis: observations in 78 patients. *Neurology.* Jul 25, 2000;55(2):296–298.

49. Amato AA, Griggs RC. Treatment of idiopathic inflammatory myopathies. *Curr Opin Neurol.* Oct 2003;16(5):569–575.

50. Froehling DA, Silverstein MD, Mohr DN, Beatty CW. Does this dizzy patient have a serious form of vertigo? *JAMA.* 1994;271(5):385–388.

51. Strupp M, Arbusow V. Acute vestibulopathy. *Curr Opin Neurol.* 2001;14(1):11–20.

52. Yardley L, Beech S, Zander L, Evans T, Weinman J. A randomized controlled trial of exercise therapy for dizziness and vertigo in primary care [see comments]. *Br J Gen Pract.* 1998;48(429):1136–1140.

53. Kim JS. Pure lateral medullary infarction: clinical-radiological correlation of 130 acute, consecutive patients. *Brain.* 2003;126:1864–1872.

54. Nelles G, Contois KA, Valente SL, Jacobs DH, Kaplan JD, Pessin MS. Recovery following lateral medullary infarction. *Neurology.* 1998;50(5):1418–1422.

55. Thorp MA, Shehab ZP, Bance ML, Rutka JA, Equilibrium A-HCoHa. The AAO-HNS Committee on Hearing and Equilibrium guidelines for the diagnosis and evaluation of therapy in Ménière's disease: have they been applied in the published literature of the last decade? *Clin Otolaryngol Allied Sci.* Jun 2003;28(3):173–176.

56. Carey J. Intratympanic gentamicin for the treatment of Ménière's disease and other forms of peripheral vertigo. *Otolaryngol Clin North Am.* Oct 2004;37(5):1075–1090.

57. Cohen-Kerem R, Kisilevsky V, Einarson TR, Kozer E, Koren G, Rutka JA. Intratympanic gentamicin for Ménière's disease: a meta-analysis. *Laryngoscope.* Dec 2004;114(12):2085–2091.

58. Ervin SE. Ménière's disease: identifying classic symptoms and current treatments. *AAOHN J.* Apr 2004;52(4):156–158.

59. James A, Thorp M. Ménière's disease [update of *Clin Evid.* 2003 Jun;(9):565–573; PMID: 12967379]. *Clin Evid.* Jun 2004(11):664–672.

60. Minor LB, Schessel DA, Carey JP. Ménière's disease. *Curr Opin Neurol.* Feb 2004;17(1):9–16.

61. Neuhauser H, Lempert T. Vertigo and dizziness related to migraine: a diagnostic challenge [see comment]. *Cephalalgia.* Feb 2004;24(2):83–91.

62. Boyev KP. Ménière's disease or migraine? The clinical significance of fluctuating hearing loss with vertigo [see comment]. *Arch Otolaryngol Head Neck Surg.* May 2005;131(5):457–459.

63. Ropper AH, Brown RJ. *Adams and Victor's Principles of Neurology.* 8th ed. New York, NY: McGraw-Hill; 2005.

64. Peigue-Lafeuille H, Croquez N, Laurichesse H, et al. Enterovirus meningitis in adults in 1999–2000 and evaluation of clinical management. *J Med Virol.* May 2002;67(1):47–53.

65. McDonald WI, Compston A, Edan G, et al. Recommended diagnostic criteria for multiple sclerosis: guidelines from the International Panel on the diagnosis of multiple sclerosis. *Ann Neurol.* Jul 2001;50(1):121–127.

66. Thompson AJ, Montalban X, Barkhof F, et al. Diagnostic criteria for primary progressive multiple sclerosis: a position paper. *Ann Neurol.* Jun 2000;47(6):831–835.

67. Confavreux C, Vukusic S, Adeleine P. Early clinical predictors and progression of irreversible disability in multiple sclerosis: an amnesic process. *Brain.* Apr 2003;126(pt 4):770–782.

68. Wenning GK, Tison F, Ben Shlomo Y, Daniel SE, Quinn NP. Multiple system atrophy: a review of 203 pathologically proven cases. *Mov Disord.* Mar 1997;12(2):133–147.

69. Wenning GK, Ben-Shlomo Y, Hughes A, Daniel SE, Lees A, Quinn NP. What clinical features are most useful to distinguish definite multiple system atrophy from Parkinson's disease? *J Neurol Neurosurg Psychiatry.* Apr 2000;68(4):434–440.

70. Ben-Shlomo Y, Wenning GK, Tison F, Quinn NP. Survival of patients with pathologically proven multiple system atrophy: a meta-analysis. *Neurology.* Feb 1997;48(2):384–393.

71. Price RW. Neurological complications of HIV infection. *Lancet.* Aug 17 1996;348(9025):445–452.

72. Boulton AJ, Vinik AI, Arezzo JC, et al. Diabetic neuropathies: a statement by the American Diabetes Association. *Diabetes Care.* Apr 2005;28(4):956–962.

73. Poncelet AN. Diabetic polyneuropathy. Risk factors, patterns of presentation, diagnosis, and treatment. *Geriatrics.* Jun 2003;58(6):16–18, 24–25, 30.

74. Vinik AI, Park TS, Stansberry KB, Pittenger GL. Diabetic neuropathies. *Diabetologia.* Aug 2000;43(8):957–973.

75. Brown DL, Frank JE. Diagnosis and management of syphilis. *Am Fam Physician.* Jul 15 2003;68(2):283–290.

76. Conde-Sendin MA, Amela-Peris R, Aladro-Benito Y, Maroto AA. Current clinical spectrum of neurosyphilis in immunocompetent patients. *Eur Neurol.* 2004;52(1):29–35.

77. Bataller L, Dalmau J. Paraneoplastic neurological syndromes: approaches to diagnosis and treatment. *Semin Neurol.* Jun 2003;23(2):215–224.

78. Darnell RB, Posner JB. Paraneoplastic syndromes involving the nervous system. *N Engl J Med.* Oct 16 2003;349(16):1543–1554.

79. Dalmau JO, Posner JB. Paraneoplastic syndromes. *Arch Neurol.* Apr 1999;56(4):405–408.

80. Wood BH, Bilclough JA, Bowron A, Walker RW. Incidence and prediction of falls in Parkinson's disease: a prospective multidisciplinary study. *J Neurol Neurosurg Psychiatry.* Jun 2002;72(6):721–725.

81. Samii A, Nutt JG, Ransom BR. Parkinson's disease. *Lancet.* May 29 2004;363(9423):1783–1793.

82. Tillerson JL, Cohen AD, Philhower J, Miller GW, Zigmond MJ, Schallert T. Forced limb-use effects on the behavioral and neurochemical effects of 6-hydroxy-dopamine. *J Neurosci.* Jun 15 2001;21(12):4427–4435.

83. Jankovic J, Kapadia AS. Functional decline in Parkinson disease. *Arch Neurol.* Oct 2001;58(10):1611–1615.

84. Marras C, Rochon P, Lang AE. Predicting motor decline and disability in Parkinson disease: a systematic review. *Arch Neurol.* Nov 2002;59(11):1724–1728.

85. Zaida DJ, Alexander MK. Falls in the elderly: identifying and managing peripheral neuropathy. *Nurse Pract.* Mar 2001;26(3):86–88.

86. Richardson JK, Ashton-Miller JA. Peripheral neuropathy: an often-overlooked cause of falls in the elderly. *Postgrad Med.* Jun 1996;99(6):161–172.

87. Bromberg MB. An approach to the evaluation of peripheral neuropathies. *Semin Neurol.* Jun 2005;25(2):153–159.

88. Borrell E. Hypokinetic movement disorders. *J Neurosci Nurs.* Oct 2000;32(5):254–255.

89. Litvan I, Mangone CA, McKee A, et al. Natural history of progressive supranuclear palsy (Steele-Richardson-Olszewski syndrome) and clinical predictors of survival: a clinicopathological study. *J Neurol Neurosurg Psychiatry.* Jun 1996;60(6):615–620.

90. Litvan I, Bhatia KP, Burn DJ, et al. Movement Disorders Society Scientific Issues Committee report: SIC Task Force appraisal of clinical diagnostic criteria for parkinsonian disorders. *Mov Disord.* May 2003;18(5):467–486.

91. Perrin RG, Laxton AW. Metastatic spine disease: epidemiology, pathophysiology, and evaluation of patients. *Neurosurg Clin N Am.* Oct 2004;15(4):365–373.

92. Hosono N, Ueda T, Tamura D, Aoki Y, Yoshikawa H. Prognostic relevance of clinical symptoms in patients with spinal metastases. *Clin Orthop Relat Res.* Jul 2005(436):196–201.

93. Simon RP, Aminoff MJ, Greenberg DA. *Clinical Neurology.* 4th ed. Stamford, CT: Appleton and Lange; 1999.

94. Taroni F, DiDonato S. Pathways to motor incoordination: the inherited ataxias. *Nat Rev Neurosci.* Aug 2004;5(8):641–655.

95. Goodman CC, Boissonnault WG. *Pathology: Implications for the Physical Therapist.* Philadelphia, PA: W. B. Saunders; 1998.

96. Granger CV, Clark GS. Functional status and outcomes of stroke rehabilitation. *Topics Geriatrics.* Mar 1994;9(3):72–84.

97. Shelton FD, Volpe BT, Reding M. Motor impairment as a predictor of functional recovery and guide to rehabilitation treatment after stroke. *Neurorehabil Neural Repair.* 2001;15(3):229–237.

98. Bruns J, Hauser WA. The epidemiology of traumatic brain injury: a review. *Epilepsia.* 2003;44(Suppl. 10):2–10.

99. Das-Gupta R, Turner-Stokes L. Traumatic brain injury. *Disabil Rehabil.* 2002;24(13):654–665.

100. Hukkelhoven CWPM, Steyerberg EW, Rampen AJJ, et al. Patient age and outcome following severe traumatic brain injury: an analysis of 5600 patients. *J Neurosurg.* 2003;99:666–673.

101. Ferro JM. Vasculitis of the central nervous system. *J Neurol.* Dec 1998;245(12):766–776.

102. Baloh RW, Honrubia V. *Clinical Neurophysiology of the Vestibular System.* 3rd ed. New York: Oxford University Press; 2001.

103. Saeed AB, Shuaib A, Al-Sulaiti G, Emery D. Vertebral artery dissection: warning symptoms, clinical features and prognosis in 26 patients. *Can J Neurol Sci.* 2000;27:292–296.

104. Haldeman S, Kohlbeck FJ, McGregor M. Unpredictability of cerebrovascular ischemia associated with cervical spine manipulation therapy: a review of sixty-four cases after cervical spine manipulation [comment]. *Spine.* 2002;27(1):49–55.

105. Baloh RW. Episodic vertigo: central nervous system causes. *Curr Opin Neurobiol.* 2002;15:17–21.

106. Haldeman S, Kohlbeck FJ, McGregor M. Risk factors and precipitating neck movements causing vertebrobasilar artery dissection after cervical trauma and spinal manipulation. *Spine.* 1999;24(8):785–794.

107. Hurwitz EL, Aker PD, Adams AH, Meeker WC, Shekelle PG. Manipulation and mobilization of the cervical spine. A systematic review of the literature [see comment]. *Spine.* Aug 1 1996;21(15):1746–1759; discussion 1759–1760.

108. Cote P, Kreitz BG, Cassidy JD, Thiel H. The validity of the extension-rotation test as a clinical screening procedure before neck manipulation: a secondary analysis. [see comments]. *J Manipulative Physiol Thera.* 1996;19(3):159–164.

109. Childs JD, Flynn TW, Fritz J, et al. Screening for vertebrobasilar insufficiency in patients with neck pain: manual therapy decision-making in the presence of uncertainty. *J Orthop Sports Phys Ther.* 2005;35:300–306.

CHAPTER 29

Sensory Abnormalities

■ *Bernadette M. Currier, PT, DPT, MS, NCS* ■ *Michelle G. Prettyman, PT, DPT, MS*

Description of the Symptom

This chapter describes pathology that may lead to sensory abnormalities. Sensation refers to the registration of an incoming, or afferent, nerve impulse. Sensory organs, such as the eyes, nose, mouth, ears, and skin, transmit information to the brain to allow us to perceive diverse stimuli.

The sensory systems are:

- *Auditory:* the detection of sound or pressure waves in the air
- *Gustatory:* the sense of taste
- *Olfactory:* the sense of smell
- *Proprioceptive:* the detection of joint or limb position in space
- *Tactile:* the detection of changes in pressure, temperature, vibration, and other stimuli for the skin
- *Visual:* the detection of light
- *Vestibular:* the perception of movement and orientation in space.

This chapter discusses abnormalities that may affect each of these sensory systems, except the vestibular system. Conditions affecting the vestibular system are discussed in Chapter 30.

Special Concerns

Sensory abnormalities accompanied by:

- A new onset of neurological symptoms, including:
  - Loss of balance
  - Falls
  - Severe headache
  - Impaired speech
  - Paresis
  - Change in mental status
  - Nausea and vomiting
- Abnormal blood pressure, heart rate, respiratory rate, or oxygen saturation
- Changes in edema, skin color, and temperature

CHAPTER PREVIEW: Conditions That May Lead to Sensory Abnormalities

T Trauma

AUDITORY ABNORMALITIES	GUSTATORY ABNORMALITIES	OLFACTORY ABNORMALITIES
COMMON		
Perilymph fistula 596	Not applicable	Not applicable
UNCOMMON		
Perforated tympanum 596	Not applicable	Not applicable
RARE		
Not applicable	Middle ear surgery 591	Not applicable

I Inflammation

AUDITORY ABNORMALITIES	GUSTATORY ABNORMALITIES	OLFACTORY ABNORMALITIES
COMMON		
Not applicable	Not applicable	Not applicable
UNCOMMON		
Not applicable	**Aseptic** Bell's palsy 583	Not applicable
	Septic Herpes zoster oticus (Ramsay Hunt syndrome) 588	
RARE		
Aseptic Not applicable	Not applicable	Not applicable
Septic Neurosyphilis (tabes dorsalis, syphilitic spinal sclerosis, progressive locomotor ataxia) 594 Otosyphilis 595		

PROPRIOCEPTIVE ABNORMALITIES	TACTILE ABNORMALITIES	VISUAL ABNORMALITIES
Benign paroxysmal positional vertigo 583 Ligament sprains 590 Traumatic brain injury 601	Brachial plexus injury 584 Carpal tunnel syndrome 584 Thoracic outlet syndrome 600	Detached retina 587
Spinal cord injuries: • Brown-Sequard syndrome 598 • Central cord syndrome 598 • Conus medullaris syndrome 598 • Traumatic spinal cord injury 599	Hydromyelia (syringomyelia) 588 Spinal cord injuries: • Brown-Sequard syndrome 598 • Central cord syndrome 598 • Conus medullaris syndrome 598 • Traumatic spinal cord injury 599	Not applicable
Not applicable	Not applicable	Not applicable

PROPRIOCEPTIVE ABNORMALITIES	TACTILE ABNORMALITIES	VISUAL ABNORMALITIES
Aseptic Not applicable **Septic** Labyrinthitis and neuronitis 589	Not applicable	Not applicable
Not applicable	**Aseptic** Multiple sclerosis 591 **Septic** Herpes zoster 588	**Aseptic** Behçet's disease 583 Progressive multifocal leukoencephalopathy 597 Systemic lupus erythematosus 599 **Septic** Not applicable
Not applicable	**Aseptic** Acute demyelinating polyneuropathy (Guillain-Barré syndrome) 581 Transverse myelitis 601 **Septic** Tropical spastic paraparesis 601	**Aseptic** Neuromyelitis optica 592 **Septic** Klüver-Bucy syndrome 589 Rickettsial diseases, including Rocky Mountain spotted fever 598

M Metabolic

AUDITORY ABNORMALITIES	GUSTATORY ABNORMALITIES	OLFACTORY ABNORMALITIES
COMMON		
Not applicable	Not applicable	Drug toxicity 587
UNCOMMON		
Not applicable	Not applicable	Not applicable
RARE		
Not applicable	Not applicable	Neurosarcoidosis 594

Va Vascular

AUDITORY ABNORMALITIES	GUSTATORY ABNORMALITIES	OLFACTORY ABNORMALITIES
COMMON		
Vasculitis (giant cell arteritis, temporal arteritis, cranial arteritis) 603	Vasculitis (giant cell arteritis, temporal arteritis, cranial arteritis) 603	Not applicable
UNCOMMON		
Not applicable	Not applicable	Not applicable
RARE		
Not applicable	Lateral medullary syndrome (Wallenberg's syndrome) 589	Not applicable

De Degenerative

AUDITORY ABNORMALITIES	GUSTATORY ABNORMALITIES	OLFACTORY ABNORMALITIES
COMMON		
Otosclerosis 595 Presbycusis 597	Not applicable	Not applicable

PROPRIOCEPTIVE ABNORMALITIES	TACTILE ABNORMALITIES	VISUAL ABNORMALITIES
Not applicable	Neuropathies: • Diabetes mellitus 593 • Peripheral neuropathy 593 Vitamin B_{12} deficiency 604	Not applicable
Not applicable	Not applicable	Cerebral beriberi (Korsakoff's amnesic syndrome, Wernicke-Korsakoff syndrome) 586
Not applicable	Paraneoplastic syndromes 596	Neurotoxicity 594

PROPRIOCEPTIVE ABNORMALITIES	TACTILE ABNORMALITIES	VISUAL ABNORMALITIES
Vasculitis (giant cell arteritis, temporal arteritis, cranial arteritis) 603	Migraine 591	Cerebral aneurysm 585 Cerebral arteriosclerosis 586 Orthostatic hypotension 594 Stroke (cerebrovascular accident) 599 Vasculitis (giant cell arteritis, temporal arteritis, cranial arteritis) 603
Not applicable	Arteriovenous malformation 583 Transient ischemic attack 600	Not applicable
Not applicable	Cavernous malformation 585	Idiopathic intracranial hypertension 588

PROPRIOCEPTIVE ABNORMALITIES	TACTILE ABNORMALITIES	VISUAL ABNORMALITIES
Not applicable	Not applicable	Cataracts 585 Glaucoma 587 Macular degeneration 590 Retinitis 597

(continued)

Degenerative *(continued)*

AUDITORY ABNORMALITIES	GUSTATORY ABNORMALITIES	OLFACTORY ABNORMALITIES
UNCOMMON		
Not applicable	Not applicable	Not applicable
RARE		
Not applicable	Not applicable	Not applicable

Tu Tumor

AUDITORY ABNORMALITIES	GUSTATORY ABNORMALITIES	OLFACTORY ABNORMALITIES
COMMON		
Malignant Primary, such as: • Brain primary tumors 602 *Malignant Metastatic:* Not applicable *Benign:* Not applicable	*Malignant Primary, such as:* • Brain primary tumors 602 *Malignant Metastatic:* Not applicable *Benign:* Not applicable	*Malignant Primary, such as:* • Brain primary tumors 602 *Malignant Metastatic:* Not applicable *Benign:* Not applicable
UNCOMMON		
Not applicable	Not applicable	Not applicable
RARE		
Malignant Primary, such as: • Brain metastases 602 • Nasopharyngeal carcinoma 602 *Malignant Metastatic:* Not applicable *Benign:* Not applicable	*Malignant Primary, such as:* • Nasopharyngeal carcinoma 602 • Oropharyngeal carcinoma 602 *Malignant Metastatic:* Not applicable *Benign:* Not applicable	*Malignant Primary, such as:* • Angiomatosis (Von Hippel-Lindau disease) 581 • Brain metastases 602 • Nasopharyngeal carcinoma 602 *Malignant Metastatic:* Not applicable *Benign:* Not applicable

Co Congenital

AUDITORY ABNORMALITIES	GUSTATORY ABNORMALITIES	OLFACTORY ABNORMALITIES
COMMON		
Not applicable	Not applicable	Not applicable
UNCOMMON		
Not applicable	Not applicable	Not applicable

PROPRIOCEPTIVE ABNORMALITIES	TACTILE ABNORMALITIES	VISUAL ABNORMALITIES
Not applicable	Not applicable	Blepharospasm 584
Not applicable	Not applicable	Progressive supranuclear palsy (Richardson-Steele-Olszewski syndrome) 597

PROPRIOCEPTIVE ABNORMALITIES	TACTILE ABNORMALITIES	VISUAL ABNORMALITIES
Malignant Primary, such as: • Brain primary tumors 602 *Malignant Metastatic:* Not applicable *Benign:* Not applicable	*Malignant Primary, such as:* • Brain primary tumors 602 *Malignant Metastatic:* Not applicable *Benign:* Not applicable	*Malignant Primary, such as:* • Brain primary tumors 602 *Malignant Metastatic:* Not applicable *Benign:* Not applicable
Not applicable	Not applicable	Not applicable
Malignant Primary: Not applicable *Malignant Metastatic, such as:* • Brain metastases 602 • Spinal metastases 603 • Spinal primary tumors 603 *Benign:* Not applicable	*Malignant Primary:* Not applicable *Malignant Metastatic, such as:* • Brain metastases 602 • Spinal metastases 603 • Spinal primary tumors 603 *Benign:* Not applicable	*Malignant Primary:* Not applicable *Malignant Metastatic, such as:* • Brain metastases 602 *Benign, such as:* • Retinoblastoma 603

PROPRIOCEPTIVE ABNORMALITIES	TACTILE ABNORMALITIES	VISUAL ABNORMALITIES
Not applicable	Not applicable	Not applicable
Not applicable	Neuropathies: • Hereditary motor and sensory neuropathies 593 Tethered spinal cord syndrome 600	Not applicable

(continued)

Congenital *(continued)*

AUDITORY ABNORMALITIES	GUSTATORY ABNORMALITIES	OLFACTORY ABNORMALITIES
RARE		
Not applicable	Not applicable	Not applicable

Ne Neurogenic/Psychogenic

AUDITORY ABNORMALITIES	GUSTATORY ABNORMALITIES	OLFACTORY ABNORMALITIES
COMMON		
Not applicable	Not applicable	Anorexia nervosa 582
UNCOMMON		
Ménière's disease 590 Neurological complications of acquired immunodeficiency syndrome 592	Not applicable	Not applicable
RARE		
Not applicable	Not applicable	Not applicable

Notes: (1) These are estimates of relative incidence because few data are available for the less common conditions. (2) See additional characterization of auditory, gustatory, olfactory, proprioceptive, tactile, and visual abnormalities in the overview section that follows this preview table.

Overview of Sensory Abnormalities

Auditory Abnormalities

The auditory system is responsible for the reception and processing of sound. Although this system is most commonly associated with hearing, its anatomical proximity to the vestibular system indicates the need to examine both systems in the event of hearing loss. (Diagnosis of dizziness and vertigo is discussed in Chapter 27.) Decline in hearing acuity may result from conductive (external or middle ear), sensorineural (cochlea or cochlear nerve), or central (nuclei, auditory areas of temporal lobes) pathologies.

Slow-onset loss of high-pitched sounds is most common in sensorineural problems and loss of low-pitched sounds in conductive problems. Additional symptoms suggesting cochlear (sensorineural) problems are heightened perception of loudness, defects in clarity and abnormalities in music tones. Reports of ringing in the ears or tinnitus and other unusual sounds, such as buzzing, roaring, hissing, pulsating, or chirping sounds, suggest auditory inner or middle ear problems and nonauditory problems. The presence of tinnitus and dizziness following a recent course of antibiotics or exposure to toxins is symptomatic of drug toxicity. Finally, symptoms suggesting an auditory perception problem may include auditory illusions, hyperacusis (abnormal sensitivity to sound), and paracusis (repeating sounds). A sudden decline in hearing acuity with fever, or change in consciousness warrants immediate medical attention.

Gustatory Abnormalities

The gustatory system is responsible for the sensation of salty, sweet, and bitter qualities of taste for caloric nutrition and prevention of spoiled food ingestion. The sense of smell, additional

PROPRIOCEPTIVE ABNORMALITIES	TACTILE ABNORMALITIES	VISUAL ABNORMALITIES
Not applicable	Not applicable	Arnold-Chiari malformation (Chiari malformation) 582 Gaucher's disease 587 Machado-Joseph disease 590

PROPRIOCEPTIVE ABNORMALITIES	TACTILE ABNORMALITIES	VISUAL ABNORMALITIES
Not applicable	Anxiety disorder/panic attacks 582 Neuropathies: • Alcohol abuse 592	Not applicable
Not applicable	Complex regional pain syndrome 586 Conversion disorder 586	Not applicable
Not applicable	Restless legs syndrome 597	Not applicable

taste receptors beyond the tongue (palate, pharynx, larynx), and somatosensory (temperature, stinging) sensation serve as further sources of taste identification, discrimination, and protection. Gustatory symptoms necessitate assessment of both taste and smell with careful attention to elimination of the redundant system.

Ageusia, the total loss of taste, is infrequent due to the contributions from olfactory and somatosensory systems. More commonly, gustatory symptoms are described as distorted, dulled, foul taste to typically pleasurable foods, or intensified taste. Disturbed sense of taste may have a slow onset related to oral and dental problems or tumor development. More immediate alterations to taste are experienced in trauma and inflammatory processes.

Olfactory Abnormalities

The olfactory system participates in the chemosensory appreciation of smell for digestive function and quality of life. Sensations of smell and taste are functionally and anatomically linked, resulting in equivocal subjective clinical reports. Symptoms of declined or absent sense of smell (hyposmia and anosmia, respectively) may be influenced by peripheral or central processing deficits of olfactory and/or gustatory systems. Loss of olfactory function is most consistent with a loss of ability to identify and distinguish odors. The loss of taste identification is a qualitative characteristic most suggestive of cranial nerve I (olfactory nerve). The trigeminal nerve also serves a qualitative odor function for irritants, such as ammonia. Careful selection of various odors used for clinical testing in the absence of cognitive deficits permits differentiation between cranial nerves.

Neurological pathology and clinical test reliability may be masked in the presence of sinus or respiratory infection, and symptoms of infection must be ruled out. Pathologies along the central olfactory pathways may result in impaired unilateral or bilateral smell, odorous hallucinations, distorted sense of smell (dysosmia), or increased olfactory acuity (hyperosmia). The loss of olfactory discrimination, olfactory agnosia, is associated with thalamic nuclei and temporal lobe problems of sudden onset most likely with trauma and stroke or slow onset more typical of tumor or autoimmune pathologies.

Proprioceptive Abnormalities

Proprioception involves a network of receptors within muscle, tendon, and joint; dorsal column ascending spinal pathways; and distributed central networks for the interpretation of position and movement. Symptoms of disordered limb movement (incoordination), posture, and balance suggest proprioceptive peripheral or central pathology. Disordered limb movement may present as temporal and spatial problems including movement path, target accuracy, alternating movements, and bimanual function.

Clinical testing for proprioceptive loss may be performed to identify loss of peripheral receptor and sensory nerve distributions as well as for spinal pathology classification. Clinical tests that indicate failure of position and movement awareness confirm involvement of the proprioceptive system without specificity of location. Observed movement abnormalities of limbs or trunk with proprioceptive clinical test failure may reflect the implicit nature of proprioception and add little to identifying the pathology of the subcortical processing or the cortical sensory areas. The implicit and intimate nature of proprioception to movement contributes to a lack of clinical tests and preference for use of tactile sensation to assist with diagnosis of pathologies above the spinal cord. Position and movement awareness symptoms that are reported clinically should be considered particularly important if they are characterized by sudden onset, accompanied by vital sign abnormalities, or coexisting with paresis with hyperreflexia.

Tactile Abnormalities

Tactile sensation requires function of multiple receptive fields in the skin, transmission centrally, and interpretation in a distributed network from brainstem to primary sensory cortex. Pathologies affecting the sensory receptors, peripheral sensory nerves, spinal pathways, and cerebral connections may all contribute to clinical symptoms affecting touch, temperature, pressure, vibration, pain, and perception of tactile information. Slow and fast onset of tactile symptoms may be described as paresthesia (abnormal spontaneous sensation, burning, tingling, pins and needles), dysesthesia (unpleasant sensation produced by normally painless stimuli), or numbness. Specific touch-related symptoms are anesthesia (total loss of touch), hypesthesia (partial loss), and hyperesthesia (increased touch sensitivity).

Anatomical arrangements of peripheral and spinal paths allow direct relationships between tactile impairments and pathology to be made. Patterns of tactile, pain, temperature, and pressure loss or symptoms that correspond to a specific peripheral sensory nerve or spinal-level dermatome permit identification of pathological location. Sudden onset of pattern-specific tactile sensory loss is most common in trauma. However, slow-onset sensory loss can be described in imprecise bilateral distributions that do not correlate with anatomical distribution and are more suggestive of metabolic, tumor, inflammatory, or degenerative pathologies. Sensory loss mapped with the medial lemniscal and anterior and lateral spinothalamic pathways may reveal patterns of spinal cord pathology and assist in classifying the injury. In the presence of cognitive function, clinical tactile tests can reveal problems with two-point discrimination, stereognosis, graphesthesia and other tactile perceptions suggesting pathology of the thalamic or sensory cortical areas. Intermittent tactile symptoms may be suggestive of seizure or transient ischemic episodes. Slow onset of sensory loss without *Red Flags* signifies degenerative, metabolic, autoimmune, or tumor causes. Sudden onset of tactile symptoms with Red Flags indicates a possibly serious pathology and medical care is indicated. Tactile symptoms in the presence of motor symptoms and hyperreflexia suggest pathology at or above the spinal cord. Subjective reports of pain, as one aspect of tactile sensation, are covered extensively in other chapters. Note, however, that although pain is an important sensation discussed elsewhere, pain may also be representative of nervous system pathology.

Visual Abnormalities

Vision is a complex sensory system utilized and depended on for function. The complexity is represented by the elaborate sensory receptor arrangement in the eye and its links with other neural networks governing motor control, posture, and equilibrium, as well as parallel processing pathways. Classification of visual symptoms by visual acuity, oculomotor, and visual perceptual categories assists with identifying pathology. Abnormality in visual acuity tested in the presence of cognition and consciousness indicates problems in the visual receptors. Abnormalities in visual acuity found on the Snellen chart indicate pathology of the lens or fovea complex, whereas problems with blindness or visual fields represent optic nerve or central pathway pathologies. Oculomotor signs include reflexes (pupillary, vestibulo-ocular, oculocephalic) and eye movement (cranial nerve and supranuclear), which if abnormal require further testing to differentiate cranial nerve, vestibular system, or central pathology. Symptoms of unilateral small pupil and ptosis indicate Horner's syndrome.

Vision participates in the perception of static and dynamic aspects of objects and the environment for function. Ventral temporal and dorsal parietal lobe neural networks from the occipital lobe participate in perception and represent an extensive cortical area at risk for pathology and contribution to visual symptoms affecting limb and mobility functions. As with the other sensations, sudden onset of visual disturbances with other neurological symptoms, unstable vital signs, or fever demands immediate medical attention. Conversely, slow onset of gradual decline in visual acuity or perception is less urgent and typical of degenerative, metabolic, and autoimmune processes.

> **Description of Conditions That May Lead to Sensory Abnormalities**

■ Acute Demyelinating Polyneuropathy (Guillain-Barré Syndrome)

Chief Clinical Characteristics
This presentation typically involves progressive paresthesias described as numbness, tingling, and prickling, and weakness over the course of several days to a few weeks. Lower extremities in

a distal to proximal pattern are usually affected first, followed by upper extremities. In the majority of cases, a mild gastrointestinal or respiratory infection precedes symptoms. Muscles of the trunk and cranium may be affected following muscles of the limbs later in the disease process.

Background Information
Symptoms are thought to result from an immunologic reaction causing demyelination of peripheral nerves, and in severe cases, axonal degeneration as well. In addition to clinical presentation, differential diagnosis is established by the presence of only a few lymphocytes and an increase in protein in cerebrospinal fluid as well as electromyographic findings of reduction in amplitudes of muscle action potentials, slowed conduction velocity, conduction block in motor nerves, prolonged distal latencies, and prolonged or absent F responses. Standard treatment includes administration of intravenous immune globulin and plasma exchange. The majority of individuals recover completely or almost completely within a few weeks to a few months; however, the presence of axonal degeneration increases the regeneration time period to 6 to 18 months. Three percent to 5% of individuals with this condition do not survive.[1]

■ Angiomatosis (Von Hippel-Lindau Disease)

Chief Clinical Characteristics
This presentation commonly includes headaches, problems with balance and walking, dizziness, weakness of the limbs, vision problems, and high blood pressure.

Background Information
This condition is a rare, genetic multisystem condition characterized by the abnormal growth of tumors in certain parts of the body (angiomatosis). Tumors of the central nervous system are benign, are comprised of a nest of blood vessels, and are called hemangioblastomas (or angiomas in the eye). Hemangioblastomas may develop in the brain, the retina of the eye, and other areas of the nervous system. Other types of tumors develop in the adrenal glands, the kidneys, or the pancreas. Cysts (fluid-filled sacs) and/or tumors (benign or cancerous) may develop around the hemangioblastomas and cause the symptoms listed

above. Specific symptoms vary among individuals and depend on the size and location of the tumors. Individuals with this condition are also at a higher risk than normal for certain types of cancer, especially kidney cancer. Treatment varies according to the location and size of the tumor and its associated cyst. In general, the objective is to treat the tumors when they are causing symptoms but are still small. Treatment of most cases usually involves surgical resection. Certain tumors can be treated with focused high-dose irradiation. Individuals with this condition need careful monitoring by a physician and/or medical team familiar with the condition.

■ Anorexia Nervosa

Chief Clinical Characteristics

This presentation involves impaired ability to smell, decreased rapid visual information processing, abnormal perception of body schema, cold body temperature, and dryness or yellowing of skin. Symptoms of mood disturbance are often present and are associated with sequelae of starvation.

Background Information

The diagnostic features of anorexia nervosa are that the individual refuses to maintain a minimally normal body weight, is intensely afraid of gaining weight, and exhibits a significant disturbance in the perception of the body shape or size. In addition, postmenarchal women with this condition are commonly amenorrheic. Treatment primarily consists of psychotherapy to address underlying cognitive and behavioral correlates of this condition. The standardized mortality ratio is high.[2]

■ Anxiety Disorder/Panic Attacks

Chief Clinical Characteristics

This presentation typically includes repeated panic or anxiety attacks. Symptoms include increased heart rate and respiratory rate, pupil dilation, and trembling and sweating with feelings of fear and dread. The symptoms usually subside in 15 to 30 minutes.

Background Information

This condition is a nonspecific syndrome and can be due to a variety of medical or psychiatric syndromes or observed as part of a drug withdrawal or drug intoxication effect. The diagnosis of an anxiety condition is based on criteria from the DSM-IV-TR.[3] Anxiety conditions are classified into specific categories. One category, panic condition, has dizziness as one of its features. Panic condition is defined by recurrent attacks with at least four of the following features: increased heart rate, sweating, trembling or shaking, dyspnea, sensation of choking, chest pain or discomfort, nausea or abdominal distress, feelings of dizziness, fear of losing control, fear of dying, paresthesias, and chills or hot flashes. The etiology of anxiety conditions includes genetic factors, social and psychological factors, and physiological and biochemical abnormalities.[4] Treatment includes cognitive-behavioral therapy, relaxation exercises and pharmacologic treatment.[4] The course of this condition is variable; most individuals maintain normal social lives. Clinicians are encouraged to consider referral of individuals suspected of having this condition to a mental health specialist for evaluation and treatment.

■ Arnold-Chiari Malformation (Chiari Malformation)

Chief Clinical Characteristics

This presentation may include visual or swallowing disturbances in combination with pain in the occipital or posterior cervical areas, downbeating nystagmus, progressive ataxia, progressive spastic quadriparesis, or cervical syringomyelia.[5,6]

Background Information

This condition encompasses a number of congenital abnormalities at the base of the brain, including extension of the cerebellar tissue or displacement of the medulla and fourth ventricle into the cervical canal.[5] This condition has two main types. Individuals with the more common form of this condition, Type I, often remain asymptomatic until adolescence or adult life.[5] Type II is primarily seen in infants and young children. Please see the pediatric section of this textbook for a more complete description of this type. Diagnosis is made by magnetic resonance imaging, computed tomography, myelography, or some combination of these tests.[6] Treatment varies depending on clinical progression, and may include surgical intervention such as an upper cervical laminectomy or enlargement of the foramen magnum. Even with surgery symptoms may persist or progress.[5]

■ Arteriovenous Malformation

Chief Clinical Characteristics

This presentation may be characterized by seizures and severe headache. Hemorrhage may result in paresis, ataxia, dyspraxia, dizziness, tactile and proprioceptive disturbances, visual disturbances, aphasia, paresthesias, and cognitive deficits.[1]

Background Information

This condition is caused by a tangle of arteries and veins that cause abnormal communication within the vasculature. Approximately 12% of the 300,000 individuals in the United States with this condition are symptomatic. This condition is caused by a developmental abnormality that likely arises during embryonic or fetal development. Neurological damage occurs due to reduction of oxygen delivery, hemorrhage, or compression of nearby structures of the brain or spinal cord. Computed tomography, magnetic resonance imaging, and arteriography confirm the diagnosis. Ligation and embolization may be used to reduce the size of the lesion prior to surgical excision, which is the preferred method of treatment. Stereotactic radiation and proton beam therapy are alternative approaches to invasive methods of intervention. Up to 90% of individuals who experience a hemorrhagic arteriovenous malformation survive.[1]

■ Behçet's Disease

Chief Clinical Characteristics

This presentation may include bilateral pyramidal signs (signs related to lesions of upper motor neurons or descending pyramidal tracts, such as a positive Babinski sign or hyperreflexia), headache, memory loss, hemiparesis, cerebellar ataxia, balance deficits, sphincter dysfunction, or cranial nerve palsies. In addition to these neurological signs individuals with this condition also may present with arthritis; renal, gastrointestinal, vascular, and cardiac diseases; and genital, oral, and cutaneous ulcerations.[7]

Background Information

Mean age of onset is in the third decade of life. Diagnostic criteria according to an international study group include presence of recurrent oral ulceration, recurrent genital ulceration, eye lesions, skin lesions, papulopustular lesions, and/or a positive pathergy test.[1,7] Medical treatment typically consists of corticosteroids and immunosuppressants. Neurological symptoms tend to clear within weeks, but can sometimes recur or result in permanent deficits.[1] Onset before the age of 25 and male sex indicate a poorer prognosis.

■ Bell's Palsy

Chief Clinical Characteristics

This presentation typically involves unilateral facial paralysis and is characterized by acute drooping of the eyelid and/or corner of the mouth, drooling, impairment of taste, and dryness of the eye with or without excessive tearing that progresses within 48 hours. Tactile sensation is intact. Facial paralysis is commonly unilateral, though in rare cases may present bilaterally. All three quadrants of the face are affected. Long-term facial paralysis may lead to synkinesis (imbalance of muscular activation), resulting in significant facial distortion.[8]

Background Information

This condition is caused by an idiopathic inflammation of the facial nerve, likely due to a viral infection, commonly herpes simplex. Diagnosis utilizes clinical examination to rule out other causes of facial weakness; for example, facial weakness due to cortical or subcortical lesions is associated with impaired sensation and the frontalis and levator palpebrae muscles are weakened, but not paralyzed. Treatment involves antiviral and anti-inflammatory medications and physical therapy to address paralysis and symmetry of motion and to prevent synkineses.[8–11] Natural recovery of facial motor control occurs within 3 to 6 months in 94% of patients with incomplete paralysis, but residual synkinesis and weakness often remain in those with complete palsies.[9]

■ Benign Paroxysmal Positional Vertigo

Chief Clinical Characteristics

This presentation commonly involves dizziness or vertigo (typically described as a spinning sensation), light-headedness, imbalance, and nausea. Symptoms are precipitated by a position change of the head relative to gravity, such as getting out of bed, rolling over in bed, or looking up.[12,13]

Background Information

This condition is thought to occur when free-floating debris becomes trapped in the semicircular canal (canalithiasis) or becomes adhered to the cupula (cupulolithiasis), rendering the semicircular canal sensitive to gravity and thus changes in head position rather than head motion. The etiology of benign paroxysmal positional vertigo is unknown in most cases, but is associated with head trauma, vestibular neuritis, and vertebrobasilar ischemia, and can occur after ear surgery or prolonged bed rest.[14] This condition occurs more often in the elderly, and tends to recur in up to 15% of cases within 1 year and 50% of cases within 40 months.[15] The diagnosis is confirmed with the Hallpike maneuver, in which the head is rotated 45 degrees and tilted back while hanging off the end of the table. This position will elicit torsional and vertical nystagmus when the vertical semicircular canals are involved. Duration of vertigo while in the Hallpike position will determine if the individual has *canalithiasis* (short duration, <1 minute) or *cupulolithiasis* (long duration, >1 minute). Turning the head while supine will elicit horizontal nystagmus and vertigo when the horizontal (lateral) semicircular canals are involved. Nonsurgical treatment consisting of a series of positional changes to move the debris out of the canals, known as the canalith repositioning maneuver, can be very successful.[14,16–20] In recalcitrant cases, the offending canal can be plugged surgically.[21]

■ Blepharospasm

Chief Clinical Characteristics

This presentation includes excessive involuntary closure of the eyelids primarily due to spasmodic contraction of the orbicularis oculi muscles. Severity of symptoms ranges from frequent blinking to functional blindness.

Background Information

The majority of cases of this condition are idiopathic. Diagnosis is made by clinical presentation. Treatment includes psychotherapy, biofeedback, drugs, and surgery. Botulinum toxin A is the most effective form of treatment.

■ Brachial Plexus Injury

Chief Clinical Characteristics

This presentation is characterized by upper extremity weakness and sensory loss related to damage of the brachial plexus, a network of nerves that conducts signals from the spine to the shoulder, arm, and hand. Associated symptoms include hyporeflexia and hypotonicity.

Background Information

Injuries are often traumatic; the most common are stretch injuries occurring during the birth process. This condition can be classified in terms of mechanism of injury, closed (motor vehicle accident) vs. open (intraoperative injury and gunshot wounds); location of injury (spinal nerve root, trunk, cord, peripheral nerve); or type of nerve damage.[22] The four types of nerve damage are avulsion, the most severe type, in which the nerve is torn from the spinal root; rupture, in which the nerve is torn midsubstance; neuroma, in which the injured nerve has scarred, causing a conduction block; and neurapraxia or stretch, in which the nerve has been damaged but not torn. Diagnosis of injury and localization of the lesion require clinical investigation, electrodiagnostic study, and imaging.[22,23] Management differs depending on type and severity of injury. Open injuries with vascular damage should be explored operatively immediately. In the absence of clinical or electrophysiological recovery after 2 to 4 months, gunshot wounds without vascular compromise should undergo surgical intervention. Spontaneous recovery occurs in many closed injures; therefore, surgical intervention is delayed 4 to 5 months.[22] Outcomes are favorable in patients who have less severe nerve damage and those who undergo early operation when indicated.[22] Despite residual weakness and impaired functional use of the extremity, the majority of patients report satisfaction with their quality of life postinjury and/or post–surgical repair.[24]

■ Carpal Tunnel Syndrome

Chief Clinical Characteristics

Presentation of decreased grip strength and difficulty performing tasks requiring grasp or manipulation of objects are preceded by initial report of pain and numbness/tingling in the palmar aspect of the thumb, index finger, middle finger, and radial half of the ring finger with radiation up the forearm.[25]

Background Information

This condition results from compression of the median nerve as it passes through the carpal tunnel. It is associated with repetitive stress, such as typing or performing assembly line tasks. Differential diagnosis includes cervical radiculopathy or compression of the median nerve proximal to the carpal tunnel. Diagnosis is achieved through use of special tests (eg, Phalen's sign, monofilament testing, and provocative tests) and via electromyography and nerve conduction velocity tests.[26] Treatment consists of splinting, pharmacologic management of inflammation and pain, modalities, stretching and strengthening, ergonomic modifications, and surgery if indicated.[27] Nonsurgical care including physical therapy is emphasized first, and it is most effective in those with mild impairment. If nonsurgical management fails, surgery is usually recommended. In those with severe forms of this condition who have been properly diagnosed, 70% report complete satisfaction with pain relief. However, residual weakness and reoccurrence may occur.[25]

■ **Cataracts**

Chief Clinical Characteristics

This presentation can be characterized by gradual central greater than peripheral vision loss that results in myopia, loss of contrast sensitivity, and blurred and foggy vision.

Background Information

This condition occurs when the normally clear lens opacifies, causing edema and shrinkage.[28] Eventually, the opacification can result in a milky sac that can dislocate either anteriorly or posteriorly through the lens. Posterior dislocations may result in improved light perception. This condition commonly affects both eyes, although one eye is usually more affected. It may occur as a primary disease process related to age-related degeneration, secondary to another medical condition, or congenitally. Age and family history are the strongest predictors of developing the age-related form of the condition.[29] Treatment typically involves surgical interventions to the lens.

■ **Cavernous Malformation**

Chief Clinical Characteristics

This presentation includes symptoms that are dependent on the neuroanatomical location affected. Symptoms often consist of paresthesias, visual disturbances, headaches, and seizures.

Background Information

This condition is a rare disorder of the vascular system of the brain where a blood-filled mass, or hemangioma, forms. This condition is frequently inherited in an autosomal dominant pattern. Diagnosis is made on clinical manifestations and magnetic resonance imaging findings of clusters of vessels with a rim of hypodensity on T_1-weighted images.[1] For individuals with this condition who experience neurological symptoms, treatment is symptomatic and supportive. Surgical removal or radiation may be performed.[1] Individuals with prior hemorrhage and infratentorial location of the hemangioma have a poorer prognosis.[30]

■ **Cerebral Aneurysm**

Chief Clinical Characteristics

This presentation may involve loss of balance in combination with a whole host of other neurological symptoms and signs that depend on the affected cerebral tissue, including visual and proprioceptive loss. Any associated signs or symptoms may not be reported due to the fact that this condition is typically asymptomatic prior to rupture. However, if the aneurysm results in a mass effect, ischemia, or hemorrhage, then neurological signs and symptoms are dependent on the affected location.[1,31,32]

Background Information

There has been some description of genetic factors in this condition.[31] Cigarette smoking, hypertension, and heavy alcohol use have all been found to be correlated with increased risk of aneurysm development.[31,32] Factors associated with increased risk of rupture include size of aneurysm, location in the posterior circulation, and a previous history of aneurismal subarachnoid hemorrhage.[33,34] Definitive diagnosis is based on catheter angiography; however, magnetic resonance angiography, magnetic resonance imaging, and computed tomography may aid in the diagnosis. Unruptured aneurysms are sometimes surgically treated.

Aneurysm size, location, and prior history of a subarachnoid hemorrhage help to determine if the risk of surgical treatment is worth the potential benefits. Most aneurysms that have hemorrhaged must be treated surgically. Patients with a previous rupture are at an 11 times greater risk of having a second intracranial aneurysm rupture. When aneurysms do rupture, many patients die within 1 month of the rupture, and those who survive often have residual neurological deficits.[31]

■ Cerebral Arteriosclerosis

Chief Clinical Characteristics

This presentation includes visual disturbances, headache, and facial pain.

Background Information

Thickening and hardening of the artery walls in the brain lead to the development of this condition. Diagnosis is established by computed tomography or magnetic resonance imaging of the brain. Treatment includes lifestyle modification, pharmacotherapy, and surgery. Cerebral arteriosclerosis can result in ischemic or hemorrhagic stroke, thus causing neurological impairments.[1]

■ Cerebral Beriberi (Korsakoff's Amnesic Syndrome, Wernicke-Korsakoff Syndrome)

Chief Clinical Characteristics

This presentation involves ophthalmoparesis, nystagmus, ataxia, and confusion, as well as impaired learning and memory. Other common symptoms include peripheral neuropathy, postural hypotension, syncope, impaired olfactory discrimination, mild hypothermia, and confabulation.[5]

Background Information

This condition is due to a thiamine deficiency that results in a diffuse decrease in cerebral glucose utilization. It is most commonly observed in individuals who abuse alcohol and have nutritional deficiencies, although it is not limited to this population.[5] Diagnosis can be made by blood tests to examine thiamine levels. Neuroimaging may show slowed brain activity as well as lesions in the medial thalamus and periaqueductal region.[5] Medical treatment involves the immediate administration of thiamine. Once thiamine has been administered, the reversal of symptoms should begin to occur within hours to days with variable degrees of recovery. Memory has been shown to have the poorest return, and mortality rates of up to 17% have been reported.[5]

■ Complex Regional Pain Syndrome

Chief Clinical Characteristics

This presentation typically includes a traumatic onset of severe pain accompanied by allodynia, hyperalgesia, and trophic, vasomotor, and sudomotor changes in later stages. This condition is characterized by disproportionate responses to painful stimuli.

Background Information

This regional neuropathic pain disorder presents either without direct nerve trauma (Type I) or with direct nerve trauma (Type II) in any region of the body.[35] This condition may precipitate due to an event distant to the affected area. Thermography may confirm associated sympathetic dysfunction. Treatment for this condition includes physical therapy for desensitization, prevention of secondary complications and restoration of mobility, pharmacotherapeutics for pain reduction, and surgical intervention such as sympathectomy. Prognosis is primarily dependent on timely detection of the disease and rate of progression.[1]

■ Conversion Disorder

Chief Clinical Characteristics

This presentation can be characterized by motor or sensory deficits, seizures or convulsions, or blindness or deafness. Symptoms usually appear suddenly and abate in less than 2 weeks.

Background Information

This condition is one type of somatoform disorder in which psychological stress becomes translated into physical problems. The DSM-IV-TR defines conversion disorder by symptoms that simulate a neurological or other medical condition that involves voluntary muscles or sensory organs excluding pain and sexual functions.[1] Clinical findings include patterns of sensory loss that do not follow normal patterns from neurological insults and symptoms that disappear when a patient is distracted or thinks that no one is watching. Patients often have a history of emotional disturbance, stress, or traumatic event. Differential diagnosis is based on clinical findings. It is helpful to treat the patient as though he or she has had an illness and is now in the process of recovery.[1] Cognitive and behavioral therapies may be effective in treating underlying psychological issues. Prognosis is variable with differing degrees of recovery in days to months. Good prognostic factors include acute onset of symptoms, short duration of symptoms, healthy premorbid functioning, higher intelligence, absence of coexisting psychopathology, and presence of an identifiable stressor. Poor prognostic symptoms include pseudoseizures, age greater than 40, and long-lasting severe disability.[36]

■ **Detached Retina**

Chief Clinical Characteristics
This presentation typically involves new onset of visual disturbances such as flashes or floaters in the visual field, accompanied by central or side visual field loss and occasionally severe vitreal hemorrhage.[37]

Background Information
This condition occurs when the retina demonstrates breaks. Breaks commonly occur in areas of high adhesion, such as about the vasculature. This condition may occur spontaneously, as a result of trauma or other forms of eye pathology, or as a result of metabolic disease such as diabetes mellitus. Prompt ophthalmic evaluation is necessary if this condition is suspected. Surgical interventions may be considered to address this condition, including scleral buckling, vitrectomy, and pneumatic retinopexy.

■ **Drug Toxicity**

Chief Clinical Characteristics
This presentation involves tinnitus (fluctuating or constant) and hearing loss (mild to complete deafness) if the cochlea is involved; vertigo, vomiting, nystagmus, and imbalance if the vestibular system is involved unilaterally; and headache, ear fullness, oscillopsia, an inability to tolerate head movement, a wide-based gait, difficulty walking in the dark, a feeling of unsteadiness and actual unsteadiness while moving, imbalance to the point of being unable to walk, light-headedness, and severe fatigue in bilateral involvement.

Background Information
The severity, type, and particular combination of symptoms are variable, depending on the drug exposure, whether it is unilateral or bilateral, the speed of onset, and the individual. A slow unilateral loss may produce few symptoms, since the brain can compensate through other mechanisms, whereas a fast bilateral loss can produce significant disability. The key diagnostic feature is a history of drug or chemical exposure. Treatment involves removing exposure to the medication if possible, and vestibular habituation and balance exercises.

■ **Gaucher's Disease**

Chief Clinical Characteristics
This presentation commonly includes slowly progressive mental decline, seizures, ataxia, and, upon later development, weakness with spasticity and splenomegaly and deficits in lateral gaze.[1]

Background Information
This condition is a rare disorder, although it is prevalent among the Ashkenazi Jewish population.[38] The disease is an autosomal genetic disorder in which glucocerebroside accumulates in the spleen, liver, lungs, bone marrow, and brain due to a deficiency in an enzyme.[1] There are three types of Gaucher's disease. The most common, type 1, is characterized by no central nervous system involvement. In type 2, infants have extensive and progressive neurological damage.[38] Type 3 is less common and is associated with less severe neurological symptoms.[38] Diagnosis is established by clinical presentation, laboratory tests that show an increase in total acid phosphatase, and biopsy of bone marrow that is positive for Gaucher cells. Enzyme replacement therapy is standard for most patients with types 1 and 3. However, there is no effective treatment for the severe brain damage that may occur in patients with types 2 and 3. Prognosis for patients with type 2 disease is poor with death within the first 2 years of life. For type 3 disease, symptoms typically present in childhood and death occurs by age 10 to 15 years.[1]

■ **Glaucoma**

Chief Clinical Characteristics
This presentation includes gradual loss of visual acuity, which classically occurs from peripheral to central within the visual field.

Background Information
This condition occurs when optic nerve fibers are lost in the retinal nerve fiber layer secondary to elevated intraocular pressure.[39] Clinical assessment of the retina usually confirms the diagnosis, but many other imaging modalities are now available to evaluate the retina and optic nerve for individuals suspected of having this condition. Management of this condition currently focuses on controlling intraocular pressure, since this finding is the only known risk factor for developing the condition.

■ Herpes Zoster

Chief Clinical Characteristics
This presentation typically includes an exquisitely painful rash or blisters along a specific dermatomal pattern accompanied by flu-like symptoms. Sensory and motor losses within spinal segmental distributions may occur, although this is rare. Individuals with this condition also demonstrate a previous history of varicella exposure or infection. Pain associated with this condition may be disproportionate to the extent of skin irritation. The initial presentation of this condition may be confused with radiculopathy due to the distribution of symptoms. The presence of the rash, extreme pain, general malaise, and unclear association with spinal movement aids in differential diagnosis.

Background Information
The virus remains dormant in the spinal ganglia until its reactivation during a period of stress, infection, or physical exhaustion. Treatment includes the administration of antiviral agents as soon as the zoster eruption is noted, ideally within 48 to 72 hours. If timing is greater than 3 days, treatment is aimed at controlling pain and pruritus and minimizing the risk of secondary infection.[40]

■ Herpes Zoster Oticus (Ramsay Hunt Syndrome)

Chief Clinical Characteristics
This presentation commonly includes intense ear pain; a rash around the ear, mouth, face, neck, and scalp; and paralysis of facial nerves. Other symptoms may include hearing loss, vertigo, and tinnitus. Taste loss in the tongue and dry mouth and eyes may also occur.

Background Information
This condition is a common complication of herpes zoster. This condition is an infection caused by the spread of varicella-zoster virus, which is the virus that causes chickenpox, to facial nerves. This condition occurs in people who have had chickenpox and represents a reactivation of the dormant varicella-zoster virus. When treatment is needed, medications such as antiviral drugs or corticosteroids may be prescribed. Vertigo also may be treated with the drug diazepam.

■ Hydromyelia (Syringomyelia)

Chief Clinical Characteristics
This presentation involves insidious onset of symptoms including upper and lower extremity weakness and numbness and, less commonly, pain. Trauma usually precedes the onset on symptoms, but the time frame for subsequent development of weakness and sensory changes is variable.

Background Information
This condition is caused by an abnormal widening of the central canal of the spinal cord, leading to the accumulation of cerebrospinal fluid and hydrocephalus. Differential diagnosis must be made between hydromyelia and other disorders such as syringomyelia, spinal cord tumor, and spinal arteriovenous malformation. Magnetic resonance imaging and electromyography are used to confirm the diagnosis of this condition. Surgery may be indicated to decrease or eliminate the symptoms. Prognosis is variable.

■ Idiopathic Intracranial Hypertension

Chief Clinical Characteristics
This presentation includes headaches, visual disturbances, dizziness, or tinnitus.[41]

Background Information
Diagnostic criteria include presence of symptoms that reflect generalized intracranial hypertension or papilledema, elevated intracranial pressure (>250 mm H_2O per lumbar puncture), normal cerebrospinal fluid composition, absence of lesions on magnetic resonance imaging or computed tomography, and

no other cause identified.[42] Also known as pseudotumor cerebri or benign intracranial hypertension, this condition is characterized by increased intracranial pressure without associated space-occupying lesions or hydrocephalus. Approximately one-third of individuals with idiopathic intracranial hypertension recover within 6 months following repeated lumbar punctures and drainage of cerebrospinal fluid to maintain the pressure at near normal or normal levels. Weight reduction and surgical gastric placation are effective forms of treatment.[1]

■ Klüver-Bucy Syndrome

Chief Clinical Characteristics

This presentation typically involves oral exploratory behavior, tactile exploratory behavior, and hypersexuality, with additional symptoms and signs that may include visual agnosia, decreased attention, seizures, and dementia.

Background Information

This condition arises from medial temporal lobe dysfunction, and it may be associated with many different etiologies including herpes encephalitis, traumatic brain injury, and Pick's disease. This condition is diagnosed clinically by the presence of the above cluster of symptoms. Treatment is symptomatic and primarily through pharmacologic means. Prognosis is poor.[1]

■ Labyrinthitis and Neuronitis

Chief Clinical Characteristics

This presentation may be characterized by a relatively sudden onset of severe, constant rotary vertigo (made worse by head movement) that resolves after days or weeks.[43,44] This condition is associated with spontaneous nystagmus, postural imbalance, and nausea without accompanying cochlear or neurological symptoms.[44] The specific presentation varies depending on the site of the infection. If the vestibular system is affected, the symptoms will include dizziness and difficulty with vision and/or balance. If the inflammation affects the cochlea, this condition will produce disturbances in hearing, such as tinnitus or hearing loss. The symptoms can be mild or severe, temporary or permanent, depending on the severity of the infection.

Background Information

The etiology is a bacterial or viral infection causing inflammation of the vestibular nerve (neuronitis) or the labyrinth (labyrinthitis). The terms are often used interchangeably because it is difficult to distinguish neuronitis from labyrinthitis.[43] The diagnostic hallmark is unilateral hyporesponsiveness with caloric testing.[44] Regardless of the type of infection, the treatment consists of destroying the bacteria by means of antibiotics. If the labyrinthitis is caused by a break in the membranes separating the middle and inner ears, surgery may also be required to repair the membranes to prevent a recurrence of the disease. Residual vertigo can be reduced with vestibular habituation exercises.[45]

■ Lateral Medullary Syndrome (Wallenberg's Syndrome)

Chief Clinical Characteristics

This presentation can include nystagmus, oscillopsia, vertigo, nausea, vomiting, impairment of pain and thermal sense over half of the body, ipsilateral Horner syndrome including miosis, ptosis, anhidrosis, hoarseness, dysphagia, ipsilateral paralysis of palate and vocal cord with a diminished gag reflex, vertical diplopia or sensation of tilting vision, ipsilateral ataxia of limbs, loss of balance to ipsilateral side, and impaired sensation of ipsilateral half of the face.[1,46,47]

Background Information

In 75% of cases, onset is sudden. Main etiologic factors associated with this condition include large-vessel infarction, arterial dissection, small-vessel infarction, cardiac embolism, tumor, hemorrhage, and other unknown factors. The most typical cause is occlusion of the vertebral artery, with the posterior inferior cerebellar artery being involved to a lesser degree. A thorough history, clinical examination, and magnetic resonance imaging may confirm the diagnosis. An emergency response is required for individuals experiencing the new onset of symptoms. Residual symptoms include balance deficits (most common), dysphagia, dizziness, and numbness, which may be addressed with physical, occupational, and speech therapy.

■ Ligament Sprains

Chief Clinical Characteristics

This presentation includes decreased proprioception and balance following a ligament sprain to the lower extremity.

Background Information

Functional instability is especially common following ankle and knee sprains, and proprioceptive loss is thought to be a contributory factor. Damage to joint capsule and muscle stretch receptors leads to proprioceptive loss. Diagnosis of proprioceptive loss following an ankle sprain is made by clinical assessment; an individual's ability to identify joint position in space without additional sensory input grossly determines the degree of proprioceptive loss. Proprioception and balance can be restored to varying degrees fusing therapeutic exercises that challenge balance.[48,49] Residual high-level balance deficits are common.[49]

■ Machado-Joseph Disease

Chief Clinical Characteristics

This presentation may involve visual impairments such as nystagmus in combination with slowly progressive ataxia, rigidity, dystonia, weakness in the hands and feet, and difficulty with respiration and swallowing.

Background Information

This condition is genetic, with an autosomal dominant pattern of inheritance and onset of symptoms in adolescence or young adulthood. Differential diagnosis includes Parkinson's disease and multiple system atrophy. The presence of ataxia decreases the likelihood of Parkinson's, and the early age of onset and visual symptoms decrease the likelihood of multiple system atrophy. Diagnosis is established by clinical symptoms and magnetic resonance imaging findings of reduced width of superior and middle cerebellar peduncles, atrophy of the frontal and temporal lobes, and decreased size of the pons and globus pallidus. There is no treatment for this condition, and prognosis is poor.[1]

■ Macular Degeneration

Chief Clinical Characteristics

This presentation involves gradual loss of central vision, which impairs the ability to read with preservation of peripheral vision.

Background Information

This condition consists of wet and dry forms. In the dry form, cellular debris (drusen) may accumulate between the choroid and retina. In the wet form, blood vessels may grow from behind the choroid, which may lead to retinal detachment.[50] Examination reveals central scotomata and an alteration of the retina around the maculae. Treatment to delay progression or possibly improve vision includes visual aids and medication. This condition worsens with time and eventually may lead to blindness.[1]

■ Ménière's Disease

Chief Clinical Characteristics

This presentation is characterized by recurrent episodic spontaneous attacks of vertigo (exacerbated by head movements and accompanied by nausea and vomiting), fluctuating sensorineural hearing loss, aural fullness, and tinnitus.[44,51–58] In the late stages the symptoms are more severe, hearing loss is less likely to fluctuate, and tinnitus and aural fullness may be more constant. Sudden unexplained falls without loss of consciousness or vertigo (drop attacks) may occur. Attacks can be preceded by an aura consisting of a sense of fullness in the ear, increasing tinnitus and a decrease in hearing,[56] but can also occur without warning. The typical duration of an attack is 2 to 3 hours, ranging from minutes to hours in length. Attacks can be single or multiple, with short or long intervening periods of remission during which the individual may be asymptomatic.

Background Information

The cause of this condition is thought to be overproduction or underabsorption of endolymph (endolymphatic hydrops), resulting in distortion of the membranous labyrinth. Ruptures of the membranous labyrinth, autoimmune disease processes, and viral infection are among other proposed causes.[58] Appropriate tests include caloric testing to determine amount of vestibular asymmetry; audiometry, which often shows a low-frequency loss rather than a high-frequency one; and exclusion of other causes (typically with gadolinium-enhanced magnetic resonance imaging). The head thrust test can be negative despite caloric asymmetry. Restricting salt intake and using diuretics may be useful in over half of individuals with this condition. Approximately 10% of individuals with this condition will have persistent vertigo and require other forms of treatment. These include surgery to decompress or drain the endolymphatic sac, selective vestibular neurectomy or labyrinthectomy, and intratympanic injections of aminoglycosides such as gentamicin[53] to reduce or abolish vestibular function on the affected side.

■ Middle Ear Surgery

Chief Clinical Characteristics
This presentation involves decreased taste perception following middle ear surgery.

Background Information
Disorders of taste are related to intraoperative insult to the facial nerve. Electrogustometry and chemical taste tests are used to diagnose taste disorders. No specific treatment is indicated. Approximately 30% of individuals with taste disorders following middle ear surgery recover completely.[59]

■ Migraine

Chief Clinical Characteristics
This presentation often includes a severe pulsating and throbbing unilateral headache that may switch sides, associated with nausea, vomiting, diarrhea, abdominal cramps, polyuria, sweating, facial pallor, photophobia, or phonophobia. This is a chronic condition of recurring attacks of transient focal neurological symptoms, headaches, or both.[60] Not only is this process responsible for producing headaches, the condition can also interfere with the function of other body systems, resulting in the characteristic presentation.[61] Migraines are preceded by aura in 20% of cases.[62] Even in individuals who commonly experience them, auras may not accompany every headache. Auras can be visual, somatosensory, olfactory, or involve speech disturbances. The location of headache may switch sides from episode to episode.

Background Information
The pathophysiology of this condition is very complex. Current theories postulate that a cascade of events occurs involving vasodilation of meningeal blood vessels, irritation of perivascular sensory nerves, and stimulation of brainstem nuclei. Additionally, extrinsic factors such as hormonal fluctuations, fatigue, or anxiety may be triggers that initiate the pathophysiological cascade. This condition also has a strong familial tendency and begins at a young age, suggesting that genetic factors may predispose individuals to migraine attacks. The use of neuroimaging is not indicated in individuals with migraine symptoms and a normal neurological exam. Certain pharmaceutical agents, such as triptans and ergots, are effective in preventing migraine attacks from becoming too severe.[63] Other medications can be considered to prevent migraine attacks. A complete discussion of headache diagnosis is included in Chapter 7.

■ Multiple Sclerosis

Chief Clinical Characteristics
This presentation may include paresthesias, weakness, spasticity, hypertonicity, hyperreflexia, positive Babinski, incoordination, optic neuritis, ataxia, vertigo, dysarthria, diplopia, bladder incontinence, tremor, balance deficits, falls, and cognitive deficits.[1]

Background Information
This condition may present as relapsing-remitting, primary progressive, or secondary progressive. The disease occurs most frequently in women between the ages of 20 and 40 years. Only a small number of children or individuals between 50 and 60 years are diagnosed with this condition.[1] This condition was originally thought to be secondary to environmental and genetic factors, but evidence suggests an autoimmune response to a viral infection, which subsequently targets myelin.[1] The diagnosis may be confirmed by a thorough history, physical examination, magnetic resonance imaging, analysis of cerebrospinal fluid, and evoked potentials.[1,64,65] Life expectancy and cause of mortality are similar for all types of this condition.[1] Clinical characteristics that are associated with a longer time interval for progression of disability include female sex, younger age of onset, relapsing-remitting type, complete recovery after the first relapse, and longer time interval between first and second exacerbation.[66] Medical management may include the use of methylprednisolone, prednisone, cyclophosphamide, immunosuppressant treatment, and betainterferon.[1] Physical, occupational, and speech therapy may be indicated to prevent secondary sequelae and to

optimize functional activity and mobility. Some individuals may benefit from psychology/ psychiatry and social support as the disease progresses.

Neurological Complications of Acquired Immunodeficiency Syndrome

Chief Clinical Characteristics

This presentation is variable and dependent on the affected neuroanatomical structures in an individual with acquired immunodeficiency syndrome.[67]

Background Information

This condition may be categorized by:

1. Meningitic symptoms including headache, malaise, and fever (such as secondary to meningitis, cryptococcal meningitis, tuberculous meningitis, and human immunodeficiency virus headache)
2. Focal cerebral symptoms including hemiparesis, aphasia, apraxia, sensory deficits, homonymous hemianopia, cranial nerve involvement, balance deficits, incoordination, and/or ataxia (such as secondary to cerebral toxoplasmosis, primary central nervous system lymphoma, and progressive multifocal leukoencephalopathy)
3. Diffuse cerebral symptoms that involve cognitive deficits, altered level of consciousness, hyperreflexia, Babinski sign, presence of primitive reflexes (such as secondary to postinfectious encephalomyelitis, acquired immunodeficiency dementia complex, cytomegalovirus encephalitis)
4. Myelopathy associated with gait difficulties, spasticity, ataxia, balance deficits, and hyperreflexia (such as secondary to herpes zoster myelitis, vacuolar myelopathy that occurs with acquired immunodeficiency syndrome dementia complex)
5. Peripheral involvement associated with sensory changes, weakness, balance deficits, and pain (such as secondary to peripheral neuropathy, acute and chronic inflammatory demyelinating polyneuropathies).[1,67]

Abnormal neurological findings are observed during a clinical examination in approximately one-third of patients with acquired immunodeficiency syndrome, however on autopsy most individuals with this condition have abnormalities within the nervous system.[1] Diagnosis of the variable neurological complications associated with this condition may be confirmed with laboratory tests, cerebrospinal fluid cultures, imaging, nerve conduction studies, and physical examination.[1,67,68] Treatment appears to be limited primarily to the use of antiviral medications.[67] Physical and occupational therapy may be indicated to address equipment needs and caregiver/patient training related to functional mobility.

Neuromyelitis Optica

Chief Clinical Characteristics

This presentation involves acute to subacute onset of blindness in one or both eyes and/or transverse myelitis. Blindness and transverse myelitis can exist in isolation or combination.

Background Information

This condition occurs when demyelinating and/or necrotizing lesions form in one or both optic nerves and in the spinal cord. Differential diagnosis especially includes acute disseminated encephalomyelitis, subacute necrotic myelopathy, and a variant form of multiple sclerosis. High-dose corticosteroids and alkylating agents are used to treat this condition. Prognosis is poor; factors placing individuals at higher risk of earlier morbidity or mortality include older age at onset and relapse during the first 2 years of the disease.[69]

NEUROPATHIES

Alcohol Abuse

Chief Clinical Characteristics

This presentation can be characterized by slowly progressive sensory disturbances in a distal to proximal pattern in an individual with history of alcohol abuse. Loss of pain sensation and painful burning sensations are among the most common sensory symptoms.

Background Information

This condition can be caused by the toxic effect of ethanol or its metabolites on the central and peripheral nervous system. Primary treatment is directed to reducing alcohol abuse behaviors. Prognosis depends on the course of the disease, in which neuropathy will continue to progress with continued alcohol abuse.

■ Diabetes Mellitus

Chief Clinical Characteristics

This presentation is variable, including manifestations such as acute diabetic mononeuropathies, which may include involvement of peripheral nerves (including cranial nerves)[1]; multiple mononeuropathies and radiculopathies, which may include unilateral or asymmetric pain, low back pain with or without symptoms in the leg, weakness, atrophy, diminished or absent deep tendon reflexes, and sensory deficits[1]; distal polyneuropathy, the most common diabetic neuropathy, which consists of chronic, symmetric, distal sensory deficits (eg, numbness and tingling), diminished or absent deep tendon reflexes, balance deficits, and weakness[1]; and autonomic neuropathy, which may involve resting tachycardia, orthostatic hypotension, sexual impotence, exercise intolerance, abnormal sweating, pupil abnormalities, weakness, sensory deficits, and gastroparesis.[1,68,70,71]

Background Information

Approximately 15% to 20% of people with diabetes may present with the signs and symptoms of this condition.[1,70] However, approximately 50% will have neuropathic symptoms and may have abnormalities in nerve conduction testing.[1] Commonly considered a metabolic disorder, this condition may be a result of vascular complications disrupting the supply of nutrients to the nerves.[68,72] A thorough history, physical examination (specifically including the assessment of deep tendon reflexes and sensory examination), electromyography/nerve conduction testing, and laboratory screen helps to differentiate other causes of neuropathy.[70,71] Treatment consists of maintaining a normal range of blood glucose levels.[1,69,71] In addition, individuals with this condition may prevent complications by completing visual inspection of the skin and routine podiatry care.[71] Medications may help to control symptoms such as paresthesias or pain.[1,68] Additional management may include consultations with an orthotist to ensure proper fitting of foot wear and physical therapy to minimize disability by addressing impairments associated with limitations in functional mobility.[72]

■ Hereditary Motor and Sensory Neuropathies

Chief Clinical Characteristics

This presentation includes distal sensory abnormalities, such as numbness and tingling of the feet, and muscle weakness of distal musculature. Individuals affected with hereditary neuropathies may also report sweating and dizziness upon standing.

Background Information

Hereditary neuropathies include hereditary motor and sensory neuropathy, hereditary sensory neuropathy, hereditary motor neuropathy, and hereditary sensory and autonomic neuropathy. The majority of all hereditary neuropathies are Charcot-Marie-Tooth neuropathy. Inherited polyneuropathies are caused by genetic abnormalities. Diagnosis is made by nerve conduction and electromyographic studies. Prognosis for hereditary sensory neuropathies is poor due to intractable pain.[73] Prognosis for hereditary motor and sensory neuropathies has also been found to be unfavorable due to slowing of conduction velocity with age.[74]

■ Peripheral Neuropathy

Chief Clinical Characteristics

This presentation may be characterized by sensory alterations, falls, loss of balance, weakness, as well as diminished or absent deep tendon reflexes, fasciculations, syncope, abnormal sweating, orthostatic hypotension, resting tachycardia, and trophic changes.[1,75]

Background Information

The patterns of peripheral neuropathies are variable and may present as polyneuropathy, polyradiculopathy, neuronopathy, mononeuropathy, mononeuropathy multiplex, and plexopathy.[1] Some of the etiologies associated with peripheral neuropathies include trauma, inflammation (eg, herpes zoster, Lyme disease, human immunodeficiency virus, Guillain-Barré syndrome), metabolic causes (eg, diabetes mellitus, uremia), nutritional causes (eg, vitamin B deficiencies commonly associated with alcohol abuse, eating disorders, and individuals with malabsorption syndromes), congenital and idiopathic causes (eg, aging or unknown causes), and toxic etiology (eg, exposure to lead, arsenic, thallium; chemotherapeutic drugs such as vincristine, cisplatin).[75] Twenty percent of individuals over the age of 60 are affected by a type of peripheral neuropathy.[76] The diagnosis of the specific disorder may be differentiated by the pattern of peripheral neuropathy and temporal features. The diagnosis may be confirmed after completing a thorough history, physical examination, gait assessment, balance assessment, laboratory testing, and electromyography/nerve conduction testing.[1,77] Treatment and prognosis will vary depending on the etiology and severity of this condition.

■ Neurosarcoidosis

Chief Clinical Characteristics
This presentation may be characterized by facial palsy; impaired taste, sight, smell, or swallowing; vertigo; loss of sensation in a stocking/glove pattern; and weakness in a distal greater than proximal distribution.[1]

Background Information
This condition is a manifestation of sarcoidosis with central and/or peripheral nervous system involvement. It is characterized by formation of granulomas in the central nervous system. The lesion consists of lymphocytes and mononuclear phagocytes surrounding a non-caseating epithelioid cell granuloma. These granulomas represent an autoimmune response to central nervous system tissues. This condition includes 5% of individuals with sarcoidosis. The diagnosis is established by the presence of clinical features, along with clinical and biopsy evidence of sarcoid granulomas in tissues outside the nervous system. Approximately two-thirds of individuals experience this illness only once, whereas the remainder experience chronic relapses. Primary treatment for neurosarcoidosis is the administration of corticosteroids.

■ Neurosyphilis (Tabes Dorsalis, Syphilitic Spinal Sclerosis, Progressive Locomotor Ataxia)

Chief Clinical Characteristics
This presentation can be characterized by hemiparesis, ataxia, aphasia, gait instability, falls, neuropathy, personality and cognitive changes, seizures, diplopia, visual impairments, hearing loss, psychotic disorders, loss of bowel/bladder function, pain, hyporeflexia, and hypotonia.[78,79]

Background Information
Treponema pallidum infects the human host by way of contact with contaminated body fluids or lesions.[78] This spirochete is responsible for the diagnosis of syphilis; however, when *T. pallidum* is present within the central nervous system the individual is diagnosed with neurosyphilis.[79] This condition occurs in approximately 10% of individuals with untreated syphilis, and in 81% of these cases it presents as meningovascular, meningeal, or general paresis. Treatment includes use of various forms of penicillin or alternative choices for those allergic to penicillin[78] and may involve rehabilitative therapies depending on the individual's activity limitations or participation restrictions. A better prognosis has been observed for individuals treated during early neurosyphilis.[79]

■ Neurotoxicity

Chief Clinical Characteristics
This presentation includes limb weakness or numbness; loss of memory, vision, and/or intellect; headache; behavioral problems; and sexual dysfunction.

Background Information
This condition occurs when exposure to natural or artificial toxins alters the normal activity of the nervous system. This can eventually disrupt or kill neurons. It results from exposure to substances used in chemotherapy, radiation treatment, drug therapies, and organ transplants, as well as exposure to heavy metals, foods, or pesticides. Diagnosis is supported by clinical presentation and lab tests for detection of the toxic substance. Treatment is prioritized at removal of the offending toxin. Prognosis varies greatly depending on the level of exposure and individual's comorbid medical conditions.

■ Orthostatic Hypotension

Chief Clinical Characteristics
This presentation commonly involves dizziness, light-headedness, and blurred vision that generally occur after sudden standing. In more severe forms of this condition, individuals may

experience seizures, transient ischemic attacks, or syncope.

Background Information
This condition is caused by a sudden decrease of greater than 20 mm Hg in systolic blood pressure or greater than 10 mm Hg in diastolic blood pressure, which occurs when a person assumes a standing position. It may be caused by hypovolemia resulting from the excessive use of diuretics, vasodilators, or other types of vasoactive medications (eg, calcium channel blockers and beta blockers), dehydration, or prolonged bed rest. Other factors to consider include the individual's neurological status and hemorrhagic/hypovolemic states. The condition may be associated with Addison's disease, atherosclerosis, diabetes, and certain neurological conditions including Shy-Drager syndrome and other dysautonomias. Hypovolemia due to medications is reversed by adjusting the dosage or by discontinuing the medication. If prolonged bed rest is the cause, improvement may occur by sitting up with increasing frequency each day. In some cases, physical counterpressure such as compression hose or whole-body inflatable suits may be required. Dehydration is treated with salt and fluids. Individuals with this condition can be instructed to rise slowly from bed in the mornings or when moving from a sitting to standing position. Symptoms usually dissipate when the individual is placed in a semirecumbent or supine position, although some individuals may progress to frank syncope. In this case, the clinician should be prepared to activate the emergency medical system.

■ Otosclerosis

Chief Clinical Characteristics
This presentation includes hearing loss as the most frequent symptom. The loss may appear very gradually. Many people with otosclerosis first notice that they cannot hear low-pitched sounds or a whisper. In addition to hearing loss, some people with otosclerosis may experience dizziness, balance problems, or tinnitus.

Background Information
Otosclerosis is the abnormal growth of bone of the middle ear. The cause of otosclerosis is not fully understood, but it may be hereditary. Audiograms and tympanograms are useful in the diagnosis of otosclerosis. Surgery is often the form of treatment, in which a stapedectomy will be performed to bypass the diseased bone with a prosthesis that allows sound waves to be passed to the inner ear. In milder cases in which surgery is not indicated, a hearing aid may be used. With either form of treatment, there may be residual mild hearing loss.

■ Otosyphilis

Chief Clinical Characteristics
This presentation may involve severe episodic vertigo, fluctuating hearing loss, low-frequency hearing loss in the early stages of the disease, and flat audiometric patterns in the later stages of the disease.[80,81] The hearing loss is usually bilateral in most individuals; the loss in speech discrimination is usually out of proportion to the speech reception threshold. Vestibular disturbances could be present in as many as 80% of individuals with this condition. This condition's presentation is similar to that of Ménière's disease.

Background Information
Otosyphilis is caused by the spirochete *Treponema pallidum*. Both congenital and acquired forms of syphilis infection can lead to this condition with subsequent degeneration of the audiovestibular system. Histopathological findings are identical for both the congenital and acquired forms. The underlying syphilis infection causes meningoneurolabyrinthitis in the early congenital form and in the acute period of the secondary and tertiary acquired forms. It causes temporal bone osteitis with secondary involvement of the membranous labyrinth in the late congenital, late latent, and tertiary syphilis stages. Endolymphatic hydrops and degenerative changes in the sensory and neural structures are seen in both the congenital and acquired forms. Poor prognosis is indicated by endolymphatic sac obstruction by microgummata. The goal of treatment is to halt the progression of the disease. Treatment includes antibiotic and steroidal anti-inflammatory medication, and the medication of choice differs with the clinical stage of the disease.

■ Paraneoplastic Syndromes

Chief Clinical Characteristics

This presentation commonly includes visual, tactile, and hearing deficits in combination with a variety of different neurological symptoms and signs in an individual with cancer. Specific neurological symptoms and signs depend on the location of involvement of the central or peripheral nervous system.

Background Information

Paraneoplastic encephalomyelitis and focal encephalitis may present with ataxia, vertigo, balance deficits, nystagmus, nausea, vomiting, cranial nerve palsies, seizures, sensory neuropathy, anxiety, depression, cognitive changes, and hallucinations. For individuals presenting with ataxia, dysarthria, dysphagia, and diplopia, paraneoplastic cerebellar degeneration may be suspected. Paraneoplastic opsoclonus/myoclonus tends to affect both children and adults with signs and symptoms including hypotonia, ataxia, irritability, truncal ataxia, gait difficulty, balance deficits, and frequent falls. Stiff-man syndrome presents with spasms and fluctuating rigidity of axial musculature, legs and possibly shoulders, upper extremities, and neck. Paraneoplastic sensory neuropathy presents with asymmetric, progressive sensory alterations involving the limbs, trunk, and face, sensorineural hearing loss, autonomic dysfunction, and pain. Other conditions in this category include vasculitis, Lambert-Eaton myasthenia syndrome, myasthenia gravis, dermatomyositis, neuromyotonia, and various neuropathies.[1,82] These conditions result from an immune-mediated response to the presence of tumor or metastases. Antibodies or T-cells respond to the presence of the tumor, but also attack normal cells of the nervous system.[83,84] Over 60% of individuals present with this condition prior to the discovery of the cancer.[82] The underlying tumor is treated according to the type of cancer. Additional treatment is dependent on this condition's type and may include steroids, plasmapheresis, immunotherapy, chemotherapy, radiation, or cyclophosphamide.[82] Physical, occupational, and speech therapy may be indicated to address functional limitations.

■ Perforated Tympanum

Chief Clinical Characteristics

This presentation can be characterized by loss of hearing, tinnitus, and occasionally clear, pustular, or bloody discharge.

Background Information

This condition can result from a temporal skull fracture, foreign body obstruction, or loud explosion. Diagnosis is made by visual inspection through an otoscope. Spontaneous closure often occurs within 2 months. If the tympanum does not close spontaneously, surgical repair, in which thin paper patches are placed over the tympanum to support healing, is indicated. Complete restoration of hearing following surgical intervention is probable.

■ Perilymph Fistula

Chief Clinical Characteristics

This presentation may involve dizziness, vertigo, imbalance, nausea, and vomiting.[44] Some individuals with this condition experience ringing or fullness in the ears, and many notice a hearing loss. Most people with fistulas find that their symptoms get worse with changes in altitude (elevators, airplanes, travel over mountain passes) or air pressure (weather changes), as well as with exertion and activity.

Background Information

The cause of this condition is a tear or defect in the oval or round window in one or both ears, allowing pressure changes in the middle ear to stimulate the inner ear and cause symptoms. Head trauma via a direct blow and whiplash injury, barotrauma sustained during diving, weightlifting, and childbirth are among common causes. This condition also may be present from birth or may result from chronic, severe ear infections. Clinical tests suggestive of a fistula include reproduction of symptoms during a Valsalva maneuver or when applying pressure to the external auditory canal. The definitive diagnosis is made by direct visualization during tympanotomy. Surgical repair with grafting is indicated if symptoms persist despite nonsurgical care consisting of activity restriction aimed at avoiding lifting, straining (Valsalva maneuver), bending over, and changes in pressure.

■ Presbycusis

Chief Clinical Characteristics

This presentation includes the loss of hearing that gradually occurs in most individuals as they grow older. The loss associated with presbycusis is usually greater for high-pitched sounds.

Background Information

This condition is most often due to a gradual loss of sensory receptors in the inner ear. Decreasing exposure to loud noises is the best way to prevent this condition. Using a hearing aid after the development of this condition is often helpful. The degree to which hearing can be restored is dependent on the extent of loss.

■ Progressive Multifocal Leukoencephalopathy

Chief Clinical Characteristics

This presentation commonly involves cortical blindness, visual field defects, hemiparesis with progression to quadriparesis, aphasia, ataxia, dysarthria, personality changes, and impaired intellect evolving over a period of days to weeks.

Background Information

This condition is most likely due to viral infection of the central nervous system, which then causes widespread demyelinative lesions primarily of the cerebral hemispheres. Diagnosis is made by computed tomography and magnetic resonance imaging to localize the lesions. Treatment for individuals with acquired immunodeficiency syndrome consists of antiretroviral drug combinations and can lead to slower progression or even remission. Currently, no treatment exists to impair disease progression in individuals with this condition who do not have acquired immunodeficiency syndrome.[1]

■ Progressive Supranuclear Palsy (Richardson-Steele-Olszewski Syndrome)

Chief Clinical Characteristics

This presentation classically includes vertical gaze palsy, prominent instability, and falls within the first year of disease onset.[85] *Other characteristics may include rigidity, akinesia, dysarthria, dysphagia, and mild dementia. Falls were found to be the most commonly reported symptom with the majority of falls occurring in a backward direction.*[86] *Difficulty with voluntary vertical eye movements (usually downward) and involuntary saccades are relatively early features. The disease progresses to the point at which all voluntary eye movements are lost.*

Background Information

Some patients may not demonstrate difficulties with ocular movements for 1 to 3 years after disease onset. Most cases are sporadic; however, a pattern of inheritance compatible with autosomal dominant transmission has been described.[1] Diagnosis is based on clinical presentation, which includes a gradually progressive disorder with age of onset at 40 years or older, vertical supranuclear palsy, and postural instability with falls within the first year of disease onset.[87] Medical treatment is typically unsuccessful, because the majority of these patients are not responsive to levodopa therapy aimed at addressing the extrapyramidal features of the disease.[88] Physical and occupational therapy are used to maintain mobility and address safety issues related to the progression of imbalance. The disease course is progressive with a mean survival time of 5.6 years.[86] Older age at disease onset, early onset of falls, incontinence, dysarthria, dysphagia, insertion of a percutaneous gastrostomy, and diplopia have all been described as being predictive of shorter survival time.[86]

■ Restless Legs Syndrome

Chief Clinical Characteristics

This presentation includes complaints of unpleasant sensations located in the legs, which commonly leads to additional problems such as sleep disturbances and depression.

Background Information

Etiology of restless legs syndrome is unknown, but commonly occurs with pregnancy, iron depletion, uremia, polyneuropathy, spinal disorders, and rheumatoid arthritis. Diagnosis is based on subjective reports. Active movement, massage, or cold compressions can provide temporary relief, and dopaminergic treatment can provide longer term relief. There is no cure however, and symptoms progressively worsen with age.[89]

■ Retinitis

Chief Clinical Characteristics

This presentation typically involves decreased vision at night or in reduced light, loss of peripheral vision, and near blindness in advanced cases.

Background Information

This condition is a progressive degeneration of the retina, affecting rods more frequently than cones. Tests to determine the integrity of the retina confirm the diagnosis, including slit lamp examination, intraocular pressure determination, and eye ultrasound. There is no known effective treatment for this slowly progressive condition, but sunglasses may protect the retina and antioxidants may have a preventive effect.

■ Rickettsial Diseases, Including Rocky Mountain Spotted Fever

Chief Clinical Characteristics

This presentation typically includes visual disturbances, a rash that occurs on the palms of hands and soles of feet, headache, nausea, fever, and myalgias.[90] Initial symptoms begin within 2 to 14 days of infection and last approximately 2 to 3 weeks.

Background Information

Rocky Mountain spotted fever is the most common type of this condition in the United States. It is transmitted by a variety of tick, and is common in Long Island, Tennessee, Virginia, North Carolina, and Maryland.[1] Like malaria, rickettsiae in the blood vessels cause vascular injury, which forms the basis for central nervous system damage. Diagnosis is based on clinical signs and symptoms and confirmed by skin biopsy. Treatment consists of the use of doxycycline or chloramphenicol. The mortality rate in untreated cases is 20% to 25%.[91]

SPINAL CORD INJURIES

■ Brown-Sequard Syndrome

Chief Clinical Characteristics

This presentation can be characterized by ipsilateral loss of strength and tactile discrimination, position, and vibration sense, with contralateral hemianesthesia to pain and temperature secondary to spinal cord injury, disk herniation, tumor, ischemia, or inflammatory disorder.[92,93]

Background Information

This condition occurs secondary to lateral hemisection of the spinal cord, usually below

the cervical enlargement, disrupting ipsilateral corticospinal and dorsal column tracts and contralateral projections of the spinothalamic tract.[5] Medical management consists of diagnosis via imaging, appropriate medical care in the acute care setting, surgical decompression of spinal cord if indicated, and multidisciplinary rehabilitation.[94] Outcome is favorable in most patients following surgical decompression of disk herniation or tumor, demonstrating vast improvement in motor function with minimal residual sensory deficits.[93]

■ Central Cord Syndrome

Chief Clinical Characteristics

This presentation commonly involves presentation of profound weakness of the arms and hands, and to a lesser extent the legs, commonly due to traumatic spinal cord injury. Associated sensory loss below the level of the lesion and/or sphincter dysfunction may occur.

Background Information

Damage to the more centrally located ascending and descending spinal tracts results in this characteristic presentation of motor and sensory loss. Medical management consists of diagnosis via imaging, appropriate medical care in the acute care setting, reduction of fracture and/or surgical decompression of spinal cord, and multidisciplinary rehabilitation.[95] Many individuals with central cord syndrome recover the ability to walk, but impairment of fine motor control in the hands often remains.[96]

■ Conus Medullaris Syndrome

Chief Clinical Characteristics

This presentation typically involves weakness of the lower extremities in association with hyperreflexia, bowel/bladder dysfunction, sexual dysfunction, and sensory loss in a dermatomal pattern of the sacral segments.[5]

Background Information

The presentation of weakness with upper motor neuron symptoms is secondary to injury to the conus medullaris, most commonly due to trauma (vertebral body fracture of acute disk herniations of the thoracolumbar junction).[97] Diagnosis and treatment involve clinical examination, imaging, and surgical investigation, decompression, fusion, and fixation if indicated. Improvement in spinal cord function, bladder function, and nerve root recovery following surgical intervention occurs in more than half of the patients following surgical intervention.[98]

■ Traumatic Spinal Cord Injury

Chief Clinical Characteristics

This presentation is characterized by loss of sensation in a dermatomal pattern, hypertonicity, spasticity, hyperreflexia, and sphincter dysfunction in combination with muscle weakness. Specific syndromes (discussed below) have characteristic presentations secondary to the location of the lesion.

Background Information

Insult to the spinal cord results from fractured bone, displaced disk material, or a foreign object transecting or injuring the cord. Imaging is used to identify the cause of injury and direct surgical stabilization or intervention. Motor vehicle accidents and falls are the most common etiology of this condition.[99] Physical examination of strength and sensation is used to assign a score from the American Spinal Injury Association.[100] Injuries are classified in terms of neurological level (ie, most rostral segment where myotomal and dermatomal function is spared) and extent as either complete (total lack of sensory or motor function below level of injury) or incomplete (some motor or sensory function spared below the level of injury). Cervical locations of injury result in tetraplegia and may cause paralysis or weakness of the respiratory musculature, requiring mechanical ventilation and/or respiratory strengthening.[101] Thoracic or lumbar locations of injury result in paraplegia. Cauda equina syndrome occurs following injury inferior to the conus medullaris. Treatment consists of medical management, multidisciplinary rehabilitation, equipment prescription, and prevention of pressure ulcers, contractures, and further complications. Individuals with incomplete forms of this condition may continue to recover strength and function, while individuals with complete forms of this condition have a poor prognosis for recovery and instead use compensatory techniques and

equipment. Individuals with this condition require adequate follow-up medical care to prevent secondary impairments.[102] Acute forms of this condition constitute a medical emergency.

■ Stroke (Cerebrovascular Accident)

Chief Clinical Characteristics

This presentation may include a wide range of symptoms that correspond to specific areas of the brain that are affected. The initial symptoms can include numbness or weakness, especially on one side of the body or face; visual disturbances, confusion or aphasia; balance deficits or falls; or sudden severe headache with no known cause.

Background Information

This condition occurs when blood flow to the brain is interrupted either by blockage (ischemia or infarction) or from hemorrhagic disruption. A thrombosis or embolic occlusion of an artery causes an ischemic type of this condition. A hemorrhagic type of this condition can be caused by arteriovenous malformation, hypertension, aneurysm, neoplasm, drug abuse and trauma. This condition is the most common and disabling neurological disorder in adults and occurs in 114 of every 100,000 people.[103] This condition is diagnosed using clinical presentation and positive findings on computed tomography and magnetic resonance imaging. Medication, surgery, and interdisciplinary therapy are the most common treatments for this condition. The prognosis for recovery is predicted by the magnitude of initial deficit. Factors that are associated with poor outcomes include coma, poor cognition, severe aphasia, severe hemiparesis with little return within 1 month, visual perceptual disorders, depression, and incontinence after 2 weeks.[104,105]

■ Systemic Lupus Erythematosus

Chief Clinical Characteristics

This presentation can include abnormal vision, swallowing, taste, hearing, changes in mood or thinking, and seizures in combination with fatigue, joint pain, and swelling affecting the hands, feet, knees, and shoulders.

Background Information

This condition affects mostly women of childbearing age. It is a chronic autoimmune disorder that can affect any organ system, including skin, joints, kidneys, brain, heart, lungs, and blood. Microinfarcts in the cerebral cortex and brainstem, which lead to destructive and proliferative changes in capillaries and arterioles, are primarily responsible for central nervous system manifestations. Hypertension and endocarditis can also predispose an affected individual to development of neurological abnormalities. Multiple sclerosis is a disease that may be mistaken for this condition, especially if the central nervous system manifestations include visual dysfunction. The diagnosis is confirmed by the presence of skin lesions; heart, lung, or kidney involvement; laboratory abnormalities including low red or white cell counts, low platelet counts, or positive ANA and anti-DNA antibody tests.[106] Treatment involves corticosteroid medication.

■ Tethered Spinal Cord Syndrome

Chief Clinical Characteristics

This presentation typically includes back pain associated with neurological deficits and bowel and bladder dysfunction.[107] The most common manifestations of this condition are worsening in motor function of the lower extremities (and less likely the upper extremities), changes in muscle tone and deep tendon reflexes, progressive loss of articular dexterity, progressively worsening scoliosis or kyphosis, and back or leg pain.[108]

Background Information

This condition occurs commonly in children, but also can present in undiagnosed adults. Magnetic resonance imaging confirms the diagnosis, with a low-lying (caudally positioned) conus medullaris present. Surgical resection of a thickened filum terminale is a common treatment.

■ Thoracic Outlet Syndrome

Chief Clinical Characteristics

This presentation can be characterized by swelling or puffiness in the arm or hand; bluish discoloration of the hand; a feeling of heaviness in the arm or hand; deep, boring toothache-like pain in the neck and shoulder region that seems to increase at night; easily fatigued arms and hands; superficial vein distention in the hand; paresthesias along the inside forearm and the palm; muscle weakness with difficulty gripping and performing fine motor tasks of the hand; atrophy of the muscles of the palm; cramps of the muscles on the inner forearm; pain in the arm and hand; and tingling and numbness in the neck, shoulder region, arm, and hand.

Background Information

There are three types of this condition, which can coexist or occur independently: compression of the subclavian vein, compression of the subclavian artery, and a primary neurological syndrome. Multiple anatomical anomalies can lead to thoracic outlet syndrome, including an incomplete cervical rib, a taut fibrous band passing from the transverse process of C7 to the first rib, and a complete rib that articulates with the first rib, or anomalies of the position and insertion of the anterior and medial scalene muscles. Diagnosis includes physical examination tests (eg, Adson's test, extremity abducted stress test, costoclavicular sign), radiology of the cervical spine, and nerve conduction and electromyography studies. Nonsurgical approaches to treatment include exercise, stretches, modalities, and analgesic medication. Surgery is indicated if pain is persistent and severe neurogenic or vascular features of the syndrome exist. Prognosis for decreased pain and improved function is good for the majority of individuals with this condition.

■ Transient Ischemic Attack

Chief Clinical Characteristics

This presentation can include numbness or weakness in the face, arm, or leg, especially on one side of the body; confusion or difficulty in talking or understanding speech; trouble seeing in one or both eyes; and difficulty with walking, dizziness, or loss of balance and coordination.

Background Information

This condition is a transient stroke that lasts only a few minutes. It occurs when the blood supply to part of the brain is briefly interrupted. Symptoms of this condition, which usually occur suddenly, are similar to those of stroke but do not last as long. Most symptoms disappear within an hour, although they may persist for up to 24 hours. Because it is impossible to differentiate between symptoms from this condition and acute stroke, individuals should assume that all stroke-like symptoms signal a medical emergency. A prompt evaluation (within 60 minutes) is necessary to identify the cause of this condition and determine appropriate therapy. Depending on the individual's medical history and the results of a medical examination, the doctor may recommend drug therapy or surgery to reduce the risk of stroke. Antiplatelet medications, particularly aspirin, are a standard treatment for individuals suspected of having this condition and who also are at risk for stroke, including individuals with atrial fibrillation.

■ Transverse Myelitis

Chief Clinical Characteristics

This presentation involves the gradual development of sensory changes, back or neck pain, weakness, and/or bowel and bladder dysfunction over the course of several hours to weeks.

Background Information

This condition occurs when inflammation affects the spinal cord, but the brain can be affected as well. Inflammation can result from viral infections, abnormal immune reactions, or ischemia, or present as an idiopathic form. Diagnosis is established by exclusion through imaging and blood tests. The first line of treatment requires accurate diagnosis of the underlying pathology and decreasing inflammation in the acute stage, usually by way of corticosteroid medication. Physical therapy is indicated to address secondary impairments and provide supportive therapy. Recovery from transverse myelitis usually begins within 2 to 12 weeks of the onset of symptoms and may continue for up to 2 years. The majority of recovery occurs within the first 3 to 6 months. About one-third of people affected with transverse myelitis experience good or full recovery from their symptoms, regaining the ability to ambulate. Another one-third is left with significant deficits, while the remaining one-third demonstrates no recovery at all. Prognosis varies between recovery without relapse to a permanent presence of symptoms, with the primary poor prognostic factors being pain in the midthoracic region or an abrupt, severe onset of symptoms.[1]

■ Traumatic Brain Injury

Chief Clinical Characteristics

This presentation typically includes dysequilibrium in the presence of cognitive changes, altered level of consciousness, seizures, nausea, vomiting, coma, dizziness, headache, pupillary changes, tinnitus, weakness, incoordination, behavioral changes, spasticity, hypertonicity, cranial nerve lesions, and sensory and motor deficits.[1,109]

Background Information

This condition can be classified as mild, moderate, or severe based on Glasgow Coma Scale, length of coma, and duration of post-traumatic amnesia.[109] Magnetic resonance imaging may be used to confirm the diagnosis.[68] Treatment initiated at the scene of the accident and during the acute phase is focused on medical stabilization.[110] Low Glasgow Coma Scale, longer length of coma, longer duration of post-traumatic amnesia, and older age tend to be associated with poor outcomes.[111] Optimal rehabilitation is interdisciplinary and customized to address the specific individuals' disablement.

■ Tropical Spastic Paraparesis

Chief Clinical Characteristics

This presentation commonly involves slowly progressive paresis of the lower extremities, sphincter dysfunction early in the disease course, paresthesias, and uncoordinated movements.[1]

Background Information

The retrovirus human T-cell leukemia virus type 1 causes a chronic infective-inflammatory disease of the spinal cord, which results in the symptoms of this condition. Diagnosis is confirmed by the presence of the serum of the antibodies to human T-cell leukemia virus type 1 in the cerebrospinal fluid. Magnetic resonance imaging also reveals thinness of the spinal cord. Treatment is primarily symptomatic with focus on improved urinary function and decreased spasticity. Steroidal medications and gamma globulin may be used. The majority of individuals with this disease survive.[112]

TUMORS

■ Brain Metastases

Chief Clinical Characteristics

This presentation may include headaches, seizures, dysphagia, weakness, cognitive changes, behavioral changes, dizziness, vomiting, alterations in the level of consciousness, ataxia, aphasia, nystagmus, visual disturbances, dysarthria, balance deficits, falls, lethargy, and incoordination.[1,113]

Background Information

The majority of individuals with brain metastases have been previously diagnosed with a primary tumor; however, a small percentage of individuals are diagnosed concomitantly with brain metastases and the primary tumor. The most common cancers resulting in subsequent brain metastases include lung, breast, melanoma, colorectal, and genitourinary tract. The new onset of neurological symptoms after a primary tumor warrants the use of imaging such as magnetic resonance imaging or computed tomography to confirm the diagnosis. Treatment may include corticosteroids, brain irradiation, surgery, chemotherapy, radiotherapy, and rehabilitative therapies. The prognosis is poor with death typically occurring within 6 months.

■ Brain Primary Tumors

Chief Clinical Characteristics

This presentation may include headaches, seizures, dysphagia, weakness, cognitive changes, behavioral changes, dizziness, vomiting, alterations in the level of consciousness, ataxia, aphasia, nystagmus, visual disturbances, dysarthria, balance deficits, falls, lethargy, and incoordination.[1,69]

Background Information

Glioblastoma multiforme, astrocytoma, oligodendroglioma, metastatic tumors, primary central nervous system lymphomas, ganglioglioma, neuroblastoma, meningioma, arachnoid cysts, hemangioblastoma, medulloblastoma, and acoustic neuroma/schwannoma are some of the more common brain tumors. Specific diagnoses for brain tumors may be confirmed with imaging and biopsy. Treatment is variable depending on the type, size, and location of the tumor and may include surgical resection, chemotherapy, radiation,

corticosteroids, and rehabilitative therapies. Prognosis is also variable and depends on the type and grade of tumor, severity of compression, and duration of compression.

■ Nasopharyngeal Carcinoma

Chief Clinical Characteristics

This presentation may include facial pain combined with headaches, palpable mass in the head or neck, bloody nasal discharge, chronic unilateral nasal congestion, unilateral hearing loss or frequent ear infections, or cranial nerve signs.

Background Information

Nasopharyngeal tumors usually develop in the wall of the nasopharynx. The relatively large amount of space to occupy in this region of the body results in a late onset of presenting symptoms and diagnostic delay. This may result in a poorer prognosis related to advanced tumor development and increased potential for metastatic spread. The diagnosis is confirmed with fused positron emission tomography–computed tomography and head/neck magnetic resonance imaging. Treatment typically depends on cancer staging, ranging from surgical resection and radiation therapy to chemotherapy.

■ Oropharyngeal Carcinoma

Chief Clinical Characteristics

This presentation may involve facial pain combined with hoarseness, throat pain, change in tongue sensation, pain in the tongue, and lump in the neck region, dysphagia, dyspnea, coughing, or hemoptysis.

Background Information

Up to 90% of oropharyngeal carcinomas are squamous cell carcinomas, or abnormal collections of squamous cells on histological observation. Lower patient socioeconomic status, patient and clinician delay in recognizing the health condition, lack of indirect laryngoscopy performed on physical examination, failure to inspect the site of the tumor, and clinician failure to consider tumor or infection as potential causes of symptoms are associated with overlooking this disease process. In turn, overlooking this disease process results in reduced prognosis.[114] Computed tomography and magnetic resonance imaging can further confirm the diagnosis. Treatment typically depends on cancer staging, ranging from surgical resection and radiation therapy to chemotherapy.[115]

■ Retinoblastoma

Chief Clinical Characteristics

This presentation may include leukocoria (white reflection from the retina of the eye) and strabismus (more commonly known as "cross eyes").

Background Information

Retinoblastoma is a rare childhood tumor that is diagnosed by funduscopy most commonly between 1 and 2 years of age. Sixty percent of cases are unilateral, while the remainder are bilateral. Treatment typically involves laser therapy, chemotherapy, cryotherapy, and brachytherapy. More severe cases occasionally require external beam radiotherapy. Prognosis is excellent.[116]

■ Spinal Metastases

Chief Clinical Characteristics

This presentation can involve spasticity, weakness, sensory alterations, bowel and bladder incontinence, neck pain, back pain, radicular pain, atrophy, cerebellar signs, balance deficits, falls, and cranial nerve involvement.[1,69,117]

Background Information

This condition is the most frequent neoplasm involving the spine.[117] The most common types and locations of primary tumors that result in spinal metastases include breast, lung, lymphoma, prostate, kidney, gastrointestinal tract, and thyroid.[1,118] The diagnosis is confirmed with gadolinium enhanced magnetic resonance imaging and computed tomography.[1,117] Treatment is variable depending on the tumor and may include surgical resection, chemotherapy, radiation, corticosteroids, and rehabilitative therapies.[1] Although the long-term prognosis is poor, individuals without paresis and pain and who are still ambulatory have longer survival rates.[118]

■ Spinal Primary Tumors

Chief Clinical Characteristics

This presentation may include spasticity, weakness, sensory alterations, bowel/bladder incontinence, back pain, radicular pain, atrophy, ataxia, balance deficits, and falls.[7]

Background Information

Types of this condition include astrocytomas, ependymomas, hemangioblastoma, myeloma, neurofibroma, lymphoma, metastasis, meningioma, schwannoma, and astrocytoma. Extradural tumors, such as meningiomas, produce a rapid onset of symptoms, with weakness being predominant. Intramedullary tumors, or ependymomas, astrocytomas, and hemangioblastomas, present with slowly progressive symptoms, of which loss of pain and temperature sensation is usually the first. The first test to diagnose brain and spinal column tumors is a neurological examination. Special imaging techniques (computed tomography, magnetic resonance imaging, positron emission tomography) are also employed. Specific diagnoses may be confirmed with imaging and biopsy. Treatment is variable depending on the type, size, and location of the tumor and may include surgical resection, chemotherapy, radiation, corticosteroids, and rehabilitative therapies. Prognosis is variable and depends on the type and grade of tumor, severity of compression, and duration of compression.

■ Vasculitis (Giant Cell Arteritis, Temporal Arteritis, Cranial Arteritis)

Chief Clinical Characteristics

This presentation can be characterized by headaches, psychiatric syndromes, dementia, peripheral or cranial nerve involvement, pain, seizures, hypertension, hemiparesis, balance deficits, neuropathies, myopathies, organ involvement, fever, and weight loss.[1,69,119]

Background Information

This condition is the result of an immune-mediated response resulting in the inflammation of vascular structures.[1,119] It includes a variety of disorders such as giant cell/temporal arteritis (which is the most common form), primary angiitis of the central nervous system, Takayasu's disease, periarteritis nodosa, Kawasaki disease, Churg-Strauss syndrome, Wegener's granulomatosis, and secondary vasculitis associated with systemic lupus erythematous, rheumatoid arthritis, and scleroderma.[119] The diagnosis is confirmed through history, physical examination, laboratory testing, angiography, biopsy, and imaging.[1,69,119] Corticosteroids, cytotoxic agents, intravenous immunoglobulin, and plasmapheresis may be used in the treatment of vasculitis.[69,119] Prognosis is variable and depends on the specific underlying disorder. For example, giant cell arteritis is typically self-limiting within 1 to 2 years; however, death usually occurs within 1 year for individuals with primary angiitis of the central nervous system.[119]

Vitamin B₁₂ Deficiency

Chief Clinical Characteristics

This presentation involves paresthesias in a stocking and glove distribution, weakness, impaired memory, irritability, and depression.

Background Information

Nutritional deficiency and gastrointestinal dysfunction cause this condition. Clinical evidence of disease, low serum vitamin B₁₂ levels, and measurements of metabolites such as methylmalonic acid and homocysteine confirm the diagnosis. Anemia is often associated with this condition. Treatment includes oral or parenteral vitamin B₁₂ replacement. Repeated measurement of serum vitamin B₁₂, methylmalonic acid, and homocysteine levels should be performed every 2 to 3 months after initiating treatment. If this condition is associated with severe anemia, marked improvement should be seen within a few weeks.[120]

References

1. Victor M, Ropper AH. *Adams and Victor's Principles of Neurology.* 7th ed. New York, NY: McGraw-Hill; 2001.
2. Birmingham CL, Su J, Hlynsky JA, Goldner EM, Gao M. The mortality rate from anorexia nervosa. *Int J Eat Disord.* Sep 2005;38(2):143–146.
3. American Psychiatric Association. *Diagnostic and Statistical Manual of Mental Disorders, Text Revision.* 4th ed. Washington, DC: American Psychiatric Association; 2000.
4. Halgin RP, Whitbourne SK. *Abnormal Psychology. The Human Experience of Psychological Disorders.* 2nd ed. Madison, WI: Brown and Benchmark; 1997.
5. Ropper AH, Brown RJ. *Adams and Victor's Principles of Neurology.* 8th ed. New York, NY: McGraw-Hill; 2005.
6. Steinbok P. Clinical features of Chiari I malformations. *Childs Nerv Syst.* May 2004;20(5):329–331.
7. Al-Otaibi LM, Porter SR, Poate TW. Behcet's disease: a review. *J Dent Res.* Mar 2005;84(3):209–222.
8. Nakamura K, Toda N, Sakamaki K, Kashima K, Takeda N. Biofeedback rehabilitation for prevention of

9. Allen D, Dunn L. Acyclovir or valacyclovir for Bell's palsy (idiopathic facial paralysis). *Cochrane Database Syst Rev.* 2004(3):CD001869.
10. VanSwearingen JM, Brach JS. Validation of a treatment-based classification system for individuals with facial neuromotor disorders. *Phys Ther.* Jul 1998;78(7): 678–689.
11. Ramsey MJ, DerSimonian R, Holtel MR, Burgess LP. Corticosteroid treatment for idiopathic facial nerve paralysis: a meta-analysis. *Laryngoscope.* Mar 2000;110 (3 pt 1):335–341.
12. Fitzgerald DC. Head trauma: hearing loss and dizziness [see comment]. *J Trauma-Injury Infect Crit Care.* 1996;40(3):488–496.
13. Herdman S, ed. *Vestibular Rehabilitation.* 2nd ed. Philadelphia, PA: F. A. Davis; 2000.
14. Hilton M, Pinder D. The Epley (canalith repositioning) manoeuvre for benign paroxysmal positional vertigo. [update of *Cochrane Database Syst Rev.* 2002;(1): CD003162; PMID: 11869655]. *Cochrane Database Syst Rev.* 2004(2):CD003162.
15. Nunez RA, Cass SP, Furman JM. Short- and long-term outcomes of canalith repositioning for benign paroxysmal positional vertigo. *Otolaryngol Head Neck Surg.* 2000;122:647–652.
16. Froehling DA, Bowen JM, Mohr DN, et al. The canalith repositioning procedure for the treatment of benign paroxysmal positional vertigo: a randomized controlled trial. *Mayo Clinic Proc.* Jul 2000;75(7):695–700.
17. Parnes LS, Agrawal SK, Atlas J. Diagnosis and management of benign paroxysmal positional vertigo (BPPV). *CMAJ.* Sep 30 2003;169(7):681–693.
18. Tusa RJ. Benign paroxysmal positional vertigo. *Curr Neurol Neurosci Rep.* Sep 2001;1(5):478–485.
19. Dornhoffer JL, Colvin GB. Benign paroxysmal positional vertigo and canalith repositioning: clinical correlations. *Am J Otol.* Mar 2000;21(2):230–233.
20. Cohen HS, Jerabek J. Efficacy of treatments for posterior canal benign paroxysmal positional vertigo. *Laryngoscope.* Apr 1999;109(4):584–590.
21. Agrawal SK, Parnes LS. Human experience with canal plugging. *Ann NY Acad Sci.* Oct 2001;942:300–305.
22. Dubuisson AS, Kline DG. Brachial plexus injury: a survey of 100 consecutive cases from a single service. *Neurosurgery.* Sep 2002;51(3):673–682; discussion 682–683.
23. Kim DH, Cho YJ, Tiel RL, Kline DG. Outcomes of surgery in 1019 brachial plexus lesions treated at Louisiana State University Health Sciences Center. *J Neurosurg.* May 2003;98(5):1005–1016.
24. Choi PD, Novak CB, Mackinnon SE, Kline DG. Quality of life and functional outcome following brachial plexus injury. *J Hand Surg [Am].* Jul 1997;22(4):605–612.
25. Katz JN, Simmons BP. Clinical practice. Carpal tunnel syndrome. *N Engl J Med.* Jun 6 2002;346(23):1807–1812.
26. MacDermid JC, Wessel J. Clinical diagnosis of carpal tunnel syndrome: a systematic review. *J Hand Ther.* Apr–Jun 2004;17(2):309–319.
27. Goodyear-Smith F, Arroll B. What can family physicians offer patients with carpal tunnel syndrome other than surgery? A systematic review of nonsurgical management. *Ann Fam Med.* May–Jun 2004;2(3):267–273.
28. Quillen DA. Common causes of vision loss in elderly patients. *Am Fam Physician.* Jul 1999;60(1):99–108.

synkinesis after facial palsy. *Otolaryngol Head Neck Surg.* Apr 2003;128(4):539–543.

29. Klein R, Peto T, Bird A, Vannewkirk MR. The epidemiology of age-related macular degeneration. *Am J Ophthalmol.* Mar 2004;137(3):486–495.

30. Sage MR, Blumbergs PC. Cavernous haemangiomas (angiomas) of the brain. *Australas Radiol.* May 2001; 45(2):247–256.

31. Schievink WI. Intracranial aneurysms. *N Engl J Med.* Jan 2 1997;336(1):28–40.

32. Vogel T, Verreault R, Turcotte JF, Kiesmann M, Berthel M. Intracerebral aneurysms: a review with special attention to geriatric aspects. *J Gerontol A Biol Sci Med Sci.* Jun 2003;58(6):520–524.

33. Consensus statement on the definition of orthostatic hypotension, pure autonomic failure, and multiple system atrophy. The Consensus Committee of the American Autonomic Society and the American Academy of Neurology. *Neurology.* May 1996;46(5):1470.

34. Unruptured intracranial aneurysms—risk of rupture and risks of surgical intervention. International Study of Unruptured Intracranial Aneurysms Investigators. *N Engl J Med.* Dec 10 1998;339(24):1725–1733.

35. Merskey H, Bogduk N. *Classification of Chronic Pain: Descriptions of Chronic Pain Syndromes and Definitions of Pain Terms.* Seattle, WA: IASP Press; 1994.

36. Krem MM. Motor conversion disorders reviewed from a neuropsychiatric perspective. *J Clin Psychiatry.* Jun 2004;65(6):783–790.

37. D'Amico DJ. Clinical practice. Primary retinal detachment. *N Engl J Med.* Nov 27 2008;359(22):2346–2354.

38. Mankin HJ, Rosenthal DI, Xavier R. Gaucher disease. New approaches to an ancient disease. *J Bone Joint Surg Am.* May 2001;83-A(5):748–762.

39. Sharma P, Sample PA, Zangwill LM, Schuman JS. Diagnostic tools for glaucoma detection and management. *Surv Ophthalmol.* Nov 2008;53 Suppl1:S17–32.

40. Chen TM, George S, Woodruff CA, Hsu S. Clinical manifestations of varicella-zoster virus infection. *Dermatol Clin.* Apr 2002;20(2):267–282.

41. Galvin JA, Van Stavern GP. Clinical characterization of idiopathic intracranial hypertension at the Detroit Medical Center. *J Neurol Sci.* 2004;30(223(2)):157–160.

42. Friedman DI, Jacobson DM. Diagnostic criteria for idiopathic intracranial hypertension. *Neurology.* 2002;59:1492–1495.

43. Froehling DA, Silverstein MD, Mohr DN, Beatty CW. Does this dizzy patient have a serious form of vertigo? *JAMA.* 1994;271(5):385–388.

44. Strupp M, Arbusow V. Acute Vestibulopathy. *Curr Opin Neurol.* 2001;14(1):11–20.

45. Yardley L, Beech S, Zander L, Evans T, Weinman J. A randomized controlled trial of exercise therapy for dizziness and vertigo in primary care [see comments]. *Br J Gen Pract.* 1998;48(429):1136–1140.

46. Kim JS. Pure lateral medullary infarction: clinical-radiological correlation of 130 acute, consecutive patients. *Brain.* 2003;126:1864–1872.

47. Nelles G, Contois KA, Valente SL, Jacobs DH, Kaplan JD, Pessin MS. Recovery following lateral medullary infarction. *Neurology.* 1998;50(5):1418–1422.

48. Reider B, Arcand MA, Diehl LH, et al. Proprioception of the knee before and after anterior cruciate ligament reconstruction. *Arthroscopy.* Jan 2003;19(1):2–12.

49. Rose A, Lee RJ, Williams RM, Thomson LC, Forsyth A. Functional instability in noncontact ankle ligament injuries. *Br J Sports Med.* Oct 2000;34(5):352–358.

50. de Jong PT. Age-related macular degeneration. *N Engl J Med.* Oct 5 2006;355(14):1474–1485.

51. Thorp MA, Shehab ZP, Bance ML, Rutka JA, Equilibrium A-HCoHa. The AAO-HNS Committee on Hearing and Equilibrium guidelines for the diagnosis and evaluation of therapy in Meniere's disease: have they been applied in the published literature of the last decade? *Clin Otolaryngol Allied Sci.* Jun 2003;28(3):173–176.

52. Carey J. Intratympanic gentamicin for the treatment of Meniere's disease and other forms of peripheral vertigo. *Otolaryngol Clin North Am.* Oct 2004;37(5):1075–1090.

53. Cohen-Kerem R, Kisilevsky V, Einarson TR, Kozer E, Koren G, Rutka JA. Intratympanic gentamicin for Meniere's disease: a meta-analysis. *Laryngoscope.* Dec 2004;114(12):2085–2091.

54. Ervin SE. Meniere's disease: identifying classic symptoms and current treatments. *AAOHN J.* Apr 2004; 52(4):156–158.

55. James A, Thorp M. Meniere's disease [update of *Clin Evid.* 2003 Jun;(9):565–573; PMID: 12967379]. *Clin Evid.* Jun 2004(11):664–672.

56. Minor LB, Schessel DA, Carey JP. Meniere's disease. *Curr Opin Neurol.* Feb 2004;17(1):9–16.

57. Neuhauser H, Lempert T. Vertigo and dizziness related to migraine: a diagnostic challenge [see comment]. *Cephalalgia.* Feb 2004;24(2):83–91.

58. Boyev KP. Meniere's disease or migraine? The clinical significance of fluctuating hearing loss with vertigo. [see comment]. *Arch Otolaryngol Head Neck Surg.* May 2005;131(5):457–459.

59. Just T, Homoth J, Graumuller S, Pau HW. [Taste disorders and recovery of the taste function after middle ear surgery]. *Laryngorhinootologie.* Jul 2003;82(7):494–500.

60. Spierings ELH. Mechanisms of migraine and Actions of Antimigraine Medications. *Med Clin North Am.* 2001;85(4):943–958.

61. Ferrari MD. Migraine. *Lancet.* Apr 4 1998;351(9108): 1043–1051.

62. Marks DR, Rapoport AM. Diagnosis of migraine. *Semin Neurol.* 1997;17(4):303–306.

63. Maizels M. Headache evaluation and treatment by primary care physicians in an emergency department in the era of triptans. *Arch Intern Med.* 2001;161:1969–1973.

64. McDonald WI, Compston A, Edan G, et al. Recommended diagnostic criteria for multiple sclerosis: guidelines from the International Panel on the Diagnosis of Multiple Sclerosis. *Ann Neurol.* Jul 2001;50(1):121–127.

65. Thompson AJ, Montalban X, Barkhof F, et al. Diagnostic criteria for primary progressive multiple sclerosis: a position paper. *Ann Neurol.* Jun 2000;47(6):831–835.

66. Confavreux C, Vukusic S, Adeleine P. Early clinical predictors and progression of irreversible disability in multiple sclerosis: an amnesic process. *Brain.* Apr 2003; 126(Pt 4):770–782.

67. Price RW. Neurological complications of HIV infection. *Lancet.* Aug 17 1996;348(9025):445–452.

68. Lindsay KW, Bone I, Callander, R. *Neurology and Neurosurgery Illustrated.* 3rd ed. New York, NY: Churchill Livingstone; 1997.

69. Bergamaschi R, Ghezzi A. Devic's neuromyelitis optica: clinical features and prognostic factors. *Neurol Sci.* Nov 2004;25(suppl 4):S364–367.

70. Boulton AJ, Vinik AI, Arezzo JC, et al. Diabetic neuropathies: a statement by the American Diabetes Association. *Diabetes Care.* Apr 2005;28(4):956–962.

71. Poncelet AN. Diabetic polyneuropathy. Risk factors, patterns of presentation, diagnosis, and treatment. *Geriatrics.* Jun 2003;58(6):16–18, 24–25, 30.

72. Vinik AI, Park TS, Stansberry KB, Pittenger GL. Diabetic neuropathies. *Diabetologia.* Aug 2000;43(8):957–973.

73. Mitsumoto H, Wilbourn AJ. Causes and diagnosis of sensory neuropathies: a review. *J Clin Neurophysiol.* Nov 1994;11(6):553–567.

74. Rossi LN, Lutschg J, Meier C, Vassella F. Hereditary motor sensory neuropathies in childhood. *Dev Med Child Neurol.* Feb 1983;25(1):19–31.

75. Zaida DJ, Alexander MK. Falls in the elderly: identifying and managing peripheral neuropathy. *Nurse Pract.* Mar 2001;26(3):86–88.

76. Richardson JK, Ashton-Miller JA. Peripheral neuropathy: an often-overlooked cause of falls in the elderly. *Postgrad Med.* Jun 1996;99(6):161–172.

77. Bromberg MB. An approach to the evaluation of peripheral neuropathies. *Semin Neurol.* Jun 2005;25(2):153–159.

78. Brown DL, Frank JE. Diagnosis and management of syphilis. *Am Fam Physician.* Jul 15 2003;68(2):283–290.

79. Conde-Sendin MA, Amela-Peris R, Aladro-Benito Y, Maroto AA. Current clinical spectrum of neurosyphilis in immunocompetent patients. *Eur Neurol.* 2004;52(1):29–35.

80. Fayad JN, Linthicum FH, Jr. Temporal bone histopathology case of the month: otosyphilis. *Am J Otol.* Mar 1999;20(2):259–260.

81. Klemm E, Wollina U. Otosyphilis: report on six cases. *J Eur Acad Dermatol Venereol.* Jul 2004;18(4):429–434.

82. Bataller L, Dalmau J. Paraneoplastic neurologic syndromes: approaches to diagnosis and treatment. *Semin Neurol.* Jun 2003;23(2):215–224.

83. Darnell RB, Posner JB. Paraneoplastic syndromes involving the nervous system. *N Engl J Med.* Oct 16 2003;349(16):1543–1554.

84. Dalmau JO, Posner JB. Paraneoplastic syndromes. *Arch Neurol.* Apr 1999;56(4):405–408.

85. Borrell E. Hypokinetic movement disorders. *J Neurosci Nurs.* Oct 2000;32(5):254–255.

86. Litvan I, Mangone CA, McKee A, et al. Natural history of progressive supranuclear palsy (Steele-Richardson-Olszewski syndrome) and clinical predictors of survival: a clinicopathological study. *J Neurol Neurosurg Psychiatry.* Jun 1996;60(6):615–620.

87. Litvan I, Bhatia KP, Burn DJ, et al. Movement Disorders Society Scientific Issues Committee report: SIC Task Force appraisal of clinical diagnostic criteria for parkinsonian disorders. *Mov Disord.* May 2003;18(5):467–486.

88. Kompoliti K, Goetz CG, Boeve BF, et al. Clinical presentation and pharmacological therapy in corticobasal degeneration. *Arch Neurol.* Jul 1998;55(7):957–961.

89. Trenkwalder C, Paulus W, Walters AS. The restless legs syndrome. *Lancet Neurol.* Aug 2005;4(8):465–475.

90. Bratton RL, Corey R. Tick-borne disease. *Am Fam Physician.* Jun 15, 2005;71(12):2323–2330.

91. Kirkland KB, Wilkinson WE, Sexton DJ. Therapeutic delay and mortality in cases of Rocky Mountain spotted fever. *Clin Infect Dis.* May 1995;20(5):1118–1121.

92. Kobayashi N, Asamoto S, Doi H, Sugiyama H. Brown-Sequard syndrome produced by cervical disc herniation: report of two cases and review of the literature. *Spine J.* Nov–Dec 2003;3(6):530–533.

93. Najjar MW, Baeesa SS, Lingawi SS. Idiopathic spinal cord herniation: a new theory of pathogenesis. *Surg Neurol.* Aug 2004;62(2):161–170; discussion 170–171.

94. Ellger T, Schul C, Heindel W, Evers S, Ringelstein EB. Idiopathic spinal cord herniation causing progressive Brown-Sequard syndrome. *Clin Neurol Neurosurg.* Jun 2006;108(4):388–391.

95. Yamazaki T, Yanaka K, Fujita K, Kamezaki T, Uemura K, Nose T. Traumatic central cord syndrome: analysis of factors affecting the outcome. *Surg Neurol.* Feb 2005;63(2):95–99; discussion 99–100.

96. Dvorak MF, Fisher CG, Hoekema J, et al. Factors predicting motor recovery and functional outcome after traumatic central cord syndrome: a long-term follow-up. *Spine.* Oct 15 2005;30(20):2303–2311.

97. Harrop JS, Hunt GE, Jr., Vaccaro AR. Conus medullaris and cauda equina syndrome as a result of traumatic injuries: management principles. *Neurosurg Focus.* Jun 15 2004;16(6):e4.

98. Rahimi-Movaghar V, Vaccaro AR, Mohammadi M. Efficacy of surgical decompression in regard to motor recovery in the setting of conus medullaris injury. *J Spinal Cord Med.* 2006;29(1):32–38.

99. Jackson AB, Dijkers M, Devivo MJ, Poczatek RB. A demographic profile of new traumatic spinal cord injuries: change and stability over 30 years. *Arch Phys Med Rehabil.* Nov 2004;85(11):1740–1748.

100. McDonald JW, Sadowsky C. Spinal-cord injury. *Lancet.* Feb 2 2002;359(9304):417–425.

101. Gutierrez CJ, Harrow J, Haines F. Using an evidence-based protocol to guide rehabilitation and weaning of ventilator-dependent cervical spinal cord injury patients. *J Rehabil Res Dev.* Sep–Oct 2003;40(5 suppl 2):99–110.

102. Bloemen-Vrencken JH, de Witte LP, Post MW. Follow-up care for persons with spinal cord injury living in the community: a systematic review of interventions and their evaluation. *Spinal Cord.* Aug 2005;43(8):462–475.

103. Goodman CC, Boissonnault WG. *Pathology: Implications for the Physical Therapist.* Philadelphia, PA: W.B. Saunders; 1998.

104. Granger CV, Clark GS. Functional status and outcomes of stroke rehabilitation. *Topics Geriatrics.* Mar 1994;9(3):72–84.

105. Shelton FD, Volpe BT, Reding M. Motor impairment as a predictor of functional recovery and guide to rehabilitation treatment after stroke. *Neurorehabil Neural Repair.* 2001;15(3):229–237.

106. Fauci AS, Haynes B, Katz P. The spectrum of vasculitis: clinical, pathologic, immunologic and therapeutic considerations. *Ann Intern Med.* Nov 1978;89(5 pt 1):660–676.

107. Iskandar BJ, Fulmer BB, Hadley MN, Oakes WJ. Congenital tethered spinal cord syndrome in adults [see comment]. *J Neurosurg.* 1998;88(6):958–961.

108. Di Rocco C, Peter JC. Management of tethered spinal cord. *Surgical Neurol.* 1997;48(4):320–322.

109. Bruns J, Hauser WA. The epidemiology of traumatic brain injury: a review. *Epilepsia.* 2003;44(Suppl. 10):2–10.

110. Das-Gupta R, Turner-Stokes L. Traumatic brain injury. *Disabil Rehabil.* 2002;24(13):654–665.

111. Hukkelhoven CWPM, Steyerberg EW, Rampen AJJ, et al. Patient age and outcome following severe traumatic brain injury: an analysis of 5600 patients. *J Neurosurg.* 2003;99:666–673.

112. Maloney EM, Cleghorn FR, Morgan OS, et al. Incidence of HTLV-I-associated myelopathy/tropical spastic paraparesis (HAM/TSP) in Jamaica and Trinidad. *J Acquir Immune Defic Syndr Hum Retrovirol.* Feb 1 1998;17(2):167–170.

113. Tosoni A, Ermani M, Brandes AA. The pathogenesis and treatment of brain metastases: a comprehensive review. *Crit Rev Oncol Hematol.* 2004;52:199–215.

114. Alho OP, Teppo H, Mantyselka P, Kantola S. Head and neck cancer in primary care: presenting symptoms and the effect of delayed diagnosis of cancer cases. *CMAJ.* Mar 14 2006;174(6):779–784.

115. Beil CM, Keberle M. Oral and oropharyngeal tumors. *Eur J Radiol.* Jun 2008;66(3):448–459.

116. Aerts I, Lumbroso-Le Rouic L, Gauthier-Villars M, Brisse H, Doz F, Desjardins L. Retinoblastoma. *Orphanet J Rare Dis.* 2006;1:31.

117. Perrin RG, Laxton AW. Metastatic spine disease: epidemiology, pathophysiology, and evaluation of patients. *Neurosurg Clin N Am.* Oct 2004;15(4):365–373.

118. Hosono N, Ueda T, Tamura D, Aoki Y, Yoshikawa H. Prognostic relevance of clinical symptoms in patients with spinal metastases. *Clin Orthop Relat Res.* Jul 2005(436):z196–201.

119. Ferro JM. Vasculitis of the central nervous system. *J Neurol.* Dec 1998;245(12):766–776.

120. Oh R, Brown DL. Vitamin B12 deficiency. *Am Fam Physician.* Mar 1 2003;67(5):979–986.

CHAPTER 30

Abnormal Movement

■ *Claire Smith, PT, DPT, NCS* ■ *Beth E. Fisher, PT, PhD*

Description of the Symptom

The chapter describes pathology that may lead to "abnormal movement." Because abnormal movement is associated with a wide spectrum of movement abnormalities, it is most appropriate to first describe normal movement. Normal movement is characterized as accurate/precise, coordinated, smooth, effortless, and purposeful/intentional. Additionally, normal movement is manifested as a countless variety of possible movements. Simply stated, abnormal movement then is any movement that lacks any or all of those characteristics.

With brain injury or disease, the areas of the brain that control the cognitive, visual, and motor functions involved in movement may be injured, resulting in a weakening or absence of the many functions required for purposeful movement and/or the development of abnormal patterns of posture and movement that

are incompatible with the performance of normal activities.

Special Concerns

■ A change in one's prior abnormal movement presentation, including but not limited to:
  ■ Increase or decrease of tremor
  ■ Worsening incoordination
  ■ Decrease in accuracy of movement
  ■ Decrease in movement speed
■ A new onset of abnormal movement not associated with the original purpose of the physical therapy visit. This may include:
  ■ Change in motor control of face, eyes, arm, leg, trunk
  ■ Tremor
  ■ Difficulty talking
  ■ Loss of coordination
  ■ Loss of balance

CHAPTER PREVIEW: Conditions That May Lead to Abnormal Movement

T Trauma

COMMON

Encephalopathy 618
Traumatic brain injury 628

UNCOMMON

Not applicable

RARE

Not applicable

I Inflammation

COMMON

Aseptic
Vasculitis (giant cell arteritis, temporal arteritis, cranial arteritis) 629

Septic
Not applicable

Inflammation *(continued)*

UNCOMMON

Aseptic
Behçet's disease 613
Multiple sclerosis 621

Septic
Not applicable

RARE

Aseptic
Miller Fisher syndrome 620
Multifocal motor neuropathy 621
Neuromyotonia (Isaac syndrome, Isaac-Merten syndrome,
   continuous muscle fiber activity syndrome, quantal squander syndrome) 623
Opsoclonus myoclonus (Kinsbourne syndrome, myoclonic encephalopathy
   of infants, dancing eyes–dancing feet syndrome, opsoclonus-myoclonus-ataxia syndrome) 624
Paraneoplastic syndromes 624
Progressive multifocal leukoencephalopathy 626

Septic
Acute disseminated encephalomyelitis 612
Encephalitis 617
Neurosyphilis (tabes dorsalis, syphilitic spinal sclerosis, progressive locomotor ataxia) 623

M Metabolic

COMMON

Drug toxicity 616

UNCOMMON

Not applicable

RARE

Cerebral beriberi (Korsakoff's amnesic syndrome, Wernicke-Korsakoff syndrome) 614
Fahr's syndrome (familial idiopathic basal ganglia calcification,
   bilateral striopallidodentate calcinosis) 618
Niemann-Pick disease (types C and D only) 623
Tardive dyskinesia 627
Whipple's disease (intestinal lipodystrophy) 629
Wilson's disease 630

Va Vascular

COMMON

Binswanger's disease (subcortical arteriosclerotic encephalopathy, subcortical dementia) 613
Hypoxia (cerebral hypoxia, anoxia) 619
Stroke (cerebrovascular accident) 627

UNCOMMON

Arteriovenous malformation 612
Cerebral aneurysm 614
Cerebral arteriosclerosis 614

RARE

Moyamoya disease 621

De Degenerative

COMMON

Dementia with Lewy bodies 615
Dysgraphia 616

UNCOMMON

Blepharospasm 613
Huntington's disease 619
Mitochondrial myopathies 620
Parkinson's disease 625

RARE

Choreoacanthocytosis (Levine-Critchley syndrome, neuroacanthocytosis) 614
Corticobasal degeneration 615
Creutzfeldt-Jakob disease 615
Dyssynergia cerebellaris myoclonica (Ramsey Hunt syndrome I, dyssynergia cerebellaris progressiva, dentate cerebellar ataxia, dentatorubral atrophy, primary dentatum atrophy) 617
Friedreich's ataxia 618
Hallervorden-Spatz syndrome (neurodegeneration with brain iron accumulation, pantothenate kinase-associated neurodegeneration) 618
Multiple system atrophy (striatonigral degeneration, olivopontocerebellar atrophy, Shy-Drager syndrome) 622
Primary lateral sclerosis 626
Progressive supranuclear palsy (Richardson-Steele-Olszewski syndrome) 626
Spinocerebellar ataxia (spinocerebellar atrophy, spinocerebellar degeneration) 627

Tu Tumor

COMMON

Not applicable

UNCOMMON

Not applicable

RARE

Malignant Primary, such as:
• Brain primary tumors 628
• Spinal primary tumors 629
Malignant Metastatic, such as:
• Brain metastases 628
• Spinal metastases 628
Benign:
Not applicable

Co Congenital

COMMON

Hydrocephalus 619

UNCOMMON

Dystonia 617

Congenital *(continued)*

RARE

Arnold-Chiari malformation (Chiari malformation) 612
Bulbospinal muscular atrophy (Kennedy's disease, X-linked bulbospinal neuronopathy) 613
Kearns-Sayre syndrome 620
Myoclonus 622
Paroxysmal choreoathetosis 625
Pelizaeus-Merzbacher disease 626

Ne Neurogenic/Psychogenic

COMMON

Depression 616

UNCOMMON

Neurological complications of acquired immunodeficiency syndrome 622

RARE

Hemifacial spasm 619
Normal pressure hydrocephalus 624

Note: These are estimates of relative incidence because few data are available for the less common conditions.

Overview of Abnormal Movement

The term *movement disorders* refers to neurological syndromes involving abnormal excess or paucity of movement, often due to basal ganglia dysfunction. Phenotypically, they appear as involuntary or semivoluntary movements. A first-pass approach to distinguishing movement disorders of the basal ganglia is to subdivide them into:

1. Hypokinesias (paucity of movement)
2. Hyperkinesias (excess of movement).

Hypokinesias include bradykinesia and akinesia. Also, *apraxia* is the inability to perform learned movements to command or imitation. The group of hyperkinesias is diverse. *Incoordination* involves abnormalities of intended (volitional) movement, while *tremor* includes more or less involuntary and rhythmic oscillatory movement produced by alternating or irregularly synchronous contractions of reciprocally innervated muscles. Tremors are characterized by whether they occur with movement (*intention tremors*) or at rest (*resting tremors*). *Ataxia* is defined as an inability to coordinate muscle activity during voluntary movement, so that smooth movements occur. It is most often due to disorders of the cerebellum or the posterior columns of the spinal cord and may involve the limbs, head, or trunk. *Chorea* involves involuntary, purposeless, arrhythmic movements of a forcible, rapid, jerky type, while *athetosis* is the inability to sustain any body part in one position. Relatively slow, sinuous, purposeless movements that have a tendency to flow into one another interrupt the maintained postures in athetosis. *Ballismus* includes an uncontrollable, poorly patterned flinging movement on an entire limb.

Dystonia is a persistent attitude or posture in an extreme of athetoid movement, produced by cocontraction of agonist and antagonist muscles in one region of the body. Dystonias may be further classified based on the number and innervation of the muscles involved. *Focal dystonia* occurs in one body part, *segmental dystonia* occurs in muscles innervated by a single segmental level of the spinal cord, and *generalized dystonia* involves most or all body parts. Finally, *myoclonus* is the shock-like contraction(s) of a group of muscles, irregular in rhythm and amplitude, and, with few exceptions, asynchronous and asymmetrical in distribution.

The impairments of motor function that result from lesions in various parts of the nervous system may be subdivided into:

1. Paralysis (or paresis) due to involvement of lower motor neurons
2. Paralysis due to involvement of upper motor (corticospinal) neurons
3. Apraxic or nonparalytic disturbances of purposeful movement due to involvement of association pathways in the cerebrum
4. Involuntary movements and abnormalities of posture due to disease of the basal ganglia
5. Abnormalities of coordination due to lesions of the cerebellum.[1] Careful characterization of the type of movement abnormality is critical to arrive at a diagnosis of its underlying cause and to accurately communicate the observed movement abnormality with another health care provider.

Description of Conditions That May Lead to Abnormal Movement

■ Acute Disseminated Encephalomyelitis

Chief Clinical Characteristics
This presentation may involve confusion, somnolence, and convulsion in its encephalitic form. Initial symptoms of the myelitic form include weakness and sensory impairments.[1]

Background Information
This condition is a demyelinating disease of the central nervous system,[2] which may be due to an immune-mediated complication of infection.[1] The presence of upper motor neuron signs, cerebrospinal fluid pleocytosis and elevated protein, and multiple white matter lesions demonstrated on magnetic resonance imaging supports the diagnosis.[3] Definitive diagnosis requires a brain biopsy. The primary goal of treatment is to suppress the immune response; thus high-dose corticosteroids are generally administered over a course of 3 to 5 days.[3] The prognosis is variable depending on the severity of the disease and acuity of the diagnosis.

■ Arnold-Chiari Malformation (Chiari Malformation)

Chief Clinical Characteristics
This presentation may include visual or swallowing disturbances in combination with pain in the occipital or posterior cervical areas, downbeating nystagmus, progressive ataxia, progressive spastic quadriparesis, or cervical syringomyelia.[4,5]

Background Information
This condition encompasses a number of congenital abnormalities at the base of the brain, including extension of the cerebellar tissue or displacement of the medulla and fourth ventricle into the cervical canal.[4] This condition has two main types. Individuals with the more common form of this condition, Type I, often remain asymptomatic until adolescence or adult life.[4] Type II is primarily seen in infants and young children. Please see the pediatric section of this textbook for a more complete description of this type of the disease. Diagnosis is made by magnetic resonance imaging, computed tomography, myelography, or some combination of these tests.[5] Treatment varies depending on clinical progression and may include surgical intervention such as an upper cervical laminectomy or enlargement of the foramen magnum. Even with surgery symptoms may persist or progress.[4]

■ Arteriovenous Malformation

Chief Clinical Characteristics
This presentation may be characterized by seizures and severe headache. Hemorrhage may result in paresis, ataxia, dyspraxia, dizziness, tactile and proprioceptive disturbances, visual disturbances, aphasia, paresthesias, and cognitive deficits.[1]

Background Information
This condition is caused by a tangle of arteries and veins that cause abnormal communication within the vasculature. Approximately 12% of the 300,000 individuals in the United States with this condition are symptomatic. This condition is caused by a developmental abnormality that likely arises during embryonic or fetal development. Neurological damage occurs due to reduction of oxygen delivery, hemorrhage, or compression of nearby structures of the brain or spinal cord.

Computed tomography, magnetic resonance imaging, and arteriography confirm the diagnosis. Ligation and embolization may be used to reduce the size of the lesion prior to surgical excision, which is the preferred method of treatment. Stereotactic radiation and proton beam therapy are alternative approaches to invasive methods of intervention. Up to 90% of individuals who experience a hemorrhagic arteriovenous malformation survive.[1]

■ Behçet's Disease

Chief Clinical Characteristics
This presentation may include bilateral pyramidal signs (signs related to lesions of upper motor neurons or descending pyramidal tracts, such as a positive Babinski sign or hyperreflexia), headache, memory loss, hemiparesis, cerebellar ataxia, balance deficits, sphincter dysfunction, or cranial nerve palsies. In addition to these neurological signs individuals with this condition also may present with arthritis; renal, gastrointestinal, vascular, and cardiac diseases; and genital, oral, and cutaneous ulcerations.[6]

Background Information
Mean age of onset is in the third decade of life. Diagnostic criteria according to an international study group include presence of recurrent oral ulceration, recurrent genital ulceration, eye lesions, skin lesions, papulopustular lesions, and/or a positive pathergy test.[1,6] Medical treatment typically consists of corticosteroids and immunosuppressants. Neurological symptoms tend to clear within weeks, but can sometimes recur or result in permanent deficits.[1] Negative prognostic factors include onset before the age of 25 and male sex.

■ Binswanger's Disease (Subcortical Arteriosclerotic Encephalopathy, Subcortical Dementia)

Chief Clinical Characteristics
This presentation involves small-stepped gait, slowed motor function with perseveration, deficits in executive function, slow information processing, and impaired memory. Other symptoms include dysarthria, dysphagia, urinary disturbances, and lateral homonymous hemianopias.[4,7,8]

Background Information
This condition is a type of vascular dementia that results from multiple strokes and demyelination of the central white matter.[4,7] Diagnosis is made by neuroimaging, specifically computed tomography and magnetic resonance imaging.[7] Medical management includes drug therapy targeted at improving core symptoms and delaying disease progression, as well as secondary prevention of stroke by decreasing hypertension.[8,9]

■ Blepharospasm

Chief Clinical Characteristics
This presentation includes excessive involuntary closure of the eyelids primarily due to spasmodic contraction of the orbicularis oculi muscles. Severity of symptoms ranges from frequent blinking to functional blindness.

Background Information
The majority of cases of this condition are idiopathic. Diagnosis is made by clinical presentation. Treatment includes psychotherapy, biofeedback, drugs, and surgery. Botulinum toxin A is the most effective form of treatment.

■ Bulbospinal Muscular Atrophy (Kennedy's Disease, X-Linked Bulbospinal Neuronopathy)

Chief Clinical Characteristics
This presentation can be characterized by severe, diffuse muscle cramping and fasciculations, muscle weakness in a limb-girdle distribution, and postural hand tremor. Other symptoms include variable bulbar muscle weakness, gynecomastia, premature muscle exhaustion, and hyporeflexia or areflexia.[10,11]

Background Information
This condition is a rare, x-linked, progressive neuromuscular disorder that is usually seen in males between 30 and 50 years old. Diagnosis is made by clinical features, electrophysiological study, and genetic testing.[10] There is currently no proven treatment for this disease, but genetic counseling is recommended upon diagnosis.[12] This condition is usually associated with a normal life span, but individuals may experience significant disability.[10]

■ Cerebral Aneurysm

Chief Clinical Characteristics

This presentation may involve loss of balance in combination with a whole host of other neurological symptoms and signs that depend on the affected cerebral tissue, including visual and proprioceptive loss. Any associated signs or symptoms may not be reported due to the fact that this condition is typically asymptomatic prior to rupture. However, if the aneurysm results in a mass effect, ischemia, or hemorrhage, then neurological signs and symptoms are dependent on the affected location.[1,13,14]

Background Information

There has been some description of genetic factors in this condition.[13] Cigarette smoking, hypertension, and heavy alcohol use have all been found to be correlated with increased risk of aneurysm development.[13,14] Factors associated with increased risk of rupture include size of aneurysm, location in the posterior circulation, and a previous history of aneurismal subarachnoid hemorrhage.[15,16] Definitive diagnosis is based on catheter angiography; however, magnetic resonance angiography, magnetic resonance imaging, and computed tomography may aid in the diagnosis. Unruptured aneurysms are sometimes surgically treated. Aneurysm size, location, and prior history of a subarachnoid hemorrhage help to determine if the risk of surgical treatment is worth the potential benefits. Most aneurysms that have hemorrhaged must be treated surgically. Patients with a previous rupture are at an 11 times greater risk of having a second intracranial aneurysm rupture. When aneurysms do rupture, many patients die within one month of the rupture, and those who survive often have residual neurological deficits.[13]

■ Cerebral Arteriosclerosis

Chief Clinical Characteristics

This presentation includes visual disturbances, headache, and facial pain.

Background Information

Thickening and hardening of the artery walls in the brain leads to the development of this condition. Diagnosis is established by computed tomography or magnetic resonance imaging of the brain. Treatment includes lifestyle modification, pharmacotherapy, and surgery. Cerebral arteriosclerosis can result in ischemic or hemorrhagic stroke, thus causing neurological impairments.[1]

■ Cerebral Beriberi (Korsakoff's Amnesic Syndrome, Wernicke-Korsakoff Syndrome)

Chief Clinical Characteristics

This presentation involves ophthalmoparesis, nystagmus, ataxia, and confusion, as well as impaired learning and memory. Other common symptoms include peripheral neuropathy, postural hypotension, syncope, impaired olfactory discrimination, mild hypothermia, and confabulation.[4]

Background Information

This condition is due to a thiamine deficiency that results in a diffuse decrease in cerebral glucose utilization. It is most commonly observed in individuals who abuse alcohol and have nutritional deficiencies, although it is not limited to this population.[4] Diagnosis can be made by blood tests to examine thiamine levels. Neuroimaging may show slowed brain activity as well as lesions in the medial thalamus and periaqueductal region.[4] Medical treatment involves the immediate administration of thiamine. Once thiamine has been administered, the reversal of symptoms should begin to occur within hours to days with variable degrees of recovery. Memory has been shown to have the poorest return, and mortality rates of up to 17% have been reported.[4]

■ Choreoacanthocytosis (Levine-Critchley Syndrome, Neuroacanthocytosis)

Chief Clinical Characteristics

This presentation commonly includes chorea, motor or vocal tics, dystonia, orofacial dyskinesias, and parkinsonism. Seizures, cognitive impairment, psychosis, paranoia, and personality changes are also seen with this diagnosis, along with hyporeflexia and distal myopathy due to denervation of muscles.[17–19]

Background Information

This condition is a rare, autosomal recessive disorder that typically has its onset during the third and fourth decades of life.[19] This neurodegenerative disorder is associated with acanthocytes, aberrant spiky or thorny red blood cells, as well as atrophy and gliosis of the caudate, putamen, and globus pallidus.[18] Diagnosis is made by a combination of tests, including clinical features, lab work demonstrating acanthocytosis, neuroimaging, and genetic testing to rule out Huntington's disease.[17] There is currently no effective, longterm treatment, although verapamil has been found to provide temporary reduction of symptoms. Life expectancy is reduced, and suicidal action or ideation is not uncommon due to cognitive impairments.[19]

■ Corticobasal Degeneration

Chief Clinical Characteristics
This presentation typically includes limb ideomotor apraxia and unilateral parkinsonism that is unresponsive to levodopa, gait disturbances, tremor, postural instability, and dementia.[20,21]

Background Information
A proposed set of criteria for the diagnosis of this condition includes core features of:

1. Insidious onset and progressive course
2. No identifiable cause
3. Cortical dysfunction (ideomotor apraxia, alien-limb phenomenon, cortical sensory loss, visual or sensory hemineglect, constructional apraxia, focal or asymmetric myoclonus, apraxia of speech or nonfluent aphasia)
4. Extrapyramidal dysfunction (rigidity which does not respond to levodopa therapy and dystonia).[22]

This condition is a sporadic disease with an average age of onset of 63 years.[21] There have been reports of familial cases; however, for most cases there is no known cause.[20] Diagnosis is suggested based on clinical presentation. A definitive diagnosis can only be made postmortem. Medical treatment is not typically successful; it has been found that only about 24% of these patients will respond to levodopa therapy aimed at addressing the extrapyramidal features of the disease.[23] Physical and occupational therapy are used to maintain mobility and address safety issues related to the progression of imbalance. Mean survival is 7.9 years with a range of 2.5 to 12.5 years.[21] Early presence of bilateral parkinsonism or frontal lobe signs indicates a less favorable prognosis.[21]

■ Creutzfeldt-Jakob Disease

Chief Clinical Characteristics
This presentation may involve rapidly progressive dementia, cerebellar ataxia, balance deficits, myoclonus, cortical blindness, pyramidal signs, extrapyramidal signs, and akinetic mutism.[24]

Background Information
Different forms of this condition have been described including sporadic, iatrogenic, and variant. Sporadic and iatrogenic forms of this condition typically affect older individuals, whereas the variant form affects younger individuals.[25] The early stages of the variant form are characterized by psychiatric symptoms, including depression and anxiety.[25] The condition is rare and affects only one to two people per million worldwide per year.[24,25] It is caused by a conformational change of the normal prion protein, which is encoded by human chromosome 20, to a disease-related prion protein. Diagnosis is suggested by a thorough history and physical examination, electroencephalography, and cerebrospinal fluid analysis.[25] Computed tomography and magnetic resonance imaging are typically normal in sporadic and iatrogenic forms and help to exclude other diagnoses.[24,26] Diagnosis for all forms of this condition is confirmed postmortem.[26] There is no proven treatment.[25,26] Death in the sporadic and iatrogenic forms occurs in a matter of months, at a mean age of 66 years.[25] Mean duration of illness in the variant form is 14 months.[25]

■ Dementia with Lewy Bodies

Chief Clinical Characteristics
This presentation can be characterized by fluctuating cognitive dysfunction, particularly visuospatial problems and executive dysfunction, visual hallucinations, and parkinsonism features such as masked facies, autonomic dysfunction, rigidity, and bradykinesia. Other signs and symptoms may include postural instability, falls, sleep disturbances, memory problems, syncope, transient loss of consciousness, and sensitivity to antipsychotic and anti-Parkinson medications.[27]

Background Information
This progressive condition is the second most common dementia after Alzheimer's disease.[27]

The specific etiology of this condition is unknown. The characteristic Lewy bodies are eosinophilic inclusion bodies found within the cytoplasm of neurons in the cerebral cortex and limbic system.[27] A thorough clinical examination, laboratory screen, and imaging are important to rule out other causes of dementia. The definitive diagnosis for this condition is made postmortem; however, it appears that the use of single-photon emission computed tomography and positron emission tomography may be useful in the identification of occipital hypoperfusion, which may be associated with the visual hallucinations.[27,28] Management includes caregiver education to assist in minimizing factors that may contribute to problematic behaviors. Medication therapy may be indicated, but should be monitored closely due to potential exacerbation of symptoms.[27] Life expectancy for individuals with this condition is similar to that of Alzheimer's disease. The average survival time is between 6 and 8 years from the onset of dementia.[27,29]

■ Depression

Chief Clinical Characteristics

This presentation may involve slowness of movement that can progress to the point of catatonia, intensely dysphoric mood, appetite loss, insomnia or hypersomnia, social withdrawal, loss of motivation, helplessness, hostility, and agitation.[4]

Background Information

The origin of this condition is not fully understood and genetic, biochemical, neuroanatomical and psychosocial factors all appear to play a role.[30] For a clinical diagnosis, the following criteria from the DSM-IV-TR[31] must be met: at least five of the following symptoms, during the same 2-week period, representing a change from previous functioning: depressed mood; diminished interest or pleasure; significant weight loss or gain; insomnia or hypersomnia; psychomotor agitation or delay; fatigue or loss of energy; feelings of worthlessness; diminished ability to think or concentrate, indecisiveness; recurrent thoughts of death, suicidal ideation, suicide attempt, or specific plan for suicide. In addition symptoms must cause clinically significant distress or impairment of

functioning and are not better accounted for by bereavement. The best approach to treatment for depression is a combination of psychotherapy and antidepressant medications.[32] This condition responds well to treatment—approximately 70% to 80% of treated patients have significant reduction in symptoms. However, approximately 20% of patients who are chronically depressed have recurrent and severe depressive episodes.[33]

■ Drug Toxicity

Chief Clinical Characteristics

This presentation involves tinnitus (fluctuating or constant) and hearing loss (mild to complete deafness) if the cochlea is involved; vertigo, vomiting, nystagmus and imbalance if the vestibular system is involved unilaterally; and headache, ear fullness, oscillopsia, an inability to tolerate head movement, a wide-based gait, difficulty walking in the dark, a feeling of unsteadiness and actual unsteadiness while moving, imbalance to the point of being unable to walk, lightheadedness, and severe fatigue in bilateral involvement.

Background Information

The severity, type, and particular combination of symptoms are variable, depending on the drug exposure, whether it is unilateral or bilateral, the speed of onset, and the individual. A slow unilateral loss may produce minimal symptoms, since the brain can compensate through other mechanisms, whereas a fast bilateral loss can produce significant disability. The key diagnostic feature is a history of drug or chemical exposure. Treatment involves removing exposure to the medication, if possible, and vestibular habituation and balance exercises.

■ Dysgraphia

Chief Clinical Characteristics

This presentation typically includes distorted or incorrect writing, including inappropriately sized or spaced letters. Individuals with this condition may also demonstrate incorrect or odd spelling.[4,34]

Background Information

In adults, dysgraphia is frequently seen in, but not limited to, patients with delirium, dementia of Alzheimer's type, or after traumatic brain injury or stroke.[34,35] Assessment and diagnosis can be made by having patients write to dictation and perform letter copying; however, the underlying cause of the dysgraphia should also be determined by clinical exam and ancillary testing.[34] Treatment varies, but may include therapy for motoric control of writing movements. Some patients may also benefit from computer training to allow communication without handwriting. Prognosis is variable due to the wide array of possible causes.

■ Dyssynergia Cerebellaris Myoclonica (Ramsay Hunt Syndrome I, Dyssynergia Cerebellaris Progressiva, Dentate Cerebellar Ataxia, Dentatorubral Atrophy, Primary Dentatum Atrophy)

Chief Clinical Characteristics
This presentation involves the clinical triad of action myoclonus, progressive ataxia, and epilepsy with cognitive impairment. Tremor typically begins in one extremity and progresses throughout the body.[36,37]

Background Information
This is a rare syndrome that is caused by degeneration of the olivodentatorubral system with a typical onset in early adulthood.[37] Diagnosis is made by clinical presentation as well as neurophysiological and radiologic findings, including atrophy of the dentate nucleus.[4,37] Treatment is symptomatic for myoclonus and seizures, and may include the prescription of drugs such as valproate and acetazolamid.[36] The disease is progressive and ataxic symptoms may not be present for up to 20 years after onset.[4]

■ Dystonia

Chief Clinical Characteristics
This presentation can be characterized by involuntary muscle contractions causing repetitive movements or abnormal postures. The abnormal posturing can be generalized, occurring in the hands, feet, head, trunk, and/or face; or focal, limited to one area of the body.

Background Information
The most frequent cause of this condition is drug intoxication; however, it can also be idiopathic, due to an autosomal dominant trait, or secondary to a vascular, traumatic, infectious, or toxic brain insult.[4,38] Diagnosis is made by clinical presentation or genetic testing in the case of hereditary forms of this condition. Treatment for generalized forms of this condition has shown only fair success and includes levodopa therapy, calcium channel blockers, anticonvulsants, and anxiolytics. Positive results have been reported for the implantation of deep brain stimulation to the globus pallidus in severe, generalized forms of this condition.[38] In focal forms of this condition, the most effective treatment is botulinum toxin injections to the affected muscles.[4,39] Rehabilitation strategies should focus on the orthopedic and neurological complications that can occur as a result of this condition.[40] Improvement is usually limited, although a small percentage have spontaneous remission.[39] Occasionally, this condition can increase in intensity or progress to other body parts.[4]

■ Encephalitis

Chief Clinical Characteristics
This presentation includes confusion, delirium, convulsions, problems with speech or hearing, memory loss, hallucinations, drowsiness, and coma. Loss of balance and/or falls may be present.

Background Information
Encephalitis is an inflammation of nerve cells in the brain. This term usually refers to the viral form, although bacterial, parasitic, and fungal agents also can cause this condition. Up to 20,000 new cases of viral forms of this condition are reported annually in the United States. Diagnosis is established by clinical presentation suggesting dysfunction of the cerebrum, brainstem, or cerebellum, cellular reaction and elevated protein in spinal fluid, and possible demonstration of diffuse edema or enhancement of the brain on magnetic resonance imaging or computed tomography. Treatment is primarily pharmacologic, with drugs such as corticosteroids, antiviral agents, and anticonvulsants. The majority of individuals with encephalitis do recover, but irreversible brain damage and death can result.[1]

ABNORMAL MOVEMENT

■ Encephalopathy

Chief Clinical Characteristics

This presentation commonly includes neuromyoclonus, nystagmus, ataxia, and tremor. Altered mental state, loss of memory, personality changes, dementia, and seizures are possible signs. Additional symptoms include muscle atrophy and weakness. Patients may also present with a progressive loss of consciousness resulting in coma.[4,41]

Background Information

Encephalopathy involves diffuse disease of the brain that alters brain function or structure. The numerous causes of encephalopathy include cirrhosis of the liver, severe hypertension, thiamine deficiency, infection, metabolic or mitochondrial dysfunction, toxin exposure, trauma, or lack of oxygen to the brain.[41] Diagnosis is made by numerous studies due to the variable causes of encephalopathy. These tests include blood work, cerebrospinal fluid examination, electroencephalography, and neuroimaging studies.[42] Treatment is symptomatic and varies according to the cause of encephalopathy. Even with treatment, encephalopathy can cause permanent brain damage and, in some cases, may be fatal.[4]

■ Fahr's Syndrome (Familial Idiopathic Basal Ganglia Calcification, Bilateral Striopallidodentate Calcinosis)

Chief Clinical Characteristics

This presentation may involve features of parkinsonism, such as chorea, athetosis, rigidity, dystonia, and tremor in addition to cognitive impairments, cerebellar impairments, gait and balance disorder, psychiatric features, pain, pyramidal signs (such as weakness, hyperreflexia in the deep tendon reflexes, hypertonia, clonus, and/or a positive Babinski sign), sensory changes, and speech disorder.[43]

Background Information

This condition occurs due to bilateral symmetric calcification of the basal ganglia with or without calcification of the dentate nucleus. The disease has been described as both familial and nonfamilial.[1] Diagnosis is established using computed tomography or magnetic resonance imaging of the brain; however, computed tomography has been found to be more

sensitive for identifying calcium deposits.[44] Treatment aimed at minimizing calcium deposits has been unsuccessful.[45] Individuals with this condition may be responsive to levodopa for treatment of their parkinsonian features.[1]

■ Friedreich's Ataxia

Chief Clinical Characteristics

This presentation can be characterized by the onset of progressive gait and limb ataxia in childhood to early adulthood. Associated symptoms include loss of vibration sense and proprioception, absent deep tendon reflexes, weakness, dysarthria, and sensorineural hearing loss. Often, cardiac hypertrophy, diabetes mellitus, and optic atrophy are also present.[4,46,47]

Background Information

This autosomal recessive condition is caused by a genetic mutation, resulting in a progressive loss of large myelinated sensory axons, followed by degeneration of the posterior columns and spinocerebellar and pyramidal tracts.[4,48] Magnetic resonance imaging may show atrophic changes characteristic of the disorder, and should be performed along with genetic testing and electrocardiography for definitive diagnosis. There is currently no medical treatment to slow or stop disease progression, but individuals with this condition may benefit from surgical intervention to correct foot and spine deformities and allow for improved mobility. Average lifetime survival is 25 to 30 years of age.[4,48]

■ Hallervorden-Spatz Syndrome (Neurodegeneration With Brain Iron Accumulation, Pantothenate Kinase-Associated Neurodegeneration)

Chief Clinical Characteristics

This presentation includes dystonia, parkinsonism, choreoathetosis, spasticity, cognitive impairment, corticospinal tract involvement, optic atrophy, and pigmentary retinopathy.[49]

Background Information

This rare, inherited disorder results from a genetic mutation in the iron regulatory pathways, resulting in excessive iron accumulation in the basal ganglia.[49,50] Diagnosis is made by magnetic resonance imaging, which shows characteristic abnormalities in the basal ganglia, known as the "eye of the tiger" sign. Pathological studies may also show brown discoloration, iron pigmentation, and gliosis in the globus pallidus and substantia nigra.[49] There is no cure or effective treatment for the condition, but patients may benefit from rehabilitation therapies to decrease disability as the disease follows its progressive course of degeneration.[50]

■ Hemifacial Spasm

Chief Clinical Characteristics
This presentation typically involves involuntary paroxysmal contractions of the muscles innervated by the facial nerve. These contractions can range in severity and may affect the orbicularis oculi, orbicularis oris, platysma, and/or other superficial muscles of the ipsilateral hemiface.[39]

Background Information
The exact pathophysiology of this condition is currently unknown, but it may be due to a hyperexcitable facial motor nucleus or compression of the facial nerve.[39] Diagnosis is made by observation and clinical history. Currently, the two most widely used treatments are microvascular decompression of the facial nerve at the pons and intramuscular injections of botulinum toxin type A.[39,51] This condition is a chronic disease and spontaneous recovery rarely occurs.[39]

■ Huntington's Disease

Chief Clinical Characteristics
This presentation involves progressive chorea of the entire body, emotional disturbances such as behavior and personality changes, and dementia.[4,52,53]

Background Information
This autosomal dominant genetic disorder causes selective neurodegeneration, most commonly in the neostriatum. Diagnosis is made by genetic testing.[53] There is currently no treatment to slow or stop the progression of this condition; care is focused on symptom management and optimization of functioning.[53] The prognosis for Huntington's disease is poor, and individuals usually experience very rapid decline. On average, patients survive for 15 to 20 years after initial diagnosis,

but require high levels of care and supervision during those years.[53]

■ Hydrocephalus

Chief Clinical Characteristics
This presentation commonly includes frontal lobe signs such as slowness of mental response, inattentiveness, distractibility, perseveration, inability to sustain complex cognitive function, and incontinence. Other symptoms include gait deterioration, frequent falls, occipital or frontal headaches, nausea and vomiting, diplopia, and lethargy. Advanced stages are associated with coma and extensor posturing.

Background Information
Intracranial pressure can be increased due to many mechanisms including a cerebral or extracerebral mass, generalized brain swelling, increased venous pressure, obstruction to the flow and absorption of cerebrospinal fluid, or volume expansion of cerebrospinal fluid.[1] Magnetic resonance imaging and the presence of papilledema are commonly used to establish the diagnosis of hydrocephalus. Medical treatment may include restriction of fluid intake and drugs with an osmotic effect, or the addition of diuretics.[54] Surgical treatment depends on the chronicity of the hydrocephalus. The acute form of this condition is considered fatal and is emergently treated via lumbar puncture or ventricular catheter.[54] The chronic form of this condition is treated with placement of a ventricular shunt or with surgical removal of a mass if that is the cause of the hydrocephalus. Although surgical procedures for hydrocephalus have a high success rate and a good prognosis, it is common to have shunt complications such as infection, occlusion, and over- or underdrainage. Thus, patients who have been treated for this condition must continue to be medically managed and educated regarding the indications of shunt compromise.

■ Hypoxia (Cerebral Hypoxia, Anoxia)

Chief Clinical Characteristics
This presentation includes a wide variety of symptoms that depend on the condition's severity. Mild hypoxia without loss of consciousness may present with inattentiveness, poor judgment,

ABNORMAL MOVEMENT

and motor incoordination. More severe levels of hypoxia can result in seizures and/or coma. Post-hypoxic neurological symptoms include dementia, parkinsonian syndrome, choreoathetosis, cerebellar ataxia, intention or action myoclonus, or a Korsakoff amnesic state.[4]

Background Information
This condition occurs as a result of a decrease of oxygen supply to the brain. It has numerous causes, including cardiac arrest, drowning, strangulation, aspiration, choking, carbon monoxide poisoning, and complications of general anesthesia. Pure hypoxia produces damage in areas susceptible to reduced oxygen delivery such as the hippocampi and the cerebellum. This condition is often seen along with ischemia, producing complex patterns of cerebral damage.[4] Diagnosis and determination of the cause of hypoxia may require magnetic resonance imaging, electrocardiography, laboratory studies, electroencephalography, and evoked potentials.[4,55] Treatment is directed at prevention of further hypoxic injury. Outcomes vary, depending on cause and severity of hypoxia, and range from full recovery to coma or even death. The longer an individual with this condition is unconscious, the lower the likelihood of a meaningful recovery.[4]

■ **Kearns-Sayre Syndrome**

Chief Clinical Characteristics
This presentation commonly includes a classic triad of symptoms, involving progressive external ophthalmoplegia, retinal pigmentary degeneration, and heart block. Common additional findings include cerebellar dysfunction, myopathy, ataxia, sensorineural hearing loss, mental retardation, growth hormone deficit with dwarfism, hypoparathyroidism, and diabetes mellitus.[56,57]

Background Information
Etiology has not been established; however this rare, sporadic mitochondrial disorder is thought to occur via a mutation in either the ovum or zygote.[56] Diagnosis is established with a combination of clinical, radiologic, pathological, biochemical, and molecular studies. Mitochondrial deoxyribonucleic acid analysis and histological verification of the presence of ragged red fibers may be helpful in determining diagnosis.[56] Treatment is

mostly symptomatic and supportive, although cardiac symptoms may be managed with medication. This condition is a slowly progressive disorder and prognosis is often determined by the degree of heart conduction impairment.[58]

■ **Miller Fisher Syndrome**

Chief Clinical Characteristics
This presentation can be characterized by an acute onset of the classic triad of ophthalmoplegia, ataxia, and areflexia. Additional symptoms include mydriasis, sensory loss, facial palsy, bulbar palsy, dysesthesia, weakness, and urinary incontinence.[59]

Background Information
This condition is thought to be a variant form of acute demyelinating polyneuropathy (Guillain-Barré syndrome) and is usually preceded by infectious gastrointestinal or respiratory symptoms approximately 8 days before onset of symptoms.[59] Diagnosis is based on clinical presentation. In addition, elevated cerebrospinal fluid protein values and electrophysiological examination demonstrating conduction block or axonal damage on limbs of normal strength can help reinforce the diagnosis.[60] Plasmapheresis and administration of intravenous immunoglobulins have both been found to be helpful in decreasing recovery time.[60] The natural course of recovery in individuals with this condition is good with minimal disability seen 6 months after onset.[59]

■ **Mitochondrial Myopathies**

Chief Clinical Characteristics
This presentation typically involves a combination of exercise intolerance, ataxia, seizures, myoclonus, headaches, small strokes, ophthalmoplegia, deafness, muscle cramps and/or slowly progressive myopathy with proximal greater than distal involvement. Other less common symptoms that may be seen include dementia, lactic acidosis, ptosis, and cardiac conduction defects.[4,61]

Background Information
This condition refers to a large group of disorders that result from a mutation in the mitochondrial genome, resulting in damage to the mitochondria. These disorders include

Kearns-Sayre syndrome, myoclonus epilepsy with ragged red fibers, mitochondrial encephalomyopathy with lactic acidosis and stroke-like episodes, as well as other childhood-onset disorders.[4] A combination of clinical picture, histological findings of ragged red fibers, elevated serum lactate, and possible family history contribute to the diagnosis of this condition.[4] There is no specific treatment, but new research shows that patients may benefit from physical therapy for submaximal exercise training.[63] Most patients experience lifelong progression of the disease and prognosis varies according to the type of disease and amount of involvement.[4]

■ Moyamoya Disease

Chief Clinical Characteristics
This presentation may include unsteady gait, involuntary movement, weakness, speech and sensory impairments, headache, seizures, impaired mental development, visual disturbances, and nystagmus.[4]

Background Information
This rare condition results from progressive occlusion of the arteries of the circle of Willis.[4] Diagnosis is based on clinical findings and results of magnetic resonance imaging and magnetic resonance angiography. Images will demonstrate the occlusion of the circle of Willis as well as secondary cerebral infarction, white matter lesions, atrophy, and hemorrhage.[62] Treatment options include revascularization surgery and medical treatment to prevent hypertension and further strokes.[63] Rehabilitative therapies are used to treat functional deficits that the patient may incur from a stroke, secondary to the progression of the disease. Outcome depends on the severity of secondary complications and presence of subsequent occlusion.

■ Multifocal Motor Neuropathy

Chief Clinical Characteristics
This presentation includes progressive, asymmetrical weakness, muscle atrophy, cramps, and fasciculations that develop slowly over several years. Other symptoms include wrist and foot drop, grip weakness, reduced tendon reflexes in affected areas, and occasional cranial or phrenic nerve involvement.

Background Information
This condition is thought to be immunologically mediated, although the exact mechanism is unknown.[64] Diagnosis is made by the presence of definite motor conduction block with normal sensory nerve conduction on electrophysiological study.[65] Medical treatment is intravenous immunoglobulin therapy.[65,66] This condition has a slow, progressive course of deterioration of muscle strength, but the disease generally does not cause severe disability or death.[65,66]

■ Multiple Sclerosis

Chief Clinical Characteristics
This presentation may include paresthesias, weakness, spasticity, hypertonicity, hyperreflexia, positive Babinski sign, incoordination, optic neuritis, ataxia, vertigo, dysarthria, diplopia, bladder incontinence, tremor, balance deficits, falls, and cognitive deficits.[1]

Background Information
This condition may present as relapsing-remitting, primary progressive, or secondary progressive. The disease occurs most frequently in women between the ages of 20 and 40 years. Only a small number of children or individuals between 50 and 60 years of age are diagnosed with this condition.[1] This condition was originally thought to be secondary to environmental and genetic factors, but evidence suggests an autoimmune response to a viral infection, which subsequently targets myelin.[1] The diagnosis may be confirmed by a thorough history, physical examination, magnetic resonance imaging, analysis of cerebrospinal fluid, and evoked potentials.[1,67,68] Life expectancy and cause of mortality are similar for all types of this condition.[1] Clinical characteristics that are associated with a longer time interval for progression of disability include female sex, younger age of onset, relapsing-remitting type, complete recovery after the first relapse, and longer time interval between first and second exacerbation.[69] Medical management may include the use of methylprednisolone, prednisone, cyclophosphamide, immunosuppressant treatment, and betainterferon.[1] Physical, occupational, and speech therapy may be indicated to prevent secondary sequelae and to optimize functional activity

and mobility. Some individuals may benefit from psychology/psychiatry and social support as the disease progresses.

■ Multiple System Atrophy (Striatonigral Degeneration, Olivopontocerebellar Atrophy, Shy-Drager Syndrome)

Chief Clinical Characteristics

This presentation involves tremor, rigidity, akinesia, and/or postural imbalance along with signs of cerebellar, pyramidal, and autonomic dysfunction. Autonomic symptoms such as orthostatic hypotension, dry mouth, loss of sweating, impotence, and urinary incontinence or retention are the initial feature in 41% of individuals, with 74% to 97% of individuals developing some degree of autonomic dysfunction during the course of the disease.[70] This condition is a combination of parkinsonian and non-parkinsonian symptoms and signs.

Background Information

Diagnostic criteria are based on the clinical presentation, which includes poor response to levodopa, presence of autonomic features, presence of speech or bulbar problems, absence of dementia, absence of toxic confusion, and presence of falls.[71] The disease course ranges between 0.5 and 24 years after diagnosis with a mean survival time of 6.2 years.[72] This condition is a progressive condition of the central and autonomic nervous systems that rarely occurs without orthostatic hypotension. There are three types of this condition. The parkinsonian-type includes symptoms of Parkinson's disease such as slow movement, stiff muscles, and tremor. The cerebellar type causes problems with coordination and speech. The combined type includes symptoms of both parkinsonism and cerebellar failure. Older age at onset is associated with a shorter survival time.[72] Average age of onset is 54 years, with mean age at death being 60.3 years.[70] Most individuals with this condition receive a trial of levodopa although only a minority respond.[70] Additional treatment addresses symptoms and involves physical and occupational therapy to maintain mobility and address safety issues related to the progression of imbalance.

■ Myoclonus

Chief Clinical Characteristics

This presentation includes sudden, brief, shock-like, involuntary movements that are caused by muscular contraction or inhibition.[73,74]

Background Information

This condition may be caused by many different processes, including epileptic forms, essential and heredofamilial forms, myoclonic dementias, myoclonus with cerebellar disease, metabolic and toxic disorders, and focal and spinal forms of myoclonus.[4,73] This condition may originate from numerous structures, including the cerebral cortex, subcortical structures, brainstem, spinal cord, and peripheral nerves.[74] Diagnosis is made by a combination of clinical picture, clinical neurophysiology testing, basic ancillary testing, and, if necessary, advanced testing for rare and specific diagnoses.[73] Treatment varies according to the etiology and primarily includes treatment of the underlying cause or antimyoclonic pharmacologic treatment.[73,74] Prognosis also varies depending on the cause of this condition, with some cases being very transient in nature and others resulting in progressive, significant disability.[4,73]

■ Neurological Complications of Acquired Immunodeficiency Syndrome

Chief Clinical Characteristics

This presentation is variable and dependent on the affected neuroanatomical structures in an individual with acquired immunodeficiency syndrome.[75]

Background Information

This condition may be categorized by:

1. Meningitic symptoms including headache, malaise, and fever (such as secondary to meningitis, cryptococcal meningitis, tuberculous meningitis, and human immunodeficiency virus headache)

2. Focal cerebral symptoms including hemiparesis, aphasia, apraxia, sensory deficits, homonymous hemianopia, cranial nerve involvement, balance deficits, incoordination, and/or ataxia (such as secondary to cerebral toxoplasmosis, primary central nervous system lymphoma, and progressive multifocal leukoencephalopathy)

3. Diffuse cerebral symptoms that involve cognitive deficits, altered level of consciousness, hyperreflexia, Babinski sign, presence of primitive reflexes (such as secondary to postinfectious encephalomyelitis, acquired immunodeficiency dementia complex, cytomegalovirus encephalitis)
4. Myelopathy associated with gait difficulties, spasticity, ataxia, balance deficits, and hyperreflexia (such as secondary to herpes zoster myelitis, vacuolar myelopathy that occurs with acquired immunodeficiency syndrome dementia complex)
5. Peripheral involvement associated with sensory changes, weakness, balance deficits, and pain (such as secondary to peripheral neuropathy, acute and chronic inflammatory demyelinating polyneuropathies).[1,75]

Abnormal neurological findings are observed during a clinical examination in approximately one-third of patients with acquired immunodeficiency syndrome; however, on autopsy most individuals with this condition have abnormalities within the nervous system.[1] Diagnosis of the variable neurological complications associated with this condition may be confirmed with laboratory tests, cerebrospinal fluid cultures, imaging, nerve conduction studies, and physical examination.[1,26,75] Treatment appears to be limited primarily to the use of antiviral medications.[75] Physical and occupational therapy may be indicated to address equipment needs and caregiver/patient training related to functional mobility.

■ Neuromyotonia (Isaac Syndrome, Isaac-Merten Syndrome, Continuous Muscle Fiber Activity Syndrome, Quantal Squander Syndrome)

Chief Clinical Characteristics
This presentation commonly involves intermittent or continuous muscle contraction, slow relaxation following muscle contraction, cramps, stiffness, and hyperhidrosis. These symptoms are commonly seen in conjunction with peripheral neuropathy.[76,77]

Background Information
This condition is an antibody-mediated potassium channel disorder, in which the suppression of these voltage-gated channels results in

hyperexcitability of the peripheral nerve.[76] It is a rare, usually acquired disease that is often seen with myasthenia gravis and is most likely due to an autoimmune or paraneoplastic origin.[77] Electrophysiological study is used in diagnosis and will show myokymic and neuromyotonic discharges.[76] Muscle activity persists throughout sleep and anesthesia, but can be blocked by curare.[4] Symptomatic relief has been demonstrated with anticonvulsant drugs such as phenytoin and carbamazepine, and research has also shown successful outcomes with plasmapharesis.[78]

■ Neurosyphilis (Tabes Dorsalis, Syphilitic Spinal Sclerosis, Progressive Locomotor Ataxia)

Chief Clinical Characteristics
This presentation can be characterized by hemiparesis, ataxia, aphasia, gait instability, falls, neuropathy, personality and cognitive changes, seizures, diplopia, visual impairments, hearing loss, psychotic disorders, loss of bowel/bladder function, pain, hyporeflexia, and hypotonia.[79,80]

Background Information
Treponema pallidum infects the human host by way of contact with contaminated body fluids or lesions.[79] This spirochete is responsible for the diagnosis of syphilis; however, when *T. pallidum* is present within the central nervous system the individual is diagnosed with neurosyphilis.[80] This condition occurs in approximately 10% of individuals with untreated syphilis, and in 81% of these cases it presents as meningovascular, meningeal, and general paresis. Treatment includes use of various forms of penicillin or alternative choices for those allergic to penicillin[79] and may involve rehabilitative therapies depending on the individual's activity limitations or participation restrictions. A better prognosis has been observed for individuals treated during early neurosyphilis.[80]

■ Niemann-Pick Disease (Types C and D Only)

Chief Clinical Characteristics
This presentation includes ataxia, dystonia, vertical gaze palsy, dysarthria, and seizures. Often the presenting feature is a psychotic episode.[4,81]

Background Information

This condition is an autosomal recessive lipid storage disorder that results in impaired cholesterol transport and excessive glycosphingolipid storage.[82] There are four types of Niemann-Pick disease; types A and B are seen only in children and are not discussed here. Types C and D have a variable age of onset ranging from childhood to late teens or even early adulthood. Individuals with types C and D demonstrate an enlarged spleen and liver, as well as progressive neurological dysfunction.[81] Diagnosis is made by a combination of studies, including filipin staining of cultured fibroblasts, cholesterol esterification studies, and DNA mutation analysis.[81] Unfortunately, there is no effective treatment for types C and D of this condition. Many patients who are diagnosed in childhood live well into adult years, and overall prognosis depends on the severity of the disease.[81]

■ Normal Pressure Hydrocephalus

Chief Clinical Characteristics

This presentation is characterized by progressive difficulty in walking characterized by diminished cadence, widened base, short steps, and en bloc turning (requiring more than 3 steps to make a 90-degree turn). Movements involving the axial musculature appear awkward and apraxic. Progression involves impairment in mental function and sphincter incontinence.

Background Information

Symptoms are caused by increased pressure on the brain, specifically the frontal lobe, due to an abnormal increase in cerebrospinal fluid secondary to trauma, infection, space-occupying lesion, or unknown cause. It is most common in the elderly, but can occur in people of any age. Symptoms must be differentiated from disorders with similar presentation such as Alzheimer's, Parkinson's, and Creutzfeldt-Jakob diseases.[83] Diagnosis involves the clinical presentation combined with imaging to identify ventricular enlargement, intracranial pressure monitoring, and neuropsychological testing.[83] Treatment entails shunt placement to drain cerebrospinal fluid and regular follow-up by a physician to monitor shunt function. Without treatment, symptoms continue to worsen. With shunt placement, 60%

of individuals with this condition improve significantly, and 30% will completely recover and return to premorbid levels of function. Others have residual gait, sphincteric, and cognitive deficits.[84]

■ Opsoclonus Myoclonus (Kinsbourne Syndrome, Myoclonic Encephalopathy of Infants, Dancing Eyes–Dancing Feet Syndrome, Opsoclonus-Myoclonus-Ataxia Syndrome)

Chief Clinical Characteristics

This presentation includes irregular, rapid eye movements (opsoclonus) and brief, shock-like muscle spasms (myoclonus), as well as staggering, falling, ataxia, drooling, decreased muscle tone, and an inability to sleep.[85]

Background Information

This autoimmune disorder is commonly found in association with the presence of neoplasm, the most common types being neuroblastoma in children, and breast and small-cell lung cancer in adults.[4] Diagnosis is made by a combination of clinical presentation, the possible presence of neoplasm, the presence of anti-Hu antibodies, mild pleocytosis on cerebrospinal fluid, and positive serologic tests in children without tumors.[4] Treatment includes adrenocorticotropic hormone, corticosteroid, and intravenous immunoglobulin therapy, and, when present, tumor resection and adjuvant treatment such as chemotherapy and radiation.[4,85] There is good response to drug and surgical treatment, but relapse is common and many patients report residual neurological symptoms.[4,85]

■ Paraneoplastic Syndromes

Chief Clinical Characteristics

This presentation includes dizziness in combination with a variety of different neurological symptoms and signs in an individual with cancer. Specific neurological symptoms and signs depend on the location of involvement of the central or peripheral nervous system.

Background Information

Paraneoplastic encephalomyelitis and focal encephalitis may present with ataxia, vertigo, balance deficits, nystagmus, nausea, vomiting, cranial nerve palsies, seizures, sensory neuropathy, anxiety, depression, cognitive changes, and hallucinations. For individuals presenting with ataxia, dysarthria, dysphagia, and diplopia, paraneoplastic cerebellar degeneration may be suspected. Paraneoplastic opsoclonus/myoclonus tends to affect both children and adults with signs and symptoms including hypotonia, ataxia, irritability, truncal ataxia, gait difficulty, balance deficits, and frequent falls. Stiff-man syndrome presents with spasms and fluctuating rigidity of axial musculature, legs and possibly shoulders, upper extremities, and neck. Paraneoplastic sensory neuropathy presents with asymmetric, progressive sensory alterations involving the limbs, trunk, and face, sensorineural hearing loss, autonomic dysfunction, and pain. Other conditions in this category include vasculitis, Lambert-Eaton myasthenia syndrome, myasthenia gravis, dermatomyositis, neuromyotonia, and various neuropathies.[1,86] These conditions result from an immune-mediated response to the presence of tumor or metastases. Antibodies or T-cells respond to the presence of the tumor, but also attack normal cells of the nervous system.[87,88] Over 60% of individuals present with this condition prior to the discovery of the cancer.[86] The underlying tumor is treated according to the type of cancer. Additional treatment is dependent on this condition's type and may include steroids, plasmapheresis, immunotherapy, chemotherapy, radiation, or cyclophosphamide.[86] Physical, occupational, and speech therapy may be indicated to address functional limitations.

■ Parkinson's Disease

Chief Clinical Characteristics

This presentation commonly involves resting tremor, bradykinesia, rigidity, and postural instability. Falls are a common problem in individuals with this condition, with up to 68% falling within a 1-year period and approximately 50% of these individuals falling multiple times within that same year.[89] Other common signs and symptoms include festination, freezing, micrographia, hypophonia (hypokinetic dysarthria), akinesia, masked facies, drooling, difficulty turning over in bed, dystonia, dyskinesia, dementia, and depression.[1]

Background Information

This condition occurs due to the depletion or injury of dopamine-producing cells in substantia nigra pars compacta. Clinical signs and symptoms are not typically present until after approximately 80% of dopamine-producing cells are lost. The definitive diagnosis is made post-mortem. However, a clinically definitive diagnosis may be made with the presence of at least two of the three criteria—asymmetric resting tremor, bradykinesia, or rigidity—and a positive response to anti-Parkinson medications.[1,90] Imaging may be useful to exclude vascular involvement. Medical management may include use of dopamine agonists, levodopa, and other medications to address nonmotor symptoms, such as depression, constipation, autonomic symptoms, and sexual dysfunction. Surgical management also may be considered, including deep brain stimulation or pallidotomy.[90] Forced use or higher intensity, challenging activities may provide a neuroprotective benefit for individuals with early forms of this condition.[91] With the high incidence of depression, consultation with a psychologist or psychiatrist may be warranted. Individuals with a late onset tend to progress more rapidly.[92,93] Poor prognostic indicators for disability include initial presentation without tremor, early dependence, dementia, balance impairments, older age, and the postural instability/gait difficulty dominant type.[92,93]

■ Paroxysmal Choreoathetosis

Chief Clinical Characteristics

This presentation includes discrete episodes of abnormal involuntary movements of the limbs, trunk, and facial muscles. Some patients report lingering muscle stiffness following the attacks.[94] The episodes of choreoathetosis may be provoked by startle, sudden movement, hyperventilation, alcohol, coffee, fatigue, or prolonged exercise. They vary in duration from 10 seconds to up to 4 hours at a time, and may occur dozens of times per day or only occasionally.[4]

Background Information

The exact pathological mechanism of this condition is unknown, but it is thought that the disorder may be genetically linked, or due to a secondary cause such as neurological or metabolic disease.[4,94] Individuals with this condition tend to respond well to antiepileptic drugs and, overall, this condition has been shown to spontaneously improve as patients move into adulthood.[94]

■ Pelizaeus-Merzbacher Disease

Chief Clinical Characteristics

This presentation commonly includes deterioration of coordination, motor abilities, and intellectual function.

Background Information

Severity and onset of the disease range widely, depending on the type of genetic mutation, and extend from the mild, adult-onset spastic paraplegia to the severe form with onset at infancy and death in early childhood.[95] This condition is an X-linked disease caused by a mutation in the gene that controls the production of a myelin protein called proteolipid protein.[95] Genetic diagnostic testing is the definitive method for diagnosing this condition.[96] There is no cure for this condition. Therefore, treatment is based on symptoms and includes physical therapy, orthotics, and antispasticity agents with a goal of minimizing the development of joint contractures, dislocations, and kyphoscoliosis.[97] Individuals with severe forms of this condition experience progressive deterioration until death. Individuals with the adult-onset form with spasticity may have a nearly normal life span.[4]

■ Primary Lateral Sclerosis

Chief Clinical Characteristics

This presentation includes spastic paraparesis of voluntary muscles with associated upper motor neuron signs in the absence of lower motor neuron signs. Onset of difficulty with gait, balance, and leg weakness appears in the fifth to sixth decade of life and may progress to affect upper extremity and facial musculature.

Background Information

Imaging, cerebrospinal fluid analysis, and electromyographic studies confirm the diagnosis. In particular, this condition is differentiated from the more severe amyotrophic lateral sclerosis only after a period of 3 years from onset to ensure the absence of lower motor neuron signs.[1] Treatment for this condition addresses symptom management. Physical therapy is indicated to prevent immobility. This condition is not fatal and progression of symptoms varies; some individuals maintain ambulatory status throughout life while others become wheelchair-bound.

■ Progressive Multifocal Leukoencephalopathy

Chief Clinical Characteristics

This presentation commonly involves cortical blindness, visual field defects, hemiparesis with progression to quadriparesis, aphasia, ataxia, dysarthria, personality changes and impaired intellect evolving over a period of days to weeks.

Background Information

This condition is most likely due to viral infection of the central nervous system, which then causes widespread demyelinative lesions primarily of the cerebral hemispheres. Diagnosis is made by computed tomography and magnetic resonance imaging to localize the lesions. Treatment for individuals with acquired immunodeficiency syndrome consists of antiretroviral drug combinations and can lead to slower progression or even remission. Currently, no treatment exists to impair disease progression in individuals with this condition but without acquired immunodeficiency syndrome.[1]

■ Progressive Supranuclear Palsy (Richardson-Steele-Olszewski Syndrome)

Chief Clinical Characteristics

This presentation classically includes vertical gaze palsy, prominent instability, and falls within the first year of disease onset.[98] Other characteristics may include rigidity, akinesia, dysarthria, dysphagia, and mild dementia. Falls were found to be the most commonly reported symptom with the majority of falls being backwards falls.[99] Difficulty with voluntary vertical eye movements (usually downward) and involuntary saccades are relatively early features. The disease generally progresses to the point at which all voluntary eye movements are lost.

Background Information

Some patients may not demonstrate difficulties with ocular movements for 1 to 3 years after disease onset. Most cases are sporadic; however, a pattern of inheritance compatible with autosomal dominant transmission has been described.[1] Diagnosis is based on clinical presentation, which includes a gradually progressive disorder with age of onset at 40 years or older, vertical supranuclear palsy, and postural instability with falls within the first year of disease onset.[100] Medical treatment is typically unsuccessful, because the majority of patients are not responsive to the levodopa therapy aimed at addressing the extrapyramidal features of the disease.[23] Physical and occupational therapy are used to maintain mobility and address safety issues related to the progression of imbalance. The disease course is progressive with a mean survival time of 5.6 years.[99] Older age at disease onset, early onset of falls, incontinence, dysarthria, dysphagia, insertion of a percutaneous gastrostomy, and diplopia have all been described as being predictive of shorter survival time.[99]

■ Spinocerebellar Ataxia (Spinocerebellar Atrophy, Spinocerebellar Degeneration)

Chief Clinical Characteristics

This presentation can be characterized by ataxia, incoordination, supranuclear ophthalmoplegia, slow saccades, optic atrophy, dysarthria, balance deficits, falls, tremor, myoclonus, chorea, nystagmus, dementia, amyotrophy, and peripheral neuropathy.[101,102]

Background Information

This condition refers to a group of progressive, neurodegenerative, autosomal dominant disorders affecting the cerebellum, brainstem, and spinal cord. Twelve variants have been identified including SCA 1, 2, 3, 6, 7, 8, 10, 12, 14, 17, FGF10-SCA, and dentatorubral-pallidoluysian atrophy.[102] The disorders occur due to expansions of CAG triplet repeats that are subsequently transcribed into long polyglutamine tracts. Diagnosis is confirmed by deoxyribonucleic acid testing. There is no current medical treatment for the various forms of this condition.[101,102] Individuals with this condition may benefit from physical, occupational, and speech therapy to address activity limitations and participation restrictions.

■ Stroke (Cerebrovascular Accident)

Chief Clinical Characteristics

This presentation may include a wide range of symptoms that correspond to specific areas of the brain that are affected, potentially including visual disturbances. The initial symptoms can include numbness or weakness, especially on one side of the body or face; confusion or aphasia; balance deficits or falls; or sudden severe headache with no known cause.

Background Information

This condition occurs when blood flow to the brain is interrupted either by blockage (ischemia or infarction) or from hemorrhagic disruption. A thrombosis or embolic occlusion of an artery causes an ischemic type of this condition. A hemorrhagic type of this condition can be caused by arteriovenous malformation, hypertension, aneurysm, neoplasm, drug abuse, and trauma. This condition is the most common and disabling neurological disorder in adults and occurs in 114 of every 100,000 people.[30] This condition is diagnosed using clinical presentation and positive findings on computed tomography and magnetic resonance imaging. Medication, surgery, and interdisciplinary therapy are the most common treatments for this condition. The prognosis for recovery is predicted by the magnitude of initial deficit. Factors that are associated with poor outcomes include coma, poor cognition, severe aphasia, severe hemiparesis with little return within 1 month, visual perceptual disorders, depression, and incontinence after 2 weeks.[103,104]

■ Tardive Dyskinesia

Chief Clinical Characteristics

This presentation includes choreoathetoid dyskinesia, which can occur in the face, trunk, and limbs. These dyskinesias have been described as repetitive, stereotyped, rhythmic movements, and are most commonly seen in the mouth or tongue.[4]

Background Information

These symptoms develop as a side effect of exposure to or withdrawal from neuroleptic-antipsychotic drugs. This condition develops in 20% of patients treated with neuroleptic medications, with a higher risk in the elderly population.[105] Excess dopamine is thought to play a role in etiology. Diagnosis is based on clinical examination and history of prior treatment with neuroleptic medications. No treatment for this condition has been proven to be effective and the best current treatment is prevention.[106,107] Improvement or resolution of the symptoms is more favorable when there is early detection, lower drug exposure, use of atypical instead of typical antipsychotic medications, younger age, and longer follow-up.[105,108]

■ Traumatic Brain Injury

Chief Clinical Characteristics

This presentation typically includes disequilibrium in the presence of cognitive changes, altered level of consciousness, seizures, nausea, vomiting, coma, dizziness, headache, pupillary changes, tinnitus, weakness, incoordination, behavioral changes, spasticity, hypertonicity, cranial nerve lesions, and sensory and motor deficits.[1,109]

Background Information

This condition can be classified as mild, moderate, or severe based on Glasgow Coma Scale, length of coma, and duration of post-traumatic amnesia.[109] Magnetic resonance imaging may be used to confirm the diagnosis.[26] Treatment initiated at the scene of the accident and during the acute phase is focused on medical stabilization. It should be initiated during the acute phase in order to minimize complications.[110] Low Glasgow Coma Scale, longer length of coma, longer duration of post-traumatic amnesia, and older age tend to be associated with poor outcomes.[111] Optimal rehabilitation is interdisciplinary and customized to address the specific individuals' needs

TUMORS

■ Brain Metastases

Chief Clinical Characteristics

This presentation may include headaches, seizures, dysphagia, weakness, cognitive changes, behavioral changes, dizziness, vomiting, alterations in the level of consciousness, ataxia, aphasia, nystagmus, visual disturbances, dysarthria, balance deficits, falls, lethargy, and incoordination.[1,112]

Background Information

The majority of individuals with brain metastases have been previously diagnosed with a primary tumor; however, a small percentage of individuals are diagnosed concomitantly with brain metastases and the primary tumor. The most common cancers resulting in subsequent brain metastases include lung, breast, melanoma, colorectal, and genitourinary tract. The new onset of neurological symptoms after a primary tumor warrants the use of imaging such as magnetic resonance imaging or computed tomography to confirm the diagnosis. Treatment may include corticosteroids, brain irradiation, surgery, chemotherapy, radiotherapy, and rehabilitative therapies. The prognosis is poor with death typically occurring within 6 months.

■ Brain Primary Tumors

Chief Clinical Characteristics

This presentation may include headaches, seizures, dysphagia, weakness, cognitive changes, behavioral changes, dizziness, vomiting, alterations in the level of consciousness, ataxia, aphasia, nystagmus, visual disturbances, dysarthria, balance deficits, falls, lethargy, and incoordination.[1,26]

Background Information

Glioblastoma multiforme, astrocytoma, oligodendroglioma, metastatic tumors, primary central nervous system lymphomas, ganglioglioma, neuroblastoma, meningioma, arachnoid cysts, hemangioblastoma, medulloblastoma, and acoustic neuroma/schwannoma are some of the more common brain tumors. Specific diagnoses for brain tumors may be confirmed with imaging and biopsy. Treatment is variable depending on the type, size, and location of the tumor and may include surgical resection, chemotherapy, radiation, corticosteroids, and rehabilitative therapies. Prognosis is also variable and depends on the type and grade of tumor, severity of compression, and duration of compression.

■ Spinal Metastases

Chief Clinical Characteristics

This presentation can involve spasticity, weakness, sensory alterations, bowel and bladder incontinence, neck pain, back pain, radicular pain, atrophy, cerebellar signs, balance deficits, falls, and cranial nerve involvement.[1,26,113]

Background Information

This condition is the most frequent neoplasm involving the spine.[113] The most common types and locations of primary tumors that result in spinal metastases include breast, lung, lymphoma, prostate, kidney, gastrointestinal tract, and thyroid.[1,114] The diagnosis is confirmed with gadolinium enhanced magnetic resonance imaging and computed tomography.[1,113] Treatment is variable depending on the tumor and may include surgical resection, chemotherapy, radiation, corticosteroids, and rehabilitative therapies.[1] Although the long-term prognosis is poor, individuals without paresis and pain and who are still ambulatory have longer survival rates.[114]

■ Spinal Primary Tumors

Chief Clinical Characteristics

This presentation may include spasticity, weakness, sensory alterations, bowel/bladder incontinence, back pain, radicular pain, atrophy, cerebellar signs, balance deficits, falls, and cranial nerve involvement.[1]

Background Information

Types of this condition include astrocytomas, ependymomas, hemangioblastoma, myeloma, neurofibroma, lymphoma, metastasis, meningioma, schwannoma, and astrocytoma. Extradural tumors, such as meningiomas, produce a rapid onset of symptoms, with weakness being predominant. Intramedullary tumors, or ependymomas, astrocytomas and hemangioblastomas, present with slowly progressive symptoms, of which loss of pain and temperature sensation is usually the first. The first test to diagnose brain and spinal column tumors is a neurological examination. Special imaging techniques (computed tomography, magnetic resonance imaging, and positron emission tomography) are also employed. Specific diagnoses may be confirmed with imaging and biopsy. Treatment is variable depending on the type, size, and location of the tumor and may include surgical resection, chemotherapy, radiation, corticosteroids, and rehabilitative therapies. Prognosis is variable and depends on the type and grade of tumor, severity of compression, and duration of compression.

■ Vasculitis (Giant Cell Arteritis, Temporal Arteritis, Cranial Arteritis)

Chief Clinical Characteristics

This presentation can be characterized by headaches, psychiatric syndromes, dementia, peripheral or cranial nerve involvement, pain, seizures, hypertension, hemiparesis, balance deficits, neuropathies, myopathies, organ involvement, fever, and weight loss.[1,26,115]

Background Information

This condition is the result of an immune-mediated response resulting in the inflammation of vascular structures.[1,115] It includes a variety of disorders such as giant cell/temporal arteritis (which is the most common form), primary angiitis of the central nervous system, Takayasu's disease, periarteritis nodosa, Kawasaki disease, Churg-Strauss syndrome, Wegener's granulomatosis, and secondary vasculitis associated with systemic lupus erythematous, rheumatoid arthritis, and scleroderma.[115] The diagnosis is confirmed through history, physical examination, laboratory testing, angiography, biopsy, and imaging.[1,26,115] Corticosteroids, cytotoxic agents, intravenous immunoglobulin, and plasmapheresis may be used in the treatment of vasculitis.[26,115] Prognosis is variable and depends on the specific underlying disorder. For example, giant cell arteritis is typically self-limiting within 1 to 2 years; however, death usually occurs within 1 year for individuals with primary angiitis of the central nervous system.[115]

■ Whipple's Disease (Intestinal Lipodystrophy)

Chief Clinical Characteristics

This presentation includes dementia, personality changes, ataxia, myoclonus, nystagmus, and visual loss. The presentation also includes weight loss, arthropathy, diarrhea, and abdominal pain. Some individuals may experience a low-grade fever, lymphadenopathy, hyperpigmentation, hypotension, peripheral edema, cardiac murmurs, occult bleeding, and myalgia.[116]

Background Information

This systemic disease is rare and is thought to be caused by the bacteria *Tropheryma whipplei*.[116] Diagnosis is determined by biopsy of the duodenum, cerebrospinal fluid, cardiac-valve tissue, lymph nodes, and/or synovial tissue.[116,117] Recommended treatment includes antibiotic therapy until subsequent biopsies are negative.[116,117] If left untreated, this condition may be fatal; however, when treated with antibiotic medications the prognosis is good. Relapses may occur and tend to be more common in those with central nervous system involvement.[116,117]

■ Wilson's Disease

Chief Clinical Characteristics

This presentation commonly involves liver dysfunction followed by neurological symptoms such as tremor, rigidity, drooling, difficulty with speech, and abrupt personality change.

Background Information

Symptoms of Wilson's disease usually appear in childhood or young adult life[118] with a frequency of 1 in 30,000.[119] This condition is an autosomal recessive disorder in which excessive amounts of copper accumulate in the body, especially in eye membranes (causing a golden brown Kayser-Fleischer ring), nailbeds, and kidney.[26] The gene abnormality has been located on chromosome 13, which causes a deficiency in ceruloplasmin. In the central nervous system, cavitation and neuronal loss occur within the putamen and globus pallidus. This condition is diagnosed based on clinical findings supported by biochemical evidence of low ceruloplasmin, elevated unbound serum copper, high urinary copper excretion, positive liver biopsy and copper metabolism tests, and T_2-weighted magnetic resonance imaging that shows thalamus and putamen hyperintensity.[26] Treatment consists of low-copper diet and a chelating agent (usually penicillamine).[26] With adequate treatment, the life span is normal. If left untreated in children, death is predicted in 2 years from hepatic and renal failure. In untreated adults, death is predicted in 10 years.[26]

References

1. Victor M, Ropper AH. *Adams and Victor's Principles of Neurology.* 7th ed. New York, NY: McGraw-Hill; 2001.
2. Garg RK. Acute disseminated encephalomyelitis. *Postgrad Med J.* Jan 2003;79(927):11–17.
3. Foreman PJ. Summary and discussion—patient #32. October 16, 2008. http://www.bcm.edu/neurology/challeng/pat32/summary.html. Accessed August 28, 2005.

4. Ropper AH, Brown RJ. *Adams and Victor's Principles of Neurology.* 8th ed. New York, NY: McGraw-Hill; 2005.
5. Steinbok P. Clinical features of Chiari I malformations. *Childs Nerv Syst.* May 2004;20(5):329–331.
6. Al-Otaibi LM, Porter SR, Poate TW. Behcet's disease: a review. *J Dent Res.* Mar 2005;84(3):209–222.
7. Loeb C. Binswanger's disease is not a single entity. *Neurol Sci.* Dec 2000;21(6):343–348.
8. Roman GC. Vascular dementia revisited: diagnosis, pathogenesis, treatment, and prevention. *Med Clin North Am.* May 2002;86(3):477–499.
9. Roman GC, Erkinjuntti T, Wallin A, Pantoni L, Chui HC. Subcortical ischaemic vascular dementia. *Lancet Neurol.* Nov 2002;1(7):426–436.
10. Meriggioli MN, Rowin J, Sanders DB. Distinguishing clinical and electrodiagnostic features of X-linked bulbospinal neuronopathy. *Muscle Nerve.* Dec 1999; 22(12):1693–1697.
11. Sperfeld AD, Karitzky J, Brummer D, et al. X-linked bulbospinal neuronopathy: Kennedy disease. *Arch Neurol.* Dec 2002;59(12):1921–1926.
12. Greenland KJ, Zajac JD. Kennedy's disease: pathogenesis and clinical approaches. *Intern Med J.* May 2004; 34(5):279–286.
13. Schievink WI. Intracranial aneurysms. *N Engl J Med.* Jan 2 1997;336(1):28–40.
14. Vogel T, Verreault R, Turcotte JF, Kiesmann M, Berthel M. Intracerebral aneurysms: a review with special attention to geriatric aspects. *J Gerontol A Biol Sci Med Sci.* Jun 2003;58(6):520–524.
15. Consensus statement on the definition of orthostatic hypotension, pure autonomic failure, and multiple system atrophy. The Consensus Committee of the American Autonomic Society and the American Academy of Neurology. *Neurology.* May 1996;46(5):1470.
16. Unruptured intracranial aneurysms—risk of rupture and risks of surgical intervention. International Study of Unruptured Intracranial Aneurysms Investigators. *N Engl J Med.* Dec 10 1998;339(24):1725–1733.
17. Aasly J, Skandsen T, Ro M. Neuroacanthocytosis—the variability of presenting symptoms in two siblings. *Acta Neurol Scand.* Nov 1999;100(5):322–325.
18. Bohlega S, Riley W, Powe J, Baynton R, Roberts G. Neuroacanthocytosis and aprebetalipoproteinemia. *Neurology.* Jun 1998;50(6):1912–1914.
19. Rubio JP, Danek A, Stone C, et al. Chorea-acanthocytosis: genetic linkage to chromosome 9q21. *Am J Hum Genet.* Oct 1997;61(4):899–908.
20. Mahapatra RK, Edwards MJ, Schott JM, Bhatia KP. Corticobasal degeneration. *Lancet Neurol.* Dec 2004; 3(12):736–743.
21. Wenning GK, Litvan I, Jankovic J, et al. Natural history and survival of 14 patients with corticobasal degeneration confirmed at postmortem examination. *J Neurol Neurosurg Psychiatry.* Feb 1998;64(2):184–189.
22. Boeve BF, Lang AE, Litvan I. Corticobasal degeneration and its relationship to progressive supranuclear palsy and frontotemporal dementia. *Ann Neurol.* 2003;54 (suppl 5):S15–19.
23. Kompoliti K, Goetz CG, Boeve BF, et al. Clinical presentation and pharmacological therapy in corticobasal degeneration. *Arch Neurol.* Jul 1998;55(7):957–961.
24. Collinge J. Molecular neurology of prion disease. *J Neurol Neurosurg Psychiatry.* Jul 2005;76(7):906–919.

25. Knight RS, Will RG. Prion diseases. *J Neurol Neurosurg Psychiatry.* Mar 2004;75(suppl 1):i36–42.

26. Lindsay KW, Bone I, Callander R. *Neurology and Neurosurgery Illustrated.* 3rd ed. New York, NY: Churchill Livingstone; 1997.

27. Geldmacher DS. Dementia with Lewy bodies: diagnosis and clinical approach. *Cleve Clin J Med.* Oct 2004; 71(10):789–790, 792–784, 797–788 passim.

28. Small GW. Neuroimaging as a diagnostic tool in dementia with Lewy bodies. *Dement Geriatr Cogn Disord.* 2004;17(suppl 1):25–31.

29. Walker Z, Allen RL, Shergill S, Mullan E, Katona CL. Three years survival in patients with a clinical diagnosis of dementia with Lewy bodies. *Int J Geriatr Psychiatry.* Mar 2000;15(3):267–273.

30. Goodman CC, Boissonnault WG. *Pathology: Implications for the physical therapist.* Philadelphia, PA: W. B. Saunders; 1998.

31. American Psychiatric Association. *Diagnostic and Statistical Manual of Mental Disorders, Text Revision.* 4th ed. Washington, DC: American Psychiatric Association; 2000.

32. Aronson SC, Ayres VE. Depression: A treatment algorithm for the family physician. *Hospital Physician.* 2000(July):21–44.

33. Halgin RP, Whitbourne SK. *Abnormal Psychology: The Human Experience of Psychological Disorders.* 2nd ed. New York, NY: William C. Brown; 1997.

34. Hughes JC, Graham N, Patterson K, Hodges JR. Dysgraphia in mild dementia of Alzheimer's type. *Neuropsychologia.* Apr 1997;35(4):533–545.

35. Baranowski SL, Patten SB. The predictive value of dysgraphia and constructional apraxia for delirium in psychiatric inpatients. *Can J Psychiatry.* Feb 2000;45(1):75–78.

36. Baig SM. Acetazolamide therapy improves action myoclonus in Ramsay Hunt Syndrome. *J Neurol Sci.* Jan 1997;145(1):123–124.

37. Wiest G, Mueller C, Wessely P, Steinhoff N, Trattnig S, Deecke L. Oculomotor abnormalities in Dyssynergia cerebellaris myoclonica. *Acta Otolaryngol Suppl.* 1995;520(pt 2):392–394.

38. Trost M. Dystonia update. *Curr Opin Neurol.* Aug 2003; 16(4):495–500.

39. Costa J, Espirito-Santo C, Borges A, et al. Botulinum toxin type A therapy for blepharospasm. *Cochrane Database Syst Rev.* 2005(1):CD004900.

40. Konrad C, Vollmer-Haase J, Anneken K, Knecht S. Orthopedic and neurological complications of cervical dystonia—review of the literature. *Acta Neurol Scand.* Jun 2004;109(6):369–373.

41. Custodio CM, Basford JR. Delayed postanoxic encephalopathy: a case report and literature review. *Arch Phys Med Rehabil.* Mar 2004;85(3):502–505.

42. Sommerfield AJ, Stimson R, Campbell IW. Hashimoto's encephalopathy presenting as an acute medical emergency. *Scott Med J.* Nov 2004;49(4):155–156.

43. Manyam BV, Walters AS, Narla KR. Bilateral striopallidodentate calcinosis: clinical characteristics of patients seen in a registry. *Mov Disord.* Mar 2001;16(2):258–264.

44. Manyam BV, Bhatt MH, Moore WD, Devleschoward AB, Anderson DR, Calne DB. Bilateral striopallidodentate calcinosis: cerebrospinal fluid, imaging, and electrophysiological studies. *Ann Neurol.* Apr 1992;31(4): 379–384.

45. Manyam BV. What is and what is not 'Fahr's disease.' *Parkinsonism Relat Disord.* Mar 2005;11(2):73–80.

46. Albin RL. Dominant ataxias and Friedreich ataxia: an update. *Curr Opin Neurol.* Aug 2003;16(4):507–514.

47. Hart PE, Lodi R, Rajagopalan B, et al. Antioxidant treatment of patients with Friedreich ataxia: four-year follow-up. *Arch Neurol.* Apr 2005;62(4):621–626.

48. Delatycki MB, Ioannou PA, Churchyard AJ. Friedreich ataxia: from genes to therapies? *Med J Aust.* May 2 2005;182(9):439.

49. Thomas M, Hayflick SJ, Jankovic J. Clinical heterogeneity of neurodegeneration with brain iron accumulation (Hallervorden-Spatz syndrome) and pantothenate kinase-associated neurodegeneration. *Mov Disord.* Jan 2004;19(1):36–42.

50. Vasconcelos OM, Harter DH, Duffy C, et al. Adult Hallervorden-Spatz syndrome simulating amyotrophic lateral sclerosis. *Muscle Nerve.* Jul 2003;28(1):118–122.

51. Defazio G, Abbruzzese G, Girlanda P, et al. Botulinum toxin A treatment for primary hemifacial spasm: a 10-year multicenter study. *Arch Neurol.* Mar 2002;59(3):418–420.

52. de Boo GM, Tibben A, Lanser JB, et al. Early cognitive and motor symptoms in identified carriers of the gene for Huntington disease. *Arch Neurol.* Nov 1997;54(11): 1353–1357.

53. Rosas HD, Feigin AS, Hersch SM. Using advances in neuroimaging to detect, understand, and monitor disease progression in Huntington's disease. *NeuroRx.* Apr 2004;1(2):263–272.

54. Arriada N, Sotelo J. Review: treatment of hydrocephalus in adults. *Surg Neurol.* Dec 2002;58(6):377–384; discussion 384.

55. Torbey MT, Geocadin R, Bhardwaj A. Brain arrest neurological outcome scale (BrANOS): predicting mortality and severe disability following cardiac arrest. *Resuscitation.* Oct 2004;63(1):55–63.

56. Chu BC, Terae S, Takahashi C, et al. MRI of the brain in the Kearns-Sayre syndrome: report of four cases and a review. *Neuroradiology.* Oct 1999;41(10):759–764.

57. Gross-Jendroska M, Schatz H, McDonald HR, Johnson RN. Kearns-Sayre syndrome: a case report and review. *Eur J Ophthalmol.* Jan–Mar 1992;2(1):15–20.

58. Polak PE, Zijlstra F, Roelandt JR. Indications for pacemaker implantation in the Kearns-Sayre syndrome. *Eur Heart J.* Mar 1989;10(3):281–282.

59. Mori M, Kuwabara S, Fukutake T, Yuki N, Hattori T. Clinical features and prognosis of Miller Fisher syndrome. *Neurology.* Apr 24 2001;56(8):1104–1106.

60. Li H, Yuan J. Miller Fisher syndrome: toward a more comprehensive understanding. *Chin Med J (Engl).* Mar 2001;114(3):235–239.

61. Cejudo P, Bautista J, Montemayor T, et al. Exercise training in mitochondrial myopathy: a randomized controlled trial. *Muscle Nerve.* Sep 2005;32(3):342–350.

62. Hasuo K, Mihara F, Matsushima T. MRI and MR angiography in moyamoya disease. *J Magn Reson Imaging.* Jul–Aug 1998;8(4):762–766.

63. Sakamoto T, Kawaguchi M, Kurehara K, Kitaguchi K, Furuya H, Karasawa J. Risk factors for neurological deterioration after revascularization surgery in patients with moyamoya disease. *Anesth Analg.* Nov 1997;85(5): 1060–1065.

64. Nobile-Orazio E, Cappellari A, Priori A. Multifocal motor neuropathy: current concepts and controversies. *Muscle Nerve.* Jun 2005;31(6):663–680.

65. Van Asseldonk JT, Franssen H, Van den Berg-Vos RM, Wokke JH, Van den Berg LH. Multifocal motor neuropathy. *Lancet Neurol.* May 2005;4(5):309–319.

66. Nagale SV, Bosch EP. Multifocal motor neuropathy with conduction block: current issues in diagnosis and treatment. *Semin Neurol.* Sep 2003;23(3):325–334.

67. McDonald WI, Compston A, Edan G, et al. Recommended diagnostic criteria for multiple sclerosis: guidelines from the International Panel on the diagnosis of multiple sclerosis. *Ann Neurol.* Jul 2001;50(1):121–127.

68. Thompson AJ, Montalban X, Barkhof F, et al. Diagnostic criteria for primary progressive multiple sclerosis: a position paper. *Ann Neurol.* Jun 2000;47(6):831–835.

69. Confavreux C, Vukusic S, Adeleine P. Early clinical predictors and progression of irreversible disability in multiple sclerosis: an amnesic process. *Brain.* Apr 2003; 126(pt 4):770–782.

70. Wenning GK, Tison F, Ben Shlomo Y, Daniel SE, Quinn NP. Multiple system atrophy: a review of 203 pathologically proven cases. *Mov Disord.* Mar 1997;12(2):133–147.

71. Wenning GK, Ben-Shlomo Y, Hughes A, Daniel SE, Lees A, Quinn NP. What clinical features are most useful to distinguish definite multiple system atrophy from Parkinson's disease? *J Neurol Neurosurg Psychiatry.* Apr 2000;68(4):434–440.

72. Ben-Shlomo Y, Wenning GK, Tison F, Quinn NP. Survival of patients with pathologically proven multiple system atrophy: a meta-analysis. *Neurology.* Feb 1997; 48(2):384–393.

73. Caviness JN, Brown P. Myoclonus: current concepts and recent advances. *Lancet Neurol.* Oct 2004;3(10):598–607.

74. Agarwal P, Frucht SJ. Myoclonus. *Curr Opin Neurol.* Aug 2003;16(4):515–521.

75. Price RW. Neurological complications of HIV infection. *Lancet.* Aug 17 1996;348(9025):445–452.

76. Arimura K, Sonoda Y, Watanabe O, et al. Isaacs' syndrome as a potassium channelopathy of the nerve. *Muscle Nerve.* 2002;(suppl 11):S55–58.

77. Van Parijs V, Van den Bergh PY, Vincent A. Neuromyotonia and myasthenia gravis without thymoma. *J Neurol Neurosurg Psychiatry.* Sep 2002;73(3):344–345.

78. Hayat GR, Kulkantrakorn K, Campbell WW, Giuliani MJ. Neuromyotonia: autoimmune pathogenesis and response to immune modulating therapy. *J Neurol Sci.* Dec 1 2000;181(1–2):38–43.

79. Brown DL, Frank JE. Diagnosis and management of syphilis. *Am Fam Physician.* Jul 15 2003;68(2): 283–290.

80. Conde-Sendin MA, Amela-Peris R, Aladro-Benito Y, Maroto AA. Current clinical spectrum of neurosyphilis in immunocompetent patients. *Eur Neurol.* 2004;52(1): 29–35.

81. Imrie J, Vijayaraghaven S, Whitehouse C, et al. Niemann-Pick disease type C in adults. *J Inherit Metab Dis.* Oct 2002;25(6):491–500.

82. Jin LW, Shie FS, Maezawa I, Vincent I, Bird T. Intracellular accumulation of amyloidogenic fragments of a myloid-beta precursor protein in neurons with Niemann-Pick type C defects is associated with endosomal abnormalities. *Am J Pathol.* Mar 2004;164(3):975–985.

83. Relkin N, Marmarou A, Klinge P, Bergsneider M, Black PM. Diagnosing idiopathic normal-pressure hydrocephalus. *Neurosurgery.* Sep 2005;57(3 suppl):S4–16; discussion ii–v.

84. Hebb AO, Cusimano MD. Idiopathic normal pressure hydrocephalus: a systematic review of diagnosis and outcome. *Neurosurgery.* Nov 2001;49(5):1166–1184; discussion 1184–1166.

85. Tate ED, Allison TJ, Pranzatelli MR, Verhulst SJ. Neuroepidemiologic trends in 105 US cases of pediatric opsoclonus-myoclonus syndrome. *J Pediatr Oncol Nurs.* Jan–Feb 2005;22(1):8–19.

86. Bataller L, Dalmau J. Paraneoplastic neurological syndromes: approaches to diagnosis and treatment. *Semin Neurol.* Jun 2003;23(2):215–224.

87. Darnell RB, Posner JB. Paraneoplastic syndromes involving the nervous system. *N Engl J Med.* Oct 16 2003;349(16):1543–1554.

88. Dalmau JO, Posner JB. Paraneoplastic syndromes. *Arch Neurol.* Apr 1999;56(4):405–408.

89. Wood BH, Bilclough JA, Bowron A, Walker RW. Incidence and prediction of falls in Parkinson's disease: a prospective multidisciplinary study. *J Neurol Neurosurg Psychiatry.* Jun 2002;72(6):721–725.

90. Samii A, Nutt JG, Ransom BR. Parkinson's disease. *Lancet.* May 29 2004;363(9423):1783–1793.

91. Tillerson JL, Cohen AD, Philhower J, Miller GW, Zigmond MJ, Schallert T. Forced limb-use effects on the behavioral and neurochemical effects of 6-hydroxydopamine. *J Neurosci.* Jun 15, 2001;21(12): 4427–4435.

92. Jankovic J, Kapadia AS. Functional decline in Parkinson disease. *Arch Neurol.* Oct 2001;58(10): 1611–1615.

93. Marras C, Rochon P, Lang AE. Predicting motor decline and disability in Parkinson disease: a systematic review. *Arch Neurol.* Nov 2002;59(11):1724–1728.

94. Huang YG, Chen YC, Du F, et al. Topiramate therapy for paroxysmal kinesigenic choreoathetosis. *Mov Disord.* Jan 2005;20(1):75–77.

95. Berger J, Moser HW, Forss-Petter S. Leukodystrophies: recent developments in genetics, molecular biology, pathogenesis and treatment. *Curr Opin Neurol.* Jun 2001;14(3):305–312.

96. Regis S, Grossi S, Lualdi S, Biancheri R, Filocamo M. Diagnosis of Pelizaeus-Merzbacher disease: detection of proteolipid protein gene copy number by real-time PCR. *Neurogenetics.* May 2005;6(2):73–78.

97. Aicardi J. The inherited leukodystrophies: a clinical overview. *J Inherit Metab Dis.* 1993;16(4):733–743.

98. Borrell E. Hypokinetic movement disorders. *J Neurosci Nurs.* Oct 2000;32(5):254–255.

99. Litvan I, Mangone CA, McKee A, et al. Natural history of progressive supranuclear palsy (Steele-Richardson-Olszewski syndrome) and clinical predictors of survival: a clinicopathological study. *J Neurol Neurosurg Psychiatry.* Jun 1996;60(6):615–620.

100. Litvan I, Bhatia KP, Burn DJ, et al. Movement Disorders Society Scientific Issues Committee report: SIC Task Force appraisal of clinical diagnostic criteria for Parkinsonian disorders. *Mov Disord.* May 2003;18(5): 467–486.

101. Simon RP, Aminoff MJ, Greenberg DA. *Clinical Neurology.* 4th ed. Stamford, CT: Appleton and Lange; 1999.

102. Taroni F, DiDonato S. Pathways to motor incoordination: the inherited ataxias. *Nat Rev Neurosci.* Aug 2004; 5(8):641–655.

103. Granger CV, Clark GS. Functional status and outcomes of stroke rehabilitation. *Topics Geriatrics.* Mar 1994; 9(3):72–84.

104. Shelton FD, Volpe BT, Reding M. Motor impairment as a predictor of functional recovery and guide to rehabilitation treatment after stroke. *Neurorehabil Neural Repair.* 2001;15(3):229–237.

105. Casey DE. Tardive dyskinesia. *West J Med.* Nov 1990;153(5):535–541.

106. Tammenmaa IA, Sailas E, McGrath JJ, Soares-Weiser K, Wahlbeck K. Systematic review of cholinergic drugs for neuroleptic-induced tardive dyskinesia: a meta-analysis of randomized controlled trials. *Prog Neuropsychopharmacol Biol Psychiatry.* Nov 2004;28(7):1099–1107.

107. Soares KV, McGrath JJ. The treatment of tardive dyskinesia—a systematic review and meta–analysis. *Schizophr Res.* Aug 23 1999;39(1):1–16; discussion 17–18.

108. Simpson GM. The treatment of tardive dyskinesia and tardive dystonia. *J Clin Psychiatry.* 2000;61(suppl 4): 39–44.

109. Bruns J, Hauser WA. The epidemiology of traumatic brain injury: a review. *Epilepsia.* 2003;44(suppl 10):2–10.

110. Das-Gupta R, Turner-Stokes L. Traumatic brain injury. *Disability and Rehabilitation.* 2002;24(13):654–665.

111. Hukkelhoven CWPM, Steyerberg EW, Rampen AJJ, et al. Patient age and outcome following severe traumatic brain injury: an analysis of 5600 patients. *J Neurosurg.* 2003;99:666–673.

112. Tosoni A, Ermani M, Brandes AA. The pathogenesis and treatment of brain metastases: a comprehensive review. *Critical Reviews in Oncology/Hematology.* 2004;52:199–215.

113. Perrin RG, Laxton AW. Metastatic spine disease: epidemiology, pathophysiology, and evaluation of patients. *Neurosurg Clin N Am.* Oct 2004;15(4): 365–373.

114. Hosono N, Ueda T, Tamura D, Aoki Y, Yoshikawa H. Prognostic relevance of clinical symptoms in patients with spinal metastases. *Clin Orthop Relat Res.* Jul 2005(436):196–201.

115. Ferro JM. Vasculitis of the central nervous system. *J Neurol.* Dec 1998;245(12):766–776.

116. Marth T, Raoult D. Whipple's disease. *Lancet.* Jan 18 2003;361(9353):239–246.

117. Mahnel R, Marth T. Progress, problems, and perspectives in diagnosis and treatment of Whipple's disease. *Clin Exp Med.* Sep 2004;4(1):39–43.

118. Greenberg DA, Aminoff MJ, Simon RP. *Clinical Neurology.* 5th ed. New York, NY: McGraw-Hill; 2002.

119. Gow PJ, Smallwood RA, Angus PW, Smith AL, Wall AJ, Sewell RB. Diagnosis of Wilson's disease: an experience over three decades. *Gut.* Mar 2000;46(3):415–419.

CHAPTER **31**

Problems of Cognition, Communication, and Behavior

■ *Julie Hershberg, PT, DPT, NCS*

Description of the Symptom

This chapter describes pathology that may lead to problems with cognition, communication, and behavior. These types of problems are often observed together with central nervous system pathology. Disturbances of cognition include difficulty with problem solving and making sound judgments, organizing information, and memory. Cognitive problems can range from difficulty attending to a task to being in a comatose state.

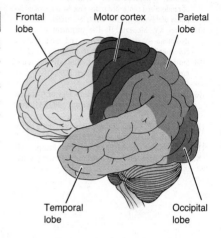

Frontal lobe / Motor cortex / Parietal lobe / Temporal lobe / Occipital lobe

Functions of Selected Brain Structures

BRAIN STRUCTURE	FUNCTION(S)
Frontal lobe Broca's area (left hemisphere)	Initiation, judgment, memory, impulse control, sequencing, social behavior Expressive language
Parietal lobe	Sensory integration, awareness of body image and environment
Temporal lobe Wernicke's area (left hemisphere)	Long-term memory, auditory processing Processing of speech
Occipital lobe	Visual field, color discrimination
Motor cortex (motor homunculus) Somatosensory cortex (sensory homunculus) Visual cortex Auditory cortex	Contralateral control of movement Contralateral perception of sensation Contralateral perception of vision Bilateral reception of auditory input

Special Concerns

■ Problems with cognition, communication, or behavior of sudden onset or rapid progression
■ Any problems that occur after trauma or are present during or soon after a viral or bacterial infection that have not yet been discussed with a physician
■ Problems with behavior that cause potential harm to the patient or others

CHAPTER PREVIEW: Conditions That May Lead to Problems with Cognition, Communication, and Behavior

Trauma

COMMON

Epilepsy/seizure disorder 645
Traumatic brain injury 658

UNCOMMON

Hypoxia (cerebral hypoxia, anoxia) 648

RARE

Not applicable

Inflammation

COMMON

Aseptic
Multiple sclerosis 650

Septic
Encephalitis 644
Encephalopathy 645
Meningitis:
• Bacterial meningitis 649
• Viral meningitis 649

UNCOMMON

Aseptic
Systemic lupus erythematosus 657

Septic
Acute disseminated encephalomyelitis 638
Cysticercosis 643
Lyme disease (tick paralysis) 649
Neurological complications of acquired immunodeficiency syndrome 652
Reye's syndrome 655
Rickettsial diseases, including Rocky Mountain spotted fever 656

RARE

Aseptic
Behçet's disease 640
Paraneoplastic syndromes 653

Septic
Klüver-Bucy syndrome 648
Malaria 649
Neurosyphilis (tabes dorsalis, syphilitic spinal sclerosis, progressive locomotor ataxia) 652
Progressive multifocal leukoencephalopathy 655
Subacute sclerosing panencephalitis (Dawson's disease) 657
Whipple's disease (intestinal lipodystrophy) 660

M Metabolic

COMMON

Cushing's syndrome (hypercortisolism) 643
Neurotoxicity 653

UNCOMMON

Not applicable

RARE

Cerebral beriberi (Korsakoff's amnesic syndrome, Wernicke-Korsakoff syndrome) 641
Mitochondrial myopathies 650

Va Vascular

COMMON

Stroke (cerebrovascular accident) 657
Transient ischemic attack 658

UNCOMMON

Arteriovenous malformation 639
Cerebral aneurysm 641
Multi-infarct dementia/vascular dementia 650

RARE

Cavernous malformation 641
Gerstmann's syndrome 646
Moyamoya disease 650

De Degenerative

COMMON

Alzheimer's disease 638
Dementia with Lewy bodies 643
Parkinson's disease 654

UNCOMMON

Binswanger's disease (subcortical arteriosclerotic encephalopathy, subcortical dementia) 640
Corticobasal degeneration 642
Frontotemporal dementia 646
Progressive supranuclear palsy (Richardson-Steele-Olszewski syndrome) 655

RARE

Creutzfeldt-Jakob disease 643
Multiple system atrophy (striatonigral degeneration, olivopontocerebellar atrophy, Shy-Drager syndrome) 651
Pick's disease 655

Tu Tumor

COMMON

Malignant Primary:
Not applicable
Malignant Metastatic:
Not applicable
Benign, such as:
• Neurofibromatosis 651

Tumor *(continued)*

UNCOMMON

Malignant Primary, such as:
• Brain primary tumors 659
Malignant Metastatic, such as:
• Brain metastases 659
Benign:
Not applicable

RARE

Malignant Primary, such as:
• Spinal primary tumors 659
Malignant Metastatic, such as:
• Spinal metastases 659
Benign:
Not applicable

Co Congenital

COMMON

Attention deficit hyperactivity disorder 639
Dyslexia (developmental reading disorder) 644
Huntington's disease 647

UNCOMMON

Choreoacanthocytosis (Levine-Critchley syndrome, neuroacanthocytosis) 642

RARE

Fahr's syndrome (familial idiopathic basal ganglia calcification, bilateral striopallidodentate calcinosis) 645
Gaucher's disease 646
Hallervorden-Spatz syndrome (neurodegeneration with brain iron accumulation, pantothenate kinase-associated neurodegeneration) 647
Hereditary spastic paraplegia (familial spastic paralysis) 647
Niemann-Pick disease (types C and D only) 653
Pelizaeus-Merzbacher disease 654
Tuberous sclerosis 658
Wilson's disease 660

Ne Neurogenic/Psychogenic

COMMON

Anxiety disorder/panic attacks 639
Bipolar disorder (manic depression) 640
Depression 644
Hydrocephalus 647
Sleep apnea 656

UNCOMMON

Paranoia, delusional disorder 654
Schizophrenia 656

(continued)

Neurogenic/Psychogenic *(continued)*

RARE
Conversion disorder 642
Hypersomnia 648
Narcolepsy 651
Tourette's syndrome 658

Note: These are estimates of relative incidence because few data are available for the less common conditions.

Overview of Problems with Cognition, Communication, and Behavior

Though often not the primary symptoms leading to a physical therapy visit, problems with cognition, communication, and behavior often are the first indicators of neurological insult and are thus important in the differential diagnosis process. Problems with cognition, communication, and behavior invariably are caused by cerebral cortex pathology. Symptoms are distinctly related to the part of the cortex involved and assist in the differential diagnosis process. If the frontal lobes are involved, prevalent signs and symptoms include hemiparesis, apathy, alterations in personality and behavior, inability to sequence motor tasks, perseveration, inattention, abulia, Broca's aphasia, and prominent grasp and suck reflexes. Lesions in the temporal cortex may cause memory and learning impairments and lesions on the left side also often cause Wernicke's aphasia and visual agnosia. Parietal lobe dysfunction includes hemisensory loss, agnosia, visual-perceptual disorders, and neglect.[1]

Problems with communication include difficulties with comprehension or production of spoken or written language. Receptive or Wernicke's aphasia denotes a difficulty with comprehension characterized by frequent word substitutions, impaired repetition and naming, and excessive talking. Expressive or Broca's aphasia is used to describe difficulty with conveying thoughts or ideas through words. Global aphasia results from damage to all language areas of the brain and includes impairments in both comprehension and expression. The most common cause of aphasia is a stroke. It can also result from traumatic brain injury, brain tumor, or any other insult affecting the language areas of the brain.[2]

Common problems with behavior or mood include anxiety, depression, and impaired control of emotion.[2] A patient or family member may report the patient has decreased initiative, personality changes, emotional lability, reduced range of mental activity, aggression, or social inappropriateness.[3]

Description of Conditions That May Lead to Problems with Cognition, Communication, and Behavior

■ Acute Disseminated Encephalomyelitis

Chief Clinical Characteristics
This presentation may involve confusion, somnolence, and convulsion in its encephalitic form. Initial symptoms of the myelitic form include weakness and sensory impairments.[2]

Background Information
This condition is a demyelinating disease of the central nervous system,[4] which may be due to an immune-mediated complication of infection.[2] The presence of upper motor neuron signs, cerebrospinal fluid pleocytosis and elevated protein, and multiple white matter lesions demonstrated on magnetic resonance imaging supports the diagnosis.[5] Definitive diagnosis requires a brain biopsy. The primary goal of treatment is to suppress the immune response; thus high-dose corticosteroids are generally administered over a course of 3 to 5 days.[5] The prognosis is variable depending on the severity of the disease and acuity of the diagnosis.

■ Alzheimer's Disease

Chief Clinical Characteristics
This presentation includes progressive memory loss, language deterioration, poor judgment, confusion, restlessness, and mood swings.

Background Information

This condition is the most common neurodegenerative disorder that causes cognitive decline in persons over the age of 60 years[6] with prevalence rates from 3% to nearly 50% in persons between ages 65 and 85 years.[7] The anatomical pathology of this condition is characterized by progressive accumulation of amyloid plaques and neurofibrillary tangles in the cortex that lead to destruction of nervous tissue.[2] Diagnosis is made based on clinical presentation and cognitive testing. There is no cure for this condition at this time and medical treatment is largely symptomatic using psychotropic medications and behavioral interventions; cholinesterase inhibitors for early stages of the disease; and N-methyl-D-aspartate antagonists for later stages of the disease. This condition is a progressive disease, but its course can vary from 5 to 20 years.[8] Most deaths result from respiratory or cardiovascular compromise.[2]

■ **Anxiety Disorder/Panic Attacks**

Chief Clinical Characteristics
This presentation typically includes repeated panic or anxiety attacks. Symptoms include increased heart rate and respiratory rate, pupil dilation, and trembling and sweating with feelings of fear and dread. The symptoms usually subside in 15 to 30 minutes.

Background Information

This condition is a nonspecific syndrome and can be due to a variety of medical or psychiatric syndromes or observed as part of a drug withdrawal or drug intoxication effect. The diagnosis of an anxiety condition is based on criteria from the DSM-IV-TR.[9] Anxiety conditions are classified into specific categories. One category, panic condition, has dizziness as one of its features. Panic condition is defined by recurrent attacks with at least four of the following features: increased heart rate, sweating, trembling or shaking, dyspnea, sensation of choking, chest pain or discomfort, nausea or abdominal distress, feelings of dizziness, fear of losing control, fear of dying, paresthesias, and chills or hot flashes. The etiology of anxiety conditions includes genetic factors, social and psychological factors, and physiological and biochemical abnormalities.[10] Treatment includes cognitive-behavioral therapy, relaxation exercises and pharmacologic treatment.[10] The course of this condition is variable; most individuals maintain normal social lives. Clinicians are encouraged to consider referral of individuals suspected of having this condition to a mental health specialist for evaluation and treatment.

■ **Arteriovenous Malformation**

Chief Clinical Characteristics
This presentation may be characterized by seizures and severe headache. Hemorrhage may result in paresis, ataxia, dyspraxia, dizziness, tactile and proprioceptive disturbances, visual disturbances, aphasia, paresthesias, and cognitive deficits.[2]

Background Information

This condition is caused by a tangle of arteries and veins that cause abnormal communication within the vasculature and approximately 12% of the 300,000 individuals in the United States with this condition are symptomatic. This condition is caused by a developmental abnormality that likely arises during embryonic or fetal development. Neurological damage occurs due to reduction of oxygen delivery, hemorrhage, or compression of nearby structures of the brain or spinal cord. Computed tomography, magnetic resonance imaging, and arteriography confirm the diagnosis. Ligation and embolization may be used to reduce the size of the lesion prior to surgical excision, which is the preferred method of treatment. Stereotactic radiation and proton beam therapy are alternative approaches to invasive methods of intervention. Up to 90% of individuals who experience a hemorrhagic arteriovenous malformation survive.[2]

■ **Attention Deficit Hyperactivity Disorder**

Chief Clinical Characteristics
This presentation includes distractibility, forgetfulness, restlessness, and impulsivity.[11]

Background Information

Diagnosis is based on DSM-IV criteria[12] and a thorough patient and family history. DSM-IV-TR criteria include having inattention and hyperactivity-impulsivity symptoms for at least 6 months; symptoms present in at least two settings; some symptoms present before age 7; and clinically significant impairment in education, work, or socially. This condition is prevalent in 1.7% to 16% of the pediatric population.[13] The etiology of this condition involves genetic and environmental factors. Several genes appear to be associated because of their affect on dopamine receptors, dopamine transport, and dopamine beta-hydroxylase. Environmental factors may also play a role, including pregnancy and delivery problems, family dysfunction, and poorer socioeconomic status. Treatment includes medication and behavioral intervention. This condition can be well controlled with treatment and the prognosis is excellent for individuals who have no major comorbidities, have individualized medication management, have received family education regarding the diagnosis and treatment, and whose associated learning disorders or emotional problems have been addressed.[13]

■ Behçet's Disease

Chief Clinical Characteristics
This presentation may include bilateral pyramidal sign (signs related to lesions of upper motor neurons or descending pyramidal tracts, such as a positive Babinski sign or hyperreflexia), headache, memory loss, hemiparesis, cerebellar ataxia, balance deficits, sphincter dysfunction, or cranial nerve palsies. In addition to these neurological signs individuals with this condition also may present with arthritis; renal, gastrointestinal, vascular, and cardiac diseases; and genital, oral, and cutaneous ulcerations.[14]

Background Information
Mean age of onset is in the third decade of life. Diagnostic criteria according to an international study group include presence of recurrent oral ulceration, recurrent genital ulceration, eye lesions, skin lesions, papulopustular lesions, and/or a positive pathergy test.[2,14] Medical treatment typically consists of corticosteroids and immunosuppressants. Neurological symptoms tend to clear within weeks, but can sometimes recur or result in permanent deficits.[2] Onset before the age of 25 and male sex indicate a poorer prognosis.

■ Binswanger's Disease (Subcortical Arteriosclerotic Encephalopathy, Subcortical Dementia)

Chief Clinical Characteristics
This presentation involves small-stepped gait, slowed motor function with perseveration, deficits in executive function, slow information processing, and impaired memory. Other symptoms include dysarthria, dysphagia, urinary disturbances, and lateral homonymous hemianopias.[15–17]

Background Information
This condition is a type of vascular dementia that results from multiple strokes and demyelination of the central white matter.[15,17] Diagnosis is made by neuroimaging, specifically computed tomography and magnetic resonance imaging.[15] Medical management includes drug therapy targeted at improving core symptoms and delaying disease progression, as well as secondary prevention of stroke by decreasing hypertension.[16,18]

■ Bipolar Disorder (Manic Depression)

Chief Clinical Characteristics
This presentation typically involves episodes of clinical depression and episodes of mania. The episodes of mania involve flight of ideas, hyperactivity, increased appetite, and poor judgment.

Background Information
Diagnosis is based on criteria from the DSM-IV-TR.[12] Manic episodes are characterized as having at least 1 week of profound mood disturbance with elation, irritability, or expansiveness. In addition, three or more of the following symptoms are present: grandiosity; diminished need for sleep; racing thoughts or flight of ideas; distractibility; increased level of goal-focused activity at home, at work, or sexually; and excessive pleasurable activities, often with painful consequences. The disturbance in mood must be sufficient to cause impairment at work or danger to the patients or others. Estimates of prevalence range from 1% to 1.6% of the population in the United States.[19] The cause of this condition is incompletely understood, although it is acknowledged that genetic and environmental factors are responsible. Pharmacologic treatment is the mainstay

of managing bipolar disorder. This condition is associated with 80% to 90% relapse and recurrence rates.[19] Poor prognosis is associated with high degrees of neuroticism, long duration before treatment, positive family history, and the presence of depression-provoking circumstances.[2] Suicide is a risk for all patients with bipolar disorder with approximately 25% of patients attempting suicide and 11% of patients dying by suicide.[19]

■ Cavernous Malformation

Chief Clinical Characteristics
This presentation includes symptoms that are dependent on the neuroanatomical location affected. Symptoms often consist of paresthesias, mood and cognitive changes, visual disturbances, headaches, and seizures.

Background Information
This condition is a rare disorder of the vascular system of the brain where a blood-filled mass, or hemangioma, forms. This condition is frequently inherited in an autosomal dominant pattern. Diagnosis is made on clinical manifestations and magnetic resonance imaging findings of clusters of vessels with a rim of hypdensity on T_1-weighted images.[2] For individuals with this condition who experience neurological symptoms, treatment is symptomatic and supportive. Surgical removal or radiation may be performed.[2] Individuals with prior hemorrhage and infratentorial location of the hemangioma have a poorer prognosis.[21]

■ Cerebral Aneurysm

Chief Clinical Characteristics
This presentation may involve mood and cognitive changes in combination with other neurological symptoms and signs that depend on the affected cerebral tissue, including visual and proprioceptive loss. Any associated signs or symptoms may not be reported due to the fact that this condition is typically asymptomatic prior to rupture. However, if the aneurysm results in a mass effect, ischemia, or hemorrhage, then neurological signs and symptoms are dependent on the affected location.[2,22,23]

Background Information
There has been some description of genetic factors in this condition.[22] Cigarette smoking, hypertension, and heavy alcohol use have all

been found to be correlated with increased risk of aneurysm development.[22,23] Factors associated with increased risk of rupture include size of aneurysm, location in the posterior circulation, and a previous history of aneurismal subarachnoid hemorrhage.[24,25] Definitive diagnosis is based on catheter angiography; however, magnetic resonance angiography, magnetic resonance imaging, and computed tomography may aid in the diagnosis. Unruptured aneurysms are sometimes surgically treated. Aneurysm size, location, and prior history of a subarachnoid hemorrhage help to determine if the risk of surgical treatment is worth the potential benefits. Most aneurysms that have hemorrhaged must be treated surgically. Patients with a previous rupture are at an 11 times greater risk of having a second intracranial aneurysm rupture. When aneurysms do rupture, many patients die within one month of the rupture, and those who survive often have residual neurological deficits.[22]

■ Cerebral Beriberi (Korsakoff's Amnesic Syndrome, Wernicke-Korsakoff Syndrome)

Chief Clinical Characteristics
This presentation involves ophthalmoparesis, nystagmus, ataxia, and confusion, as well as impaired learning and memory. Other common symptoms include peripheral neuropathy, postural hypotension, syncope, impaired olfactory discrimination, mild hypothermia, and confabulation.[17]

Background Information
This condition is due to a thiamine deficiency that results in a diffuse decrease in cerebral glucose utilization. It is most commonly observed in individuals who abuse alcohol and have nutritional deficiencies, although it is not limited to this population.[17] Diagnosis can be made by blood tests to examine thiamine levels. Neuroimaging may show slowed brain activity as well as lesions in the medial thalamus and periaqueductal region.[17] Medical treatment involves the immediate administration of thiamine. Once thiamine has been administered, the reversal of symptoms should begin to occur within hours to days with variable degrees of recovery. Memory has been shown to have the poorest return, and mortality rates of up to 17% have been reported.[17]

■ Choreoacanthocytosis (Levine-Critchley Syndrome, Neuroacanthocytosis)

Chief Clinical Characteristics
This presentation commonly includes chorea, motor or vocal tics, dystonia, orofacial dyskinesias, and parkinsonism. Seizures, cognitive impairment, psychosis, paranoia, and personality changes are also seen with this diagnosis, along with hyporeflexia and distal myopathy due to denervation of muscles.[26–28]

Background Information
This condition is a rare, autosomal recessive disorder that typically has its onset during the third and fourth decades of life.[28] This neurodegenerative disorder is associated with acanthocytes, aberrant spiky or thorny red blood cells, as well as atrophy and gliosis of the caudate, putamen, and globus pallidus.[27] Diagnosis is made by a combination of tests, including clinical features, lab work demonstrating acanthocytosis, neuroimaging, and genetic testing to rule out Huntington's disease.[26] There is currently no effective, long-term treatment, although verapamil has been found to provide temporary reduction of symptoms. Life expectancy is reduced, and suicidal action or ideation is not uncommon due to cognitive impairments.[28]

■ Conversion Disorder

Chief Clinical Characteristics
This presentation can be characterized by motor or sensory deficits, seizures or convulsions, or blindness or deafness. Symptoms usually appear suddenly and abate in less than 2 weeks.

Background Information
This condition is one type of somatoform disorder in which psychological stress becomes translated into physical problems. The DSM-IV-TR defines conversion disorder by symptoms that simulate a neurological or other medical condition that involves voluntary muscles or sensory organs excluding pain and sexual functions.[2] Clinical findings include patterns of sensory loss that do not follow normal patterns from neurological insults and symptoms that disappear when a patient is distracted or thinks that no one is watching. Patients often have a history of emotional disturbance, stress, or traumatic

event. Differential diagnosis is based on clinical findings. It is helpful to treat the patient as though he or she has had an illness and is now in the process of recovery.[2] Cognitive and behavioral therapies may be effective in treating underlying psychological issues. Prognosis is variable with differing degrees of recovery in days to months. Good prognostic factors include acute onset of symptoms, short duration of symptoms, healthy premorbid functioning, higher intelligence, absence of coexisting psychopathology, and presence of an identifiable stressor. Poor prognostic symptoms include pseudoseizures, age greater than 40, and long-lasting severe disability.[29]

■ Corticobasal Degeneration

Chief Clinical Characteristics
This presentation typically includes limb ideomotor apraxia and unilateral parkinsonism that is unresponsive to levodopa, gait disturbances, tremor, postural instability, and dementia.[30,31]

Background Information
A proposed set of criteria for the diagnosis of this condition includes core features of:

1. Insidious onset and progressive course
2. No identifiable cause
3. Cortical dysfunction (ideomotor apraxia, alien-limb phenomenon, cortical sensory loss, visual or sensory hemineglect, constructional apraxia, focal or asymmetric myoclonus, apraxia of speech or nonfluent aphasia), and
4. Extrapyramidal dysfunction (rigidity which does not respond to levodopa therapy and dystonia).[32]

This condition is a sporadic disease with an average age of onset of 63 years.[31] There have been reports of familial cases; however, for most cases there is no known cause.[30] Diagnosis is made based on clinical presentation. A definitive diagnosis can only be made postmortem. Medical treatment is not typically successful; it has been found that only about 24% of these patients will respond to levodopa therapy aimed at addressing the extrapyramidal features of the disease.[33] Physical and occupational therapy are used to maintain mobility and address safety issues related to the progression of imbalance. Mean survival is

7.9 years with a range of 2.5 to 12.5 years.[31] Early presence of bilateral parkinsonism or frontal lobe signs indicates a less favorable prognosis.[31]

■ Creutzfeldt-Jakob Disease

Chief Clinical Characteristics

This presentation may involve rapidly progressive dementia, cerebellar ataxia, balance deficits, myoclonus, cortical blindness, pyramidal signs, extrapyramidal signs, and akinetic mutism.[34]

Background Information

Different forms of this condition have been described including sporadic, iatrogenic, and variant. Sporadic and iatrogenic forms of this condition typically affect older individuals; whereas the variant form affects younger individuals.[35] The early stages of the variant form are characterized by psychiatric symptoms, including depression and anxiety.[35] The condition is rare and affects only one to two people per million worldwide per year.[34,35] It is caused by a conformational change of the normal prion protein which is encoded by human chromosome 20 to a disease-related prion protein. Diagnosis is suggested by a thorough history and physical examination, electroencephalography, and cerebrospinal fluid analysis.[35] Computed tomography and magnetic resonance imaging are typically normal in sporadic and iatrogenic forms and help to exclude other diagnoses.[1,34] Diagnosis for all forms of this condition is only confirmed postmortem.[1] There is no proven treatment.[1,35] Death in sporadic and iatrogenic forms occurs in a matter of months with death occurring at a mean age of 66 years.[35] Mean duration of illness in the variant form is 14 months.[35]

■ Cushing's Syndrome (Hypercortisolism)

Chief Clinical Characteristics

This presentation includes severe weakness of the proximal limb and girdle muscles often manifested by difficulty climbing stairs or rising from a low chair. Additional signs and symptoms include fatigue, obesity of the upper body (including the hallmark feature of a moon-shaped face), easy bruising and bluish-red stretch marks, high blood pressure, elevated blood glucose, memory loss, and depression.[36,37] *Women with this condition may show an increased growth of facial and body hair and irregularity of menstruation.*

Background Information

This rare endocrine disorder is caused by chronic exposure of the body's tissues to excess levels of cortisol due to medications or tumors of the pituitary or adrenal gland. Diagnosis is confirmed by laboratory evidence of excessive cortisol in the urine and blood.[36,37] Treatment is achieved through decreasing cortisol levels via medication, surgery, or radiation. Most individuals with this condition show significant improvement in symptom presentation with treatment. However, in some individuals, residual symptoms may persist and some kinds of tumors may recur.

■ Cysticercosis

Chief Clinical Characteristics

This presentation commonly involves seizures, headache, motor deficits, and psychiatric symptoms.[38] In children headache and vomiting are seen in about a third of cases.[39]

Background Information

Cysticercosis is more prevalent in immigrants in California, New Mexico, and Texas than elsewhere in the United States. This condition is the most frequent parasitosis of the central nervous system and occurs when a person ingests *Taenia solium* eggs by fecal-oral contamination. The larvae become established as viable cysts, which are eventually destroyed by cellular response and later appear as a residual calcification.[2] The diagnosis is confirmed with the presence of multiple calcified lesions in the cortex as shown in computed tomography or magnetic resonance imaging, positive histological findings, and direct visualization of the parasite by funduscopic examination. Treatment for cysticercosis includes anticysticercal drugs and corticosteroids for cerebral edema. If a large cyst obstructs the flow of cerebrospinal fluid, surgical removal of the cyst or a shunt becomes necessary.[2] Prognosis is most favorable for patients with one lesion.

■ Dementia with Lewy Bodies

Chief Clinical Characteristics

This presentation can be characterized by fluctuating cognitive dysfunction, particularly visuospatial problems and executive dysfunction, visual hallucinations, and parkinsonism features such as masked facies, autonomic dysfunction, rigidity, and bradykinesia. Other signs and symptoms may include postural instability, falls, sleep disturbances, memory problems, syncope, transient loss of consciousness, and sensitivity to antipsychotic and anti-Parkinson medications.[40]

Background Information

This progressive condition is the second most common dementia after Alzheimer's disease.[40] The specific etiology of this condition is unknown. The characteristic Lewy bodies are eosinophilic inclusion bodies found within the cytoplasm of neurons in the cerebral cortex and limbic system.[40] A thorough clinical examination, laboratory screen, and imaging are important to rule out other causes of dementia. The definitive diagnosis for this condition is made postmortem; however, it appears that the use of single-photon emission computed tomography and positron emission tomography may be useful in the identification of occipital hypoperfusion which may be associated with the visual hallucinations.[40,41] Management includes caregiver education to assist in minimizing factors that may contribute to problematic behaviors. Medication therapy may be indicated, but should be monitored closely due to potential exacerbation of symptoms.[40] Life expectancy for individuals with this condition is similar that of Alzheimer's disease. The average survival time is between 6 and 8 years from the onset of dementia.[40,42]

■ Depression

Chief Clinical Characteristics

This presentation may involve slowness of movement that can progress to the point of catatonia, intensely dysphoric mood, appetite loss, insomnia or hypersomnia, social withdrawal, loss of motivation, helplessness, hostility, and agitation.

Background Information

The origin of this condition is not fully understood and genetic, biochemical, neuroanatomical and psychosocial factors all appear to play a role.[43] For a clinical diagnosis, the following criteria from the DSM-IV-TR[12] must be met: at least five of the following symptoms, during the same 2-week period, representing a change from previous functioning: depressed mood;

diminished interest or pleasure; significant weight loss or gain; insomnia or hypersomnia; psychomotor agitation or delay; fatigue or loss of energy; feelings of worthlessness; diminished ability to think or concentrate, indecisiveness; recurrent thoughts of death, suicidal ideation, suicide attempt, or specific plan for suicide. In addition symptoms must cause clinically significant distress or impairment of functioning and are not better accounted for by bereavement. The best approach to treatment for depression is a combination of psychotherapy and antidepressant medications.[44] This condition responds well to treatment—approximately 70% to 80% of treated patients have significant reduction in symptoms. However, approximately 20% of patients who are chronically depressed have recurrent and severe depressive episodes.[11]

■ Dyslexia (Developmental Reading Disorder)

Chief Clinical Characteristics

This presentation is characterized by an inability to read, write, and spell words with the preservation of intelligence, motivation, and schooling necessary to accomplish these tasks.[45] *During early school years individuals with dyslexia may experience difficulty copying and naming colors and frequent reversal of letters.*[2]

Background Information

This condition occurs in approximately 5% to 10% of the school-age population[46] and is commonly familial with a sex-linked recessive pattern. This condition may also be present in children with congenital developmental abnormalities or after brain injury.[2] Neurophysiological studies suggest abnormal cortical organization in the language areas of the brain.[46] The diagnosis is based on clinical presentation of symptoms, family history, and school-based testing. Treatment for dyslexia includes referral to special education or special tutoring for intensive individualized training.[46] Most children with dyslexia do not spontaneously remit or catch up to peers in reading ability.[47]

■ Encephalitis

Chief Clinical Characteristics

This presentation includes confusion, delirium, convulsions, problems with speech or hearing, memory loss, hallucinations, drowsiness, and coma. Loss of balance and/or falls may be present.

Background Information

Encephalitis is an inflammation of nerve cells in the brain. This term usually refers to the viral form, although bacterial, parasitic, and fungal agents also can cause this condition. Up to 20,000 new cases of viral forms of this condition are reported annually in the United States. Diagnosis is established by clinical presentation suggesting dysfunction of the cerebrum, brainstem, or cerebellum, cellular reaction and elevated protein in spinal fluid, and possible demonstration of diffuse edema or enhancement of the brain on magnetic resonance imaging or computed tomography. Treatment is primarily pharmacologic, with drugs such as corticosteroids, antiviral agents, and anticonvulsants. The majority of individuals with encephalitis do recover, but irreversible brain damage and death can result.[2]

■ Encephalopathy

Chief Clinical Characteristics

This presentation commonly includes neuromyoclonus, nystagmus, ataxia, and tremor. Altered mental state, loss of memory, personality changes, dementia, and seizures are possible signs. Additional symptoms include muscle atrophy and weakness. Patients may also present with a progressive loss of consciousness resulting in coma.[17,48]

Background Information

Encephalopathy involves diffuse disease of the brain that alters brain function or structure. The numerous causes of encephalopathy include cirrhosis of the liver, severe hypertension, thiamine deficiency, infection, metabolic or mitochondrial dysfunction, toxin exposure, trauma, or lack of oxygen to the brain.[48] Diagnosis is made by numerous studies due to the variable causes of encephalopathy. These tests include blood work, cerebrospinal fluid examination, electroencephalography, and neuroimaging studies.[49] Treatment is symptomatic and varies according to the cause of encephalopathy. Even with treatment, encephalopathy can cause permanent brain damage and, in some cases, may be fatal.[17]

■ Epilepsy/Seizure Disorder

Chief Clinical Characteristics

This presentation is variable and can range from abnormal sensations or behavior to convulsions, muscles spasms, and loss of consciousness. Specific cognitive symptoms include problems with perception, attention, emotion, and memory.[50]

Background Information

According to the International League Against Epilepsy an epileptic seizure is defined as "a transient occurrence of signs and/or symptoms due to abnormal excessive or synchronous neuronal activity in the brain."[50] The diagnosis of epilepsy includes a history of at least one seizure with the "associated neurobiologic, cognitive, psychological, and social disturbances."[50] Seizures are also classified into different categories based on presentation and electroencephalogram features. Approximately 1% of the U.S. population will have epilepsy before 20 years of age, although the incidence increases slightly after age 60.[2] Most seizures can be controlled pharmacologically with antiepileptic drugs. Surgical treatment is indicated in patients with recurrent seizures that arise from a single focus and prevent a normal lifestyle.[51] The prognosis for a patient with epilepsy depends on the cause of the seizures and treatment. Remission occurs in only 16% to 43% of patients with partial seizures.[55] Less favorable prognosis is also associated with multiple seizure types, associated neurological deficits, and behavioral or psychiatric disturbances.[52]

■ Fahr's Syndrome (Familial Idiopathic Basal Ganglia Calcification, Bilateral Striopallidodentate Calcinosis)

Chief Clinical Characteristics

This presentation may involve features of parkinsonism, such as chorea, athetosis, rigidity, dystonia, and tremor in addition to cognitive impairments, cerebellar impairments, gait and balance disorders, psychiatric features, pain, pyramidal signs (such as weakness, hyperreflexia in the deep tendon reflexes, hypertonia, clonus, and/or a positive Babinski sign), sensory changes and speech disorders.[53]

Background Information

This condition occurs due to bilateral symmetric calcification of the basal ganglia with or without calcification of the dentate nucleus. The disease has been described as both familial and nonfamilial.[2] Diagnosis is established using computed tomography or magnetic resonance imaging of the brain; however, computed tomography has been found to be more sensitive for identifying calcium deposits.[54] Treatment aimed at minimizing calcium deposits has been unsuccessful.[55] Individuals with this condition may be responsive to levodopa for treatment of their parkinsonian features.[2]

■ Frontotemporal Dementia

Chief Clinical Characteristics

This presentation can be characterized by apathy, perseveration, poor judgment, aphasia, bizarre affect, and disengagement.[2]

Background Information

With frontotemporal dementia, progression of symptoms ranges from a few years to 10 years and the average age at onset is 59 years. This condition is distinguished from Alzheimer's disease by earlier onset and more prominent behavioral rather than cognitive impairments.[7] Prevalence is 81 per 100,000 persons ages 45 to 64 years.[56] The cause of this disease is unknown, but recent evidence has suggested that an abnormality of chromosome 17 may be responsible.[57] Diagnosis is based on clinical presentation, and magnetic resonance imaging and computed tomography are useful to distinguish it from focal neurological insults. Effective treatment is not well characterized. Speech language therapy may be helpful to maintain or improve spared function and most pharmacologic treatments are investigative at this time. Prognosis is poor for those patients with this condition who also develop motor neuron diseases in which dysphagia is present in late stages.[58]

■ Gaucher's Disease

Chief Clinical Characteristics

This presentation commonly includes slowly progressive mental decline, seizures, ataxia, and, upon later development, weakness with spasticity and splenomegaly and deficits in lateral gaze.[2]

Background Information

This condition is a rare disorder, although it is prevalent among the Ashkenazi Jewish population.[59] The disease is an autosomal genetic disorder in which glucocerebroside accumulates in the spleen, liver, lungs, bone marrow, and the brain due to a deficiency in an enzyme.[2] There are three types of Gaucher's disease. The most common, type 1, is characterized by no central nervous system involvement. In type 2, infants have extensive and progressive neurological damage.[59] Type 3 is less common and is associated with less severe neurological symptoms.[59] Diagnosis is established by clinical presentation, laboratory tests that show an increase in total acid phosphatase, and biopsy of bone marrow that is positive for Gaucher cells. Enzyme replacement therapy is standard for most patients with types 1 and 3. However, there is no effective treatment for the severe brain damage that may occur in patients with types 2 and 3. Prognosis for patients with type 2 disease is poor with death within the first 2 years of life. For type 3 disease, symptoms typically present in childhood and death occurs by age 10 to 15 years.[2]

■ Gerstmann's Syndrome

Chief Clinical Characteristics

This presentation commonly includes a distinct collection of symptoms including agraphia, dysgraphia, dyscalculia, finger agnosia, and aphasia.[2] Children may also manifest behavioral problems.[60]

Background Information

The cause of the developmental form of this disorder in children is not known. In adults, this syndrome may result from damage to the dominant or left parietal lobe caused by stroke, tumor, or trauma. Magnetic resonance imaging will usually demonstrate a lesion of the angular gyrus in the left parietal lobe.[61] The underlying cause in adults should be treated appropriately; rehabilitation may help diminish symptoms. Prognosis for adults with this condition is dependent on the underlying cause and usually improves with time and therapy.[62]

■ Hallervorden-Spatz Syndrome (Neurodegeneration with Brain Iron Accumulation, Pantothenate Kinase-Associated Neurodegeneration)

Chief Clinical Characteristics

This presentation includes dystonia, parkinsonism, choreoathetosis, spasticity, cognitive impairment, corticospinal tract involvement, optic atrophy, and pigmentary retinopathy.[63]

Background Information

This rare, inherited disorder results from a genetic mutation in the iron regulatory pathways, resulting in excessive iron accumulation in the basal ganglia.[63,64] Diagnosis is made by magnetic resonance imaging, which shows characteristic abnormalities in the basal ganglia, known as the "eye of the tiger" sign. Pathological studies may also show brown discoloration, iron pigmentation, and gliosis in the globus pallidus and substantia nigra.[63] There is no cure or effective treatment for the condition, but patients may benefit from rehabilitation therapies to decrease disability as the disease follows its progressive course of degeneration.[64]

■ Hereditary Spastic Paraplegia (Familial Spastic Paralysis)

Chief Clinical Characteristics

This presentation includes insidious, progressive difficulty with walking due to bilateral, symmetric lower extremity spastic weakness. Patients may report tripping, stumbling, and falling, as well as urinary urgency.[65]

Background Information

This condition can be divided into two types. The complicated form of this condition is indicated by the presence of neurological abnormalities such as dementia, mental retardation, epilepsy, extrapyramidal disturbance, ataxia, deafness, retinopathy, optic neuropathy, peripheral neuropathy, and skin lesions. The uncomplicated form is indicated by the absence of these features.[66] This condition is a group of inherited disorders with a primary pathological feature of axonal degeneration of the distal ends of the longest ascending and descending tracts, resulting in the characteristic spasticity.[65,66] Diagnosis is made by the presence of symptoms of gait disturbance, neurological findings of corticospinal tract deficits in the lower extremities, family history or genetic testing, and exclusion of any other disorders that could account for the symptoms.[65] Current treatment is limited to decreasing muscle spasticity through exercise and medication. Physical therapy is beneficial for the maintenance and improvement of muscle flexibility, muscle strength, gait, and cardiovascular fitness.[65] Prognosis varies, and those with an onset after adolescence are more likely to have insidious worsening.[65]

■ Huntington's Disease

Chief Clinical Characteristics

This presentation involves progressive chorea of the entire body, emotional disturbances such as behavior and personality changes, and dementia.[17,67,68]

Background Information

This autosomal dominant genetic disorder causes selective neurodegeneration, most commonly in the neostriatum. Diagnosis is made by genetic testing.[68] There is currently no treatment to slow or stop the progression of this condition; care is focused on symptom management and optimization of functioning.[68] The prognosis for Huntington's disease is poor, and individuals usually experience very rapid decline. On average, patients survive for 15 to 20 years after initial diagnosis, but require high levels of care and supervision during those years.[68]

■ Hydrocephalus

Chief Clinical Characteristics

This presentation commonly includes frontal lobe signs such as slowness of mental response, inattentiveness, distractibility, perseveration, inability to sustain complex cognitive function, and incontinence. Other symptoms include gait deterioration, frequent falls, occipital or frontal headaches, nausea and vomiting, diplopia, and lethargy. Advanced stages are associated with coma and extensor posturing.

Background Information

Intracranial pressure can be increased due to many mechanisms including a cerebral or extracerebral mass, generalized brain swelling, increased venous pressure, obstruction to the flow and absorption of cerebrospinal fluid, or volume expansion of cerebrospinal fluid.[2] Magnetic resonance imaging and the presence of papilledema are commonly used to establish the diagnosis of hydrocephalus. Medical treatment may include restriction of fluid intake and drugs with an osmotic effect, or the addition of diuretics.[69] Surgical treatment depends on the chronicity of the hydrocephalus. The acute form of this condition is considered fatal and is emergently treated via lumbar puncture or ventricular catheter.[69] The chronic form of this condition is treated with placement of a ventricular shunt or with surgical removal of a mass if that is the cause of the hydrocephalus. Although surgical procedures for hydrocephalus have a high success rate and a good prognosis, it is common to have shunt complications such as infection, occlusion, and over- or underdrainage. Thus, patients who have been treated for this condition must continue to be medically managed and educated regarding the indications of shunt compromise.

■ Hypersomnia

Chief Clinical Characteristics

This presentation can involve recurrent episodes of excessive daytime sleepiness or prolonged nighttime sleep. Individuals with this condition nap repeatedly during the day and may demonstrate anxiety, increased irritation, decreased energy, restlessness, slow thinking, slow speech, loss of appetite, hallucinations, and memory difficulty.

Background Information

This condition typically affects adolescents and young adults.[70] It may be caused by another sleep disorder (such as narcolepsy or sleep apnea), dysfunction of the autonomic nervous system, or drug or alcohol abuse. In some cases this condition results from a tumor, head trauma, or other injury to the central nervous system, especially localized to the mesencephalon and the floor and walls of the third ventricle.[1] Diagnosis is based on clinical presentation and classified according to DSM-IV criteria.[12] Treatment involves medication. The prognosis for persons with hypersomnia depends on the cause of the disorder. This condition can have serious consequences, such as automobile accidents caused by falling asleep while driving.[70]

■ Hypoxia (Cerebral Hypoxia, Anoxia)

Chief Clinical Characteristics

This presentation includes a wide variety of symptoms that depend on the condition's severity. Mild hypoxia without loss of consciousness may present with inattentiveness, poor judgment, and motor incoordination. More severe levels of hypoxia can result in seizures and/or coma. Post-hypoxic neurological symptoms include dementia, parkinsonian syndrome, choreoathetosis, cerebellar ataxia, intention or action myoclonus, or a Korsakoff amnesic state.[17]

Background Information

This condition occurs as a result of a decrease of oxygen supply to the brain. It has numerous causes, including cardiac arrest, drowning, strangulation, aspiration, choking, carbon monoxide poisoning, and complications of general anesthesia. Pure hypoxia produces damage in areas susceptible to reduced oxygen delivery such as the hippocampi and the cerebellum. This condition is often seen along with ischemia, producing complex patterns of cerebral damage.[17] Diagnosis and determination of the cause of hypoxia may require magnetic resonance imaging, electrocardiography, laboratory studies, electroencephalography, and evoked potentials.[17,71] Treatment is directed at prevention of further hypoxic injury. Outcomes vary, depending on cause and severity of hypoxia, and range from full recovery to coma or even death. The longer an individual with this condition is unconscious, the lower the likelihood of a meaningful recovery.[17]

■ Klüver-Bucy Syndrome

Chief Clinical Characteristics

This presentation typically involves oral exploratory behavior, tactile exploratory behavior, and hypersexuality, with additional symptoms and signs that may include visual agnosia, decreased attention, seizures, and dementia.

Background Information

This condition arises from medial temporal lobe dysfunction, and it may be associated with many different etiologies including herpes encephalitis, traumatic brain injury, and Pick's disease. This condition is diagnosed clinically by the presence of the above cluster of symptoms. Treatment is symptomatic and primarily through pharmacologic means. Prognosis is poor.[2]

■ Lyme Disease (Tick Paralysis)

Chief Clinical Characteristics

This presentation can include fluctuating signs or symptoms such as headache, neck stiffness, nausea, vomiting, malaise, fever, pain, fatigue, and presence of a "bull's-eye" rash.[2] Over time, additional symptoms may include sensory changes, irritability, cognitive changes, depression, behavioral changes, seizures, ataxia, chorea movements, pain, weakness, balance deficits, arthritis, and cranial nerve involvement.[1,2]

Background Information

Borrelia burgdorferi, an organism that infects ticks, is responsible for the transmission of this condition to a human host.[2] The diagnosis is confirmed with a thorough history, clinical assessment, enzyme-linked immunosorbent assay, and Western blot or immunoblot analysis. In addition, magnetic resonance imaging or computed tomography may reveal multifocal or periventricular cerebral lesions.[2] Medical management includes treatment with oral tetracycline, penicillin, or intravenous ceftriaxone.[2] Many individuals experience full recovery with treatment; however, residual deficits may persist for individuals with chronic Lyme disease.[2]

■ Malaria

Chief Clinical Characteristics

This presentation commonly involves fever, tachycardia, and sweating. Neurological symptoms that characterize cerebral malaria present in about 2% to 6% of cases and may include confusion, focal neurological deficits, convulsions, and coma.[2,72]

Background Information

Cases of malaria are most common in tropical areas.[72] Malaria is transmitted by bites from infected female mosquitoes usually at dusk and during the night. The protozoan infects red blood cells, which then adhere to blood vessels and block capillaries. Diagnosis is made by clinical presentation and the presence of plasmodia in red blood cells.[7] Treatment for malaria involves quinine, chloroquine, and related antimalarial drugs.[2] This condition is

managed easily if diagnosed promptly; it follows a serious course in 12% of patients.[72] Once coma is present, 20% to 30% of patients do not survive.[2]

MENINGITIS

■ Bacterial Meningitis

Chief Clinical Characteristics

This presentation includes acute symptoms such as fever, severe headache, neck stiffness, seizures, changes in consciousness, facial and ocular palsies, positive Kernig and Brudzinski signs, and possible hemiparesis, which may lead to falls. Chronic symptoms include hydrocephalus, vomiting, immobility, impaired alertness, hemiplegia, decorticate or decerebrate posturing, cortical blindness, stupor, or coma.[17]

Background Information

Bacterial meningitis results from an infection and inflammation of the meninges surrounding the brain and spinal cord. Lumbar puncture for spinal fluid pressure and cerebrospinal fluid culture, blood cultures, and radiologic studies confirm the diagnosis.[17] This condition is considered a medical emergency. Medical management includes maintenance of blood pressure, treatment for septic shock, and administration of intravenous antibiotics for 10 to 14 days.[17] Prognosis depends on the strain of bacteria; approximately 5% to 15% of patients with bacterial meningitis do not survive.[17] Residual effects after the infection resolves are variable and patients with pneumococcal and *H. influenzae* bacterial meningitis are more likely to have lasting neurological deficits.[17]

■ Viral Meningitis

Chief Clinical Characteristics

This presentation can be characterized by an acute onset of fever, headache, and neck stiffness. Drowsiness, lethargy, and irritability may occur, but overall symptoms tend to be relatively mild.[17] Although not a common presenting sign, falls or imbalance may occur due to drowsiness and lethargy.

Background Information

This condition is an infection and inflammation of the meninges surrounding the brain and spinal cord. Also known as aseptic meningitis, this condition is most commonly caused by the echovirus or coxsackie virus.[17] Cerebrospinal fluid analysis and blood work are used to determine the diagnosis.[73] There is no specific treatment, although supportive care may include administration of analgesics. This condition is rarely fatal and most patients demonstrate a full recovery.[17]

■ Mitochondrial Myopathies

Chief Clinical Characteristics
This presentation typically involves a combination of exercise intolerance, ataxia, seizures, myoclonus, headaches, small strokes, ophthalmoplegia, deafness, muscle cramps and/or slowly progressive myopathy with proximal greater than distal involvement. Other less common symptoms that may be seen include dementia, lactic acidosis, ptosis, and cardiac conduction defects.[17,74]

Background Information
This condition refers to a large group of disorders that result from a mutation in the mitochondrial genome, resulting in damage to the mitochondria. These disorders include Kearns-Sayre syndrome, myoclonus epilepsy with ragged red fibers, mitochondrial encephalomyopathy with lactic acidosis and stroke-like episodes, as well as other childhood-onset disorders.[17] A combination of clinical picture, histological findings of ragged red fibers, elevated serum lactate, and possible family history contribute to the diagnosis of this condition.[17] There is no specific treatment, but new research shows that patients may benefit from physical therapy for submaximal exercise training.[74] Most patients experience lifelong progression of the disease, and prognosis varies according to the type of disease and amount of involvement.[17]

■ Moyamoya Disease

Chief Clinical Characteristics
This presentation may include unsteady gait, involuntary movement, weakness, speech and sensory impairments, headache, seizures, impaired mental development, visual disturbances, and nystagmus.[17]

Background Information
This rare condition results from progressive occlusion of the arteries of the circle of Willis.[17] Diagnosis is based upon clinical findings and results of magnetic resonance imaging and magnetic resonance angiography. Images will demonstrate the occlusion of the circle of Willis as well as secondary cerebral infarction, white matter lesions, atrophy, and hemorrhage.[75] Treatment options include revascularization surgery and medical treatment to prevent hypertension and further strokes.[76] Rehabilitative therapies are used to treat functional deficits that the patient may incur from a stroke secondary to the progression of the disease. Outcome depends on the severity of secondary complications and presence of subsequent occlusion.

■ Multi-Infarct Dementia/Vascular Dementia

Chief Clinical Characteristics
This presentation includes confusion, memory impairment, aphasia, and agnosia that occur in a progressive stepwise and patchy pattern.[11,77]

Background Information
More men than women are affected with peak incidence between the ages of 60 and 75 years. This condition occurs when a series of small strokes gradually leads to mental decline.[1] Diagnosis is obtained from the history and confirmed by magnetic resonance imaging or computed tomography. Treatment emphasizes prevention of additional brain damage by controlling high blood pressure. Prognosis is generally poor. Early treatment and management of blood pressure may prevent progression of the disorder.[77]

■ Multiple Sclerosis

Chief Clinical Characteristics
This presentation may include paresthesias, weakness, spasticity, hypertonicity, hyperreflexia, positive Babinski sign, incoordination, optic neuritis, ataxia, vertigo, dysarthria, diplopia, bladder incontinence, tremor, balance deficits, falls, and cognitive deficits.[2]

Background Information
This condition may present as relapsing-remitting, primary progressive, or secondary progressive. The disease occurs most frequently in women between the ages of 20 and 40 years. Only a small number of children or individuals between 50 and 60 years of age are

diagnosed with this condition.[2] This condition was originally thought to be secondary to environmental and genetic factors, but evidence suggests an autoimmune response to a viral infection, which subsequently targets myelin.[2] The diagnosis may be confirmed by a thorough history, physical examination, magnetic resonance imaging, analysis of cerebrospinal fluid, and evoked potentials.[2,78,79] Life expectancy and cause of mortality are similar for all types of this condition.[2] Clinical characteristics that are associated with a longer time interval for progression of disability include female sex, younger age of onset, relapsing-remitting type, complete recovery after the first relapse, and longer time interval between first and second exacerbation.[80] Medical management may include the use of methylprednisolone, prednisone, cyclophosphamide, immunosuppressant treatment, and betainterferon.[2] Physical, occupational, and speech therapy may be indicated to prevent secondary sequelae and to optimize functional activity and mobility. Some individuals may benefit from psychology/psychiatry and social support as the disease progresses.

■ Multiple System Atrophy (Striatonigral Degeneration, Olivopontocerebellar Atrophy, Shy-Drager Syndrome)

Chief Clinical Characteristics
This presentation involves tremor, rigidity, akinesia, and/or postural imbalance along with signs of cerebellar, pyramidal, and autonomic dysfunction. Autonomic symptoms such as orthostatic hypotension, dry mouth, loss of sweating, impotence, and urinary incontinence or retention are the initial feature in 41% of individuals, with 74% to 97% of individuals developing some degree of autonomic dysfunction during the course of the disease.[81] This condition is a combination of parkinsonian and non-parkinsonian symptoms and signs.

Background Information
Diagnostic criteria are based on the clinical presentation, which includes poor response to levodopa, presence of autonomic features, presence of speech or bulbar problems, absence of dementia, absence of toxic confusion, and presence of falls.[82] The disease course ranges between 0.5 and 24 years after diagnosis with a

mean survival time of 6.2 years.[83] This condition is a progressive condition of the central and autonomic nervous systems that rarely occurs without orthostatic hypotension. There are three types of this condition. The parkinsonian-type includes symptoms of Parkinson's disease such as slow movement, stiff muscles, and tremor. The cerebellar type causes problems with coordination and speech. The combined type includes symptoms of both parkinsonism and cerebellar failure. Older age at onset is associated with a shorter survival time.[83] Average age of onset is 54 years, with mean age at death being 60.3 years.[81] Most individuals with this condition receive a trial of levodopa although only a minority respond.[81] Additional treatment addresses symptoms and involves physical and occupational therapy to maintain mobility and address safety issues related to the progression of imbalance.

■ Narcolepsy

Chief Clinical Characteristics
This presentation includes excessive daytime sleepiness; cataplexy, or the sudden loss of voluntary muscle tone; vivid hallucinations during sleep onset or upon awakening; and brief episodes of total paralysis at the beginning or end of sleep.

Background Information
This condition is hypothesized to result from a genetic predisposition, abnormal neurotransmitter functioning and sensitivity, and abnormal immune predisposition.[2] Prevalence is 1:2000[1] with onset between the ages of 15 and 35.[2] Diagnosis is based on the clinical presentation. Treatment for narcolepsy includes strategically placed naps and medication.[84] With individualized treatment, most patients are able to function in daily activities.

■ Neurofibromatosis

Chief Clinical Characteristics
This presentation depends on the type of neurofibromatosis. Neurofibromatosis type 1 (NF1, Von Recklinghausen's disease) may include café au lait spots, neurofibromas, pathological fractures, syringomyelia, scoliosis, stroke, neoplasms, learning difficulties, and hyperactivity. Neurofibromatosis type 2 (NF2) is characterized by bilateral vestibular schwannomas, progressive

hearing loss, and possible intracranial or intraspinal neoplasms.[1,2]

Background Information

This condition is an autosomal dominant disorder on chromosome 17 (NF1) and 22 (NF2), respectively. The tumors in NF1 occur due to the excessive proliferation of cells within the meninges, vascular system, skin, viscera, peripheral, and central nervous systems.[1,2] The tumors in NF2 arise from the posterior nerve roots. Depending on the type of this condition the diagnosis may be confirmed by a thorough family history, the presence of six or more café au lait spots, imaging, and genetic testing. If indicated, the tumors that result from this condition may be surgically removed.[1] Both forms of this condition are progressive and the prognosis varies depending on the severity of lesions.[2]

■ Neurological Complications of Acquired Immunodeficiency Syndrome

Chief Clinical Characteristics

This presentation is variable and dependent upon the affected neuroanatomical structures in an individual with acquired immunodeficiency syndrome.[85]

Background Information

This condition may be categorized by:

1. Meningitic symptoms including headache, malaise, and fever (such as secondary to meningitis, cryptococcal meningitis, tuberculous meningitis, and human immunodeficiency virus headache)
2. Focal cerebral symptoms including hemiparesis, aphasia, apraxia, sensory deficits, homonymous hemianopia, cranial nerve involvement, balance deficits, incoordination, and/or ataxia (such as secondary to cerebral toxoplasmosis, primary central nervous system lymphoma, and progressive multifocal leukoencephalopathy)
3. Diffuse cerebral symptoms that involve cognitive deficits, altered level of consciousness, hyperreflexia, Babinski sign, presence of primitive reflexes (such as secondary to postinfectious encephalomyelitis, acquired immunodeficiency dementia complex, cytomegalovirus encephalitis)
4. Myelopathy associated with gait difficulties, spasticity, ataxia, balance deficits, and hyperreflexia (such as secondary to herpes zoster myelitis, vacuolar myelopathy that occurs with acquired immunodeficiency syndrome dementia complex)
5. Peripheral involvement associated with sensory changes, weakness, balance deficits, and pain (such as secondary to peripheral neuropathy, acute and chronic inflammatory demyelinating polyneuropathies).[2,85]

Abnormal neurological findings are observed during a clinical examination in approximately one-third of patients with acquired immunodeficiency syndrome; however, on autopsy most individuals with this condition have abnormalities within the nervous system.[2] Diagnosis of the variable neurological complications associated with this condition may be confirmed with laboratory tests, cerebrospinal fluid cultures, imaging, nerve conduction studies, and physical examination.[1,2,85] Treatment appears to be limited primarily to the use of antiviral medications.[85] Physical and occupational therapy may be indicated to address equipment needs and caregiver/patient training related to functional mobility.

■ Neurosyphilis (Tabes Dorsalis, Syphilitic Spinal Sclerosis, Progressive Locomotor Ataxia)

Chief Clinical Characteristics

This presentation can be characterized by hemiparesis, ataxia, aphasia, gait instability, falls, neuropathy, personality and cognitive changes, seizures, diplopia, visual impairments, hearing loss, psychotic disorders, loss of bowel/bladder function, pain, hyporeflexia, and hypotonia.[86,87]

Background Information

Treponema pallidum infects the human host by way of contact with contaminated body fluids or lesions.[86] This spirochete is responsible for the diagnosis of syphilis; however, when *T. pallidum* is present within the central nervous system the individual is diagnosed with neurosyphilis.[87] This condition occurs in approximately 10% of individuals with untreated syphilis, and in 81% of these cases it presents as meningovascular, meningeal, or general paresis. Treatment includes use of various forms of penicillin or alternative choices for those allergic to penicillin[86] and may involve rehabilitative therapies depending on the individual's activity limitations or participation restrictions. A better prognosis has been observed for individuals treated during early neurosyphilis.[87]

■ Neurotoxicity

Chief Clinical Characteristics
This presentation includes limb weakness or numbness; loss of memory, vision, and/or intellect; headache; behavioral problems; and sexual dysfunction.

Background Information
This condition occurs when exposure to natural or artificial toxins alters the normal activity of the nervous system, eventually leading to disruption or death of neurons. It results from exposure to substances use inchemotherapy, radiation treatment, drug therapies, and organ transplants, as well as eposure to heavy metals, foods, or pesticides. Diagnosis is supported by clinical presentation and lab tests for detection of the toxic substance. Treatment is prioritized at removal of the offending toxin. Prognosis varies greatly depending upon the level of exposure and individual's comorbid medical conditions.

■ Niemann-Pick Disease (Types C and D Only)

Chief Clinical Characteristics
This presentation includes ataxia, dystonia, vertical gaze palsy, dysarthria, and seizures. Often the presenting feature is a psychotic episode.[17,88]

Background Information
This condition is an autosomal recessive lipid storage disorder that results in impaired cholesterol transport and excessive glycosphingolipid storage.[89] There are four types of Niemann-Pick disease: types A and B are seen only in children and are not discussed here. Types C and D have a variable age of onset ranging from childhood to late teens or even early adulthood. Individuals with types C and D demonstrate an enlarged spleen and liver, as well as progressive neurological dysfunction.[88] Diagnosis is made by a combination of studies, including filipin staining of cultured fibroblasts, cholesterol esterification studies, and DNA mutation analysis.[91] Unfortunately, there is no effective treatment for types C and D of this condition. Many patients who are diagnosed in childhood live well into adult years, and overall prognosis depends on the severity of the disease.[88]

■ Paraneoplastic Syndromes

Chief Clinical Characteristics
This presentation includes dizziness in combination with a variety of different neurological symptoms and signs in an individual with cancer. Specific neurological symptoms and signs depend on the location of involvement of the central or peripheral nervous system.

Background Information
Paraneoplastic encephalomyelitis and focal encephalitis may present with ataxia, vertigo, balance deficits, nystagmus, nausea, vomiting, cranial nerve palsies, seizures, sensory neuropathy, anxiety, depression, cognitive changes, and hallucinations. For individuals presenting with ataxia, dysarthria, dysphagia, and diplopia, paraneoplastic cerebellar degeneration may be suspected. Paraneoplastic opsoclonus/myoclonus tends to affect both children and adults with signs and symptoms including hypotonia, ataxia, irritability, truncal ataxia, gait difficulty, balance deficits, and frequent falls. Stiff-man syndrome presents with spasms and fluctuating rigidity of axial musculature, legs and possibly shoulders, upper extremities, and neck. Paraneoplastic sensory neuropathy presents with asymmetric, progressive sensory alterations involving the limbs, trunk, and face, sensorineural hearing loss, autonomic dysfunction, and pain. Other conditions in this category include vasculitis, Lambert-Eaton myasthenia syndrome, myasthenia gravis, dermatomyositis, neuromyotonia, and various neuropathies.[2,90] These conditions result from an immune-mediated response to the presence of tumor or metastases. Antibodies or T-cells respond to the presence of the tumor, but also attack normal cells of the nervous system.[91,92] Over 60% of individuals present with this condition prior to the discovery of the cancer.[90] The underlying tumor is treated according to the type of cancer. Additional treatment is dependent on this condition's type and may include steroids, plasmapheresis, immunotherapy, chemotherapy, radiation, or cyclophosphamide.[90] Physical, occupational, and speech therapy may be indicated to address functional limitations.

■ Paranoia, Delusional Disorder

Chief Clinical Characteristics

This presentation is characterized by delusions. The delusions can be one of several types such as being followed (persecutory type), having a disease (somatic type), being loved at a distance (erotomanic type), having an unfaithful sexual partner (jealous type), and possessing inflated worth, power, identity, or knowledge (grandiose type).[2] Age at onset is usually middle or late adulthood, and the course is variable.

Background Information

The cause of this condition is unknown, but familial transmission is suspected. Diagnosis is defined by the DSM-IV-TR[12] with the following criteria: one or more nonbizarre (could occur in everyday life) delusions for at least 1 month; hallucinations not as prominent as in schizophrenia; functioning is not markedly impaired and behavior is not obviously bizarre; and mood episodes are brief. Psychotherapy and medication are often indicated for treatment of this condition. The course of this condition is variable, with improvement of delusional symptoms in 10%, remission in 33% to 50%, and persisting symptoms in 30% to 40% of cases. Patients with the acute and jealous subtypes may have a better prognosis.[93]

■ Parkinson's Disease

Chief Clinical Characteristics

This presentation commonly involves resting tremor, bradykinesia, rigidity, and postural instability. Falls are a common problem in individuals with this condition, with up to 68% falling within a 1-year period and approximately 50% of these individuals falling multiple times within that same year.[94] Other common signs and symptoms include festination, freezing, micrographia, hypophonia (hypokinetic dysarthria), akinesia, masked facies, drooling, difficulty turning over in bed, dystonia, dyskinesia, dementia, and depression.[2]

Background Information

This condition occurs due to the depletion or injury of dopamine-producing cells in substantia nigra pars compacta. Clinical signs and symptoms are not typically present until after approximately 80% of dopamine-producing cells are lost. The definitive diagnosis is made post-mortem. However, a clinically definitive diagnosis may be made with the presence of at least two of the three criteria—asymmetric resting tremor, bradykinesia, or rigidity—and a positive response to anti-Parkinson medications.[2,95] Imaging may be useful to exclude vascular involvement. Medical management may include use of dopamine agonists, levodopa, or other medications to address nonmotor symptoms, such as depression, constipation, autonomic symptoms, and sexual dysfunction. Surgical management also may be considered, including deep brain stimulation or pallidotomy.[95] Forced use or higher intensity, challenging activities may provide a neuroprotective benefit for individuals with early forms of this condition.[96] With the high incidence of depression, consultation with a psychologist or psychiatrist may be warranted. Individuals with a late onset tend to progress more rapidly.[97,98] Poor prognostic indicators for disability include initial presentation without tremor, early dependence, dementia, balance impairments, older age, and the postural instability/gait difficulty dominant type.[97,98]

■ Pelizaeus-Merzbacher Disease

Chief Clinical Characteristics

This presentation commonly includes deterioration of coordination, motor abilities, and intellectual function.

Background Information

Severity and onset of the disease range widely, depending on the type of genetic mutation, and extend from the mild, adult-onset spastic paraplegia to the severe form with onset at infancy and death in early childhood.[99] This condition is an X-linked disease caused by a mutation in the gene that controls the production of a myelin protein called proteolipid protein.[99] Genetic diagnostic testing is the definitive method for diagnosing this condition.[100] There is no cure for this condition. Therefore, treatment is based on symptoms and includes physical therapy, orthotics, and antispasticity agents with goals to minimize the development of joint contractures, dislocations, and kyphoscoliosis.[101] Individuals with severe forms of this condition experience progressive deterioration until death. Individuals with the adult-onset form with spasticity may have nearly normal life span.[17]

■ Pick's Disease

Chief Clinical Characteristics

This presentation includes a gradual onset of difficulty with memory, apathy, poor concentration, personality changes, and disturbances of speech. The disease usually affects individuals, more commonly women, between the ages of 40 and 60.[1]

Background Information

Individuals with this condition typically have atrophy of the frontal and temporal lobes, as evidenced on magnetic resonance imaging. Computed tomography and single photon emission computed tomography reveal anterior hypoperfusion.[1] On microscopic inspection, argyrophilic inclusion bodies (Pick bodies) are found within the cytoplasm of cells taken from the frontotemporal cortex.[1] The cause of the disease is unknown, though genetics are thought to play a role. Often, this condition is described as a subtype of frontotemporal dementia.[102] There is no cure or specific treatment for this condition and its progression cannot be slowed. However, some of the symptoms of the disease may be treated effectively pharmacologically.[103] The course of this condition involves an inevitable progressive deterioration that lasts approximately 2 to 5 years.[2]

■ Progressive Multifocal Leukoencephalopathy

Chief Clinical Characteristics

This presentation commonly involves cortical blindness, visual field defects, hemiparesis with progression to quadriparesis, aphasia, ataxia, dysarthria, personality changes and impaired intellect evolving over a period of days to weeks.

Background Information

This condition is most likely due to viral infection of the central nervous system, which then causes widespread demyelinative lesions primarily of the cerebral hemispheres. Diagnosis is made by computed tomography and magnetic resonance imaging to localize the lesions. Treatment for individuals with acquired immunodeficiency syndrome consists of antiretroviral drug combinations and can lead to slower progression or even remission. Currently, no treatment exists to impair disease progression in individuals with this condition but without acquired immunodeficiency syndrome.[2]

■ Progressive Supranuclear Palsy (Richardson-Steele-Olszewski Syndrome)

Chief Clinical Characteristics

This presentation classically includes vertical gaze palsy, prominent instability, and falls within the first year of disease onset.[104] *Other characteristics may include rigidity, akinesia, dysarthria, dysphagia, and mild dementia. Falls were found to be the most commonly reported symptom with the majority of falls being backwards falls.*[105] *Difficulty with voluntary vertical eye movements (usually downward) and involuntary saccades are relatively early features. The disease generally progresses to the point at which all voluntary eye movements are lost.*

Background Information

Some patients may not demonstrate difficulties with ocular movements for 1 to 3 years after disease onset. Most cases are sporadic; however, a pattern of inheritance compatible with autosomal dominant transmission has been described.[2] Diagnosis is based on clinical presentation, which includes a gradually progressive disorder with age of onset at 40 years or older, vertical supranuclear palsy, and postural instability with falls within the first year of disease onset.[106] Medical treatment is typically unsuccessful, because the majority of these patients are not responsive to levodopa therapy aimed at addressing the extrapyramidal features of the disease.[33] Physical and occupational therapy are used to maintain mobility and address safety issues related to the progression of imbalance. The disease course is progressive with a mean survival time of 5.6 years.[105] Older age at disease onset, early onset of falls, incontinence, dysarthria, dysphagia, insertion of a percutaneous gastrostomy, and diplopia have all been described as being predictive of shorter survival time.[105]

■ Reye's Syndrome

Chief Clinical Characteristics

This presentation involves persistent or recurrent vomiting, listlessness, personality changes such as irritability or combativeness, disorientation or confusion, delirium, convulsions, and loss of consciousness.[8]

PROBLEMS OF COGNITION, COMMUNICATION, AND BEHAVIOR

Background Information

Reye's syndrome primarily presents in children, although it can occur at any age.[107] The cause of this condition is unclear, but it commonly occurs during recovery from a viral infection or 3 to 5 days after the onset. There is an increased risk of the disease if aspirin was taken during the course of the illness.[107] This condition causes an acute increase of pressure within the brain and massive accumulations of fat in the liver and other organs. Diagnosis is made on clinical presentation and by the presence of cerebral edema.[107] Treatment is primarily aimed at reducing brain swelling, reversing the metabolic injury, preventing complications in the lungs, and anticipating cardiac arrest. The fatality rate for this condition is approximately 30%, with the worst prognosis for children under 5 years of age.[107]

■ Rickettsial Diseases, Including Rocky Mountain Spotted Fever

Chief Clinical Characteristics

This presentation typically includes visual disturbances, a rash that occurs on the palms of hands and soles of feet, headache, nausea, fever and myalgias.[108] Initial symptoms begin within 2 to 14 days of infections and last approximately 2 to 3 weeks.

Background Information

Rocky Mountain spotted fever is the most common type of this condition in the United States. It is transmitted by a variety of tick, and is common in Long Island, Tennessee, Virginia, North Carolina and Maryland.[2] Like malaria, rickettsiae in the blood vessels cause vascular injury, which forms the basis for central nervous system damage. Diagnosis is based on clinical signs and symptoms and confirmed by skin biopsy. Treatment consists of the use of doxycycline or chloramphenicol. The mortality rate in untreated cases is 20% to 25%.[109]

■ Schizophrenia

Chief Clinical Characteristics

This presentation can be characterized by hallucinations, delusions, disorganized speech, and negative symptoms such as flat affect, decreased initiation, and decreased spontaneity in conversation. Most marked deterioration in patients occurs within the first 5 to 10 years of the disease followed by a time of relative stability (though not often a return to baseline).

Background Information

Diagnosis of schizophrenia is made on clinical presentation and according to DSM-IV-TR criteria[12]: The patient must have experienced at least two of the following symptoms for at least 1 month of a 6-month period causing significant social or occupational problems: delusions, hallucinations, disorganized speech, disorganized or catatonic behavior, or negative symptoms. The incidence peaks during adolescent years with a 1% worldwide lifetime prevalence.[110] The cause of this condition is not known, but genetic and neurodevelopmental factors may play a role, as well as neurotransmitter and metabolic activity in different areas of the cortex.[2] Treatment involves use of antipsychotic medications. The prognosis is guarded, because full recovery is unusual. Poor prognosis is associated with early onset of symptoms, family history, and prominent negative symptoms. Individuals with this condition also have a 4% to 10% risk of committing suicide.[110] With pharmacologic treatment and psychiatric management, 60% of patients return to home and some social activity.[2]

■ Sleep Apnea

Chief Clinical Characteristics

This presentation is characterized by brief breathing disturbances during sleep that occur repeatedly throughout the night. The hallmark symptom of the disorder is excessive daytime sleepiness. Additional symptoms of sleep apnea include loud snoring, irritability, forgetfulness, mood or behavior changes, anxiety, and depression.[111]

Background Information

The most common type of sleep apnea is obstructive sleep apnea, with mechanical causes such as obesity or enlarged tonsils.[1] Central sleep apnea is the result of impairment in respiratory control of breathing often caused by brainstem medullary infarction or following cervical/foramen magnum surgery.[1] The prevalence of sleep apnea is between approximately 2% and 4%, with higher incidence in the elderly.[111] Diagnosis is made based on clinical presentation. Most treatment regimens begin with lifestyle changes, such as avoiding alcohol and medications that relax the central nervous system, weight management, and quitting smoking. If these conservative methods are inadequate, continuous positive airway pressure is recommended. In extreme cases surgical procedures can be used to remove tissue and widen the airway.[2] If untreated, sleep apnea can lead to hypertension with right heart failure secondary to pulmonary hypertension, which can become life threatening.[1]

■ Stroke (Cerebrovascular Accident)

Chief Clinical Characteristics

This presentation may include a wide range of symptoms that correspond to specific areas of the brain that are affected, potentially including visual disturbances. The initial symptoms can include numbness or weakness, especially on one side of the body or face; confusion or aphasia; balance deficits or falls; or sudden severe headache with no known cause.

Background Information

This condition occurs when blood flow to the brain is interrupted either by blockage (ischemia or infarction) or from hemorrhagic disruption. A thrombosis or embolic occlusion of an artery causes an ischemic type of this condition. A hemorrhagic type of this condition can be caused by arteriovenous malformation, hypertension, aneurysm, neoplasm, drug abuse and trauma. This condition is the most common and disabling neurological disorder in adults and occurs in 114 of every 100,000 people.[43] This condition is diagnosed using clinical presentation and positive findings on computed tomography and magnetic resonance imaging. Medication, surgery and interdisciplinary therapy are the most common treatments for this condition. The prognosis for recovery is predicted by the magnitude of initial deficit. Factors that are associated with poor outcomes include coma, poor cognition, severe aphasia, severe hemiparesis with little return within 1 month, visual perceptual disorders, depression, and incontinence after 2 weeks.[112,113]

■ Subacute Sclerosing Panencephalitis (Dawson's Disease)

Chief Clinical Characteristics

This presentation may involve progressive stages of abnormal behavior, irritability, intellectual deterioration, and memory loss, followed by involuntary movements and seizures.

Background Information

This condition primarily presents in children younger than 10 years, and since the introduction of the measles vaccine it has become very rare.[2] It is an infection of the central nervous system caused by an altered form of the measles virus that triggers changes in the white and gray matter primarily of the hemispheres and brainstem.[2] The annual incidence is between 0.1 and 5 per one million children.[114] Diagnosis is made using the clinical presentation, elevated measles antibody titers, and typical electroencephalographic changes.[2] Patients with this condition have shown stabilization of disease and delay in clinical progression after therapy with immunomodulator and antiviral medications. When not treated, this condition is almost always fatal. Death usually occurs between 1 and 3 years after onset, although some spontaneous remissions (up to 5%) have been reported.[115]

■ Systemic Lupus Erythematosus

Chief Clinical Characteristics

This presentation can include abnormal vision, swallowing, taste, hearing, or changes in mood or thinking, and seizures in combination with fatigue, joint pain, and swelling affecting the hands, feet, knees, and shoulders.

Background Information

This condition affects mostly women of childbearing age. It is a chronic autoimmune disorder that can affect any organ system, including skin, joints, kidneys, brain, heart, lungs, and blood. Microinfarcts in the cerebral cortex and brainstem, which lead to destructive and proliferative changes in capillaries and arterioles, are primarily responsible for central nervous system manifestations. Hypertension and endocarditis can also predispose an affected individual to development of neurological abnormalities. Multiple sclerosis is a disease that may be mistaken for this condition, especially if the central nervous system manifestations include visual dysfunction. The diagnosis is confirmed by the presence of skin lesions, heart, lung, or kidney involvement, laboratory abnormalities including low red or white cell counts, low platelet counts, or positive ANA and anti-DNA antibody tests.[116] Treatment involves corticosteroid medication.

■ Tourette's Syndrome

Chief Clinical Characteristics
This presentation involves motor and vocal tics, inappropriate and involuntary obscene speech and gestures, and anger control problems that begin before 21 years of age.[7] Many children with this condition experience additional neurobehavioral problems including inattention and obsessive-compulsive symptoms.[117]

Background Information
This condition may be inherited and appears to be due to a neurotransmitter disturbance. Its incidence is 0.5 in 1,000 and occurs more commonly in males than females.[117] It is diagnosed by presentation of tics for over a year and onset prior to age 18 according to DSM-IV-TR guidelines.[12] Currently all treatment is symptomatic with medication and behavioral therapy.[7] This condition is considered chronic, but tic severity on average peaks in adolescence and wanes thereafter.[118]

■ Transient Ischemic Attack

Chief Clinical Characteristics
This presentation can include numbness or weakness in the face, arm, or leg, especially on one side of the body; confusion or difficulty in talking or understanding speech; trouble seeing in one or both eyes; and difficulty with walking, dizziness, or loss of balance and coordination.

Background Information
This condition is a transient stroke that lasts only a few minutes. It occurs when the blood supply to part of the brain is briefly interrupted. Symptoms of this condition, which usually occur suddenly, are similar to those of stroke but do not last as long. Most symptoms disappear within an hour, although they may persist for up to 24 hours. Because it is impossible to differentiate between symptoms from this condition and acute stroke, individuals should assume that all stroke-like symptoms signal a medical emergency. A prompt evaluation (within 60 minutes) is necessary to identify the cause of this condition and determine appropriate therapy. Depending on the individual's medical history and the results of a medical examination, the doctor may recommend

drug therapy or surgery to reduce the risk of stroke. Antiplatelet medications, particularly aspirin, are a standard treatment for individuals suspected of this condition and who also are at risk for stroke, including individuals with atrial fibrillation.

■ Traumatic Brain Injury

Chief Clinical Characteristics
This presentation typically includes dysequilibrium in the presence of cognitive changes, altered level of consciousness, seizures, nausea, vomiting, coma, dizziness, headache, pupillary changes, tinnitus, weakness, incoordination, behavioral changes, spasticity, hypertonicity, cranial nerve lesions, and sensory and motor deficits.[2,119]

Background Information
This condition can be classified as mild, moderate, or severe based on Glasgow Coma Scale, length of coma, and duration of post-traumatic amnesia.[119] Magnetic resonance imaging may be used to confirm the diagnosis.[1] Treatment initiated at the scene of the accident and during the acute phase is focused on medical stabilization. It should be initiated during the acute phase in order to minimize complications.[120] Low Glasgow Coma Scale, longer length of coma, longer duration of post-traumatic amnesia, and older age tend to be associated with poor outcomes.[121] Optimal rehabilitation is interdisciplinary and customized to address the specific individuals' disablement.

■ Tuberous Sclerosis

Chief Clinical Characteristics
This presentation includes seizures, mental retardation, behavior problems, and skin abnormalities.

Background Information
This condition is a genetic disease that causes benign tumors to grow in the brain and on other vital organs such as the kidneys, heart, eyes, lungs, and skin.[122] Limited hyperplasia of ectodermal and mesodermal cells during development causes the tumors.[2] The inheritance is autosomal dominant in approximately 50% of cases and due to mutations in the other cases. The estimated prevalence of the disease is 1:10,000.[123] The presence of seizures and angiofibromas is diagnostic. Angiofibromas are

pink or skin-colored papules commonly observed in the nasolabial folds and on the cheeks and chin.[2] In addition, computed tomography may show subependymal areas of calcium deposits, and magnetic resonance imaging will reveal uncalcified subependymal tubers. Treatment includes anticonvulsant therapy for seizures and surgical removal of symptomatic lesions. This condition shows a wide variety of clinical expressions depending on the location of the tumors. Approximately 30% of severely affected infants are thought to die before age 5, and 50% to 75% die before attaining adult age.[2]

TUMORS

■ Brain Metastases

Chief Clinical Characteristics
This presentation may include headaches, seizures, dysphagia, weakness, cognitive changes, behavioral changes, dizziness, vomiting, alterations in the level of consciousness, ataxia, aphasia, nystagmus, visual disturbances, dysarthria, balance deficits, falls, lethargy, and incoordination.[2,20]

Background Information
The majority of individuals with brain metastases have been previously diagnosed with a primary tumor; however, a small percentage of individuals are diagnosed concomitantly with brain metastases and the primary tumor. The most common cancers resulting in subsequent brain metastases include lung, breast, melanoma, colorectal, and genitourinary tract. The new onset of neurological symptoms after a primary tumor warrants the use of imaging such as magnetic resonance imaging or computed tomography to confirm the diagnosis. Treatment may include corticosteroids, brain irradiation, surgical resection, chemotherapy, radiotherapy, and rehabilitative therapies. The prognosis is poor with death typically occurring within 6 months.

■ Brain Primary Tumors

Chief Clinical Characteristics
This presentation may include headaches, seizures, dysphagia, weakness, cognitive changes, behavioral changes, dizziness, vomiting, alterations in the level of consciousness, ataxia, aphasia, nystagmus, visual disturbances,

dysarthria, balance deficits, falls, lethargy, and incoordination.[1,2]

Background Information
Glioblastoma multiforme, astrocytoma, oligodendroglioma, metastatic tumors, primary central nervous system lymphomas, ganglioglioma, neuroblastoma, meningioma, arachnoid cysts, hemangioblastoma, medulloblastoma, and acoustic neuroma/schwannoma are some of the more common brain tumors. Specific diagnoses for brain tumors may be confirmed with imaging and biopsy. Treatment is variable depending on the type, size, and location of the tumor and may include surgical resection, chemotherapy, radiation, corticosteroids, and rehabilitative therapies. Prognosis is also variable and depends on the type and grade of tumor, severity of compression, and duration of compression.

■ Spinal Metastases

Chief Clinical Characteristics
This presentation can involve spasticity, weakness, sensory alterations, bowel and bladder incontinence, neck pain, back pain, radicular pain, atrophy, cerebellar signs, balance deficits, falls, and cranial nerve involvement.[1,2,124]

Background Information
This condition is the most frequent neoplasm involving the spine.[124] The most common types and locations of primary tumors that result in spinal metastases include breast, lung, lymphoma, prostate, kidney, gastrointestinal tract, and thyroid.[2,125] The diagnosis is confirmed with gadolinium-enhanced magnetic resonance imaging and computed tomography.[2,124] Treatment is variable depending on the tumor and may include surgical resection, chemotherapy, radiation, corticosteroids, and rehabilitative therapies.[2] Although the long-term prognosis is poor, individuals without paresis, pain, and who are still ambulatory have longer survival rates.[125]

■ Spinal Primary Tumors

Chief Clinical Characteristics
This presentation may include spasticity, weakness, sensory alterations, bowel/bladder incontinence, back pain, radicular pain,

atrophy, cerebellar signs, balance deficits, falls, and cranial nerve involvement.[2]

Background Information

Types of this condition include myeloma, neurofibroma, lymphoma, metastasis, meningioma, schwannoma, and astrocytoma. The first test to diagnose brain and spinal column tumors is a neurological examination. Special imaging techniques (computed tomography, magnetic resonance imaging, and positron emission tomography) are also employed. Specific diagnoses may be confirmed with imaging and biopsy. Treatment is variable depending on the type, size, and location of the tumor and may include surgical resection, chemotherapy, radiation, corticosteroids, and rehabilitative therapies. Prognosis is variable and depends on the type and grade of tumor, severity of compression, and duration of compression.

■ Whipple's Disease (Intestinal Lipodystrophy)

Chief Clinical Characteristics

This presentation includes dementia, personality changes, ataxia, myoclonus, nystagmus, and visual loss. The presentation also includes weight loss, arthropathy, diarrhea, and abdominal pain. Some individuals may experience a low-grade fever, lymphadenopathy, hyperpigmentation, hypotension, peripheral edema, cardiac murmurs, occult bleeding, and myalgia.[126]

Background Information

This systemic disease is rare and is thought to be caused by the bacteria *Tropheryma whipplei*.[126] Diagnosis is determined by biopsy of the duodenum, cerebral spinal fluid, cardiac-valve tissue, lymph nodes, and/or synovial tissue.[126,127] Recommended treatment includes antibiotic therapy until subsequent biopsies are negative.[126,127] If left untreated, this condition may be fatal; however, when treated with antibiotic medications the prognosis is good. Relapses may occur and tend to be more common in those with central nervous system involvement.[126,127]

■ Wilson's Disease

Chief Clinical Characteristics

This presentation commonly involves liver dysfunction followed by neurological symptoms *such tremor, rigidity, drooling, difficulty with speech, and abrupt personality change.*

Background Information

Symptoms of Wilson's disease usually appear in childhood or young adult life[7] with a frequency of 1 in 30,000.[128] This condition is an autosomal recessive disorder in which excessive amounts of copper accumulate in the body especially in eye membranes (causing a golden brown Kayser-Fleischer ring), nailbeds, and kidney.[1] The gene abnormality has been located on chromosome 13, which causes a deficiency in ceruloplasmin. In the central nervous system, cavitation and neuronal loss occur within the putamen and globus pallidus. This condition is diagnosed on clinical findings supported by biochemical evidence of low ceruloplasmin, elevated unbound serum copper, high urinary copper excretion, positive liver biopsy and copper metabolism tests, and T_2-weighted magnetic resonance imaging that shows thalamus and putamen hyperintensity.[1] Treatment consists of low-copper diet and a chelating agent (usually penicillamine).[1] With adequate treatment, the life span is normal. If left untreated in children, death is predicted in 2 years from hepatic and renal failure. In untreated adults, death is predicted in 10 years.[1]

References

1. Lindsay KW, Bone I, Callander R. *Neurology and Neurosurgery Illustrated.* 3rd ed. New York, NY: Churchill Livingstone; 1997.
2. Victor M, Ropper AH. *Adams and Victor's Principles of Neurology.* 7th ed. New York, NY: McGraw-Hill; 2001.
3. O'Sullivan SB, Schmitz TJ. *Physical Rehabilitation: Assessment and Treatment.* 4th ed. Philadelphia, PA: F. A. Davis; 2001.
4. Garg RK. Acute disseminated encephalomyelitis. *Postgrad Med J.* Jan 2003;79(927):11–17.
5. Foreman PJ. Summary and discussion—patient #32. October 16, 2008. http://www.bcm.edu/neurology/challeng/pat32/summary.html. Accessed August 28, 2005.
6. Hamdy RC. Alzheimer's disease: an overview. *South Med J.* Jul 2001;94(7):661–662.
7. Greenberg DA, Aminoff MJ, Simon RP. *Clinical Neurology.* 5th ed. New York, NY: McGraw-Hill; 2002.
8. National Institute of Neurological Disorders and Stroke. NINDS Alzheimer's Disease Information Page. March 27, 2009. http://www.ninds.nih.gov/disorders/alzheimers disease/alzheimersdisease.htm. Accessed August 28, 2005.
9. American Psychiatric Association. *Diagnostic and Statistical Manual of Mental Disorders. Text Revision.* 4th ed. Washington, DC: American Psychiatric Association; 2000.
10. Halgin RP, Whitbourne SK. *Abnormal Psychology. The Human Experience of Psychological Disorders.* 2nd ed. Madison: Brown and Benchmark; 1997.

11. Halgin RP, Whitbourne SK. *Abnormal Psychology: The Human Experience of Psychological Disorders.* 2nd ed. New York, NY: William C Brown; 1997.

12. American Psychiatric Association. *Diagnostic and Statistical Manual of Mental Disorders.* 4th ed. Washington, DC: American Psychiatric Association; 1994.

13. Goldman LS, Genel M, Bezman RJ, Slanetz PJ. Diagnosis and treatment of attention-deficit/hyperactivity disorder in children and adolescents. Council on Scientific Affairs, American Medical Association. *JAMA.* Apr 8 1998;279(14):1100–1107.

14. Al-Otaibi LM, Porter SR, Poate TW. Behcet's disease: a review. *J Dent Res.* Mar 2005;84(3):209–222.

15. Loeb C. Binswanger's disease is not a single entity. *Neurol Sci.* Dec 2000;21(6):343–348.

16. Roman GC. Vascular dementia revisited: diagnosis, pathogenesis, treatment, and prevention. *Med Clin North Am.* May 2002;86(3):477–499.

17. Ropper AH, Brown RJ. *Adams and Victor's Principles of Neurology.* 8th ed. New York, NY: McGraw-Hill; 2005.

18. Roman GC, Erkinjuntti T, Wallin A, Pantoni L, Chui HC. Subcortical ischaemic vascular dementia. *Lancet Neurol.* Nov 2002;1(7):426–436.

19. Hilty DM, Brady KT, Hales RE. A review of bipolar disorder among adults. *Psychiatr Serv.* Feb 1999;50(2):201–213.

20. Tosoni A, Ermani M, Brandes AA. The pathogenesis and treatment of brain metastases: a comprehensive review. *Crit Rev Oncol Hematol.* 2004;52:199–215.

21. Sage MR, Blumbergs PC. Cavernous haemangiomas (angiomas) of the brain. *Australas Radiol.* May 2001;45(2):247–256.

22. Schievink WI. Intracranial aneurysms. *N Engl J Med.* Jan 2, 1997;336(1):28–40.

23. Vogel T, Verreault R, Turcotte JF, Kiesmann M, Berthel M. Intracerebral aneurysms: a review with special attention to geriatric aspects. *J Gerontol A Biol Sci Med Sci.* Jun 2003;58(6):520–541.

24. Consensus statement on the definition of orthostatic hypotension, pure autonomic failure, and multiple system atrophy. The Consensus Committee of the American Autonomic Society and the American Academy of Neurology. *Neurology.* May 1996;46(5):1470.

25. Unruptured intracranial aneurysms—risk of rupture and risks of surgical intervention. International Study of Unruptured Intracranial Aneurysms Investigators. *N Engl J Med.* Dec 10, 1998;339(24):1725–1733.

26. Aasly J, Skandsen T, Ro M. Neuroacanthocytosis—the variability of presenting symptoms in two siblings. *Acta Neurol Scand.* Nov 1999;100(5):322–325.

27. Bohlega S, Riley W, Powe J, Baynton R, Roberts G. Neuroacanthocytosis and aprebetalipoproteinemia. *Neurology.* Jun 1998;50(6):1912–1914.

28. Rubio JP, Danek A, Stone C, et al. Chorea-acanthocytosis: genetic linkage to chromosome 9q21. *Am J Hum Genet.* Oct 1997;61(4):899–908.

29. Krem MM. Motor conversion disorders reviewed from a neuropsychiatric perspective. *J Clin Psychiatry.* Jun 2004;65(6):783–790.

30. Mahapatra RK, Edwards MJ, Schott JM, Bhatia KP. Corticobasal degeneration. *Lancet Neurol.* Dec 2004;3(12):736–743.

31. Wenning GK, Litvan I, Jankovic J, et al. Natural history and survival of 14 patients with corticobasal de-

generation confirmed at postmortem examination. *J Neurol Neurosurg Psychiatry.* Feb 1998;64(2):184–189.

32. Boeve BF, Lang AE, Litvan I. Corticobasal degeneration and its relationship to progressive supranuclear palsy and frontotemporal dementia. *Ann Neurol.* 2003;54 (suppl 5):S15–19.

33. Kompoliti K, Goetz CG, Boeve BF, et al. Clinical presentation and pharmacological therapy in corticobasal degeneration. *Arch Neurol.* Jul 1998;55(7):957–961.

34. Collinge J. Molecular neurology of prion disease. *J Neurol Neurosurg Psychiatry.* Jul 2005;76(7):906–919.

35. Knight RS, Will RG. Prion diseases. *J Neurol Neurosurg Psychiatry.* Mar 2004;75(suppl 1):i36–42.

36. Arnaldi G, Angeli A, Atkinson AB, et al. Diagnosis and complications of Cushing's syndrome: a consensus statement. *J Clin Endocrinol Metab.* Dec 2003;88 (12):5593–5602.

37. Orth DN. Cushing's syndrome. *N Engl J Med.* Mar 23 1995;332(12):791–803.

38. Garcia HH, Gonzalez AE, Gilman RH. Diagnosis, treatment and control of Taenia solium cysticercosis. *Curr Opin Infect Dis.* Oct 2003;16(5):411–419.

39. Singhi P, Singhi S. Neurocysticercosis in children. *J Child Neurol.* Jul 2004;19(7):482–492.

40. Geldmacher DS. Dementia with Lewy bodies: diagnosis and clinical approach. *Cleve Clin J Med.* Oct 2004;71 (10):789–790, 792–794, 797–798 passim.

41. Small GW. Neuroimaging as a diagnostic tool in dementia with Lewy bodies. *Dement Geriatr Cogn Disord.* 2004;17(suppl 1):25–31.

42. Walker Z, Allen RL, Shergill S, Mullan E, Katona CL. Three years survival in patients with a clinical diagnosis of dementia with Lewy bodies. *Int J Geriatr Psychiatry.* Mar 2000;15(3):267–273.

43. Goodman CC, Boissonnault WG. *Pathology: Implications for the Physical Therapist.* Philadelphia, PA: W. B. Saunders; 1998.

44. Aronson SC, Ayres VE. Depression: A treatment algorithm for the family physician. *Hospital Physician.* 2000(July):21–44.

45. Shaywitz SE. Dyslexia. *N Engl J Med.* Jan 29 1998; 338(5):307–312.

46. Olitsky SE, Nelson LB. Reading disorders in children. *Pediatr Clin North Am.* Feb 2003;50(1):213–224.

47. Shaywitz SE, Fletcher JM, Holahan JM, et al. Persistence of dyslexia: the Connecticut Longitudinal Study at adolescence. *Pediatrics.* Dec1999;104(6):1351–1359.

48. Custodio CM, Basford JR. Delayed postanoxic encephalopathy: a case report and literature review. *Arch Phys Med Rehabil.* Mar 2004;85(3):502–505.

49. Sommerfield AJ, Stimson R, Campbell IW. Hashimoto's encephalopathy presenting as an acute medical emergency. *Scott Med J.* Nov 2004;49(4):155–156.

50. Fisher RS, van Emde Boas W, Blume W, et al. Epileptic seizures and epilepsy: definitions proposed by the International League Against Epilepsy (ILAE) and the International Bureau for Epilepsy (IBE). *Epilepsia.* Apr 2005;46(4):470–472.

51. Wiebe S. Randomized controlled trials of epilepsy surgery. *Epilepsia.* 2003;44(suppl 7):38–43.

52. Sander JW. The natural history of epilepsy in the era of new antiepileptic drugs and surgical treatment. *Epilepsia.* 2003;44(suppl 1):17–20.

53. Manyam BV, Walters AS, Narla KR. Bilateral striopallidodentate calcinosis: clinical characteristics of patients seen in a registry. *Mov Disord.* Mar 2001;16(2): 258–264.

54. Manyam BV, Bhatt MH, Moore WD, Devleschoward AB, Anderson DR, Calne DB. Bilateral striopallidodentate calcinosis: cerebrospinal fluid, imaging, and electrophysiological studies. *Ann Neurol.* Apr 1992;31(4):379–384.

55. Manyam BV. What is and what is not "Fahr's disease." *Parkinsonism Relat Disord.* Mar 2005;11(2):73–80.

56. Ratnavalli E, Brayne C, Dawson K, Hodges JR. The prevalence of frontotemporal dementia. *Neurology.* Jun 11 2002;58(11):1615–1621.

57. Kertesz A. Frontotemporal dementia/Pick's disease. *Arch Neurol.* Jun 2004;61(6):969–971.

58. Kertesz A, McMonagle P, Blair M, Davidson W, Munoz DG. The evolution and pathology of frontotemporal dementia. *Brain.* Sep 2005;128(pt 9):1996–2005.

59. Mankin HJ, Rosenthal DI, Xavier R. Gaucher disease. New approaches to an ancient disease. *J Bone Joint Surg Am.* May 2001;83-A(5):748–762.

60. Suresh PA, Sebastian S. Developmental Gerstmann's syndrome: a distinct clinical entity of learning disabilities. *Pediatr Neurol.* Apr 2000;22(4):267–278.

61. Benton AL. Gerstmann's syndrome. *Arch Neurol.* May 1992;49(5):445–447.

62. National Institute of Neurological Disorders and Stroke. NINDS Gerstmann's syndrome information page. July, 2, 2008. http://www.ninds.nih.gov/disorders/gerstmanns/gerstmanns.htm. Accessed August 28, 2005.

63. Thomas M, Hayflick SJ, Jankovic J. Clinical heterogeneity of neurodegeneration with brain iron accumulation (Hallervorden-Spatz syndrome) and pantothenate kinase-associated neurodegeneration. *Mov Disord.* Jan 2004;19(1):36–42.

64. Vasconcelos OM, Harter DH, Duffy C, et al. Adult Hallervorden-Spatz syndrome simulating amyotrophic lateral sclerosis. *Muscle Nerve.* Jul 2003;28(1):118–122.

65. Fink JK. Advances in the hereditary spastic paraplegias. *Exp Neurol.* Nov 2003;184(suppl 1):S106–110.

66. Park SY, Ki CS, Kim HJ, et al. Mutation analysis of SPG4 and SPG3A genes and its implication in molecular diagnosis of Korean patients with hereditary spastic paraplegia. *Arch Neurol.* Jul 2005;62(7):1118–1121.

67. de Boo GM, Tibben A, Lanser JB, et al. Early cognitive and motor symptoms in identified carriers of the gene for Huntington disease. *Arch Neurol.* Nov 1997;54(11): 1353–1357.

68. Rosas HD, Feigin AS, Hersch SM. Using advances in neuroimaging to detect, understand, and monitor disease progression in Huntington's disease. *NeuroRx.* Apr 2004;1(2):263–272.

69. Arriada N, Sotelo J. Review: treatment of hydrocephalus in adults. *Surg Neurol.* Dec 2002;58(6):377–384; discussion 384.

70. National Institute of Neurological Disorders and Stroke. NINDS hypersomnia information page. June 23, 2008. http://www.ninds.nih.gov/disorders/hypersomnia/hypersomnia.htm. Accessed August 28, 2005.

71. Torbey MT, Geocadin R, Bhardwaj A. Brain arrest neurological outcome scale (BrANOS): predicting mortality and severe disability following cardiac arrest. *Resuscitation.* Oct 2004;63(1):55–63.

72. Croft A. Extracts from "Clinical Evidence." Malaria: prevention in travellers. *BMJ.* Jul 15, 2000;321(7254): 154–160.

73. Peigue-Lafeuille H, Croquez N, Laurichesse H, et al. Enterovirus meningitis in adults in 1999–2000 and evaluation of clinical management. *J Med Virol.* May 2002;67(1):47–53.

74. Cejudo P, Bautista J, Montemayor T, et al. Exercise training in mitochondrial myopathy: a randomized controlled trial. *Muscle Nerve.* Sep 2005;32(3):342–350.

75. Hasuo K, Mihara F, Matsushima T. MRI and MR angiography in moyamoya disease. *J Magn Reson Imaging.* Jul–Aug 1998;8(4):762–766.

76. Sakamoto T, Kawaguchi M, Kurehara K, Kitaguchi K, Furuya H, Karasawa J. Risk factors for neurological deterioration after revascularization surgery in patients with moyamoya disease. *Anesth Analg.* Nov 1997;85(5): 1060–1065.

77. National Institute of Neurological Disorders and Stroke. NINDS Multi-infarct dementia information page. March 27, 2009. http://www.ninds.nih.gov/disorders/multi_infarct_dementia/multi_infarct_dementia.htm. Accessed August 28, 2005.

78. McDonald WI, Compston A, Edan G, et al. Recommended diagnostic criteria for multiple sclerosis: guidelines from the International Panel on the diagnosis of multiple sclerosis. *Ann Neurol.* Jul 2001;50(1): 121–127.

79. Thompson AJ, Montalban X, Barkhof F, et al. Diagnostic criteria for primary progressive multiple sclerosis: a position paper. *Ann Neurol.* Jun 2000;47(6):831–835.

80. Confavreux C, Vukusic S, Adeleine P. Early clinical predictors and progression of irreversible disability in multiple sclerosis: an amnesic process. *Brain.* Apr 2003; 126(pt 4):770–782.

81. Wenning GK, Tison F, Ben Shlomo Y, Daniel SE, Quinn NP. Multiple system atrophy: a review of 203 pathologically proven cases. *Mov Disord.* Mar 1997;12(2): 133–147.

82. Wenning GK, Ben-Shlomo Y, Hughes A, Daniel SE, Lees A, Quinn NP. What clinical features are most useful to distinguish definite multiple system atrophy from Parkinson's disease? *J Neurol Neurosurg Psychiatry.* Apr 2000;68(4):434–440.

83. Ben-Shlomo Y, Wenning GK, Tison F, Quinn NP. Survival of patients with pathologically proven multiple system atrophy: a meta-analysis. *Neurology.* Feb 1997;48(2):384–393.

84. National Institute of Neurological Disorders and Stroke. NINDS narcolepsy information page. March 4, 2009. http://www.ninds.nih.gov/disorders/narcolepsy/narcolepsy.htm. Accessed August 28, 2005.

85. Price RW. Neurological complications of HIV infection. *Lancet.* Aug 17 1996;348(9025):445–452.

86. Brown DL, Frank JE. Diagnosis and management of syphilis. *Am Fam Physician.* Jul 15, 2003;68(2): 283–290.

87. Conde-Sendin MA, Amela-Peris R, Aladro-Benito Y, Maroto AA. Current clinical spectrum of neurosyphilis in immunocompetent patients. *Eur Neurol.* 2004;52 (1):29–35.

88. Imrie J, Vijayaraghaven S, Whitehouse C, et al. Niemann-Pick disease type C in adults. *J Inherit Metab Dis.* Oct 2002;25(6):491–500.

89. Jin LW, Shie FS, Maezawa I, Vincent I, Bird T. Intracellular accumulation of amyloidogenic fragments of amyloid-beta precursor protein in neurons with Niemann-Pick type C defects is associated with endosomal abnormalities. *Am J Pathol.* Mar 2004;164(3): 975–985.

90. Bataller L, Dalmau J. Paraneoplastic neurologic syndromes: approaches to diagnosis and treatment. *Semin Neurol.* Jun 2003;23(2):215–224.

91. Darnell RB, Posner JB. Paraneoplastic syndromes involving the nervous system. *N Engl J Med.* Oct 16 2003;349(16):1543–1554.

92. Dalmau JO, Posner JB. Paraneoplastic syndromes. *Arch Neurol.* Apr 1999;56(4):405–408.

93. Guryanova I. Delusional disorder. http://www.emedicine.com/med/topic3351.htm. Accessed August 28, 2005.

94. Wood BH, Bilclough JA, Bowron A, Walker RW. Incidence and prediction of falls in Parkinson's disease: a prospective multidisciplinary study. *J Neurol Neurosurg Psychiatry.* Jun 2002;72(6):721–725.

95. Samii A, Nutt JG, Ransom BR. Parkinson's disease. *Lancet.* May 29, 2004;363(9423):1783–1793.

96. Tillerson JL, Cohen AD, Philhower J, Miller GW, Zigmond MJ, Schallert T. Forced limb-use effects on the behavioral and neurochemical effects of 6-hydroxydopamine. *J Neurosci.* Jun 15, 2001;21(12): 4427–4435.

97. Jankovic J, Kapadia AS. Functional decline in Parkinson disease. *Arch Neurol.* Oct 2001;58(10):1611–1615.

98. Marras C, Rochon P, Lang AE. Predicting motor decline and disability in Parkinson disease: a systematic review. *Arch Neurol.* Nov 2002;59(11): 1724–1728.

99. Berger J, Moser HW, Forss-Petter S. Leukodystrophies: recent developments in genetics, molecular biology, pathogenesis and treatment. *Curr Opin Neurol.* Jun 2001;14(3):305–312.

100. Regis S, Grossi S, Lualdi S, Biancheri R, Filocamo M. Diagnosis of Pelizaeus-Merzbacher disease: detection of proteolipid protein gene copy number by real-time PCR. *Neurogenetics.* May 2005;6(2):73–78.

101. Aicardi J. The inherited leukodystrophies: a clinical overview. *J Inherit Metab Dis.* 1993;16(4):733–743.

102. Hodges JR, Davies RR, Xuereb JH, et al. Clinicopathological correlates in frontotemporal dementia. *Ann Neurol.* Sep 2004;56(3):399–406.

103. Kertesz A. Pick complex: an integrative approach to frontotemporal dementia: primary progressive aphasia, corticobasal degeneration, and progressive supranuclear palsy. *Neurologist.* Nov 2003;9(6): 311–317.

104. Borrell E. Hypokinetic movement disorders. *J Neurosci Nurs.* Oct 2000;32(5):254–255.

105. Litvan I, Mangone CA, McKee A, et al. Natural history of progressive supranuclear palsy (Steele-Richardson-Olszewski syndrome) and clinical predictors of survival: a clinicopathological study. *J Neurol Neurosurg Psychiatry.* Jun 1996;60(6):615–620.

106. Litvan I, Bhatia KP, Burn DJ, et al. Movement Disorders Society Scientific Issues Committee report: SIC Task Force appraisal of clinical diagnostic criteria for Parkinsonian disorders. *Mov Disord.* May 2003;18 (5):467–486.

107. Belay ED, Bresee JS, Holman RC, Khan AS, Shahriari A, Schonberger LB. Reye's syndrome in the United States from 1981 through 1997. *N Engl J Med.* May 6 1999;340(18):1377–1382.

108. Bratton RL, Corey R. Tick-borne disease. *Am Fam Physician.* Jun 15 2005;71(12):2323–2330.

109. Kirkland KB, Wilkinson WE, Sexton DJ. Therapeutic delay and mortality in cases of Rocky Mountain spotted fever. *Clin Infect Dis.* May 1995;20(5): 1118–1121.

110. Buckley PF, Dayem M, Parker G, Weisser L. Schizophrenia today: what do we know—and how sure are we? *J Psychiatr Pract.* Jul 2001;7(4):244–246.

111. Redline S, Strohl KP. Recognition and consequences of obstructive sleep apnea hypopnea syndrome. *Clin Chest Med.* Mar 1998;19(1):1–19.

112. Granger CV, Clark GS. Functional status and outcomes of stroke rehabilitation. *Topics Geriatrics.* Mar 1994; 9(3):72–84.

113. Shelton FD, Volpe BT, Reding M. Motor impairment as a predictor of functional recovery and guide to rehabilitation treatment after stroke. *Neurorehabil Neural Repair.* 2001;15(3):229–237.

114. Yaqub BA. Subacute sclerosing panencephalitis (SSPE): early diagnosis, prognostic factors and natural history. *J Neurol Sci.* Aug 1996;139(2):227–234.

115. National Institute of Neurological Disorders and Stroke. NINDS subacute sclerosing panencephalitis information page. March 16, 2009. http://www.ninds.nih. gov/disorders/subacute_panencephalitis/subacute_ panencephalitis.htm. Accessed August 28, 2005.

116. Fauci AS, Haynes B, Katz P. The spectrum of vasculitis: clinical, pathologic, immunologic and therapeutic considerations. *Ann Intern Med.* Nov 1978;89(5 pt 1):660–676.

117. Eapen V, Fox-Hiley P, Banerjee S, Robertson M. Clinical features and associated psychopathology in a Tourette syndrome cohort. *Acta Neurol Scand.* Apr 2004; 109(4):255–260.

118. National Institute of Neurological Disorders and Stroke. NINDS Tourette syndrome information page. July 15, 2008. http://www.ninds.nih.gov/disorders/ tourette/tourette.htm. Accessed August 28, 2008.

119. Bruns J, Hauser WA. The epidemiology of traumatic brain injury: a review. *Epilepsia.* 2003;44(suppl 10):2–10.

120. Das-Gupta R, Turner-Stokes L. Traumatic brain injury. *Disability and Rehabilitation.* 2002;24(13):654–665.

121. Hukkelhoven CWPM, Steyerberg EW, Rampen AJJ, et al. Patient age and outcome following severe traumatic brain injury: an analysis of 5600 patients. *J Neurosurg.* 2003;99:666–673.

122. National Institute of Neurological Disorders and Stroke. NINDS tuberous sclerosis information page. September 9, 2008. http://www.ninds.nih.gov/disorders/ tuberous_sclerosis/tuberous_sclerosis.htm. Accessed August 28, 2005.

123. Lendvay TS, Marshall FF. The tuberous sclerosis complex and its highly variable manifestations. *J Urol.* May 2003;169(5):1635–1642.

124. Perrin RG, Laxton AW. Metastatic spine disease: epidemiology, pathophysiology, and evaluation of patients. *Neurosurg Clin N Am.* Oct 2004;15(4): 365–373.

125. Hosono N, Ueda T, Tamura D, Aoki Y, Yoshikawa H. Prognostic relevance of clinical symptoms in patients with spinal metastases. *Clin Orthop Relat Res.* Jul 2005(436):196–201.

126. Marth T, Raoult D. Whipple's disease. *Lancet.* Jan 18 2003;361(9353):239–246.

127. Mahnel R, Marth T. Progress, problems, and perspectives in diagnosis and treatment of Whipple's disease. *Clin Exp Med.* Sep 2004;4(1):39–43.

128. Gow PJ, Smallwood RA, Angus PW, Smith AL, Wall AJ, Sewell RB. Diagnosis of Wilson's disease: an experience over three decades. *Gut.* Mar 2000;46(3):415–419.

CHAPTER **32**

Stiffness

■ *Claire Smith, PT, DPT, NCS* ■ *Beth E. Fisher, PT, PhD*

Description of the Symptom

This chapter describes pathology that may lead to stiffness of the body. Stiffness is both an objective event that can be perceived by a clinician and a subjective phenomenon that is perceived by the individual. The increased resistance to movement a therapist feels while passively moving a limb of his or her patient might be described as stiffness. Additionally, *stiff* might refer to a patient's description of how the limbs feel when he or she attempts to actively move or bend. Subjective stiffness may arise from issues with motor sequencing and recruitment, coordination, and the length of passive structures.

Special Concerns

■ A change in prior level of stiffness, including but not limited to:
  ■ Increase in spasticity
  ■ Change in resting muscle tone
■ A new onset of stiffness not associated with original purpose of the physical therapy visit. This may include:
  ■ Spasticity
  ■ Clonus
  ■ Rigidity
  ■ Hypertonicity
  ■ Hypotonicity
  ■ Stiffness that is not of musculoskeletal origin

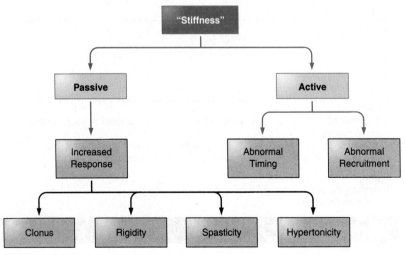

Conceptual overview of conditions that lead to stiffness

CHAPTER PREVIEW: Conditions That May Lead to Stiffness

T Trauma

COMMON

Overuse syndromes (repetitive motion disorders, cumulative trauma disorders, repetitive stress injuries) 675
Traumatic brain injury 678
Traumatic spinal cord injury 678
Whiplash injury (whiplash-associated disorder) 680

UNCOMMON

Not applicable

RARE

Not applicable

I Inflammation

COMMON

Aseptic
Encephalitis 670
Meningitis:
• Bacterial meningitis 673
• Viral meningitis 674
Vasculitis (giant cell arteritis, temporal arteritis, cranial arteritis) 679

Septic
Not applicable

UNCOMMON

Aseptic
Behçet's disease 669

Septic
Not applicable

RARE

Aseptic
Neuromyotonia (Isaac syndrome, Isaac-Merten syndrome, continuous muscle fiber activity syndrome, quantal squander syndrome) 675
Opsoclonus myoclonus (Kinsbourne syndrome, myoclonic encephalopathy of infants, dancing eyes–dancing feet syndrome, opsoclonus-myoclonus-ataxia syndrome) 675

Septic
Acute disseminated encephalomyelitis 669
Lyme disease (tick paralysis) 673

M Metabolic

COMMON

Not applicable

UNCOMMON

Neuroleptic malignant syndrome 675

Metabolic *(continued)*

RARE

Fahr's syndrome (familial idiopathic basal ganglia calcification, bilateral striopallidodentate calcinosis) 671
Gaucher's disease 671
Wilson's disease 680

Va Vascular

COMMON

Stroke (cerebrovascular accident) 677

UNCOMMON

Cerebral aneurysm 669
Spinal cord infarction (vascular myelopathy) 677

RARE

Not applicable

De Degenerative

COMMON

Dementia with Lewy bodies 670
Parkinson's disease 676

UNCOMMON

Huntington's disease 672

RARE

Choreoacanthocytosis (Levine-Critchley syndrome, neuroacanthocytosis) 670
Hallervorden-Spatz syndrome (neurodegeneration with brain iron accumulation, pantothenate
  kinase-associated neurodegeneration) 672
Hereditary spastic paraplegia (familial spastic paralysis) 672
Machado-Joseph disease 673
Multiple system atrophy (striatonigral degenerative, olivopontocerebellar atrophy, Shy-Drager
  syndrome) 674
Primary lateral sclerosis 676
Stiff-person syndrome 677

Tu Tumor

COMMON

Not applicable

UNCOMMON

Malignant Primary:
Not applicable
Malignant Metastatic:
Not applicable
Benign, such as:
• Hydromyelia (syringomyelia) 672

(continued)

Tumor *(continued)*

RARE

Malignant Primary, such as:
- Brain primary tumors 679
- Spinal primary tumors 679

Malignant Metastatic, such as:
- Brain metastases 678
- Spinal metastases 679

Benign:
Not applicable

Co   Congenital

COMMON

Not applicable

UNCOMMON

Not applicable

RARE

Paroxysmal choreoathetosis 676

Ne   Neurogenic/Psychogenic

COMMON

Epilepsy/seizure disorder 671

UNCOMMON

Myotonia congenital 674

RARE

Not applicable

Note: These are estimates of relative incidence because few data are available for the less common conditions.

Overview of Stiffness

Clinical assessment of stretch reflex dysfunction has generally been a key assessment of "stiffness" and has focused on spasticity. The precise definition of *spasticity* is a velocity-dependent increase in the tonic stretch reflex with exaggerated tendon jerks resulting from hyperexcitability of the stretch reflex as one component of the upper motor neuron syndrome.[1,2] In addition to increased stretch reflexes, hypertonicity, defined as increased resistance to passive movement, and paresis are other signs collectively called the *upper motor neuron syndrome.* Upper motor neuron syndrome results from damage to descending motor pathways at cortical, brainstem, or spinal cord levels.

The pathophysiological basis of these passive processes is incompletely understood. The changes in muscle tone (hypertonicity) probably result from alterations in the balance of inputs from reticulospinal and other descending pathways to the motor and interneuronal circuits of the spinal cord, and the absence of an intact corticospinal system. Loss of descending tonic or phasic excitatory and inhibitory inputs to the spinal motor apparatus, alterations in the segmental balance of excitatory and inhibitory control, denervation supersensitivity, and neuronal sprouting may be observed. Once hypertonicity is established, the chronically shortened muscle may develop physical changes, such as shortening and contracture, that further contribute to muscle stiffness. The pathophysiological mechanisms causing the increase in stretch reflexes in spasticity also are not well understood.[3]

Spasticity is a form of muscle overactivity. Spasticity is often used as an umbrella term to describe other forms of muscle overactivity that often occur. However, each of the following represents a distinct pathophysiological mechanism and it is inaccurate to interchange these terms even though it is commonly done in the clinic (particularly the terms *spasticity* and *hypertonicity*).[2] Other forms of muscle overactivity that may be part of the upper motor neuron syndrome are:

- Spasms, or strong and sustained contractions of muscles, which are often painful
- Increased reflexes, in which the normal reflexes (such as knee extension in response to tapping) are greatly exaggerated
- Clonus, which refers to self-sustaining oscillating movements around a joint elicited with quick stretch
- Hypertonicity, or an abnormal increase in resting muscle tension
- Rigidity, which describes involuntary bidirectional non–velocity-dependent resistance to movement.

Description of Conditions That May Lead to Stiffness

■ **Acute Disseminated Encephalomyelitis**

Chief Clinical Characteristics
This presentation may involve confusion, somnolence, and convulsion in its encephalitic form. Individuals with this condition may report headache and neck stiffness. Initial symptoms of the myelitic form include weakness and sensory impairments.[2]

Background Information
This condition is a demyelinating disease of the central nervous system,[4] which may be due to an immune-mediated complication of infection.[2] The presence of upper motor neuron signs, cerebrospinal fluid pleocytosis and elevated protein, and multiple white matter lesions demonstrated on magnetic resonance imaging supports the diagnosis.[5] Definitive diagnosis requires a brain biopsy. The primary goal of treatment is to suppress the immune response; thus high-dose corticosteroids are generally

administered over a course of 3 to 5 days.[5] The prognosis is variable depending on the severity of the disease and acuity of the diagnosis.

■ **Behçet's Disease**

Chief Clinical Characteristics
This presentation may include bilateral pyramidal signs (eg, weakness, hyperreflexia in the deep tendon reflexes, hypertonia, clonus, and/or a positive Babinski sign), headache, memory loss, hemiparesis, cerebellar ataxia, balance deficits, sphincter dysfunction, or cranial nerve palsies. In addition to these neurological signs individuals with this condition also may present with arthritis; renal, gastrointestinal, vascular, and cardiac diseases; and genital, oral, and cutaneous ulcerations.[6]

Background Information
Mean age of onset is in the third decade of life. Diagnostic criteria according to an international study group include presence of recurrent oral ulceration, recurrent genital ulceration, eye lesions, skin lesions, papulopustular lesions, and/or a positive pathergy test.[2,6] Medical treatment typically consists of corticosteroids and immunosuppressants. Neurological symptoms tend to clear within weeks, but can sometimes recur or result in permanent deficits.[2] Negative prognostic factors include onset before the age of 25 and male sex.

■ **Cerebral Aneurysm**

Chief Clinical Characteristics
This presentation may involve loss of balance in combination with a whole host of other neurological symptoms and signs that depend on the affected cerebral tissue, including visual and proprioceptive loss. Any associated signs or symptoms may not be reported due to the fact that this condition is typically asymptomatic prior to rupture. However, if the aneurysm results in a mass effect, ischemia, or hemorrhage, then neurological signs and symptoms are dependent on the affected location.[2,7,8]

Background Information
There has been some description of genetic factors in this condition.[7] Cigarette smoking, hypertension, and heavy alcohol use have all been found to be correlated with increased risk of aneurysm development.[7,8] Factors associated with increased risk of rupture include size of

aneurysm, location in the posterior circulation, and a previous history of aneurismal subarachnoid hemorrhage.[9,10] Definitive diagnosis is based on catheter angiography; however, magnetic resonance angiography, magnetic resonance imaging, and computed tomography may aid in the diagnosis. Unruptured aneurysms are sometimes surgically treated. Aneurysm size, location, and prior history of a subarachnoid hemorrhage help to determine if the risk of surgical treatment is worth the potential benefits. Most aneurysms that have hemorrhaged must be treated surgically. Patients with a previous rupture are at an 11 times greater risk of having a second intracranial aneurysm rupture. When aneurysms do rupture, many patients die within one month of the rupture, and those who survive often have residual neurological deficits.[7]

■ Choreoacanthocytosis (Levine-Critchley Syndrome, Neuroacanthocytosis)

Chief Clinical Characteristics
This presentation commonly includes chorea, motor or vocal tics, dystonia, orofacial dyskinesias, and parkinsonism. Seizures, cognitive impairment, psychosis, paranoia, and personality changes are also seen with this diagnosis, along with hyporeflexia and distal myopathy due to denervation of muscles.[11–13]

Background Information
This condition is a rare, autosomal recessive disorder that typically has its onset during the third and fourth decades of life.[13] This neurodegenerative disorder is associated with acanthocytes, aberrant spiky or thorny red blood cells, as well as atrophy and gliosis of the caudate, putamen, and globus pallidus.[12] Diagnosis is made by a combination of tests, including clinical features, lab work demonstrating acanthocytosis, neuroimaging, and genetic testing to rule out Huntington's disease.[11] There is currently no effective, long-term treatment, although verapamil has been found to provide temporary reduction of symptoms. Life expectancy is reduced, and suicidal action or ideation is not uncommon due to cognitive impairments.[13]

■ Dementia with Lewy Bodies

Chief Clinical Characteristics
This presentation can be characterized by fluctuating cognitive dysfunction, particularly visuospatial problems and executive dysfunction, visual hallucinations, and parkinsonism features such as masked facies, autonomic dysfunction, rigidity, and bradykinesia. Other signs and symptoms may include postural instability, falls, sleep disturbances, memory problems, syncope, transient loss of consciousness, and sensitivity to antipsychotic and anti-Parkinson medications.[14]

Background Information
This progressive condition is the second most common dementia after Alzheimer's disease.[14] The specific etiology of this condition is unknown. The characteristic Lewy bodies are eosinophilic inclusion bodies found within the cytoplasm of neurons in the cerebral cortex and limbic system.[14] A thorough clinical examination, laboratory screen, and imaging are important to rule out other causes of dementia. The definitive diagnosis for this condition is made postmortem; however, it appears that the use of single-photon emission computed tomography and positron emission tomography may be useful in the identification of occipital hypoperfusion which may be associated with the visual hallucinations.[14,15] Management includes caregiver education to assist in minimizing factors that may contribute to problematic behaviors. Medication therapy may be indicated, but should be monitored closely due to potential exacerbation of symptoms.[14] Life expectancy for individuals with this condition is similar to that of Alzheimer's disease. The average survival time is between 6 and 8 years from the onset of dementia.[14,16]

■ Encephalitis

Chief Clinical Characteristics
This presentation includes confusion, delirium, convulsions, problems with speech or hearing, memory loss, hallucinations, drowsiness, and coma. Headache or back stiffness may be present.

Background Information
Encephalitis is an inflammation of nerve cells in the brain. This term usually refers to the viral form, although bacterial, parasitic, and fungal agents also can cause this condition. Up to 20,000 new cases of viral forms of this

condition are reported annually in the United States. Diagnosis is established by clinical presentation suggesting dysfunction of the cerebrum, brainstem, or cerebellum, cellular reaction and elevated protein in spinal fluid, and possible demonstration of diffuse edema or enhancement of the brain on magnetic resonance imaging or computed tomography. Treatment is primarily pharmacologic, with drugs such as corticosteroids, antiviral agents, and anticonvulsants. The majority of individuals with encephalitis do recover, but irreversible brain damage and death can result.[2]

■ Epilepsy/Seizure Disorder

Chief Clinical Characteristics

This presentation is variable and can range from abnormal sensations or behavior to convulsions, muscles spasms, and loss of consciousness. Specific cognitive symptoms include problems with perception, attention, emotion, and memory.[17]

Background Information

According to the International League Against Epilepsy an epileptic seizure is defined as "a transient occurrence of signs and/or symptoms due to abnormal excessive or synchronous neuronal activity in the brain."[17] The diagnosis of epilepsy includes a history of at least one seizure with the "associated neurobiological, cognitive, psychological, and social disturbances."[17] Seizures are also classified into different categories based on presentation and electroencephalogram features. Approximately 1% of the U.S. population will have epilepsy before 20 years of age, although the incidence increases slightly after age 60.[2] Most seizures can be controlled pharmacologically with antiepileptic drugs. Surgical treatment is indicated in patients with recurrent seizures that arise from a single focus and prevent a normal lifestyle.[18] The prognosis for a patient with epilepsy depends on the cause of the seizures and treatment. Remission occurs in only 16% to 43% of patients with partial seizures.[19] Less favorable prognosis is also associated with multiple seizure types, associated neurological deficits, and behavioral or psychiatric disturbance.[19]

■ Fahr's Syndrome (Familial Idiopathic Basal Ganglia Calcification, Bilateral Striopallidodentate Calcinosis)

Chief Clinical Characteristics

This presentation may involve features of parkinsonism, such as chorea, athetosis, rigidity, dystonia, and tremor in addition to cognitive impairments, cerebellar impairments, gait and balance disorder, psychiatric features, pain, pyramidal signs, such as weakness, hyperreflexia in the deep tendon reflexes, hypertonia, clonus, and/or a positive Babinski, sensory changes and speech disorder.[20]

Background Information

This condition occurs due to bilateral symmetric calcification of the basal ganglia with or without calcification of the dentate nucleus. The disease has been described as both familial and nonfamilial.[2] Diagnosis is established using computed tomography or magnetic resonance imaging of the brain; however, computed tomography has been found to be more sensitive for identifying calcium deposits.[21] Treatment aimed at minimizing calcium deposits has been unsuccessful.[22] Individuals with this condition may be responsive to levodopa for treatment of their parkinsonian features.[2]

■ Gaucher's Disease

Chief Clinical Characteristics

This presentation commonly includes slowly progressive mental decline, seizures, ataxia, and, upon later development, weakness with spasticity and splenomegaly and deficits in lateral gaze.[2]

Background Information

This condition is a rare disorder, although it is prevalent among the Ashkenazi Jewish population.[23] The disease is an autosomal genetic disorder in which glucocerebroside accumulates in the spleen, liver, lungs, bone marrow, and brain due to a deficiency in an enzyme.[2] There are three types of Gaucher's disease. The most common, type 1, is characterized by no central nervous system involvement. In type 2, infants have extensive and progressive neurological damage.[23] Type 3 is less common and is associated with less severe neurological symptoms.[23] Diagnosis is established by clinical presentation, laboratory tests that show increase in total acid phosphatase and biopsy of bone marrow that is positive for Gaucher cells. Enzyme replacement therapy is standard for most patients with types 1 and 3. However, there is no effective treatment for the severe brain damage that may occur in patients with types 2 and 3. Prognosis for patients with type 2 disease is poor with death within the first 2 years of life. For type 3 disease, symptoms typically present in childhood and death occurs by age 10 to 15 years.[2]

■ Hallervorden-Spatz Syndrome (Neurodegeneration with Brain Iron Accumulation, Pantothenate Kinase-Associated Neurodegeneration)

Chief Clinical Characteristics
This presentation includes dystonia, parkinsonism, choreoathetosis, spasticity, cognitive impairment, corticospinal tract involvement, optic atrophy, and pigmentary retinopathy.[24]

Background Information
This rare, inherited disorder results from a genetic mutation in the iron regulatory pathways, resulting in excessive iron accumulation in the basal ganglia.[24,25] Diagnosis is made by magnetic resonance imaging, which shows characteristic abnormalities in the basal ganglia, known as the "eye of the tiger" sign. Pathological studies may also show brown discoloration, iron pigmentation, and gliosis in the globus pallidus and substantia nigra.[24] There is no cure or effective treatment for the condition, but patients may benefit from rehabilitation therapies to decrease disability as the disease follows its progressive course of degeneration.[25]

■ Hereditary Spastic Paraplegia (Familial Spastic Paralysis)

Chief Clinical Characteristics
This presentation includes insidious, progressive difficulty with walking due to bilateral, symmetric lower extremity spastic weakness. Patients may report tripping, stumbling, and falling, as well as urinary urgency.[26]

Background Information
This condition can be divided into two types. The complicated form of this condition is indicated by the presence of neurological abnormalities such as dementia, mental retardation, epilepsy, extrapyramidal disturbance, ataxia, deafness, retinopathy, optic neuropathy, peripheral neuropathy, and skin lesions. The uncomplicated form is indicated by the absence of these features.[27] This condition is a group of inherited disorders with a primary pathological feature of axonal degeneration of the distal ends of the longest ascending and descending tracts, resulting in the characteristic spasticity.[26,27] Diagnosis is made by the presence of symptoms of gait disturbance, neurological findings of corticospinal tract deficits in the lower extremities, family history or genetic testing, and exclusion of any other disorders that could account for the symptoms.[26] Current treatment is limited to decreasing muscle spasticity through exercise and medication. Physical therapy is beneficial for the maintenance and improvement of muscle flexibility, muscle strength, gait, and cardiovascular fitness.[26] Prognosis varies, and those with an onset after adolescence are more likely to have insidious worsening.[26]

■ Huntington's Disease

Chief Clinical Characteristics
This presentation involves progressive chorea of the entire body, emotional disturbances such as behavior and personality changes, and dementia.[28–30]

Background Information
This autosomal dominant genetic disorder causes selective neurodegeneration, most commonly in the neostriatum. Diagnosis is made by genetic testing.[30] There is currently no treatment to slow or stop the progression of this condition; care is focused on symptom management and optimization of functioning.[30] The prognosis for Huntington's disease is poor, and individuals usually experience very rapid decline. On average, patients survive for 15 to 20 years after initial diagnosis, but require high levels of care and supervision during those years.[30]

■ Hydromyelia (Syringomyelia)

Chief Clinical Characteristics
This presentation involves insidious onset of symptoms including upper and lower extremity weakness and numbness, lower extremity

stiffness, and less commonly, pain. Trauma usually precedes the onset of symptoms, but the time frame for subsequent development of these symptoms is variable.

Background Information
This condition is caused by an abnormal widening of the central canal of the spinal cord, leading to the accumulation of cerebrospinal fluid and hydrocephalus. Differential diagnosis must be made between hydromyelia and other disorders such as syringomyelia, spinal cord tumor, and spinal arteriovenous malformation. Magnetic resonance imaging and electromyography are used to confirm the diagnosis of this condition. Surgery may be indicated to decrease or eliminate the symptoms. Prognosis is variable.

■ Lyme Disease (Tick Paralysis)

Chief Clinical Characteristics
This presentation can include fluctuating signs or symptoms such as headache, neck stiffness, nausea, vomiting, malaise, fever, pain, fatigue, and presence of a "bull's-eye" rash.[2] Over time, additional symptoms may include sensory changes, irritability, cognitive changes, depression, behavioral changes, seizures, ataxia, chorea movements, pain, weakness, balance deficits, arthritis, and cranial nerve involvement.[2,31]

Background Information
Borrelia burgdorferi, an organism that infects ticks, is responsible for the transmission of this condition to a human host.[2] The diagnosis is confirmed with a thorough history, clinical assessment, enzyme-linked immunosorbent assay, and Western blot or immunoblot analysis. In addition, magnetic resonance imaging or computed tomography may reveal multifocal or periventricular cerebral lesions.[2] Medical management includes treatment with oral tetracycline, penicillin, or intravenous ceftriaxone.[2] Many individuals experience full recovery with treatment; however, residual deficits may persist for individuals with chronic Lyme disease.[2]

■ Machado-Joseph Disease

Chief Clinical Characteristics
This presentation may involve visual impairments such as nystagmus in combination with slowly progressive ataxia, rigidity, dystonia, weakness in the hands and feet, and difficulty with respiration and swallowing.

Background Information
This condition is genetic, with an autosomal dominant pattern of inheritance and onset of symptoms in adolescence or young adulthood. Differential diagnosis includes Parkinson's disease and multiple system atrophy. The presence of ataxia decreases the likelihood of Parkinson's, and the early age of onset and visual symptoms decrease the likelihood of multiple system atrophy. Diagnosis is established by clinical symptoms and magnetic resonance imaging findings of reduced width of superior and middle cerebellar peduncles, atrophy of the frontal and temporal lobes, and decreased size of the pons and globus pallidus. There is no treatment for this condition, and prognosis is poor.[2]

MENINGITIS

■ Bacterial Meningitis

Chief Clinical Characteristics
This presentation includes acute symptoms such as fever, severe headache, neck stiffness, seizures, changes in consciousness, facial and ocular palsies, positive Kernig and Brudzinski signs, and possible hemiparesis, which may lead to falls. Chronic symptoms include hydrocephalus, vomiting, immobility, impaired alertness, hemiplegia, decorticate or decerebrate posturing, cortical blindness, stupor, or coma.[29]

Background Information
Bacterial meningitis results from an infection and inflammation of the meninges surrounding the brain and spinal cord. Lumbar puncture for spinal fluid pressure and cerebrospinal fluid culture, blood cultures, and radiologic studies confirm the diagnosis.[29] This condition is considered a medical emergency. Medical management includes maintenance of blood pressure, treatment for septic shock, and administration of intravenous antibiotics for 10 to 14 days [29] Prognosis depends on the strain of bacteria; approximately 5% to 15% of patients with bacterial meningitis do not survive.[29] Residual effects after the infection resolves are variable and patients with pneumococcal and *H. influenzae* bacterial meningitis are more likely to have lasting neurological deficits.[29]

■ Viral Meningitis

Chief Clinical Characteristics

This presentation can be characterized by an acute onset of fever, headache, and neck stiffness. Drowsiness, lethargy, and irritability may occur, but overall symptoms tend to be relatively mild.[29] Although not a common presenting sign, falls or imbalance may occur due to drowsiness and lethargy.

Background Information

This condition is an infection and inflammation of the meninges surrounding the brain and spinal cord. Also known as aseptic meningitis, this condition is most commonly caused by the echovirus or coxsackie virus.[29] Cerebrospinal fluid analysis and blood work are used to determine the diagnosis.[32] There is no specific treatment, although supportive care may include administration of analgesics. This condition is rarely fatal and most patients demonstrate a full recovery.[29]

■ Multiple System Atrophy (Striatonigral Degeneration, Olivopontocerebellar Atrophy, Shy-Drager Syndrome)

Chief Clinical Characteristics

This presentation involves tremor, rigidity, akinesia, and/or postural imbalance along with signs of cerebellar, pyramidal, and autonomic dysfunction. Autonomic symptoms such as orthostatic hypotension, dry mouth, loss of sweating, impotence, and urinary incontinence or retention are the initial feature in 41% of individuals, with 74% to 97% of individuals developing some degree of autonomic dysfunction during the course of the disease.[33] This condition is a combination of parkinsonian and non-parkinsonian symptoms and signs.

Background Information

Diagnostic criteria are based on the clinical presentation, which includes poor response to levodopa, presence of autonomic features, presence of speech or bulbar problems, absence of dementia, absence of toxic confusion, and presence of falls.[34] The disease course ranges between 0.5 and 24 years after diagnosis with a mean survival time of 6.2 years.[35] This condition is a progressive condition of the central and autonomic nervous systems that rarely occurs without orthostatic hypotension. There are three types of this condition. The parkinsonian-type includes symptoms of Parkinson's disease such as slow movement, stiff muscles, and tremor. The cerebellar type causes problems with coordination and speech. The combined type includes symptoms of both parkinsonism and cerebellar failure. Older age at onset is associated with a shorter survival time.[35] Average age of onset is 54 years, with mean age at death being 60.3 years.[33] Most individuals with this condition receive a trial of levodopa although only a minority respond.[33] Additional treatment addresses symptoms and involves physical and occupational therapy to maintain mobility and address safety issues related to the progression of imbalance.

■ Myotonia Congenital

Chief Clinical Characteristics

This presentation includes impaired relaxation of a muscle after forceful voluntary contraction. Individuals with this condition may also experience some degree of hypertrophy of involved muscle groups.[29]

Background Information

There are many different variants of this condition, all of which are thought to be the result of mutations in the genes coding for skeletal muscle sodium channels and chloride channels.[36] Of the different types, the two most common are Thomsen's disease and Becker's disease. Thomsen's disease begins early in life and is characterized by myotonia, muscular hypertrophy, a nonprogressive course, and dominant inheritance. Becker's disease is recessive, with a later onset in life, and patients present with more severe myotonia and hypertrophy, and often with weakness and atrophy of the forearm and neck muscles.[29] Becker's disease typically has a progressive course until about 30 years of age. Medical management may include quinidine sulfate, procainamide, or mexiletine to relieve myotonia. Patients may also benefit from what is known as the "warm-up effect," which refers to repeated contractions of a muscle that can reduce or abolish myotonia. This effect is short lived and wears off after approximately 5 minutes of rest.[29]

■ Neuroleptic Malignant Syndrome

Chief Clinical Characteristics
This presentation can be characterized by severe muscle rigidity, changes in mental status such as confusion and delirium, high fever, diaphoresis, dysphagia, incontinence, and autonomic dysfunction.

Background Information
This condition is a rare, but potentially fatal disorder that is caused by a complication of treatment with neuroleptic medication.[37] The pathophysiology of this condition is unknown, but is thought to be related to a dopaminergic transmission block in the basal ganglia and hypothalamus.[37] Diagnosis is made by a temperature of 38°C or higher, rigidity, mental status and autonomic changes, and laboratory findings, as well as a recent history of exposure to antipsychotic medication. The best treatment for this condition is prevention, including early recognition of symptoms and prompt discontinuation of the causal agent. Medical management of this condition in its acute form includes fluid replacement, reduction of temperature, and monitoring of cardiac, pulmonary, and renal functions. Patients may also benefit from electroconvulsive therapy and the introduction of dopamine agonists and/or dantrolene. The clinical course varies, and most patients eventually experience a total resolution of symptoms.

■ Neuromyotonia (Isaac Syndrome, Isaac-Merten Syndrome, Continuous Muscle Fiber Activity Syndrome, Quantal Squander Syndrome)

Chief Clinical Characteristics
This presentation commonly involves intermittent or continuous muscle contraction, slow relaxation following muscle contraction, cramps, stiffness, and hyperhidrosis. These symptoms are commonly seen in conjunction with peripheral neuropathy.[38,39]

Background Information
This condition is an antibody-mediated potassium channel disorder, in which the suppression of these voltage-gated channels results in hyperexcitability of the peripheral nerve.[38] It is a rare, usually acquired disease that is often seen with myasthenia gravis and is most likely due to an autoimmune or paraneoplastic origin.[39] Electrophysiological study is used in diagnosis and will show myokymic and neuromyotonic discharges.[38] Muscle activity persists throughout sleep and anesthesia, but can be blocked by curare.[29] Symptomatic relief has been demonstrated with anticonvulsant drugs such as phenytoin and carbamazepine, and research has also shown successful outcomes with plasmapharesis.[40]

■ Opsoclonus Myoclonus (Kinsbourne Syndrome, Myoclonic Encephalopathy of Infants, Dancing Eyes–Dancing Feet Syndrome, Opsoclonus-Myoclonus-Ataxia Syndrome)

Chief Clinical Characteristics
This presentation includes irregular, rapid eye movements (opsoclonus) and brief, shock-like muscle spasms (myoclonus), as well as staggering, falling, ataxia, drooling, decreased muscle tone, and an inability to sleep.[41]

Background Information
This autoimmune disorder is commonly found in association with the presence of neoplasm, the most common types being neuroblastoma in children, and breast and small-cell lung cancer in adults.[29] Diagnosis is made by a combination of clinical presentation, the possible presence of neoplasm, the presence of anti-Hu antibodies, mild pleocytosis on cerebrospinal fluid, and positive serologic tests in children without tumors.[29] Treatment includes adrenocorticotropic hormone, corticosteroid, and intravenous immunoglobulin therapy, and, when present, tumor resection and adjuvant treatment such as chemotherapy and radiation.[29,41] There is good response to drug and surgical treatment, but relapse is common and many patients report residual neurological symptoms.[29,41]

■ Overuse Syndromes (Repetitive Motion Disorders, Cumulative Trauma Disorders, Repetitive Stress Injuries)

Chief Clinical Characteristics
This presentation includes pain, tingling, numbness, swelling, erythema, loss of flexibility, and/or weakness in the affected body area.[42]

Background Information

Overuse syndromes are a group of disorders that result from the performance of repetitive motions. Common pathologies that are associated with this condition include carpal tunnel syndrome, trigger finger, and epicondylitis.[42] In addition, bursitis, tendonitis, and tenosynovitis may occur at numerous different locations throughout the body, depending on the type of activity performed. Treatment varies, but usually begins with stopping the motions or activities that cause the symptoms. Physical therapy is often indicated for stretching, strengthening, splinting, and therapeutic modalities such as ice and ultrasound. Further medical management may include analgesics, corticosteroids, and even surgery.[42] If this condition is suspected, the reader is encouraged to review the appropriate chapter discussing diagnosis of pain within the affected body region.

■ Parkinson's Disease

Chief Clinical Characteristics

This presentation commonly involves resting tremor, bradykinesia, rigidity, and postural instability. Falls are a common problem in individuals with this condition, with up to 68% falling within a 1-year period and approximately 50% of these individuals falling multiple times within that same year.[43] Other common signs and symptoms include festination, freezing, micrographia, hypophonia (hypokinetic dysarthria), akinesia, masked facies, drooling, difficulty turning over in bed, dystonia, dyskinesia, dementia, and depression.[2]

Background Information

This condition occurs due to the depletion or injury of dopamine-producing cells in substantia nigra pars compacta. Clinical signs and symptoms are not typically present until after approximately 80% of dopamine-producing cells are lost. The definitive diagnosis is made post-mortem. However, a clinically definitive diagnosis may be made with the presence of at least two of the three criteria—asymmetric resting tremor, bradykinesia, or rigidity—and a positive response to anti-Parkinson medications.[2,44] Imaging may be useful to exclude vascular involvement. Medical management may include use of dopamine agonists, levodopa, and other medications to address nonmotor symptoms, such as depression, constipation,

autonomic symptoms, and sexual dysfunction. Surgical management also may be considered, including deep brain stimulation or pallidotomy.[44] Forced use or higher intensity, challenging activities may provide a neuroprotective benefit for individuals with early forms of this condition.[45] With the high incidence of depression, consultation with a psychologist or psychiatrist may be warranted. Individuals with a late onset tend to progress more rapidly.[46,47] Poor prognostic indicators for disability include initial presentation without tremor, early dependence, dementia, balance impairments, older age, and the postural instability/gait difficulty dominant type.[46,47]

■ Paroxysmal Choreoathetosis

Chief Clinical Characteristics

This presentation includes discrete episodes of abnormal involuntary movements of the limbs, trunk, and facial muscles. Some patients report lingering muscle stiffness following the attacks.[48] The episodes of choreoathetosis may be provoked by startle, sudden movement, hyperventilation, alcohol, coffee, fatigue, or prolonged exercise. They vary in duration from 10 seconds to up to 4 hours at a time, and may occur dozens of times per day or only occasionally.[29]

Background Information

The exact pathological mechanism of this condition is unknown, but it is thought that the disorder may be genetically linked, or due to a secondary cause such as neurological or metabolic disease.[29,48] Individuals with this condition tend to respond well to antiepileptic drugs and, overall, this condition has been shown to spontaneously improve as patients move into adulthood.[48]

■ Primary Lateral Sclerosis

Chief Clinical Characteristics

This presentation includes spastic paraparesis of voluntary muscles with associated upper motor neuron signs in the absence of lower motor neuron signs. Onset of difficulty with gait, balance, and leg weakness appears in the fifth to sixth decade of life and may progress to affect upper extremity and facial musculature.

Background Information

Imaging, cerebrospinal fluid analysis, and electromyographic studies confirm the diagnosis. In particular, this condition is differentiated from the more severe amyotrophic lateral sclerosis only after a period of 3 years from onset to ensure the absence of lower motor neuron signs.[2] Treatment for this condition addresses symptom management. Physical therapy is indicated to prevent immobility. This condition is not fatal and progression of symptoms varies; some individuals maintain ambulatory status throughout life while others become wheelchair-bound.

■ Spinal Cord Infarction (Vascular Myelopathy)

Chief Clinical Characteristics
This presentation depends on the location of the infarction. The most common anterior spinal artery syndrome presents with bilateral, incomplete motor paralysis and loss of pinprick and temperature sensation below the level of the lesion, loss of deep tendon reflexes, sphincter paralysis, acute complaint of back pain, and spared proprioception. Onset of symptoms occurs over the course of minutes to hours.

Background Information
Most forms of this condition are insidious, or secondary to aortic surgery or rupture, atherosclerosis, aneurysm, or an acute deficit of perfusion. Diagnosis is often difficult at initial presentation, because magnetic resonance imaging may be negative. Repeat magnetic resonance imaging may show T_2 hyperintensity secondary to edema.[49] This condition has a severe prognosis with often permanent disability. Prognosis for recovery of ambulation is inversely correlated with the severity of motor deficit at onset.[50] Physical therapy interventions address weakness, spasticity, and mobility and ambulation deficits.

■ Stiff-Person Syndrome

Chief Clinical Characteristics
This presentation typically involves progressive, painful muscle stiffness and rigidity along with spontaneous and reflex muscle spasms. These symptoms are seen primarily in the axial and proximal limb muscles and can cause walking to become very slow and awkward. Individuals with this condition also commonly present with exaggerated lumbar lordosis secondary to involvement of the lumbar paraspinal muscles.[51]

Background Information
This rare, chronic condition is thought to be the result of an autoimmune process that results in continuous motor unit activity.[2] Stiff-person syndrome is characterized by an insidious onset and follows a progressive course for months to years before it stabilizes. Diagnosis of this condition is made by clinical picture, the demonstration of continuous muscle activity in affected muscles despite an effort to relax, and enhanced exteroceptive reflexes. Many patients also present with antibodies to glutamic acid decarboxylase, but the role of these antibodies is not yet fully understood. Treatment options include diazepam or baclofen, as well as immune-directed therapy such as plasma exchange, corticosteroids, or intravenous immunoglobulin.[29,51]

■ Stroke (Cerebrovascular Accident)

Chief Clinical Characteristics
This presentation may include a wide range of symptoms that correspond to specific areas of the brain that are affected, potentially including visual disturbances. The initial symptoms can include numbness or weakness, especially on one side of the body or face; confusion or aphasia; balance deficits or falls; or sudden severe headache with no known cause.

Background Information
This condition occurs when blood flow to the brain is interrupted either by blockage (ischemia or infarction) or from hemorrhagic disruption. A thrombosis or embolic occlusion of an artery causes an ischemic type of this condition. A hemorrhagic type of this condition can be caused by arteriovenous malformation, hypertension, aneurysm, neoplasm, drug abuse and trauma. This condition is the most common and disabling neurological disorder in adults and occurs in 114 of every 100,000 people.[52] This condition is diagnosed using clinical presentation and positive findings on computed tomography and magnetic resonance imaging. Medication, surgery and interdisciplinary therapy are the most common treatments for this condition. The prognosis for recovery is predicted by the magnitude of initial deficit. Factors that are associated with poor outcomes include coma, poor cognition, severe aphasia, severe hemiparesis with little return within 1 month, visual perceptual disorders, depression, and incontinence after 2 weeks.[53,54]

■ Traumatic Brain Injury

Chief Clinical Characteristics

This presentation typically includes disequilibrium in the presence of cognitive changes, altered level of consciousness, seizures, nausea, vomiting, coma, dizziness, headache, pupillary changes, tinnitus, weakness, incoordination, behavioral changes, spasticity, hypertonicity, cranial nerve lesions, and sensory and motor deficits.[2,55]

Background Information

This condition can be classified as mild, moderate, or severe based on Glasgow Coma Scale, length of coma, and duration of post-traumatic amnesia.[55] Magnetic resonance imaging may be used to confirm the diagnosis.[31] Treatment initiated at the scene of the accident and during the acute phase is focused on medical stabilization. It should be initiated during the acute phase in order to minimize complications.[56] Low Glasgow Coma Scale, longer length of coma, longer duration of post-traumatic amnesia, and older age tend to be associated with poor outcomes.[57] Optimal rehabilitation is interdisciplinary and customized to address the specific individuals' needs.

■ Traumatic Spinal Cord Injury

Chief Clinical Characteristics

This presentation is characterized by loss of sensation in a dermatomal pattern, hypertonicity, spasticity, hyperreflexia, and sphincter dysfunction in combination with muscle weakness. Specific syndromes (discussed below) have characteristic presentations secondary to the location of the lesion.

Background Information

Insult to the spinal cord results from fractured bone, displaced disk material, or a foreign object transecting or injuring the cord. Imaging is used to identify the cause of injury and direct surgical stabilization or intervention. Motor vehicle accidents and falls are the most common etiology of this condition.[58] Physical examination of strength and sensation is used to assign a score from the American Spinal Injury Association.[59] Injuries are classified in terms of neurological level (ie, most rostral segment where myotomal and dermatomal function is spared) and extent as either complete

(total lack of sensory or motor function below level of injury) or incomplete (some motor or sensory function spared below the level of injury). Cervical locations of injury result in tetraplegia and may cause paralysis or weakness of the respiratory musculature, requiring mechanical ventilation and/or respiratory strengthening.[60] Thoracic or lumbar locations of injury result in paraplegia. Treatment consists of medical management, multidisciplinary rehabilitation, equipment prescription, and prevention of pressure ulcers, contractures, and further complications. Individuals with incomplete forms of this condition may continue to recover strength and function, while individuals with complete forms of this condition have a poor prognosis for recovery and instead use compensatory techniques and equipment. Individuals with this condition require adequate follow-up medical care to prevent secondary impairments.[61] Acute forms of this condition constitute a medical emergency.

TUMORS

■ Brain Metastases

Chief Clinical Characteristics

This presentation may include headaches, seizures, dysphagia, weakness, cognitive changes, behavioral changes, dizziness, vomiting, alterations in the level of consciousness, ataxia, aphasia, nystagmus, visual disturbances, dysarthria, balance deficits, falls, lethargy, and incoordination.[2,62]

Background Information

The majority of individuals with brain metastases have been previously diagnosed with a primary tumor; however, a small percentage of individuals are diagnosed concomitantly with brain metastases and the primary tumor. The most common cancers resulting in subsequent brain metastases include lung, breast, melanoma, colorectal, and genitourinary tract. The new onset of neurological symptoms after a primary tumor warrants the use of imaging such as magnetic resonance imaging or computed tomography to confirm the diagnosis. Treatment may include corticosteroids, brain irradiation, surgery, chemotherapy, radiotherapy, and rehabilitative therapies. The prognosis is poor with death typically occurring within 6 months.

STIFFNESS

◼ Brain Primary Tumors

Chief Clinical Characteristics

This presentation may include headaches, seizures, dysphagia, weakness, cognitive changes, behavioral changes, dizziness, vomiting, alterations in the level of consciousness, ataxia, aphasia, nystagmus, visual disturbances, dysarthria, balance deficits, falls, lethargy, and incoordination.[2,31]

Background Information

Glioblastoma multiforme, astrocytoma, oligodendroglioma, metastatic tumors, primary central nervous system lymphomas, ganglioglioma, neuroblastoma, meningioma, arachnoid cysts, hemangioblastoma, medulloblastoma, and acoustic neuroma/schwannoma are some of the more common brain tumors. Specific diagnoses for brain tumors may be confirmed with imaging and biopsy. Treatment is variable depending on the type, size, and location of the tumor and may include surgical resection, chemotherapy, radiation, corticosteroids, and rehabilitative therapies. Prognosis is also variable and depends on the type and grade of tumor, severity of compression, and duration of compression.

◼ Spinal Metastases

Chief Clinical Characteristics

This presentation can involve spasticity, weakness, sensory alterations, bowel and bladder incontinence, neck pain, back pain, radicular pain, atrophy, cerebellar signs, balance deficits, falls, and cranial nerve involvement.[2,31,63]

Background Information

This condition is the most frequent neoplasm involving the spine.[63] The most common types and locations of primary tumors that result in spinal metastases include breast, lung, lymphoma, prostate, kidney, gastrointestinal tract, and thyroid.[2,64] The diagnosis is confirmed with gadolinium enhanced magnetic resonance imaging and computed tomography.[2,63] Treatment is variable depending on the tumor and may include surgical resection, chemotherapy, radiation, corticosteroids, and rehabilitative therapies.[2] Although the long-term prognosis is poor, individuals without paresis and pain and who are still ambulatory have longer survival rates.[64]

◼ Spinal Primary Tumors

Chief Clinical Characteristics

This presentation may include spasticity, weakness, sensory alterations, bowel/bladder incontinence, back pain, radicular pain, atrophy, cerebellar signs, balance deficits, falls, and cranial nerve involvement.[56]

Background Information

Types of this condition include ependymoma, hemangioblastoma, myeloma, neurofibroma, lymphoma, metastasis, meningioma, schwannoma, and astrocytoma. Extradural tumors, such as meningiomas, produce a rapid onset of symptoms, with weakness being predominant. Intramedullary tumors, or ependymomas, astrocytomas and hemangioblastomas, present with slowly progressive symptoms, of which loss of pain and temperature sensation is usually the first. The first test to diagnose brain and spinal column tumors is a neurological examination. Special imaging techniques (computed tomography, magnetic resonance imaging, and positron emission tomography) are also employed. Specific diagnoses may be confirmed with imaging and biopsy. Treatment is variable depending on the type, size, and location of the tumor and may include surgical resection, chemotherapy, radiation, corticosteroids, and rehabilitative therapies. Prognosis is variable and depends on the type and grade of tumor, severity of compression, and duration of compression.

◼ Vasculitis (Giant Cell Arteritis, Temporal Arteritis, Cranial Arteritis)

Chief Clinical Characteristics

This presentation can be characterized by headaches, psychiatric syndromes, dementia, peripheral or cranial nerve involvement, pain, seizures, hypertension, hemiparesis, balance deficits, neuropathies, myopathies, organ involvement, fever, and weight loss.[2,31,65]

Background Information

This condition is the result of an immune-mediated response resulting in the inflammation of vascular structures.[2,65] It includes a variety of disorders such as giant cell/temporal arteritis (which is the most common form),

STIFFNESS

primary angiitis of the central nervous system, Takayasu's disease, periarteritis nodosa, Kawasaki disease, Churg-Strauss syndrome, Wegener's granulomatosis, and secondary vasculitis associated with systemic lupus erythematous, rheumatoid arthritis, and scleroderma.[65] The diagnosis is confirmed through history, physical examination, laboratory testing, angiography, biopsy, and imaging.[2,31,65] Corticosteroids, cytotoxic agents, intravenous immunoglobulin, and plasmapheresis may be used in the treatment of vasculitis.[31,65] Prognosis is variable and depends on the specific underlying disorder. For example, giant cell arteritis is typically self-limiting within 1 to 2 years; however, death usually occurs within 1 year for individuals with primary angiitis of the central nervous system.[65]

■ Whiplash Injury (Whiplash-Associated Disorder)

Chief Clinical Characteristics

This presentation commonly involves dizziness in combination with neck pain, stiffness, headache, abnormal sensations such as burning or prickling, or shoulder or back pain.[66] *Whiplash is characterized by a collection of symptoms that occur following damage to the neck, usually because of sudden extension and flexion such as might happen in an automobile accident.*

Background Information

Cervicocephalic kinesthesia is adversely affected and may be responsible for this condition.[67–69] In addition, some people experience cognitive, somatic, or psychological conditions such as memory loss, concentration impairment, nervousness/irritability, sleep disturbances, fatigue, or depression. Symptoms such as neck pain may be present directly after the injury or may be delayed for several days. The condition may include injury to intervertebral joints, disks, and ligaments, cervical muscles, and nerve roots. The trauma may dislodge otoconia in the inner ear, leading to benign paroxysmal positional vertigo, and concerns of dizziness upon change of position.[70] The need for radiographs can be determined through a careful history; they are not always necessary.[71] Otolaryngologic evaluation may reveal abnormal findings suggestive of central and/or

peripheral vestibular involvement.[72,73] Treatment for individuals with an acute whiplash may include pain medications, physical therapy modalities, nonsteroidal anti-inflammatory drugs, antidepressants, muscle relaxants, and use of a cervical collar. Range of motion and strengthening exercises are key aspects of long-term management. Treatment for decreased kinesthetic awareness involves eye–head–neck–trunk coordination exercises.[74]

■ Wilson's Disease

Chief Clinical Characteristics

This presentation commonly involves liver dysfunction followed by neurological symptoms such as tremor, rigidity, drooling, difficulty with speech and abrupt personality change.

Background Information

Symptoms of Wilson's disease usually appear in childhood or young adult life[75] with a frequency of 1 in 30,000.[76] This condition is an autosomal recessive disorder in which excessive amounts of copper accumulate in the body especially in eye membranes (causing a golden brown Kayser-Fleischer ring), nailbeds, and kidney.[31] The gene abnormality has been located on chromosome 13, which causes a deficiency in ceruloplasmin. In the central nervous system, cavitation and neuronal loss occur within the putamen and globus pallidus. This condition is diagnosed based on clinical findings supported by biochemical evidence of low ceruloplasmin, elevated unbound serum copper, high urinary copper excretion, positive liver biopsy and copper metabolism tests, and T_2-weighted magnetic resonance imaging that shows thalamus and putamen hyperintensity.[31] Treatment consists of low-copper diet and a chelating agent (usually penicillamine).[31] With adequate treatment, the life span is normal. If left untreated in children, death is predicted in 2 years from hepatic and renal failure. In untreated adults, death is predicted in 10 years.[31]

References

1. Lance R, Link ME, Padua M, Clavell LE, Johnson G, Knebel A. Comparison of different methods of obtaining orthostatic vital signs. *Clin Nurs Res.* Nov 2000;9(4):479–491.
2. Victor M, Ropper AH. *Adams and Victor's Principles of Neurology.* 7th ed. New York, NY: McGraw-Hill; 2001.

3. Thilmann AF, Fellows SJ, Garms E. The mechanism of spastic muscle hypertonus. Variation in reflex gain over the time course of spasticity. *Brain.* Feb 1991;114 (pt 1A):233–244.

4. Garg RK. Acute disseminated encephalomyelitis. *Postgrad Med J.* Jan 2003;79(927):11–17.

5. Foreman PJ. Summary and discussion—patient #32. October 16, 2008. http://www.bcm.edu/neurology/challeng/pat32/summary.html. Accessed August 28, 2005.

6. Al-Otaibi LM, Porter SR, Poate TW. Behcet's disease: a review. *J Dent Res.* Mar 2005;84(3):209–222.

7. Schievink WI. Intracranial aneurysms. *N Engl J Med.* Jan 2, 1997;336(1):28–40.

8. Vogel T, Verreault R, Turcotte JF, Kiesmann M, Berthel M. Intracerebral aneurysms: a review with special attention to geriatric aspects. *J Gerontol A Biol Sci Med Sci.* Jun 2003;58(6):520–524.

9. Consensus statement on the definition of orthostatic hypotension, pure autonomic failure, and multiple system atrophy. The Consensus Committee of the American Autonomic Society and the American Academy of Neurology. *Neurology.* May 1996;46(5):1470.

10. Unruptured intracranial aneurysms—risk of rupture and risks of surgical intervention. International Study of Unruptured Intracranial Aneurysms Investigators. *N Engl J Med.* Dec 10, 1998;339(24):1725–1733.

11. Aasly J, Skandsen T, Ro M. Neuroacanthocytosis—the variability of presenting symptoms in two siblings. *Acta Neurol Scand.* Nov 1999;100(5):322–325.

12. Bohlega S, Riley W, Powe J, Baynton R, Roberts G. Neuroacanthocytosis and aprebetalipoproteinemia. *Neurology.* Jun 1998;50(6):1912–1914.

13. Rubio JP, Danek A, Stone C, et al. Chorea-acanthocytosis: genetic linkage to chromosome 9q21. *Am J Hum Genet.* Oct 1997;61(4):899–908.

14. Geldmacher DS. Dementia with Lewy bodies: diagnosis and clinical approach. *Cleve Clin J Med.* Oct 2004;71(10):789–790, 792–794, 797–798 passim.

15. Small GW. Neuroimaging as a diagnostic tool in dementia with Lewy bodies. *Dement Geriatr Cogn Disord.* 2004;17(suppl 1):25–31.

16. Walker Z, Allen RL, Shergill S, Mullan E, Katona CL. Three years survival in patients with a clinical diagnosis of dementia with Lewy bodies. *Int J Geriatr Psychiatry.* Mar 2000;15(3):267–273.

17. Fisher RS, van Emde Boas W, Blume W, et al. Epileptic seizures and epilepsy: definitions proposed by the International League Against Epilepsy (ILAE) and the International Bureau for Epilepsy (IBE). *Epilepsia.* Apr 2005; 46(4):470–472.

18. Wiebe S. Randomized controlled trials of epilepsy surgery. *Epilepsia.* 2003;44(suppl 7):38–43.

19. Sander JW. The natural history of epilepsy in the era of new antiepileptic drugs and surgical treatment. *Epilepsia.* 2003;44(suppl 1):17–20.

20. Manyam BV, Walters AS, Narla KR. Bilateral striopallidodentate calcinosis: clinical characteristics of patients seen in a registry. *Mov Disord.* Mar 2001;16(2):258–264.

21. Manyam BV, Bhatt MH, Moore WD, Devleschoward AB, Anderson DR, Calne DB. Bilateral striopallidodentate calcinosis: cerebrospinal fluid, imaging, and electrophysiological studies. *Ann Neurol.* Apr 1992; 31(4):379–384.

22. Manyam BV. What is and what is not "Fahr's disease." *Parkinsonism Relat Disord.* Mar 2005;11(2):73–80.

23. Mankin HJ, Rosenthal DI, Xavier R. Gaucher disease. New approaches to an ancient disease. *J Bone Joint Surg Am.* May 2001;83-A(5):748–762.

24. Thomas M, Hayflick SJ, Jankovic J. Clinical heterogeneity of neurodegeneration with brain iron accumulation (Hallervorden-Spatz syndrome) and pantothenate kinase-associated neurodegeneration. *Mov Disord.* Jan 2004;19(1):36–42.

25. Vasconcelos OM, Harter DH, Duffy C, et al. Adult Hallervorden-Spatz syndrome simulating amyotrophic lateral sclerosis. *Muscle Nerve.* Jul 2003; 28(1):118–122.

26. Fink JK. Advances in the hereditary spastic paraplegias. *Exp Neurol.* Nov 2003;184(suppl 1):S106–110.

27. Park SY, Ki CS, Kim HJ, et al. Mutation analysis of SPG4 and SPG3A genes and its implication in molecular diagnosis of Korean patients with hereditary spastic paraplegia. *Arch Neurol.* Jul 2005;62(7):1118–1121.

28. de Boo GM, Tibben A, Lanser JB, et al. Early cognitive and motor symptoms in identified carriers of the gene for Huntington disease. *Arch Neurol.* Nov 1997; 54(11):1353–1357.

29. Ropper AH, Brown RJ. *Adams and Victor's Principles of Neurology.* 8th ed. New York, NY: McGraw-Hill; 2005.

30. Rosas HD, Feigin AS, Hersch SM. Using advances in neuroimaging to detect, understand, and monitor disease progression in Huntington's disease. *NeuroRx.* Apr 2004;1(2):263–272.

31. Lindsay KW, Bone I, Callander R. *Neurology and Neurosurgery Illustrated.* 3rd ed. New York, NY: Churchill Livingstone; 1997.

32. Peigue-Lafeuille H, Croquez N, Laurichesse H, et al. Enterovirus meningitis in adults in 1999–2000 and evaluation of clinical management. *J Med Virol.* May 2002;67(1):47–53.

33. Wenning GK, Tison F, Ben Shlomo Y, Daniel SE, Quinn NP. Multiple system atrophy: a review of 203 pathologically proven cases. *Mov Disord.* Mar 1997;12(2):133–147.

34. Wenning GK, Ben-Shlomo Y, Hughes A, Daniel SE, Lees A, Quinn NP. What clinical features are most useful to distinguish definite multiple system atrophy from Parkinson's disease? *J Neurol Neurosurg Psychiatry.* Apr 2000;68(4):434–440.

35. Ben-Shlomo Y, Wenning GK, Tison F, Quinn NP. Survival of patients with pathologically proven multiple system atrophy: a meta-analysis. *Neurology.* Feb 1997; 48(2):384–393.

36. Pusch M. Myotonia caused by mutations in the muscle chloride channel gene CLCN1. *Hum Mutat.* Apr 2002; 19(4):423–434.

37. Assion HJ, Heinemann F, Laux G. Neuroleptic malignant syndrome under treatment with antidepressants? A critical review. *Eur Arch Psychiatry Clin Neurosci.* 1998;248(5):231–239.

38. Arimura K, Sonoda Y, Watanabe O, et al. Isaacs' syndrome as a potassium channelopathy of the nerve. *Muscle Nerve.* 2002;(suppl 11):S55–58.

39. Van Parijs V, Van den Bergh PY, Vincent A. Neuromyotonia and myasthenia gravis without thymoma. *J Neurol Neurosurg Psychiatry.* Sep 2002;73(3):344–345.

40. Hayat GR, Kulkantrakorn K, Campbell WW, Giuliani MJ. Neuromyotonia: autoimmune pathogenesis and response to immune modulating therapy. *J Neurol Sci.* Dec 1, 2000;181(1–2):38–43.

41. Tate ED, Allison TJ, Pranzatelli MR, Verhulst SJ. Neuro-epidemiologic trends in 105 US cases of pediatric opsoclonus-myoclonus syndrome. *J Pediatr Oncol Nurs.* Jan–Feb 2005;22(1):8–19.

42. Goodyear-Smith F, Arroll B. What can family physicians offer patients with carpal tunnel syndrome other than surgery? A systematic review of nonsurgical management. *Ann Fam Med.* May–Jun 2004;2(3): 267–273.

43. Wood BH, Bilclough JA, Bowron A, Walker RW. Incidence and prediction of falls in Parkinson's disease: a prospective multidisciplinary study. *J Neurol Neurosurg Psychiatry.* Jun 2002;72(6):721–725.

44. Samii A, Nutt JG, Ransom BR. Parkinson's disease. *Lancet.* May 29, 2004;363(9423):1783–1793.

45. Tillerson JL, Cohen AD, Philhower J, Miller GW, Zigmond MJ, Schallert T. Forced limb-use effects on the behavioral and neurochemical effects of 6-hydroxydopamine. *J Neurosci.* Jun 15 2001;21(12):4427–4435.

46. Jankovic J, Kapadia AS. Functional decline in Parkinson disease. *Arch Neurol.* Oct 2001;58(10):1611–1615.

47. Marras C, Rochon P, Lang AE. Predicting motor decline and disability in Parkinson disease: a systematic review. *Arch Neurol.* Nov 2002;59(11):1724–1728.

48. Huang YG, Chen YC, Du F, et al. Topiramate therapy for paroxysmal kinesigenic choreoathetosis. *Mov Disord.* Jan 2005;20(1):75–77.

49. Masson C, Pruvo JP, Meder JF, et al. Spinal cord infarction: clinical and magnetic resonance imaging findings and short term outcome. *J Neurol Neurosurg Psychiatry.* Oct 2004;75(10):1431–1435.

50. Cheshire WP, Santos CC, Massey EW, Howard JF, Jr. Spinal cord infarction: etiology and outcome. *Neurology.* Aug 1996;47(2):321–330.

51. Gerschlager W, Brown P. Effect of treatment with intravenous immunoglobulin on quality of life in patients with stiff-person syndrome. *Mov Disord.* May 2002;17(3):590–593.

52. Goodman CC, Boissonnault WG. *Pathology: Implications for the Physical Therapist.* Philadelphia, PA: W. B. Saunders; 1998.

53. Granger CV, Clark GS. Functional status and outcomes of stroke rehabilitation. *Topics Geriatrics.* Mar 1994;9(3):72–84.

54. Shelton FD, Volpe BT, Reding M. Motor impairment as a predictor of functional recovery and guide to rehabilitation treatment after stroke. *Neurorehabil Neural Repair.* 2001;15(3):229–237.

55. Bruns J, Hauser WA. The epidemiology of traumatic brain injury: a review. *Epilepsia.* 2003;44(suppl 10):2–10.

56. Das-Gupta R, Turner-Stokes L. Traumatic brain injury. *Disability and Rehabilitation.* 2002;24(13):654–665.

57. Hukkelhoven CWPM, Steyerberg EW, Rampen AJJ, et al. Patient age and outcome following severe traumatic brain injury: an analysis of 5600 patients. *J Neurosurg.* 2003;99:666–673.

58. Jackson AB, Dijkers M, Devivo MJ, Poczatek RB. A demographic profile of new traumatic spinal cord injuries: change and stability over 30 years. *Arch Phys Med Rehabil.* Nov 2004;85(11):1740–1748.

59. McDonald JW, Sadowsky C. Spinal-cord injury. *Lancet.* Feb 2, 2002;359(9304):417–425.

60. Gutierrez CJ, Harrow J, Haines F. Using an evidence-based protocol to guide rehabilitation and weaning of ventilator-dependent cervical spinal cord injury patients. *J Rehabil Res Dev.* Sep–Oct 2003;40(5 suppl 2):99–110.

61. Bloemen-Vrencken JH, de Witte LP, Post MW. Follow-up care for persons with spinal cord injury living in the community: a systematic review of interventions and their evaluation. *Spinal Cord.* Aug 2005;43(8):462–475.

62. Tosoni A, Ermani M, Brandes AA. The pathogenesis and treatment of brain metastases: a comprehensive review. *Crit Rev Oncol Hematol.* 2004;52:199–215.

63. Perrin RG, Laxton AW. Metastatic spine disease: epidemiology, pathophysiology, and evaluation of patients. *Neurosurg Clin N Am.* Oct 2004;15(4):365–373.

64. Hosono N, Ueda T, Tamura D, Aoki Y, Yoshikawa H. Prognostic relevance of clinical symptoms in patients with spinal metastases. *Clin Orthop Relat Res.* Jul 2005(436):196–201.

65. Ferro JM. Vasculitis of the central nervous system. *J Neurol.* Dec 1998;245(12):766–776.

66. Herdman S, ed. *Vestibular Rehabilitation.* 2nd ed. Philadelphia, PA: F. A. Davis; 2000.

67. Revel M, Andre-Deshays C, Minguet M. Cervicocephalic kinesthetic sensibility in patients with cervical pain. *Arch Phys Med Rehabil.* 1991;72(5):288–291.

68. Treleaven J, Jull G, Sterling M. Dizziness and unsteadiness following whiplash injury: characteristic features and relationship with cervical joint position error. *J Rehabil Med.* 2003;35(1):36–43.

69. Wrisley DM, Sparto PJ, Whitney SL, Furman JM. Cervicogenic dizziness: a review of diagnosis and treatment. *J Orthop Sports Phys Ther.* 2000;30(12):755–766.

70. Parnes LS, Agrawal SK, Atlas J. Diagnosis and management of benign paroxysmal positional vertigo (BPPV). *CMAJ.* Sep 30, 2003;169(7):681–693.

71. Stiell IG, Wells GA, Vandemheen KL, et al. The Canadian C-spine rule for radiography in alert and stable trauma patients [comment]. *JAMA.* 2001;286(15):1841–1848.

72. Oosterveld WJ, Kortschot HW, Kingma GG, de Jong HA, Saatci MR. Electronystagmographic findings following cervical whiplash injuries. *Acta Otolaryngol.* 1991;111:201–205.

73. Toglia JU. Acute flexion-extension injury of the neck: electronystagmographic study of 309 patients. *Neurology.* 1976;26:808–814.

74. Revel M, Minguet M, Gregoy P, Vaillant J, Manuel JL. Changes in cervicocephalic kinesthesia after a proprioceptive rehabilitation program in patients with neck pain: a randomized controlled study. *Arch Phys Med Rehabil.* 1994;75(8):895–899.

75. Greenberg DA, Aminoff MJ, Simon RP. *Clinical Neurology.* 5th ed. New York, NY: McGraw-Hill; 2002.

76. Gow PJ, Smallwood RA, Angus PW, Smith AL, Wall AJ, Sewell RB. Diagnosis of Wilson's disease: an experience over three decades. *Gut.* Mar 2000;46(3):415–419.

CHAPTER 33

Weakness

Katherine J. Sullivan, PT, PhD, FAHA ▪ *Katherine M. Weimer, PT, DPT, NCS*

Description of the Symptom

This chapter describes pathology that may lead to weakness. Weakness is the inability of muscles to generate force to generate the age-related functional activities. Strength is the capacity of skeletal muscle to develop the amount of force needed to provide the musculoskeletal mobility and stability required for functional performance.[1] Impairment in strength result in the symptom of weakness.

Special Concerns

■ A sudden onset of rapidly evolving weakness or progressive change in strength in combination with any of the following:
  ■ Abnormal reflexes
  ■ Cranial nerve signs
  ■ Visual disturbances
  ■ Language disturbances
  ■ Changes in level of consciousness
  ■ Confusion or other cognitive changes
■ Weakness accompanied by numbness or tingling
■ Weakness with paresthesias that are progressive and in a radicular pattern
■ Weakness accompanied by changes in bowel and bladder function
■ Weakness accompanied by signs or symptoms of systemic illness such as fever, diaphoresis, and anxiousness
■ Weakness accompanied by lower motor neuron disease signs such as fasciculations and noticeable atrophy
■ Weakness accompanied by severe, localized pain or generalized muscle pain

CHAPTER PREVIEW: Conditions That May Lead to Weakness

T │ Trauma

COMMON

(continued)

Trauma *(continued)*

UNCOMMON

Bell's palsy 689
Brachial plexus injuries:
• Dejerine-Klumpke palsy (Klumpke's palsy) 690
• Erb-Duchenne palsy (Erb's palsy) 690
Hydromyelia (syringomyelia) 693

RARE

Locked-in syndrome 696

I Inflammation

COMMON

Aseptic
Not applicable

Septic
Poliomyelitis (undeveloped countries) 704
Rheumatoid arthritis 705

UNCOMMON

Aseptic
Behçet's disease 689
Multiple sclerosis 698
Neuropathies:
• Chronic inflammatory demyelinating polyneuropathy 700
• Multifocal motor neuropathy 701
Systemic lupus erythematosus 707

Septic
Neurological complications of acquired immunodeficiency syndrome 699
Poliomyelitis (most developed countries) 704

RARE

Aseptic
Acute demyelinating polyneuropathy (Guillain-Barré syndrome) 687
Critical illness polyneuropathy 691
Inflammatory myopathies:
• Dermatomyositis 694
• Inclusion body myositis 694
• Polymyositis 694
Lambert-Eaton myasthenic syndrome 695
Lyme disease (tick paralysis) 696
Miller Fisher syndrome 697
Neurosarcoidosis 702
Transverse myelitis 709

Septic
Botulism 689
Neurosyphilis (tabes dorsalis, syphilitic spinal sclerosis, progressive locomotor ataxia) 703
Tropical spastic paralysis 710

M Metabolic

COMMON

Neuropathies:
• Diabetes mellitus-induced neuropathies 701

UNCOMMON

Mitochondrial myopathies 697
Toxic myopathy 709

RARE

Cushing's syndrome (hypercortisolism) 691
Glycogen storage diseases (glycogenosis, Pompe's disease, McArdle's disease, Cori's disease) 693
Lipid storage diseases of muscle 696
Myasthenia gravis 699
Neuropathies:
• Toxic neuropathy 702
Neurotoxicity 703
Thyrotoxic myopathy (Graves' disease) 708

Va Vascular

COMMON

Stroke (cerebrovascular accident) 707

UNCOMMON

Arteriovenous malformation 688
Spinal cord infarction (vascular myelopathy) 705
Transient ischemic attack 709

RARE

Moyamoya disease 697
Normal pressure hydrocephalus 703
Vasculitis (giant cell arteritis, temporal arteritis, cranial arteritis) 711

De Degenerative

COMMON

Deconditioning 692

UNCOMMON

Not applicable

RARE

Amyotrophic lateral sclerosis (Lou Gehrig disease) 688
Parry-Romberg syndrome 703
Post-polio syndrome 704
Primary lateral sclerosis 705

Tu Tumor

COMMON

Not applicable

(continued)

WEAKNESS

Tumor *(continued)*

UNCOMMON

Malignant Primary, such as:
• Brain primary tumors 710
Malignant Metastatic, such as:
Not applicable
Benign:
Not applicable

RARE

Malignant Primary, such as:
• Spinal primary tumors 711
Malignant Metastatic, such as:
• Brain metastases 710
• Spinal metastases 711
Benign, such as:
• Angiomatosis (Von Hippel-Lindau disease) 688

Co Congenital

COMMON

Not applicable

UNCOMMON

Muscular dystrophy 698
Tethered spinal cord syndrome 707

RARE

Arnold-Chiari malformation (Chiari malformation) 688
Bulbospinal muscular atrophy (Kennedy's disease, X-linked bulbospinal neuronopathy) 691
Familial periodic paralysis 692
Friedreich's ataxia 692
Hereditary spastic paraplegia (familial spastic paralysis) 693
Kearns-Sayre syndrome 695
Machado-Joseph disease 696
Monomelic amyotrophy (benign focal amyotrophy, Hirayama syndrome, O'Sullivan-McLeod syndrome) 697
Neuropathies:
• Hereditary motor and sensory neuropathies 701
Pelizaeus-Merzbacher disease 704
Spinal muscular atrophy (Werdnig-Hoffmann disease, Kugelberg-Welander disease) 707

Ne Neurogenic/Psychogenic

COMMON

Not applicable

UNCOMMON

Hysterical paralysis 694

RARE

Todd's paralysis 708

Note: These are estimates of relative incidence because few data are available for the less common conditions.

Overview of Weakness

Weakness, the inability to generate force, can result from pathological disease conditions that affect the nervous system or motor unit. In addition, factors such as age, disuse, immobilization, and musculoskeletal trauma can have a direct and immediate effect on muscle function that can result in weakness.[1] Weakness must be differentiated from generalized fatigue. Individuals with conditions that cause fatigue may describe themselves as feeling weak or lacking strength. Fatigue may be associated with poor physical health, psychological health, or sleep disorders. In some cases, such as multiple sclerosis, fatigue can be primarily associated with the disease state or may be a secondary complication of functioning daily with a degenerative neurological disease that results in progressive weakness.

Individuals who may have weakness that is directly related to impairments in strength will often report changes in functional ability. Inability to come to a standing position or clear the foot during walking or an increased incidence of falls may be related to changes in lower extremity strength. Inability to manipulate items with the hands, problems reaching overhead, and changes in ability to lift and carry loads may be related to changes in upper extremity strength.

Weakness of pathological origin can result from involvement of the central nervous system, peripheral nervous system, or the muscle itself. Therefore, it is common to determine if the pattern of weakness and the associated neurological signs are consistent with an upper motor neuron or lower motor neuron syndrome, neuromuscular transmission disorder, or myopathic disease.[2] An upper motor neuron syndrome indicates disease or injury of the central nervous system in which weakness is accompanied by hyperreflexia (increased deep tendon reflexes). A lower motor neuron syndrome indicates disease or injury of the peripheral nervous system in which weakness is accompanied by hyporeflexia (decrease in deep tendon reflexes). Neuromuscular transmission disorders are characterized by fluctuating weakness, particularly of muscles with high metabolic demands such as cranial nerve or postural muscles with normal to reduced muscle tone and no sensory loss. Myopathic disorders are diseases that affect muscle fibers; therefore, weakness is most noticeable in proximal muscle groups with no sensory loss and normal tendon reflexes until later in the disease course when tendon reflexes may be depressed.

Description of Conditions That May Lead to Weakness

■ Acute Demyelinating Polyneuropathy (Guillain-Barré Syndrome)

Chief Clinical Characteristics

This presentation typically involves progressive paresthesias described as numbness, tingling, and prickling, and weakness over the course of several days to a few weeks. Lower extremities in a distal to proximal pattern are usually affected first, followed by upper extremities. Muscles of the trunk and face may be affected. If paralysis progresses to respiratory muscles, a ventilator may be required. In the majority of cases, a mild gastrointestinal or respiratory infection precedes symptoms.

Background Information

Symptoms are a result of immunologic reaction causing demyelination of peripheral nerves, and in severe cases, axonal degeneration as well. In addition to clinical presentation, differential diagnosis is established by the presence of increased lymphocytes and an increase in protein in cerebrospinal fluid as well as electromyographic findings of reduction in amplitudes of muscle action potentials, slowed conduction velocity, conduction block in motor nerves, and prolonged distal latencies. Standard treatment includes administration of intravenous immune globulin and plasma exchange. The majority of individuals recover completely or almost completely within a few weeks to a few months; however, the presence of axonal degeneration increases the regeneration time period to 6 to 18 months. Three percent to 5% of individuals with this condition do not survive.[3]

WEAKNESS

■ Amyotrophic Lateral Sclerosis (Lou Gehrig Disease)

Chief Clinical Characteristics

This presentation includes weakness that can begin in the muscles of the lower or upper limbs, trunk, face or throat. People affected will complain of difficulty walking or running, writing, speakiing clearly, or swallowing. The disease advances rapidly with death usually occuring within 5 years due to respiratory failure.

Background Information

A hallmark of this condition is the presence of weakness accompanied by fasciculations (muscle fiber twitching) and hyperreflexia of one or more segmental reflexes. ALS is a degenerative disease that affects the pyramidal cells of the motor cortex and the motor neurons in the brainstem and spinal cord. The presentation of hyperreflexia with weakness, atrophy, and fasciculation is due to the progressive and relentless death of upper and lower motor neurons throughout the nervous system. Sensation, cognitive function, and bowel and bladder control are not affected. While there are some familial variants, the majority of cases are idiopathic, thought to be related to a possible toxic exposure.

■ Angiomatosis (Von Hippel-Lindau Disease)

Chief Clinical Characteristics

This presentation commonly includes headaches, problems with balance and walking, dizziness, weakness of the limbs, vision problems, and high blood pressure.

Background Information

This condition is a rare, genetic multisystem condition characterized by the abnormal growth of tumors in certain parts of the body (angiomatosis). Tumors of the central nervous system are benign, are comprised of a nest of blood vessels, and are called hemangioblastomas (or angiomas in the eye). Hemangioblastomas may develop in the brain, the retina of the eye, and other areas of the nervous system. Other types of tumors develop in the adrenal glands, the kidneys, or the pancreas. Cysts (fluid-filled sacs) and/or tumors (benign or cancerous) may develop around the hemangioblastomas and cause the symptoms

listed above. Specific symptoms vary among individuals and depend on the size and location of the tumors. Individuals with this condition are also at a higher risk than normal for certain types of cancer, especially kidney cancer. Treatment varies according to the location and size of the tumor and its associated cyst. In general, the objective is to treat the tumors when they are causing symptoms but are still small. Treatment of most cases usually involves surgical resection. Certain tumors can be treated with focused high-dose irradiation. Individuals with this condition need careful monitoring by a physician and/or medical team familiar with the condition.

■ Arnold-Chiari Malformation (Chiari Malformation)

Chief Clinical Characteristics

This presentation may include visual or swallowing disturbances in combination with pain in the occipital or posterior cervical areas, downbeating nystagmus, progressive ataxia, progressive spastic quadriparesis, or cervical syringomyelia.[4,5]

Background Information

This condition encompasses a number of congenital abnormalities at the base of the brain, including extension of the cerebellar tissue or displacement of the medulla and fourth ventricle into the cervical canal.[4] This condition has two main types. Individuals with the more common form of this condition, Type I, often remain asymptomatic until adolescence or adult life.[4] Type II is primarily seen in infants and young children. Please see the pediatric section of this textbook for a more complete description of this type. Diagnosis is made by magnetic resonance imaging, computed tomography, myelography, or some combination of these tests.[5] Treatment varies depending on clinical progression, and may include surgical intervention such as an upper cervical laminectomy or enlargement of the foramen magnum. Even with surgery symptoms may persist or progress.[4]

■ Arteriovenous Malformation

Chief Clinical Characteristics

This presentation may be characterized by weakness, seizures and severe headache. Hemorrhage may result in paresis, ataxia, dyspraxia, dizziness, tactile and proprioceptive disturbances, visual disturbances, aphasia, paresthesias, and cognitive deficits.[3]

Background Information

This condition is caused by a tangle of arteries and veins caused by a developmental abnormality that likely arises during embryonic or fetal development. Approximately 12% of the 300,000 individuals in the United States with this condition are symptomatic. Neurological damage occurs due to reduction of oxygen delivery, hemorrhage, or compression of nearby structures of the brain or spinal cord due to the tangle of vessels. Computed tomography, magnetic resonance imaging, and arteriography confirm the diagnosis. Ligation and embolization may be used to reduce the size of the lesion prior to surgical excision, which is the preferred method of treatment. Stereotactic radiation and proton beam therapy are alternative approaches to invasive methods of intervention. Up to 90% of individuals who experience a hemorrhagic arteriovenous malformation survive.[3]

■ Behçet's Disease

Chief Clinical Characteristics

This presentation may include bilateral pyramidal signs (signs related to lesions of upper motor neurons or descending pyramidal tracts, such as a positive Babinski sign or hyperreflexia), headache, memory loss, hemiparesis, cerebellar ataxia, balance deficits, sphincter dysfunction, or cranial nerve palsies. In addition to these neurological signs individuals with this condition also may present with arthritis; renal, gastrointestinal, vascular, and cardiac diseases; and genital, oral, and cutaneous ulcerations.[6]

Background Information

Mean age of onset is in the third decade of life. Diagnostic criteria according to an international study group include presence of recurrent oral ulceration, recurrent genital ulceration, eye lesions, skin lesions, papulopustular lesions, and/or a positive pathergy test.[3,6] Medical treatment typically consists of corticosteroids and immunosuppressants. Neurological symptoms tend to clear within weeks, but can sometimes recur or result in permanent deficits.[3] Onset before the age of 25 and male sex indicate a poorer prognosis.

■ Bell's Palsy

Chief Clinical Characteristics

This presentation typically involves unilateral facial paralysis and is characterized by acute drooping of the eyelid and/or corner of the mouth, drooling, impairment of taste, and dryness of the eye with or without excessive tearing that progresses within 48 hours. Tactile sensation is intact. Facial paralysis is commonly unilateral, though in rare cases may present bilaterally. All three quadrants of the face are affected. Long-term facial paralysis may lead to synkinesis (imbalance of muscular activation), resulting in significant facial distortion.[7]

Background Information

This condition is caused by an idiopathic inflammation of the facial nerve, likely due to a viral infection, commonly herpes simplex. Diagnosis utilizes clinical examination to rule out other causes of facial weakness; for example, facial weakness due to cortical or subcortical lesions is associated with impaired sensation and the frontalis and levator palpebrae muscles are weakened, but not paralyzed. Treatment involves antiviral and anti-inflammatory medications and physical therapy to address paralysis and symmetry of motion and to prevent synkineses.[7-10] Natural recovery of facial motor control occurs within 3 to 6 months in 94% of patients with incomplete paralysis, but residual synkinesis and weakness often remains in those with complete palsies.[8]

■ Botulism

Chief Clinical Characteristics

This presentation involves nausea and vomiting, followed by rapid onset and progression of diplopia, blurred vision, ptosis, dysphagia, flaccid descending paralysis, and possible progression to respiratory failure. There are no central neurological manifestations or sensory impairments.[11,12]

Background Information

Botulism toxin affects the function of cranial nerve musculature, skeletal muscle, and the diaphragm by preventing the release of acetylcholine from synaptic terminals, thus blocking neuromuscular transmission.[12] The foodborne variety of this condition is the most common variant, followed by infant, wound, and intestinal. Differential diagnosis especially includes stroke, Guillain-Barré syndrome, and myasthenia gravis.[13] Rapid diagnosis via clinical examination and administration of botulism antitoxin result in decreased mortality and shorter length of hospital stay.[11] A longer interval between onset and treatment, ventilatory failure, and complete paralysis are poor prognostic indicators.[11,13] The majority of patients who do not receive the antitoxin will die.[13]

BRACHIAL PLEXUS INJURIES

■ Dejerine-Klumpke Palsy (Klumpke's Palsy)

Chief Clinical Characteristics
This presentation commonly includes weakness in the ulnar nerve distribution with associated sensory loss in the C8–T1 dermatome.

Background Information
This condition refers to paralysis of the lower brachial plexus that results from maximal abduction of the shoulder.[14] True forms of this condition are rare.[14] Diagnosis of injury and localization of the lesion require clinical investigation and electrodiagnostic study.[15] There is a poorer prognosis for recovery with Dejerine-Klumpke palsy compared to Erb's palsy or total brachial plexus palsy resulting from the birth process, with most individuals with this condition requiring surgical intervention.[16]

■ Erb-Duchenne Palsy (Erb's Palsy)

Chief Clinical Characteristics
This presentation includes profound weakness of the scapular muscles and deltoid with loss of sensation in the dermatomal distribution of the C5 and C6 dermatomes. The typical resting posture is the arm held in shoulder adduction with fingers pointing backward (waiter's tip position). Distal strength of the upper extremity remains intact.

Background Information
This condition refers to paralysis of the upper brachial plexus in response to an excessive separation or stretch of the neck and shoulder such as from a sliding injury or stretch during the birth process.[14] Diagnosis of injury and localization of the lesion require clinical investigation and electrodiagnostic study.[15] Many infants improve or recover strength by 3 to 4 months of age with a 90% to 100% recovery of function.[14] If spontaneous recovery does not occur, surgical intervention is indicated. Physical therapy is indicated to maintain range of motion and strength.[16]

■ Traumatic Brachial Plexus Injury

Chief Clinical Characteristics
This presentation includes upper extremity weakness and sensory loss related to damage of the brachial plexus, a network of nerves that conducts signals from the spine to the shoulder, arm, and hand. Associated symptoms include hyporeflexia, and hypotonicity.

Background Information
Injuries to the brachial plexus are often due to trauma, the most common of which are stretch injuries occurring during the birth process. Brachial plexus injuries can be classified in terms of mechanism of injury, closed (motor vehicle accident) versus open (intraoperative injury and gunshot wounds); location of injury (spinal nerve root, trunk, cord, peripheral nerve); or type of nerve damage.[15] There are four types of nerve damage: avulsion is the most severe type, in which the nerve is torn from the spinal root; rupture, in which the nerve is torn midsubstance; neuroma, in which the injured nerve has scarred, causing a conduction block; and neurapraxia or stretch, in which the nerve has been damaged but not torn. Diagnosis of injury and localization of the lesion require clinical investigation, electrodiagnostic study, and imaging.[15,17] Management of brachial plexus injuries differs depending on type and severity of injury. Open injuries with vascular damage should be explored operatively immediately. In the absence of clinical or electrophysiological recovery after 2 to 4 months, gunshot wounds without vascular compromise should undergo surgical intervention. Spontaneous recovery occurs in many closed injures; therefore, surgical intervention is delayed 4 to 5 months.[15] Outcomes are favorable in patients who have less severe nerve damage and those who undergo early operation when indicated.[15] Despite

residual weakness and impaired functional use of the extremity, the majority of patients report satisfaction with their quality of life postinjury and/or postsurgical repair.[18]

Bulbospinal Muscular Atrophy (Kennedy's Disease, X-Linked Bulbospinal Neuronopathy)

Chief Clinical Characteristics

This presentation can be characterized by severe, diffuse muscle cramping and fasciculations, muscle weakness in a limb-girdle distribution, and postural hand tremor. Other symptoms include variable bulbar muscle weakness, gynecomastia, premature muscle exhaustion, and hyporeflexia or areflexia.[19,20]

Background Information

This condition is a rare, x-linked, progressive neuromuscular disorder that is usually seen in males between 30 and 50 years old. Diagnosis is made by clinical features, electrophysiological study, and genetic testing.[19] There is currently no proven treatment for this disease, but genetic counseling is recommended upon diagnosis.[21] This condition is usually associated with a normal life span, but individuals may experience significant disability.[19]

Cervical Spondylotic Myelopathy

Chief Clinical Characteristics

This presentation can be characterized by weakness and sensory loss to light touch, vibration, and position sense occurring in a radicular pattern in the upper extremity. Presentation of associated signs of upper and lower extremity paresis, hypertonia, and hyperreflexia indicates involvement of the corticospinal tract.[4]

Background Information

This condition is caused by spondylitic changes in the cervical spine that compress the cord. It occurs in middle to late age and is more common in men than women. Upon clinical examination, patients will have cervical spine abnormalities, crepitus, restricted range of motion, pain, and abnormal reflexes.[3] Diagnosis involves clinical history and examination, use of imaging, electrophysiological testing, and use of additional diagnostic tests to rule out competing diagnosis. Management is controversial. Many individuals with this condition can be

successfully managed with conservative treatment including anti-inflammatory medication and physical therapy.[22] In severe disease, with significantly narrowed canal and severe neurological compromise, surgical decompression is indicated and patients have the potential to recover strength and function and to decrease pain.[22,23]

Critical Illness Polyneuropathy

Chief Clinical Characteristics

This condition is characterized by symmetric limb muscle weakness, often sparing cranial nerve musculature, with hyporeflexia or areflexia, sensory loss, and involvement of the phrenic nerve with resultant diaphragm weakness.[24] Patients are often unable to wean from mechanical ventilation after the acute presenting illness has resolved.[25]

Background Information

This condition is estimated to be present in 25% to 50% of patients in surgical and medical intensive care units. It generally occurs in the presence of sepsis, systemic inflammatory response syndrome, and multiorgan failure within the first 2 to 5 days.[25] Electrodiagnostic investigation confirms the presence of denervation consistent with sensorimotor axonal polyneuropathy.[24] Critical medical care may include intubation, physical therapy, prevention of pressure ulcers and compression neuropathies, and psychological support. There is no proven treatment for this condition.[24] Roughly half of patients with mild forms of this condition who survive the initial causative illness completely return to the previous level of function.[25] However, many continue to have persistent functional disabilities, reduced quality of life, and restrictions in participation 1 year after onset.[26] Therefore, intensive interdisciplinary rehabilitation is crucial to reduce disability and achieve autonomy and social participation.[25,26]

Cushing's Syndrome (Hypercortisolism)

Chief Clinical Characteristics

This presentation includes severe weakness of the proximal limb and girdle muscles often manifested by difficulty climbing stairs or rising from a low chair. Additional signs and symptoms include fatigue, obesity of the upper body (including the hallmark feature of a moon-shaped face), easy bruising and bluish-red stretch marks, high blood pressure, elevated blood glucose, memory loss, and depression.[27,28] Women with this condition may show an increased growth of facial and body hair and irregularity of menstruation.

Background Information

This rare endocrine disorder is caused by chronic exposure of the body's tissues to excess levels of cortisol due to medications or tumors of the pituitary or adrenal gland. Diagnosis is confirmed by laboratory evidence of excessive cortisol in the urine and blood.[27,28] Treatment is achieved through decreasing cortisol levels via medication, surgery, or radiation. Most individuals with this condition show significant improvement in symptom presentation with treatment. However, in some individuals, residual symptoms may persist and some kinds of tumors may recur.

■ Deconditioning

Chief Clinical Characteristics

This presentation commonly involves a gradual onset of muscle weakness and limited endurance following immobilization, bed rest, or a period of reduced physical activity. The etiology may or may not include another condition that caused the initial reduction in physical activity level.

Background Information

Deconditioning involves decreased functioning related to impairments spanning multiple body systems. The physiological maladaptations underlying deconditioning include effects on the cardiovascular, skeletal muscle, bone, immune, endocrine, and peripheral and central nervous systems. This condition typically responds to a gradually progressive exercise program. Specific improvements noted at the body systems level will depend on the mode of training selected. The physical therapist should be sensitive to the potential presence of comorbid conditions that may affect the ability to initiate and progress the exercise program. Additional consultation with other health care providers may be necessary depending on the extent and etiology of deconditioning, in order to optimize the safety of the exercise program.[29]

■ Familial Periodic Paralysis

Chief Clinical Characteristics

This presentation involves a rapid onset of severe weakness and paralysis usually after a period of fasting, carbohydrate load, or rest after a bout of strenuous exercise. Between episodes, the affected muscles usually function normally but myopathy may remain. Familial periodic paralyses are channelopathies causing underexcitability of the sarcolemma and resultant paralysis.[30]

Background Information

Four types of familial periodic paralysis can be clinically delineated: hyperkalemic, hypokalemic, paramyotonia congenita, and Anderson-Tawil syndrome.[31] Clinical differentiation is based on age of onset, duration and severity of attack, precipitating factors, and associated symptoms such as persisting proximal weakness in hypokalemia-induced forms of this condition, paramyotonia of the hands and face in paramyotonia congenita, and ventricular arrhythmia and dysmorphic features in Anderson-Tawil syndrome.[32] Diagnosis is supported with genetic testing, electromyography, serum creatine kinase, and muscle biopsy. Prevention of attacks is achieved via dietary management, pharmaceutical prophylactics, and avoidance of precipitating factors. Patients with familial periodic paralysis benefit from mild-to-moderate intensity regular exercise to counter progressive weakness that persists between attacks, maintain health, and prevent future onset of attacks.

■ Friedreich's Ataxia

Chief Clinical Characteristics

This presentation can be characterized by the onset of progressive gait and limb ataxia in childhood to early adulthood. Associated symptoms include loss of vibration sense and proprioception, absent deep tendon reflexes, weakness, dysarthria, and sensorineural hearing loss. Often, cardiac hypertrophy, diabetes mellitus, and optic atrophy are also present.[4,33,34]

Background Information

This autosomal recessive condition is caused by a genetic mutation resulting in a progressive loss of large myelinated sensory axons, followed by degeneration of the posterior column and spinocerebellar and pyramidal tracts.[4,35] Magnetic resonance imaging may show atrophic changes characteristic of the disorder, and should be performed along with genetic testing and electrocardiography for definitive diagnosis. There is currently no medical treatment to slow or stop disease progression, but individuals with this condition may benefit from surgical intervention to correct foot and spine deformities and allow for improved mobility. Average lifetime survival is 25 to 30 years of age.[4,35]

■ Glycogen Storage Diseases (Glycogenosis, Pompe's Disease, McArdle's Disease, Cori's Disease)

Chief Clinical Characteristics

This presentation typically involves benign truncal and proximal limb myopathy or exercise-induced severe myalgia, cramping, and fatigue in adults.[36]

Background Information

This condition refers to a group of 11 autosomal recessive diseases of glycogen storage affecting the liver, heart, and skeletal muscle.[37] Pathophysiology is due to inherited deficiencies of enzymes that regulate the synthesis or degradation of glycogen.[38] The many variants of this condition differ in the age of presentation from infancy to adulthood and predominance of presenting symptoms, such as proximal weakness in Pompe's disease, mixed proximal and distal weakness in Cori's disease, and cramping and fatigue after exercise in McArdle's disease.[39] Diagnosis involves electromyography, blood studies, and muscle biopsy. Treatment consists of dietary therapy, enzyme replacement, activity modification, and symptom-based care. The prognosis for individuals with glycogenoses varies according to the variant, onset, and severity of symptoms. Serious long-term complications such as nephropathy, cirrhosis, cardiomyopathy, and progressive myopathy are a major concern.[38] This condition is characterized by slow progressive weakness over years that eventually results in death secondary to failure of respiratory musculature.

■ Hereditary Spastic Paraplegia (Familial Spastic Paralysis)

Chief Clinical Characteristics

This presentation includes insidious, progressive difficulty with walking due to bilateral, symmetric lower extremity spastic weakness. Patients may report tripping, stumbling, and falling, as well as urinary urgency.[40]

Background Information

This condition can be divided into two types. The complicated form of this condition is indicated by the presence of neurological abnormalities such as dementia, mental retardation, epilepsy, extrapyramidal disturbance, ataxia, deafness, retinopathy, optic neuropathy, peripheral neuropathy, and skin lesions. The uncomplicated form is indicated by the absence of these features.[41] This condition is a group of inherited disorders with a primary pathological feature of axonal degeneration of the distal ends of the longest ascending and descending tracts, resulting in the characteristic spasticity.[40,41] Diagnosis is made by the presence of symptoms of gait disturbance, neurological findings of corticospinal tract deficits in the lower extremities, family history or genetic testing, and exclusion of any other disorders that could account for the symptoms.[40] Current treatment is limited to decreasing muscle spasticity through exercise and medication. Physical therapy is beneficial for the maintenance and improvement of muscle flexibility, muscle strength, gait, and cardiovascular fitness.[40] Prognosis varies, and those with an onset after adolescence are more likely to have insidious worsening.[40]

■ Hydromyelia (Syringomyelia)

Chief Clinical Characteristics

This presentation involves insidious onset of symptoms including upper and lower extremity weakness and numbness, and less commonly, pain. Trauma usually precedes the onset on symptoms, but the time frame for subsequent development of weakness and sensory changes is variable.

Background Information

This condition is caused by an abnormal widening of the central canal of the spinal cord, leading to the accumulation of cerebrospinal fluid and hydrocephalus. Differential diagnosis must be made between hydromyelia and other disorders such as syringomyelia, spinal cord tumor, and spinal arteriovenous malformation. Magnetic resonance imaging and electromyography are used to confirm the diagnosis of this condition. Surgery may be indicated to decrease or eliminate the symptoms. Prognosis is variable.

■ Hysterical Paralysis

Chief Clinical Characteristics

This presentation commonly includes a varied presentation of weakness associated with sensory loss, but no change in sphincter tone or reflexes.[42]

Background Information

This condition is a type of conversion disorder. The presentation of nonorganic loss of motor function is often precipitated by a traumatic event.[43] All diagnostic testing, such as imaging, laboratory investigation, and electrodiagnostic testing, fails to identify dysfunction. Inconsistencies in history, physical examination, and presentation following traumatic event should lead to suspicion of hysterical paralysis.[42] The DSM-IV-TR criteria must be met to fulfill the diagnosis of conversion disorder. Intervention includes treatment of any underlying depression or anxiety disorders as well as behavior-oriented therapy and biofeedback.[43] With proper psychological intervention and discussion of physical findings and discrepancies with the patient, prognosis for full recovery of function is excellent, and 98% of patients/clients will demonstrate recovery within 1 year.[43]

INFLAMMATORY MYOPATHIES
■ Dermatomyositis

Chief Clinical Characteristics

This presentation typically involves patchy, bluish-purple (heliotrope) discolorations of face, neck, shoulders, upper chest, elbows, knees, knuckles, and back often preceding or coinciding with onset of symmetrical truncal or proximal limb weakness. Individuals with this condition have difficulty arising from a chair, climbing stairs, and lifting objects. Progression of weakness occurs in a *proximal to distal pattern.[3] Associated symptoms include muscle ache and tenderness, fatigue, discomfort, weight loss, and low-grade fever.*

Background Information

This condition is an inflammatory myopathy with a severe onset, affecting children and adults, and females more often than males. Diagnostic criteria include typical changes upon muscle biopsy, electrodiagnostic abnormalities characteristic of myopathy, and skin lesion/rash.[3] Pharmacologic treatment with steroids, immunosuppressants, and intravenous immunoglobulin is often combined with physical therapy to preserve muscle function and prevent secondary impairments.[44] Most cases respond to therapy. Individuals with concomitant cardiac or pulmonary involvement have a poorer prognosis

■ Inclusion Body Myositis

Chief Clinical Characteristics

This presentation may include onset of proximal and distal muscle weakness that may asymmetrically affect the extremities, with common early involvement of the knee extensor, ankle dorsiflexor, and wrist and finger flexor greater than extensor muscle groups.[45]

Background Information

Isolated erector spinae weakness may cause "droopy neck syndrome." Dysphagia is common in individuals with this condition. The mean age of onset is 55 to 60 years, and approximately 80% of individuals with this condition begin to demonstrate symptoms and signs after age 50 years.[46] The histopathological hallmark of this condition is protein aggregates consisting of inclusion bodies within affected muscle fibers. Pathophysiology is unclear, although roles for degeneration and humoral immunity have been suggested. This condition typically is unresponsive to immunosuppressive agents, and optimal treatment remains unclear. Severe disease results in significant disability, but is rarely fatal.

■ Polymyositis

Chief Clinical Characteristics

This presentation is characterized by onset of subacute or chronic and symmetrical

weakness of proximal and trunk muscles, resulting in difficulty arising from a chair, climbing stairs, and carrying objects. Polymyositis most commonly occurs in young adulthood. Progression occurs in a proximal to distal pattern. Associated symptoms include difficulty swallowing, muscle tenderness, and an absence of dermatitis.

Background Information
Diagnostic criteria for this condition include weakness evolving over weeks to months sparing facial and eye muscles manifested in patients 18 years and older; absence of rash; no family history of neuromuscular, endocrine, or neurogenic disease; no exposure to myotoxic drugs; and exclusion of other myopathies via clinical examination, muscle biopsy, and exclusion of myopathies commonly associated with another autoimmune disease or viral infection (ie, Crohn's disease, myasthenia gravis, or human immunodeficiency virus or acquired immunodeficiency syndrome).[47] Treatment involves steroidal, immunosuppressive, and/or intravenous immunoglobulin medications. However, the optimal therapeutic regimen remains unclear.[44] Physical therapy is indicated to prevent muscle atrophy and contractures. Prognosis is variable. Severe disease not responsive to therapy results in significant disability, but is rarely fatal.

■ Kearns-Sayre Syndrome

Chief Clinical Characteristics
This presentation commonly includes a classic triad of symptoms, involving progressive external ophthalmoplegia, retinal pigmentary degeneration, and heart block. Common additional findings include cerebellar dysfunction, myopathy, ataxia, sensorineural hearing loss, mental retardation, growth hormone deficit with dwarfism, hypoparathyroidism, and diabetes mellitus.[48,49]

Background Information
Etiology has not been established, however this rare, sporadic mitochondrial disorder is thought to occur via a mutation in either the ovum or zygote.[48] Diagnosis is established with a combination of clinical, radiologic, pathological, biochemical, and molecular studies. Mitochondrial deoxyribonucleic acid

analysis and histological verification of the presence of ragged red fibers may be helpful in determining diagnosis.[48] Treatment is mostly symptomatic and supportive, although cardiac symptoms may be managed with medication. This condition is a slowly progressive disorder and prognosis is often determined by the degree of heart conduction impairment.[50]

■ Lambert-Eaton Myasthenic Syndrome

Chief Clinical Characteristics
This presentation includes insidious onset of symmetrical weakness in the trunk, pelvic girdle, lower extremities, and shoulder girdle. Report of a perception of increased strength after a few muscle contractions, followed by weakness after prolonged exertion, is characteristic of this condition. Additional symptoms include paresthesias, aching pain, dry mouth, constipation, difficult micturition, and impotence.[3] This presentation initially includes difficulty rising from a chair, climbing stairs, and walking.

Background Information
The pathological process of this condition involves a defect in the release of acetylcholine from presynaptic nerve terminals due to a loss of voltage-sensitive calcium channels on the presynaptic motor nerve channel. Approximately two-thirds of the known cases are associated with cancer.[3] Of those, small-cell lung cancer is the most prevalent. This condition is also associated with autoimmune diseases. The syndrome of symmetrical weakness and easily fatigable proximal muscles combined with dry mouth and aching pain suggests the diagnosis. Differential diagnosis especially includes amyotrophic lateral sclerosis, multiple sclerosis, polymyositis, and myasthenia gravis. The Tensilon test is the primary method used to distinguish myasthenia gravis from this condition. Treatment of the underlying pathological process, usually a tumor or autoimmune disease, is the first goal, followed by administration of cholinesterase inhibitors and immunosuppressants.[3] Prognosis varies depending on the association with a tumor or autoimmune disease, with the prognosis being worse in the presence of a tumor.

■ Lipid Storage Diseases of Muscle

Chief Clinical Characteristics

This presentation involves progressive myopathy, with or without cardiomyopathy, appearing late in infancy, childhood, or adult life.[3]

Background Information

Myopathy results from a deficit in the metabolism of fatty acids, secondary to carnitine deficiency. There are many variants of carnitine deficiency. Primary systemic carnitine deficiency is autosomal recessive, presenting with progressive myopathy and cardiomyopathy that is fatal if untreated.[51] Carnitine palmitoyltransferase deficiency is autosomal recessive, presenting in teenage males, with myalgia, cramps, weakness, and stiffness often precipitated by sustained exercise or fasting.[52] Weakness may occur in any muscle group without warning. Myopathy due to secondary systemic carnitine deficiency results from dietary deprivation or impaired hepatic and renal function.[3] Diagnosis may include laboratory investigation, muscle biopsy, and electrodiagnostic testing used to rule out competing diagnoses.[51] Treatment involves dietary modifications, medication, and education. Prognosis is variable depending on type of deficiency and severity of myopathy.

■ Locked-In Syndrome

Chief Clinical Characteristics

This presentation includes complete paralysis of all voluntary muscles characterized by tetraplegia, paralysis of lower cranial nerves, anarthria, and paralysis of horizontal gaze sparing only vertical gaze and blinking.[53] Cognition and sensation are spared.

Background Information

This condition is a rare neurological disorder caused by a lesion to the ventral pons due to obstruction of the basilar artery, traumatic brain injury, tumor, central pontine myelinolysis, or medication overdose.[53] It is crucial to discern this condition from a minimally conscious state or vegetative state, because in the latter condition the patient is not conscious and aware. The standard of care consists of long-term multidisciplinary rehabilitation. The prognosis for those with locked-in syndrome is poor. The vast majority of individuals do not return to premorbid levels of function. However, with rehabilitation, many recover swallowing, improve motor and sphincter control, and/or are able to communicate verbally or through devices.[53]

■ Lyme Disease (Tick Paralysis)

Chief Clinical Characteristics

This presentation can include fluctuating signs or symptoms such as headache, neck stiffness, nausea, vomiting, malaise, fever, pain, fatigue, and presence of a "bull's-eye" rash.[3] Over time, additional symptoms may include sensory changes, irritability, cognitive changes, depression, behavioral changes, seizures, ataxia, chorea movements, pain, weakness, balance deficits, arthritis, and cranial nerve involvement.[3,54]

Background Information

Borrelia burgdorferi, an organism that infects ticks, is responsible for the transmission of this condition to a human host.[3] The diagnosis is confirmed with a thorough history, clinical assessment, enzyme-linked immunosorbent assay, and Western blot or immunoblot analysis. In addition, magnetic resonance imaging or computed tomography may reveal multifocal or periventricular cerebral lesions.[3] Medical management includes treatment with oral tetracycline, penicillin, or intravenous ceftriaxone.[3] Many individuals experience full recovery with treatment; however, residual deficits may persist for individuals with chronic Lyme disease.[3]

■ Machado-Joseph Disease

Chief Clinical Characteristics

This presentation may involve visual impairments such as nystagmus in combination with slowly progressive ataxia, rigidity, dystonia, weakness in the hands and feet, and difficulty with respiration and swallowing.

Background Information

This condition is genetic, with an autosomal dominant pattern of inheritance and onset of symptoms in adolescence or young adulthood. Differential diagnosis includes Parkinson's disease and multiple system atrophy. The presence of ataxia decreases the likelihood of Parkinson's, and the early age of onset and visual symptoms decrease the likelihood of multiple system atrophy. Diagnosis is established by clinical symptoms and magnetic resonance imaging findings of reduced width of superior and middle cerebellar peduncles, atrophy of the frontal and temporal lobes, and decreased size of the pons and globus pallidus. There is no treatment for this condition, and prognosis is poor.[3]

■ Miller Fisher Syndrome

Chief Clinical Characteristics

This presentation can be characterized by an acute onset of the classic triad of ophthalmoplegia, ataxia, and areflexia. Additional symptoms include mydriasis, sensory loss, facial palsy, bulbar palsy, dysesthesia, weakness, and urinary incontinence.[55]

Background Information

This condition is thought to be a variant form of acute demyelinating polyneuropathy (Guillain-Barré syndrome) and is usually preceded by infectious gastrointestinal or respiratory symptoms approximately 8 days before onset of symptoms.[55] Diagnosis is based on clinical presentation. In addition, elevated cerebrospinal fluid protein values and electrophysiological examination demonstrating conduction block or axonal damage on limbs of normal strength can help reinforce the diagnosis.[56] Plasmapheresis and administration of intravenous immunoglobulins have both been found to be helpful in decreasing recovery time.[56] The natural course of recovery in individuals with this condition is good with minimal disability seen 6 months after onset.[55]

■ Mitochondrial Myopathies

Chief Clinical Characteristics

This presentation typically involves a combination of exercise intolerance, ataxia, seizures, myoclonus, headaches, small strokes, ophthalmoplegia, deafness, muscle cramps, and/or slowly progressive myopathy with proximal greater than distal involvement. Other less common symptoms that may be seen include dementia, lactic acidosis, ptosis, and cardiac conduction defects.[4,57]

Background Information

This condition refers to a large group of disorders that result from a mutation in the mitochondrial genome, resulting in damage to the mitochondria. These disorders include Kearns-Sayre syndrome, myoclonus epilepsy with ragged red fibers, mitochondrial encephalomyopathy with lactic acidosis and stroke-like episodes, as well as other childhood-onset disorders.[4] A combination of clinical picture, histological findings of ragged red fibers, elevated serum lactate, and possible family history contributes to the diagnosis of this condition.[4] There is no specific treatment, but new research shows that patients may benefit from physical therapy for submaximal exercise training.[57] Most patients experience lifelong progression of the disease, and prognosis varies according to the type of disease and amount of involvement.[4]

■ Monomelic Amyotrophy (Benign Focal Amyotrophy, Hirayama Syndrome, O'Sullivan-McLeod Syndrome)

Chief Clinical Characteristics

This presentation typically involves slowly progressive unilateral weakness and atrophy restricted to one limb (more commonly arm/hand than leg/foot) followed by a period of stabilization of symptoms. Sensation is intact.

Background Information

This condition usually occurs in males between the ages of 15 and 25 and is more frequently seen in Asia, particularly in Japan and India.[58] Pathophysiology is unknown, but this condition is thought to be due to a degeneration of the lower motor neuron. Diagnosis is made through history, clinical presentation, electromyographic evidence of denervation and polyphasics in the affected limb, and possible imaging evidence of muscle atrophy. Differential diagnosis particularly includes spinal muscular atrophy, amyotrophic lateral sclerosis, and post-polio syndrome. Clinical presentation can delineate specific syndromes of this condition, such as O'Sullivan-McLeod syndrome and Hirayama syndrome.[59] Treatment consists of muscle strengthening exercises and training in hand coordination. Weakness continues to progress slowly over a period of months to years before reaching a plateau. Recovery of strength and function is possible, but residual weakness remains.[58]

■ Moyamoya Disease

Chief Clinical Characteristics

This presentation may include weakness of an arm, a leg, or arm and leg unilaterally in combination with unsteady gait, involuntary movement, speech and sensory impairments, headache, seizures, impaired mental development, visual disturbances, and nystagmus.[4]

Background Information
This rare condition results from progressive occlusion of the arteries of the circle of Willis.[4] Diagnosis is based upon clinical findings and results of magnetic resonance imaging and magnetic resonance angiography. Images will demonstrate the occlusion of the circle of Willis as well as secondary cerebral infarction, white matter lesions, atrophy, and hemorrhage.[60] Treatment options include revascularization surgery and medical treatment to prevent hypertension and further strokes.[61] Rehabilitative therapies are used to treat functional deficits that the patient may incur from a stroke secondary to the progression of the disease. Outcome depends on the severity of secondary complications and presence of subsequent occlusion.

■ Multiple Sclerosis

Chief Clinical Characteristics
This presentation may include weakness, paresthesias, spasticity, hypertonicity, hyperreflexia, positive Babinski sign, incoordination, optic neuritis, ataxia, vertigo, dysarthria, diplopia, bladder incontinence, tremor, balance deficits, falls, and cognitive deficits.[3]

Background Information
This condition may present as relapsing-remitting, primary progressive, or secondary progressive. The disease occurs most frequently in women between the ages of 20 and 40 years. Only a small number of children or individuals between 50 and 60 years of age are diagnosed with this condition.[3] This condition was originally thought to be secondary to environmental and genetic factors, but evidence suggests an autoimmune response to a viral infection, which subsequently targets myelin.[3] The diagnosis may be confirmed by a thorough history, physical examination, magnetic resonance imaging, analysis of cerebrospinal fluid, and evoked potentials.[3,62,63] Life expectancy and cause of mortality are similar for all types of this condition.[3] Clinical characteristics that are associated with a longer time interval for progression of disability

include female sex, younger age of onset, relapsing-remitting type, complete recovery after the first relapse, and longer time interval between first and second exacerbation.[64] Medical management may include the use of methylprednisolone, prednisone, cyclophosphamide, immunosuppressant treatment, and beta interferon.[3] Physical, occupational, and speech therapy may be indicated to prevent secondary sequelae and to optimize functional activity and mobility. Some individuals may benefit from psychology/psychiatry and social support as the disease progresses.

■ Muscular Dystrophy

Chief Clinical Characteristics
This presentation can be characterized by a symmetric distribution of muscular weakness and atrophy, intact sensation, preservation of cutaneous reflexes, and a strong familial incidence.

Background Information
This group of conditions involves purely degenerative muscular diseases of the hereditary type. The various types of muscular dystrophies are classified by distribution of dominant weakness, varying in age of presentation, severity of weakness and debility, and prognosis for life expectancy. Duchenne muscular dystrophy is an X-linked recessive disorder, occurring predominantly in males. This condition is characterized by proximal weakness, pseudohypertrophy, and Gower's sign (difficulty rising from the ground); this condition is usually diagnosed in the first 3 to 6 years of life. Becker-type muscular dystrophy has a similar presentation, however onset is much later (average age 12 years), with individuals remaining ambulatory well into adulthood. Emery-Dreifuss muscular dystrophy presents in the second to third decade; this phenotype includes proximal weakness, joint contractures, and cardiac arrhythmias. Difficulty raising arms above the head, muscular atrophy, and winging of the scapulae presenting between 6 and 20 years of life are characteristic of facioscapulohumeral muscular dystrophy. Limb girdle muscular dystrophies can present in the first to fifth decade of life, with a characteristic presentation involving primarily proximal weakness (scapulohumeral and pelvifemoral), but may initially present or

progress to include distal weakness, joint contractures, and cardiac involvement. Additional dystrophies include oculopharyngeal, distal muscular dystrophies, congenital muscular dystrophies, and myotonic dystrophy. Diagnosis requires laboratory studies, deoxyribonucleic acid analysis, clinical examination, and family history when available. There is no specific treatment. Medical management consists of nutritional support, pharmacologic management to retard progression or manage symptoms, and physical therapy to protect range of motion, strength, and function. Supportive care and equipment recommendations are also provided. The prognosis varies depending on the type of dystrophy; the life expectancy of individuals with Duchenne type is usually limited to late adolescence, whereas those with the scapulohumeral type live into the seventh or eighth decade.

■ Myasthenia Gravis

Chief Clinical Characteristics
This presentation is characterized by weakness that worsens during periods of activity and improves after periods of rest. Patients present with variable degrees of weakness, ranging from ptosis or diplopia to critical respiratory weakness. Muscles that control speech, facial expression, mastication, swallowing, breathing, and neck and limb movements may be involved.[65]

Background Information
This condition is caused by autoimmune mediated acetylcholine receptor damage, resulting in a deficit in neuromuscular transmission. Diagnosis is achieved through clinical observation of skeletal muscle weakness increased by exercise and relieved by rest, improvement with anticholinesterase medications, electrophysiological evidence of limited neuromuscular transmission, and the presence of circulating acetylcholine receptor antibodies. Medications are used to improve function of the neuromuscular junction and alter the immune response, but have significant side effects. Thymectomy and plasmapheresis are other possible therapeutic interventions.[66] With treatment, most patients with myasthenia gravis recover control of the affected musculature; however, some weakness may remain or relapse.

■ Neurological Complications of Acquired Immunodeficiency Syndrome

Chief Clinical Characteristics
This presentation is variable and dependent on the affected neuroanatomical structures in an individual with acquired immunodeficiency syndrome.[67]

Background Information
This condition may be categorized by:

1. Meningitic symptoms including headache, malaise, and fever (such as secondary to meningitis, cryptococcal meningitis, tuberculous meningitis, and human immunodeficiency virus headache)
2. Focal cerebral symptoms including hemiparesis, aphasia, apraxia, sensory deficits, homonymous hemianopia, cranial nerve involvement, balance deficits, incoordination, and/or ataxia (such as secondary to cerebral toxoplasmosis, primary central nervous system lymphoma, and progressive multifocal leukoencephalopathy)
3. Diffuse cerebral symptoms that involve cognitive deficits, altered level of consciousness, hyperreflexia, Babinski sign, presence of primitive reflexes (such as secondary to postinfectious encephalomyelitis, acquired immunodeficiency dementia complex, cytomegalovirus encephalitis)
4. Myelopathy associated with gait difficulties, spasticity, ataxia, balance deficits, and hyperreflexia (such as secondary to herpes zoster myelitis, vacuolar myelopathy that occurs with acquired immunodeficiency syndrome dementia complex)
5. Peripheral involvement associated with sensory changes, weakness, balance deficits, and pain (such as secondary to peripheral neuropathy, acute and chronic inflammatory demyelinating polyneuropathies).[3,68]

Abnormal neurological findings are observed during a clinical examination in approximately one-third of patients with acquired immunodeficiency syndrome; however, on autopsy most individuals with this condition have abnormalities within the nervous system.[3] Diagnosis of the variable neurological complications associated with this condition may be confirmed with laboratory tests, cerebrospinal fluid cultures, imaging, nerve conduction studies, and physical examination.[3,54,67] Treatment appears to be limited primarily to the use of antiviral medications.[67] Physical and occupational therapy may be indicated to address equipment needs and caregiver/patient training related to functional mobility.

NEUROPATHIES

■ Carpal Tunnel Syndrome

Chief Clinical Characteristics

This presentation typically involves weakness of grip strength and difficulty performing tasks requiring grasp or manipulation of objects, which is preceded by initial report of pain and numbness/tingling in the palmar aspect of the thumb, index finger, middle finger, and radial half of the ring finger with radiation up the forearm.[68]

Background Information

This condition results from compression of the median nerve as it passes through the carpal tunnel. It is associated with repetitive stress, such as typing or performing assembly line tasks. Differential diagnosis includes cervical radiculopathy or compression of the median nerve proximal to the carpal tunnel. Diagnosis is achieved through use of special tests (eg, Phalen's sign, monofilament testing, and provocative tests) and via electromyography and nerve conduction velocity tests.[69] Treatment consists of splinting, pharmacologic management of inflammation and pain, modalities, stretching and strengthening, ergonomic modifications, and surgery if indicated.[70] Nonsurgical care including physical therapy is emphasized first, and it is most effective in those with mild impairment. If nonsurgical management fails, surgery is usually recommended. In those individuals with severe forms of this condition who have been properly diagnosed, 70% report complete satisfaction with pain relief. However, residual weakness and reoccurrence may occur.[68]

■ Chronic Inflammatory Demyelinating Polyneuropathy

Chief Clinical Characteristics

This presentation is characterized by symmetrical distal progressive weakness and impaired sensation in the legs and hands, progressing in a distal to proximal pattern. Presentation of tingling, numbness, weakness, areflexia, and abnormal sensation in a young adult male or female raises the index of clinical suspicion for this condition.[71]

Background Information

This condition is caused by damage to the myelin sheath of the peripheral nerves. Diagnosis requires acute onset of progressive weakness of the limbs, sensory dysfunction with hyporeflexia or areflexia, elevated cerebrospinal fluid protein, and demyelinative features on electromyography-nerve conduction velocity studies. Pharmacologic management involves anti-inflammatories, immunosuppressive agents, intravenous immunoglobulin therapy, and plasmapheresis.[71] Physical therapy is indicated to improve strength, mobility, and endurance and to prevent secondary impairments.[72] Early diagnosis and treatment is essential to prevent axonal loss. The course varies among individuals, from spontaneous recovery to bouts of recovery and relapse. Recovery is seen in patients with a relapsing-remitting course, young onset, and early treatment. Individuals with axonal loss, chronic progressive course with combined sensory and motor presentation, older age at onset, and/or diabetes have a poor prognosis for recovery of function.[73,74]

■ Compression Neuropathy

Chief Clinical Characteristics

This presentation can be characterized by weakness that is often preceded by a lengthy history of pain, paresthesias, and numbness in the distribution of a specific peripheral nerve. Associated lower motor neuron signs of hyporeflexia, atrophy, and fasciculations may occur, as well as trophic skin changes with severe compression neuropathies.

Background Information

This group of conditions is often called mononeuropathy simplex, referring to a single peripheral nerve. The distribution of sensorimotor symptoms is specific to the compressed nerve. The most common form of this condition is carpal tunnel syndrome, in which the medial nerve is compressed at the wrist. Other upper extremity neuropathies include interdigital, ulnar, radial, and thoracic outlet syndrome. Lower extremity compression neuropathies include peroneal, femoral, saphenous, lateral femoral cutaneous, and obturator nerve lesions, as well as tarsal tunnel syndrome. Diagnosis involves clinical examination, detailed history, and often electrodiagnostic testing. Prognosis for recovery of sensation and strength is poor in the presence of lower motor neuron signs and trophic changes, indicating long-standing compression. However, if diagnosed early, prognosis for recovery of sensation and strength is good. Treatment includes accurate diagnosis, removal of compression via physical therapy intervention or surgery, and preventative interventions to preclude recurrence of the neuropathy.

■ Diabetes Mellitus-Induced Neuropathies

Chief Clinical Characteristics
This presentation is variable, including manifestations such as acute diabetic mononeuropathies, which may include involvement of cranial nerves (eg, oculomotor or abducens nerve involvement) or peripheral nerves[3]; multiple mononeuropathies and radiculopathies, which may include unilateral or asymmetric pain, low back pain with or without symptoms in leg, weakness, atrophy, diminished or absent deep tendon reflexes, and sensory deficits[3]; distal polyneuropathy, the most common diabetic neuropathy, which consists of chronic, symmetric, distal sensory deficits (eg, numbness and tingling), diminished or absent deep tendon reflexes, balance deficits, and weakness[3]; and autonomic neuropathy, which may involve resting tachycardia, orthostatic hypotension, sexual impotence, exercise intolerance, abnormal sweating, pupil abnormalities, weakness, sensory deficits, and gastroparesis.[3,54,75,76]

Background Information
Approximately 15% to 20% of people with diabetes may present with the clinical signs and symptoms of this condition.[3,75] However, approximately 50% will have neuropathic symptoms and may have abnormalities in nerve conduction testing.[3] Commonly considered a metabolic disorder, this condition may be a result of vascular complications disrupting the supply of nutrients to the nerves.[54,77] A thorough history, physical examination (specifically including the assessment of deep tendon reflexes and sensory examination), electromyography/nerve conduction testing, and laboratory screen helps to differentiate other causes of neuropathy.[75,76] Treatment consists of maintaining a normal range of blood glucose levels.[3,75,76] In addition, individuals with this condition may prevent complications by completing visual inspection of the skin and routine podiatry care.[76] Medications may help to control symptoms such as paresthesias or pain.[3,54] Additional management may include consultations with an orthotist to ensure proper fitting of foot wear and physical therapy to minimize disability by addressing impairments associated with limitations in functional mobility.[77]

■ Hereditary Motor and Sensory Neuropathies

Chief Clinical Characteristics
This presentation includes distal sensory abnormalities, such as numbness and tingling of the feet, and muscle weakness of distal musculature. Individuals affected with hereditary neuropathies may also report sweating and dizziness upon standing.

Background Information
Hereditary neuropathies include hereditary motor and sensory neuropathy, hereditary sensory neuropathy, hereditary motor neuropathy, and hereditary sensory and autonomic neuropathy. The majority of all hereditary neuropathies are Charcot-Marie-Tooth neuropathy. Inherited polyneuropathies are caused by genetic abnormalities. Diagnosis is made by nerve conduction and electromyographic studies. Prognosis for hereditary sensory neuropathies is poor due to intractable pain.[78] Prognosis for hereditary motor and sensory neuropathies has also been found to be unfavorable due to slowing of conduction velocity with age.[79]

■ Multifocal Motor Neuropathy

Chief Clinical Characteristics
This presentation includes progressive, asymmetrical weakness, muscle atrophy, cramps,

and fasciculations that develop slowly over several years. Other symptoms include wrist and foot drop, grip weakness, reduced tendon reflexes in affected areas, and occasional cranial or phrenic nerve involvement.

Background Information

This condition is thought to be immunologically mediated, although the exact mechanism is unknown.[80] Diagnosis is made by the presence of definite motor conduction block with normal sensory nerve conduction on electrophysiological study.[81] Medical treatment is intravenous immunoglobulin therapy.[81,82] This condition has a slow, progressive course of deterioration of muscle strength, but the disease generally does not cause severe disability or death.[81,82]

■ Peripheral Neuropathies

Chief Clinical Characteristics

This presentation includes weakness and sensory changes along the distribution of a peripheral nerve. Other potential signs and symptoms may include impaired balance, diminished or absent deep tendon reflexes, fasciculations, syncope, abnormal sweating, orthostatic hypotension, resting tachycardia, and trophic changes.[3,83]

Background Information

The patterns of this condition are variable and may present as polyneuropathy, polyradiculopathy, neuronopathy, mononeuropathy, mononeuropathy multiplex, and plexopathy.[3] Some of the etiologies associated with peripheral neuropathies include trauma, inflammation (eg, acute demyelinating polyneuropathy [Guillain-Barré syndrome], herpes zoster, Lyme's disease, human immunodeficiency virus), metabolic (eg, diabetes mellitus, uremia), nutritional (eg, vitamin B deficiencies commonly associated with alcohol abuse, eating disorders, and individuals with malabsorption syndromes), hereditary, idiopathic (eg, aging or unknown causes), and toxic (eg, exposure to lead, arsenic, or thallium or to chemotherapeutic drugs such as vincristine, cisplatin).[83] Twenty percent of individuals over the age of 60 are affected by a type of peripheral neuropathy.[84] The diagnosis of the specific disorder may be differentiated by the pattern of peripheral

neuropathy and temporal features. The diagnosis may be confirmed after completing a thorough history, physical examination, laboratory testing, and possibly electromyography/nerve conduction testing.[3,85] Treatment and prognosis will vary depending on the etiology and severity.

■ Toxic Neuropathy

Chief Clinical Characteristics

This presentation can involve onset of weakness, sensory deficits, and hyporeflexia in a distal to proximal polyneuropathy pattern following exposure to a toxic agent.[86] Presentation of weakness is often preceded by abnormal changes in sensation, often hyperalgesia.

Background Information

This condition may be caused by drugs, organic compounds found in solvents and glues, heavy metals (ie, lead, arsenic, thallium, gold), and plant or animal toxins. Most forms of this condition are primarily sensory or sensorimotor in nature.[2] Forms of this condition that are associated with weakness at onset can be due to lead (often presenting as distal upper extremity weakness) or ingestion of plant or shellfish toxins. Electrodiagnostic testing and histopathological analysis identify axonal damage. Effective medical management involves supportive care and removal or avoidance of the offending toxin. The majority of cases of this condition are self-limited and improve after removal of the toxic agent.[86]

■ Neurosarcoidosis

Chief Clinical Characteristics

This presentation may be characterized by facial palsy, impaired taste, sight, smell or swallowing; vertigo; loss of sensation in a stocking/glove pattern; and weakness in a distal greater than proximal distribution.[3]

Background Information

This condition is a manifestation of sarcoidosis with central and/or peripheral nervous system involvement. It is characterized by formation of granulomas in the central nervous system. The lesion consists of lymphocytes and mononuclear phagocytes surrounding a noncaseating epithelioid cell granuloma. These granulomas represent an autoimmune response to central nervous system tissues. This condition includes 5% of individuals with sarcoidosis. The diagnosis is established by the presence of clinical features, along with clinical and biopsy evidence of sarcoid granulomas in tissues outside the nervous system. Approximately two-thirds of individuals experience this illness only once, whereas the remainder experience chronic relapses. Primary treatment for neurosarcoidosis is the administration of corticosteroids.

■ Neurosyphilis (Tabes Dorsalis, Syphilitic Spinal Sclerosis, Progressive Locomotor Ataxia)

Chief Clinical Characteristics
This presentation can be characterized by hemiparesis, ataxia, aphasia, gait instability, falls, neuropathy, personality and cognitive changes, seizures, diplopia, visual impairments, hearing loss, psychotic disorders, loss of bowel/bladder function, pain, hyporeflexia, and hypotonia.[87,88]

Background Information
Treponema pallidum infects the human host by way of contact with contaminated bodily fluids or lesions.[87] This spirochete is responsible for the diagnosis of syphilis; however, when *T. pallidum* is present within the central nervous system the individual is diagnosed with neurosyphilis.[88] This condition occurs in approximately 10% of individuals with untreated syphilis, and in 81% of these cases it presents as meningovascular, meningeal, and general paresis. Treatment includes use of various forms of penicillin or alternative choices for those allergic to penicillin[87] and may involve rehabilitative therapies depending on the individual's activity limitations or participation restrictions. A better prognosis has been observed for individuals treated during early neurosyphilis.[88]

■ Neurotoxicity

Chief Clinical Characteristics
This presentation includes limb weakness or numbness, loss of memory, vision, and/or intellect, headache, behavioral problems, and sexual dysfunction.

Background Information
This condition occurs when exposure to natural or artificial toxins alters the normal activity of the nervous system. This can eventually disrupt or kill neurons. It results from exposure to substances used in chemotherapy, radiation treatment, drug therapies, and organ transplants, as well as exposure to heavy metals, foods, or pesticides. Diagnosis is supported by clinical presentation and lab tests for detection of the toxic substance. Treatment is prioritized at removal of the offending toxin. Prognosis varies greatly depending on the level of exposure and individual's comorbid medical conditions.

■ Normal Pressure Hydrocephalus

Chief Clinical Characteristics
This presentation is characterized by progressive difficulty in walking characterized by diminished cadence, widened base, short steps, and en bloc turning (requiring more than 3 steps to make a 90-degree turn). Movements involving the axial musculature appear awkward and apraxic. Progression involves impairment in mental function and sphincter incontinence.

Background Information
Symptoms are caused by increased pressure on the brain, specifically the frontal lobe, due to an abnormal increase in cerebrospinal fluid secondary to trauma, infection, space-occupying lesion, or unknown cause. It is most common in the elderly, but can occur in people of any age. Symptoms must be differentiated from disorders with similar presentation such as Alzheimer's, Parkinson's, and Creutzfeldt-Jakob diseases.[89] Diagnosis involves the clinical presentation combined with imaging to identify ventricular enlargement, intracranial pressure monitoring, and neuropsychological testing.[89] Treatment entails shunt placement to drain cerebrospinal fluid and regular follow-up by a physician to monitor shunt function. Without treatment, symptoms continue to worsen. With shunt placement, 60% of individuals with this condition improve significantly, and 30% will completely recover and return to premorbid levels of function. Others have residual gait, sphincteric, and cognitive deficits.[90]

■ Parry-Romberg Syndrome

Chief Clinical Characteristics
This presentation involves atrophy of one side of the face, head, and associated structures. The left side of the face is usually affected.

Individuals may also report difficulties involving the tongue, lips, and salivary glands. Headaches, facial pain, and seizures may occur.

Background Information
This condition is a rare disease. Exact etiology is unknown, although possible causes do include trophic malfunction of the cervical sympathetic nervous system or viral or *Borrelia* infection.[91] Diagnosis is established by clinical presentation along with radiology reports revealing deficient root development or root resorption, and histological studies demonstrating atrophy of the epidermis and infiltrates of lymphocytes and monocytes. Treatment is symptomatic and may include facial plastic surgery after the disease process has stopped. This disease is a degenerative process with a poor prognosis.

■ Pelizaeus-Merzbacher Disease

Chief Clinical Characteristics
This presentation commonly includes deterioration of strength, coordination, motor abilities, and intellectual function.

Background Information
Severity and onset of the disease range widely, depending on the type of genetic mutation, and extends from the mild, adult-onset spastic paraplegia to the severe form with onset at infancy and death in early childhood.[92] This condition is an X-linked disease caused by a mutation in the gene that controls the production of a myelin protein called proteolipid protein.[92] Genetic diagnostic testing is the definitive method for diagnosing this condition.[93] There is no cure. Therefore, treatment is based on symptoms and includes physical therapy, orthotics, and antispasticity agents with goals to minimize the development of joint contractures, dislocations, and kyphoscoliosis.[94] Individuals with severe forms of this condition experience progressive deterioration until death. Individuals with the adult-onset form with spasticity may have nearly normal life span.[4]

■ Poliomyelitis

Chief Clinical Characteristics
This presentation typically involves acute, asymmetrical, flaccid paralysis with associated LMN signs of hyporeflexia and atrophy, *accompanied by signs and symptoms of systemic infection including fever, nausea, vomiting, pain, and respiratory distress.[3]*

Background Information
The incidence of poliomyelitis has been nearly eradicated in the United States, but outbreaks continue in some areas of Africa, Southeast Asia, and India. This mainly affects children and immunocompromised individuals. The virus that causes this condition selectively attacks the anterior horn motor neurons as well as cranial nerve motor nuclei, resulting in denervation and further Wallerian degeneration.[3] In individuals who survive the initial insult, recovery of strength via neuronal sprouting may occur, resulting in giant motor units. Paralysis may be reversed; however, the patient is at risk for post-polio syndrome sequelae later in life. Physical therapy is indicated for supportive care, prevention of secondary impairments, and education on prevention of exacerbations of post-polio syndrome.[3]

■ Post-Polio Syndrome

Chief Clinical Characteristics
This presentation usually includes debilitating and slowly progressive muscle weakness. Associated symptoms include atrophy, myalgia, fasciculations, cramps, respiratory insufficiency, bulbar muscle dysfunction, and sleep apnea.[95]

Background Information
This condition affects an average of 50% of survivors of poliomyelitis approximately 35 years after the initial onset.[96] The syndrome slowly progresses in a stepwise course. Severity of weakness is correlated to severity of acute weakness and disability from original infection. Pathophysiology is unknown, but a common hypothesis purports that over time, excess metabolic stress on remaining motor neurons causes dropout of new nerve terminals and eventually death of the motor neurons.[97] Diagnosis is attained through exclusion of other causes using laboratory studies, electromyography, imaging, and a history of acute poliomyelitis infection.[95] Treatment is achieved through lifestyle changes for energy conservation, weight loss, and use of assistive devices, pharmacologic agents to ameliorate fatigue, and

nonfatiguing exercise. Low-intensity, alternate-day, interval-strength, and cardiovascular exercise is indicated to combat fatigue, weakness, and myalgias as long as care is taken to avoid overwork.[95]

■ Primary Lateral Sclerosis

Chief Clinical Characteristics
This presentation includes spastic paraparesis of voluntary muscles with associated upper motor neuron signs in the absence of lower motor neuron signs. Onset of difficulty with gait, balance, and leg weakness appears in the fifth to sixth decade of life and may progress to affect upper extremity and facial musculature.

Background Information
Imaging, cerebrospinal fluid analysis, and electromyographic studies confirm the diagnosis. In particular, this condition is differentiated from the more severe amyotrophic lateral sclerosis only after a period of 3 years from onset to ensure the absence of lower motor neuron signs.[3] Treatment for this condition addresses symptom management. Physical therapy is indicated to prevent immobility. This condition is not fatal. Progression of symptoms varies; some individuals maintain ambulatory status throughout life while others become wheelchair bound.

■ Rheumatoid Arthritis

Chief Clinical Characteristics
This presentation may be characterized by muscle weakness that is either generalized or more focal in proximal muscles. Typically, this condition presents with joint pains. Leg pain (18%) and leg numbness (14%) have been reported in people with this condition.[98]

Background Information
Women are twice as likely as men to be affected. Symptoms associated with this progressive inflammatory joint disease are caused by synovial membrane thickening and cytokine production in synovial fluid. Blood tests confirm the diagnosis if rheumatoid factor is detected. Typical radiographic findings include disk space narrowing, facet erosion, and end-plate erosion.[98] Steroidal, nonsteroidal, and biological medications

have been widely used in the treatment of this condition.[98]

■ Spinal Cord Infarction (Vascular Myelopathy)

Chief Clinical Characteristics
This presentation depends on the location of the infarction. The most common anterior spinal artery syndrome presents with bilateral, incomplete motor paralysis and loss of pinprick and temperature sensation below the level of the lesion, loss of deep tendon reflexes, sphincter paralysis, acute complaint of back pain, and spared proprioception. Onset of symptoms occurs over the course of minutes to hours.

Background Information
Most forms of this condition are insidious, or secondary to aortic surgery, aortic rupture, atherosclerosis, aneurysm, or an acute deficit of perfusion. Diagnosis is often difficult at initial presentation, because magnetic resonance imaging may be negative. Repeat magnetic resonance imaging may show T_2 hyperintensity secondary to edema.[99] This condition has a poor prognosis with often permanent disability. Prognosis for recovery of ambulation is inversely correlated with the severity of motor deficit at onset.[100] Physical therapy interventions address weakness, spasticity, and mobility and ambulation deficits.

SPINAL CORD INJURIES
■ Brown-Sequard Syndrome

Chief Clinical Characteristics
This presentation can be characterized by ipsilateral loss of strength and tactile discrimination, position, and vibration sense, with contralateral hemianesthesia to pain and temperature secondary to spinal cord injury, disk herniation, tumor, ischemia, or inflammatory disorder.[101,102]

Background Information
This condition occurs secondary to lateral hemisection of the spinal cord, usually below the cervical enlargement, disrupting ipsilateral corticospinal and dorsal column tracts and contralateral projections of the spinothalamic tract.[4] Medical management consists of diagnosis via imaging, appropriate

medical care in the acute care setting, surgical decompression of spinal cord if indicated, and multidisciplinary rehabilitation.[103] Outcome is favorable in most patients following surgical decompression of disk herniation or tumor, demonstrating vast improvement in motor function with minimal residual sensory deficits.[102]

■ Central Cord Syndrome

Chief Clinical Characteristics

This presentation commonly involves presentation of profound weakness of the arms and hands, and to a lesser extent the legs, commonly due to traumatic spinal cord injury. Associated sensory loss below the level of the lesion and/or sphincter dysfunction may occur.

Background Information

Damage to the more centrally located ascending and descending spinal tracts results in this characteristic presentation of motor and sensory loss. Medical management consists of diagnosis via imaging, appropriate medical care in the acute care setting, reduction of fracture and/or surgical decompression of spinal cord, and multidisciplinary rehabilitation.[104] Many individuals with central cord syndrome recover the ability to walk, but impairment of fine motor control in the hands often remains.[105]

■ Conus Medullaris Syndrome

Chief Clinical Characteristics

This presentation typically involves weakness of the lower extremities in association with hyperreflexia, bowel/bladder dysfunction, sexual dysfunction, and sensory loss in a dermatomal pattern of the sacral segments.[4]

Background Information

The presentation of weakness with upper motor neuron symptoms is secondary to injury to the conus medullaris, most commonly due to trauma (vertebral body fracture of acute disk herniations of the thoracolumbar junction).[106] Diagnosis and treatment involve clinical examination, imaging, and surgical investigation, decompression, fusion, and fixation if indicated. Improvement in spinal cord function, bladder function, and nerve root recovery

following surgical intervention occurs in more than half of the patients following surgical intervention.[107]

■ Traumatic Spinal Cord Injury

Chief Clinical Characteristics

This presentation is characterized by loss of sensation in a dermatomal pattern, hypertonicity, spasticity, hyperreflexia, and sphincter dysfunction in combination with muscle weakness. Specific syndromes have characteristic presentations secondary to the location of the lesion.

Background Information

Insult to the spinal cord results from fractured bone, displaced disk material, or a foreign object transecting or injuring the cord. Imaging is used to identify the cause of injury and direct surgical stabilization or intervention. Motor vehicle accidents and falls are the most common etiology of this condition.[108] Physical examination of strength and sensation is used to assign a score from the American Spinal Injury Association.[109] Injuries are classified in terms of neurological level (ie, most rostral segment where myotomal and dermatomal function is spared) and extent as either complete (total lack of sensory or motor function below level of njury) or incomplete (some motor or sensory function spared below the level of injury). Cervical locations of injury result in tetraplegia and may cause paralysis or weakness of the respiratory musculature, requiring mechanical ventilation and/or respiratory strengthening.[110] Thoracic or lumbar locations of injury result in paraplegia. Treatment consists of medical management, multidisciplinary rehabilitation, equipment prescription, and prevention of pressure ulcers, contractures, and further complications. Individuals with incomplete forms of this condition may continue to recover strength and function, while individuals with complete forms of this condition have a poor prognosis for recovery and instead use compensatory techniques and equipment. Individuals with this condition require adequate follow-up medical care to prevent secondary impairments.[111] Acute forms of this condition constitute a medical emergency.

■ Spinal Muscular Atrophy (Werdnig-Hoffmann Disease, Kugelberg-Welander Disease)

Chief Clinical Characteristics

This presentation is characterized by profound weakness and hypotonia in infancy, early childhood, or adolescence associated with an autosomal dominant genetic disorder. Deep tendon reflexes are absent, but sphincter tone and sensation are intact.

Background Information

This condition is the most common neuromuscular disease in children.[112] Onset of spinal muscular atrophy I (Werdnig-Hoffmann disease) occurs in infancy and is always fatal. Onset of spinal muscular atrophy II is between 6 and 18 months, as noted by the child's ability to sit but not stand or walk. Spinal muscular atrophy III (Kugelberg-Welander disease) is the mildest form with onset any time after age 18 months to early adulthood. Earlier onset is associated with more severity and shorter life expectancy.[113] Individuals with spinal muscular atrophy will lose function over time. There is no cure for spinal muscular atrophy. Therefore, treatment includes therapy to preserve mobility and reduce disability as the disease progresses. The most common cause of death is respiratory failure.[114]

■ Stroke (Cerebrovascular Accident)

Chief Clinical Characteristics

This presentation may include a wide range of symptoms that correspond to specific areas of the brain that are affected, potentially including weakness or numbness, especially on one side of the body or face, confusion, aphasia, balance deficits or falls, visual disturbances, or sudden severe headache with no known cause.

Background Information

This condition occurs when blood flow to the brain is interrupted either by blockage (ischemia or infarction) or from hemorrhagic disruption. A thrombosis or embolic occlusion of an artery causes an ischemic type of this condition. A hemorrhagic type of this condition can be caused by arteriovenous malformation, hypertension, aneurysm, neoplasm, drug abuse or trauma. This condition is the most common and disabling neurological disorder in adults and occurs in 114 of every 100,000 people.[115] This condition is diagnosed using clinical presentation and positive findings on computed tomography or magnetic resonance imaging. Medication, surgery, and interdisciplinary therapy are the most common treatments for this condition. The prognosis for recovery is predicted by the magnitude of initial deficit. Factors that are associated with poor outcomes include coma, poor cognition, severe aphasia, severe hemiparesis with little return within 1 month, visual perceptual disorders, depression, and incontinence after 2 weeks.[116,117]

■ Systemic Lupus Erythematosus

Chief Clinical Characteristics

This presentation can include abnormal vision, swallowing, taste, hearing, changes in mood or thinking, and seizures in combination with fatigue, joint pain, and swelling affecting the hands, feet, knees, and shoulders.

Background Information

This condition affects mostly women of childbearing age. It is a chronic autoimmune disorder that can affect any organ system, including skin, joints, kidneys, brain, heart, lungs, and blood. Microinfarcts in the cerebral cortex and brainstem, which lead to destructive and proliferative changes in capillaries and arterioles, are primarily responsible for central nervous system manifestations. Hypertension and endocarditis can also predispose an affected individual to development of neurological abnormalities. Multiple sclerosis is a disease that may be mistaken for this condition, especially if the central nervous system manifestations include visual dysfunction. The diagnosis is confirmed by the presence of skin lesions; heart, lung, or kidney involvement; and laboratory abnormalities including low red or white cell counts, low platelet counts, or positive ANA and anti-DNA antibody tests.[118] Treatment involves corticosteroid medication.

■ Tethered Spinal Cord Syndrome

Chief Clinical Characteristics

This presentation typically includes back pain, associated with neurological deficits, and bowel and bladder dysfunction.[119] The most common manifestations of this condition are worsening in motor function of the lower extremities (and

WEAKNESS

less likely the upper extremities), changes in muscle tone and deep tendon reflexes, progressive loss of articular dexterity, progressively worsening scoliosis or kyphosis, and back or leg pain.[120]

Background Information

This condition occurs commonly in children, but also can present in undiagnosed adults. Magnetic resonance imaging confirms the diagnosis, with a low-lying (caudally positioned) conus medullaris present. Surgical resection of a thickened filum terminale is a common treatment.

■ Thoracic Outlet Syndrome

Chief Clinical Characteristics

This presentation can be characterized by swelling or puffiness in the arm or hand; bluish discoloration of the hand; a feeling of heaviness in the arm or hand; deep, boring toothache-like pain in the neck and shoulder region that seems to increase at night; easily fatigued arms and hands; superficial vein distention in the hand; paresthesias along the inside forearm and the palm; muscle weakness with difficulty gripping and performing fine motor tasks of the hand; atrophy of the muscles of the palm; cramps of the muscles on the inner forearm; pain in the arm and hand; and tingling and numbness in the neck, shoulder region, arm, and hand.

Background Information

There are three types of this condition which can coexist or occur independently: compression of the subclavian vein, compression of the subclavian artery, and a primary neurological syndrome. Multiple anatomical anomalies can lead to thoracic outlet syndrome including an incomplete cervical rib, a taut fibrous band passing from the transverse process of C7 to the first rib, a complete rib that articulates with the first rib, or anomalies of the position and insertion of the anterior and medial scalene muscles. Diagnosis includes physical examination tests (ie, Adson's test, extremity abducted stress test, costoclavicular sign), radiology of the cervical spine, and nerve conduction and electromyography studies. Nonsurgical approaches to treatment include exercise, stretches, modalities, and analgesic medication. Surgery is indicated if pain is persistent and severe neurogenic or vascular features of the syndrome exist. Prognosis for

decreased pain and improved function is good for the majority of individuals with this condition.

■ Thyrotoxic Myopathy (Graves' Disease)

Chief Clinical Characteristics

This presentation includes progressive weakness, wasting of the pelvic girdle and shoulder muscles, fatigue, and heat intolerance. Physical acts such as climbing stairs may be difficult. Individuals with this condition may develop muscle damage to the eyes and eyelids, which may affect mobility of the eye muscles, and temporary, but severe, attacks of muscle weakness known as periodic paralysis.

Background Information

This condition is a rare neuromuscular disorder that may accompany hyperthyroidism (Graves' disease) caused by overproduction of the thyroid hormone thyroxine. It is more common in middle-aged men and in individuals of Asian descent.[121] This condition is difficult to diagnose because reflexes, electromyography, muscle enzymes, and muscle biopsy are usually normal. Myopathy often improves as a result of restoring normal thyroid function via medications, surgery, or radioiodine therapy.[122] Complete or partial removal of the thyroid may be required in severe cases. With treatment, muscle weakness often improves or may be reversed.

■ Todd's Paralysis

Chief Clinical Characteristics

This presentation includes partial or complete paralysis on one side of the body following a seizure.

Background Information

This condition is rare and its etiology is unknown. Diagnosis is made by clinical presentation and exclusion of competing diagnoses, particularly stroke or a transient ischemic attack via magnetic resonance imaging or computed tomography. Treatment is symptomatic, because recovery spontaneously occurs, usually within 48 hours. Prognosis is excellent for recovery of hemiparesis. However, specific etiology of the seizures will determine prognosis for resolution of seizures and this condition.[3]

■ Toxic Myopathy

Chief Clinical Characteristics

This presentation can be characterized by generalized or local weakness, with or without muscle pain, associated neuropathy, or systemic illness following exposure or ingestion of a toxic substance.

Background Information

The presentation of this condition varies for each toxin or drug. Toxic substances produce myopathy via various mechanisms. Primary etiology relates to directly damaging the muscle cell. Secondary etiology occurs via electrolyte disturbances, excessive energy requirements, or inadequate delivery of oxygen and nutrients due to muscle compression and ischemia.[123] This group of conditions is classified according to presentation, histopathological features, pathogenetic mechanism, or type of toxin. Diagnosis relies on laboratory testing, electrodiagnostic investigation, and often muscle biopsy.[124] Treatment involves removal of the toxic agent, supportive physical therapy to prevent secondary impairments and recover strength, and pharmacologic intervention. Prognosis is often good with early diagnosis and removal of the toxic agent; however, when myopathy progresses to involve respiratory and swallowing function or if the toxin affects other organs including the kidney, prognosis for full recovery is poor.[124,125]

■ Transient Ischemic Attack

Chief Clinical Characteristics

This presentation can include weakness or numbness in the face, arm, or leg, especially on one side of the body; confusion or difficulty in talking or understanding speech; trouble seeing in one or both eyes; and difficulty with walking, dizziness, or loss of balance and coordination.

Background Information

This condition is a transient stroke that lasts only a few minutes. It occurs when the blood supply to part of the brain is briefly interrupted. Symptoms of this condition, which usually occur suddenly, are similar to those of stroke but do not last as long. Most symptoms disappear within an hour, although they may persist for up to 24 hours. Because it is impossible to differentiate symptoms from this condition and acute stroke, individuals should assume that all stroke-like symptoms signal a medical emergency. A prompt evaluation (within 60 minutes) is necessary to identify the cause of this condition and determine appropriate therapy. Depending on the individual's medical history and the results of a medical examination, the doctor may recommend drug therapy or surgery to reduce the risk of stroke. Antiplatelet medications, particularly aspirin, are a standard treatment for individuals suspected of this condition and who also are at risk for stroke, including individuals with atrial fibrillation.

■ Transverse Myelitis

Chief Clinical Characteristics

This presentation involves the gradual development of weakness and sensory changes below the level of the lesion, back or neck pain, and/or bowel and bladder dysfunction over the course of several hours to weeks.

Background Information

This condition occurs when inflammation affects the spinal cord, but the brain can be affected as well. Inflammation can result from viral infections, abnormal immune reactions, or ischemia or present as an idiopathic form. Diagnosis is established by exclusion through imaging and blood tests. The first line of treatment requires accurate diagnosis of the underlying pathology and decreasing inflammation in the acute stage, usually by way of corticosteroid medication. Physical therapy is indicated to address secondary impairments and provide supportive therapy. Recovery from transverse myelitis usually begins within 2 to 12 weeks of the onset of symptoms and may continue for up to 2 years. The majority of recovery occurs within the first 3 to 6 months. About one-third of people affected with transverse myelitis experience good or full recovery from their symptoms, regaining the ability to ambulate. Another one-third is left with significant deficits, while the remaining one-third demonstrates no recovery at all. Prognosis varies between recovery without relapse to a permanent presence of symptoms, with the primary poor prognostic factors being pain in the midthoracic region or an abrupt, severe onset of symptoms.[3]

■ Traumatic Brain Injury

Chief Clinical Characteristics

This presentation typically includes weakness in the presence of cognitive changes, altered level of consciousness, seizures, nausea, vomiting, coma, dizziness, headache, pupillary changes, tinnitus, dysequilibrium, incoordination, behavioral changes, spasticity, hypertonicity, cranial nerve lesions, and sensory and motor deficits.[3,126]

Background Information

This condition can be classified as mild, moderate, or severe based on Glasgow Coma Scale, length of coma, and duration of post-traumatic amnesia.[126] Magnetic resonance imaging may be used to confirm the diagnosis.[54] Treatment initiated at the scene of the accident and during the acute phase is focused on medical stabilization. It should be initiated during the acute phase in order to minimize complications.[127] Low Glasgow Coma Scale, longer length of coma, longer duration of post-traumatic amnesia, and older age tend to be associated with poor outcomes.[128] Optimal rehabilitation is interdisciplinary and customized to address the specific individuals' disablement.

■ Tropical Spastic Paralysis

Chief Clinical Characteristics

This presentation commonly involves slowly progressive paresis of the lower extremities, sphincter dysfunction early in the disease course, paresthesias, and uncoordinated movements.[3]

Background Information

The retrovirus human T-cell leukemia virus type 1 causes a chronic infective-inflammatory disease of the spinal cord, which results in the symptoms of this condition. Diagnosis is confirmed by the presence of the serum of the antibodies to human T-cell leukemia virus type 1 in the cerebrospinal fluid. Magnetic resonance imaging also reveals thinness of the spinal cord. Treatment is primarily symptomatic with focus on improved urinary function and decreased spasticity. Steroidal medications and gamma globulin may be used. The majority of individuals with this disease survive.[129]

TUMORS

■ Brain Metastases

Chief Clinical Characteristics

This presentation may include weakness, headaches, seizures, dysphagia, cognitive changes, behavioral changes, dizziness, vomiting, alterations in the level of consciousness, ataxia, aphasia, nystagmus, visual disturbances, dysarthria, balance deficits, falls, lethargy, and incoordination.[3,130]

Background Information

The majority of individuals with brain metastases have been previously diagnosed with a primary tumor; however, a small percentage of individuals are diagnosed concomitantly with brain metastases and the primary tumor. The most common cancers resulting in subsequent brain metastases include lung, breast, melanoma, colorectal, and genitourinary tract. The new onset of neurological symptoms after a primary tumor warrants the use of imaging such as magnetic resonance imaging or computed tomography to confirm the diagnosis. Treatment may include corticosteroids, brain irradiation, surgery, chemotherapy, radiotherapy, and rehabilitative therapies. The prognosis is poor with death typically occurring within 6 months.

■ Brain Primary Tumors

Chief Clinical Characteristics

This presentation may include weakness, headaches, seizures, dysphagia, cognitive changes, behavioral changes, dizziness, vomiting, alterations in the level of consciousness, ataxia, aphasia, nystagmus, visual disturbances, dysarthria, balance deficits, falls, lethargy, and incoordination.[3,54]

Background Information

Glioblastoma multiforme, astrocytoma, oligodendroglioma, metastatic tumors, primary central nervous system lymphomas, ganglioglioma, neuroblastoma, meningioma, arachnoid cysts, hemangioblastoma, medulloblastoma, and acoustic neuroma/schwannoma are some of the more common brain tumors. Specific diagnoses for brain tumors may be confirmed with imaging and biopsy. Treatment is variable depending on the type, size, and location of the tumor and may include surgical resection, chemotherapy, radiation, corticosteroids, and rehabilitative therapies. Prognosis is also variable and depends on the type and grade of tumor, severity of compression, and duration of compression.

■ Spinal Metastases

Chief Clinical Characteristics
This presentation can involve spasticity, weakness, sensory alterations, bowel and bladder incontinence, neck pain, back pain, radicular pain, atrophy, cerebellar signs, balance deficits, falls, and cranial nerve involvement.[3,54,131]

Background Information
This condition is the most frequent neoplasm involving the spine.[131] The most common types and locations of primary tumors that result in spinal metastases include breast, lung, lymphoma, prostate, kidney, gastrointestinal tract, and thyroid.[3,132] The diagnosis is confirmed with gadolinium enhanced magnetic resonance imaging and computed tomography.[3,131] Treatment is variable depending on the tumor and may include surgical resection, chemotherapy, radiation, corticosteroids, and rehabilitative therapies.[3] Although the long-term prognosis is poor, individuals without paresis or pain and who are still ambulatory have longer survival rates.[132]

■ Spinal Primary Tumors

Chief Clinical Characteristics
This presentation may include spasticity, weakness, sensory alterations, bowel/bladder incontinence, back pain, radicular pain, atrophy, cerebellar signs, balance deficits, falls, and cranial nerve involvement.[3]

Background Information
Types of this condition include ependymoma, hemangioblastoma, myeloma, neurofibroma, lymphoma, metastasis, meningioma, schwannoma, and astrocytoma. Extradural tumors, such as meningiomas, produce a rapid onset of symptoms, with weakness being predominant. Intramedullary tumors, or ependymomas, astrocytomas, and hemangioblastomas, present with slowly progressive symptoms, of which loss of pain and temperature

sensation are usually the first. The first test to diagnose brain and spinal column tumors is a neurological examination. Special imaging techniques (computed tomography, magnetic resonance imaging, positron emission tomography) are also employed. Specific diagnoses may be confirmed with imaging and biopsy. Treatment is variable depending on the type, size, and location of the tumor and may include surgical resection, chemotherapy, radiation, corticosteroids, and rehabilitative therapies. Prognosis is variable and depends on the type and grade of tumor, severity of compression, and duration of compression.

■ Vasculitis (Giant Cell Arteritis, Temporal Arteritis, Cranial Arteritis)

Chief Clinical Characteristics
This presentation can be characterized by headaches, psychiatric syndromes, dementia, peripheral or cranial nerve involvement, pain, seizures, hypertension, hemiparesis, balance deficits, neuropathies, myopathies, organ involvement, fever, and weight loss.[3,54,133]

Background Information
This condition is the result of an immune-mediated response resulting in the inflammation of vascular structures.[3,133] It includes a variety of disorders such as giant cell/temporal arteritis (which is the most common form), primary angiitis of the central nervous system, Takayasu's disease, periarteritis nodosa, Kawasaki disease, Churg-Strauss syndrome, Wegener's granulomatosis, and secondary vasculitis associated with systemic lupus erythematous, rheumatoid arthritis, and scleroderma.[133] The diagnosis is confirmed through history, physical examination, laboratory testing, angiography, biopsy, and imaging.[3,54,133] Corticosteroids, cytotoxic agents, intravenous immunoglobulin, and plasmapheresis may be used in the treatment of vasculitis.[54,133] Prognosis is variable and depends on the specific underlying disorder. For example, giant cell arteritis is typically self-limiting within 1 to 2 years; however, death usually occurs within 1 year for individuals with primary angiitis of the central nervous system.[133]

WEAKNESS

References

1. Harris BA, Watkins MP. Adaptations to strength training. In: Frontera W, Dawson D, Slovik D, eds. *Exercise in Rehabilitation Medicine.* Champaign, IL: Human Kinetics; 2005.

2. Greenberg DA, Aminoff MJ, Simon RP. *Clinical Neurology.* 5th ed. New York, NY: McGraw-Hill; 2002.

3. Victor M, Ropper AH. *Adams and Victor's Principles of Neurology.* 7th ed. New York, NY: McGraw-Hill; 2001.

4. Ropper AH, Brown RJ. *Adams and Victor's Principles of Neurology.* 8th ed. New York, NY: McGraw-Hill; 2005.

5. Steinbok P. Clinical features of Chiari I malformations. *Childs Nerv Syst.* May 2004;20(5):329–331.

6. Al-Otaibi LM, Porter SR, Poate TW. Behcet's disease: a review. *J Dent Res.* Mar 2005;84(3):209–222.

7. Nakamura K, Toda N, Sakamaki K, Kashima K, Takeda N. Biofeedback rehabilitation for prevention of synkinesis after facial palsy. *Otolaryngol Head Neck Surg.* Apr 2003;128(4):539–543.

8. Allen D, Dunn L. Acyclovir or valacyclovir for Bell's palsy (idiopathic facial paralysis). *Cochrane Database Syst Rev.* 2004(3):CD001869.

9. VanSwearingen JM, Brach JS. Validation of a treatment-based classification system for individuals with facial neuromotor disorders. *Phys Ther.* Jul 1998;78(7):678–689.

10. Ramsey MJ, DerSimonian R, Holtel MR, Burgess LP. Corticosteroid treatment for idiopathic facial nerve paralysis: a meta-analysis. *Laryngoscope.* Mar 2000;110 (3 pt 1):335–341.

11. Robinson RF, Nahata MC. Management of botulism. *Ann Pharmacother.* Jan 2003;37(1):127–131.

12. Horowitz BZ. Botulinum toxin. *Crit Care Clin.* Oct 2005;21(4):825–839, viii.

13. Shapiro RL, Hatheway C, Swerdlow DL. Botulism in the United States: a clinical and epidemiologic review. *Ann Intern Med.* Aug 1 1998;129(3):221–228.

14. Kay SP. Obstetrical brachial palsy. *Br J Plast Surg.* Jan 1998;51(1):43–50.

15. Dubuisson AS, Kline DG. Brachial plexus injury: a survey of 100 consecutive cases from a single service. *Neurosurgery.* Sep 2002;51(3):673–682; discussion 682–683.

16. Winfree CJ. Peripheral nerve injury evaluation and management. *Curr Surg.* Sep–Oct 2005;62(5):469–476.

17. Kim DH, Cho YJ, Tiel RL, Kline DG. Outcomes of surgery in 1019 brachial plexus lesions treated at Louisiana State University Health Sciences Center. *J Neurosurg.* May 2003;98(5):1005–1016.

18. Choi PD, Novak CB, Mackinnon SE, Kline DG. Quality of life and functional outcome following brachial plexus injury. *J Hand Surg [Am].* Jul 1997;22(4):605–612.

19. Meriggioli MN, Rowin J, Sanders DB. Distinguishing clinical and electrodiagnostic features of X-linked bulbospinal neuronopathy. *Muscle Nerve.* Dec 1999;22(12): 1693–1697.

20. Sperfeld AD, Karitzky J, Brummer D, et al. X-linked bulbospinal neuronopathy: Kennedy disease. *Arch Neurol.* Dec 2002;59(12):1921–1926.

21. Greenland KJ, Zajac JD. Kennedy's disease: pathogenesis and clinical approaches. *Intern Med J.* May 2004; 34(5):279–286.

22. Fouyas IP, Statham PF, Sandercock PA. Cochrane review on the role of surgery in cervical spondylotic radiculomyelopathy. *Spine.* Apr 1 2002;27(7):736–747.

23. Kadanka Z, Mares M, Bednanik J, et al. Approaches to spondylotic cervical myelopathy: conservative versus

24. surgical results in a 3-year follow-up study. *Spine.* Oct 15, 2002;27(20):2205–2210; discussion 2210–2211.

24. Green DM. Weakness in the ICU: Guillain-Barré syndrome, myasthenia gravis, and critical illness polyneuropathy/myopathy. *Neurologist.* Nov 2005;11(6): 338–347.

25. van Mook WN, Hulsewe-Evers RP. Critical illness polyneuropathy. *Curr Opin Crit Care.* Aug 2002; 8(4):302–310.

26. van der Schaaf M, Beelen A, de Vos R. Functional outcome in patients with critical illness polyneuropathy. *Disabil Rehabil.* Oct 21, 2004;26(20):1189–1197.

27. Arnaldi G, Angeli A, Atkinson AB, et al. Diagnosis and complications of Cushing's syndrome: a consensus statement. *J Clin Endocrinol Metab.* Dec 2003;88(12): 5593–5602.

28. Orth DN. Cushing's syndrome. *N Engl J Med.* Mar 23 1995;332(12):791–803.

29. Thijssen DH, Maiorana AJ, O'Driscoll G, Cable NT, Hopman MT, Green DJ. Impact of inactivity and exercise on the vasculature in humans. *Eur J Appl Physiol.* Mar 2010;108(5):845–875.

30. Lehmann-Horn F, Jurkat-Rott K, Rudel R. Periodic paralysis: understanding channelopathies. *Curr Neurol Neurosci Rep.* Jan 2002;2(1):61–69.

31. Cannon SC. An expanding view for the molecular basis of familial periodic paralysis. *Neuromuscul Disord.* Aug 2002;12(6):533–543.

32. Miller TM, Dias da Silva MR, Miller HA, et al. Correlating phenotype and genotype in the periodic paralyses. *Neurology.* Nov 9, 2004;63(9):1647–1655.

33. Albin RL. Dominant ataxias and Friedreich ataxia: an update. *Curr Opin Neurol.* Aug 2003;16(4):507–514.

34. Hart PE, Lodi R, Rajagopalan B, et al. Antioxidant treatment of patients with Friedreich ataxia: four-year follow-up. *Arch Neurol.* Apr 2005;62(4):621–626.

35. Delatycki MB, Ioannou PA, Churchyard AJ. Friedreich ataxia: from genes to therapies? *Med J Aust.* May 2 2005;182(9):439.

36. DiMauro S, Lamperti C. Muscle glycogenoses. *Muscle Nerve.* Aug 2001;24(8):984–999.

37. DiMauro S, Bruno C. Glycogen storage diseases of muscle. *Curr Opin Neurol.* Oct 1998;11(5):477–484.

38. Wolfsdorf JI, Crigler JF, Jr. Effect of continuous glucose therapy begun in infancy on the long-term clinical course of patients with type I glycogen storage disease. *J Pediatr Gastroenterol Nutr.* Aug 1999;29(2):136–143.

39. Quinlivan R, Beynon RJ, Martinuzzi A. Pharmacological and nutritional treatment for McArdle disease (glycogen storage disease type V). *Cochrane Database Syst Rev.* 2008(2):CD003458.

40. Fink JK. Advances in the hereditary spastic paraplegias. *Exp Neurol.* Nov 2003;184(suppl 1):S106–110.

41. Park SY, Ki CS, Kim HJ, et al. Mutation analysis of SPG4 and SPG3A genes and its implication in molecular diagnosis of Korean patients with hereditary spastic paraplegia. *Arch Neurol.* Jul 2005;62(7):1118–1121.

42. Yugue I, Shiba K, Ueta T, Iwamoto Y. A new clinical evaluation for hysterical paralysis. *Spine.* Sep 1, 2004; 29(17):1910–1913; discussion 1913.

43. Letonoff EJ, Williams TR, Sidhu KS. Hysterical paralysis: a report of three cases and a review of the literature. *Spine.* Oct 15 2002;27(20):E441–445.

44. Choy EH, Hoogendijk JE, Lecky B, Winer JB. Immunosuppressant and immunomodulatory treatment for

dermatomyositis and polymyositis. *Cochrane Database Syst Rev.* 2005(3):CD003643.

45. Lin HC, Barkhaus PE, Collins MP, Collins MJP. Inclusion body myositis. http://emedicine.medscape.com/article/1172746-overview. Accessed January 3, 2010.

46. Lotz BP, Engel AG, Nishino H, Stevens JC, Litchy WJ. Inclusion body myositis. Observations in 40 patients. *Brain.* Jun 1989;112 (pt 3):727–747.

47. Dalakas MC. Inflammatory disorders of muscle: progress in polymyositis, dermatomyositis and inclusion body myositis. *Curr Opin Neurol.* Oct 2004; 17(5):561–567.

48. Chu BC, Terae S, Takahashi C, et al. MRI of the brain in the Kearns-Sayre syndrome: report of four cases and a review. *Neuroradiology.* Oct 1999;41(10):759–764.

49. Gross-Jendroska M, Schatz H, McDonald HR, Johnson RN. Kearns-Sayre syndrome: a case report and review. *Eur J Ophthalmol.* Jan–Mar 1992;2(1):15–20.

50. Polak PE, Zijlstra F, Roelandt JR. Indications for pacemaker implantation in the Kearns-Sayre syndrome. *Eur Heart J.* Mar 1989;10(3):281–282.

51. Vielhaber S, Feistner H, Weis J, et al. Primary carnitine deficiency: adult onset lipid storage myopathy with a mild clinical course. *J Clin Neurosci.* Nov 2004; 11(8):919–924.

52. Deschauer M, Wieser T, Zierz S. Muscle carnitine palmitoyltransferase II deficiency: clinical and molecular genetic features and diagnostic aspects. *Arch Neurol.* Jan 2005;62(1):37–41.

53. Leon-Carrion J, van Eeckhout P, Dominguez-Morales R. The locked-in syndrome: a syndrome looking for a therapy. *Brain Inj.* Jul 2002;16(7):555–569.

54. Lindsay KW, Bone I, Callander R. *Neurology and Neurosurgery Illustrated.* 3rd ed. New York, NY: Churchill Livingstone; 1997.

55. Mori M, Kuwabara S, Fukutake T, Yuki N, Hattori T. Clinical features and prognosis of Miller Fisher syndrome. *Neurology.* Apr 24 2001;56(8):1104–1106.

56. Li H, Yuan J. Miller Fisher syndrome: toward a more comprehensive understanding. *Chin Med J (Engl).* Mar 2001;114(3):235–239.

57. Cejudo P, Bautista J, Montemayor T, et al. Exercise training in mitochondrial myopathy: a randomized controlled trial. *Muscle Nerve.* Sep 2005;32(3):342–350.

58. De Freitas MR, Nascimento OJ. Benign monomelic amyotrophy: a study of twenty-one cases. *Arq Neuropsiquiatr.* Sep 2000;58(3B):808–813.

59. Petiot P, Gonon V, Froment JC, Vial C, Vighetto A. Slowly progressive spinal muscular atrophy of the hands (O'Sullivan-McLeod syndrome): clinical and magnetic resonance imaging presentation. *J Neurol.* Aug 2000; 247(8):654–655.

60. Hasuo K, Mihara F, Matsushima T. MRI and MR angiography in moyamoya disease. *J Magn Reson Imaging.* Jul–Aug 1998;8(4):762–766.

61. Sakamoto T, Kawaguchi M, Kurehara K, Kitaguchi K, Furuya H, Karasawa J. Risk factors for neurologic deterioration after revascularization surgery in patients with moyamoya disease. *Anesth Analg.* Nov 1997;85(5): 1060–1065.

62. McDonald WI, Compston A, Edan G, et al. Recommended diagnostic criteria for multiple sclerosis: guidelines from the International Panel on the diagnosis of multiple sclerosis. *Ann Neurol.* Jul 2001;50(1): 121–127.

63. Thompson AJ, Montalban X, Barkhof F, et al. Diagnostic criteria for primary progressive multiple sclerosis: a position paper. *Ann Neurol.* Jun 2000;47(6):831–835.

64. Confavreux C, Vukusic S, Adeleine P. Early clinical predictors and progression of irreversible disability in multiple sclerosis: an amnesic process. *Brain.* Apr 2003; 126(Pt 4):770–782.

65. Scherer K, Bedlack RS, Simel DL. Does this patient have myasthenia gravis? *JAMA.* Apr 20 2005;293(15): 1906–1914.

66. Graves M, Katz JS. Myasthenia gravis. *Curr Treat Options Neurol.* Mar 2004;6(2):163–171.

67. Price RW. Neurological complications of HIV infection. *Lancet.* Aug 17 1996;348(9025):445–452.

68. Katz JN, Simmons BP. Clinical practice. Carpal tunnel syndrome. *N Engl J Med.* Jun 6 2002;346(23):1807–1812.

69. MacDermid JC, Wessel J. Clinical diagnosis of carpal tunnel syndrome: a systematic review. *J Hand Ther.* Apr–Jun 2004;17(2):309–319.

70. Goodyear-Smith F, Arroll B. What can family physicians offer patients with carpal tunnel syndrome other than surgery? A systematic review of nonsurgical management. *Ann Fam Med.* May–Jun 2004;2(3):267–273.

71. European Federation of Neurological Societies/ Peripheral Nerve Society Guideline on management of chronic inflammatory demyelinating polyradiculoneuropathy. Report of a joint task force of the European Federation of Neurological Societies and the Peripheral Nerve Society. *J Peripher Nerv Syst.* Sep 2005; 10(3):220–228.

72. Garssen MP, Bussmann JB, Schmitz PI, et al. Physical training and fatigue, fitness, and quality of life in Guillain-Barre syndrome and CIDP. *Neurology.* Dec 28 2004;63(12):2393–2395.

73. Hattori N, Misu K, Koike H, et al. Age of onset influences clinical features of chronic inflammatory demyelinating polyneuropathy. *J Neurol Sci.* Feb 15 2001; 184(1):57–63.

74. Bouchard C, Lacroix C, Plante V, et al. Clinicopathologic findings and prognosis of chronic inflammatory demyelinating polyneuropathy. *Neurology.* Feb 1999;52(3): 498–503.

75. Boulton AJ, Vinik AI, Arezzo JC, et al. Diabetic neuropathies: a statement by the American Diabetes Association. *Diabetes Care.* Apr 2005;28(4):956–962.

76. Poncelet AN. Diabetic polyneuropathy. Risk factors, patterns of presentation, diagnosis, and treatment. *Geriatrics.* Jun 2003;58(6):16–18, 24–25, 30.

77. Vinik AI, Park TS, Stansberry KB, Pittenger GL. Diabetic neuropathies. *Diabetologia.* Aug 2000;43(8):957–973.

78. Mitsumoto H, Wilbourn AJ. Causes and diagnosis of sensory neuropathies: a review. *J Clin Neurophysiol.* Nov 1994;11(6):553–567.

79. Rossi LN, Lutschg J, Meier C, Vassella F. Hereditary motor sensory neuropathies in childhood. *Dev Med Child Neurol.* Feb 1983;25(1):19–31.

80. Nobile-Orazio E, Cappellari A, Priori A. Multifocal motor neuropathy: current concepts and controversies. *Muscle Nerve.* Jun 2005;31(6):663–680.

81. Van Asseldonk JT, Franssen H, Van den Berg-Vos RM, Wokke JH, Van den Berg LH. Multifocal motor neuropathy. *Lancet Neurol.* May 2005;4(5):309–319.

82. Nagale SV, Bosch EP. Multifocal motor neuropathy with conduction block: current issues in diagnosis and treatment. *Semin Neurol.* Sep 2003;23(3):325–334.

83. Zaida DJ, Alexander MK. Falls in the elderly: identifying and managing peripheral neuropathy. *Nurse Pract.* Mar 2001;26(3):86–88.

84. Richardson JK, Ashton-Miller JA. Peripheral neuropathy: an often-overlooked cause of falls in the elderly. *Postgrad Med.* Jun 1996;99(6):161–172.

85. Bromberg MB. An approach to the evaluation of peripheral neuropathies. *Semin Neurol.* Jun 2005;25(2): 153–159.

86. Grogan PM, Katz JS. Toxic neuropathies. *Neurol Clin.* May 2005;23(2):377–396.

87. Brown DL, Frank JE. Diagnosis and management of syphilis. *Am Fam Physician.* Jul 15, 2003;68(2):283–290.

88. Conde-Sendin MA, Amela-Peris R, Aladro-Benito Y, Maroto AA. Current clinical spectrum of neurosyphilis in immunocompetent patients. *Eur Neurol.* 2004;52(1): 29–35.

89. Relkin N, Marmarou A, Klinge P, Bergsneider M, Black PM. Diagnosing idiopathic normal-pressure hydrocephalus. *Neurosurgery.* Sep 2005;57(3 suppl):S4–16; discussion ii–v.

90. Hebb AO, Cusimano MD. Idiopathic normal pressure hydrocephalus: a systematic review of diagnosis and outcome. *Neurosurgery.* Nov 2001;49(5):1166–1184; discussion 1184–1186.

91. Kurian K, Shanmugam S, Mathew B, Elongavan A. Facial hemiatrophy—a report of 5 cases. *Indian J Dent Res.* Oct–Dec 2003;14(4):238–245.

92. Berger J, Moser HW, Forss-Petter S. Leukodystrophies: recent developments in genetics, molecular biology, pathogenesis and treatment. *Curr Opin Neurol.* Jun 2001; 14(3):305–312.

93. Regis S, Grossi S, Lualdi S, Biancheri R, Filocamo M. Diagnosis of Pelizaeus-Merzbacher disease: detection of proteolipid protein gene copy number by real-time PCR. *Neurogenetics.* May 2005;6(2):73–78.

94. Aicardi J. The inherited leukodystrophies: a clinical overview. *J Inherit Metab Dis.* 1993;16(4):733–743.

95. Jubelt B, Agre JC. Characteristics and management of postpolio syndrome. *JAMA.* Jul 26, 2000;284(4):412–414.

96. Stolwijk-Swuste JM, Beelen A, Lankhorst GJ, Nollet F. The course of functional status and muscle strength in patients with late-onset sequelae of poliomyelitis: a systematic review. *Arch Phys Med Rehabil.* Aug 2005;86(8):1693–1701.

97. Agre JC, Rodriquez AA, Tafel JA. Late effects of polio: critical review of the literature on neuromuscular function. *Arch Phys Med Rehabil.* Oct 1991;72(11):923–931.

98. Kawaguchi Y, Matsuno H, Kanamori M, Ishihara H, Ohmori K, Kimura T. Radiologic findings of the lumbar spine in patients with rheumatoid arthritis, and a review of pathologic mechanisms. *J Spinal Disord Tech.* Feb 2003;16(1):38–43.

99. Masson C, Pruvo JP, Meder JF, et al. Spinal cord infarction: clinical and magnetic resonance imaging findings and short term outcome. *J Neurol Neurosurg Psychiatry.* Oct 2004;75(10):1431–1435.

100. Cheshire WP, Santos CC, Massey EW, Howard JF, Jr. Spinal cord infarction: etiology and outcome. *Neurology.* Aug 1996;47(2):321–330.

101. Kobayashi N, Asamoto S, Doi H, Sugiyama H. Brown-Sequard syndrome produced by cervical disc herniation: report of two cases and review of the literature. *Spine J.* Nov–Dec 2003;3(6):530–533.

102. Najjar MW, Baeesa SS, Lingawi SS. Idiopathic spinal cord herniation: a new theory of pathogenesis. *Surg Neurol.* Aug 2004;62(2):161–170; discussion 170–171.

103. Ellger T, Schul C, Heindel W, Evers S, Ringelstein EB. Idiopathic spinal cord herniation causing progressive Brown-Sequard syndrome. *Clin Neurol Neurosurg.* Jun 2006;108(4):388–391.

104. Yamazaki T, Yanaka K, Fujita K, Kamezaki T, Uemura K, Nose T. Traumatic central cord syndrome: analysis of factors affecting the outcome. *Surg Neurol.* Feb 2005;63(2):95–99; discussion 99–100.

105. Dvorak MF, Fisher CG, Hoekema J, et al. Factors predicting motor recovery and functional outcome after traumatic central cord syndrome: a long-term follow-up. *Spine.* Oct 15, 2005;30(20):2303–2311.

106. Harrop JS, Hunt GE, Jr., Vaccaro AR. Conus medullaris and cauda equina syndrome as a result of traumatic injuries: management principles. *Neurosurg Focus.* Jun 15 2004;16(6):e4.

107. Rahimi-Movaghar V, Vaccaro AR, Mohammadi M. Efficacy of surgical decompression in regard to motor recovery in the setting of conus medullaris injury. *J Spinal Cord Med.* 2006;29(1):32–38.

108. Jackson AB, Dijkers M, Devivo MJ, Poczatek RB. A demographic profile of new traumatic spinal cord injuries: change and stability over 30 years. *Arch Phys Med Rehabil.* Nov 2004;85(11):1740–1748.

109. McDonald JW, Sadowsky C. Spinal-cord injury. *Lancet.* Feb 2, 2002;359(9304):417–425.

110. Gutierrez CJ, Harrow J, Haines F. Using an evidence-based protocol to guide rehabilitation and weaning of ventilator-dependent cervical spinal cord injury patients. *J Rehabil Res Dev.* Sep–Oct 2003;40(5 suppl 2):99–110.

111. Bloemen-Vrencken JH, de Witte LP, Post MW. Follow-up care for persons with spinal cord injury living in the community: a systematic review of interventions and their evaluation. *Spinal Cord.* Aug 2005;43(8):462–475.

112. Hirtz D, Iannaccone S, Heemskerk J, Gwinn-Hardy K, Moxley R, 3rd, Rowland LP. Challenges and opportunities in clinical trials for spinal muscular atrophy. *Neurology.* Nov 8 2005;65(9):1352–1357.

113. Bertini E, Burghes A, Bushby K, et al. 134th ENMC International Workshop: Outcome Measures and Treatment of Spinal Muscular Atrophy, 11–13 February 2005, Naarden, The Netherlands. *Neuromuscul Disord.* Nov 2005;15(11):802–816.

114. Russman BS, Buncher CR, White M, Samaha FJ, Iannaccone ST. Function changes in spinal muscular atrophy II and III. The DCN/SMA Group. *Neurology.* Oct 1996;47(4):973–976.

115. Goodman CC, Boissonnault WG. *Pathology: Implications for the Physical Therapist.* Philadelphia, PA: W. B. Saunders; 1998.

116. Granger CV, Clark GS. Functional status and outcomes of stroke rehabilitation. *Topics Geriatrics.* Mar 1994;9(3):72–84.

117. Shelton FD, Volpe BT, Reding M. Motor impairment as a predictor of functional recovery and guide to rehabilitation treatment after stroke. *Neurorehabil Neural Repair.* 2001;15(3):229–237.

118. Fauci AS, Haynes B, Katz P. The spectrum of vasculitis: clinical, pathologic, immunologic and therapeutic considerations. *Ann Intern Med.* Nov 1978;89(5 pt 1): 660–676.

119. Iskandar BJ, Fulmer BB, Hadley MN, Oakes WJ. Congenital tethered spinal cord syndrome in adults [see comment]. *J Neurosurg.* 1998;88(6):958–961.

120. Di Rocco C, Peter JC. Management of tethered spinal cord. *Surg Neurol.* 1997;48(4):320–322.

121. Ali AS, Akavaram NR. Neuromuscular disorders in thyrotoxicosis. *Am Fam Physician.* Sep 1980;22(3):97–102.

122. Abraham P, Avenell A, Park CM, Watson WA, Bevan JS. A systematic review of drug therapy for Graves' hyperthyroidism. *Eur J Endocrinol.* Oct 2005;153(4):489–498.

123. Sieb JP, Gillessen T. Iatrogenic and toxic myopathies. *Muscle Nerve.* Feb 2003;27(2):142–156.

124. Walsh RJ, Amato AA. Toxic myopathies. *Neurol Clin.* May 2005;23(2):397–428.

125. Guis S, Mattei JP, Liote F. Drug-induced and toxic myopathies. *Best Pract Res Clin Rheumatol.* Dec 2003; 17(6):877–907.

126. Bruns J, Hauser WA. The epidemiology of traumatic brain injury: a review. *Epilepsia.* 2003;44(suppl 10):2–10.

127. Das-Gupta R, Turner-Stokes L. Traumatic brain injury. *Disabil Rehabil.* 2002;24(13):654–665.

128. Hukkelhoven CWPM, Steyerberg EW, Rampen AJJ, et al. Patient age and outcome following severe traumatic brain injury: an analysis of 5600 patients. *J Neurosurg.* 2003;99:666–673.

129. Maloney EM, Cleghorn FR, Morgan OS, et al. Incidence of HTLV-I-associated myelopathy/tropical spastic paraparesis (HAM/TSP) in Jamaica and Trinidad. *J Acquir Immune Defic Syndr Hum Retrovirol.* Feb 1 1998; 17(2):167–170.

130. Tosoni A, Ermani M, Brandes AA. The pathogenesis and treatment of brain metastases: a comprehensive review. *Crit Rev Oncol Hematol.* 2004;52:199–215.

131. Perrin RG, Laxton AW. Metastatic spine disease: epidemiology, pathophysiology, and evaluation of patients. *Neurosurg Clin N Am.* Oct 2004;15(4):365–373.

132. Hosono N, Ueda T, Tamura D, Aoki Y, Yoshikawa H. Prognostic relevance of clinical symptoms in patients with spinal metastases. *Clin Orthop Relat Res.* Jul 2005(436):196–201.

133. Ferro JM. Vasculitis of the central nervous system. *J Neurol.* Dec 1998;245(12):766–776.

WEAKNESS

CHAPTER 34

Case Demonstration: Inability to Stand

■ *Chris A. Sebelski, PT, DPT, OCS, CSCS*

NOTE: This case demonstration was developed using the diagnostic process described in Chapter 4 and demonstrated in Chapter 5. The reader is encouraged to use this diagnostic process in order to ensure thorough clinical reasoning. If additional elaboration is required on the information presented in this chapter, please consult Chapters 4 and 5.

THE DIAGNOSTIC PROCESS

Step 1 Identify the patient's chief concern.

Step 2 Identify *barriers to communication.*

Step 3 Identify *special concerns.*

Step 4 Create a symptom timeline and sketch the anatomy (if needed).

Step 5 Create a diagnostic hypothesis list considering all possible forms of *remote* and *local* pathology that could cause the patient's chief concern.

Step 6 Sort the diagnostic hypothesis list by epidemiology and specific case characteristics.

Step 7 Ask specific questions to rule specific conditions or pathological categories less likely.

Step 8 Re-sort the diagnostic hypothesis list based on the patient's responses to specific questioning.

Step 9 Perform tests to differentiate among the remaining diagnostic hypotheses.

Step 10 Re-sort the diagnostic hypothesis list based on the patient's responses to specific tests.

Step 11 Decide on a diagnostic impression.

Step 12 Determine the appropriate patient disposition.

Case Description

Mrs. RS is an 82-year-old retired teacher who lives alone in a single-story ranch-style home on a 3-acre property. She has been widowed for 10 years and has four grown children.

Though unsure of the exact timeline, it seems that during the past 6 months, she has noted increasing difficulty standing up after sitting on a low couch, getting around her house, and pulling weeds in her garden nearby the house. She has a history of three falls in the past 6 months, none of which has been associated with serious injury. She presents to the session with her son who drove her and is in the waiting room. Mrs. RS does drive short distances from her home, maintains her own checking account, and attends two routine weekly functions with her friends. She has refused any assistive device and holds onto her son's arm as she enters the clinic.

When asked why she was falling and having trouble getting around, Mrs. RS replied that her "legs don't work like they used to" and she rubs her thighs as she says this. She states she is slow to get up and get going in the morning as she feels that her "legs need to wake up," and she reports nonspecific intermittent "pains." If her son walks too fast, then she does sometimes get short of breath. She does wear glasses and saw an ophthalmologist this past year for a "routine checkup." She also wears one hearing aid while in "social settings." Mrs. RS states she is in "good health" and denies a personal history of cardiac disease, respiratory pathology, or cancer. She denies alcohol or recreational drug use and is a nonsmoker.

Current daily medications include Lipitor, a multivitamin, a fish oil dietary supplement, and 81 mg baby aspirin.

STEP #1: Identify the patient's chief concern.

● **Difficulty standing, walking around her house, and gardening**

STEP #2: Identify *barriers to communication.*

● **Age of patient and environment.** Although this patient has communicated clearly her needs and appears to be forthcoming with information and challenges, she is a fall risk. If needed, the therapist should be prepared to have clear conversations regarding the patient's safety and her ability to continue to live independently. These types of conversations are challenging and require heightened sensitivity by the therapist.

Teaching Comments: A thorough examination should include an exploration of the relationship of the phrase "my legs don't work like they used to" and the onset of pain. This information will appropriately adapt the breadth and depth of the examination.

STEP #3: Identify *special concerns.*
• Insidious onset of weakness associated with pain.

STEP #4: Create a symptom timeline and sketch the anatomy (if needed).

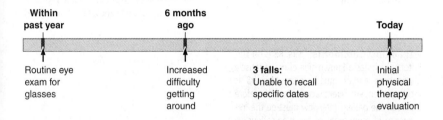

Within past year	6 months ago		Today
Routine eye exam for glasses	Increased difficulty getting around	**3 falls:** Unable to recall specific dates	Initial physical therapy evaluation

STEP #5: Create a diagnostic hypothesis list considering all possible forms of *remote* and *local* pathology that could cause the patient's chief concern.

T   Trauma

    Compression neuropathy of femoral nerve
    Hydromyelia (syringomyelia)
    Spinal cord compression/radicular pain
    Spinal cord injuries

I   Inflammation

    Aseptic
    Chronic inflammatory demyelinating
      polyneuropathy

    Inflammatory myopathies:
    • Dermatomyositis
    • Inclusion body myositis
    • Polymyositis
    Lambert-Eaton myasthenic syndrome
    Lyme disease (tick paralysis)
    Multifocal motor neuropathy
    Multiple sclerosis
    Rheumatoid arthritis of lumbar spine,
      hips, knees
    Systemic lupus erythematosus

STEP #6: Sort the diagnostic hypothesis list by epidemiology and specific case characteristics.

T   Trauma

    Compression neuropathy of femoral nerve
    Hydromyelia (syringomyelia)
    Spinal cord compression/radicular pain
    ~~Spinal cord injuries~~ (no mechanism of injury)

I   Inflammation

    Aseptic
    ~~Chronic inflammatory demyelinating~~
      ~~polyneuropathy~~ (typically symmetrical
      distal to proximal weakness)
    Inflammatory myopathies:
    • Dermatomyositis
    • Inclusion body myositis
    • ~~Polymyositis~~ (age of patient)
    Lambert-Eaton myasthenic syndrome
    Lyme disease (tick paralysis)
    ~~Multifocal motor neuropathy~~ (time course)
    ~~Multiple sclerosis~~ (age of patient)
    Rheumatoid arthritis of lumbar spine, hips,
      knees
    ~~Systemic lupus erythematosus~~ (age of patient)

Septic

Septic arthritis of lumbar spine, hips, knees

M Metabolic

Diabetic neuropathy

Medication toxicity/toxic myopathy

Mitochondrial myopathies

Myasthenia gravis

Toxic myopathy

Septic

Septic arthritis of lumbar spine, hips, knees

M Metabolic

~~Diabetic neuropathy~~ (no history of diabetes mellitus)

~~Medication toxicity~~ (per patient report, her medications are managed by her internist every 6 months)

~~Mitochondrial myopathies~~ (patient age not common for age of onset)

~~Myasthenia gravis~~ (patient age not common for age of onset)

~~Toxic myopathy~~ (typically distal to proximal presentation, no exposure to toxic agent)

Teaching Comments: Mrs. RS is on Lipitor, which has a known side effect of muscle weakness and/or muscle pain. Mrs. RS is being seen via direct access and therefore part of the patient interview must be the frequency of monitoring of her medications by her internist. In response to this questioning, she states she sees her MD every 6 months.

Va Vascular

Arteriovenous malformation
Normal pressure hydrocephalus
Transient ischemic attack/stroke

Vasculitis

De Degenerative

Deconditioning
Lumbar spine disk herniation with
   radiculopathy
Primary lateral sclerosis
Progressive supranuclear palsy

Tu Tumor

Malignant Primary, such as:
• Brain tumor
Malignant Metastatic, such as:
• Brain metastases
• Spinal metastases
Benign:
Not applicable

Co Congenital

Familial spastic paraplegia

Va Vascular

Arteriovenous malformation
Normal pressure hydrocephalus
~~Transient ischemic attack/stroke~~ (time course of symptoms)

Vasculitis

De Degenerative

Deconditioning
Lumbar spine disk herniation with
   radiculopathy
~~Primary lateral sclerosis~~ (age of onset)
~~Progressive supranuclear palsy~~ (time course, age of onset, no visual disturbance)

Tu Tumor

Malignant Primary, such as:
• Brain tumor
Malignant Metastatic, such as:
• Brain metastases
• Spinal metastases
Benign:
Not applicable

Co Congenital

Familial spastic paraplegia

Ne Neurogenic/Psychogenic

Depression
Hysterical paralysis
Hypochondriasis

Ne Neurogenic/Psychogenic

Depression
Hysterical paralysis
~~Hypochondriasis~~ (may be less likely to
cause falling)

STEP #7: Ask specific questions to rule specific conditions or pathological categories less likely.

- **Do you have numbness or tingling in your legs?** *No.* With this answer, several pathologies that have neurological origins move to less likely on the list.

- **When you use your low back, hips, or knees in an activity, do they hurt and feel weak?** *No.* Rules less likely primary pathology of the lumbar spine, hips, and knees.

- **Have you noticed feeling ill recently?** *No.* Rules less likely conditions that are associated with a prodromal illness.

- **Do you have problems with grasping or holding objects?** *No.* Rules less likely conditions associated with upper extremity weakness.

STEP #8: Re-sort the diagnostic hypothesis list based on the patient's responses to specific questioning.

T Trauma

~~Compression neuropathy of femoral nerve~~
(denies sensory symptoms)
~~Hydromyelia (syringomyelia)~~ (denies
sensory symptoms)
~~Spinal cord compression/radicular pain~~
(denies sensory symptoms, low back pain)

I Inflammation

Aseptic
~~Inflammatory myopathies:~~
- ~~Dermatomyositis~~ (no upper extremity
weakness)
- ~~Inclusion body myositis~~ (no upper
extremity weakness)
~~Lambert-Eaton myasthenic syndrome~~
(denies sensory symptoms)
~~Lyme disease (tick paralysis)~~ (denies sensory
symptoms, denies recent illness, no
presence of rash)
~~Rheumatoid arthritis of lumbar spine, hips,
knees~~ (denies low back, hip, and knee pain)

Septic
~~Septic arthritis of lumbar spine, hips, knees~~
(denies low back, hip, and knee pain)

M Metabolic
Not applicable

Va Vascular
~~Arteriovenous malformation~~ (no reports of
recent illness, performs high cognitive
functions independently including
managing checking account and driving)
~~Normal pressure hydrocephalus~~ (performs
high cognitive functions independently
including managing checking account
and driving)
~~Vasculitis~~ (denies recent illness)

De Degenerative
Deconditioning
~~Lumbar spine disk herniation with
radiculopathy~~ (denies sensory symptoms,
low back pain)

Tu Tumor
Malignant Primary, such as:
- ~~Brain tumor~~ (no reports of recent illness,
performs high cognitive functions
independently including managing
checking account and driving)
Malignant Metastatic, such as:
- ~~Brain metastases~~ (no reports of recent
illness, performs high cognitive functions
independently including managing
checking account and driving)
- ~~Spine metastases~~ (denies low back pain)
Benign:
Not applicable

Co Congenital
~~Familial spastic paraplegia~~ (patient age of
onset not typical)

Ne Neurogenic/Psychogenic
Depression
~~Hysterical paralysis~~ (denies sensory
symptoms)

STEP #9: Perform tests to differentiate among the remaining diagnostic hypotheses.

- **Observation.** The demeanor of the patient was observed to be calm and with clear answers during questioning. Affect appeared appropriate, reducing the likelihood of depression as a primary cause for the patient's self-reported functional deficits.

Teaching Comments: Due to the prevalence of neurological disorders on the differential diagnosis list that could have signs via cognitive changes, the clinician may choose to utilize a clinical exam tool such as the Mini-Mental Status Examination. Although this tool is not diagnostic of a particular pathology, it does assist with screening for cognitive loss.[1]

- **Manual muscle tests of the muscles innervated by the lumbar plexus and femoral nerve:** iliopsoas: 5/5 bilaterally; quadriceps: 4/5 bilaterally, suggesting a role for deconditioning as a cause of the patient's self-reported functional deficits.
- **Neurological exam.** No asymmetries to light touch within the lower extremities. Deep tendon reflexes: 2+ throughout the upper/lower extremities.
- **Temperature.** 97.8°F.

Teaching Comments: Several physiological factors play a role in the change of baseline body temperature in older adults. Temperature testing requires multiple tests in similar conditions, similar time frame and via the same method in order to increase the accuracy.[2]

STEP #10: Re-sort the diagnostic hypothesis list based on the patient's responses to specific tests.

- Deconditioning

STEP #11: Decide on a diagnostic impression.

- Deconditioning

STEP #12: Determine the appropriate patient disposition.

- Initiate physical therapy treatment for Mrs. RS to address diagnostic impression; inform primary internist of visit and plan of care.

Case Outcome

Mrs. RS gave several cues of functional changes with inability to achieve a sitting or standing position or ascend/descend stairs without upper extremity assistance. Only partial data from the physical exam is given as it directly relates to the differential diagnostic list. Further manual muscle testing of the proximal lower extremities found an asymmetrical nonmyotomal pattern of weakness of the gluteal muscles, quadriceps, hamstrings, and calf musculature. Based on her functional concerns and the American College of Sports Medicine's recommendations for strength training in older adults, the plan of care for Mrs. RS consisted of a progressive resistance training program involving the lower extremity major muscle groups and balance activities.[3] The exercise prescription was for 8 to 12 repetitions per exercise. Mrs. RS was seen initially 2 days a week at a clinic with a home exercise program on a third day. After 3 weeks, her sessions in the clinic were reduced to one time a week due to transportation challenges. At the 10th week of care (13 visits), she was discharged to her home program. Significant improvement was noted in her Timed Up and Go test, manual muscle testing, and self-reported quality of life measures including fall risk and perceived activity level.

References

1. Crum RM, Anthony JC, Bassett SS, Folstein MF. Population-based norms for the Mini-Mental State Examination by age and educational level. *JAMA.* May 12, 1993;269(18):2386–2391.
2. Kenney WL, Munce TA. Invited review: aging and human temperature regulation. *J Appl Physiol.* Dec 2003; 95(6):2598–2603
3. Chodzko-Zajko WJ, Proctor DN, et al. American College of Sports Medicine position stand. Exercise and physical activity for older adults. *Med Sci Sports Exerc.* 2009;41 (7):1510–1530.

CHAPTER 35

Palpitations

■ *Jesus F. Dominguez, PT, PhD*

Description of the Symptom

This chapter describes pathology that may lead to palpitations. The term *palpitations* refers to an uncomfortable awareness of the heartbeat, usually associated with a cardiac dysrhythmia. The individual may report noticing a forceful, rapid, irregular, or slow heartbeat and may experience associated symptoms that include light-headedness, shortness of breath, chest discomfort, or frank syncope.

Special Concerns

The therapist should be prepared to administer basic life support interventions or activate the emergency medical system should an individual present with palpitations in association with any of the following:

■ Significant shortness of breath, chest discomfort, light-headedness, or presyncopal symptoms (faintness, dizziness, weakness, etc)

■ Marked hypertension (>220/110) or hypotension (<90/60 in an individual who is typically normotensive)

■ Occurring suddenly (paroxysmal) and lasting longer than 15 to 20 minutes with associated symptoms

Individuals who experience palpitations and who also have a family history of sudden death represent a high-risk population. These individuals merit special consideration and the therapist should initiate a timely referral to the appropriate health care provider for definitive assessment.

Overview of Palpitations

Palpitations are a conscious awareness of one's own heartbeat. The sensation may be described as a pounding, racing, or irregular heartbeat and can usually be felt in the chest, throat, or neck. Often, the individual reports a *fluttering in the chest* or a *skipped beat*.

CHAPTER PREVIEW: Conditions That May Lead to Palpitations

T Trauma

COMMON

Exercise 731

UNCOMMON

Obstructive sleep apnea 734

RARE

Postsurgical repair of congenital heart disease 737

I Inflammation

COMMON

Aseptic
Not applicable

Septic
Fever 731

(continued)

PALPITATIONS

Inflammation (*continued*)

UNCOMMON

Aseptic
Cardiomyopathies:
- Arrhythmogenic right ventricular cardiomyopathy 727
- Dilated cardiomyopathy 727
- Hypertrophic cardiomyopathy (hypertrophic obstructive cardiomyopathy) 728
- Restrictive cardiomyopathy 728

Septic
Not applicable

RARE

Aseptic
Mastocytosis 733

Septic
Pericarditis 736

M Metabolic

COMMON

Central nervous system stimulants 728:
- Caffeine 729
- Ephedrine (herbal ephedra) 729
- Nicotine 729
Dehydration/hypovolemia 730
Menopause 733
Pregnancy 737

UNCOMMON

Anemia 725
Cocaine and other illicit stimulants 729
Electrolyte imbalance 731
Hyperthyroidism/thyrotoxicosis 732
Hypoglycemia 732
Side effect of medications 738:
- Alpha-1 blockers 738
- Beta blockers 738
- Beta-2 agonists 738
- Digoxin 739
- Lasix 739
- Nitrates and calcium channel blockers 739
- Potassium supplement 739

RARE

Not applicable

Va Vascular

COMMON

Congestive heart failure 729
Coronary artery/atherosclerotic heart disease 730

Vascular *(continued)*

UNCOMMON
Orthostatic hypotension (postural orthostatic tachycardia syndrome) 735
Pulmonary hypertension 737

RARE
Pulmonary embolus 737

De Degenerative

COMMON
Not applicable

UNCOMMON
Pacemaker/automatic implantable cardioverter defibrillator failure 735

RARE
Sick sinus syndrome 738

Tu Tumor

COMMON
Not applicable

UNCOMMON
Not applicable

RARE
Malignant Primary:
Not applicable
Malignant Metastatic:
Not applicable
Benign, such as:
• Myxoma 734
• Pheochromocytoma 736

Co Congenital

COMMON
Not applicable

UNCOMMON
Aortic insufficiency (aortic regurgitation) 727
Mitral valve prolapse 734

RARE
Wolff-Parkinson-White syndrome (pre-excitation syndrome) 739

Ne Neurogenic/Psychogenic

COMMON
Anxiety/panic disorder 726
Muscular fasciculations 734

(continued)

Neurogenic/Psychogenic *(continued)*

UNCOMMON
Vasovagal syncope (neurocardiogenic syncope, common faint) 739

RARE
Not applicable

Note: These are estimates of relative incidence because few data are available for the less common conditions.

Palpitations may be precipitated by anxiety, fever, lack of sleep, caffeine, certain medications, cocaine and other amphetamines, hyperthyroidism, anemia, and vigorous exercise. More serious causes include abnormalities of the heart valves, electrical conduction system, and myocardial tissue, as well as coronary artery disease and heart failure. These latter pathologies often lead to the development of more complex cardiac dysrhythmias. Palpitations may occur as isolated, transient events or in association with more serious symptoms such as dizziness, light-headedness, shortness of breath, chest discomfort, and syncope.

Palpitations occur in most individuals, even in the absence of underlying heart disease. In general, clinical experience suggests that they are most often due to cardiac dysrhythmias or anxiety.[1,2] Although the majority of these episodes represent little risk to health, some cardiac dysrhythmias can lead to sudden death. With experience, the therapist can develop critical skills that allow a distinction to be made between benign palpitations and more serious conditions that place the patient's life at risk. Normal sinus rhythm may usually be inferred when the pulse is noted to be regular and within the range of 60 to 100 beats per minute (bpm), although atrial flutter with a fixed ventricular response, 2° atrioventricular block Type II, or accelerated atrioventricular junctional rhythm cannot be ruled out by this method alone. A regular pulse that is >100 bpm typically indicates a tachycardia (either sinus, ventricular, or supraventricular), whereas one that is <60 bpm can be associated with sinus bradycardia, atrioventricular junctional rhythm, 2° atrioventricular block, or complete heart block. Because of its irregularly irregular pattern, atrial fibrillation is usually identifiable with a reasonable degree of certainty by palpation of the patient's pulse. However, the definitive assessment tool for identifying a particular dysrhythmia is the electrocardiographic (ECG) monitor. In practice, most physical therapy settings may not have immediate access to an ECG monitor. For that reason, assessment of palpitations by physical therapists should be based on subjective data and pertinent physical findings (ie, the severity of symptoms and the associated hemodynamic consequences).

This chapter was written with the premise that few, if any, patients who experience palpitations will seek advice from a physical therapist prior to consultation with a physician. The more likely scenario is one in which the patient is being seen by a therapist for another health issue and happens to mention these symptoms during the course of treatment. The patient should always be encouraged to report symptoms of palpitations to a physician for definitive evaluation and management, or more appropriately, the therapist may inform the physician directly. Furthermore, reporting of palpitations by an individual with a family history of sudden death necessitates timely medical referral. Figure 35-1, which is a flowchart adapted from Bates,[3] demonstrates examples of pulse rates and the most likely associated cardiac rhythms. Box 35-1 presents key clinical findings noted by Abbott[1] in patients with palpitations and their suggested diagnoses. Both references provide the physical therapist with general guidelines for dysrhythmia identification in the absence of ECG monitoring and likely precipitating diagnoses. However, the therapist is reminded that the guidelines are not intended to supersede assessment of symptom severity and hemodynamic status in guiding the appropriate course of action.

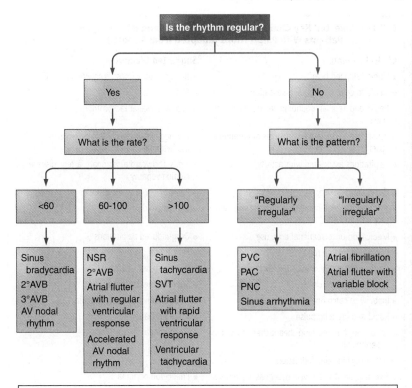

FIGURE 35-1 Flowchart depicting the most likely cardiac dysrhythmias associated with palpitations distinguished on the basis of pulse rate and regularity. (Adapted from Bates.[3])

Description of Conditions That May Lead to Palpitations

■ Anemia

Chief Clinical Characteristics

This presentation includes a rapid and regular pulse, suggesting the presence of sinus tachycardia. Associated symptoms include lethargy, cold skin, depression, easy fatigability, shortness of breath, and cognitive impairment.[4]

Background Information

This condition involves a decrease in the oxygen-carrying capacity of blood secondary to:

1. A decrease in the erythrocyte (red blood cell) content of blood,

2. A diminished content of hemoglobin per erythrocyte, or

3. A combination of both.[5]

It can arise from failed synthesis, premature destruction, hemorrhage, or deficiencies in iron, vitamin B_{12}, or folic acid. Other conditions that render the patient susceptible to anemia include recent major surgery (eg, orthopedic and cardiopulmonary surgeries), pregnancy, lesions of the gastrointestinal tract, sickle cell trait, and cancer.[6] The resultant reduction in the blood's oxygen-carrying capacity initiates a reflex sinus tachycardia in attempts to maintain adequate tissue oxygenation while blood pressure is usually within the normal resting range.[7] If this condition is

---

BOX 35-1 **Selected Key Clinical Findings and Their Suggested Diagnoses in Patients With Palpitations (adapted from Abbott[1])**

Clinical Findings	Suggested Diagnoses
• Single "skipped beat"	• Benign ectopy (most likely PACs or PVCs)
• Single forceful or pounding sensation	• PVC
• Rapid and regular pounding in the neck and chest	• Supraventricular tachycardia
• Palpitations associated with stress or emotional upset	• Psychogenic or catecholamine-sensitive dysrhythmia
• Palpitations associated with activity	• Sinus tachycardia, coronary artery disease, or cardiomyopathy
• Generalized anxiety	• Panic attack or panic disorder
• Thyromegaly, heat intolerance, tremors, sweating, exophthalmos	• Hyperthyroidism
• Medication or recreational drug use	• Drug-induced palpitations
• Pericardial friction rub	• Pericarditis
• Cardiac murmur or midsystolic click	• Valvular heart disease
• Palpitations since childhood	• Supraventricular tachycardia
• Inability to catch one's breath	• PVCs or ventricular tachycardia
• Rapid and irregular pulse	• Atrial fibrillation
• Loud snoring, morning headaches, systemic hypertension	• Sleep apnea
• Lethargy, cold skin, depression	• Anemia
• Sweating, headache, severe hypertension, feelings of doom	• Pheochromocytoma
• Third heart sound, shortness of breath, peripheral edema	• Congestive heart failure

---

suspected, the patient should be referred to his or her primary care practitioner for further evaluation. The diagnosis is confirmed by routine blood testing. Treatment involves addressing the underlying cause of anemia, including iron supplementation.

■ **Anxiety/Panic Disorder**

Chief Clinical Characteristics

This condition is characterized by an acute increase in heartbeat that is both rapid and forceful. The pulse is typically rapid and regular and associated with a discrete period of intense fear or discomfort during which several predictable symptoms develop and peak in intensity within 10 minutes. These symptoms can include palpitations, sweating or flushing, muscle tension, headaches, insomnia, changes in appetite, nausea, vomiting, diarrhea, edginess, and irritability.[8]

Background Information

The body's response to this condition is usually short-lived and subsides when the individual is reassured or the stressful stimulus is removed. Although anxiety or stress is perceived by many areas of the brain, the integrated response ultimately leads to elevation of plasma cortisol and catecholamine levels. Both hormones are responsible for raising blood pressure and cardiac output by increasing heart rate, cardiac contractile force, and vasoconstriction. The response leads to a general state of arousal and prepares the individual for useful defensive behavior (ie, the "fight-or-flight" response). In the absence of other adverse symptoms or underlying cardiovascular pathology, palpitations due to stress pose no serious risk and the therapist should reinforce this in the mind of the patient. Disabling cases of this condition should be referred to the appropriate health care provider and may include pharmacologic and psychological therapy.

■ Aortic Insufficiency (Aortic Regurgitation)

Chief Clinical Characteristics
This presentation often involves weakness, significant lethargy, and severe dyspnea. Isolated systolic hypertension is often noted on assessment of blood pressure. An early symptom is an awareness of the heartbeat due to increased stroke volume as a result of elevated end-diastolic volume. The heartbeat may be described as forceful or uncomfortable. Patients with this condition may also present with anginal symptoms because of the reduced coronary perfusion associated with decreased diastolic pressure. Other symptoms include exertional dyspnea, orthopnea, paroxysmal nocturnal dyspnea, and palpitations. In chronic forms of this condition, there is a rapid runoff of blood back into the left ventricle during cardiac diastole that results in a low peripheral diastolic pressure. A wide pulse pressure is also present secondary to the elevated systolic pressure created by enhanced stroke volume and the low diastolic blood pressure created by the retrograde flow of blood.

Background Information
A common clinical finding during cardiac auscultation is a diastolic murmur typically heard best along the left sternal border, although it can be heard over the right second intercostal space as well.[9] The murmur of the acute form of this condition is short and low frequency in nature. The murmur of this condition in its chronic state is high in frequency, has a blowing quality, and tends to be of longer duration than in the acute form. There also appears to be an association between aortic insufficiency combined with ventricular septal defect and an increased incidence of dysrhythmias.[10] The palpitations are often the result of resting sinus tachycardia in response to peripheral hypotension. This condition is a disorder of the aortic valve in which the annulus or leaflets weaken or balloon, leading to retrograde flow of blood from the aorta into the left ventricle during diastole. It may be the result of any condition that weakens the valve leaflets or annulus, including congenital valvular defects (eg, bicuspid aortic valve), rheumatic fever, endocarditis, Marfan's syndrome, hypertension, aortic dissection, Reiter's syndrome, ankylosing spondylitis, syphilis, or Ehlers-Danlos syndrome. Diagnosis and assessment of severity are made on the basis of echocardiography and angiography. Patients should be referred to their medical practitioner if this condition is suspected and the therapist should be prepared to administer cardiopulmonary resuscitation or activate the emergency medical system if the palpitations are associated with other signs or symptoms of significant hemodynamic instability.

CARDIOMYOPATHIES

■ Arrhythmogenic Right Ventricular Cardiomyopathy

Chief Clinical Characteristics
This presentation includes dyspnea on exertion, paroxysmal (of sudden onset) nocturnal dyspnea, orthopnea, angina, palpitations, and syncope. This variant's presentation can also range from asymptomatic to signs and symptoms of heart failure, fatigue, lightheadedness, syncope, and palpitations that may be associated with sweating.

Background Information
The palpitations may be due to single premature ventricular contractions, atrial fibrillation, or ventricular tachycardia. Diagnosis is made by biopsy and typically reveals replacement of myocardial tissue with fibrous connective tissue and fat deposits.[11] In some instances, the rhythm may deteriorate into pulseless ventricular fibrillation and the patient will lose consciousness. Cardiopulmonary resuscitation, use of an automated external defibrillator if available, and activation of the emergency medical system are warranted.

■ Dilated Cardiomyopathy

Chief Clinical Characteristics
This presentation involves dyspnea on exertion, paroxysmal nocturnal dyspnea, orthopnea, angina, palpitations, and syncope. This variant is distinguished by the appreciation of pulmonary crackles (secondary to pulmonary edema), a weak or laterally displaced cardiac point of maximal impulse, sacral/pretibial/ankle edema, and sudden significant weight gain. Associated symptoms may include general fatigue/tiredness,

shortness of breath, chest discomfort, and palpitations.[12]

Background Information

Several predisposing conditions have been linked to the development of this condition, including atherosclerotic heart disease, genetic/familial inheritance, viral infection, excessive alcohol consumption, pregnancy, and autoimmune disease.[13] This condition often progresses to congestive heart failure. The specific rhythm disturbance noted as palpitations may be atrial fibrillation, ventricular ectopy/ventricular tachycardia, or atrioventricular heart block. In rare cases, the rhythm may deteriorate into ventricular fibrillation and the patient will lose consciousness. Immediate basic life support, including use of an automatic external defibrillator if available, should be administered while the emergency medical system is being activated.

■ Hypertrophic Cardiomyopathy (Hypertrophic Obstructive Cardiomyopathy)

Chief Clinical Characteristics

This presentation can include dyspnea on exertion, paroxysmal nocturnal dyspnea, orthopnea, angina, palpitations, and syncope. This variant also includes progressive shortness of breath, chest discomfort, chronic palpitations, and syncope typically manifesting in early adulthood (mid-20s) and should be considered in young athletes who present with these symptoms. A harsh systolic murmur heard best along the left sternal border may be appreciated upon auscultation. With dynamic auscultation, the therapist will note that the murmur's intensity increases when the patient is asked to perform and hold a Valsalva maneuver and decreases when the patient resumes normal breathing.[13]

Background Information

A decrease in the intensity of the murmur is also noted when the patient is asked to move from a standing position to a squatting position. In both cases, a larger left ventricular end-diastolic volume is associated with a diminished murmur intensity. Dysrhythmias associated with this condition can be of supraventricular or ventricular origin and can lead to hemodynamic compromise. This condition accounts for more than 50% of all sudden death cases in young individuals below the age of 25 years.[14] Young patients with suspicious symptoms and in whom a previously undiagnosed harsh holosystolic murmur is heard along the right upper sternal border and cardiac apex should be referred to their physician for further evaluation prior to initiating vigorous physical exercise. The therapist is reminded that a preexisting primary diagnosis of cardiomyopathy requires careful and direct patient monitoring.[15] If palpitations are associated with hemodynamic compromise or collapse, the emergency medical system should be activated immediately.

■ Restrictive Cardiomyopathy

Chief Clinical Characteristics

This presentation typically involves dyspnea on exertion, paroxysmal nocturnal dyspnea, orthopnea, angina, palpitations, and syncope. This variant can be characterized by shortness of breath, fatigue/lethargy, peripheral edema, and the presence of abdominal ascites. In some patients, Kussmaul's sign (a rise in jugular venous distension upon inspiration) is also noted and suggests reduced right ventricular compliance.

Background Information

Most often the source of this form of palpitations is atrial fibrillation or atrioventricular heart block secondary to infiltrative involvement of the cardiac conduction system.[13] With the latter rhythm disturbance, the therapist may note the patient's pulse to be significantly bradycardic (<60 bpm) and the patient may report light-headedness or presyncopal aura. Diagnosis is made on the basis of clinical findings and diagnostic procedures such as echocardiography, angiography, and endomyocardial biopsy. In the event of palpitations with hemodynamic compromise, the emergency medical system should be activated immediately.

CENTRAL NERVOUS SYSTEM STIMULANTS

Chief Clinical Characteristics

This presentation typically includes an increased heart rate, which is sensed by the individual as a rapid or bounding pulse.[16] In most cases, the rhythm is a sinus tachycardia and the pulse is noted to be rapid and regular, although some reentrant tachyarrhythmias may be associated with an irregular pulse.

Background Information

If the tachyarrhythmia is pronounced, diastolic filling will be significantly impaired and the pulse may be absent, causing the patient to rapidly become hemodynamically unstable. Common substances that cause this condition include:

■ Caffeine

This substance is a neuronal stimulant that occurs naturally in various food products, including coffee, tea, and cocoa. It is known to be a competitive antagonist of adenosine receptors, potentiate increased intracellular calcium release, and reduce AV nodal refractoriness, all of which can contribute to the genesis of dysrhythmias.[17] In low doses (<250 mg), caffeine is known to elicit elation, peacefulness, and pleasantness, whereas at high doses (>500 mg), it can lead to the emergence of unfavorable side effects, including anxiety, irritability, palpitations, and nausea.[18]

■ Ephedrine (Herbal Ephedra)

This alkaloid substance possesses adrenergic properties that include shortening of the cardiac refractory period, increased chronotropy, increased inotropy, and increased peripheral resistance as a result of vasoconstriction.[19] Common side effects of ephedra include hypertension associated with palpitations, tachycardia, or both.

■ Nicotine

This substance acts in a manner similar to the endogenous neurotransmitter acetylcholine to stimulate postsynaptic neurons of the autonomic nervous system. However, its effects are longer lasting than acetylcholine because it is not degraded by cholinesterases. In the event of palpitations associated with hemodynamic instability, administration of basic life support measures should be provided immediately and activation of the emergency medical system is warranted. Careful attention to the patient's dietary habits and smoking history during the

interview process will alert the therapist to the habitual use of these stimulants as a possible cause of the palpitations. Subsequent recommendations to reduce or even eliminate these substances from the diet and lifestyle are often beneficial in minimizing or eliminating future episodes.

■ Cocaine and Other Illicit Stimulants

Chief Clinical Characteristics

This presentation typically involves palpitations, hypertension, shortness of breath, agitation, bizarre and/or erratic behavior, and chest discomfort. Often, the patient's pupils become dilated and he or she may report a history of chronic nose bleeding (this latter finding is the result of nasal septum and vascular deterioration).

Background Information

Careful questioning during the initial interview may provide clues to the patient's use of cocaine or other sympathomimetic drugs. Classified as a sympathomimetic drug, cocaine simulates a state of heightened sympathetic activity by stimulating the release of epinephrine and norepinephrine from the adrenal medulla and blocking the reuptake of norepinephrine at preganglionic synaptic nerve endings.[20] It is known to induce dose-dependent increases in heart rate and systolic and diastolic blood pressure.[21] The palpitations are often driven by cocaine-induced sinus tachycardia, but heart rhythm may deteriorate into ventricular tachycardia and ventricular fibrillation. Palpitations may range from a self-limiting episode to sudden death. In the event of the latter, the emergency medical system should be activated and the therapist should begin to render basic life support measures. Exercise is contraindicated in patients who present with signs/symptoms suspicious for acute cocaine intoxication.

■ Congestive Heart Failure

Chief Clinical Characteristics

This presentation includes a wide variety of palpitation symptoms from slow and forceful to rapid and weak. Associated symptoms may include shortness of breath, chest discomfort, or light-headedness/syncope. Various physical findings, such as peripheral/pretibial edema, pulmonary crackles, an auscultated S_3 cardiac sound, cyanosis, and sudden and dramatic *weight gain, provide clues to the presence of this condition.*

Background Information

In patients with this condition who present with palpitations, the dysrhythmias can originate from either the ventricles or supraventricular structures (eg, atrial fibrillation). However, ventricular dysrhythmias may be more likely to result in sudden death. In this condition's chronic form, several factors contribute to the development of episodic dysrhythmias. These include mechanical stretch of cardiomyocytes leading to hyperirritability and spontaneous discharge, abnormal intracellular calcium handling, and repolarization abnormalities.[22] Electrolyte balance is typically upset in these individuals, both as a result of chronic fluid retention and the depletion of certain electrolytes by various medications used to treat the condition (eg, potassium-depleting diuretics). The use of digoxin to improve cardiac contractility in these patients may in some cases precipitate bradycardia, secondary to slowing of the electrical conduction through the atrioventricular node, or tachycardia, secondary to enhancement of automaticity in Purkinje fibers. By communicating with the patient's physician, the therapist plays a crucial role during titration of the patient's medical regimen. Definitive diagnosis is made by echocardiography or angiography. As with atherosclerotic heart disease, supplemental oxygen prescribed by the patient's physician can improve symptoms and suppress the palpitations in some cases. However, if the patient becomes unstable, the emergency medical system should be activated.

■ Coronary Artery/Atherosclerotic Heart Disease

Chief Clinical Characteristics

This presentation can include a pulse that is noted to range from bradycardic to tachycardic during an ischemic event.[23] Individuals with this condition may also experience symptoms of angina, often described as substernal chest discomfort, pressure, heaviness, squeezing, or burning that radiates to the shoulders, arms (left greater than right), neck, jaw, and epigastrium.

Background Information

With decreased myocardial oxygen supply (or increased demand in the case of exertion),

vulnerable myocardial cells become ischemic, hyperirritable, and discharge spontaneously, driving abnormal cardiac rhythms. The ectopic rhythm can be supraventricular or ventricular in origin, tachycardic or bradycardic (in the case of complete heart block), and is difficult to differentiate on the basis of palpation alone. In the elderly population, heart block and sinus bradycardia are the most common dysrhythmias, followed by premature atrial and ventricular beats, with atrial fibrillation being the most common sustained rhythm.[24] In cases of tachyarrhythmias, the resulting increase in myocardial oxygen demand may escalate the condition from one of transient ischemia to one of frank infarction and the episode may become life threatening. Use of sublingual nitroglycerin or supplemental oxygen prescribed by the patient's physician may resolve minor episodes and the palpitations usually subside. However, if the patient becomes unstable during episodes of palpitations with associated angina pectoris, activation of the emergency medical system is warranted. The therapist should be prepared to administer basic life support measures (including the use of an automated external defibrillator if warranted) while awaiting advanced cardiac life support assistance.

■ Dehydration/Hypovolemia

Chief Clinical Characteristics

This presentation involves increased heart rate and augmentation of cardiac contractile force often described by the patient as a fast and bounding pulse. Associated symptoms may include lethargy, poor concentration, tremors, light-headedness, constipation, and dry mouth.

Background Information

In most cases, the rhythm is sinus tachycardia and the therapist will note a rapid but regular pulse that may be slightly diminished in strength. If this condition is profound, the therapist may note cyanosis of the lips, sunken eyes, cold extremities, failure of skin to bounce back when it is lightly pinched and released, confusion, and syncope. Dehydration due to sweat loss and/or inadequate fluid replacement during physical exertion can lead to a significant decrease in central blood volume. Reflexively, the sympathetic nervous system increases heart rate and contractile force to maintain mean arterial pressure. The magnitude of the tachycardic response is highly correlated with the severity of hypovolemia. Older patients tend to be at higher risk for dehydration as age-related decreases in total body water, sensitivity to aldosterone and antidiuretic hormone, and thirst perception render them more vulnerable.[25] This condition can be avoided by reminding the patient to drink fluids during exercise sessions in the clinic, especially if the exercise is aerobic and will be maintained at high intensity for greater than 20 to 30 minutes. Mild hypovolemia necessitates fluid replacement, which may be accomplished by having the patient lie in a semirecumbent position and drink water as the therapist monitors signs and symptoms. More severe cases of hypovolemia associated with unstable signs/symptoms usually require activation of the emergency medical system and administration of intravenous fluids.

■ **Electrolyte Imbalance**

Chief Clinical Characteristics
This presentation may involve symptoms of palpitations often associated with lethargy, shortness of breath, chest discomfort, lightheadedness, and syncope.

Background Information
This condition (in particular, hypokalemia and hyperkalemia) may result from dehydration, hemorrhage, hypovolemia, use of potassium-depleting medications (eg, thiazide diuretics), and excessive potassium supplementation. Deviation of electrolyte values from normal ranges may predispose the patient to life-threatening dysrhythmias. For example, hypokalemia (<4 mmol/L) is significantly associated with serious ventricular dysrhythmias, including ventricular tachycardia and ventricular fibrillation.[26] Hyperkalemia is also correlated with the generation of severe dysrhythmias, purportedly by altering acid–base balance and cardiac myocyte function.[27] Ventricular rhythm disturbances will significantly impair cardiac output and may lead to hemodynamic collapse. The therapist will note absent pulses, and cardiopulmonary resuscitation should be initiated while the emergency medical system is being activated. Electrolyte imbalance can be confirmed by routine blood tests and the therapist should refer the patient to the primary care physician for assessment if the condition is suspected.

■ **Exercise**

Chief Clinical Characteristics
This presentation typically involves a pulse that increases gradually and appropriately for the intensity of the exercise bout. When the exercise bout is terminated, the pulse gradually returns to resting values. Assessment of the blood pressure will typically reveal elevated systolic values that are appropriate for the intensity of physical exertion (eg, 10 to 12 mm Hg increase for every metabolic equivalent increase in workload).

Background Information
In response to the metabolic demands placed on the cardiopulmonary system by activities involving the contraction of large muscle groups, cardiac output will increase. This is primarily accomplished by enhanced cardiac automaticity and contractility, yielding a substantial increase in heart rate and a moderate increase in stroke volume. To the individual who is typically sedentary or otherwise unaccustomed to exercise, the resultant sinus tachycardia and vigorous force of cardiac contraction may be felt as a rapid or pounding pulse. The response is mediated by enhanced sympathetic outflow and circulating catecholamines involved in the "fight-or-flight" response and does not typically lead to any adverse consequences in the absence of underlying organic heart disease. This is a normal response to exertion and will subside with cessation of the exercise bout. No emergency intervention is warranted.

■ **Fever**

Chief Clinical Characteristics
This presentation may include a rapid or bounding pulse that can often be felt in the area of the temples (eg, a pounding headache). These features can also be appreciated by palpating the patient's pulse and noting a rapid, regular rhythm that is most suggestive of sinus tachycardia. This presentation may be associated with an acute pattern of fever and malaise.

Background Information
An assessment of temperature usually confirms the presence of fever and identifies it as a

possible contributor to the palpitations. Fever, typically a core temperature >98.6°F, is a systemic response to invading microorganisms or other inflammatory processes. It is primarily regulated by a cluster of neurons in the hypothalamus that act as a physiological thermostat. During febrile states, the autonomic nervous system and inflammatory mediators act to increase heart rate and route blood to the body's surface for heat exchange as well as to support the increased metabolic rate of inflammatory cells.[28] In most cases, this condition precludes the patient from participating in exercise until the process resolves. Fever lasting longer than 3 to 4 days typically indicates the need for referral to an appropriate health care practitioner.

■ Hyperthyroidism/Thyrotoxicosis

Chief Clinical Characteristics

This presentation often includes hypertension, dyspnea (ie, orthopnea, exertional dyspnea, and paroxysmal nocturnal dyspnea), and rapid, bounding palpitations that may lead to feelings of dizziness or light-headedness. Atrial fibrillation is not common before the age of 50 but is present in up to 20% of older patients.[29] Associated signs and symptoms include nervousness, heat intolerance, fatigue, weight loss despite increased appetite, sweating, tremors, and exophthalmos.[30] In some individuals, a goiter may also be present (Fig. 35-2).

Background Information

The most common dysrhythmia associated with this condition is sinus tachycardia, although supraventricular dysrhythmias

(particularly atrial fibrillation) can occur and may pose a serious health risk for individuals with known coronary artery disease or history of stroke.[31] Individuals with this condition often fail to exhibit the expected decrease in heart rate during sleep, with little or no difference between resting heart rate during the waking and sleeping hours. Monitoring heart rate during sleep is often helpful in confirming this finding. Palpitations in individuals with this condition are typically chronic, felt during resting states, and exaggerated with activity. This condition is characterized by overactivity of the thyroid gland and primarily results in elevated levels of thyroid hormones in the bloodstream, while thyrotoxicosis refers to the clinical syndrome resulting from hyperthyroidism. Typical etiologies include Graves' disease (often associated with exophthalmos), excessive thyroid hormone replacement therapy, toxic adenoma, thyroiditis, goiter, and use of amiodarone or iodine-containing radiographic contrast agents. Thyroid hormones are known to enhance myocardial contractility and elevate the body's metabolic rate, leading to arterial vasodilation and possible hypotension. A reflex tachycardia may ensue to counteract the hypotension. If this condition is suspected, the individual should be referred to a medical practitioner for definitive assessment. The diagnosis is made on the basis of blood tests that indicate elevated thyroid hormone levels. Management of this condition may include pharmacologic administration of iodine, antithyroid medications, and surgical thyroidectomy.

■ Hypoglycemia

Chief Clinical Characteristics

This presentation can be characterized by a pulse that is noted to be tachycardic but regular. The suspicion of hypoglycemia can be quickly confirmed by asking the patient (if diabetic) to utilize his or her personal glucose monitor (or the facility's monitor) if available. Associated signs and symptoms often include headache, slurred speech, dizziness, feelings of "vagueness," impaired motor function, anxiety, sweating, shakiness, pallor, increased systolic blood pressure, disorientation, weakness, and palpitations.[32]

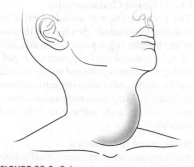

FIGURE 35-2 Goiter.

Background Information

The rhythm is usually a reflex tachycardia in response to the hypoglycemic state. Low blood glucose (hypoglycemia) in patients with diabetes may result from excess ingestion of insulin/oral hypoglycemic agents or insufficient food intake in relation to insulin/oral hypoglycemic dose. In people who do not have diabetes, this condition may result from insufficient caloric intake/ starvation or an abnormal increase in physical activity or exercise in the absence of proper nutrition. The onset of signs and symptoms typically occurs when blood sugar falls below 50 mg/dL, and findings can be divided into two categories: those related to the activation of the autonomic nervous system and those caused by altered cerebral function. The condition can be readily reversed by having the patient immediately ingest a source of concentrated carbohydrate such as sugar, honey, candy, or orange juice. Vital signs should be monitored until they return to normal values. The therapist should be prepared to administer supportive care or activate the emergency medical system should the patient lapse into a diabetic coma (typically preceded by convulsions and unresponsiveness). Individuals with this condition related to diabetes mellitus should be reminded to check blood glucose levels periodically and to avoid exercising during the peak insulin effect to prevent episodes of hypoglycemia.

■ Mastocytosis

Chief Clinical Characteristics

This presentation may include rash, itchy skin, abdominal discomfort, diarrhea, nausea and vomiting, bone pain, ulcers, skin lesions, severe hypotension, fainting, and bronchiolar constriction with labored breathing during an anaphylactic reaction. Palpitations may also be associated with the increased release of histamine.[33]

Background Information

Typically, the underlying rhythm is sinus tachycardia and the pulse is felt to be rapid and regular. Symptoms typically stem from excessive release of histamine (a vasoactive chemical released by mast cells during the normal allergic reaction to an antigen or allergen). Mastocytosis can occur in two forms. Individuals with cutaneous mastocytosis (urticaria pigmentosa) typically present with dark brown lesions on the skin that may become itchy if rubbed or scratched. Systemic mastocytosis is confirmed by taking a tissue biopsy (eg, bone marrow) and examining it for the presence of increased mast cell counts. This condition is a term for a group of disorders characterized by an overabundance of mast cells (especially plentiful in the skin and digestive tract). In both forms, the mast cells are triggered to release chemotactic agents by the presence of an allergen.[34] Antihistamine medications and epinephrine are useful as a first-line treatment for an acute episode and the patient should be reminded to avoid the triggering source if known. The therapist should monitor the patient for signs of hypotension and presyncope and be prepared to administer supportive care. In the event of severe anaphylactic shock, the therapist should activate the emergency medical system.

■ Menopause

Chief Clinical Characteristics

This presentation can be characterized by a rapid pulse that may be associated with depression/moodiness/irritability, shortness of breath, numbness or tingling of extremities, hot flashes, sleeplessness, loss of appetite, poor concentration, and early morning awakenings.[35]

Background Information

The palpitations associated with menopause are generally benign and self-limiting. There is strong evidence to suggest that hormonal changes accompanying menopause likely contribute to increased incidence of palpitations, likely mediated by the effects of estradiol on electrophysiological parameters.[36] The palpitations may be secondary to altered autonomic control of cardiovascular function in the presence of altered hormonal balance. It has been reported that the female sex hormones slow electrical conduction within the right atrium, prolong the refractory period of atrial tissue, and slow the propagation of electrical conduction through the atrioventricular node.[37] Referral to a physician for evaluation of palpitations is made primarily on the basis of the severity of symptoms and the presence of clinical findings that suggest cardiovascular compromise during episodes.

Mitral Valve Prolapse

Chief Clinical Characteristics

This presentation can include palpitations, chest pain, shortness of breath, fatigue, and light-headedness and may cause periodic syncopal episodes in a small subset of patients.[38] Most individuals with this condition are asymptomatic. Upon cardiac auscultation, a midsystolic click is often heard best over the fifth intercostal space at the midclavicular line, often followed by a late systolic murmur in the presence of mitral valve regurgitation.

Background Information

The palpitations are usually supraventricular in origin and occur paroxysmally. The pulse is typically rapid and regular, although very rapid rates may be difficult to palpate. The palpitation episodes commonly are self-limiting and last several minutes (less often, they may last for hours) during which the patient may experience the other associated symptoms. The diagnosis is confirmed by echocardiography, which usually reveals exaggerated systolic bowing beyond the mitral annulus of one or both valve leaflets. Individuals with this condition may be instructed to cough forcefully or perform a Valsalva maneuver, bearing down against a closed glottis, during episodes of palpitations in an effort to convert the abnormal rhythm through parasympathetic vagal mediation. Quite often, individuals with this condition are also prescribed calcium channel blockers or beta blockers to suppress the occurrence of palpitations. Occasionally, the tachycardia may be prolonged and immediate medical intervention is usually warranted, especially if the patient has underlying coronary artery disease and becomes hemodynamically unstable.

Muscular Fasciculations

Chief Clinical Characteristics

This presentation commonly involves muscular twitching localized to the neck or chest musculature that may be misinterpreted as palpitations.

Background Information

This condition can be quickly identified by observation of rapid muscular contractions, during which examination of the pulse will reveal that the fasciculations and pulse are not coincident. Spontaneously discharging motor units that are visible as rapid muscular contractions cause this condition. The spontaneous discharges may be secondary to vigorous sympathetic activity or in response to any neural irritant.[39] In the absence of neurological disorders, this condition is typically benign. Although this condition can be bothersome, the patient should be assured that the twitching is not associated with any adverse physiological consequences and no treatment is required.

Myxoma

Chief Clinical Characteristics

This presentation typically includes dyspnea, orthopnea, and paroxysmal nocturnal dyspnea in combination with dizziness/light-headedness, palpitations, and syncope.[40] Cardiac auscultation may reveal a mid-diastolic murmur as the myxoma encroaches on the mitral opening during ventricular filling, as well as a tumor plop heard in mid- to late diastole.

Background Information

A myxoma is a primary, most often benign, intracardiac tumor composed of connective tissue surrounded by a mucopolysaccharide coat and anchored to the endocardium. Although rare, the vast majority (>75%) of myxomas form in the left atrium, and if a murmur is present, it is heard best at the fifth intercostal space, midclavicular line. This condition is more common in females than males and involves a generally friable lesion with small fragments that often break free from the main tumor. The site of embolization depends on the cardiac chamber location and the presence of an intracardiac shunt. Larger left atrial myxomas usually interfere with normal cardiac function and significantly obstruct blood flow through the mitral valve. Auscultatory findings suggest, but do not confirm, the presence of an intracardiac tumor and should prompt the therapist to refer the patient to a physician for definitive assessment. The diagnosis is usually confirmed by echocardiography.

Obstructive Sleep Apnea

Chief Clinical Characteristics

This presentation typically involves snoring loudly, morning headaches, systemic hypertension, and daytime somnolence. Individuals with this condition are aroused from sleep continuously throughout the night up to 40 to 60 times per hour and often experience acute shortness of breath and palpitations. The palpitations can be slow or rapid, and the patient may often experience a slight sense of anxiety or restlessness.[41]

Background Information

Several conditions often associated with sleep apnea include obesity, a short thick neck, enlarged adenoids, reduced tone of the soft palate, a deviated nasal septum, and nasal polyps. Individuals with clinical findings suggestive of Pickwickian syndrome—characterized by obesity, alveolar hypoventilation, pulmonary hypertension, cyanosis, daytime somnolence, secondary polycythemia, and right-sided heart failure with peripheral edema—should also be evaluated for the occurrence of obstructive sleep apnea. An opportunity to engage the patient's spouse or significant other during the interview process usually reveals a history of loud snoring and frequent apneic episodes throughout the night. Individuals with this condition rarely attain the deep stages of sleep (rapid eye movement sleep) because of constant hypoxic arousal and, thus, they are sleep deprived. The origin of this condition may be central (cessation of respiratory muscle effort leading to absence of airflow), obstructive (upper airway obstruction), or mixed (airflow and inspiratory efforts stop early in the episode). There may be an associated impairment of cardiac autonomic function characterized by a rise in sympathetic tone accompanied by a withdrawal of parasympathetic activity.[42] Chronic forms of this condition can eventually lead to significant pulmonary hypertension and *cor pulmonale*. The use of a pulse oximeter during the activity assessment is warranted for patients suspected of having sleep apnea, because it often reveals exercise-induced hemoglobin desaturation. If pulmonary hypertension is suggested by history and physical findings in individuals suspected of having this condition, referral to a physician is necessary for further testing, which often includes monitored sleep studies and echocardiography.

■ Orthostatic Hypotension (Postural Orthostatic Tachycardia Syndrome)

Chief Clinical Characteristics

This presentation can include dizziness, lightheadedness, palpitations, shortness of breath, chest discomfort, urinary incontinence, and syncope when assuming a more vertical position.

Background Information

Orthostatic hypotension is defined as a drop in systolic and/or diastolic blood pressure when going from the supine position to sitting or standing. The accepted criteria is a drop of ≥ 20 mm Hg in systolic pressure and/or a drop of ≥ 10 mm Hg in diastolic pressure within 3 minutes of standing.[43] In some patients, a reflex tachycardia (usually an increase in heart rate of ≥ 30 bpm) is noted as the sympathetic nervous system attempts to compensate for the drop in arterial pressure, termed *postural orthostatic tachycardia syndrome* (POTS).[44] Absence of a heart rate increase in the presence of hypotension may imply a more serious neurological component to the disorder. Other factors to consider when evaluating a patient for orthostatic hypotension include the patient's neurological status, prescription of vasoactive medications (eg, calcium channel blocker and beta-blocker medications), prolonged bed rest, and hemorrhagic/hypovolemic states. A tilt table test is most often the initial evaluative procedure for symptoms suggestive of this condition. Patients should be instructed to rise slowly from bed in the morning (eg, sitting at the edge of the bed and performing ankle/calf exercises) or when going from a sitting/squatting to standing position. Symptoms usually dissipate when the patient is placed in a semirecumbent or supine position, although some patients may progress to frank syncope. In this case, the therapist should be prepared to activate the emergency medical system if the patient fails to regain consciousness spontaneously.

■ Pacemaker/Automatic Implantable Cardioverter Defibrillator Failure

Chief Clinical Characteristics

This presentation involves palpitations described as an irregular heart rhythm with a pulse that is usually bradycardic and either regular or irregular, suggesting that the pacemaker is failing to either sense or support the abnormal heart rhythm. If failure of an automatic implantable cardioverter defibrillator occurs in an individual who reports palpitations, the pulse is noted to be tachycardic and regular. Associated symptoms in either case may include lethargy, light-headedness, shortness of breath, and presyncope/syncope.[45]

Background Information

Loss of capture, or the failure of a pacemaker to elicit a cardiac contraction (primarily ventricular), is an uncommon but potentially life-threatening complication of cardiac pacing. This is often caused by movement or dislodgement of the lead wire or physical damage to the lead wire itself. This results in failure of the pacemaker to stimulate ventricular contraction after sensing a missed beat/abnormal rhythm or failing to sense the abnormality altogether. Automatic implantable cardioverter defibrillator malfunction may also involve displacement or damage of a lead wire or failure of the device. When working with an individual who has a permanent pacemaker implanted, the therapist should be aware of the pacemaker's programmed pace rate. This information is readily available from patients' pacemaker identification cards, which should be carried with them at all times. Palpation of a carotid or radial pulse rate that is slower than the documented paced rate should alert the therapist to the possibility of pacemaker failure. Knowing the programmed threshold rate of an individual's automatic implantable cardioverter defibrillator allows the therapist to prescribe exercise intensities that maintain the heart rate below the threshold rate to avoid inadvertent electrical discharge. In the event of inappropriate discharge or function, the automatic implantable cardioverter defibrillator can be disabled temporarily by placing a large magnet over it while the emergency medical system is being activated. Likewise, if the individual becomes symptomatically unstable, the therapist should be prepared to administer basic life support and activate the emergency medical system.

■ Pericarditis

Chief Clinical Characteristics

This presentation is characterized by chest pain and fever as the hallmark symptoms. The chest pain almost always has a mechanical component in that it is aggravated by coughing, sneezing, deep inspiration, and lying supine. This characteristic distinguishes the condition from angina. The sensation of palpitations may also be reported.[1,46] A pericardial friction rub that is likened to two pieces of leather rubbing against one another may be heard during cardiac auscultation. Asking the patient to momentarily hold his or her breath while auscultating helps to distinguish a pericardial from a pleural friction rub (the latter would disappear upon breath-holding).

Background Information

This condition can be either aseptic (eg, post-myocardial infarction, radiation-induced, drug-induced, or connective tissue disease) or septic (eg, viral, pyogenic bacteria, or tuberculosis). Pericarditis is often self-limiting, but individuals with this condition should be referred to their primary care physician for supportive care that may include prescription of anti-inflammatory or antibiotic medication.

■ Pheochromocytoma

Chief Clinical Characteristics

This presentation typically includes sweating, headache, pallor, anxiety, palpitations, severe hypertension, and feelings of imminent death.[47]

Background Information

This condition is caused by a rare tumor that arises from tissue in the chromaffin cells of the adrenal glands. The tumor causes excessive production and release of epinephrine and norepinephrine from the adrenal glands, leading to an enhanced sympathetic state. Among their various effects, both epinephrine and norepinephrine act on *alpha-1* adrenergic receptors in the vasculature and *beta-1* adrenergic receptors in myocardial tissue to elicit vasoconstriction and enhance myocardial contractility and automaticity, respectively. Pheochromocytoma may induce the release of large amounts of hormones after trauma or surgery and can lead to life-threatening complications if unrecognized. Typically, bouts of hypertension are cyclical in nature but can last indefinitely. In cases of marked hypertension or protracted periods of palpitations, the therapist should initiate referral to the primary medical practitioner. The diagnosis is suggested by blood and urine tests that reveal elevated levels of epinephrine and norepinephrine in the circulation. Computed tomography or magnetic resonance imaging usually detects the adrenal tumor and confirms the diagnosis.

■ Postsurgical Repair of Congenital Heart Disease

Chief Clinical Characteristics

This presentation can be characterized by palpitations, light-headedness, and dizziness months to years after surgical intervention to repair congenital heart disease. In symptomatic patients, the presence of a surgical scar over the precordium or report of heart surgery during the intake interview often suggests the possibility of this syndrome.

Background Information

The development of atrial tachyarrhythmias (most commonly, atrial fibrillation) is a recognized phenomenon that occurs in some patients with this condition, including atrial septal defect, ventricular septal defect, and tetralogy of Fallot.[48] The mechanism for tachyarrhythmias often involves direct trauma to cardiac tissue during the surgical procedure, rendering some cells susceptible to hyperirritability and spontaneous depolarization. The symptoms may appear soon after the procedure or remain latent for prolonged periods. Further evaluation by a primary care physician is usually indicated.

■ Pregnancy

Chief Clinical Characteristics

This presentation includes a rapid and bounding pulse often associated with shortness of breath, and there may be an increase in the occurrence of symptoms to term.[49] At times, the palpitations may precipitate dizziness, presyncope, or frank syncope.[50]

Background Information

Episodes are usually benign and self-limiting. Significant changes occur in hormonal and hemodynamic function during pregnancy that predispose women to the development of dysrhythmias. Changes in hormone levels during pregnancy (particularly progesterone) have been associated with enhanced sympathetic activity and the precipitation of dysrhythmias.[36] The enhanced maternal blood volume and associated increase in stroke volume may lead to the sensation of a forceful, bounding pulse in some patients. The type of dysrhythmia associated with palpitations is often sinus tachycardia or supraventricular tachycardia. Only very rarely is atrial fibrillation or ventricular tachycardia the source of the dysrhythmia.[51] Patients who are pregnant and report palpitations associated with symptoms of cardiovascular instability should be referred to their primary care physician for evaluation. In the event of cardiovascular compromise, supportive interventions and activation of the emergency medical system may be necessary.

■ Pulmonary Embolus

Chief Clinical Characteristics

This condition may involve an acute onset of nonspecific dyspnea, hemoptysis, and chest discomfort, as well as tachypnea, wheezing, cyanosis, syncope, and tachycardia manifested as palpitations.[52] Individuals with this condition quite frequently feel great anxiety and may have a sense of impending doom. With large pulmonary emboli, jugular venous distension may be observed and an S_3 sound may be heard at the cardiac apex.

Background Information

This condition is usually the result of dislodgement of a portion of a venous thrombus that ultimately lodges in small branches of the pulmonary arterial tree. Risk factors include surgery, trauma, immobilization, obesity, stroke, cancer, spinal cord injury, pregnancy/oral contraceptives, increasing age, and prolonged placement of indwelling central venous catheters. An individual in whom this condition is suspected must receive immediate medical attention. The therapist should activate the emergency medical system and be prepared to administer basic life support should the individual become unstable.

■ Pulmonary Hypertension

Chief Clinical Characteristics

This presentation commonly includes shortness of breath, fatigue, chest discomfort, palpitations, and syncope.[53] Physical findings mimic those of right-sided heart failure, such as jugular venous distension, peripheral edema, abdominal ascites, and an S_3 sound that is heard on auscultation. These latter signs are associated with the development of cor pulmonale.

Background Information

This condition is associated with thickening and hypertrophy of the medial layer of the pulmonary arteries that ultimately involves intimal layer proliferation. Eventually, mean pulmonary arterial pressure exceeds 25 mm Hg, while pulmonary capillary wedge pressure remains below 15 mm Hg.[54] Use of a pulse oximeter during the initial activity assessment typically reveals hemoglobin desaturation suggestive of significant pulmonary hypertension with impaired oxygenation, although it is usually diagnosed by echocardiography and right-sided cardiac catheterization. If this condition is suspected, the individual should be referred to his or her primary care physician for further evaluation.

■ Sick Sinus Syndrome

Chief Clinical Characteristics
This presentation may vary from significant vagotonia to severe tachycardia-bradycardia syndrome during which the patient may feel very rapid palpitations and become symptomatic during the subsequent and prolonged bradycardic episodes. Associated symptoms may include light-headedness, anxiety, shortness of breath, and syncope. Palpation of the pulse usually reveals a paroxysmal episode of rapid pulse followed by a period of slow pulse that may be cyclical or erratic in nature.

Background Information
This condition refers to a wide range of disorders of the conduction system of the heart including failed sinoatrial node impulse generation and impaired internodal conduction.[55] In some cases, there is histological evidence of sclero-degenerative changes within the cardiac conduction pathways. The source of the tachyarrhythmia is usually supraventricular, but ventricular dysrhythmias may result in the event of sinus arrest. Medical treatment usually consists of antiarrhythmic therapy and often a cardiac pacemaker is necessary to prevent untoward consequences in the event of complete sinus arrest. In a previously undiagnosed patient, noting a cyclic or erratic acceleration and deceleration of the pulse associated with symptoms warrants timely referral to the physician. In extreme cases of symptomatic forms of this condition, the therapist should be prepared to administer supportive therapy if needed and activate the emergency medical system as appropriate.

SIDE EFFECT OF MEDICATIONS

Chief Clinical Characteristics
This presentation may be characterized by palpitations ranging from a slow, bounding to a rapid, weak pulse and is associated with various prescribed and over-the-counter medications.

Background Information
The following medications in particular may cause this presentation:

■ Alpha-1 Blockers

Alpha-1 blockers lower blood pressure by blocking *alpha-1* receptors located in vascular smooth muscle to cause vasodilation, while *angiotensin-converting enzyme inhibitors* block the conversion of angiotensin I to angiotensin II (an extremely potent vasoconstrictor). Both classes of medications may result in significantly lowered blood pressure that can precipitate a reflex tachycardic response from the heart that is felt as palpitations by the patient. One of the clinical signs associated with this phenomenon is a very rapid pulse in the presence of marked hypotension.

■ Beta Blockers

These act to block *beta-1* (selective) or both *beta-1* and *beta-2* (non-selective) receptors (*beta-1* found primarily in cardiac tissue and *beta-2* primarily in vascular and bronchial tissue). The important cardiac effects result in a slowing of the heart rate and a reduction in the force of contraction. One of the first signs of excessive beta blockade is a marked sinus bradycardia with associated symptoms of unusual fatigue, shortness of breath (especially with non-selective beta blockers), light-headedness, or syncope.[56]

■ Beta-2 Agonists

Beta-2 agonists (medications that act on bronchiolar smooth muscle to elicit bronchodilation) are often prescribed to individuals who have asthma or other reversible airway diseases. Minor adverse side effects of *beta-2* agonist administration include headache, tremor, and palpitations and the severity of symptoms appears to be dose dependent.[57] At higher doses, there is a "spillover" effect that leads to inadvertent *beta-1* stimulation and enhanced cardiac contractility.

■ Digoxin

Digoxin is a cardiac glycoside that acts on the heart to slow electrical impulse transmission through the atrioventricular node and to increase ventricular contractile force by impairing sodium-potassium pump activity, enhancing reverse sodium-calcium exchanger activity, and increasing the sensitivity of ryanodine receptors on the sarcoplasmic reticulum to calcium-induced calcium release.[58] Individuals prescribed this medication often experience a sense of a "bounding" heartbeat, especially at night prior to falling asleep. In addition to its side effects, overdose of this medication can result in a significant slowing of the heart rate and the individual may experience associated symptoms of nausea, dizziness, light-headedness, general malaise, or syncope, suggesting digoxin toxicity.

■ Lasix

Lasix is a loop diuretic that can significantly lower plasma volume and serum potassium levels. This may lead to destabilization of the myocardial resting membrane potential, resulting in the development of serious ventricular dysrhythmias. Symptoms of excessive plasma volume loss and potassium depletion also include confusion, dizziness, and unusual fatigue.[59]

■ Nitrates and Calcium Channel Blockers

Nitrates (eg, nitroglycerin) are metabolized and converted to nitric oxide (a vascular smooth muscle relaxer) and calcium channel blockers act to prevent calcium entry into vascular smooth muscle. Both medications elicit vascular smooth muscle relaxation and can reduce arterial blood pressure. In some cases, a reflex sinus tachycardia may ensue in response to systemic hypotension and patients may experience palpitations. Individuals who present with symptoms while taking any cardioinhibitory or vasoactive medications should be referred to their primary physician for evaluation of appropriate medication dosage and should be monitored closely during treatment sessions to assess heart rate and blood pressure responses to exercise.

■ Potassium Supplement

An overdose of a potassium supplement can result in dangerously high levels of serum potassium and also precipitate life-threatening ventricular dysrhythmias. Patients taking a combination of Lasix and potassium supplement should be questioned for the presence of frequent or prolonged episodes of palpitations that may indicate electrolyte imbalance. The therapist should remind the patient to consult with their physician in cases where potassium supplementation is self-initiated.

■ Vasovagal Syncope (Neurocardiogenic Syncope, Common Faint)

Chief Clinical Characteristics

This presentation involves prodromal symptoms, which include nausea, abdominal discomfort, light-headedness, dizziness, palpitations, shortness of breath, diaphoresis, and chest pain.[60] The pulse is typically slow and regular, and blood pressure measurements may reveal hypotension.

Background Information

The precise mechanism responsible for this condition is not well understood. Individuals with this condition usually have difficulty standing for prolonged periods of time and exhibit delayed or diminished neurocardiovascular responses when assuming an upright posture. Predisposing factors include hypovolemia, anemia, sympathetic blocking medications, and antihypertensive medications. Similar to orthostatic hypotension and POTS, having the individual assume a more recumbent position and administering fluids will often cause the symptoms to abate. A tilt table test is the diagnostic procedure of choice for confirming this condition, and the individual should be referred to his or her primary care physician for definitive assessment.

■ Wolff-Parkinson-White Syndrome (Pre-Excitation Syndrome)

Chief Clinical Characteristics

This presentation ranges from asymptomatic and undiagnosed to palpitations associated with chest discomfort, shortness of breath, light-headedness, and syncope.

Background Information

The tachyarrhythmias associated with this condition are typically supraventricular in nature and include supraventricular tachycardia and atrial flutter. In some cases, the dysrhythmia may lead to severe systolic hypotension and, rarely, deterioration of cardiac rhythm into ventricular fibrillation. This is a congenital condition that results from the presence of an accessory electrical conduction pathway that connects the atria to the ventricles across the mitral or tricuspid annulus. The conduction velocity along the accessory pathway is usually faster compared to that of the normal atrioventricular nodal pathway. As a result, part of the ventricular muscle mass is depolarized prematurely by impulses traveling through the accessory pathway.[61] The diagnosis is confirmed by the clinical finding of a slurring of the initial portion of the QRS complex manifested by the *delta wave* on ECG recording. If the palpitations are prolonged and are associated with symptoms of cardiovascular instability, the therapist should be prepared to administer basic life support maneuvers and activate the emergency medical system as appropriate.

References

1. Abbott AV. Diagnostic approach to palpitations. *Am Fam Physician*. Feb 15, 2005;71(4):743–750.
2. Wexler RK, Pleister A, Raman S. Outpatient approach to palpitations. *Am Fam Physician*. July 2011;84(1):63-69.
3. Bickley LS. *Bates' Guide to Physical Examination and History Taking*. 10th ed. Philadelphia, PA: Lippincott Williams & Wilkins; 2008.
4. Ludwig H, Strasser K. Symptomatology of anemia. *Semin Oncol*. Apr 2001;28(2 suppl 8):7–14.
5. Widmaier EP, Raff H, Strang KT. *Vander, Sherman, and Luciano's Human Physiology: The Mechanisms of Body Function*. 9th ed. New York, NY: McGraw-Hill; 2004.
6. Pujade-Lauraine E, Gascon P. The burden of anaemia in patients with cancer. *Oncology*. 2004;67(suppl 1):1–4.
7. Toy P, Feiner J, Viele MK, Watson J, Yeap H, Weiskopf RB. Fatigue during acute isovolemic anemia in healthy, resting humans. *Transfusion*. Apr 2000;40(4):457–460.
8. Torpy JM, Burke AE. Generalized anxiety disorder. *JAMA*. Feb 2011;305(5):522.
9. Chatterjee K. Auscultation of cardiac murmurs. In: UpToDate, Otto CM (Ed), UpToDate, Waltham, MA, 2011.
10. Driscoll DJ, Wolfe RR, Gersony WM, et al. Cardiorespiratory responses to exercise of patients with aortic stenosis, pulmonary stenosis, and ventricular septal defect. *Circulation*. Feb 1993;87(2 suppl):102–113.
11. Sen-Chowdhry S, Lowe MD, Sporton SC, McKenna WJ. Arrhythmogenic right ventricular cardiomyopathy: clinical presentation, diagnosis, and management. *Am J Med*. Nov 1 2004;117(9):685–695.
12. Jefferies JL, Towbin JA. Dilated cardiomyopathy. *Lancet*. Feb 2010;375:752-762.
13. Lee CT, Dec WG, Lilly LS. The cardiomyopathies. In: Lilly LS, ed. *Pathophysiology of Heart Disease; A Collaborative Project of Medical Students and Faculty*. 5th ed. Baltimore, MD: Lippincott Williams & Wilkins; 2011.
14. Firoozi S, Sharma S, Hamid MS, McKenna WJ. Sudden death in young athletes: HCM or ARVC? *Cardiovasc Drugs Ther*. Jan 2002;16(1):11–17.
15. Chiu C, Sequeira IB. Diagnosis and treatment of idiopathic ventricular tachycardia. *AACN Clin Issues*. Jul–Sep 2004;15(3):449–461.
16. Shekelle PG, Hardy ML, Morton SC, et al. Efficacy and safety of ephedra and ephedrine for weight loss and athletic performance: a meta-analysis. *JAMA*. Mar 26, 2003;289(12):1537–1545.
17. Pelchovitz DJ, Goldberger JJ. Caffeine and cardiac arrhythmias; a review of the evidence. *Am J Med*. Apr 2011;124(4):284-289.
18. Kaplan GB, Greenblatt DJ, Ehrenberg BL, et al. Dose-dependent pharmacokinetics and psychomotor effects of caffeine in humans. *J Clin Pharmacol*. Aug 1997;37(8):693–703.
19. Persky AM, Berry NS, Pollack GM, Brouwer KL. Modelling the cardiovascular effects of ephedrine. *Br J Clin Pharmacol*. May 2004;57(5):552–562.
20. Maraj S, Figueredo VM, Morris DL. Cocaine and the heart. *Clin Cardiol*. 2010;33(5):264-269.
21. Foltin RW, Haney M. Intranasal cocaine in humans: acute tolerance, cardiovascular and subjective effects. *Pharmacol Biochem Behav*. May 2004;78(1):93–101.
22. Jin H, Lyon AR, Akar FG. Arrhythmia mechanisms in the failing heart. *PACE*. Aug 2008;31:1048-1056.
23. Jones I, Goode I. Percutaneous coronary intervention. *Nurs Times*. Jul 8–14, 2003;99(27):46–47.
24. Lok NS, Lau CP. Prevalence of palpitations, cardiac arrhythmias and their associated risk factors in ambulant elderly. *Int J Cardiol*. Jun 1996;54(3):231–236.
25. Collins M, Claros E. Recognizing the face of dehydration. Aug 2011;41(8):26-31.
26. Maciejewski P, Bednarz B, Chamiec T, Gorecki A, Lukaszewicz R, Ceremuzynski L. Acute coronary syndrome: potassium, magnesium and cardiac arrhythmia. *Kardiol Pol*. Nov 2003;59(11):402–407.
27. Stammers AH, Mills N, Kmiecik SA, et al. The effect of electrolyte imbalance on weaning from cardiopulmonary bypass: an experimental study. *J Extra Corpor Technol*. Dec 2003;35(4):322–325.
28. Fischler MP, Reinhart WH. [Fever: friend or enemy?] *Schweiz Med Wochenschr*. May 17 1997;127(20):864–870.
29. Boelaert K, Torlinska B, Holder RL, Franklyn JA. Older subjects with hyperthyroidism present with a paucity of symptoms and signs: a large cross-sectional study. *J Clin Endocrinol Metab*. June 2010;95(6):2715-2726.
30. Wilkins LW. *Professional Guide to Signs and Symptoms*. 6th ed. Philadelphia, PA: Lippincott Williams & Wilkins; 2010.
31. Roffi M, Cattaneo F, Topol EJ. Thyrotoxicosis and the cardiovascular system: subtle but serious effects. *Cleve Clin J Med*. Jan 2003;70(1):57–63.
32. Tesfaye N, Seaquist ER. Neuroendocrine responses to hypoglycemia. *Ann NY Acad Sci*. 2010;1212(1):12-28.

33. Barker A, Stewart RW. Case report of mastocytosis in an adult. *South Med J.* 2009;102(1):91-93.

34. Tefferi A, Pardanani A. Systemic mastocytosis: current concepts and treatment advances. *Curr Hematol Rep.* May 2004;3(3):197–202.

35. Lyndaker C, Hulton L. The influence of age on symptoms of perimenopause. *J Obstet Gynecol Neonatal Nurs.* May–Jun 2004;33(3):340–347.

36. Bruce D, Rymer J. Symptoms of the menopause. *Best Pract Res Cl Ob.* 2009;23:25-32.

37. Rosano GM, Leonardo F, Dicandia C, et al. Acute electrophysiologic effect of estradiol 17 beta in menopausal women. *Am J Cardiol.* Dec 15 2000;86(12):1385–1387, A1385–1386.

38. Hayek E, Gring CN, Griffin BP. Mitral valve prolapse. *Lancet.* Feb 2005;365:507-518.

39. Desai J, Swash M. Fasciculations: what do we know of their significance? *J Neurol Sci.* Oct 1997;152(suppl 1): S43–48.

40. Castillo JG, Silvay G. Characterization and management of cardiac tumors. *Sem Cardiothorac Vasc Anesth.* 2010;14(1):6-20.

41. Patil SP, Schneider H, Schwartz AR, Smith PL. Adult obstructive sleep apnea: pathophysiology and diagnosis. *Chest.* 2007;132:325-337.

42. Aydin M, Altin R, Ozeren A, Kart L, Bilge M, Unalacak M. Cardiac autonomic activity in obstructive sleep apnea: time-dependent and spectral analysis of heart rate variability using 24-hour Holter electrocardiograms. *Tex Heart Inst J.* 2004;31(2):132–136.

43. Low PA. Prevalence of orthostatic hypotension. *Clin Auton Res.* 2008;18(Suppl 1):8-13.

44. Johnson JN, Mack KJ, Kuntz NL, et al. Postural orthostatic tachycardia syndrome: a clinical review. *Pediatr Neurol.* Feb 2010;42(2):77-85.

45. Nanthakumar K, Dorian P, Ham M, et al. When pacemakers fail: an analysis of clinical presentation and risk in 120 patients with failed devices. *Pacing Clin Electrophysiol.* Jan 1998;21(1 pt 1):87–93.

46. Sparano DM, Parker Ward R. Pericarditis and pericardial effusion: management update. *Curr Treat Options Cardiovasc Med.* 2011;13:543-555.

47. Goldman L, Ausiello D. *Cecil Textbook of Medicine.* 22nd ed. Philadelphia, PA: Saunders; 2004.

48. Nakagawa H, Shah N, Matsudaira K, et al. Characterization of reentrant circuit in macroreentrant right atrial tachycardia after surgical repair of congenital heart disease: isolated channels between scars allow "focal" ablation. *Circulation.* Feb 6, 2001;103(5):699–709.

49. Adamson DL, Nelson-Piercy C. Managing palpitations and arrhythmias during pregnancy. *Heart.* 2007;93: 1630-1636.

50. Burkart TA, Conti JB. Cardiac arrhythmias during pregnancy. *Curr Treat Options Cardiovasc Med.* 2010;12:457-471.

51. Wolbrette D. Treatment of arrhythmias during pregnancy. *Curr Womens Health Rep.* Apr 2003;3(2): 135-139.

52. Tapson VF. Acute pulmonary embolism. *N Engl J Med.* 2008;358:1037-1052.

53. Gaile N, Hoeper MM, Humbert M, et al. Guidelines for the diagnosis and treatment of pulmonary hypertension: the task force for the diagnosis and treatment of pulmonary hypertension of the european society of cardiology (ESC) and the european respiratory society (ERS), endorsed by the international society of heart and lung transplantation (ISHLT). *Eur Heart J.* 2009;30(20):2493-2537.

54. Badesch DB, Abman SH, Simonneau G, et al. Medical therapy for pulmonary arterial hypertension: updated ACCP evidence-based clinical practice guidelines. *Chest.* 2007;131:1917-1928.

55. Scott WA. Sick sinus syndrome. In: Macdonald D, ed. *Clinical Cardiac Electrophysiology in the Young.* New York, NY: Springer; 2006.

56. Abramson MJ, Walters J, Walters EH. Adverse effects of beta-agonists: are they clinically relevant? *Am J Respir Med.* 2003;2(4):287–297.

57. Armstrong DJ, Mottram DR. Beta-2 agonists. In: Mottram DR, ed. *Drugs in Sport.* 5th ed. New York, NY: Routledge; 2011.

58. Wasserstrom A. Are we ready for a new mechanism of action underlying digitalis toxicity? *J Physiol.* Nov 2011;589:5015.

59. Ciccone CD. Medications. In: DeTurk WE, Cahalin LP, eds. *Cardiovascular and Pulmonary Physical Therapy: An Evidence-Based Approach.* New York, NY: McGraw-Hill; 2011.

60. Tan MP, Parry SW. Vasovagal syncope in the older patient. *J Am Coll Cardiol.* 2008;51(6):599-606.

61. Kulig J, Koplan BA. Wolff-Parkinson-White syndrome and accessory pathways. *Circ.* 2010;122:e480-e483.

CHAPTER 36

Persistent Cough

■ *Jeffrey S. Rodrigues, PT, DPT, CCS*

Description of the Symptom

This chapter describes pathology that may lead to a persistent cough. A persistent cough is described as one that the person is unable to stop despite basic therapeutic intervention, as in a common cold remedy. A cough is considered persistent, or chronic, after 3 weeks in duration.[1]

Special Concerns

The physical therapist should consider referral to an appropriate health care provider or be prepared to administer basic life support measures should an individual present with any of the following:

■ Tussive syncope, which is an episode of persistent coughing that becomes so severe in intensity that the person has a syncopal event
■ Productive cough that is:
  ■ Pink, frothy (suggestive of pulmonary embolism or pulmonary edema)
  ■ Bright red (suggestive of an active bleed)
  ■ Dark red (suggestive of an old bleed)
  ■ Green (suggestive of an active infection)

CHAPTER PREVIEW: Conditions That May Lead to Persistent Cough

T   Trauma

COMMON

Aspiration of a foreign object 745
Aspiration pneumonia 746
Exercise-induced bronchospasm (exercise-induced asthma) 751
Inhaled irritant or foreign object 752

UNCOMMON

Chest injury 748
Pneumothorax 754

RARE

Not applicable

I   Inflammation

COMMON

Aseptic
Asthma 746

Septic
Bronchiectasis 746
Bronchitis 748
Common cold 749
Pertussis (whooping cough) 752
Pneumonia:
• Bacterial pneumonia (community-acquired pneumonia, nursing home–acquired pneumonia) 753
• Viral pneumonia 753
Tuberculosis 757

Inflammation *(continued)*

UNCOMMON

Aseptic
Pleural effusion 753

Septic
Not applicable

RARE

Not applicable

M Metabolic

COMMON

Emphysema 750
Tobacco smoke 757

UNCOMMON

Sarcoidosis 756
Side effect of medications 756
Upper airway cough syndrome 758
Volume overload 758

RARE

Gastroesophageal reflux disease 751

Va Vascular

COMMON

Cor pulmonale 749

UNCOMMON

Congestive heart failure 749
Mitral valve stenosis/regurgitation 752
Pulmonary hypertension 755

RARE

Pulmonary embolism 755

De Degenerative

COMMON

Idiopathic pulmonary fibrosis 751

UNCOMMON

Not applicable

RARE

Not applicable

(continued)

Tu Tumor

COMMON

Not applicable

UNCOMMON

Malignant Primary, such as:
• Pulmonary carcinomas 754
Malignant Metastatic, such as:
• Metastases, including from primary kidney, breast, pancreas, and colon disease 752
Benign:
Not applicable

RARE

Not applicable

Co Congenital

COMMON

Alpha-1-antitrypsin emphysema 745
Cystic fibrosis 750

UNCOMMON

Not applicable

RARE

Not applicable

Ne Neurogenic/Psychogenic

COMMON

Not applicable

UNCOMMON

Not applicable

RARE

Psychogenic cough 754
Swallowing difficulties associated with a stroke 756

Note: These are estimates of relative incidence because few data are available for the less common conditions.

Overview of Persistent Cough

A cough is the body's defense mechanism for removing irritating substances from the bronchial airways, thus providing airway hygiene. A persistent cough can disrupt the individual's lifestyle by causing sleep disturbances and throat and voice soreness and diminish the ability to clear secretions in the future.

Two mechanisms can trigger a cough: the expiratory reflex, which serves as a defensive mechanism caused by mechanical stimulation of the larynx and causes expiratory effects, and the enhancement of mucociliary stimulation for airway clearance.[2,3] A cough is only effective as a defense mechanism down to the sixth or seventh generation of the bronchi (Fig. 36-1).[4] Some of the more common causes of a persistent cough include prolonged exposure to tobacco smoke, complications due to chest trauma, inhaled irritants, infections, inflammation of bronchial airway tissues, bronchial airway tumors, postnasal

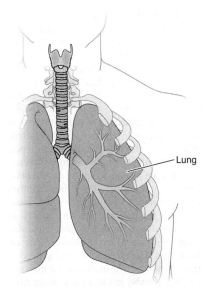

FIGURE 36-1 Generational structure of the airways in the human lung.

drip, or an underlying pulmonary or cardiac disease.

Description of Conditions That May Lead to Persistent Cough

■ Alpha-1-Antitrypsin Emphysema

Chief Clinical Characteristics

This presentation includes persistent cough combined with dyspnea on exertion, decreased exercise tolerance, prolonged expiration, wheezes and/or crackles with distant breath sounds on pulmonary auscultation, cough productive of sputum, and excessive use of accessory muscles for respiration.

Background Information

The primary pulmonary complication of alpha-1-antitrypsin (A1A) deficiency is emphysema and the most common pulmonary feature is chronic obstructive pulmonary disease.[5] This condition is a hereditary disorder characterized by low serum levels of A1A. Individuals with this deficiency are at increased risk for developing premature emphysema, often in the third and fourth decade of life.[6] Individuals with severe A1A deficiency are known to be genetically susceptible to developing emphysema, chronic bronchitis, and other respiratory symptoms. Occupational exposure to dust and chemical irritants/fumes and exposure to first- or second-hand smoke[5] will lead to early development of emphysema in the person with A1A deficiency. The persistent cough is triggered by the emphysematous changes that occur in the lungs. Medical treatment may consist of administration of A1A concentrate to keep A1A serum levels therapeutic.[6] The physical therapist's intervention should include aspects of a pulmonary rehabilitation program including airway hygiene techniques and aerobic exercises at a submaximal level.

■ Aspiration of a Foreign Object

Chief Clinical Characteristics

This presentation includes persistent cough with a slight wheeze in its mild form. In more severe cases, the presentation may include stridor, dyspnea, rapid and shallow respirations, decreased oxygen saturation, and cyanosis and may eventually lead to a syncopal event.[7] This presentation will likely involve the universal choking sign (hands at the throat).

Background Information

Aspiration of a foreign object is more common in infants and children than adults. The objects are usually accidentally aspirated. Frequently, children are misdiagnosed initially in this situation.[8] Objects aspirated in children tend to be centrally lodged, whereas objects will likely be lodged in the right main stem bronchus in adults. In a child, the main stem bronchi are more horizontally oriented and as a person becomes an adult the bronchi become more vertically orientated (the right more so than the left side). The body uses a cough as a defense mechanism to try to remove the object. In mild cases the presentation can commonly be mistaken for an asthmatic episode. Breath sounds on auscultation will be diminished or absent distal to the lodged object.[7] Aspirated objects have included items such as chewed meat, peanuts, popcorn kernels, candy, pins, pen caps, and razor blades.[9,10] Individuals with alcoholism tend to be prone to aspiration of objects and fluids when intoxicated. If the symptoms are mild, referring the individual to urgent care or an emergency department would be appropriate. If the symptoms are severe and acute, the physical therapist should activate the emergency medical system and be prepared to perform the Heimlich maneuver if the individual's status warrants. If this does not produce the object, the individual will likely need to have a bronchoscopy or surgery to remove it.

■ Aspiration Pneumonia

Chief Clinical Characteristics
This presentation is characterized by cough and associated with dyspnea, chest pain, wheezing, fever, nausea, or vomiting. The individual will present with diminished breath sounds in the areas in which the aspirated contents exist.

Background Information
Aspiration is identified as the inhalation of oropharyngeal or gastric contents into the larynx and lower respiratory tract. Aspiration pneumonia will arise after the aspiration of colonized oropharyngeal contents.[11] Commonly aspirated items include chewed food or liquids. In the elderly aspiration is common in those with dysphagia,[12] swallowing difficulties following stroke,[13] or with a decreased cough reflex. A decreased cough reflex will diminish the defensive properties of the cough and the individual will be prone to aspiration. The individual will then develop a persistent cough as the body tries to remove the aspirated contents that are directly irritating the cough receptors. The individual's oxygen saturation may be lower due to the decreased gas exchange. If the above signs and symptoms appear, the physical therapist should ascertain a recent history from the individual or family member to rule in the possibility of an aspiration pneumonia that has developed or is in the process of developing. The individual should be referred to his or her primary physician if stable. If the individual appears to be in respiratory distress, the physical therapist should activate the emergency medical system.

■ Asthma

Chief Clinical Characteristics
This presentation typically involves a chronic or intermittent persistent cough, especially in response to factors or stimuli such as pollen, dust, animal dander, environmental conditions, certain foods, and exercise.[14]

Background Information
The stimulating factor irritates the lining of the bronchial airway and a hyperadaptive response is provoked, resulting in a narrowing of the airway. This leads to an irritation of the cough receptors, which provokes a cough response. If the individual is in an area that exposes him or her to such triggers as pollen, dust, or animal dander, a prudent course of action would be to have the individual exercise in a different area away from the trigger, if possible. For example, if outdoors, move the exercise program indoors. Cold, dry air is another cause of exacerbation for individuals with this condition. Exercising in a warm, moist climate or performing activities in a pool would help to reduce triggering an asthma-induced coughing episode. Individuals who are prone to "asthma attacks," especially during exercise, should try to exercise in an area free from any airborne irritants and in a warm, moist environment. Asthma is the most common cause of persistent cough in children. If an asthma exacerbation occurs, the individual should be instructed to stop any activity, rest, and use any medically prescribed medications such as inhaled bronchodilators or corticosteroids until the symptoms subside. The physical therapist should try to alter the environment to avoid further episodes. If the individual is unable to control the situation within a reasonable amount of time, the physical therapist should be prepared to activate the emergency medical system so as to avoid progression to tussive syncope.

■ Bronchiectasis

Chief Clinical Characteristics
This presentation involves persistent cough that is productive of purulent, foul-smelling sputum with or without hemoptysis, dyspnea, fever, or pleurisy and can have digital clubbing in severe cases. Daily sputum production can range from 10 mL/day in mild cases to more than 150 mL/day in severe cases.[15] Individuals with this condition frequently have a persistent cough throughout the year and commonly have hemoptysis.

Background Information
Bronchiectasis is defined as an abnormal dilation of a bronchus that is irreversible (Fig. 36-2). The dilation can be due to an infection such as

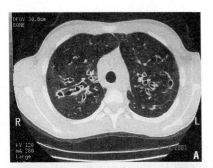

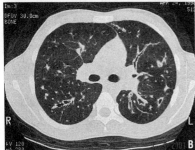

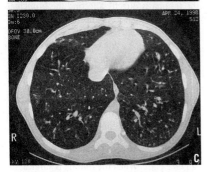

FIGURE 36-2 Computed tomography scan of a patient with bronchiectasis: (A) upper airways; (B) middle airways; (C) lower airways.

tuberculosis, inflammation due to aspiration, the presence of a tumor or foreign bodies in the airways, and genetic disorders such as cystic fibrosis. This condition is technically not a disease, but the outcome of various insults and trauma to the lungs. Regardless of the cause, an inadequate host defense mechanism and severe inflammation are the two most common factors that culminate in this condition. Chest radiography will likely demonstrate increased bronchial markings in the lower lobes and increased airway dilation. Medical treatment

commonly includes use of oral, intravenous, or aerosolized antibiotics.[15] The individual may also use mechanical devices such as the Flutter valve (VarioRaw Percutive SARL, Aubonne, Switzerland) (Fig. 36-3) or a high-frequency chest compression vest to help clear secretions. In severe cases resection of a segment, lobe, or entire lung may be necessary.[16] The physical therapist's intervention should consist of airway hygiene by percussion and vibration, postural drainage, assisted cough techniques such as the active cycle of breathing, and pulmonary rehabilitation.[17] The physical therapist should be aware of the individual's baseline signs and symptoms and note any increase in the frequency or production of sputum with the cough. The individual should be referred back to his or her primary care

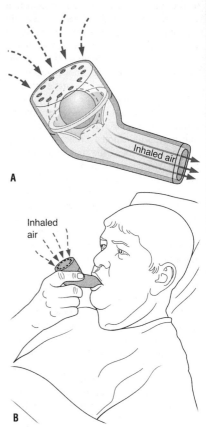

FIGURE 36-3 (A) Example of Flutter valve; (B) patient using a Flutter valve.

physician if an increase in sputum production is reported.

■ Bronchitis

Chief Clinical Characteristics

This presentation can be characterized by symptoms mimicking the upper respiratory infection of a common cold. The symptoms progress to a dry, irritating cough, fever and chest pain due to increased frequency of coughing. Its chronic form is a condition in which a persistent productive cough lasts for at least 3 months for two consecutive years.[17,18] The sputum is commonly yellow-green in color and produced in small amounts. Lung auscultation reveals expiratory wheezes and crackles.

Background Information

This condition is defined as an inflammation of the trachea and bronchial tree that results in a persistent cough. In its acute form, the cause of the cough can be irritants such as smoke, fumes/gases, or viral infections. As the condition worsens the cough becomes more productive of purulent sputum.[17] Cigarette smokers[3] and those persons exposed to significant amounts of second-hand smoke[18] are predisposed to developing chronic bronchitis. The individual with chronic bronchitis presents with persistent cough and sputum production that is typically worse in the morning and evening than during midday. These individuals can possibly develop airflow obstructions due to the constant sputum production.[3] The airflow obstruction over time will progress to reduced chest expansion, air trapping, wheezing, cyanosis, and decreased exercise tolerance.[17] The acute form of this condition can develop into its chronic form if not treated early. The physical therapist should refer an individual to his or her primary physician if the individual is exhibiting the signs and symptoms of chronic bronchitis. The physical therapist's treatment should focus on removing secretions, increasing ventilation, decreasing the work of breathing, and increasing exercise tolerance. Percussion and vibration, postural drainage, and assisted cough techniques are useful in clearing the lungs of sputum. Progressive low-level aerobic exercises can be a practical approach to increasing exercise tolerance.

■ Chest Injury

Chief Clinical Characteristics

This presentation typically involves guarding over the affected area of an injury to the thorax in combination with diminished chest wall movement and pain in and around the affected area.

Background Information

Direct trauma to the upper body including the chest wall, lungs, and throat are apparent causes of cough following a chest injury. The trauma can include a physical injury resulting from a motor vehicle accident, fall, physical assault, or penetrating wound. The trauma can also occur from surgery to the regions mentioned above. In the case of a flail chest secondary to trauma, the breathing mechanics will be altered. During inspiration the chest wall will expand, but the injured area will draw inward. During expiration the chest wall contracts, while the area of injury protrudes.[17] The reaction that causes the cough is similar in nature regardless of the origin of trauma. If the trauma is directly affecting the bronchial airway, the cough mechanism is protective in nature and the purpose is to remove the cause of the irritation. When the trauma is not directly affecting the bronchial airway (as in the case of a crush or penetrating chest wall injury), the surrounding areas will become inflamed and swollen. In this case the excess fluids can accumulate in the lungs. These excess fluids will become an irritation to the bronchial airway. The cough reaction will be to remove the fluids so that normal gas exchange can take place. When the trauma is surgical in nature, fluids will arise due to the inflammatory response of the surrounding tissues. The cough response is similar in quality to the physical trauma mentioned above. The physical therapist should be able to recognize the source of the trauma and respond accordingly. If the cause of the cough is due to direct trauma to the airways (physical or surgical), the physical therapist should suggest splinting techniques to relieve pain and give external support. If the cause of the cough is indirect trauma, the physical therapist should incorporate postural drainage, percussion, vibration, deep-breathing exercises, and assisted cough techniques in an attempt to facilitate removal of the secretions. The physical therapist should be aware of the underlying causes and physical structures present prior to administering any of the above pulmonary physical therapy techniques. Percussion and vibration directly over fractured ribs are contraindicated but encouraged around the site.[17]

■ Common Cold

Chief Clinical Characteristics
This presentation commonly involves runny nose, sneezing, fever, general body aches, and cough. An inflamed throat that has become irritated can induce this condition.

Background Information
The chronic cough can also be triggered by an upper airway cough syndrome, more commonly known as postnasal drip, from a runny nose. The direct irritation of a substance on the cough receptors in the upper airway structures can generate a cough.[19,20] It would be wise to inform the individual to return home until the symptoms dissipate and he or she is no longer potentially infectious to the physical therapist or other individuals. If the symptoms persist, or are severe, the individual should be referred to his or her primary care physician for further evaluation and treatment.

■ Congestive Heart Failure

Chief Clinical Characteristics
This presentation can be characterized by dyspnea on exertion, orthopnea, persistent cough, peripheral edema, and fatigue. On examination, individuals with this condition may exhibit systolic murmur, crackles/rales on pulmonary auscultation, a third (S_3) and/or fourth (S_4) heart sound on cardiac auscultation, jugular venous distention, or peripheral cyanosis.

Background Information
This condition is characterized by left ventricular contractile dysfunction resulting in ventricular dilation and poor contraction. Contractile dysfunction can be caused by myocardial ischemia or infarction, coronary artery disease, or bacterial/viral infection. As the heart pump fails, the blood returning to the heart from the lungs is backed up, causing overload in the pulmonary circulation, which leads to bronchial hyperreactivity. Dyspnea,

wheezing, and persistent coughing are common signs in individuals with bronchial hyperreactivity.[21] Medical treatment usually consists of a combination of vasodilators, diuretics, digoxin, beta blockers, antiarrhythmic agents, and anticoagulants.[22] Implementing a cardiac rehabilitation program would be beneficial.[23] The individual who is newly diagnosed or having an exacerbation of symptoms would begin in Phase I of a cardiac rehabilitation program as an inpatient and progress to Phase II and Phase III as an outpatient over a period of several months.

■ Cor Pulmonale

Chief Clinical Characteristics
This presentation involves chronic productive cough, dyspnea on exertion, wheezing, lower extremity edema, jugular venous distention, and in chronic cases digital clubbing.[17]

Background Information
This condition is characterized as pulmonary heart disease. The right side of the heart may become enlarged due to pulmonary hypertension, pulmonary embolism, chronic obstructive pulmonary disease, idiopathic pulmonary fibrosis, and Pickwickian syndrome.[24] The additional fluid irritates the bronchial airways, resulting in a reactive chronic cough. Medical management includes diuretics, supplemental oxygen use, and dietary salt restrictions.[17] The physical therapist should take to the role of preventing the onset of cor pulmonale by addressing the underlying cause. Aerobic exercises, mobility training, and breathing exercises could have an important effect on the above-mentioned causes. Individual education would also be beneficial, including how to monitor lower extremity edema and signs of respiratory failure. The physical therapist should be aware of any acute signs and symptoms of a severe form of this condition to the point that the individual experiences pallor, sweating, severe chest pain, weak and rapid pulse, anxiety, and diminished level of consciousness. In this situation, the physical therapist should activate the emergency medical system immediately, because these signs and symptoms suggest the condition has progressed to the point of being life threatening.

PERSISTENT COUGH

■ Cystic Fibrosis

Chief Clinical Characteristics
This presentation classically involves a chronic cough that is usually productive of sputum throughout the course of the day.

Background Information
This condition is a genetic disease in which exocrine gland function is altered. Excess mucus can be produced in the linings of the lungs, pancreatic duct, gastrointestinal tract, or other areas where exocrine glands are located.[25] An exacerbation may be due to an infectious process that commonly has the symptoms of increased cough frequency with an increase of greenish sputum, fever, malaise, and decreased appetite. The contact and irritation from increased amounts of sputum in the airways during an exacerbation will increase the frequency of the productive cough. Survival rates continue to improve in individuals with this condition, and the impact of exercise plays a significant role.[26] Aerobic[27] and anaerobic[28] exercise programs are showing significant promise for improving exercise capacity and quality of life. Physical therapists will likely be involved with more individuals with this condition as the need for exercise programs for this population becomes more common. Due to the type of exercise being performed, the frequency of coughing may increase from the loosening of the sputum in the lungs. In this instance the individual should be advised to perform a pulmonary hygiene technique of his or her choice. This may consist of postural drainage with or without percussion and vibration, assisted coughing techniques, or the use of mechanical devices such as a high-frequency chest compression vest or Flutter valve (see Fig. 36-3). If the coughing episode increases in frequency and duration without some relief, it is possible for the individual to progress to tussive syncope and/or hemoptysis (blood in the sputum). The individual and physical therapist should be advised to continue to monitor the color of the sputum for any changes to a bright red. Bright red hemoptysis is indicative of an active bleed in the lung tissue. At this point, the individual should be advised to limit pulmonary hygiene activities and try to minimize coughing and physical activity and seek medical attention, or the physical therapist should be ready to activate the emergency medical system. If the hemoptysis is a dark red, it reveals blood that had yet to be expectorated.

■ Emphysema

Chief Clinical Characteristics
This presentation typically includes reports of shortness of breath, persistent cough with sputum production, wheezing, and decreased exercise tolerance.[29] Physical examination reveals a prolonged expiratory phase during respiration, increased anterior-posterior diameter of the chest (barrel chest appearance), flattened diaphragm, and distant breath sounds on pulmonary auscultation with wheezes and/or crackles.

Background Information
This condition is the most common obstructive pulmonary disease. It is characterized as enlarged air spaces due to the disruption of the elastic fibers in the alveolar wall leading to destruction that is irreversible.[30] The emphysematous changes produce airway obstruction with impaired ventilation and gas exchange in the lungs, resulting in decreased diffusion of oxygen. A persistent cough is noted as a method of enhancing gas exchange by removing any irritating stimuli. The elastic recoil of the lungs is lost, resulting in the retention of air. A history of tobacco smoking or exposure to second-hand smoke or occupational toxins can make a person prone to developing emphysema. Medical intervention commonly consists of smoking cessation, use of bronchodilators, and limited use of supplemental oxygen. In severe cases lung volume reduction surgery may be performed to remove hyperinflated blebs or bullae. The physical therapist's treatment should include aspects of a pulmonary rehabilitation program including airway hygiene techniques, such as percussion and vibration, and postural drainage and aerobic exercises at a submaximal level. Individual education should also be included for pursed-lip breathing techniques. If the individual has undergone surgery for removal of emphysematous blebs or bullae, the physical therapist should also address any postsurgical movement dysfunction that may be affecting the individual. See

the entry for Chest Injury earlier in this chapter for reference as needed.

■ Exercise-Induced Bronchospasm (Exercise-Induced Asthma)

Chief Clinical Characteristics
This presentation can include a persistent cough that will usually occur 10 to 15 minutes into an exercise session and will then continue for up to 15 minutes after the conclusion of the exercise session.[31]

Background Information
This condition is a reaction of the bronchial airways during bouts of exercise, usually in response to a change in environmental conditions. The airway narrowing consists of increased mucus production in the airway along with spasm of the smooth muscle in the airway lining. The response has a clinical appearance similar to that of an asthmatic episode, yet the mast cells in the bronchial airway do not respond as they do during an asthma attack.[32] It occurs during prolonged exercise, and is more likely to occur when the ambient air is cold and dry.[33] The easiest way to avoid cough secondary to this condition is to remove or minimize precipitating factors. Conducting the exercise session in an area with warm, moist air will help to eliminate a primary precursor to this condition. A mild warm-up session prior to the start of vigorous exercise will help to prepare the airways for the exercise session and likely reduce the hyperreactivity of the bronchial passages. Medical treatment involves bronchodilator medications that can help reduce the bronchial reaction. These medications can include long-acting beta-adrenergic agonists such as cromone, formoterol, and salmeterol.[34] The individual who is prone to exercise-induced bronchospasm should be instructed to take the medications prior to the exercise session to prevent cough from this condition.

■ Gastroesophageal Reflux Disease

Chief Clinical Characteristics
This presentation commonly includes dysphonia, hoarseness, sore throat, gum inflammation, dental erosion, chest pain, heart burn, dyspnea, sputum production with coughing, and wheezing.[35] The cough will be more prevalent in the morning and after meals. This condition is common among individuals who are non-smokers with a normal chest radiograph and not taking angiotensin-converting enzyme inhibitors.[35]

Background Information
This condition involves retrograde movement of gastric contents into the esophagus. In individuals with this condition, persistent cough is one of the most common complaints.[36] The mechanism of cough in an individual with gastroesophageal reflux disease is from microaspiration of gastric contents or a vagally mediated esophageal-tracheobronchial reflex. Medical treatment includes vigorous acid suppression, elevating the head of the individual's bed 10 cm, weight loss, diet modification to high-protein and low-fat foods, omitting high-acid foods, antacid use prior to bedtime, and limiting food intake 2 hours prior to bedtime.[36] Referral should be made to the individual's primary physician for a 24-hour esophageal pH test. Physical therapists treating individuals with this condition in its acute form should avoid having the individual flex forward at the trunk or hips and also avoid vigorous activities in the early morning or after meals, because these situations raise the likelihood of symptom aggravation.

■ Idiopathic Pulmonary Fibrosis

Chief Clinical Characteristics
This presentation involves an irritating, non-productive cough and exertional dyspnea.[37] Lung auscultation will reveal a "Velcro"-like quality crackle most noticeable at the bases. Pulmonary function tests will demonstrate a restrictive disease pattern with decreased vital capacity, residual volume, and total lung capacity.

Background Information
This condition is a specific form of chronic fibrosing interstitial pneumonia that is limited to the lung. The "stiffness" of the lungs causes a rapid, shallow breathing pattern. This is due to a ventilation/perfusion mismatch and the individual can become hypoxic during exercise. This will lead to a worsening of the above cough and dyspnea symptoms. Pulmonary rehabilitation may help improve the quality of life and prepare the individual for possible

lung transplantation. The physical therapist should progress through the program slowly so as not to exacerbate symptoms. If the symptoms worsen to tussive syncope or increased hypoxemia, the physical therapist should activate the emergency medical system as warranted. The prognosis is poor and most individuals die within 3 to 8 years from onset of symptoms.[38]

■ Inhaled Irritant or Foreign Object

Chief Clinical Characteristics
This presentation typically involves a chronic or intermittent persistent cough in the presence of an irritant.

Background Information
The cough reaction in the airway is similar to that of an asthmatic reaction in which the irritant causes an inflammatory response. One of the most common causes of a persistent cough is inhalation of an irritant or foreign body. Some examples of inhaled irritants are smoke, odors from heavy perfume or cleaning products, and dust. Along with direct contact, the inhaled irritant can trigger a cough episode by irritating the cough receptors. The best plan of action is to remove the individual from the area where the irritant is located.

■ Metastases, Including from Primary Kidney, Breast, Pancreas, and Colon Disease

Chief Clinical Characteristics
This presentation commonly includes persistent cough, hemoptysis, dyspnea, chest discomfort, weight loss, and voice hoarseness, in association with possible symptoms related to the primary disease.

Background Information
The lungs are the most common site of metastases from other types of cancer. When tumor cells migrate from their primary site they can work their way into the circulation or lymphatic system. The lungs filter these systems. The most common cancers to metastasize to the lungs are kidney, breast, pancreas, colon, and uterus. Treatment of this condition depends on the type and extent of metastases, including surgical resection, chemotherapy, and radiation therapy.

■ Mitral Valve Stenosis/ Regurgitation

Chief Clinical Characteristics
This presentation includes persistent cough, decreased exercise tolerance, orthopnea, dyspnea on exertion, and occasionally hemoptysis in combination with a systolic murmur best heard at the apex of the heart, rales on pulmonary auscultation, a third (S_3) and/or fourth (S_4) heart sound on cardiac auscultation and jugular venous distention.

Background Information
This condition is characterized by the leaflets of the mitral valve becoming stiff and closing incompletely, usually due to the annulus (rim) of the valve being stretched. Left arterial and/or ventricular enlargement can pull and stretch on the mitral valve annulus. With this condition, the blood coming from the lungs into the left side of the heart will be slowed and can back up into the lungs, leading to volume overload in the lungs.[39] The chronic overload in the pulmonary circulation is accompanied by bronchial hyperreactivity. Symptoms of dyspnea, wheezing, and persistent coughing are common in individuals with bronchial hyperreactivity.[21] This condition usually occurs secondary to prior rheumatic fever occurring in childhood, yet the individual does not become symptomatic until the adult years. Other etiologies include coronary artery disease, bacterial endocarditis, and left ventricular dilation. Medical treatment consists of antibiotic, digitalis diuretic, and vasodilator medications. In cases of significant forms of this condition, repair or replacement of the mitral valve will be warranted. A cardiac rehabilitation program is optimal in the surgical and postsurgical management of this condition.[23] The physical therapist should be aware that the individual will be self-limiting in his or her exercise tolerance if the condition worsens.

■ Pertussis (Whooping Cough)

Chief Clinical Characteristics
This presentation is characterized by a persistent violent cough with a loud inspiratory "whoop," post-tussive vomiting, and wheezing.

Background Information
Pertussis is most common in children who have not been vaccinated against this condition,[40] but it can also affect adolescents and adults.

Adults tend to have a persistent cough for longer duration, are less likely to have a "whoop," and are more likely to wake at night due to their cough in combination with sweating attacks.[41] This condition is a respiratory illness caused by the bacterium *Bordetella pertussis*. In the United States, children are regularly vaccinated with DTaP (diphtheria and tetanus toxoids and acellular pertussis) in a five-dose series starting from 2 months of age until 4 to 6 years of age. Medical treatment for this condition includes use of antibiotic medications, such as macrolides (eg, erythromycin, azithromycin, or clarithromycin) or trimethoprim-sulfamethoxazole.[42] Individuals suspected of having this condition should be referred to their primary care physician immediately for evaluation and management. This action becomes even more pressing if there is a known outbreak of pertussis locally. The physical therapist also should self-monitor for symptoms and seek testing for *B. pertussis* if they develop.

■ Pleural Effusion

Chief Clinical Characteristics
This presentation commonly includes dyspnea, persistent cough, and pleuritic chest pain. Physical examination may reveal decreased chest expansion, diminished or absent breath sounds, dullness to percussion, and possible friction rub.

Background Information
This condition is a collection of fluid between the visceral pleura and parietal pleura that occurs as fluid production exceeds fluid absorption in the pleural space. The etiology of this condition involves congestive heart failure, atelectasis, pneumonia, impaired lymphatic drainage, and kidney or liver failure.[43] The cough is due to the excess fluid and dyspnea, which irritate the cough receptors in the bronchial airways and diminish gas exchange. The cough reflex is triggered in a response designed to remove the excess fluids. In severe cases, the individual may have a tracheal shift away from the affected side[44] and may develop mild hypoxemia. In this case the physical therapist should administer supplemental oxygen, as prescribed by a physician, to maintain oxygen saturation at a level where the individual is comfortable and maintains a calm respiratory rate. If the symptoms persist or worsen, the physical therapist should activate the emergency medical system. Except for pleural effusion caused by congestive heart failure, the medical treatment for pleural effusion is to remove the fluid by thoracocentesis or to place a chest tube.[44] If the individual has recently had a thoracocentesis performed to drain a pleural effusion, the physical therapist should be aware of the signs and symptoms of a possible pneumothorax that may have developed due to the procedure.

PNEUMONIA

■ Bacterial Pneumonia (Community-Acquired Pneumonia, Nursing Home–Acquired Pneumonia)

Chief Clinical Characteristics
This presentation usually includes persistent cough, sputum production with occasional hemoptysis, dyspnea, fatigue, and pleuritic chest pain.[45] Pulmonary auscultation will likely reveal decreased or absent breath sounds and crackles.[46]

Background Information
The onset of illness is usually abrupt. The persistent cough is produced by the increased sputum production irritating the cough receptors. Medical treatment consists of some form of penicillin or amoxicillin.[45] A physical therapist's intervention should include airway hygiene techniques such as percussion and vibration, postural drainage, assisted cough techniques, and deep-breathing exercises. Mobilizing the individual would also be beneficial in assisting to clear the lungs of sputum.

■ Viral Pneumonia

Chief Clinical Characteristics
This presentation commonly involves persistent, dry, nonproductive cough and increasing dyspnea. Chest auscultation reveals crackles or wheezes. The individual may also exhibit fever, decreased appetite, headache, and fatigue. This condition most commonly occurs after the onset of influenza or inhalation of some other airborne virus.

Background Information
This condition can be community acquired or nosocomial. The cough reflex is triggered

by stimulation of the cough receptors from the infectious material in the airways. A chest radiograph will show infiltrates in the areas affected. The aim of treatment in an individual with a viral pneumonia is to increase oxygen transportation. This includes pulmonary percussion and vibration, postural drainage, deep-breathing exercises, assisted cough techniques, and mobilizing the individual. The physical therapist should be aware of the potential for contamination or infection from one individual to another or to the physical therapist. The affected individual should be treated away from other susceptible individuals. Physical therapists should protect themselves by wearing a mask that covers their nose and mouth. The affected individual may also consider wearing a mask to protect others. Performing hand hygiene before and after treatment of an affected individual will help reduce the spread of infection.

■ Pneumothorax

Chief Clinical Characteristics

This presentation typically involves pleuritic chest pain, dyspnea, and dry cough and the individual may have absent breath sounds with hyperresonant percussion over the affected area.

Background Information

This condition is free air that leaks into the pleural space between the visceral and parietal pleura. The cough seen in an individual with this condition results from irritation of the cough receptors from the increased intrathoracic pressure. There are three main classifications of this condition. *Traumatic pneumothorax* is caused by a trauma or injury, direct or indirect, to the thorax. Common causes include gunshot wound, knife wound, and motor vehicle accidents. *Spontaneous pneumothorax* occurs as the structural integrity of the pleural tissue is weakened. The tissue becomes so weakened that a bleb or bullae can rupture, allowing air into the pleural space. Individuals with asthma, cystic fibrosis, emphysema, pulmonary infections, and empyema are likely candidates for developing a spontaneous pneumothorax. This condition can also occur in healthy individuals. Healthy individuals who smoke, have a positive family history, and males between the ages of 10 and 30 years who have a tall, thin body habitus are more prone to developing a spontaneous pneumothorax.[47] *Tension pneumothorax* is characterized by air entering the pleural space but not exiting. This condition is caused by a one-way or ball valve fistula. The ipsilateral lung becomes compressed and the mediastinum shifts contralaterally. A tension pneumothorax is a medical emergency because the individual will develop decreased cardiac output, refractory hypoxemia, and hypotension. The physical therapist will need to activate the emergency medical system. Medical treatment consists of chest tube placement to remove the trapped air. The use of high concentrations of supplemental oxygen will reabsorb the lesion four times faster than if no supplemental oxygen was used.[47] This situation may resolve without the use of a chest tube in individuals with small pneumothoraces (<15% of the hemithorax). The physical therapist should have supplemental oxygen available for use, as prescribed by the physician, during therapy sessions. If the individual appears to be in respiratory distress during a session, the physical therapist should activate the emergency medical system.

■ Psychogenic Cough

Chief Clinical Characteristics

This presentation includes dry, chronic coughing with no known somatic etiology. It is most commonly seen in children and adolescents but it also appears in adults.[48]

Background Information

This condition should be considered when medical therapies for postnasal drip, asthma, and gastroesophageal reflux disease fail.[48] In children and adolescents, school phobia, fear of rejection, and need for attention are common causes of psychogenic cough.[49] The physical therapist should refer the individual back to his or her primary physician for further evaluation and management if this condition is suspected. Treatment may consist of psychosocial intervention.

■ Pulmonary Carcinomas

Chief Clinical Characteristics

This presentation commonly includes persistent cough, hemoptysis, dyspnea, chest discomfort, weight loss, and voice hoarseness. If the individual has bronchoalveolar cell carcinoma, he or she can produce copious amounts of thin secretions.[50]

Background Information

Cigarette smoking is the primary cause of carcinoma in the lung, and exposure to asbestos is the most common occupational exposure cause for a person developing lung carcinoma.[50] There are many types of carcinoma of the bronchial airways including small-cell lung cancer (ie, oat cell carcinoma) and non–small-cell lung cancers (ie, squamous cell, adenocarcinoma, and large-cell carcinomas).[17] This condition has a strong association with rheumatoid arthritis, and may even precede joint involvement.[51] In an individual who is in the early stages of localized lung cancer, the symptoms do not vary much from the symptoms related to cigarette smoking; therefore, the individual may not seek medical attention promptly.[17] Individuals with this condition may have tumors located in the main stem or segmental bronchi, causing a cough. Pulmonary auscultation will usually reveal normal findings. Individuals suspected of having this condition should be referred to their primary care physician. Complete blood count, chest radiography, computed tomography, positron emission tomography, pulmonary function tests, ventilation/perfusion scan, and biopsy of the suspected tumor are procedures that can be performed to rule in the diagnosis. Medical treatment for the individual who is diagnosed with carcinoma of the lungs can include radiation and chemotherapy. In certain cases, surgical resection of the tumor and possibly some of the surrounding tissues may be necessary. Physical therapists should construct a therapeutic program to improve the individual's pulmonary function along with any possible complications due to the radiation or chemotherapies. This may include decreased endurance and muscle weakness due to the side effects of loss of appetite and weight loss resulting from the above treatments. Frequents rest breaks and interval training may be beneficial for the individual. Following surgery physical therapists should also address movement dysfunction related to chest trauma.

■ Pulmonary Embolism

Chief Clinical Characteristics

This presentation includes dyspnea, pleuritic chest pain, persistent cough, hemoptysis, and syncope.[52] Individuals with a history of deep venous thrombosis are susceptible. Other factors that put an individual at risk include immobility, resulting in blood stasis, endothelial injuries due to lower extremity trauma or surgery, and hypercoagulable states arising from such situations as oral contraceptive use or cancer.

Background Information

This condition is defined as a blood clot that has become lodged in a pulmonary artery and significantly inhibits or ceases blood flow to the lung tissue. The obstruction is commonly a blood clot, but this condition can also be caused by air, fat, bone marrow, foreign intravenous material, or tumor cells.[17] The persistent cough results from the irritation caused by the pulmonary congestion due to the embolism and the ensuing respiratory distress. Medical treatment will depend on the severity of the blocked pulmonary artery. In an acute case of severe disease, sudden death may occur. In the case of severe disease in which signs and symptoms appear significant and hemodynamic instability or respiratory compromise is evident, the physical therapist should activate the emergency medical system. In other cases where the signs and symptoms appear not as severe, the individual should be directed to an emergent care facility. Medical treatment includes thrombolytic medications to dissolve the clot.[52]

■ Pulmonary Hypertension

Chief Clinical Characteristics

This presentation commonly involves dyspnea on exertion, fatigue, cough, wheezing, lower extremity edema, coarse breath sounds, and angina.

Background Information

These symptoms arise from the fluid overload in the lungs and the resulting pulmonary congestion irritating the cough receptors. Pulmonary hypertension is classified as an elevation of the pulmonary artery pressure above normal.[53] This condition is classified as primary or secondary. The primary form of this condition is due to an unknown etiology.[54] Secondary disease has a known etiology and can include pulmonary vasoconstriction due to scleroderma, Eisenmenger's syndrome (a right-to-left shunt in the cardiac septum), left-sided heart failure, or other causes. Pulmonary hypertension can only be confirmed via cardiac catheterization. Medical treatment includes prostacyclins, diuretics, cardiac glycosides, supplemental oxygen,[53] and vasodilators such as sildenafil.[55] The physical therapist should be familiar with the individual's medical regime. Coordinating therapy during the peak of medical intervention will help reduce the cough symptoms and help to prevent the individual from developing an exacerbation of symptoms.

■ Sarcoidosis

Chief Clinical Characteristics
This presentation includes persistent cough, exertional dyspnea, and wheezing.

Background Information
This condition is an idiopathic systemic granulomatous disorder. The well-formed granulomas become inflamed and are usually near the connective tissue sheath of the pulmonary vessels and bronchioles and usually irritate cough receptors.[56] This condition is the most common cause of bilateral hilar adenopathy, or enlargement of the lymph nodes at the hilum. The lungs are the most frequently affected organ system. Pulmonary function tests normally demonstrate a restrictive disease pattern with lower total lung capacity, functional residual capacity, residual volume, and diffusing capacity for carbon monoxide. This condition is diagnosed by bronchoscopy and transbronchial biopsies. The individual with pulmonary sarcoidosis has a good chance of remission within 2 to 5 years from diagnosis.[56] Medical treatment usually consists of inhaled corticosteroids or glucocorticoids[57] in combination with supplemental oxygen. No emergency intervention is warranted.

■ Side Effect of Medications

Chief Clinical Characteristics
This presentation involves a chronic, dry, nonproductive cough,[58] especially in an individual with known hypertension or congestive heart failure who takes an angiotensin-converting enzyme inhibitor.

Background Information
The action of angiotensin-converting enzyme (ACE) inhibitors is arterial and venous vasodilation. The metabolism of bradykinin is affected by the ACE inhibitor and accumulates in the airways. The reactivity of the smooth muscles of the airway and the sensitivity of the cough reflex are enhanced. Some examples of common ACE inhibitors appear in Table 36-1. A thorough history will indicate whether this condition is the potential source of the persistent cough. If the cough persists to the point of adversely affecting the individual's exercise routine, then the individual may be referred to his or her physician in regards to changing to a different medication that is safe, effective, and achieves the same desired results as the ACE inhibitor. Once the ACE inhibitor is stopped, the persistent cough usually subsides within a couple of weeks.

■ Swallowing Difficulties Associated with a Stroke

Chief Clinical Characteristics
This presentation involves symptoms ranging from a persistent cough with a slight wheeze to stridor, dyspnea, rapid and shallow respirations, decreased oxygen saturation, and cyanosis. An individual with this condition who has a history of dysphagia related to stroke[7] may be prone to having a syncopal event.

TABLE 36-1 ■ **Common Angiotensin-Converting Enzyme (ACE) Inhibitor Medications**

GENERIC NAME (ALL END IN –*PRIL*)	TRADE NAME
Benazepril hydrochloride	Lotensin
Captopril	Capoten
Enalapril maleate	Vasotec
Lisinopril	Zestril, Prinivil
Quinapril hydrochloride	Accupril
Ramipril	Altace

Background Information

Dysphagia, or difficulty swallowing, is a common occurrence following a stroke.[11] Individuals with dysphagia tend to take longer to chew and swallow their food and also have a tendency to "pocket" chewed food in the mouth after swallowing.[59] This puts the individual recovering from a stroke at risk for aspirating food and liquids. In turn, individuals with this condition are at risk for developing aspiration pneumonia. The individual will respond with a cough as a defensive mechanism to remove the aspirated contents. The physical therapist treating an individual recovering from a stroke should refer the individual for evaluation of his or her swallowing.[59] The physical therapist should visualize the stroke individual's oral cavity if a persistent cough is noted, especially if it is after mealtime or after the individual has taken medications. If the symptoms become acutely severe, the physical therapist should activate the emergency medical system.

■ Tobacco Smoke

Chief Clinical Characteristics

This presentation includes a persistent, likely productive cough, dyspnea, wheezing, and decreased oxygen saturation. Individuals with this condition may have a barrel-chest appearance.

Background Information

The airway inflammation generally present in smokers causes a persistent cough, sputum production, and reactive airway disease due to the inhaled noxious stimulant. For some time now tobacco smoke has been linked to many symptoms and signs, particularly persistent cough. When airways are exposed to smoke, they become inflamed. The short-term response (cough) to tobacco smoke is a protective action. The cilia in the airway are part of the defense mechanism of the lungs. These cilia get destroyed with prolonged exposure to tobacco smoke. The long-term pathological consequences include swelling of the bronchial airways, increased mucus production, and increased airway reactivity characteristic of chronic bronchitis and chronic obstructive lung disease and the tissue destruction characteristic of emphysema.

Similar findings occur in those who are exposed to second-hand tobacco smoke. The cough reflex for those exposed to first-hand tobacco smoke becomes diminished.[60] In individuals who begin to demonstrate emphysematous changes in the lungs from first-hand tobacco smoke, cessation of smoke exposure does not undo but stabilizes the changes that had occurred.[61] The persistent cough is enhanced by the continued mucus production and therefore will not significantly dissipate. The physical therapists' treatment aim would be to improve pulmonary function through pulmonary clearance techniques, aerobic exercise, and individual education. For the individual exposed to second-hand tobacco smoke, encouragement to avoid the source of the tobacco smoke, especially during exercise treatments, would be practical. For the individual exposed to first-hand smoke, the physical therapist should alert the individual to smoking cessation programs.

■ Tuberculosis

Chief Clinical Characteristics

This presentation typically includes fever, night sweats, anorexia, weight loss, weakness, persistent cough, pleuritic chest pain, and hemoptysis.

Background Information

This condition is an infectious disease of the lungs caused by inhalation of airborne tubercle bacilli, triggering an inflammation response that, in turn, produces fluid leukocytes and macrophages. The infection can spread into extrapulmonary sites such as lymph nodes, pleura, bones, joints, kidneys, or brain. A chest radiograph will reveal infiltrates in the middle and lower zones that can irritate the cough receptors.[62] Individuals suspected of having this condition should be referred to their primary care physician immediately. Care should be taken to avoid close contact with the individual because this condition is commonly transmitted by inhalation of infected airborne particles. Medical treatment includes antituberculosis medications such as isoniazid, rifampin, pyrazinamide, ethambutol, and streptomycin. This course of treatment can last for 6 to 9 months.[62] Individuals who have this infectious disease are placed in an isolated room in the hospital. Due to the limited area in which to exercise and the necessity for isolation, the individual is prone to cardiopulmonary and physical deconditioning, disuse atrophy, and progressive dyspnea.[17] The physical therapist is often challenged with providing the individual with functional and effective exercise activities within the confines of the individual's room. Therapeutic activities and exercises using free weights or resistive bands would be practical. Bringing (and leaving) a stationary bicycle in the individual's room would address the aerobic component of an exercise program. The physical therapist should be aware that any objects used by an individual with this condition must be thoroughly cleaned with a germicidal solution prior to use by another individual because tubercle bacilli can live in sputum not exposed to sunlight for many months. If the objects are improperly cleaned, they may become vectors for disease transmission.

■ Upper Airway Cough Syndrome

Chief Clinical Characteristics

This presentation involves the sensation of "something dripping" down the back of the individual's throat or the need to clear the throat often, a condition commonly referred to as postnasal drip. This is usually due to rhinitis consisting of nasal decongestion, sneezing, or rhinorrhea, or sinusitis consisting of nasal discharge or sneezing, or a combination of both.[63]

Background Information

This condition is considered one of the most common causes of persistent cough.[64,65] The direct stimulation of the cough receptors in the upper respiratory tract triggers the cough reflex. The individual may be in an infectious state if an infection is the cause. The individual should be directed to seek advice from his or her primary care physician in regards to what medications would be most practical for his or her situation. If the affected individual is in an infectious state, the individual should be asked to refrain from continued therapy sessions until the infection has subsided to avoid infecting the physical therapist or other individuals.

■ Volume Overload

Chief Clinical Characteristics

This presentation may involve dyspnea, persistent cough, wheezes, and fatigue. Pulmonary auscultation will commonly reveal crackles.

Background Information

This is a condition in which the extracellular fluid in the body increases. Common causes of volume overload include congestive heart failure and kidney failure but can also include chronic obstructive pulmonary disease.[66] The lungs, heart, abdomen, and extremities are common places for excess fluid to accumulate. The excess fluid that collects in the lungs is similar in characteristics to a pleural effusion, cor pulmonale, congestive heart failure, or mitral valve stenosis/regurgitation, all of which lead to a persistent cough. Medical treatment generally consists of loop diuretics such as furosemide (Lasix) or Aldactone to help remove the excess fluid. The cause or location of the volume overload should dictate the physical therapist's treatment. If the cause of the volume overload is due to congestive heart failure or congestive obstructive pulmonary disease, the physical therapist should implement items from cardiac or pulmonary rehabilitation programs, respectfully. Aerobic exercises and pulmonary hygiene therapy techniques would be beneficial to the individual depending on the location of the excess fluids. The use of compression stockings or wrapping of the lower extremities, in conjunction with diuretic usage, assists in moving fluids away from the lower extremities. If the symptoms progress to limiting the individual's participation with rehabilitation, he or she should be referred to a physician for further follow-up.

References

1. Pradal M, Retornaz K, Poisson A. [Chronic cough in childhood]. *Rev Mal Respir.* Sep 2004;21(4 pt 1): 743–762.
2. Chang AB. Cough, cough receptors, and asthma in children. *Pediatr Pulmonol.* Jul 1999;28(1):59–70.
3. Morice AH, Fontana GA, Sovijarvi AR, et al. The diagnosis and management of chronic cough. *Eur Respir J.* Sep 2004;24(3):481–492.
4. Massery M, Frownfelter D. Facilitating airway clearance with coughing techniques. In: Dean E, Frownfelter DL, eds. *Principles and Practice of Cardiopulmonary Physical Therapy.* 3rd ed. St. Louis, MO: Mosby; 1996:367–416.

5. Stoller JK. Clinical features and natural history of severe alpha 1-antitrypsin deficiency. Roger S. Mitchell Lecture. *Chest.* Jun 1997;111(6 suppl):123S–128S.

6. Barker AF, Iwata-Morgan I, Oveson L, Roussel R. Pharmacokinetic study of alpha1-antitrypsin infusion in alpha1-antitrypsin deficiency. *Chest.* Sep 1997; 112(3):607–613.

7. Tokar B, Ozkan R, Ilhan H. Tracheobronchial foreign bodies in children: importance of accurate history and plain chest radiography in delayed presentation. *Clin Radiol.* Jul 2004;59(7):609–615.

8. Hilliard T, Sim R, Saunders M, Hewer SL, Henderson J. Delayed diagnosis of foreign body aspiration in children. *Emerg Med J.* Jan 2003;20(1):100–101.

9. Arya CL, Gupta R, Arora VK. Accidental condom inhalation. *Indian J Chest Dis Allied Sci.* Jan–Mar 2004;46(1):55–58.

10. Pritt B, Harmon M, Schwartz M, Cooper K. A tale of three aspirations: foreign bodies in the airway. *J Clin Pathol.* Oct 2003;56(10):791–794.

11. Marik PE. Aspiration pneumonitis and aspiration pneumonia. *N Engl J Med.* Mar 1 2001;344(9):665–671.

12. Akritidis N, Gousis C, Dimos G, Paparounas K. Fever, cough, and bilateral lung infiltrates. Achalasia associated with aspiration pneumonia. *Chest.* Feb 2003;123(2): 608–612.

13. Marik PE, Kaplan D. Aspiration pneumonia and dysphagia in the elderly. *Chest.* Jul 2003;124(1):328–336.

14. Cerny FJ, Burton HW. *Exercise Physiology for Health Care Professionals.* Champaign, IL: Human Kinetics; 2001.

15. Silverman E, Ebright L, Kwiatkowski M, Cullina J. Current management of bronchiectasis: review and 3 case studies. *Heart Lung.* Jan–Feb 2003;32(1):59–64.

16. Balkanli K, Genc O, Dakak M, et al. Surgical management of bronchiectasis: analysis and short-term results in 238 patients. *Eur J Cardiothorac Surg.* Nov 2003; 24(5):699–702.

17. Goodman CC. The respiratory system. In: Goodman CC, Boissonnault WG, eds. *Pathology: Implications for the Physical Therapist.* Philadelphia, PA: W. B. Saunders; 1998.

18. Radon K, Busching K, Heinrich J, et al. Passive smoking exposure: a risk factor for chronic bronchitis and asthma in adults? *Chest.* Sep 2002;122(3):1086–1090.

19. Pratter MR. Cough and the common cold: ACCP evidence-based clinical practice guidelines. *Chest.* Jan 2006;129(1 suppl):72S–74S.

20. Pratter MR. Chronic upper airway cough syndrome secondary to rhinosinus diseases (previously referred to as postnasal drip syndrome): ACCP evidence-based clinical practice guidelines. *Chest.* Jan 2006;129 (1 suppl):63S–71S.

21. Brunnee T, Graf K, Kastens B, Fleck E, Kunkel G. Bronchial hyperreactivity in patients with moderate pulmonary circulation overload. *Chest.* May 1993; 103(5):1477–1481.

22. Guyatt GH, Devereaux PJ. A review of heart failure treatment. *Mt Sinai J Med.* Jan 2004;71(1):47–54.

23. Cahalin LP, Ice RG, Irwin S. Program planning and implementation. In: Irwin S, ed. *Cardiopulmonary Physical Therapy.* 3rd ed. St. Louis, MO: Mosby; 1995:142–184.

24. Weitzenblum E. Chronic cor pulmonale. *Heart.* Feb 2003;89(2):225–230.

25. Orenstein DM. *Cystic Fibrosis: A Guide for Patient and Family.* 2nd ed. New York, NY: Lippincott-Raven; 1997.

26. Nixon PA, Orenstein DM, Kelsey SF. Habitual physical activity in children and adolescents with cystic fibrosis. *Med Sci Sports Exerc.* Jan 2001;33(1):30–35.

27. Turchetta A, Salerno T, Lucidi V, Libera F, Cutrera R, Bush A. Usefulness of a program of hospital-supervised physical training in patients with cystic fibrosis. *Pediatr Pulmonol.* Aug 2004;38(2):115–118.

28. Klijn PH, Terheggen-Lagro SW, Van Der Ent CK, Van Der Net J, Kimpen JL, Helders PJ. Anaerobic exercise in pediatric cystic fibrosis. *Pediatr Pulmonol.* Sep 2003;36(3):223–229.

29. Selim AJ, Ren XS, Fincke G, Rogers W, Lee A, Kazis L. A symptom-based measure of the severity of chronic lung disease: results from the Veterans Health Study. *Chest.* Jun 1997;111(6):1607–1614.

30. Jeffery PK. Comparison of the structural and inflammatory features of COPD and asthma. Giles F. Filley Lecture. *Chest.* May 2000;117(5 suppl 1):251S–260S.

31. Milgrom H, Taussig LM. Keeping children with exercise-induced asthma active. *Pediatrics.* Sep 1999; 104(3):e38.

32. McFadden ER Jr, Gilbert IA. Exercise-induced asthma. *N Engl J Med.* May 12 1994;330(19):1362–1367.

33. Anderson SD, Holzer K. Exercise-induced asthma: is it the right diagnosis in elite athletes? *J Allergy Clin Immunol.* Sep 2000;106(3):419–428.

34. Price JF. Choices of therapy for exercise-induced asthma in children. *Allergy.* 2001;56 suppl 66:12–17.

35. Fontana GA, Pistolesi M. Cough. 3: chronic cough and gastro-oesophageal reflux. *Thorax.* Dec 2003;58(12): 1092–1095.

36. Harding SM, Richter JE. The role of gastroesophageal reflux in chronic cough and asthma. *Chest.* May 1997; 111(5):1389–1402.

37. Hope-Gill BD, Hilldrup S, Davies C, Newton RP, Harrison NK. A study of the cough reflex in idiopathic pulmonary fibrosis. *Am J Respir Crit Care Med.* Oct 15, 2003;168(8):995–1002.

38. Selman M, Thannickal VJ, Pardo A, Zisman DA, Martinez FJ, Lynch JP 3rd. Idiopathic pulmonary fibrosis: pathogenesis and therapeutic approaches. *Drugs.* 2004;64(4):405–430.

39. Romano MA, Bolling SF. Update on mitral repair in dilated cardiomyopathy. *J Card Surg.* Sep–Oct 2004; 19(5):396–400.

40. Rivest P, Richer F, Bedard L. Difficulties associated with pertussis surveillance. *Can Commun Dis Rep.* Feb 15 2004;30(4):29–33, 36.

41. Goldrick BA. Pertussis on the rise. *Am J Nurs.* Jan 2005; 105(1):69–71.

42. Outbreaks of pertussis associated with hospitals—Kentucky, Pennsylvania, and Oregon, 2003. *MMWR.* Jan 28 2005;54(3):67–71.

43. Sahn SA. Pleural effusions. In: Polly PE, Heffner JE, eds. *Pulmonary/Respiratory Therapy Secrets.* 2nd ed. Philadelphia, PA: Hanley and Belfus; 2002:459–462.

44. Wells CL. Pulmonary pathology. In: DeTurk WE, Cahalin LP, eds. *Cardiovascular and Pulmonary Physical Therapy. An Evidence-Based Approach.* New York, NY: McGraw-Hill Medical; 2004:151–188.

45. Brandenburg JA, Marrie TJ, Coley CM, et al. Clinical presentation, processes and outcomes of care for

patients with pneumococcal pneumonia. *J Gen Intern Med.* Sep 2000;15(9):638–646.

46. Meehan TP, Chua-Reyes JM, Tate J, et al. Process of care performance, patient characteristics, and outcomes in elderly patients hospitalized with community-acquired or nursing home-acquired pneumonia. *Chest.* May 2000; 117(5):1378–1385.

47. Saavedra MT, Hanley ME. Pneumothorax. In: Polly PE, Heffner JE, eds. *Pulmonary/Respiratory Therapy Secrets.* 2nd ed. Philadelphia, PA: Hanley and Belfus; 2002: 463–466.

48. Mastrovich JD, Greenberger PA. Psychogenic cough in adults: a report of two cases and review of the literature. *Allergy Asthma Proc.* Jan–Feb 2002;23(1):27–33.

49. Bhatia MS, Chandra R, Vaid L. Psychogenic cough: a profile of 32 cases. *Int J Psychiatry Med.* 2002; 32(4):353–360.

50. Lee-Chiong TL, Matthay RA. Lung cancer. In: Polly PE, Heffner JE, eds. *Pulmonary/Respiratory Therapy Secrets.* 2nd ed. Philadelphia, PA: Hanley and Belfus; 2002: 370–379.

51. Baruch AC, Steinbronn K, Sobonya R. Pulmonary adenocarcinomas associated with rheumatoid nodules: a case report and review of the literature. *Arch Pathol Lab Med.* Jan 2005;129(1):104–106.

52. Lipson DA, Palevsky HI. Thromboembolic disease. In: Polly PE, Heffner JE, eds. *Pulmonary/Respiratory Therapy Secrets.* 2nd ed. Philadelphia, PA: Hanley and Belfus; 2002:237–247.

53. McLaughlin VV, Rich S. Pulmonary hypertension. *Curr Probl Cardiol.* Oct 2004;29(10):575–634.

54. Rubin LJ. Primary pulmonary hypertension. *N Engl J Med.* Jan 9, 1997;336(2):111–117.

55. Sastry BK, Narasimhan C, Reddy NK, Raju BS. Clinical efficacy of sildenafil in primary pulmonary hypertension: a randomized, placebo-controlled, double-blind, crossover study. *J Am Coll Cardiol.* Apr 7 2004; 43(7):1149–1153.

56. Fontenot AP. Sarcoidosis. In: Polly PE, Heffner JE, eds. *Pulmonary/Respiratory Therapy Secrets.* 2nd ed. Philadelphia, PA: Hanley and Belfus; 2002:270–273.

57. Mixides G, Guy E. Sarcoidosis confined to the airway masquerading as asthma. *Can Respir J.* Mar 2003; 10(2):114–116.

58. Franova S, Nosal'ova G, Antosova M, Nosal S. Enalapril and diltiazem co-administration and respiratory side effects of enalapril. *Physiol Res.* 2005;54(5):515–520.

59. Leder SB, Espinosa JF. Aspiration risk after acute stroke: comparison of clinical examination and fiberoptic endoscopic evaluation of swallowing. *Dysphagia.* Summer 2002;17(3):214–218.

60. Dicpinigaitis PV. Cough reflex sensitivity in cigarette smokers. *Chest.* Mar 2003;123(3):685–688.

61. Groneberg DA, Chung KF. Models of chronic obstructive pulmonary disease. *Respir Res.* 2004;5:18.

62. Small PM, Fujiwara PI. Management of tuberculosis in the United States. *N Engl J Med.* Jul 19 2001;345(3): 189–200.

63. McGarvey LP, Heaney LG, Lawson JT, et al. Evaluation and outcome of patients with chronic non-productive cough using a comprehensive diagnostic protocol. *Thorax.* Sep 1998;53(9):738–743.

64. Jaspersen D. Extra-esophageal disorders in gastroesophageal reflux disease. *Dig Dis.* 2004;22(2):115–119.

65. Philp EB. Chronic cough. *Am Fam Physician.* Oct 1, 1997;56(5):1395–1404.

66. de Leeuw PW, Dees A. Fluid homeostasis in chronic obstructive lung disease. *Eur Respir J Suppl.* Nov 2003; 46:33s–40s.

CHAPTER 37

Dyspnea

■ *Ragen L. Agler, PT, DPT, ATC*

Description of the Symptom

This chapter describes pathology that may lead to dyspnea. Dyspnea or shortness of breath refers to the inability to feel adequately oxygenated. The individual may report a smothering feeling, difficulty taking a breath, chest tightness or constriction, and/or an increased effort to breathe. The term *dyspnea* is derived from the Latin *dys-pnoea*, meaning "difficult breath."

Special Concerns
The therapist should be prepared to administer basic life support interventions or activate the emergency medical system should an individual present with dyspnea in association with any of the following:
■ Loss of consciousness
■ Chest discomfort, presyncopal episodes, or palpitations
■ An oxygen saturation of <88%
■ Cyanosis of the lips or fingernail beds
■ Marked hypertension (ie, >220/110) or hypotension (ie, <90/60) in an individual who is typically normotensive

CHAPTER PREVIEW: Conditions That May Lead to Dyspnea

T Trauma

COMMON

Chest injury 766
Exercise 769
Pneumothorax 773

UNCOMMON

Not applicable

RARE

Not applicable

I Inflammation

COMMON

Aseptic
Asthma 765
Bronchitis 766
Cardiomyopathy 766
Pericarditis 772

Septic
Bronchitis 766
Cardiomyopathy 766
Gastroesophageal reflux disease 770
Pericarditis 772

(continued)

Inflammation (continued)

COMMON

Pneumonia:
• Bacterial pneumonia (community-acquired pneumonia, nursing home–acquired pneumonia) 772
• Viral pneumonia 773

UNCOMMON

Aseptic
Allergic reaction 764
Idiopathic pulmonary fibrosis 770
Pleural effusion 772

Septic
Not applicable

RARE

Not applicable

M   Metabolic

COMMON

Emphysema 769
Mountain/altitude sickness 771
Renal failure 775
Tobacco smoke 776
Transfusion reaction 776

UNCOMMON

Anemia 764
Decompression sickness 768
Diabetic ketoacidosis 769
Pregnancy 774
Sarcoidosis 775

RARE

Cocaine toxicity 767

Va   Vascular

COMMON

Aortic aneurysm 765
Arrhythmias 765
Congestive heart failure 767
Cor pulmonale 767
Coronary artery disease 768
Mitral valve stenosis/regurgitation 771
Myocardial infarction (heart attack) 771
Pulmonary embolus 774
Pulmonary hypertension 775
Sickle cell disease/crisis 776

UNCOMMON

Not applicable

RARE

Not applicable

De Degenerative

COMMON

Deconditioning 768

UNCOMMON

Not applicable

RARE

Not applicable

Tu Tumor

COMMON

Malignant Primary:
Not applicable
Malignant Metastatic:
Not applicable
Benign, such as:
• Benign lung nodules 766

UNCOMMON

Malignant Primary, such as:
• Pulmonary carcinoma 774
Malignant Metastatic, such as:
• Metastases, including from primary kidney, breast, pancreas, and colon disease 770
Benign:
Not applicable

RARE

Not applicable

Co Congenital

COMMON

Mitral valve prolapse 770

UNCOMMON

Not applicable

RARE

Not applicable

Ne Neurogenic/Psychogenic

COMMON

Anxiety/panic disorder 764

UNCOMMON

Not applicable

RARE

Not applicable

Note: These are estimates of relative incidence because few data are available for the less common conditions.

Overview of Dyspnea

Dyspnea is a conscious awareness of one's own breathing (which is normally an unconscious event). The sensation may be described as a smothering feeling and the inability to get enough air. The individual often presents with labored breathing, a distressed anxious expression, dilated nostrils, a protrusion of the abdomen, and an expanded chest. Dyspnea is a common event that occurs in most individuals, even in the absence of pathology. It may be precipitated by vigorous exercise, anxiety, deconditioning, certain medications, seasonal allergies, and anemia. However, because dyspnea can be the symptom of a very serious medical condition, the therapist must be able to critically evaluate the cause of dyspnea and take the appropriate actions to ensure the patient's safety. In most cases, including those where the patient's initial referring condition is not that of dyspnea, the patient should be strongly encouraged to report any dyspnea to his or her primary physician to ensure that the proper medical workup is completed.

Description of Conditions That May Lead to Dyspnea

■ Allergic Reaction

Chief Clinical Characteristics
This presentation includes short quick breaths, tingling in the lips, tightness in the throat, and a rash or welt on the skin after exposure to an allergen. Patient can also present with wheezing, cough, and nausea.[1]

Background Information
When an individual is exposed to an allergen (ie, pollen, food, medication, and insect bites), the B cells produce immunoglobulin E (IgE) antibodies. These antibodies bind to the receptors of basophils and tissue mast cells. On subsequent exposures, the allergen reacts to the IgE antibody, which causes degranulation of the basophils and tissue mast cells.[1] This results in histamine release, which causes an increase in vascular permeability and smooth muscle contraction. The smooth muscle contraction causes bronchospasm, resulting in dyspnea. If the allergic reaction is serious, anaphylactic shock occurs, which is

potentially fatal. Individuals who present with shortness of breath interfering with the ability to carry on a conversation with the therapist or oxygen saturation of less than 88% should receive emergency medical attention.

■ Anemia

Chief Clinical Characteristics
This presentation includes lethargy, cold skin, depression, easy fatigability, shortness of breath, and cognitive impairment.[2]

Background Information
This condition involves a decrease in the oxygen-carrying capacity of blood secondary to (1) a decrease in the erythrocyte (red blood cell) content of blood, (2) a diminished content of hemoglobin per erythrocyte, or (3) a combination of both.[3] It can arise from failed synthesis, premature destruction, hemorrhage, or deficiencies in iron, B_{12}, or folic acid. Other conditions that render the patient susceptible to anemia include recent major surgery (eg, orthopedic and cardiopulmonary surgeries), pregnancy, lesions of the gastrointestinal tract, sickle cell trait, and cancer.[4] The resultant reduction in the blood's oxygen-carrying capacity initiates a reflex sinus tachycardia in attempts to maintain adequate tissue oxygenation while blood pressure is usually within the normal resting range.[5] If this condition is suspected, the patient should be referred to his or her primary care practitioner for further evaluation. The diagnosis is confirmed by routine blood testing. Treatment involves addressing the underlying cause of anemia, including iron supplementation.

■ Anxiety/Panic Disorder

Chief Clinical Characteristics
This condition is characterized by dyspnea with and without exertion and the inability to catch one's breath. Patients may also present with dizziness, palpitations, and unexplained weakness.[6] Pulse is typically rapid and regular and associated with a discrete period of intense fear or discomfort during which several predictable symptoms develop and peak in intensity within 10 minutes. These symptoms can include palpitations, chest pain/discomfort, feeling faint or dizzy, sweating, shaking/trembling, paresthesias, chills/hot flashes, fear of losing control, and fear of dying.[7]

Background Information

The body's response to this condition is usually short lived and subsides when the individual is reassured or the stressful stimulus is removed. Although anxiety or stress is perceived by many areas of the brain, the integrated response ultimately leads to elevation of plasma cortisol and catecholamine levels. Both hormones are responsible for raising blood pressure and cardiac output, the former directly leading to increased heart rate and force of contraction. The response leads to a general state of arousal and prepares the individual for useful defensive behavior (ie, the "fight-or-flight" response). In the absence of other adverse symptoms or underlying cardiovascular pathology, palpitations due to stress pose no serious risk and the therapist should reinforce this in the mind of the patient. Disabling cases of this condition should be referred to the appropriate health care provider and may include pharmacologic and psychological therapy.

■ Aortic Aneurysm

Chief Clinical Characteristics

This presentation can include dyspnea upon exertion. Individuals with an abdominal aortic aneurysm can also present with a pulsatile abdominal mass, abdominal pain, and abdominal rigidity.[8] Individuals with a thoracic aortic aneurysm can present with hoarseness, wheezing, coughing, hemoptysis, chest pain, back pain, or abdominal pain.[9]

Background Information

Many individuals with this condition are asymptomatic. This condition is defined as the focal dilation of the aorta with at least a 50% increase over normal arterial diameter. It is caused primarily by a degenerative process of the aortic medial layer secondary to atherosclerosis. Increased concentration of proteolytic enzymes in the aorta appears to be the cause of the aortic media degradation. X-ray, ultrasound, computed tomography, and angiography confirm the diagnosis. Individuals suspected of having this condition must be referred to their primary care physician immediately.

■ Arrhythmias

Chief Clinical Characteristics

This presentation may include shortness of breath with and without exertion. Patients can also report changes in their heartbeat or the feeling of their heart fluttering or skipping a beat, fatigue, or syncope.[10]

Background Information

This group of conditions is caused by a malfunction in the heart's electrical system.[10] A large variety of arrhythmias can occur. Many of them can result in a decrease in cardiac output. The primary concern with decreased cardiac output is dyspnea.[10] The diagnosis is confirmed with cardiac auscultation and electrocardiography. If an individual has a history of this condition and has a new onset of dyspnea, it is of critical importance for the individual to receive emergency medical attention.

■ Asthma

Chief Clinical Characteristics

This presentation typically involves dyspnea in combination with a chronic or intermittent persistent cough, especially in response to factors or stimuli such as pollen, dust, animal dander, environmental conditions, certain foods, and exercise.[11]

Background Information

The stimulating factor irritates the lining of the bronchial airway and a hyperadaptive response is provoked, resulting in a narrowing of the airway. If the individual is in an area that exposes him or her to such triggers as pollen, dust, or animal dander, a prudent course of action would be to have the individual exercise in a different area away from the trigger, if possible. For example, if outdoors, move the exercise program indoors. Cold, dry air is another cause of exacerbation for individuals with this condition. Exercising in a warm, moist climate or performing activities in a pool would help to reduce triggering an asthma-induced dyspneic episode. Individuals who are prone to "asthma attacks," especially during exercise, should try to exercise in an area free from any airborne irritants and in a warm, moist environment. If an asthma exacerbation occurs, the individual should be instructed to stop the activity, rest, and use any medically prescribed medications such as inhaled bronchodilators or corticosteroids until the symptoms subside. The physical therapist should try to alter the environment to avoid further episodes of dyspnea. If the individual is unable to control the situation within a reasonable amount of time, the physical therapist should be prepared to activate the emergency medical system.

■ Benign Lung Nodules

Chief Clinical Characteristics

This presentation includes a new onset of shortness of breath with exertion, as well as possible blood in the sputum; chest, shoulder, or back pain; and wheezing.[12,13]

Background Information

Up to 70% of solitary pulmonary nodules are benign lung tumors. Although not considered a significant health problem, these tumors can increase the patient's risk of pneumonia, atelectasis, and hemoptysis.[14] Chest x-ray and computed tomography confirm the diagnosis, and biopsy of neoplasia may be necessary to determine the tumor cell type. Treatment typically involves observation, although individuals with this condition who demonstrate bloody sputum, new onset of dyspnea, or instability of hemodynamic/oxygen transport should be referred for emergency evaluation and treatment by a physician.

■ Bronchitis

Chief Clinical Characteristics

This presentation includes shortness of breath upon exertion, frequently combined with fever, cough with sputum production, muscle aches, and fatigue. Individuals with this condition may also report a sore throat, runny or stuffy nose, and/or a headache.[15]

Background Information

Acute bronchitis—inflammation of the trachea, bronchi, or bronchioles[16]—can be associated with smoking, inhalation of dust or chemical pollutants, or infectious disease process. During an acute episode, there is a decrease in bronchial mucociliary function due to the mucous membranes being hyperemic and edematous. This leads to increased mucus production.[15] Individuals who present to the clinic with this clinical picture should be referred to their primary care physician for medical follow-up. Physical therapy intervention can continue as long as the oxygen saturation does not fall below 88%. Individuals with this condition will not have a typical physical energy level and, therefore, their ability to fully participate in physical therapy treatment may be impaired.

■ Cardiomyopathy

Chief Clinical Characteristics

This presentation can involve dyspnea with and without exertion, in addition to swelling of the extremities, abdominal distention, fatigue, dizziness, and fainting during physical activities.[17]

Background Information

There are three primary types of this condition, including restrictive, dilated, and hypertrophic.[17,18] This condition can be caused uncontrolled diabetes, drug abuse, radiation therapy, fibrosis, malignancies or autosomal dominant genetic factor. A viral, bacterial, rickettsial, metazoal, or protozoal infection also may account for this presentation. Regardless of the type of cardiomyopathy, the cardiac output is severely altered secondary to myocardial contractile disruption and arrythmias.[17,18] The diagnosis is confirmed by murmur or an S_3 heart sound on cardiac auscultation in combination with echocardiography. It is of critical importance that the emergency medical system be activated immediately if this condition is suspected. In addition, if an individual with known cardiomyopathy reports dyspnea with exertion that does not subside with rest, the emergency medical system must be activated.

■ Chest Injury

Chief Clinical Characteristics

This presentation typically involves guarding over the affected area of an injury to the thorax, in combination with diminished chest wall movement and pain in and around the affected area.

Background Information

Direct trauma to the upper body including the chest wall, lungs, and throat is an apparent cause of cough following a chest injury. The trauma can include a physical injury resulting from a motor vehicle accident, fall, physical assault, or penetrating wound. The trauma can also occur from surgery to the regions mentioned above. In the case of a flail chest secondary to trauma, the breathing mechanics will be altered. During inspiration the chest wall will expand, but the injured area will draw inward. During expiration the chest wall contracts, while the area of injury protrudes.[19] The reaction that causes the cough is similar in nature regardless of the origin of trauma. If the trauma is directly affecting the bronchial airway, the cough mechanism is protective in nature and the purpose is to remove the cause of the irritation. When the trauma is not directly affecting the bronchial airway (as in the case of a crush or penetrating chest wall injury), the surrounding areas will become inflamed and swollen. In this case the excess fluids can accumulate in the lungs. These excess fluids will become an irritation to the bronchial airway. The cough reaction will be to remove the fluids so that normal gas exchange can take place. When the trauma is surgical in nature, fluids will arise due to the inflammatory response of the surrounding tissues. The cough response is similar in quality to the physical trauma mentioned above. The physical therapist should be able to recognize the source of the trauma and respond accordingly. If the cause of the cough is due to direct trauma to the airways (physical or surgical), the physical therapist should suggest splinting techniques to relieve pain and give external support. If the cause of the cough is indirect trauma, the physical therapist should incorporate postural drainage, percussion, vibration, deep-breathing exercises, and assisted cough techniques in an attempt to facilitate removal of the secretions. The physical therapist should be aware of the underlying causes and physical structures present prior to administering any of the above pulmonary physical therapy techniques. Percussion and vibration directly over fractured ribs are contraindicated but encouraged around the site.[19]

■ **Cocaine Toxicity**

Chief Clinical Characteristics

This presentation commonly involves shortness of breath with and without exertion in association with a high blood pressure and heart rate, tremors, and sweaty skin. Psychosis can also be a common feature.[20]

Background Information

Cocaine is presently the second most abused illicit stimulant in the United States. The major effect of cocaine is the stimulation of the sympathetic nervous system. This results in an increased heart rate and increased blood pressure. The overstimulation of the sympathetic nervous system can result in abnormal heart rhythms. These arrhythmias can lead to dyspnea.[20] This diagnosis can be confirmed with a history positive for cocaine use and abuse.

■ **Congestive Heart Failure**

Chief Clinical Characteristics

This presentation can be characterized by dyspnea on exertion, orthopnea, persistent cough, peripheral edema, and fatigue. On examination, individuals with this condition may demonstrate systolic murmur, crackles/rales on pulmonary auscultation, a third (S_3) and/or fourth (S_4) heart sound on cardiac auscultation, jugular vein distention, or peripheral cyanosis.

Background Information

This condition is characterized by left ventricular contractile dysfunction resulting in ventricular dilation and poor contraction. Contractile dysfunction can be caused by myocardial ischemia or infarction, coronary artery disease, or bacterial/viral infection. As the heart pump fails, the blood returning to the heart from the lungs is backed up, causing overload in the pulmonary circulation and leading to bronchial hyperreactivity. Dyspnea, wheezing, and persistent coughing are common signs in individuals with bronchial hyperreactivity.[21] Medical treatment usually consists of a combination of vasodilators, diuretics, digoxin, beta blockers, antiarrhythmic agents, and anticoagulants.[22] Implementing a cardiac rehabilitation program would be beneficial.[23] The individual who is newly diagnosed or having an exacerbation of symptoms would begin in Phase I of a cardiac rehabilitation program and progress to Phase III over a period of several months.

■ **Cor Pulmonale**

Chief Clinical Characteristics

This presentation involves dyspnea on exertion, chronic productive cough, wheezing, lower extremity edema, jugular venous distention, and in chronic cases digital clubbing.[19]

Background Information

This condition is characterized as pulmonary heart disease. The right side of the heart may become enlarged due to pulmonary hypertension, pulmonary embolism, chronic obstructive pulmonary disease, idiopathic pulmonary fibrosis, and Pickwickian syndrome.[24] Medical management includes diuretics, supplemental oxygen use, and dietary salt restrictions.[19] The physical therapist should take to the role of preventing the onset of cor pulmonale by addressing the underlying cause. Aerobic exercises, mobility training, and breathing exercises could have an important effect on the above-mentioned causes. Individual education would also be beneficial, including how to monitor lower extremity edema and signs of respiratory failure. The physical therapist should be aware of any acute signs and symptoms of severe forms of this condition to the point that the individual experiences pallor, sweating, severe chest pain, weak and rapid pulse, anxiety, and diminished level of consciousness. In this situation, the physical therapist should activate the emergency medical system immediately, because these signs and symptoms suggest the condition has progressed to become life threatening.

■ Coronary Artery Disease

Chief Clinical Characteristics
This presentation can include dyspnea in combination with symptoms of angina, often described as substernal chest discomfort, pressure, heaviness, squeezing, or burning that radiates to the shoulders, arms (left greater than right), neck, jaw, and epigastrium.

Background Information
With decreased myocardial oxygen supply (or increased demand in the case of exertion), vulnerable myocardial cells become ischemic and hyperirritable and discharge spontaneously, driving abnormal cardiac rhythms. The ectopic rhythm can be supraventricular or ventricular in origin, tachycardic or bradycardic (in the case of complete heart block), and is difficult to differentiate on the basis of palpation alone. Arrhythmia leads to dyspnea. In cases of tachyarrhythmias, the resulting increase in myocardial oxygen demand may escalate the condition from one of transient ischemia to one of frank infarction and the episode may become life threatening. Use of sublingual nitroglycerin or supplemental oxygen prescribed by the patient's physician may resolve minor episodes. However, if the patient becomes unstable during episodes of dyspnea with associated angina pectoris, activation of the emergency medical system is warranted. The

therapist should be prepared to administer basic life support measures (including the use of an automated external defibrillator if warranted) while awaiting advanced cardiac life support assistance.

■ Decompression Sickness

Chief Clinical Characteristics
This presentation may involve short, shallow breathing after an episode of scuba diving in combination with joint pain in the ankles, knees, wrists, hips, shoulders, and elbows; headaches; confusion; pain with breathing; and itching of the face, arms, and upper torso.[25,26]

Background Information
The gas nitrogen leads to the pathology of decompression sickness. As a scuba diver descends, more nitrogen enters the tissues due to the increase in pressure. If a diver ascends slowly, the excess nitrogen can be expelled through the lungs. However, if the diver ascends too quickly, the nitrogen will come out of solution in the body fluids and tissues and convert to the gas phase, forming bubbles in the blood and tissues of the body.[26,27] These bubbles can involve the skin, muscles, and lymphatic system (Type I); the lungs, brain, and ears (Type II); or they can lead to arterial gas embolism (Type III).[25,26] It is of critical importance that the emergency medical system be activated secondary to potentially fatal consequences of this condition. Typical treatment involves supportive intervention combined with a hyperbaric chamber protocol.

■ Deconditioning

Chief Clinical Characteristics
This presentation may be characterized by shortness of breath with low-level exertion and a history of being sedentary.[28]

Background Information
Deconditioning is the result of a person being inactive. This can be caused by an illness, an injury, or a sedentary lifestyle. With exercise, the body responds with an increased heart rate and an increased respiratory rate.[28] The increased respiratory rate can lead to dyspnea.[28] Due to the fact that deconditioned individuals can present with symptoms while they exercise that could indicate a pathology, a thorough pre-exercise screening examination completed by the physical therapist will allow the therapist

to differentiate dyspnea caused by this condition from dyspnea caused by a serious pathology. In the absence of serious pathology, individuals with this condition should be assured that this is a normal response to increased physical activity and counseled in how to control symptoms by modifying the intensity of exercise and other behavioral methods as appropriate.

■ Diabetic Ketoacidosis

Chief Clinical Characteristics
This presentation typically involves confusion, agitation, dyspnea, tachycardia, and fruity breath odor.[29]

Background Information
In a fasting state in a healthy individual, the body changes from carbohydrate metabolism to fat oxidation. During this process the free fatty acids are converted to acetate, which is then turned into ketoacids.[29] This is exported from the liver to the peripheral tissues. Despite the amount of circulating glucose in an individual with insulin-dependent diabetes, the carbohydrate cannot be used secondary to a lack of insulin. This results in a maximal production of ketones, which leads to this condition.[29] Primary intervention involves prevention by timing physical activity with the insulin schedule and by maintaining a regular insulin dosing regimen. However, when present, this condition is considered a medical emergency.

■ Emphysema

Chief Clinical Characteristics
This presentation includes complaints of shortness of breath, persistent cough with sputum production, wheezing, and decreased exercise tolerance.[30] *Physical examination reveals a prolonged expiratory phase during respiration, increased anteroposterior diameter of the chest (barrel chest appearance), flattened diaphragm, and distant breath sounds on pulmonary auscultation with wheezes and/or crackles.*

Background Information
This condition is the most common obstructive pulmonary disease. It is characterized as enlarged air spaces due to disruption of the destruction of elastic fibers in the alveolar wall, which is irreversible.[31] The emphysematous changes produce airway obstruction with impaired ventilation and gas exchange in the

lungs, resulting in decreased diffusion of oxygen. The elastic recoil of the lungs is lost, resulting in retention of air. A history of smoking tobacco is common; exposure to second-hand smoke or occupational toxins also can make a person prone to developing emphysema. Medical intervention commonly consists of smoking cessation, use of bronchodilators, and limited use of supplemental oxygen. In severe cases lung volume reduction surgery may be performed to remove hyperinflated blebs or bullae. The physical therapist's treatment should include aspects of a pulmonary rehabilitation program including airway hygiene techniques such as percussion and vibration, postural drainage, and aerobic exercises at a submaximal level. Individual education about pursed-lip breathing techniques should also be included. If the individual has undergone surgery for removal of emphysematous blebs or bullae, the physical therapist should also address any postsurgical movement dysfunction that may be affecting the individual.

■ Exercise

Chief Clinical Characteristics
This presentation typically involves a breathing rate that increases gradually and appropriately for the intensity of the exercise bout. When the exercise bout is terminated, the breathing rate gradually returns to resting values. Assessment of the blood pressure will typically reveal elevated systolic values that are appropriate for the intensity of physical exertion (eg, 10 to 12 mm Hg increase for every metabolic equivalent increase in workload).

Background Information
In response to the metabolic demands placed on the cardiopulmonary system by activities involving the contraction of large muscle groups, cardiac output will increase. This is primarily accomplished by enhanced cardiac automaticity and contractility, yielding a substantial increase in heart rate that parallels this increase in respiratory rate. To the individual who is typically sedentary or otherwise unaccustomed to exercise, the resultant shortness of breath may be considered unusual and pathological. The response is mediated by enhanced sympathetic outflow and circulating catecholamines involved in the "fight-or-flight"

response and does not typically lead to any adverse consequences in the absence of underlying organic heart and lung disease. This condition is a normal response to exertion and will subside with cessation of the exercise bout. No emergency intervention is warranted.

Gastroesophageal Reflux Disease

Chief Clinical Characteristics

This presentation commonly includes dyspnea, dysphonia, hoarseness, sore throat, gum inflammation, dental erosion, chest pain, heart burn, sputum production with coughing, and wheezing.[32] The cough will be more prevalent in the morning and after meals. This condition is common among individuals who are nonsmokers with a normal chest radiograph and not taking angiotensin-converting enzyme inhibitors.[32]

Background Information

This condition involves retrograde movement of gastric contents into the esophagus. In individuals with this condition, persistent cough is one of the most common complaints.[33] The mechanism of cough in an individual with gastroesophageal reflux disease is from microaspiration of gastric contents or a vagally mediated esophageal-tracheobronchial reflex. Medical treatment includes vigorous acid suppression, elevating the head of the individual's bed 10 cm, weight loss, diet modification to high-protein and low-fat foods, omitting high-acid foods, antacid use prior to bedtime, and limiting food intake 2 hours prior to bedtime.[33] Referral should be made to the individual's primary physician for a 24-hour esophageal pH test. Physical therapists treating individuals with this condition in its acute form should avoid having the individual flex forward at the trunk or hips and also avoid vigorous activities in the early morning or after meals, because these situations raise the likelihood of symptom aggravation.

Idiopathic Pulmonary Fibrosis

Chief Clinical Characteristics

This presentation involves exertional dyspnea and an irritating, nonproductive cough.[34] Lung auscultation will reveal a "Velcro"-like quality crackle most noticeable at the bases. Pulmonary function tests will demonstrate a restrictive disease pattern with decreased vital capacity, residual volume, and total lung capacity.

Background Information

This condition is a specific form of chronic fibrosing interstitial pneumonia that is limited to the lung. The "stiffness" of the lungs causes a rapid, shallow breathing pattern. This is due to a ventilation/perfusion mismatch and the individual can become hypoxic during exercise. This will lead to a worsening of the above cough and dyspnea symptoms. Pulmonary rehabilitation may help improve the quality of life and prepare the individual for possible lung transplantation. The physical therapist should progress through the program slowly so as not to exacerbate symptoms. If the symptoms worsen to tussive syncope or increased hypoxemia, the physical therapist should activate the emergency medical system as warranted. The prognosis is poor and most individuals die within 3 to 8 years from onset of symptoms.[35]

Metastases, Including from Primary Kidney, Breast, Pancreas, and Colon Disease

Chief Clinical Characteristics

This presentation commonly includes dyspnea, hemoptysis, persistent cough, chest discomfort, weight loss, and voice hoarseness, in association with possible symptoms related to the primary disease.

Background Information

The lungs are the most common site of metastases from other types of cancer. When tumor cells migrate from their primary site they can work their way into the circulation or lymphatic system. The lungs filter these systems. The most common cancers to metastasize to the lungs are kidney, breast, pancreas, colon and uterus. Treatment of this condition depends on the type and extent of metastases, including surgical resection, chemotherapy, and radiation therapy.

Mitral Valve Prolapse

Chief Clinical Characteristics

This presentation can include shortness of breath, chest pain, palpitations, fatigue, and light-headedness and may cause periodic syncopal episodes in a small subset of patients.[36] Most individuals with this condition are asymptomatic. Upon cardiac auscultation, a midsystolic click is often heard best over the fifth intercostal space, midclavicular line, often followed by a late systolic murmur.

Background Information
The diagnosis is confirmed by echocardiography or angiography, which usually reveals exaggerated systolic bowing beyond the mitral annulus of one or both valve leaflets. Individuals with this condition may be instructed to cough forcefully or perform a Valsalva maneuver, bearing down against a closed glottis, during episodes of palpitations in an effort to break the abnormal rhythm through vagal mediation. Quite often, individuals with this condition are also prescribed calcium channel blockers or beta blockers to suppress the occurrence of palpitations. Occasionally, the tachycardia may be prolonged and immediate medical intervention is usually warranted, especially if the patient has underlying coronary artery disease and becomes hemodynamically unstable.

■ **Mitral Valve Stenosis/ Regurgitation**

Chief Clinical Characteristics
This presentation includes dyspnea on exertion, persistent cough, decreased exercise tolerance, orthopnea, and occasionally hemoptysis in combination with a systolic murmur best heard at the apex of the heart, rales on pulmonary auscultation, a third (S_3) and/or fourth (S_4) heart sound on cardiac auscultation and jugular venous distintion.

Background Information
This condition is characterized by the leaflets of the mitral valve becoming stiff and closing incompletely, usually due to the annulus (rim) of the valve being stretched. Left arterial and/or ventricular enlargement can pull and stretch on the mitral valve annulus. With this condition, the blood coming from the lungs into the left side of the heart will be slowed and can back up into the lungs, leading to volume overload in the lungs.[37] The chronic overload in the pulmonary circulation is accompanied by bronchial hyperreactivity. Symptoms of dyspnea, wheezing and persistent coughing are common in individuals with bronchial hyperreactivity.[21] This condition usually occurs secondary to prior rheumatic fever occurring in childhood, yet the individual does not become symptomatic until the adult years. Other etiologies include coronary artery disease, bacterial endocarditis, and left ventricular dilation. Medical treatment consists of antibiotic,

digitalis diuretic, and vasodilator medications. In cases of significant forms of this condition, repair or replacement of the mitral valve will be warranted. Cardiac rehabilitation program is optimal in the surgical and postsurgical management of this condition.[23] The physical therapist should be aware that the individual will be self-limiting in his or her exercise tolerance if the condition worsens.

■ **Mountain/Altitude Sickness**

Chief Clinical Characteristics
This presentation typically involves dyspnea with exertion after a hike, ski trip, or mountain climb in association with headache, difficulty sleeping, nausea, and the sensation of a bounding pulse.[38]

Background Information
As altitude increases, the atmospheric concentration of oxygen decreases.[38] For example at 8,000 and 18,000 feet there is 25% less and 50% less available oxygen compared to sea level, respectively.[39] Typical physiological response to a decrease in oxygen is an increase in respiratory rate and heart rate. As CO_2 is eliminated with each exhalation, the kidneys increase excretion of bicarbonate to maintain pH balance. However, if the respiratory rate remains high for an extended period of time (24 to 44 hours), the kidneys are unable to excrete enough bicarbonate to maintain the balance and, thus, the blood becomes alkalotic. This pH change leads to the dilation and leaking of the microvascular beds,[39] resulting in an accumulation of fluids in all body tissues. Respiratory distress may result from pulmonary edema. Physical therapists should be vigilant for this condition, since it may occur in individuals who participate in activities at lower elevations, as well. This condition is a medical emergency.

■ **Myocardial Infarction (Heart Attack)**

Chief Clinical Characteristics
This presentation often includes chest pain, left arm or shoulder pain, jaw pain, upper back pain, palpitations, and dyspnea.[40–42]

Background Information
This condition involves irreversible necrosis of the heart muscle secondary to prolonged ischemia.[40,41] Atherosclerosis is a disease

process that is primarily responsible for this condition. Plaque fissures and ruptures result from stress at the atherosclerotic lesion. These plaque ruptures are considered the major trigger for coronary thrombosis.[40–42] Strenuous physical activity or emotional stress leads to an increased sympathetic nervous system response, increased blood pressure, increased heart rate, and increased force production during ventricular contraction. In turn, this sequence of events increases the stress at the atherosclerotic lesion and causes the plaque to rupture.[40–42] During acute forms of this condition, ST-segment elevations, dynamic T-wave changes, or ST depressions may be present upon electrocardiographic analysis. Upon auscultation an S_4 gallop may be detected. If this condition is suspected, the emergency medical system (EMS) must be activated immediately to decrease the risk of sudden death. Basic life support (BLS) should be initiated immediately after the EMS system is activated. If after completing the BLS assessment of the patient's condition, the patient continues to present with an acute myocardial infarction, it is recommended that the therapist administer a baby aspirin to the patient.

■ **Pericarditis**

Chief Clinical Characteristics

This presentation is characterized by chest pain and fever as the hallmark symptoms. Chest pain almost always has a mechanical component in which it is aggravated by coughing, deep inspiration, or lying supine. This characteristic distinguishes this condition from angina. Dyspnea may be reported. Pericardial friction rub that is likened to two pieces of leather rubbing against one another may be heard during cardiac auscultation. Asking the patient to momentarily hold his or her breath while auscultating helps to distinguish friction rub from this condition and a pleural friction rub (the latter would disappear upon breath-holding).

Background Information

This condition can be either aseptic (eg, post-myocardial infarction, radiation induced, drug induced, or connective tissue disease) or septic (eg, viral, pyogenic bacteria, and tuberculosis). This condition is often self-limiting, but individuals with this condition should be referred to their primary care physician for supportive care that may include prescription of anti-inflammatory or antibiotic medication.

■ **Pleural Effusion**

Chief Clinical Characteristics

This presentation commonly includes dyspnea, persistent cough, and pleuritic chest pain. Physical examination may reveal decreased chest expansion, diminished or absent breath sounds, dullness to percussion, and possible friction rub.

Background Information

This condition is a collection of fluid between the visceral pleura and parietal pleura, which occurs as fluid production exceeds fluid absorption in the pleural space. The etiology of this condition involves congestive heart failure, atelectasis, pneumonia, impaired lymphatic drainage, and kidney or liver failure.[43] The cough is due to the excess fluid and dyspnea, which irritate the cough receptors in the bronchial airways and diminish gas exchange. The cough reflex is triggered in a response to remove the excess fluids. In severe cases, the individual may have a tracheal shift away from the affected side[44] and may develop mild hypoxemia. In this case the physical therapist should administer supplemental oxygen to maintain oxygen saturation at a level where the individual is comfortable and maintains a calm respiratory rate. Except for pleural effusion caused by congestive heart failure, the medical treatment for pleural effusion is to remove the fluid by thoracocentesis or placement of a chest tube.[44] If the individual has recently had a thoracocentesis performed to drain a pleural effusion, the physical therapist should be aware of the signs and symptoms of a possible pneumothorax that may have developed due to the procedure.

PNEUMONIA

■ **Bacterial Pneumonia (Community-Acquired Pneumonia, Nursing Home–Acquired Pneumonia)**

Chief Clinical Characteristics

This presentation usually includes dyspnea, persistent cough, sputum production with occasional hemoptysis, fatigue, and pleuritic chest pain.[45] *Pulmonary auscultation will likely reveal decreased or absent breath sounds and wheezes/crackles.*[46]

Background Information

The onset of illness is usually abrupt. Medical treatment consists of some form of penicillin or amoxicillin.[45] Physical therapists' intervention should include airway hygiene techniques such as percussion and vibration, postural drainage, assisted cough techniques, and deep-breathing exercises. Mobilizing the individual would also be beneficial in assisting to clear the lungs of sputum.

■ Viral Pneumonia

Chief Clinical Characteristics

This presentation commonly involves increasing dyspnea and persistent, dry, nonproductive cough. Chest auscultation reveals rhonchi, rales, or wheezes. The individual may also exhibit fever, decreased appetite, headache and fatigue. This condition most commonly occurs after the onset of influenza or inhalation of some other airborne virus.

Background Information

This condition can be community acquired or nosocomial. The cough reflex is triggered by stimulation of the cough receptors from the infectious material in the airways. A chest radiograph will show infiltrates in the areas affected. The aim of treatment in an individual with a viral pneumonia is to increase oxygen transportation. This includes pulmonary percussion and vibration, postural drainage, deep-breathing exercises, assisted cough techniques, and mobilizing the individual. The physical therapist should be aware of the potential for contamination or infection from one individual to another or to the physical therapist. The affected individual should be treated away from other susceptible individuals. Physical therapists should protect themselves by wearing a mask that covers their nose and mouth. The affected individual may also consider wearing a mask to protect others. Performing hand hygiene before and after treatment of an affected individual will help reduce the spread of infection.

■ Pneumothorax

Chief Clinical Characteristics

This presentation typically involves dyspnea, pleuritic chest pain, and dry cough and the individual may have absent breath sounds with hyperresonant percussion over the affected area.

Background Information

This condition is free air that leaks into the pleural space between the visceral and parietal pleura. The cough seen in an individual with this condition results from the irritation of the cough receptors from the increased intrathoracic pressure. There are three main classifications of this condition. *Traumatic pneumothorax* is caused by a trauma or injury, direct or indirect, to the thorax. Common causes include gunshot wound, knife wound and motor vehicle accidents. *Spontaneous pneumothorax* occurs as the structural integrity of the pleural tissue is weakened. The tissue becomes so weakened that a bleb or bullae can rupture, allowing air into the pleural space. Individuals with asthma, cystic fibrosis, emphysema, pulmonary infections and empyema are likely candidates for developing a spontaneous pneumothorax. This condition can also occur in healthy individuals. Healthy individuals who smoke, have a positive family history, and males between the ages of 10 and 30 years who have a tall, thin body habitus are more prone to developing a spontaneous pneumothorax.[47] *Tension pneumothorax* is characterized by air entering the pleural space but not exiting. This condition is caused by a one-way or ball valve fistula. The ipsilateral lung becomes compressed and the mediastinum shifts contralaterally. A tension pneumothorax is a medical emergency because the individual will develop decreased cardiac output, refractory hypoxemia and hypotension. The physical therapist will need to activate the emergency medical system. Medical treatment consists of chest tube placement to remove the trapped air. The use of high concentrations of supplemental oxygen will reabsorb the lesion four times faster than if no supplemental oxygen was used.[47] This situation may resolve without the use of a chest tube in individuals with small pneumothoraces (<15% of the hemithorax).

The physical therapist should have supplemental oxygen available for use during therapy sessions. If the individual appears to be in respiratory distress during a session, the physical therapist should activate the emergency medical system.

■ Pregnancy

Chief Clinical Characteristics
This presentation includes shortness of breath often associated with a rapid and bounding pulse, and there may be an increased occurrence of symptoms to term.[48] At times, the palpitations may precipitate dizziness, presyncope, or frank syncope.[49]

Background Information
Episodes of dyspnea are usually benign and self-limiting. Significant changes occur in hormonal and hemodynamic function during pregnancy that predispose women to the development of dysrhythmias and corresponding dyspnea. Changes in hormone levels during pregnancy (particularly progesterone) have been associated with enhanced sympathetic activity and the precipitation of dysrhythmias.[50] Only very rarely is atrial fibrillation or ventricular tachycardia the source of the dysrhythmia.[51] Mechanical compression of the diaphragm by way of increasing fetal volume compressing against the abdominal contents and volume overload are other factors that may cause dyspnea in individuals with this condition. Patients who are pregnant and report palpitations associated with symptoms of cardiovascular instability should be referred to their primary care physician for evaluation. In the event of cardiovascular compromise, supportive interventions and activation of the emergency medical system may necessary.

■ Pulmonary Carcinoma

Chief Clinical Characteristics
This presentation commonly includes persistent dyspnea, cough, hemoptysis, chest discomfort, weight loss, and voice hoarseness. Individuals who have bronchoalveolar cell carcinoma can produce copious amounts of thin secretions.[52]

Background Information
Cigarette smoking is the primary cause of carcinoma in the lung, and exposure to asbestos is the most common occupational exposure cause for a person developing lung carcinoma.[52] There are many types of carcinoma of the bronchial airways including small-cell lung cancer (ie, oat cell carcinoma) and non–small-cell lung cancers (ie, squamous cell, adenocarcinoma, and large-cell carcinomas).[19] This condition has a strong association with rheumatoid arthritis, and may even precede joint involvement.[53] In an individual who is in the early stages of localized lung cancer, symptoms do not vary much from the symptoms related to cigarette smoking; therefore, the individual may not seek medical attention promptly.[19] Individuals with this condition may have tumors located in the main stem or segmental bronchi, causing dyspnea and cough. Pulmonary auscultation will usually reveal normal findings. Individuals suspected of having this condition should be referred to their primary care physician. Complete blood count, chest radiography, computed tomography, positron emission tomography, pulmonary function tests, ventilation/perfusion scan, and biopsy of the suspected tumor are diagnostic. Medical treatment for the individual who is diagnosed with carcinoma of the lungs can include radiation and chemotherapy. In certain cases, surgical resection of the tumor and possibly some of the surrounding tissues may be necessary. Physical therapists should construct a therapeutic program to improve the individual's pulmonary function along with any possible complications due to the radiation or chemotherapies. This may include decreased endurance and muscle weakness due to the side effects of loss of appetite and weight loss resulting from the above treatments. Frequents rest breaks and interval training may be beneficial for the individual. Following surgery, physical therapists also should address movement dysfunction related to chest trauma.

■ Pulmonary Embolus

Chief Clinical Characteristics
This presentation includes dyspnea, pleuritic chest pain, persistent cough, hemoptysis, and syncope.[54] Individuals with a history of deep venous thrombosis are susceptible. Other factors that put an individual at risk include immobility resulting in blood stasis, endothelial injuries due to lower extremity trauma or surgery, and hypercoagulable states arising from such situations as oral contraceptive use or cancer.

Background Information

This condition is defined as a blood clot that has become lodged in a pulmonary artery and significantly inhibits or ceases blood flow to the lung tissue. The obstruction is commonly a blood clot, but this condition can also be caused by air, fat, bone marrow, foreign intravenous material, or tumor cells.[19] Medical treatment will depend on the severity of the blocked pulmonary artery. In an acute case of severe disease, sudden death may occur. In the case of severe disease in which signs and symptoms appear significant and hemodynamic instability or respiratory compromise is evident, the physical therapist should activate the emergency medical system. In other cases where the signs and symptoms appear not as severe, the individual should be directed to an emergent care facility. Medical treatment includes thrombolytic medications to dissolve the clot.[54]

■ Pulmonary Hypertension

Chief Clinical Characteristics

This presentation commonly involves dyspnea on exertion, fatigue, cough, wheezing, lower extremity edema, coarse breath sounds, and angina.

Background Information

The symptoms of this condition arise from the fluid overload in the lungs and the resulting pulmonary congestion. Pulmonary hypertension is classified as an elevation of the pulmonary artery pressure above normal.[55] The two classifications of this condition are primary and secondary. The primary form of this condition is due to an unknown etiology.[56] Secondary disease has a known etiology and can include pulmonary vasoconstriction due to scleroderma, Eisenmenger's syndrome (a right-to-left shunt in the cardiac septum), left-sided heart failure, or other causes. Pulmonary hypertension can only be confirmed via cardiac catheterization. Medical treatment includes prostacyclins, diuretics, cardiac glycosides, supplemental oxygen,[55] and vasodilators such as sildenafil.[57] The physical therapist should be familiar with the individual's medical regime. Coordinating therapy during the peak of medical intervention will help reduce the cough symptoms and help to prevent the individual from developing an exacerbation of symptoms.

■ Renal Failure

Chief Clinical Characteristics

This presentation can involve shortness of breath with exertion. Patients can also present with abdominal distention and nausea.

Background Information

This condition, which can be either acute or chronic, is the result of a glomerular or tubulointerstitial lesion.[58] It is associated with increased serum creatinine and or urea levels. The seven primary characteristics of renal failure are azotemia, acidosis, hyperkalemia, abnormal fluid volume control, hypocalcemia, anemia, and hypertension.[58–60] The abnormal control of fluid volume results in a decreased ability to concentrate the urine. This progresses to the inability to dilute urine, resulting in retention of sodium and water. This retention can lead to congestive heart failure, which is the primary cause of dyspnea in this patient population.[58] Medical treatment typically involves hemodialysis. When treating these patients, a therapist must monitor symptoms. If dyspnea worsens with activities, the primary care physician must be contacted to rule out worsening congestive heart failure.

■ Sarcoidosis

Chief Clinical Characteristics

This presentation includes persistent cough, exertional dyspnea, and wheezing.

Background Information

This condition is an idiopathic systemic granulomatous disorder. The well-formed granulomas become inflamed and are usually near the connective tissue sheath of the pulmonary vessels and bronchioles.[61] This condition is the most common cause of bilateral hilar adenopathy, or enlargement of the lymph nodes at the hilum. The lungs are the most frequently affected organ system. Pulmonary function tests normally demonstrate a restrictive disease pattern with lower total lung capacity, functional residual capacity, residual volume, and diffusing capacity for carbon monoxide. This condition is diagnosed by bronchoscopy and transbronchial biopsies. The individual with pulmonary sarcoidosis has a good chance of remission within 2 to 5 years from diagnosis.[61] Medical intervention usually consists of inhaled corticosteroids or glucocorticoids[62] in combination with supplemental oxygen. No emergency intervention is warranted.

Sickle Cell Disease/Crisis

Chief Clinical Characteristics

This presentation includes sudden, acute chest pain and shortness of breath in combination with acute abdominal and joint pain.

Background Information

This condition is the most common hereditary blood disorder.[63] It most commonly affects individuals of African indigenous descent.[63,64] It is also called hemolytic anemia due to the shortening of the life span of the red blood cell.[63,64] Patients with this disorder experience what is called sickle cell crisis. During such a crisis, the patient may develop bone crisis that results in acute sudden bone pain. Development of acute chest syndrome is possible. At the first sign of this condition, physical therapy treatment should discontinue and the patient should be referred back to his or her primary physician for follow-up and additional management.

Tobacco Smoke

Chief Clinical Characteristics

This presentation includes dyspnea, a persistent and likely productive cough, wheezing, and decreased oxygen saturation and the individual may have a barrel-chest appearance.

Background Information

The airway inflammation generally present in smokers causes the persistent cough, sputum production, and reactive airway disease that result from inhalation of a noxious stimulant. For some time now tobacco smoke has been linked to many symptoms and signs, particularly persistent cough. When airways are exposed to smoke they become inflamed. The short-term response (cough) to tobacco smoke is a protective action. The cilia in the airway are part of the defense mechanism of the lungs. These cilia get destroyed with prolonged exposure to tobacco smoke. The long-term pathological consequences include swelling of the bronchial airways, increased mucus production, and increased airway reactivity characteristic of chronic bronchitis and chronic obstructive lung disease and the tissue destruction characteristic of emphysema. Similar findings occur in those who are exposed to second-hand tobacco smoke. The cough reflex for those exposed to first-hand tobacco smoke becomes diminished.[65] In individuals who begin to demonstrate emphysematous changes in the lungs from first-hand tobacco smoke, cessation of smoke exposure does not undo but stabilizes the changes that had occurred.[66] The persistent cough therefore will not significantly dissipate. The physical therapist's treatment aim would be to improve pulmonary function through pulmonary clearance techniques, aerobic exercise, and individual education. For the individual exposed to second-hand tobacco smoke, encouragement to avoid the source of the tobacco smoke, especially during exercise treatment, would be practical. For the individual exposed to first-hand smoke, the physical therapist should alert the individual to smoking cessation programs.

Transfusion Reaction

Chief Clinical Characteristics

This presentation involves dyspnea, skin rash, fever, back pain, or dizziness within 24 hours after a transfusion.[67]

Background Information

The three types of transfusion reactions are acute hemolytic reactions, immune-mediated hemolytic reactions, and nonimmune hemolytic reactions.[67] Dyspnea related to this condition usually resolves promptly without specific treatment or complications. However, in the presence of a serious anaphylactic response, this condition can become more serious, leading to hemolysis, sepsis, and death.[67] If an individual has received a transfusion in the past 24 hours and presents with shortness of breath, wheezing, or hypotension, the therapist must assume that a serious transfusion reaction is occurring. The therapist should contact the primary care physician as well as be prepared to activate the emergency medical system if the individual's symptoms worsen.

References

1. Atkinson TP, Kaliner MA. Anaphylaxis. *Med Clin North Am.* Jul 1992;76(4):841–855.
2. Ludwig H, Strasser K. Symptomatology of anemia. *Semin Oncol.* Apr 2001;28(2 suppl 8):7–14.
3. Widmaier EP, Raff H, Strang KT. *Vander, Sherman, and Luciano's Human Physiology: The Mechanisms of Body Function.* 9th ed. New York, NY: McGraw-Hill; 2003.
4. Pujade-Lauraine E, Gascon P. The burden of anaemia in patients with cancer. *Oncology.* 2004;67(suppl 1):1–4.
5. Toy P, Feiner J, Viele MK, Watson J, Yeap H, Weiskopf RB. Fatigue during acute isovolemic anemia in healthy, resting humans. *Transfusion.* Apr 2000;40(4):457–460.
6. Rickels K, Schweizer E. The clinical presentation of generalized anxiety in primary-care settings: practical concepts of classification and management. *J Clin Psychiatry.* 1997;58(suppl 11):4–10.
7. Jeejeebhoy FM, Dorian P, Newman DM. Panic disorder and the heart: a cardiology perspective. *J Psychosom Res.* Apr–May 2000;48(4–5):393–403.
8. Ailawadi G, Eliason JL, Upchurch GR, Jr. Current concepts in the pathogenesis of abdominal aortic aneurysm. *J Vasc Surg.* Sep 2003;38(3):584–588.
9. Coady MA, Rizzo JA, Goldstein LJ, Elefteriades JA. Natural history, pathogenesis, and etiology of thoracic aortic aneurysms and dissections. *Cardiol Clin.* Nov 1999;17(4):615–635; vii.
10. Zipes DP. Specific arrhythmias: diagnosis and treatment. In: Braunwald E, ed. *Heart Disease: A Textbook of Cardiovascular Medicine.* 5th ed. Philadelphia, PA: W. B. Saunders; 1996.
11. Cerny FJ, Burton HW. *Exercise Physiology for Health Care Professionals.* Champaign, IL: Human Kinetics; 2001.
12. Hyde L, Hyde CI. Clinical manifestations of lung cancer. *Chest.* Mar 1974;65(3):299–306.
13. Seifter EJ. Clinical Oncology, Second Edition. *J Natl Cancer Inst.* Jan 3 2001;93(1):63.
14. Minna JD. Neoplasms of the lung. In: Fauci AS, Braunwald E, Isselbacher KJ, et al., eds. *Harrison's Principles of Internal Medicine.* 14th ed. New York, NY: McGraw-Hill; 1998.
15. Gonzales R, Sande MA. Uncomplicated acute bronchitis. *Ann Intern Med.* Dec 19 2000;133(12):981–991.
16. Becker KL, Appling S. Acute bronchitis. *Prim Care Pract.* Nov–Dec 1998;2(6):643–646.
17. Elliott P. Cardiomyopathy. Diagnosis and management of dilated cardiomyopathy. *Heart.* Jul 2000;84(1):106–112.
18. Roberts TG, Lilly LS. Diseases of the pericardium. In: Lilly LS, ed. *Pathophysiology of Heart Disease: A Collaborative Project of Medical Students and Faculty.* 2nd ed. Philadelphia, PA: Lippincott Williams & Wilkins; 1998.
19. Goodman CC. The respiratory system. In: Goodman CC, Boissonnault WG, eds. *Pathology: Implications for the Physical Therapist.* Philadelphia, PA: W. B. Saunders; 1998.
20. Cregler LL, Mark H. Medical complications of cocaine abuse. *N Engl J Med.* Dec 4 1986;315(23):1495–1500.
21. Brunnee T, Graf K, Kastens B, Fleck E, Kunkel G. Bronchial hyperreactivity in patients with moderate pulmonary circulation overload. *Chest.* May 1993;103(5):1477–1481.
22. Guyatt GH, Devereaux PJ. A review of heart failure treatment. *Mt Sinai J Med.* Jan 2004;71(1):47–54.
23. Cahalin LP, Ice RG, Irwin S. Program planning and implementation. In: Irwin S, ed. *Cardiopulmonary Physical Therapy.* 3rd ed. St. Louis, MO: Mosby; 1995:142–184.
24. Weitzenblum E. Chronic cor pulmonale. *Heart.* Feb 2003;89(2):225–230.
25. Hardy KR. Diving-related emergencies. *Emerg Med Clin North Am.* Feb 1997;15(1):223–240.
26. Jerrard DA. Diving medicine. *Emerg Med Clin North Am.* May 1992;10(2):329–338.
27. Campbell ES. Decompression illness in sports divers: part I. *Medscape Orthop Sports Med eJournal.* 1997;1(5).
28. Brooks GA, Fahey TD, White TP. Cardiovascular dynamics during exercise. In: Brooks GA, Fahey TD, White TP, eds. *Exercise Physiology: Human Bioenergetics and Its Applications.* 2nd ed. New York, NY: Mayfield; 1996.
29. Graber TW. Diabetes mellitus and glucose disorders. In: Rosen P, Barkins RM, eds. *Emergency Medicine: Concepts and Clinical Practice.* 4th ed. St. Louis, MO: Mosby; 1992.
30. Selim AJ, Ren XS, Fincke G, Rogers W, Lee A, Kazis L. A symptom-based measure of the severity of chronic lung disease: results from the Veterans Health Study. *Chest.* Jun 1997;111(6):1607–1614.
31. Jeffery PK. Comparison of the structural and inflammatory features of COPD and asthma. Giles F. Filley Lecture. *Chest.* May 2000;117(5 suppl 1):251S–260S.
32. Fontana GA, Pistolesi M. Cough. 3: chronic cough and gastro-oesophageal reflux. *Thorax.* Dec 2003;58(12):1092–1095.
33. Harding SM, Richter JE. The role of gastroesophageal reflux in chronic cough and asthma. *Chest.* May 1997;111(5):1389–1402.
34. Hope-Gill BD, Hilldrup S, Davies C, Newton RP, Harrison NK. A study of the cough reflex in idiopathic pulmonary fibrosis. *Am J Respir Crit Care Med.* Oct 15 2003;168(8):995–1002.
35. Selman M, Thannickal VJ, Pardo A, Zisman DA, Martinez FJ, Lynch JP, 3rd. Idiopathic pulmonary fibrosis: pathogenesis and therapeutic approaches. *Drugs.* 2004;64(4):405–430.
36. Bouknight DP, O'Rourke RA. Current management of mitral valve prolapse. *Am Fam Physician.* Jun 1, 2000;61(11):3343–3350, 3353–3344.
37. Romano MA, Bolling SF. Update on mitral repair in dilated cardiomyopathy. *J Card Surg.* Sep–Oct 2004; 19(5):396–400.
38. Zafren K, Honigman B. High-altitude medicine. *Emerg Med Clin North Am.* Feb 1997;15(1):191–222.
39. Nicolazzo PS. Acute mountain sickness: the physiology and prevention of altitude related illness. *Off-Piste The Magazine.* 2001;13.
40. Califf RM. Acute myocardial infarction and other acute ischemic syndromes. In: Braunwald E, ed. *Atlas of Heart Disease.* St. Louis, MO: Mosby; 1996.
41. Sabatine MS, O'Gara PT, Lilly LS. Acute myocardial infarction. In: Lilly LS, ed. *Pathophysiology of Heart Disease: A Collaborative Project of Medical Students and Faculty.* 2nd ed. Philadelphia, PA: Lippincott Williams & Wilkins; 1998.
42. Tavazzi L. Clinical epidemiology of acute myocardial infarction. *Am Heart J.* Aug 1999;138(2 pt 2):S48–54.
43. Sahn SA. Pleural effusions. In: Polly PE, Heffner JE, eds. *Pulmonary/Respiratory Therapy Secrets.* 2nd ed. Philadelphia, PA: Hanley and Belfus; 2002:459–462.

44. Wells CL. Pulmonary pathology. In: DeTurk WE, Cahalin LP, eds. *Cardiovascular and Pulmonary Physical Therapy. An Evidence-Based Approach.* New York, NY: McGraw-Hill Medical; 2004:151–188.

45. Brandenburg JA, Marrie TJ, Coley CM, et al. Clinical presentation, processes and outcomes of care for patients with pneumococcal pneumonia. *J Gen Intern Med.* Sep 2000;15(9):638–646.

46. Meehan TP, Chua-Reyes JM, Tate J, et al. Process of care performance, patient characteristics, and outcomes in elderly patients hospitalized with community-acquired or nursing home-acquired pneumonia. *Chest.* May 2000;117(5):1378–1385.

47. Saavedra MT, Hanley ME. Pneumothorax. In: Polly PE, Heffner JE, eds. *Pulmonary/Respiratory Therapy Secrets.* 2nd ed. Philadelphia, PA: Hanley and Belfus; 2002:463–466.

48. Choi HS, Han SS, Choi HA, et al. Dyspnea and palpitation during pregnancy. *Korean J Intern Med.* Dec 2001;16(4):247–249.

49. Shotan A, Ostrzega E, Mehra A, Johnson JV, Elkayam U. Incidence of arrhythmias in normal pregnancy and relation to palpitations, dizziness, and syncope. *Am J Cardiol.* Apr 15 1997;79(8):1061–1064.

50. Rosano GM, Rillo M, Leonardo F, Pappone C, Chierchia SL. Palpitations: what is the mechanism, and when should we treat them? *Int J Fertil Womens Med.* Mar–Apr 1997;42(2):94–100.

51. Wolbrette D. Treatment of arrhythmias during pregnancy. *Curr Womens Health Rep.* Apr 2003;3(2):135–139.

52. Lee-Chiong TL, Matthay RA. Lung cancer. In: Polly PE, Heffner JE, eds. *Pulmonary/Respiratory Therapy Secrets.* 2nd ed. Philadelphia, PA: Hanley and Belfus; 2002:370–379.

53. Baruch AC, Steinbronn K, Sobonya R. Pulmonary adenocarcinomas associated with rheumatoid nodules: a case report and review of the literature. *Arch Pathol Lab Med.* Jan 2005;129(1):104–106.

54. Lipson DA, Palevsky HI. Thromboembolic disease. In: Polly PE, Heffner JE, eds. *Pulmonary/Respiratory Therapy Secrets.* 2nd ed. Philadelphia, PA: Hanley and Belfus; 2002:237–247.

55. McLaughlin VV, Rich S. Pulmonary hypertension. *Curr Probl Cardiol.* Oct 2004;29(10):575–634.

56. Rubin LJ. Primary pulmonary hypertension. *N Engl J Med.* Jan 9 1997;336(2):111–117.

57. Sastry BK, Narasimhan C, Reddy NK, Raju BS. Clinical efficacy of sildenafil in primary pulmonary hypertension: a randomized, placebo-controlled, double-blind, crossover study. *J Am Coll Cardiol.* Apr 7 2004;43(7):1149–1153.

58. Cotran RS, Kumar V, Robbins SL. The kidney. In: Cotran RS, Kumar V, Robbins SL, eds. *Pathologic Basis of Disease.* 5th ed. Philadelphia, PA: W. B. Saunders; 1994.

59. Klahr S, Schreiner G, Ichikawa I. The progression of renal disease. *N Engl J Med.* Jun 23 1988;318(25): 1657–1666.

60. Rahman M, Smith MC. Chronic renal insufficiency: a diagnostic and therapeutic approach. *Arch Intern Med.* Sep 14 1998;158(16):1743–1752.

61. Fontenot AP. Sarcoidosis. In: Polly PE, Heffner JE, eds. *Pulmonary/Respiratory Therapy Secrets.* 2nd ed. Philadelphia, PA: Hanley and Belfus; 2002: 270–273.

62. Mixides G, Guy E. Sarcoidosis confined to the airway masquerading as asthma. *Can Respir J.* Mar 2003;10(2): 114–116.

63. Chandrasoma P, Taylor CR. Blood: structure and function. Anemias due to decreased erythropoiesis. In: Chandrasoma P, Taylor CR, eds. *Concise Pathology.* 3rd ed. New York, NY: McGraw-Hill; 1998.

64. Cotran RS, Kumar V, Robbins SL. Diseases of red cells and bleeding disorders. In: Cotran RS, Kumar V, Robbins SL, ed. *Pathologic Basis of Disease.* 5th ed. New York, NY: W.B. Saunders; 1994.

65. Dicpinigaitis PV. Cough reflex sensitivity in cigarette smokers. *Chest.* Mar 2003;123(3):685–688.

66. Groneberg DA, Chung KF. Models of chronic obstructive pulmonary disease. *Respir Res.* 2004;5:18.

67. Capon SM, Goldfinger D. Acute hemolytic transfusion reaction, a paradigm of the systemic inflammatory response: new insights into pathophysiology and treatment. *Transfusion.* Jun 1995;35(6):513–520.

CHAPTER 38

Edema

■ *Marisa Perdomo, PT, DPT*

Description of the Symptom

This chapter describes pathology that may lead to edema. Edema is enlargement of the soft tissues secondary to excess water accumulation. It can be classified as intracellular or extracellular. Intracellular edema develops when there is direct injury to tissues, causing inflammatory insult to the cell or alterations in cellular metabolism and resulting in an increase in intracellular sodium and water. Extracellular edema is an abnormal accumulation of fluid and protein molecules in the intercellular spaces of tissues.[1] Edema that develops in the arms or legs, which is the focus of this chapter, is called *peripheral edema*. Peripheral edema may be due to either a systemic dysfunction such as cardiac or renal insufficiency or an obstruction such as a blood clot or tumor. The development of edema may be associated with loss of skin mobility, loss of joint range of motion, loss of joint shape and definition, loss of muscle strength, pain, and changes in skin color, texture, and temperature.[2]

Special Concerns

■ Bilateral edema of the hands or feet; may or may not be progressive
■ Sudden onset of edema without traumatic event
■ Edema that occurs simultaneously with fever, sweats, and chills
■ Distal edema with reports of shortness of breath either with exertion or at rest
■ Calf pain and edema after trauma
■ Edematous body part with red streaks
■ Edema involving the face or arm that is present with discoloration of the chest, arm, or face; loss of carotid pulses; dysphagia; wheezing; chest pain; headaches; dizziness; or orthopnea
■ Total body edema or total quadrant edema

CHAPTER PREVIEW: Conditions That May Lead to Edema

T Trauma
COMMON
Not applicable
UNCOMMON
Lymphedemas: • Secondary lymphedema 790 Thoracic outlet syndrome 794
RARE
Not applicable

(continued)

I   Inflammation

COMMON

Aseptic
Phlebitis 793

Septic
Cellulitis 784
Erysipelas (St. Elmo's fire) 787

UNCOMMON

Not applicable

RARE

Aseptic
Angioedema 783
Lymphangiitis 789

Septic
Necrotizing fasciitis 792

M   Metabolic

COMMON

Hypothyroidism 788
Medication-induced edemas:
• Adrenergic blockers 791
• Calcium channel blockers 791
• Corticosteroids 791
• Nonsteroidal anti-inflammatory drugs 791
• Oncologic agents 791

UNCOMMON

Ascites/cirrhosis of the liver 783
Hyperthyroidism/thyrotoxicosis (myxedema) 788
Lipedema 788
Nephrotic syndrome 792
Protein energy malnutrition (kwashiorkor) 793

RARE

Not applicable

Va   Vascular

COMMON

Chronic venous insufficiency (varicose veins) 785
Congestive heart failure 787
Deep venous thrombosis 787
Post-thrombotic syndrome 793

UNCOMMON

Not applicable

RARE

Capillary leak syndrome 784
Superior vena cava syndrome 794

De **Degenerative**

COMMON

Not applicable

UNCOMMON

Not applicable

RARE

Not applicable

Tu **Tumor**

COMMON

Not applicable

UNCOMMON

Not applicable

RARE

Malignant Primary, such as:
• Lymphoma 795
Malignant Metastatic, such as:
• Metastases, including from primary breast, kidney, lung, prostate, and thyroid disease 795
Benign:
Not applicable

Co **Congenital**

COMMON

Not applicable

UNCOMMON

Not applicable

RARE

Lymphedemas:
• Primary lymphedema (Milroy's disease, Meige disease) 789

Ne **Neurogenic/Psychogenic**

COMMON

Post-stroke hand edema 793

UNCOMMON

Complex regional pain syndrome (reflex sympathetic dystrophy, causalgia) 785

RARE

Not applicable

Note: These are estimates of relative incidence because few data are available for the less common conditions.

EDEMA

Overview of Edema

Peripheral edema may be the first clinical sign of systemic and peripheral disease states. Because edema itself can cause body structure and function deficits, this sign is common among individuals who present to physical therapy with a broad variety of conditions. The first task in providing treatment to an individual with edema is to determine the underlying cause of the swelling. Physical therapy interventions may be contraindicated because treatment of the edema could potentially be life threatening.

The presentation of edema has some characteristics that are uniform across all causes, and other features that differ across causes. In the early stages of edema formation, palpation of the edematous body part causes pitting and the edema is soft. Over time, the edema may become harder to pit and may become fibrotic and brawny in nature. Skin color can vary from normal to pink (suggesting an inflammatory cause), red (suggesting an infectious cause), blue (suggesting a venous cause), or white (suggesting an arterial cause). Individuals with venous edema may develop hemosiderin stains, lipodermatosclerosis, eczema, and venous ulcers (Fig. 38-1). If infection is the cause of edema, fever and flu-like symptoms may be present. Individuals with secondary lymphedema may develop hyperkeratosis of the skin and papillomatosis (Fig. 38-2). If the etiology of edema involves the cardiovascular system, the individual also may report symptoms of fatigue, shortness of breath, orthopnea, or a sensation of abdominal fullness. Skin temperature can vary from normal to warm to cold depending on vascular involvement or the presence of an infection. The individual may report feeling pressure, tightness, fullness, pain, tingling, numbness, heaviness, achiness and hypersensitivity of the affected limb. The edema may be either painful or painless.

Although peripheral edema has various causes, the physiological mechanisms for the formation of edema are the result of alterations in Starling's law of equilibrium.[3-5] In general, the formation of peripheral edema is due to:

- an increase in capillary filtration rate that exceeds the maximum lymphatic transport capacity;
- a decrease in venous capillary and lymphatic resorption rate and a decrease in lymphatic transport capacity; or
- a combination of both.[6]

Accurate determination of the cause of edema depends on an understanding of the physiology governing fluid movement across capillary beds. Filtration and reabsorption of fluid depend on the difference between capillary blood pressure and extravascular hydrostatic pressure, the difference between the capillary and extravascular colloid osmotic pressures, and the permeability of the blood capillary wall. The sum of these pressure gradients allows for fluid movement out of the arterial capillary vessel (filtration) and reabsorption along the venous capillary vessel and the initial lymphatic vessels. Protein molecules are impermeable to the venous capillary wall and must be reabsorbed by the lymphatic vessels, thereby preventing edema formation. In a healthy lymphatic system, any increase in extracellular fluid will be removed by the lymph and venous systems. However, if the volume of interstitial fluid exceeds the maximum lymphatic transport capacity, then edema will develop. Over time, with a normal lymphatic system, the lymphatic transport capacity will "catch up" to the fluid overload and the edema will dissipate.

One key to treatment of individuals with edema is to determine whether the edema is a result of overloading the lymphatic and venous system with fluid or an impairment of venous and lymphatic resorption and transportation. For individuals with lymphatic and venous overloading, intervention is directed toward

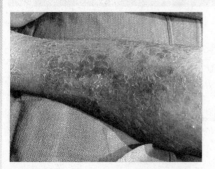

FIGURE 38-1 Venous edema (lipodermatosclerosis).

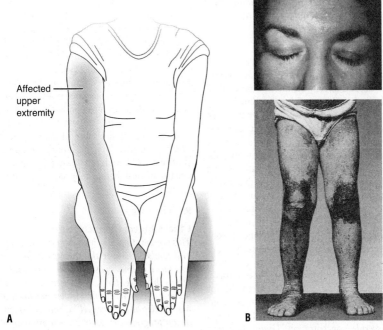

Affected
upper
extremity

A

B

FIGURE 38-2 Secondary lymphedema. Potential associated findings: (A) hyperkeratosis; (B) papillomatosis. (Insets A and B from Goldsmith, LA, Lazarus, GS, Tharp, MD. *Adult and Pediatric Dermatology: A Color Guide to Diagnosis and Treatment.* 1997. Philadelphia, FA Davis Company, with permission.)

reducing the quantity of interstitial fluid; for individuals with limited resorption and transportation, intervention is based on methods to improve pressure gradients in order to facilitate the resorption and transportation processes.

Description of Conditions That May Lead to Edema

■ Angioedema

Chief Clinical Characteristics

This presentation may include nonpitting edema that most commonly affects the face, hands, and neck; less commonly, the buttocks, genitals, and abdominal organs may be affected. Symptoms may also include tingling, paresthesias, or pruritus.[7–10]

Background Information

Causes of angioedema include drug reactions, most commonly to nonsteroidal anti-inflammatory medications and angiotensin-converting enzyme inhibitor medications;

trauma; and reactions to food.[11] There is also a hereditary form of this condition that occurs in childhood and requires lifelong attention for possible reactions. This condition is an immune-mediated disorder that is present in up to 10% of the U.S. population. It is caused by a temporary increase in capillary permeability of small blood vessels. Diagnosis is confirmed with a complete medical history and the clinical presentation of the patient. Treatment includes medications such as antihistamines, steroids, and in severe cases adrenaline.[7] Physical therapy is not indicated in patients with this condition. This condition is a medical emergency when it affects the larynx, and it requires immediate medical intervention.

■ Ascites/Cirrhosis of the Liver

Chief Clinical Characteristics

This presentation typically includes an abdomen that becomes distended or swollen. In severe cases, the edema progresses and may include bilateral lower extremities. Individuals may report increased abdominal girth, respiratory distress, and satiety.

Background Information

This condition involves excess fluid accumulation within the peritoneal cavity, and symptoms depend directly on the amount of fluid in the cavity. This condition is a clinical finding with a variety of causes. Asymptomatic liver disease is one of the most common causes. Liver disease develops as a result of portal hypertension and hypoalbuminemia, which are often associated with patients with cirrhosis of the liver. Individuals with a history of alcohol abuse and advanced cancer are at high risk for developing this condition. Ultrasonography confirms the presence of fluid in the peritoneal cavity. If fluid presence is confirmed, analysis of the fluid is necessary to differentiate from other causes such as cancer, congestive heart failure, and tuberculosis.[12] The ascetic fluid should be analyzed for serum-ascetic albumin gradient, amylase concentration, white cell count and red cell count, triglyceride concentration, Gram stain and culture, pH < 7, and cytology. Treatment depends on this condition's cause. In the majority of patients, cirrhosis leading to portal hypertension is the major cause and is managed with diuretic and dietary salt restriction.[12,13] Medications such as spironolactone and a low-dose loop diuretic are commonly prescribed.[13] However, when this condition is associated with cancer, the condition will not respond to similar treatments. Physical therapy is not indicated in patients with this condition.

■ Capillary Leak Syndrome

Chief Clinical Characteristics

This presentation typically includes recurrent episodes of peripheral edema and hypoproteinemia. Edema often includes both lower extremities and may include the face, lungs, and pericardium.[14]

Background Information

In this rare and complex condition, microvascular damage causes an increase in capillary permeability and a rapid and sudden increase in the capillary filtration rate. This condition was first noted in the literature in 1960 and can be acute or chronic in nature. In severe cases, renal damage may occur and result in hypovolemic shock. This condition is a diagnosis of exclusion. Also, a blood test should reveal the presence of serum IgG-K paraprotein. While there is no standard successful treatment approach, various pharmacologic treatments have demonstrated positive results, such as prednisone, furosemide, theophylline, loop diuretics, and terbutaine.[14] Medical management for the cause of capillary leak syndrome is necessary. Once the condition is controlled, if there is any residual peripheral edema, physical therapy may have a role in its treatment.

■ Cellulitis

Chief Clinical Characteristics

This presentation may include erythema, pain and tenderness over the infected area with associated edema, in association with possible serous drainage, fever, chills, headaches, and malaise. The skin becomes swollen and hot and may develop an "orange peel" texture as this condition progresses (Fig. 38-3). The individual may present with an increased resting heart rate and may, in extreme or severe cases, even become disoriented. The regional lymph nodes of the involved body part may become enlarged, tender or painful to palpation.[15,16]

Background Information

This condition refers to an acute inflammation of the dermis and subcutaneous tissue. It is one

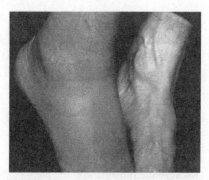

FIGURE 38-3 Cellulitis. (From Goldsmith, LA, Lazarus, GS, Tharp, MD. *Adult and Pediatric Dermatology: A Color Guide to Diagnosis and Treatment.* 1997. Philadelphia, FA Davis Company, with permission.)

of the most common bacterial skin infections typically caused by *Staphylococcus* and *Streptococcus* species.[16,17] The infective agent may enter the body through any break or opening in the skin and spread via the lymphatic system. In lower extremity cellulitis, pedal edema is an early sign. Individuals who have peripheral edema from other etiologies (eg, chronic venous insufficiency and lymphedema) are at risk for developing cellulitis. A complete blood count that indicates an elevated white blood cell count confirms the diagnosis. Tissue culture is required to identify the exact infective agents that are involved. This condition must particularly be differentiated from other forms of infection, such as necrotizing fasciitis, folliculitis, erysipelas, impetigo, and gas gangrene.[18,19] Treatment includes intravenous antibiotics. If the etiology of this condition involves systemic infection, this condition may become life threatening without proper treatment.[18]

■ Chronic Venous Insufficiency (Varicose Veins)

Chief Clinical Characteristics
This presentation includes dilated subcutaneous veins, hyperpigmentation, edema, pain, lipodermatosclerosis, and ulceration. This condition is sometimes equated with postthrombotic syndrome.[20]

Background Information
This condition may be caused by incompetent valves (reflux) in the superficial, deep, or perforating veins; obstruction; or both. As the calf contracts, the increased pressure will be transferred to the superficial veins, resulting in venous hypertension. Varicose veins are classified into "grades" based on severity. Varicose veins are described as "dilated palpable subcutaneous veins usually larger than 4 mm." Currently two classification systems are used to assess the clinical presentation of chronic venous insufficiency: the CEAP classification system and the Venous Clinical Severity Score system (Table 38-1). These classification systems attempt to incorporate the clinical signs and symptoms with the results from duplex ultrasonography to diagnose and classify the severity of this condition. Interventions for both conditions include the recommendation of compression garments, exercise (eg, walking while wearing the garments and pool exercises), and elevation of the legs.[20,21]

■ Complex Regional Pain Syndrome (Reflex Sympathetic Dystrophy, Causalgia)

Chief Clinical Characteristics
This presentation includes pain that is out of proportion to the injury, burning pain, allodynia, hyperesthesias, vasomotor changes, swelling, loss of joint range of motion, loss of skin mobility, and contractures. Edema that is associated with this condition may be pitting or nonpitting. It is usually present in the early stages and may decrease in the later stages.[22]

TABLE 38-1 ■ Criteria for the CEAP Classification and Venous Clinical Severity Score

CEAP[a] Classification		
	CATEGORY	**RECOMMENDED COURSE OF ACTION**
CEAP I	Superficial spider (reticular) veins only	No need to refer to a vascular specialist for this cosmetic problem
CEAP II	Varicose veins	Refer to vascular specialist for evaluation and management, with level of urgency increasing from routine at level II to more urgent at level V
CEAP III	Varicose veins and leg swelling	
CEAP IV	Varicose veins and evidence of venous stasis skin changes	
CEAP V	Varicose veins with healed cutaneous ulcer	
CEAP VI	Varicose veins with open cutaneous ulcer	Refer very urgently to a vascular specialist for evaluation and treatment

(continued)

EDEMA

TABLE 38-1 ■ **Criteria for the CEAP Classification and Venous Clinical Severity Score—cont'd**

		Venous Clinical Severity Score[63]		
	ABSENT (0)	**MILD (1)**	**MODERATE (2)**	**SEVERE (3)**
Pain	None	Occasional, nonlimiting, does not require analgesic medication	Daily, moderately limiting, requires occasional use of analgesic medication	Daily, severely limiting, requires regular use of analgesic medication
Varicose veins	None	Few	Multiple	Extensive
Venous edema	None	Evening ankle edema only	Afternoon edema, edema occurring above the ankle	Morning edema above the ankle requiring activity change and elevation
Skin pigmentation	None	Diffuse but limited in area and old (brown)	Diffuse over the lower one-third of the calf (gaiter area) or recent (purple)	Wide distribution (above the lower one-third of the calf) and recent
Inflammation	None	Mild cellulitis limited to region around an ulcer	Moderate cellulitis of the lower one-third of the calf	Severe cellulitis affecting the region above the lower one-third of the calf, venous eczema present
Induration	None	Focal, around the malleoli (<5 mm)	Medial or lateral lower leg, but less than the lower one-third of the leg	Entire lower one-third of the lower leg or more
Number of active ulcers	0	1	2	>2
Active ulcer duration	None	<3 months	Greater than 3 months but less than 1 year	Not healed >1 year
Active ulcer size	None	<2-cm diameter	2- to 6-cm diameter	>6-cm diameter
Compression therapy	None or not compliant	Intermittent use	Wears elastic stockings most days	Full compliance with stockings and elevation

[a]CEAP is a mnemonic that stands for clinical, etiologic, anatomical, and pathophysiological. The CEAP classification has been used to stratify subjects from large populations to ensure comparison of like individuals in clinical and research applications. Since its inception for this purpose, the CEAP classification has been simplified to guide management and referral decisions by clinicians.

Background Information

This condition is subdivided into two types: complex regional pain syndrome 1 (previously known as reflex sympathetic dystrophy), which develops after an initiating noxious event without nerve damage, and complex regional pain syndrome 2 (previously known as causalgia), which develops after injury to a nerve. Diagnosis is based on clinical signs and symptoms. Diagnostic tests such as x-ray, bone scans, and bone density tests are helpful to confirm abnormalities and can support the diagnosis. Physical therapy focuses on early mobilization of the affected joints and prevention of the sequelae of disuse, atrophy, and loss of function. However, a multidisciplinary treatment approach is critical to minimize the debilitating consequences of this condition.[22,23]

■ Congestive Heart Failure

Chief Clinical Characteristics

This presentation includes peripheral/pretibial edema in association with shortness of breath, chest discomfort, or light-headedness/syncope. Various physical findings, such as palpitations, pulmonary crackles, an auscultated S_3 cardiac sound, cyanosis, and sudden and dramatic weight gain, provide clues to the presence of this condition.

Background Information

Electrolyte balance is typically upset in individuals with this condition, as a result of both chronic fluid retention and the depletion of certain electrolytes by various medications (eg, potassium-depleting diuretics). The use of digoxin to improve cardiac contractility in these patients may in some cases precipitate bradycardia secondary to slowing of the electrical conduction through the atrioventricular node, or tachycardia secondary to enhancement of automaticity in Purkinje fibers episodes. By communicating with the patient's physician, the therapist plays a crucial role during titration of the patient's medical regimen. Definitive diagnosis is made by echocardiography or angiography. As with coronary artery disease, supplemental oxygen prescribed by the patient's physician can improve symptoms and suppress the palpitations in some cases. However, if the patient becomes unstable, the emergency medical system should be activated.

■ Deep Venous Thrombosis

Chief Clinical Characteristics

This presentation typically includes pain and swelling, warmth, skin color changes, a palpable cord, and dilation of the superficial veins. If the collateral veins are sufficient to allow for venous drainage, there will be no edema. General risk factors include a history of trauma, history of a previous deep venous thrombosis (DVT), a period of immobilization, recent surgery, cancer, intravenous chemotherapy treatment, indwelling central line, present oral contraceptive use, and medical comorbidities such as congestive heart failure, stroke, pulmonary obstructive disease, obesity, or an inherited coagulopathy. With repeated thromboses or the presence of cardiovascular comorbidities, edema distal to the clot will be present.

Background Information

The clinical presentation of this condition in the upper extremity may include sudden onset of upper extremity edema, pain, tenderness, venous distention, and skin color changes of the arm, face, supraclavicular fossa, and shoulder.[24] Risk factors for this condition in the upper extremity include use of central venous catheters such as in the delivery of chemotherapy agents, congestive heart failure, pregnancy, rigorous and repetitive activity of the upper extremities, and venous compression as in thoracic outlet syndrome (Paget-Schroetter syndrome).[24] This condition should be suspected in the lower extremity in any individual who presents with sudden onset of unilateral calf pain and swelling. The diagnosis is confirmed with Doppler ultrasound, magnetic resonance imaging, or computed tomography. D-dimer blood testing can be used as a method to rule out a DVT, thus negating the need for further testing. However, because other pathologies such as cancer, late pregnancy and sepsis produce elevated D-dimer levels, it does not discriminate specifically for a diagnosis of a DVT.[25] Early diagnosis is important because of the potential risk of a thrombus resulting in a pulmonary embolism or stroke. Treatment typically involves anticoagulants including heparin or low-molecular-weight heparin to prevent extension of the thrombus. Once sufficiently anticoagulated, the patient is transitioned to Coumadin. In addition, a compression garment, usually a knee-high garment or arm sleeve, is recommended to assist in venous return and prevent recurrence. For this condition in the lower extremity, calf exercises and a walking program are important to assist in venous return and help prevent venous stasis.

■ Erysipelas (St. Elmo's Fire)

Chief Clinical Characteristics

This presentation can be characterized by erythema, pain and tenderness over the infected area with associated edema, in association with possible serous drainage, fever, chills, headaches, vomiting, and malaise. The skin lesion associated with this condition involves clear bright red patches of skin with definite borders and raised margins as a distinct form of cellulitis (see Fig. 38-3).

Background Information

This commonly occurs in populations such as the elderly, neonates, immunocompromised individuals, and young children. Risk factors include individuals with diabetes mellitus, those with nephrotic syndrome, and those with a compromised immune system.[26] Red streaks (lymphatic streaking) may be present, indicating that the infection is spreading via the lymphatic vessels. Localized edema is present and the individual may report pain or local tenderness.[16,18,19] The most common location is the legs and face. Erysipelas is a distinct type of superficial cellulitis and therefore involves the epidermis. It can rapidly lead to a systemic toxicity and therefore requires immediate referral to a physician for individuals suspected of having this condition.[18,19] The medical diagnosis of erysipelas is usually based on clinical presentation; however, diagnostic tests such as a complete blood count with differential, a needle aspiration with culture, and a swab culture of the nose/throat may assist in differentiating this pathology from other causes. Antibiotics are required. If left untreated, this condition can lead to nephritis, abscesses, and a life-threatening systemic infection called septicemia.[16,18,19]

■ Hyperthyroidism/Thyrotoxicosis (Myxedema)

Chief Clinical Characteristics

This presentation often includes pretibial edema and dorsal foot edema (pretibial myxedema), hypertension, dyspnea (ie, orthopnea, exertional dyspnea, and paroxysmal nocturnal dyspnea), and palpitations that may lead to feelings of dizziness or light-headedness.[27] Associated signs and symptoms include nervousness, heat intolerance, fatigue, weight loss despite increased appetite, goiter, sweating, tremors, and exophthalmos.[28]

Background Information

This condition is characterized by overactivity of the thyroid gland and primarily results in elevated levels of thyroid hormones in the bloodstream; thyrotoxicosis refers to the clinical syndrome resulting from hyperthyroidism. Typical etiologies include Graves' disease (often associated with exophthalmos), excessive thyroid hormone replacement therapy, toxic adenoma, thyroiditis, goiter, amiodarone use, or use of iodine-containing radiographic contrast agents. Thyroid hormones are known to enhance myocardial contractility and elevate the body's metabolic rate, leading to arterial vasodilation and possible hypotension. If this condition is suspected, the individual should be referred to a medical practitioner for definitive assessment. The diagnosis is made on the basis of blood tests that indicate elevated thyroid hormone levels. Management of this condition may include pharmacologic administration of iodine, antithyroid medications, and surgical thyroidectomy.

■ Hypothyroidism

Chief Clinical Characteristics

This presentation may be characterized by severe fatigue in combination with edema of the eyelids, face, and dorsum of the hand. Myxedema also may be present.

Background Information

This condition develops as a result of decreased production or levels of T_4 and T_3 hormones.[3,29] This condition may be suspected if an individual presents with pretibial edema and unusual fatigue that does not improve with rest.[29,30] Lab values for thyroid-stimulating hormone are elevated and can be detected before abnormal plasma levels of T_3 and T_4 hormones are observed. Blood values for serum T_3 and free T_4 are elevated, while serum TSH is decreased and radioactive iodine uptake is increased. Thyroid hormone replacement therapy is given for individuals with this condition. In many cases, the thyroid gland is surgically removed and hormone replacement therapy is required.

■ Lipedema

Chief Clinical Characteristics

This presentation involves gradual and progressive increase in the size of bilateral lower extremities often mistaken for obesity, lymphedema, or venous dysfunction.[31] Typically this condition begins with the leg edema beginning just above the malleoli. There is no involvement of the feet (negative Stemmer sign). Palpation is tender and painful with a soft end feel, and no pitting is produced. Neither leg elevation nor diet and weight loss decrease the diameter of the legs. Typically, the individual's history is unremarkable for cellulitis and leg ulcers.

Background Information

This condition occurs in women and in some cases there are familiar tendencies. This condition involves abnormal fat deposits in the subcutaneous tissue, which cause abnormal enlargement of the lower extremities, pelvis, and buttock. The size and shape of the lower extremities are disproportionately larger when compared to the upper extremities. There are cases of all four extremities being involved; however, the more common presentation involves just the lower extremities. The majority of individuals with this condition are often misdiagnosed with lymphedema, venous insufficiency, or obesity or not diagnosed at all.[3,32–34] Diagnostic tests such as magnetic resonance imaging and computed tomography scans demonstrate the presence of subcutaneous fat and can add in ruling out competing diagnosis such as obesity and lymphedema. Manual lymphatic mobilizations, compression bandaging with short-stretch bandages, and exercise can reduce the size of the limb significantly. Strength training is highly recommended. Individuals with this condition must wear compression garments after the initial physical therapy treatment has ended. Individuals with this condition can be instructed in a home program of self-lymph drainage massage techniques, self-bandaging, and a progressive resistance training program. Maximal reduction of the extremities can take more than 1 year to achieve in some cases. In some individuals, lymphatic insufficiency develops over time and therefore the individual would be diagnosed with lipedema and secondary lymphedema. In this case, the key clinical symptom is edema of the feet and a positive Stemmer sign. Physical therapy may be indicated to help address secondary lymphedema.

■ **Lymphangiitis**

Chief Clinical Characteristics

This presentation typically includes high fever, chills, swollen lymph nodes, and pain, warmth, swelling, and red streaks along the vessels that drain to the lymph nodes.

Background Information

This condition is an inflammation of lymphatic vessels draining the body region that has an infection or is inflamed.[35] If this condition is suspected, referral to a physician is warranted. Treatment includes antibiotic medications for the infection. Septicemia can develop if the underlying infection spreads into the venous system. Physical therapy is not indicated for this condition.

LYMPHEDEMAS

■ **Primary Lymphedema (Milroy's Disease, Meige Disease)**

Chief Clinical Characteristics

This presentation can involve a distal to proximal progression of unilateral or bilateral extremity edema in an individual with possible hypoparathyroidism, yellow nails, ptosis, and webbing at the neck.[36] Most commonly, the lower extremities are involved; however, all four extremities may be affected. Initially the edema is soft and pitting, but over time the edema will progress to become hard, brawny, and indurated, and pitting can become extremely difficult. The limb can become quite large with abnormal deposition of fat cells, which leads to loss of joint spaces and a columnar-like appearance. Skin changes such as papillomatosis and hyperkeratosis and development of lymphocytes can occur.

Background Information

This condition develops as a result of a malformation of the lymph vessels or lymph nodes. This malformation occurred as the embryo was developing *in utero*. The limb is at risk for developing cellulitis, erysipelas, and fungal infections. The infections increase the lymphatic load and further increase the edema. In severe cases, elephantiasis may develop.[36,37] Hypoplasia is the most common cause of this condition. Several ages of onset are possible including at or around the time of birth (congenital lymphedema; Milroy's disease); at puberty, when it is called lymphedema praecox (Meige disease); and during adulthood (lymphedema tarde). This condition remains a diagnosis of exclusion from all other causes of peripheral edema. Lymphoscintigraphy, bioelectrical impedance, magnetic resonance imaging, and computed tomography can assist in determining the appropriate diagnosis. The individual with lymphedema will require lifelong self-treatment and physical therapy intervention if the individual experiences repeated infections or has difficulty in controlling acute exacerbations.[5,33,38–42] The most commonly accepted treatment for lymphedema includes manual lymphatic drainage techniques, use of short-stretch compression bandages or compression braces, exercise, and skin care to prevent infection. Once the limb size has been maximally reduced, the individual is fitted with an appropriate compression garment. Lymphedema requires lifelong care with a home program and replacement of compression garments every 3 to 6 months. Referral to physical therapy is necessary if the individual experiences an exacerbation of the lymphedema.

■ Secondary Lymphedema

Chief Clinical Characteristics

This presentation typically includes heaviness, achiness, tightness, tingling and numbness of the involved extremity, and painless swelling of a limb that initially fluctuates with rest or elevation but with time does not dissipate. The clinical presentation of secondary lymphedema is the same as primary lymphedema with typically only one limb affected. If the hand or foot is involved, the individual will have difficulty making a fist or curling the toes. These concerns may worsen with activity and increase in heat and humidity or during changes in elevation. The distal aspect of the limb (foot or hand) may be affected initially; however, in some cases the proximal part of the limb may swell first. The edema usually spreads distally to proximally if left untreated. Initially, pitting edema is present and palpation of the limb is soft. Chronic edema causes fibrosis to develop within the subcutaneous tissues, which may lead to a loss of skin mobility and decrease range of motion. As fibrosis develops, the edema becomes harder to pit and palpation of the limb becomes hard and firm.

Background Information

As the edema becomes indurated, the skin can develop a "peau d'orange" appearance. Over time hyperkeratosis and papillomatosis may develop. The skin may begin to break down and infections such as cellulitis and erysipelas may occur. In lower extremity lymphedema, inability to pinch the skin at the base of the metatarsal heads (positive Stemmer sign) is present.[5,40,42] If the condition is untreated, repeated infections may occur and the combination of obstruction and infection can lead to elephantiasis. The limb becomes grossly enlarged; hyperkeratosis, papillomatosis, and the development of a lymphocele may occur and result in severe disfigurement and disability. This condition occurs as a result of abnormal accumulation of protein molecules and fluid in the interstitial spaces of the body from an acquired impairment of the lymphatic system that affects reabsorption of the interstitial fluid and transportation of lymph (lymphatic drainage). Cancer surgery and radiation therapy are considered the most frequent cause of secondary lymphedema in the United States, while parasitic infection is the most common primary cause worldwide. Diagnosis of lymphedema is primarily a diagnosis of exclusion. All other causes of edema are ruled out before this diagnosis is reached. Lymphoscintigraphy, bioelectrical impedance, magnetic resonance imaging, and computed tomography can be used to assist in the diagnosis. Treatment of this condition begins first with treating any infections that might be present. Treatment may include manual lymphatic drainage mobilizations followed by compression bandages with short-stretch materials, joint range of motion, proper skin care, and exercise. Patient education regarding skin care, independent bandaging techniques, and lymph drainage massage techniques are critical in order for the individual to control the lymphedema. The individual with this condition will require lifelong self-treatment and physical therapy intervention if the individual experiences repeated infections or has difficulty in controlling acute exacerbations.[5,33,38–42]

MEDICATION-INDUCED EDEMAS

Chief Clinical Characteristics
Many medications cause varying degrees of peripheral edema.

Background Information
In these cases, the peripheral edema is not appropriate for physical therapy intervention; however, this condition may be mistaken for forms of edema, such as secondary lymphedema, that is appropriate for physical therapy intervention. Any individual who is suspected of having this condition should be referred to a physician for additional evaluation. Changing the dose and type of medication, or providing additional supportive treatment as appropriate, commonly address this condition. The following list provides an example of some of the medications that have the potential to cause peripheral edema.

ADRENERGIC BLOCKERS
These medications may promote the adverse effects of orthostatic hypotension, dizziness, syncope, and peripheral edema of bilateral feet, ankles, and legs. Typically, these agents are used in patients with hypertension or those experiencing cardiac arrhythmias. Medications in this class include bretylium and guanadrel.

CALCIUM CHANNEL BLOCKERS
These medications may cause pitting edema in bilateral feet and ankles. In some cases the edema may progress proximally. Other adverse effects such as orthostatic hypotension, dizziness, headache, and nausea may also be present. These classes of medications are used for individuals experiencing hypertension, angina pectoris, cardiac arrhythmias, atrial flutter, and fibrillation. They include dihydropyridine, benzodiazepine, verapamil, and Calan. The severity of the edema varies between each type of this class of medication taken.[43] Any individual who presents with lower extremity swelling and is taking this class of medication should be evaluated by

their cardiologist before initiating treatment for peripheral edema.

CORTICOSTEROIDS
These agents—including prednisone, dexamethasone, and Decadron—are used for a variety of pathologies including cancer and autoimmune conditions and following transplant surgeries. These medications can cause sodium and fluid retention and potassium depletion.[44] The individual will most likely present with systemic peripheral edema. Depending on the dose, the individual may present with "Cushing-like" features of the face. Physical therapy is not indicated and referral to a physician is necessary.

NONSTEROIDAL ANTI-INFLAMMATORY DRUGS
The presentation of edema with this class of medications involves peripheral edema that especially affects the bilateral feet and ankles. These medications are very commonly encountered in physical therapy practice because they are commonly prescribed for individuals with pain. This class of medications includes ibuprofen, naproxen, and iodine.

ONCOLOGIC AGENTS
Tamoxifen (Nolvadex; hormone therapy) is a selective estrogen receptor that inhibits the effects of estrogen by binding on the estrogen receptor protein in cancer cells. It is most often used for patients with breast cancer whose tumors are estrogen receptor positive. Generalized peripheral edema is occasionally reported.[44] The clinical presentation is a generalized edema that forms fairly uniformly throughout the upper and lower extremities. Docetaxel (Taxotere) is a chemotherapy agent most commonly used to treat breast cancer and non–small-cell lung cancer. Systemic edema is also referred to as fluid retention syndrome and is a common occurrence.[44] Individuals with edema associated with this medication are given steroids before infusion of docetaxel in order to minimize the systemic edema. This condition should be carefully differentiated from secondary lymphedema. Doxorubicin is a chemotherapy agent

most commonly used in the treatment of breast, bladder, liver, stomach, and lung cancer, Hodgkin's and non-Hodgkin's lymphomas, leukemia, and bone and soft-tissue sarcomas.[44] Congestive heart failure is a potential serious adverse effect; therefore, individuals receiving doxorubicin who develop any symptoms of bilateral peripheral edema with or without shortness of breath should be referred to their oncologist for cardiac evaluation. With greater heart damage the lower extremity edema becomes more proximal and may progress to involve the trunk and upper extremities. Individuals treated for a childhood cancer are at significantly higher risk for developing cardiac complications such as congestive heart failure. This risk may be further increased if radiation therapy was applied to the thorax. Therefore, if an individual with a history of a childhood cancer (such as leukemia or lymphoma) presents to physical therapy with a diagnosis of bilateral lower extremity edema, the therapist must consult with the physician to rule out any cardiac involvement.[45,46] Individuals being treated for cancer are also at risk for developing lymphedema secondary to lymph node dissection and radiation therapy. The physical therapist should be aware of the differences in clinical presentation of someone with peripheral edema caused by medications versus someone who is at risk for developing lymphedema (systemic edema with increase in fluid retention in all four extremities versus a single limb swelling).

■ Necrotizing Fasciitis
Chief Clinical Characteristics
This presentation commonly involves erythema and edema without demarcated borders; severe pain (a diagnostic symptom different from cellulitis); tense shiny skin, progressing to ischemic skin as tissue necrosis advances; clear or hemorrhagic blisters, progressing to bullae filled with gray odiferous fluid (termed dishwater pus); dry black eschar (in advanced disease); separation of necrotic tissue along fascial planes with myonecrosis; high fever and chills; decreased urinary output; change in mental status; and weakness and fatigue.

Background Information
This condition is a life-threatening infection of the fascia (plus the underlying skin and subcutaneous tissue) characterized by acute onset and rapid progression. A biopsy or examination during surgery is required in order to accurately diagnose necrotizing fasciitis. Magnetic resonance imaging may be used to assist the physician in differentiating necrotizing fasciitis from cellulitis.[17] Immediate medical attention is critical; treatment includes surgical debridement, intravenous antibiotics, and meticulous wound care.

■ Nephrotic Syndrome
Chief Clinical Characteristics
This presentation may involve bilateral lower extremity pitting edema, specifically the ankles, lower extremities, and sometimes the abdomen, eyes, and eyelids, in association with ascites, pleural effusions, and pericarditis. Individuals with this condition also may present with shortness of breath (pulmonary edema), and males may also present with edema of the scrotum and penis. In children the clinical presentation can also include facial edema and periorbital edema.[47]

Background Information
Individuals with nephrotic syndrome develop peripheral edema as a result of significant loss of plasma protein molecules from the glomerular capillaries that are excreted via urine (proteinuria). The result is a decrease in plasma protein concentration (hypoalbuminemia) and an increase in protein concentration in the urine. In addition, sodium accumulates in the extracellular tissue spaces as a result of an imbalance between sodium intake and sodium output. There are several causes of nephrotic syndrome, including cancer, drugs such as heroin, gold and captopril, systemic lupus erythematosus, diabetes mellitus, and a variety of glomerular diseases. Tests include a urinalysis, complete blood count, imaging, and a kidney biopsy, although there is no gold standard test to confirm the diagnosis.[12,48,49] Diuretics are usually the first medication provided to prevent renal sodium retention, and amiloride and furosemide aid in decreasing the peripheral edema.[50]

■ **Phlebitis**

Chief Clinical Characteristics
This presentation can be characterized by edema (inflammation) distal to the injured vein, pain, and tenderness and redness of the tissue surrounding the vein.

Background Information
This condition refers to inflammation of a vein. There are many causes, but the most common include thrombosis, chemical irritants, malignancy, indwelling catheters, and infection. Duplex ultrasonography is necessary if a larger and deeper vein is involved, whereas venography typically suffices for smaller more distal venules. If this condition is suspected, the affected body part (more commonly the lower leg) should be elevated. The underlying cause of this condition must be addressed. Treatment depends on the underlying cause, and may involve anticoagulant, antibiotic, or thrombolytic agents.[35]

■ **Post-Stroke Hand Edema**

Chief Clinical Characteristics
This presentation involves edema of the hand and wrist area that can cause pain, joint stiffness, loss of range of motion, shortening of connective tissue, and adhesions[51] in association with paralysis and dependency.

Background Information
Approximately one-half of cases of this condition are associated with shoulder-hand syndrome.[52] Hand edema in this condition that is also associated with shoulder-hand syndrome overlies the metacarpals and is accompanied by relatively little pain or tenderness. Assessment of edema is difficult and may be missed if based solely on observation[51]; for hand edema, volumetric measurements appear to be most accurate. Swelling and hand edema are common among individuals following stroke in the early stages of clinical rehabilitation, even in individuals with good hand function. Hand edema is most common among patients with severe paresis of the hand, hypertonic fingers, and hyposensibility. Treatment involves a variety of modalities, such as compression therapy, elevation, continuous passive motion, massage, and splinting. However, present research has yet to demonstrate an optimal intervention for this condition.[51,52]

■ **Post-Thrombotic Syndrome**

Chief Clinical Characteristics
This presentation typically includes pain, heaviness, and cramping, which improve with leg elevation in combination with clinical signs of edema, skin changes, hyperpigmentation, induration, redness, venous ectasia, lipodermatosclerosis, and a healed or active ulcer in an individual with history of deep venous thrombosis.[20]

Background Information
Risk factors include age, family history, prolonged standing, history of a blood clot, phlebitis, smoking, and obesity. This condition is a chronic venous insufficiency caused by a deep venous thrombosis. This syndrome is caused by a combination of events involving the thrombus, the inflammatory response, and the recanalization of the vein. These events can damage the venous valves and result in valvular incompetence leading to venous hypertension, edema, tissue hypoxia, and in severe cases venous ulcers.[53,54] Doppler ultrasound may confirm the presence of deep venous thrombosis and identify incompetent valves. However, clinical symptoms must also be present to confirm the diagnosis of this condition.[53,54] Although studies are limited, evidence supports a reduction in edema related to this condition in individuals who wore a compression garment.[20]

■ **Protein Energy Malnutrition (Kwashiorkor)**

Chief Clinical Characteristics
This presentation is characterized by edema, anorexia, general loss of interest in surroundings, and irritability. It most typically affects children between the ages of 1 and 3 who have sustained a prolonged dietary protein deficit. Edema is typically present about the abdominal region and face.

Background Information
This condition is thought to be caused by limitation in protein, micronutrient, and antioxidant content in the diet. However, predictors for the development of kwashiorkor versus related conditions that do not involve edema (ie, marasmus and marasmus kwashiorkor) remain unclear. Although this condition is classically associated with

EDEMA

children in developing countries during times of famine, it is also present in developed nations. In developed nations, children at particular risk include those living in large urban areas within low socioeconomic groups that are without the means to ensure proper nutrition or dietary education. Treatment involves correction of dietary insufficiency. Prognosis for recovery is good, although delayed treatment may result in persistent disruption of growth and development.[55]

■ Superior Vena Cava Syndrome

Chief Clinical Characteristics
This presentation involves facial, neck, and arm swelling, distention of the veins of the neck and arms, cyanosis of the chest, arms, and face, loss of venous neck pulses, dyspnea, dysphasia, wheezing, coughing, chest pain, headaches, dizziness, orthopnea, and syncope. Upon auscultation, diminished breath sounds may be present.

Background Information
This condition occurs as a result of obstruction of the venous drainage of the upper body and an increase in central venous pressure. Malignant tumors are responsible for about 90% of the syndrome and the rest are caused by aortic aneurysms, fibrotic mediastinitis, and tuberculosis.[56,57] This condition is most commonly caused by lung cancer, followed by non-Hodgkin's lymphoma and is rare in other cancers such as Hodgkin's lymphoma, acute lymphoblastic leukemia, thyroid cancer, neuroblastoma, rhabdomyosarcoma, Ewing's sarcoma, breast cancer, non–small-cell lung cancer, and germ cell tumors. The increased use of indwelling central venous catheters to administer chemotherapy agents may cause a thrombosis to develop and cause this condition.[56–60] Diagnosis includes a detailed physical examination, blood work, biopsy, and chest radiograph. The best treatment is to remove the cause or decrease the size of the obstruction.

■ Thoracic Outlet Syndrome

Chief Clinical Characteristics
This presentation can be characterized by swelling or puffiness in the arm or hand, bluish discoloration of the hand, a feeling of heaviness in the arm or hand, deep, boring toothache-like pain in the neck and shoulder region that seems to increase at night, easily fatigued arms and hands, superficial vein distention in the hand, paresthesias along the inside forearm and the palm, muscle weakness with difficulty gripping and performing fine motor tasks of the hand, atrophy of the muscles of the palm, cramps of the muscles on the inner forearm, pain in the arm and hand, and tingling and numbness in the neck, shoulder region, arm, and hand.

Background Information
Diagnosing this condition can be controversial because disagreement exists about the "types" of thoracic outlet syndrome (TOS). In general, three common types of this condition are presented in the literature, which can coexist or occur independently: compression of the subclavian vein, compression of the subclavian artery, and a primary neurological syndrome. There is also a subset of neurological TOS referred to as "disputed" neurogenic type of TOS. This type presents clinically with primarily sensory symptoms and does not typically present with definitive objective findings.[61] Multiple anatomical anomalies can lead to thoracic outlet syndrome, including an incomplete cervical rib, a taut fibrous band passing from the transverse process of C7 to the first rib, and a complete rib that articulates with the first rib, or anomalies of the position insertion of the anterior and medial scalene muscles and the pectoralis minor tendon.[61,62] Traditionally diagnosis includes physical examination tests (ie, Adson's test, extremity abducted stress test, costoclavicular sign, Roos test, Eden maneuver, and the Halstead maneuver), radiology of the cervical spine, magnetic resonance imaging, and nerve conduction and electromyography studies. Unfortunately, Adson's test is not a reliable test to rule in or rule out a diagnosis of TOS.[62] Clinical neural tissue provocation testing may provide support for a diagnosis of neurogenic TOS.[62] Nonsurgical approaches to treatment include manual therapy such as joint mobilizations, first rib mobilizations, exercise, stretches, modalities, and analgesic medication. The hand or finger edema can dissipate with the preceding physical therapy interventions. Surgery is indicated if pain is persistent and severe neurogenic or vascular

features of the syndrome exist. Prognosis for decreased pain and improved function is good for the majority of individuals with this condition.

TUMORS
■ Lymphoma
Chief Clinical Characteristics
This presentation commonly includes lymph node tenderness and swelling, weight loss, night sweats, fever, and fatigue in association with possible edema and pruritus. Bone pain, shortness of breath, cough, and abdominal pain are possible depending on the dominant sites of involvement. Clinical features may wax and wane.

Background Information
This condition refers to a whole host of malignancies affecting B and T cells. Broadly, this condition is divided among Hodgkin's and non-Hodgkin's lymphomas. Hodgkin's lymphomas are a group of five separate conditions that arise from a specific B-cell abnormality, whereas non-Hodgkin's lymphomas number approximately 30. A combination of genetic and environmental factors has been implicated in the development of this condition. Environmental factors include exposure to solvents and organic chemicals, pesticides and herbicides, wood preservatives, and radiation. In addition, states of immunocompromise, including autoimmune conditions and acquired immunodeficiency virus, have been implicated in this condition's development. Treatment depends on the type and stage of lymphoma. It generally includes radiation, chemotherapy, and biological agents.

■ Metastases, Including from Primary Breast, Kidney, Lung, Prostate, and Thyroid Disease
Chief Clinical Characteristics
This presentation involves pain or aching that is described as unrelenting, in association with fatigue and swelling that waxes and wanes. Edema may begin proximally and progress distally or may begin distally and progress proximally, and may not respond to elevation. Other clinical signs that may accompany edema include skin discoloration, loss of

joint range of motion, and venous distention. Rarely is peripheral edema the only symptom of this condition. However, it may be the symptom that brings the individual to the physician.

Background Information
This condition is caused by obstruction of lymph nodes due to a malignancy. As this condition progresses and lymph nodes become more obstructed, swelling increases and the tissue becomes fibrotic, indurated, and difficult to induce pitting. Upon further questioning, the individual may report fatigue that is usually not improved with rest and progressively worsens over time. Diagnosis includes magnetic resonance imaging, computed tomography, bone scan, ultrasound, complete blood count, and surgical biopsy as needed to identify the source of primary disease. Treatment of the underlying tumor is the primary intervention for this condition. If the peripheral edema persists even though the tumor has shrunk or has disappeared, then the individual may be diagnosed with secondary lymphedema and physical therapy may provide the appropriate intervention.

References
1. Magee DJ. Principles and concepts. In: Magee DJ, ed. *Orthopedic Physical Assessment*. 4th ed. Philadelphia, PA: W. B. Saunders; 2002:51.
2. Aukland K, Reed RK. Interstitial-lymphatic mechanisms in the control of extracellular fluid volume. *Physiol Rev.* Jan 1993;73(1):1–78.
3. Cho S, Atwood JE. Peripheral edema. *Am J Med.* Nov 2002;113(7):580–586.
4. Mortimer PS. Implications of the lymphatic system in CVI-associated edema. *Angiology.* Jan 2000;51(1):3–7.
5. Topham EJ, Mortimer PS. Chronic lower limb oedema. *Clin Med.* Jan–Feb 2002;2(1):28–31.
6. Mortimer PS, Levick JR. Chronic peripheral oedema: the critical role of the lymphatic system. *Clin Med.* Sep–Oct 2004;4(5):448–453.
7. Grattan CE. Urticaria, angio-oedema and anaphylaxis. *Clin Med.* Jan–Feb 2002;2(1):20–23.
8. Kozel MM, Bossuyt PM, Mekkes JR, Bos JD. Laboratory tests and identified diagnoses in patients with physical and chronic urticaria and angioedema: A systematic review. *J Am Acad Dermatol.* Mar 2003;48(3):409–416.
9. Muller BA. Urticaria and angioedema: a practical approach. *Am Fam Physician.* Mar 1, 2004;69(5):1123–1128.
10. Shah UK, Jacobs IN. Pediatric angioedema: ten years' experience. *Arch Otolaryngol Head Neck Surg.* Jul 1999;125(7):791–795.
11. Varadarajulu S. Urticaria and angioedema. Controlling acute episodes, coping with chronic cases. *Postgrad Med.* May 2005;117(5):25–31.

EDEMA

12. Rasool A, Palevsky PM. Treatment of edematous disorders with diuretics. *Am J Med Sci.* Jan 2000;319(1): 25–37.

13. O'Brien JG, Chennubhotla SA, Chennubhotla RV. Treatment of edema. *Am Fam Physician.* Jun 1 2005;71(11): 2111–2117.

14. Airaghi L, Montori D, Santambrogio L, Miadonna A, Tedeschi A. Chronic systemic capillary leak syndrome. Report of a case and review of the literature. *J Intern Med.* Jun 2000;247(6):731–735.

15. Cox NH. Oedema as a risk factor for multiple episodes of cellulitis/erysipelas of the lower leg: a series with community follow-up. *Br J Dermatol.* Nov 2006; 155(5):947–950.

16. Stevens DL. Treatments for skin and soft-tissue and surgical site infections due to MDR Gram-positive bacteria. *J Infect.* Sep 2009;59(suppl 1):S32–39.

17. Cox NH. Management of lower leg cellulitis. *Clin Med.* Jan–Feb 2002;2(1):23–27.

18. Stulberg DL, Penrod MA, Blatny RA. Common bacterial skin infections. *Am Fam Physician.* Jul 1, 2002;66(1): 119–124.

19. Swartz MN. Clinical practice. Cellulitis. *N Engl J Med.* Feb 26, 2004;350(9):904–912.

20. Beebe-Dimmer JL, Pfeifer JR, Engle JS, Schottenfeld D. The epidemiology of chronic venous insufficiency and varicose veins. *Ann Epidemiol.* Mar 2005;15(3):175–184.

21. Porter JM, Moneta GL. Reporting standards in venous disease: an update. International Consensus Committee on Chronic Venous Disease. *J Vasc Surg.* Apr 1995;21(4): 635–645.

22. Atkins RM. Complex regional pain syndrome. *J Bone Joint Surg Br.* Nov 2003;85(8):1100–1106.

23. Perez RS, Burm PE, Zuurmond WW, Bezemer PD, Brink HE, de Lange JJ. Physicians' assessments versus measured symptoms of complex regional pain syndrome type 1: presence and severity. *Clin J Pain.* May–Jun 2005;21(3):272–276.

24. Kommareddy A, Zaroukian MH, Hassouna HI. Upper extremity deep venous thrombosis. *Semin Thromb Hemost.* Feb 2002;28(1):89–99.

25. Fields JM, Goyal M. Venothromboembolism. *Emerg Med Clin North Am.* Aug 2008;26(3):649–683, viii.

26. Celestin R, Brown J, Kihiczak G, Schwartz RA. Erysipelas: a common potentially dangerous infection. *Acta Dermatovenerol Alp Panonica Adriat.* Sep 2007; 16(3):123–127.

27. Aronow WS. The heart and thyroid disease. *Clin Geriatr Med.* May 1995;11(2):219–229.

28. Wilkins LW. *Professional Guide to Signs and Symptoms.* 4th ed. Philadelphia, PA: Lippincott Williams & Wilkins; 2003.

29. Hierholzer K, Finke R. Myxedema. *Kidney Int Suppl.* Jun 1997;59:S82–89.

30. Lindsay RS, Toft AD. Hypothyroidism. *Lancet.* Feb 8 1997;349(9049):413–417.

31. Harwood CA, Bull RH, Evans J, Mortimer PS. Lymphatic and venous function in lipoedema. *Br J Dermatol.* Jan 1996;134(1):1–6.

32. Koss T, Lanatra N, Stiller MJ, Grossman ME. An unusual combination: lipedema with myiasis. *J Am Acad Dermatol.* Jun 2004;50(6):969–972.

33. Tiwari A, Cheng KS, Button M, Myint F, Hamilton G. Differential diagnosis, investigation, and current treatment of lower limb lymphedema. *Arch Surg.* Feb 2003; 138(2):152–161.

34. Warren AG, Janz BA, Borud LJ, Slavin SA. Evaluation and management of the fat leg syndrome. *Plast Reconstr Surg.* Jan 2007;119(1):9e–15e.

35. Venes D. *Taber's Cyclopedic Medical Dictionary.* 20th ed. Philadelphia, PA: F. A. Davis; 2005.

36. Levinson KL, Feingold E, Ferrell RE, Glover TW, Traboulsi EI, Finegold DN. Age of onset in hereditary lymphedema. *J Pediatr.* Jun 2003;142(6):704–708.

37. Foldi E, Foldi M, Clodius L. The lymphedema chaos: a lancet. *Ann Plast Surg.* Jun 1989;22(6):505–515.

38. Piso DU, Eckardt A, Liebermann A, Gutenbrunner C, Schafer P, Gehrke A. Early rehabilitation of head-neck edema after curative surgery for orofacial tumors. *Am J Phys Med Rehabil.* Apr 2001;80(4):261–269.

39. Stanton AW, Levick JR, Mortimer PS. Chronic arm edema following breast cancer treatment. *Kidney Int Suppl.* Jun 1997;59:S76–81.

40. Szuba A, Cooke JP, Yousuf S, Rockson SG. Decongestive lymphatic therapy for patients with cancer-related or primary lymphedema. *Am J Med.* Sep 2000;109(4): 296–300.

41. Wrone DA, Tanabe KK, Cosimi AB, Gadd MA, Souba WW, Sober AJ. Lymphedema after sentinel lymph node biopsy for cutaneous melanoma: a report of 5 cases. *Arch Dermatol.* Apr 2000;136(4):511–514.

42. Rockson SG. Lymphedema. *Am J Med.* Mar 2001; 110(4):288–295.

43. Andresdottir MB, van Hamersvelt HW, van Helden MJ, van de Bosch WJ, Valk IM, Huysmans FT. Ankle edema formation during treatment with the calcium channel blockers lacidipine and amlodipine: a single-centre study. *J Cardiovasc Pharmacol.* 2000;35(3 suppl 1): S25–30.

44. Skeel RT. *Handbook of Cancer Chemotherapy.* 5th ed. Philadelphia, PA: Lippincott Williams & Wilkins; 1999.

45. Lipshultz SE, Lipsitz SR, Sallan SE, et al. Chronic progressive cardiac dysfunction years after doxorubicin therapy for childhood acute lymphoblastic leukemia. *J Clin Oncol.* Apr 20 2005;23(12):2629–2636.

46. Simbre VC, Duffy SA, Dadlani GH, Miller TL, Lipshultz SE. Cardiotoxicity of cancer chemotherapy: implications for children. *Paediatr Drugs.* 2005;7(3):187–202.

47. Palmer BF, Alpern RJ. Pathogenesis of edema formation in the nephrotic syndrome. *Kidney Int Suppl.* Jun 1997;59:S21–27.

48. Andreoli TE. Edematous states: an overview. *Kidney Int Suppl.* Jun 1997;59:S2–10.

49. Vande Walle JG, Donckerwolcke RA. Pathogenesis of edema formation in the nephrotic syndrome. *Pediatr Nephrol.* Mar 2001;16(3):283–293.

50. Deschenes G, Feraille E, Doucet A. Mechanisms of oedema in nephrotic syndrome: old theories and new ideas. *Nephrol Dial Transplant.* Mar 2003;18(3):454–456.

51. Post MW, Visser-Meily JM, Boomkamp-Koppen HG, Prevo AJ. Assessment of oedema in stroke patients: comparison of visual inspection by therapists and volumetric assessment. *Disabil Rehabil.* Nov 18 2003;25(22): 1265–1270.

52. Geurts AC, Visschers BA, van Limbeek J, Ribbers GM. Systematic review of aetiology and treatment of poststroke hand oedema and shoulder-hand syndrome. *Scand J Rehabil Med.* Mar 2000;32(1):4–10.

53. Kahn SR, Ginsberg JS. Relationship between deep venous thrombosis and the postthrombotic syndrome. *Arch Intern Med.* Jan 12 2004;164(1):17–26.

54. Sieggreen M. Venous disorders: overview of current practice. *J Vasc Nurs.* Mar 2005;23(1):33–35.

55. Ahmed T, Rahman S, Cravioto A. Oedematous malnutrition. *Indian J Med Res.* Nov 2009;130(5):651–654.

56. Van Putten JW, Schlosser NJ, Vujaskovic Z, Leest AH, Groen HJ. Superior vena cava obstruction caused by radiation induced venous fibrosis. *Thorax.* Mar 2000; 55(3):245–246.

57. Wan JF, Bezjak A. Superior vena cava syndrome. *Emerg Med Clin North Am.* May 2009;27(2):243–255.

58. Brigden ML. Hematologic and oncologic emergencies. Doing the most good in the least time. *Postgrad Med.* Mar 2001;109(3):143–146, 151–154, 157–158 passim.

59. Krimsky WS, Behrens RJ, Kerkvliet GJ. Oncologic emergencies for the internist. *Cleve Clin J Med.* Mar 2002;69(3):209–210, 213–214, 216–217 passim.

60. Thirlwell C, Brock CS. Emergencies in oncology. *Clin Med.* Jul–Aug 2003;3(4):306–310.

61. Campbell WW, Landau ME. Controversial entrapment neuropathies. *Neurosurg Clin N Am.* Oct 2008;19(4): 597–608, vi–vii.

62. Sanders RJ, Hammond SL, Rao NM. Diagnosis of thoracic outlet syndrome. *J Vasc Surg.* Sep 2007;46(3): 601–604.

63. Rutherford RB, Padberg FT Jr, Comerota AJ, Kistner RL, Meissner MH, Moneta GL. Venous severity scoring: An adjunct to venous outcome assessment. *J Vasc Surg.* Jun 2000;31(6):1307–1312.

EDEMA

CHAPTER 39

Case Demonstration:
Edema and Shoulder Pain

■ *Marisa Perdomo, PT, DPT* ■ *Chris A. Sebelski, PT, DPT, OCS, CSCS*

NOTE: This case demonstration was developed using the diagnostic process described in Chapter 4 and demonstrated in Chapter 5. The reader is encouraged to use this diagnostic process in order to ensure thorough clinical reasoning. If additional elaboration is required on the information presented in this chapter, please consult Chapters 4 and 5.

THE DIAGNOSTIC PROCESS

Step 1 Identify the patient's chief concern.
Step 2 Identify *barriers to communication.*
Step 3 Identify *special concerns.*
Step 4 Create a symptom timeline and sketch the anatomy (if needed).
Step 5 Create a diagnostic hypothesis list considering all possible forms of *remote* and *local* pathology that could cause the patient's chief concern.
Step 6 Sort the diagnostic hypothesis list by epidemiology and specific case characteristics.
Step 7 Ask specific questions to rule specific conditions or pathological categories less likely.
Step 8 Re-sort the diagnostic hypothesis list based on the patient's responses to specific questioning.
Step 9 Perform tests to differentiate among the remaining diagnostic hypotheses.
Step 10 Re-sort the diagnostic hypothesis list based on the patient's responses to specific tests.
Step 11 Decide on a diagnostic impression.
Step 12 Determine the appropriate patient disposition.

Case Description

Mrs. SR is a 79-year-old Asian female referred to physical therapy by an anesthesiologist who specializes in pain management with a referral diagnosis of "left shoulder pain, decreased range of motion, and lymphedema." Her chief concern is further loss of motion and increasing pain, which she describes as "dull, achy upper arm pain" that radiates down to the left elbow and occasionally radiates up to the left side of her neck. She reports skin and muscle tightness of the anterior chest region, which prevents her from moving her arm above her head. Three cortisone injections within the past 3 weeks did not change her pain concerns or limitations. Her physician advised her to rest, but this did not seem to help the pain. Additionally, she reports occasional lower back pain and left hip pain with symptoms of general fatigue. She denies feeling more ill than usual lately.

SR was diagnosed with stage IIIC left invasive lobular carcinoma approximately 10 months prior to this physical therapy consult. Medical treatment included a left modified radical mastectomy with axillary lymph node dissection followed by Arimidex (hormonal therapy) and 5 to 6 weeks of radiation therapy. The radiated field included the left chest wall, axilla, and supraclavicular fossa. The onset of left shoulder pain began during the fourth week of radiation therapy. Present cancer treatment includes only Arimidex therapy, and she has taken an antihypertensive medication "for years." SR began physical therapy and occupational therapy toward the end of her radiation treatments.

Interventions to date included lymphedema management such as manual lymphatic drainage, compression bandaging, light exercises, and issuance of a compression garment. Physical therapy interventions included soft tissue mobilizations and general stretching and range-of-motion exercise for the left shoulder. Concurrently, she received acupuncture treatments. Unfortunately, she reported only slight improvement in her left shoulder symptoms though she did notice a decrease in the cording of her axilla.

Her husband of 50 years died of metastatic cancer 1 year prior to her diagnosis. Prior to her cancer diagnosis, SR volunteered one afternoon per week at a local cancer center. However, since completing radiation therapy she reports that she is very tired and has difficulty volunteering. SR reports that she is "out of shape" because she is now unable to perform a daily 30-minute walking routine. She lives in a large two-story home and her grown children are urging her to sell the home because it is too large for her to independently manage.

sternum (internal mammary lymph nodes) or inferior clavicular lymph node involvement. This information further increases the possibility of metastatic disease. A phone call to her oncologist and referring physician is indicated to obtain additional detailed background information, such as:

- Was chemotherapy offered? Was chemotherapy refused? (options: doxorubicin, cyclophosphamide, paclitaxel, with or without hormone therapy/Herceptin, and Arimidex)
- How many lymph nodes were positive?
- Any present metastases?
- What imaging tests were performed and what were the results?

Teaching Comments:

T: size and location of the tumor

N: number of regional lymph nodes involved

M: presence of metastases

In operable stage IIIC, the cancer (1) is found in 10 or more axillary lymph nodes, or (2) is found in the lymph nodes below the collarbone, or (3) is found in axillary lymph nodes and in lymph nodes near the breastbone. In inoperable stage IIIC, the cancer has spread to the lymph nodes above the collarbone.

Staging a malignant tumor is part of the medical diagnostic process and assists in determining the appropriate medical treatment as well as the long-term prognosis. In this case, the knowledge of a "stage IIIC" breast cancer will guide the therapist's differential diagnosis list. According to the National Cancer Institute, stage IIIC breast cancer is defined as the following: "there may be no tumor found in the breast or the tumor may be any size and may have spread to the chest wall and/or the skin of the breast. Cancer has spread to lymph nodes above or below the collarbone and may have spread to axillary lymph nodes or to lymph nodes near the breastbone. Therefore, the interpretation of the information thus far by a physical therapist may be that SR has operable stage IIIC with significant axillary node involvement and probable lymph node involvement near the

STEP #1: Identify the patient's chief concern.

- Left shoulder loss of motion, increasing pain in the left shoulder with occasional lower back pain, left hip pain, and fatigue

STEP #2: Identify *barriers to communication.*

- **Patient hesitant to discuss cancer history.** Her nonverbal behavior when answering questions regarding her breast cancer diagnosis demonstrated that the patient was not comfortable discussing the medical treatment and prognosis.

STEP #3: Identify *special concerns.*

- **Prior diagnosis of stage IIIC carcinoma.** Increases the likelihood that metastatic disease is responsible for the patient's symptoms.
- **Presentation of pain.** Lack of effect of rest on the patient's symptoms should increase the index of clinical suspicion for metastatic disease.
- **Report of concurrent fatigue and pain.** Fatigue combined with daily reports of left shoulder pain (joint pain) and the new onset of occasional hip pain is significant due to her cancer history.[1] Contextually, this combination of symptoms can be interpreted several ways:
  1. The fatigue is expected due to the age of the patient and the traditional recovery from cancer therapy.

2. The combination of fatigue + joint pain raises the possibility of metastatic disease as a potential cause of this patient's symptoms.
3. Consideration of the patient's recent social history makes it seem completely plausible that "these life events" resulted in depression-related fatigue.

Teaching Comments: Range-of-motion loss and chest wall flexibility/elasticity issues following the termination of radiation therapy are expected. Due to the inflammatory process initiated by radiation, the stimulation of fibroblasts to produce collagen can last for up to 1 year after radiation therapy.[2] Therefore, it is expected that if an individual does not actively maintain joint range of motion and soft tissue pliability following radiation, the tissues may continue to contract and result in greater loss of range of motion 6 months to 1 year after treatment than previously experienced immediately at the end of radiation therapy.[3,4]

STEP #4: Create a symptom timeline and sketch the anatomy (if needed).

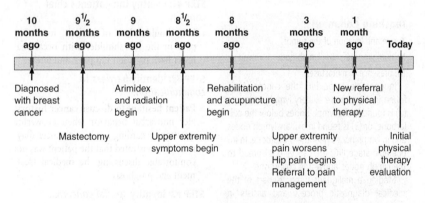

10 months ago	9½ months ago	9 months ago	8½ months ago	8 months ago	3 months ago	1 month ago	Today
Diagnosed with breast cancer		Arimidex and radiation begin		Rehabilitation and acupuncture begin		New referral to physical therapy	
	Mastectomy		Upper extremity symptoms begin		Upper extremity pain worsens / Hip pain begins / Referral to pain management		Initial physical therapy evaluation

STEP #5: Create a diagnostic hypothesis list considering all possible forms of *remote* and *local* pathology that could cause the patient's chief concern.

Causes of Edema

T   Trauma

Secondary lymphedemas:
• Radiation-induced
• Surgical lymph node dissection
Thoracic outlet syndrome

I   Inflammation

Aseptic
Angioedema

STEP #6: Sort the diagnostic hypothesis list by epidemiology and specific case characteristics.

Causes of Edema

T   Trauma

Secondary lymphedemas:
• Radiation-induced
• Surgical lymph node dissection
~~Thoracic outlet syndrome~~ (no symptoms distal to elbow)

I   Inflammation

Aseptic
~~Angioedema~~ (region of symptoms, patient age)

Lymphangiitis
Phlebitis

~~Lymphangiitis~~ (denies recent illness)
~~Phlebitis~~ (no history of recent trauma, less typical in the upper extremity)

Septic
Cellulitis
Erysipelas
Necrotizing fasciitis

Septic
Cellulitis
Erysipelas
~~Necrotizing fasciitis~~ (no recent illness)

M   Metabolic

Ascites/cirrhosis of the liver

Hyperthyroidism
Hypothyroidism

Lipedema

Medication-induced edemas:
• Angiotensin-converting enzyme inhibitors

• Antihypertensives

• Calcium channel blockers

• Chemotherapy agents
• Corticosteroids

• Nonsteroidal anti-inflammatories

• Selective and nonselective cyclooxygenase-2 inhibitors

Myxedema

Nephrotic syndrome

M   Metabolic

~~Ascites/cirrhosis of the liver~~ (less typical of the upper extremity)

Hyperthyroidism
~~Hypothyroidism~~ (not typical of the upper extremities)

~~Lipedema~~ (not typical of the upper extremities)

Medication-induced edemas:
• ~~Angiotensin-converting enzyme inhibitors~~ (patient not taking this medication)

• ~~Antihypertensives~~ (has been taking medications for many years without symptoms)

• ~~Calcium channel blockers~~ (patient not taking this medication)

• Chemotherapy agents
• ~~Corticosteroids~~ (patient not taking this medication)

• ~~Nonsteroidal anti-inflammatories~~ (patient not taking this medication)

• ~~Selective and nonselective cyclooxygenase-2 inhibitors~~ (patient not taking this medication)

~~Myxedema~~ (not typical of the upper extremities)

~~Nephrotic syndrome~~ (not typical of the upper extremities)

Va   Vascular

Capillary leak syndrome

Cardiomyopathy

Chronic venous insufficiency

Congestive heart failure

Deep venous thrombosis
Peripheral vascular disease

Post-thrombotic syndrome

Superior vena cava syndrome

Va   Vascular

~~Capillary leak syndrome~~ (not typical of the upper extremity)

~~Cardiomyopathy~~ (involvement of one extremity uncommon)

~~Chronic venous insufficiency~~ (not typical of the upper extremities)

~~Congestive heart failure~~ (involvement of one extremity uncommon)

Deep venous thrombosis
~~Peripheral vascular disease~~ (unilateral involvement of the upper extremity less common)

~~Post-thrombotic syndrome~~ (not typical of the upper extremities)

Superior vena cava syndrome

De Degenerative

Not applicable

Tu Tumor

Malignant Primary, such as:
- Lymphoma

Malignant Metastatic, such as:
- Metastases, including from primary breast, kidney, lung, prostate, and thyroid disease

Benign:

Not applicable

Co Congenital

Primary lymphatic malformation:
- Milroy's disease

- Meige disease

Non-Milroy's disease

Ne Neurogenic/Psychogenic

Complex regional pain syndrome
Post-stroke hand edema

Remote

T Trauma

Cervical disk herniation
Internal organ injuries:
- Diaphragm

- Liver
- Lung
- Spleen

Status postlaparoscopic procedure

Thoracic outlet syndrome

I Inflammation

Aseptic

Acute cholecystitis

Costochondritis (Tietze's syndrome)

Gaseous distention of the stomach

Inflammatory bowel diseases:
- Crohn's disease

- Ulcerative colitis

Rheumatoid arthritis–like diseases of the cervical spine:

De Degenerative

Not applicable

Tu Tumor

Malignant Primary, such as:
- Lymphoma

Malignant Metastatic, such as:
- Metastases, including from primary breast, kidney, lung, prostate, and thyroid disease

Benign:

Not applicable

Co Congenital

Primary lymphatic malformation:
- ~~Milroy's disease~~ (patient age, less typical of the upper extremities in isolation)

- ~~Meige disease~~ (patient age, less typical of the upper extremities in isolation)

~~Non-Milroy's disease~~ (patient age)

Ne Neurogenic/Psychogenic

Complex regional pain syndrome
~~Post-stroke hand edema~~ (no recent history of stroke)

Remote

T Trauma

Cervical disk herniation
~~Internal organ injuries:~~
- ~~Diaphragm~~ (no history of sufficient trauma)
- ~~Liver~~ (no history of sufficient trauma)
- ~~Lung~~ (no history of sufficient trauma)
- ~~Spleen~~ (no history of sufficient trauma)

~~Status postlaparoscopic procedure~~ (no recent history of laparoscopy)

Thoracic outlet syndrome

I Inflammation

Aseptic

~~Acute cholecystitis~~ (limited shoulder range of motion)

~~Costochondritis (Tietze's syndrome)~~ (no chest pain)

~~Gaseous distention of the stomach~~ (limited shoulder range of motion)

~~Inflammatory bowel diseases:~~
- ~~Crohn's disease~~ (no abdominal pain, limited shoulder range of motion)

- ~~Ulcerative colitis~~ (no abdominal pain, limited shoulder range of motion)

Rheumatoid arthritis–like diseases of the cervical spine:

- Inflammatory muscle diseases

- Psoriatic arthritis

- Scleroderma

- Systemic lupus erythematosus

Septic
Acute viral/idiopathic pericarditis
Cat-scratch disease

Cervical epidural abscess
Cervical lymphadenitis
Hepatitis

Perihepatitis (Fitz-Hugh-Curtis syndrome)

Pleuritis
Pneumonia

Subphrenic abscess
Ulcers:
- Duodenal
- Gastric

M Metabolic

Ectopic pregnancy
Osteomalacia

Va Vascular

Acute myocardial infarction
Aneurysm (such as involving the aortic or
    subclavian arteries)
Coronary artery insufficiency
Pulmonary embolus
Upper extremity deep venous thrombosis
    (Paget-Schroetter syndrome)

De Degenerative

Osteoarthritis/osteoarthrosis of the cervical
    spine

Tu Tumor

Malignant Primary, such as:
- Breast tumor
- Pancoast tumor

Malignant Metastatic:
Not applicable
Benign:
Not applicable

- ~~Inflammatory muscle diseases~~ (not
    associated with upper extremity edema)
- ~~Psoriatic arthritis~~ (not associated with
    upper extremity edema)
- ~~Scleroderma~~ (not associated with upper
    extremity edema)
- ~~Systemic lupus erythematosus~~ (not
    associated with upper extremity edema)

Septic
Acute viral/idiopathic pericarditis
~~Cat-scratch disease~~ (not typically associated
    with pain)
Cervical epidural abscess
Cervical lymphadenitis
~~Hepatitis~~ (no abdominal pain, no recent
    illness)
~~Perihepatitis (Fitz-Hugh-Curtis syndrome)~~
    (time course)
~~Pleuritis~~ (no chest pain)
~~Pneumonia~~ (no recent upper respiratory
    illness)
~~Subphrenic abscess~~ (time course)
~~Ulcers:~~
- ~~Duodenal~~ (no abdominal pain)
- ~~Gastric~~ (no abdominal pain)

M Metabolic

~~Ectopic pregnancy~~ (patient age)
~~Osteomalacia~~ (few risk factors, primary
    shoulder pain not a characteristic feature)

Va Vascular

~~Acute myocardial infarction~~ (time course)
Aneurysm (such as involving the aortic or
    subclavian arteries)
Coronary artery insufficiency
~~Pulmonary embolus~~ (time course)
~~Upper extremity deep venous thrombosis
    (Paget-Schroetter syndrome)~~ (time
    course)

De Degenerative

Osteoarthritis/osteoarthrosis of the cervical
    spine

Tu Tumor

Malignant Primary, such as:
- Breast tumor
- ~~Pancoast tumor~~ (no symptoms distal to
    the elbow)
Malignant Metastatic:
Not applicable
Benign:
Not applicable

Co Congenital

Not applicable

Ne Neurogenic/Psychogenic

Anxiety
Depression
Radiation-induced brachial plexopathy

Local

T Trauma

Axillary web syndrome
Dislocations:
- Acromioclavicular joint

- Glenohumeral joint

- Sternoclavicular joint

Fractures:
- Bankart lesion

- Bennett lesion

- Clavicle
- Hills Sachs lesion

- Proximal humerus (such as insufficiency fracture)
- Scapula
Glenohumeral joint sprain/subluxation

Glenoid labrum tear

Muscle strains:
- Levator scapula
- Pectoralis muscle group

- Rotator cuff
- Upper trapezius
Myofascial pain secondary to radiation fibrosis or mastectomy
Nerve entrapments:
- Median
- Musculocutaneous
- Radial
- Ulnar
Subacromial impingement syndrome
Thoracic outlet syndrome

Co Congenital

Not applicable

Ne Neurogenic/Psychogenic

Anxiety
Depression
~~Radiation-induced brachial plexopathy~~ (time course)

Local

T Trauma

Axillary web syndrome
Dislocations:
- ~~Acromioclavicular joint~~ (no history of sufficient trauma)
- ~~Glenohumeral joint~~ (no history of sufficient trauma)
- ~~Sternoclavicular joint~~ (no history of sufficient trauma)
Fractures:
- ~~Bankart lesion~~ (no history of sufficient trauma)
- ~~Bennett lesion~~ (no history of sufficient trauma)
- ~~Clavicle~~ (no history of sufficient trauma)
- ~~Hills Sachs lesion~~ (no history of sufficient trauma)
- Proximal humerus (such as insufficiency fracture)
- ~~Scapula~~ (no history of sufficient trauma)
~~Glenohumeral joint sprain/subluxation~~ (no history of sufficient trauma)
~~Glenoid labrum tear~~ (no history of sufficient trauma)
Muscle strains:
- Levator scapula
- ~~Pectoralis muscle group~~ (location of symptoms)
- Rotator cuff
- Upper trapezius
Myofascial pain secondary to radiation fibrosis or mastectomy
Nerve entrapments:
- Median
- Musculocutaneous
- Radial
- Ulnar
Subacromial impingement syndrome
~~Thoracic outlet syndrome~~ (no symptoms distal to elbow)

I Inflammation

Aseptic
Adhesive capsulitis
Bursitis

Chronic fatigue syndrome

Complex regional pain syndrome
Fibromyalgia

Myofascial pain syndrome
Neuralgic amyotrophy (Parsonage Turner syndrome)
Polymyalgia rheumatica

Reiter's syndrome
Rheumatoid arthritis

Rheumatoid arthritis–like diseases of the shoulder:
* Ankylosing spondylitis

* Inflammatory muscle diseases

* Psoriatic arthritis

* Scleroderma

* Systemic lupus erythematosus

Rotator cuff tendinitis

Septic
Osteomyelitis
Septic arthritis
Skeletal tuberculosis (Pott's disease)

M Metabolic
Amyloid arthropathy
Cancer-related fatigue syndrome
Gout

Hereditary neuralgic amyotrophy

Heterotopic ossification (myositis ossificans)
Medication-induced joint pain
Pseudogout

I Inflammation

Aseptic
Adhesive capsulitis
~~Bursitis~~ (symptoms began during radiation treatment)
~~Chronic fatigue syndrome~~ (this is a diagnosis of exclusion)
Complex regional pain syndrome
~~Fibromyalgia~~ (this is a diagnosis of exclusion)
Myofascial pain syndrome
~~Neuralgic amyotrophy (Parsonage Turner syndrome)~~ (time course, age)
~~Polymyalgia rheumatica~~ (unilateral symptoms uncommon)
~~Reiter's syndrome~~ (no recent illness)
~~Rheumatoid arthritis~~ (first involvement of the shoulder is uncommon)
~~Rheumatoid arthritis–like diseases of the shoulder:~~
* ~~Ankylosing spondylitis~~ (patient age, first involvement of the shoulder is uncommon)
* ~~Inflammatory muscle diseases~~ (unilateral symptoms uncommon)
* ~~Psoriatic arthritis~~ (first involvement of the shoulder is uncommon)
* ~~Scleroderma~~ (first involvement of the shoulder is uncommon)
* ~~Systemic lupus erythematosus~~ (first involvement of the shoulder is uncommon)
~~Rotator cuff tendinitis~~ (symptoms began during radiation treatment)

Septic
Osteomyelitis
Septic arthritis
~~Skeletal tuberculosis (Pott's disease)~~ (no recent illness)

M Metabolic
Amyloid arthropathy
Cancer-related fatigue syndrome
~~Gout~~ (uncommon presentation at the shoulder)
~~Hereditary neuralgic amyotrophy~~ (patient age at first presentation)
Heterotopic ossification (myositis ossificans)
Medication-induced joint pain
~~Pseudogout~~ (time course)

Va Vascular

Aneurysm (such as involving the subclavian or axillary arteries)
Avascular necrosis of the humeral head
Compartment syndrome
Deep venous thrombosis
Quadrilateral space syndrome

De Degenerative

Osteoarthritis/osteoarthrosis:
- Acromioclavicular joint
- Glenohumeral joint
- Sternoclavicular joint
Rotator cuff tear

Tu Tumor

Malignant Primary, such as:
- Breast cancer in remaining lymph nodes
- Chondrosarcoma
- Lymphoma
- Osteosarcoma
Malignant Metastatic, such as:
- Metastases, including from primary breast, kidney, lung, prostate, and thyroid disease
Benign, such as:
- Enchondroma
- Lipoma
- Osteoblastoma
- Osteochondroma
- Osteoid osteoma
- Unicameral bone cyst

Co Congenital

Not applicable

Ne Neurogenic/Psychogenic

Erb's palsy

Neuropathic arthropathy (Charcot-Marie-Tooth disease)

Va Vascular

Aneurysm (such as involving the subclavian or axillary arteries)
Avascular necrosis of the humeral head
~~Compartment syndrome~~ (time course)
~~Deep venous thrombosis~~ (time course)
~~Quadrilateral space syndrome~~ (time course)

De Degenerative

Osteoarthritis/osteoarthrosis:
- Acromioclavicular joint
- Glenohumeral joint
- Sternoclavicular joint
Rotator cuff tear

Tu Tumor

Malignant Primary, such as:
- Breast cancer in remaining lymph nodes
- ~~Chondrosarcoma~~ (patient age)
- Lymphoma
- Osteosarcoma
Malignant Metastatic, such as:
- Metastases, including from primary breast, kidney, lung, prostate, and thyroid disease
Benign, such as:
- ~~Enchondroma~~ (condition is painless)
- Lipoma
- Osteoblastoma
- ~~Osteochondroma~~ (patient age)
- ~~Osteoid osteoma~~ (patient age)
- ~~Unicameral bone cyst~~ (patient age)

Co Congenital

Not applicable

Ne Neurogenic/Psychogenic

~~Erb's palsy~~ (patient age at first symptom presentation)

~~Neuropathic arthropathy (Charcot-Marie-Tooth disease)~~ (time course)

STEP #7: Ask specific questions to rule specific conditions or pathological categories less likely.

Teaching Comments: The focus of the first session was for the clarification of arm pain and lymphedema because they were the chief concerns of SR. However, due to the barriers to communication and the cautions of the case, the interview and the examination process may take several sessions within this patient population.

- **Did your shoulder pain start during radiation treatment?** Yes, making less likely that axillary cording or any acute inflammatory condition is the source of her pathology.
- **Do you have chest pain with physical exertion?** No, ruling less likely primary cardiac pathology.
- **Do you have numbness or tingling?** No, decreasing index of clinical suspicion for cervical spine or neurogenic pathology.
- **Have you had x-ray or magnetic resonance imaging of your shoulder in the past**

3 months? No, so possibility of metastases or primary bone tumor unable to be excluded.

STEP #8: Re-sort the diagnostic hypothesis list based on the patient's responses to specific questioning.

Causes

T　Trauma

Secondary lymphedemas:
* Radiation-induced
* Surgical lymph node dissection

I　Inflammation

Aseptic

Not applicable

Septic

Cellulitis

Erysipelas

M　Metabolic

Medication-induced edemas:
* Chemotherapy agents

Hyperthyroidism

Va　Vascular

Deep venous thrombosis

~~Superior vena cava syndrome~~ (no pain with exertion)

De　Degenerative

Not applicable

Tu　Tumor

Malignant Primary, such as:
* Lymphoma

Malignant Metastatic, such as:
* Metastases, including from primary breast, kidney, lung, prostate, and thyroid disease

Benign:

Not applicable

Co　Congenital

Not applicable

Ne　Neurogenic/Psychogenic

Complex regional pain syndrome

Remote

T　Trauma

~~Cervical disk herniation~~ (no numbness and tingling)

~~Thoracic outlet syndrome~~ (no numbness and tingling)

I　Inflammation

Aseptic

Not applicable

Septic

~~Acute viral/idiopathic pericarditis~~ (no change in symptoms with physical exertion)

~~Cervical epidural abscess~~ (no numbness and tingling)

Cervical lymphadenitis

M　Metabolic

Not applicable

Va　Vascular

Aneurysm (such as involving the aortic or subclavian arteries)

~~Coronary artery insufficiency~~ (no change in symptoms with physical exertion)

De　Degenerative

Osteoarthritis/osteoarthrosis of the cervical spine

Tu　Tumor

Malignant Primary, such as:
* Breast tumor

Malignant Metastatic:

Not applicable

Benign:

Not applicable

Co　Congenital

Not applicable

Ne　Neurogenic/Psychogenic

Anxiety

Depression

Local

T　Trauma

~~Axillary web syndrome~~ (onset not coincident with radiation treatment)

Fractures:
* Proximal humerus (such as insufficiency fracture)

Muscle strains:
* Levator scapula
* Rotator cuff
* Upper trapezius

Nerve entrapments:
* Median
* Musculocutaneous

- Radial
- Ulnar

Subacromial impingement syndrome

I   Inflammation

Aseptic

Adhesive capsulitis

Complex regional pain syndrome

~~Myofascial pain syndrome~~ (secondary to radiation; onset not coincident with radiation therapy)

Septic

Osteomyelitis

Septic arthritis

M   Metabolic

Amyloid arthropathy

Cancer-related fatigue syndrome

Heterotopic ossification (myositis ossificans)

Medication-induced joint pain

Va   Vascular

Aneurysm (such as involving the subclavian or axillary arteries)

Avascular necrosis of the humeral head

De   Degenerative

Osteoarthritis/osteoarthrosis:

- Acromioclavicular joint
- Glenohumeral joint
- Sternoclavicular joint

Rotator cuff tear

Tu   Tumor

Malignant Primary, such as:

- Breast cancer in remaining lymph nodes
- Lymphoma
- Osteosarcoma

Malignant Metastatic, such as:

- Metastases, including from primary breast, kidney, lung, prostate, and thyroid disease

Benign, such as:

- Lipoma
- Osteoblastoma

Co   Congenital

Not applicable

Ne   Neurogenic/Psychogenic

Not applicable

STEP #9: Perform tests to differentiate among the remaining diagnostic hypotheses.

- **Observation of the face, neck, and shoulder.** Well-healed left axillary incision was noted with minimal cording, decreasing the index of suspicion for axillary web syndrome. Coloration and temperature of the skin was grossly normal throughout the neck and shoulders, reducing the likelihood of infection. Mild lymphedema was noted in the left shoulder axilla and left lateral chest wall, increasing the likelihood of secondary lymphedema.

- **Auscultation.** Cardiac auscultation revealed normal heart sounds, ruling less likely primary cardiac pathology. Rate and rhythm also were grossly normal, ruling less likely hyperthyroidism. Pulmonary auscultation was unremarkable for crackles, rales, or absent breath sounds, decreasing likelihood of primary pulmonary pathology.

- **Neurological tests.** Reflexes and sensation were normal throughout the upper extremities, reducing the likelihood of primary cervical spine pathology.

- **Range of motion of the cervical spine, shoulder, lumbar spine, and hip.** Cervical spine range of motion was normal without reproduction of symptoms in the right upper extremity, ruling even less likely primary cervical spine pathology. Left shoulder active and passive range of motion revealed moderately limited movement in all planes secondary to reproduction of symptoms, increasing suspicion of pathology specific to the shoulder region. Lumbar and hip ranges of motion were normal and did not change the patient's pain.

- **Palpation.** Rotator cuff tendons, acromioclavicular joint, and sternoclavicular joint were nontender.

Teaching Comments: It is probable that the soft tissue fibrosis resulting in decreased muscle length of the pectoralis major/minor and loss of skin mobility are due to radiation therapy. These soft tissue alterations can lead to altered positioning of the glenohumeral joint within the fossa. At this point in the exam, it will be difficult to determine the structural cause of the shoulder symptoms if they are musculoskeletal.

STEP #10: Re-sort the diagnostic hypothesis list based on the patient's responses to specific tests.

Causes

T   Trauma

Secondary lymphedemas:
- Radiation-induced
- Surgical lymph node dissection

I   Inflammation

Aseptic

Not applicable

Septic

~~Cellulitis~~ (no swelling, increase in skin temperature)

~~Erysipelas~~ (no change in skin color, swelling, skin temperature)

M   Metabolic

Medication-induced edemas:
- Chemotherapy agents

~~Hyperthyroidism~~ (normal cardiac rate and rhythm)

Va   Vascular

~~Deep venous thrombosis~~ (no swelling, change in skin temperature)

De   Degenerative

Not applicable

Tu   Tumor

Malignant Primary, such as:
- Lymphoma

Malignant Metastatic, such as:
- Metastases, including from primary breast, kidney, lung, prostate, and thyroid disease

Benign

Not applicable

Co   Congenital

Not applicable

Ne   Neurogenic/Psychogenic

Complex regional pain syndrome

Remote

T   Trauma

Not applicable

I   Inflammation

Aseptic

Not applicable

Septic

~~Cervical lymphadenitis~~ (no swelling)

M   Metabolic

Not applicable

Va   Vascular

Aneurysm (such as involving the aortic or subclavian arteries)

De   Degenerative

~~Osteoarthritis/osteoarthrosis of the cervical spine~~ (normal cervical range of motion without reproduction of left shoulder pain)

Tu   Tumor

Malignant Primary, such as:
- Breast tumor

Malignant Metastatic:

Not applicable

Benign

Not applicable

Co   Congenital

Not applicable

Ne   Neurogenic/Psychogenic

Anxiety
Depression

Local

T   Trauma

Fractures:
- ~~Proximal humerus (such as insufficiency fracture)~~ (shoulder range of motion)

Muscle strains:
- Levator scapula
- Rotator cuff
- Upper trapezius

Nerve entrapments:
- Median
- Musculocutaneous
- Radial
- Ulnar

Subacromial impingement syndrome

I   Inflammation

Aseptic

~~Adhesive capsulitis~~ (pattern of shoulder range-of-motion limitation)

Complex regional pain syndrome

Septic

Osteomyelitis
Septic arthritis

M Metabolic

~~Amyloid arthropathy~~ (no swelling)
Cancer-related fatigue syndrome
Heterotopic ossification (myositis ossificans)
Medication-induced joint pain

Va Vascular

Aneurysm (such as involving the subclavian or axillary arteries)
Avascular necrosis of the humeral head

De Degenerative

Osteoarthritis/osteoarthrosis:
- ~~Acromioclavicular joint~~ (joint is nontender)
- Glenohumeral joint
- ~~Sternoclavicular joint~~ (joint is nontender)
~~Rotator cuff tear~~ (negative palpation)

Tu Tumor

Malignant Primary, such as:
- Breast cancer in remaining lymph nodes
- Lymphoma
- Osteosarcoma
Malignant Metastatic, such as:
- Metastases disease, including from primary breast, kidney, lung, prostate, and thyroid disease
Benign, such as:
- Lipoma
- Osteoblastoma

Co Congenital

Not applicable

Ne Neurogenic/Psychogenic

Not applicable

STEP #11: Decide on a diagnostic impression.

The preliminary diagnostic impression is a mix of permanent structural changes, transient orthopedic impairments, and the potential serious consequences of progression of metastatic disease. The most likely conditions of those that remain include (in alphabetical order):

- **Breast cancer metastasis affecting the brachial plexus, supraclavicular lymph nodes, or remaining axillary lymph nodes.** Based on the stage of the patient's breast cancer this diagnosis should be considered present until proven otherwise. Classic clinical signs and symptoms of cancer reported

in the literature include weight loss or gain greater than 10% of body weight in 1 month, night pain, or constant pain. It is this author's experience that more common complaints include fatigue (low intensity with slow onset that steadily and gradually increases over time) that is not relieved by rest and reports of a "dull ache" that initially appears to be intermittent and then progresses to constant. Additionally, the patient currently reports occasional low back pain and hip pain. The mere presence of associated pains should also alert the clinician to the possibility of metastasis. Although the complaints of low back pain and hip pain were not the patient's chief concern as of this visit, during subsequent visits these comments will have to be examined and provocative tests completed to deduce if there is a nonmechanical versus musculoskeletal cause.

An established diagnosis of metastatic breast cancer would not preclude physical therapy; physical therapy is an acceptable intervention even in the presence of metastatic disease. The therapist must consult with the medical team to determine the structures involved that must be considered in determining ongoing physical therapy interventions. It is the remaining possibility of undetected metastatic disease of the hip and lumbar spine, and the serious consequences that accompany that diagnosis, that necessitates a formal return visit by the patient to the oncologist.

- **Cancer-related fatigue syndrome with depression-related fatigue.** Cancer-related fatigue syndrome is well documented and is a result of physical deconditioning and psychosocial factors that occur as a result of the cancer and its treatment modalities.[5,6]

- **Medication-induced arthralgia.** Arimidex is an aromatase inhibitor, which prevents estrogen from being produced in postmenopausal women. It is effective in controlling the growth of metastatic breast cancer. Presumably it has fewer side effects than Tamoxifen; however, side effects may include joint pain, stiffness, and arthritic-type complaints. Given that this patient has left shoulder pain with occasional low back and left hip pain, Arimidex could be a potential contributor to this individual's source of pain. If the joint pain is due to Arimidex or is medication induced, the patient's pain would be bilateral and involve many joints. It is therefore unlikely that this adverse effect is the primary cause of her musculoskeletal complaints. The specific complaint of left hip pain is suspicious and, based on the author's clinical experience, raises the concern for metastatic disease.

- Radiation fibrosis resulting in myofascial restrictions of the left upper extremity muscles. The underlying joints within the radiated field as identified by the radiation field tattoos will also have restriction. Finally, observation of the skin discoloration will cue the clinician to the integumentary system and its altered skin texture and mobility. The consequence of this altered mobility is scapular dyskinesia. It is frequently related to several of the remaining musculoskeletal diagnoses on the hypothesis list such as subacromial impingement, rotator cuff tendinitis/tendinosis, glenohumeral joint restriction/capsulitis, and bursitis.

STEP #12: Determine the appropriate patient disposition.

- Initiate physical therapy treatment with consultation of the oncologist.

Case Outcome

A lumbar and hip evaluation was performed and completed by the patient's third visit to physical therapy. Physical therapy could not alleviate or reproduce the patient's hip pain. Based on these findings, the physical therapist reconnected with the patient's oncologist immediately and relayed these concerns. Magnetic resonance imaging and a bone scan were ordered and findings did indicate a new metastatic lesion to the hip. The finding of a new metastatic lesion did not alter the original physical therapy plan for the upper quadrant.

References

1. Deyo RA, Diehl AK. Cancer as a cause of back pain: frequency, clinical presentation, and diagnostic strategies. *J Gen Intern Med.* May–Jun 1988;3(3):230–238.
2. O'Sullivan B, Levin W. Late radiation-related fibrosis: pathogenesis, manifestations, and current management. *Semin Radiat Oncol.* 2003;13(3):274–289.
3. Davis AM, Dische S, Gerber L, Saunders M, Leuing SF, O'Sullivan B. Measuring postirradiation subcutaneous soft-tissue fibrosis: state-of-the-art and future directions. *Semin Radiat Oncol.* 2003;13(3):203–213.
4. Bentzen SM. Preventing or reducing late side effects of radiation therapy: radiobiology meets molecular pathology. *Nature Rev Cancer.* 2006;6(9):702–713.
5. Ahlberg K, Ekman T, Gaston-Lohansson F, Mock V. Assessment and management of cancer-related fatigue in adults. *Lancet.* 2003;362:640–650.
6. Curt G. The impact of fatigue on patients with cancer: overview of FATIGUE 1 and 2. *Oncologist.* 2000;5(suppl 2):9–12.

CHAPTER 40

Failure of Wounds to Heal

■ *Rose Hamm, PT, DPT, CWS, FACCWS*

Description of the Symptom

This chapter describes pathology that may lead to wounds that fail to heal. Chronic wounds are defined as wounds that "fail to progress through a normal, orderly, and timely sequence of repair or wounds that pass through the repair process without restoring anatomic and functional results."[1] Without adequate treatment of the wound etiology and comorbidities, the composition of the wound tissue and fluid (called chronic wound fluid) will develop certain properties that inhibit healing. The length of time a wound exists is less important in determining if it is chronic than are the characteristics of the wound tissue.

Special Concerns

■ Sinus, undermining, or fistula formation
■ Bone involvement that may lead to osteomyelitis
■ Friable granulation tissue
■ Contractures
■ Deformities of adjacent joints
■ Malignant changes
■ Systemic amyloidosis
■ Calcification[2]
■ Failure to respond to standard care

CHAPTER PREVIEW: Conditions That May Lead to Failure of Wounds to Heal

T | Trauma

COMMON

Burns 818
Neuropathic wounds 825
Traumatic injury 830

UNCOMMON

Not applicable

RARE

Not applicable

I | Inflammation

COMMON

Aseptic
Bullous pemphigoid 818
Foreign body reaction 822
Pemphigus 826
Pyoderma gangrenosum 828

Septic
Cellulitis 819
Dermal viral infections 821
Fungal infection 822
Necrotizing fasciitis 825
Osteomyelitis 826

Inflammation *(continued)*

UNCOMMON

Not applicable

RARE

Not applicable

M Metabolic

COMMON

Allergic responses:
- Contact dermatitis 815
- Drug hypersensitivity syndromes 815
- Spider bites 816

UNCOMMON

Not applicable

RARE

Not applicable

Va Vascular

COMMON

Arterial insufficiency 816
Calciphylaxis 818
Chronic venous insufficiency 820
Coumadin-induced skin necrosis (warfarin-induced skin necrosis) 820
Cryoglobulinemia 821
Lymphedemas:
- Primary lymphedema (Milroy's disease, Meige disease) 822
- Secondary lymphedema 823
Martorell's ulcer 824
Raynaud's disease 829
Sickle cell disease 829
Vasculitis 830

UNCOMMON

Buerger disease (thromboangiitis obliterans) 817

RARE

Not applicable

De Degenerative

COMMON

Pressure ulcers 827

UNCOMMON

Not applicable

RARE

Not applicable

(continued)

Tu Tumor

COMMON

Not applicable

UNCOMMON

Malignant Primary, such as:
• Basal cell carcinoma 817
• Squamous cell carcinoma 829
Malignant Metastatic, such as:
• Kaposi's sarcoma 822
Benign:
Not applicable

RARE

Malignant Primary, such as:
• Cutaneous lymphoma 821
• Melanoma 824
Malignant Metastatic, such as:
• Marjolin's ulcer 824
Benign:
Not applicable

Co Congenital

COMMON

Not applicable

UNCOMMON

Not applicable

RARE

Not applicable

Ne Neurogenic/Psychogenic

COMMON

Not applicable

UNCOMMON

Factitious disorder 822

RARE

Not applicable

Note: These are estimates of relative incidence because few data are available for the less common conditions.

Overview of Wounds That Fail to Heal

A chronic wound can have any of the following characteristics:

- Necrotic and unhealthy tissue
- Impaired hemodynamics (for example, hypoxia, ischemia, or edema)
- Collagen degradation resulting in unhealthy extracellular matrix
- Rolled edges without epithelial migration as a result of senescent fibroblasts and keratinocytes that are unresponsive to normal facilitating factors
- Overgrowth of epithelium due to the lack of underlying connective tissue
- Recurrent wound deterioration as a result of superficial epithelial bridging
- Chronic inflammation resulting in lack of healthy granulation tissue
- Increased bacterial loads with or without clinical infection (pain, warmth, erythema, edema, drainage, odor)
- Presence of biofilm on the wound surface, sometimes visible as a thin opaque layer.

The four most common causes of chronic wounds are pressure, arterial insufficiency, chronic venous insufficiency, and neuropathy (sensory, motor, and/or autonomic). If these four etiologies are ruled out, atypical etiologies need to be identified so the underlying cause of the wound can be treated in addition to local wound care.

Description of Conditions That May Lead to Failure of Wounds to Heal

ALLERGIC RESPONSES

■ Contact Dermatitis

Chief Clinical Characteristics
This presentation involves erythema, edema, pruritus, and vesicular lesions in the contact area (Fig. 40-1).

Background Information
This condition occurs from direct contact of the skin with an antigen (eg, latex, metals, poisonous plants, drugs, tape) or with prolonged exposure to an irritant (eg, detergent, perfume, chemical). The antigen is bound to

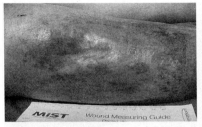

FIGURE 40-1 Contact dermatitis causes skin changes such as erythema, edema, pruritus, and vesicles.

a carrier protein and transported by Langerhans cells to T cells that become sensitive to the antigen. Upon reexposure, the T cells initiate an inflammatory response that is visible as this condition.[3] After identification and removal of the irritating substance, contact dermatitis is usually adequately managed with local treatment; however, in severe cases referral to a medical specialist is indicated. In addition to eliminating exposure to the antigen or irritant, local care involves immediate thorough washing of the exposed area with warm water and mild soap, use of topical creams (eg, steroids or antibiotics), and avoidance of tape, adhesive dressings, or nonprescription topical ointments that may exacerbate this condition. Diffuse cellulitis may develop if this condition is improperly treated.

■ Drug Hypersensitivity Syndromes

Chief Clinical Characteristics
This presentation usually includes fever, malaise, pharyngitis, small joint polyarthritis, and cervical lymphadenopathy. Skin eruptions, which occur in approximately 85% of individuals with this condition, may be eczematous eruptions with erythema, vesicles, and scales with itching; red rash or measle-like eruptions that usually begin in pressured or dependent areas and rapidly become generalized; vesicular or bullous eruptions; erythema and edema followed by hyperpigmentation at a specific site of drug injection; generalized pustules usually on the face or between skinfolds; subcutaneous nodules that are tender and erythematous, usually on the anterior legs; or wheals, welts, or hives (Fig. 40-2).

FAILURE OF WOUNDS TO HEAL

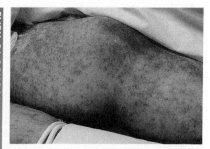

FIGURE 40-2 Drug hypersensitivity syndrome. Initial signs of drug hypersensitivity include rash or measle-like symptoms in dependent extremities.

Background Information

Symptoms usually occur 2 to 6 weeks after the first drug exposure, and the allergen is usually the drug most recently included in the individual's medications. This condition is a systemic allergic reaction to ingested drugs, which can vary in the number of involved organs, severity of symptoms, type of lesions, and number of skin eruptions. Cutaneous pathology involves immunoglobulin hypersensitivity reactions that result in destruction of the basal membrane binding the epidermis and dermis, leading to the variety of skin eruptions listed above. Medical intervention is dependent on the severity of the reaction and symptoms, including meticulous local wound care for milder cases and emergent medical care for severe cases, especially the life-threatening syndromes of toxic epidermal necrolysis and Stevens-Johnson syndrome. Individuals who exhibit signs of this condition should be referred to the physician or emergency department for immediate care.

■ Spider Bites

Chief Clinical Characteristics

This presentation commonly involves slight erythema, localized urticaria, and discomfort for 3 to 5 days for cases of minor envenomation. For cases of moderate envenomation, discomfort begins 4 to 6 hours after the bite and involves pale skin with a small blister in the center, and resolution of symptoms with topical care after 1 to 2 weeks. Cases of severe envenomation involve pain 6 to 12 hours after the bite; two tiny puncture marks with surrounding erythema; bluish and cyanotic color in a blanched ring surrounded by erythema ("bull's-eye" lesion) within a few hours; a hemorrhagic bleb that becomes several centimeters with generalized fine punctate rash; systemic symptoms of nausea, vomiting, and malaise; and subcutaneous fat necrosis that expands to 3 to 10 cm, becomes gangrenous, desiccates, and becomes eschar that requires 6 weeks to 4 months to heal.

Background Information

While many arachnids, which include spiders and scorpions, may cause reactions to bites, most necrotic skin wounds are caused by the genus *Loxosceles*.[4] Of the many species of *Loxosceles,* the brown recluse spider is the most prevalent and has the most potent venom.[5] This condition involves an inflammatory response to the venomous toxin. The resulting platelet aggregation and endothelial edema occlude the capillaries, causing ischemia and necrosis. Standard wound care is sufficient in mild cases; however, if symptoms of severe involvement occur, emergent medical care is indicated. In addition to the soft tissue and skin loss, disseminated intravascular coagulation is a complication that requires immediate medical attention.[6]

■ Arterial Insufficiency

Chief Clinical Characteristics

This presentation usually involves wounds that are located on the peripheral extremities (toes, fingers, dorsum of the forefoot or hand, interdigital spaces, or lateral malleolus where pressure areas are unable to heal) and appear as "punched-out" wounds with even, sharp demarcation of the edges. The wound is typically dry and necrotic with black sloughing periwound skin. The digits may progress from a dusky color (typical if the occlusion is an acute embolism or thrombosis) to a dark, dry, black mummified appearance if the anoxia is chronic (Fig. 40-3).

Background Information

This condition is caused by ischemia as a result of interruption of the blood flow in either the macrovascular (large, named arteries) or microvascular (arterioles and capillaries) circulation. The individual also may report claudication, defined as exercise-induced leg pain, or

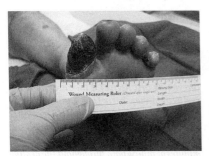

FIGURE 40-3 Arterial wound caused by arterial insufficiency.

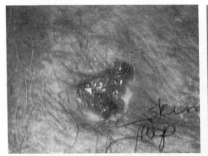

FIGURE 40-4 Nonhealing wound on the forearm was diagnosed by biopsy as a basal cell carcinoma.

resting or night pain, which occurs during the night when the blood pressure tends to be lower. Associated conditions include peripheral arterial disease, diabetes mellitus, hypertension, and acute arterial embolism after trauma or vascular/cardiovascular surgery. Screening tests that can be performed by the therapist include pulse examination, capillary refill, rubor of dependency, and ankle-brachial index. Individuals suspected of this condition should be referred to a vascular surgeon for a thorough vascular examination to determine the location and severity of the occlusion; debridement is contraindicated prior to revascularization unless infected necrotic tissue is present. Complications include infection (including osteomyelitis), failed or occluded bypass grafts with further tissue necrosis or failure to heal, and dehisced surgical incisions.

■ Basal Cell Carcinoma

Chief Clinical Characteristics

This condition is characterized by two or more of the following characteristics: persistent, nonhealing wound of more than 3 weeks' duration; red, irritated patch that may or may not cause itching and pain; pearly or translucent bump or nodule that can be any of a variety of colors (for example, red, pink, white, tan, brown, black); pink lesion with rolled edges, crusted center, and superficial blood vessels; and white, yellow, or waxy scar-like lesion with poorly defined edges (Fig. 40-4).

Background Information

This condition is the most common form of skin cancer, and it originates in the cells of the basal membrane between the dermis and

epidermis.[7] Caused almost exclusively by chronic exposure to sunlight, this condition usually occurs on the face, neck, shoulders, back, and scalp. Furthermore, people who tend to burn rather than tan, and have fair skin, light hair, or blue, gray, or green eyes are more susceptible to this condition.[8] Two specific types of this condition—ulcerating basal cell carcinoma and basalioma terebrans—can become open wounds with the risk of becoming infected. Ulcerating basal cell carcinoma is identified by hemorrhagic crusting and hard pearly edges; basalioma terebrans, by deep tissue necrosis with red granulated surfaces.[9] Individuals suspected of having this condition should be referred to a primary care physician or dermatologist for additional evaluation. Physical therapy intervention for wound management is not indicated.

■ Buerger Disease (Thromboangiitis Obliterans)

Chief Clinical Characteristics

This presentation includes pain (including resting pain), tenderness, red skin, cyanosis, thin shiny skin, and thickened malformed nails (Fig. 40-5). In addition, the hands and feet are usually cool and mildly edematous. Ulcerations are common on the toes, feet, or fingers.

Background Information

The pathology of Buerger disease is nonatherosclerotic inflammation of the small- and medium-sized peripheral arteries and veins in combination with thrombi and vasospasm of arterial segments of the feet and/or hands. This condition is most common in men who are heavy smokers. It can be differentiated from peripheral vascular disease by the presence of

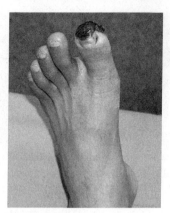

FIGURE 40-5 Gangrenous wound on the toe of a patient with Buerger disease. The wound has the appearance of an arterial wound; however, the patient is a young male in his 20s.

normal proximal pulses.[10] Individuals suspected of having this condition should be referred to a physician. Intervention includes cessation of smoking, vasodilators to prevent vasospasms, and exercise to increase blood flow to the affected extremity. Complications include gangrene, ulceration, and resulting loss of function and impairments if the disease exacerbates.

■ Bullous Pemphigoid

Chief Clinical Characteristics
This presentation involves pruritic, urticarial, papular lesions that become large flaccid bullae when serous or hemorrhagic fluid fills the space between the dermal/epidermal layers. Bullae occur most frequently on the axillae, abdomen, thighs, groin, lower legs, and flexor surfaces of the arm.

Background Information
This condition is an autoimmune disease that causes binding of immunoglobulin autoantibodies to the epidermal basement membrane, resulting in subepidermal blistering; it may be idiopathic, drug induced, or related to ultraviolet exposure.[11] Individuals suspected of having this condition should be referred to a physician for medical care, including anti-inflammatory medications, antibacterials, and immunosuppressants.[12] Local wound management is indicated after a definitive diagnosis is made and medical management has been initiated.

■ Burns

Chief Clinical Characteristics
This presentation can be characterized by different features depending on the severity of the burn. Burns are categorized as superficial (previously first degree) if they are characterized by immediate but not long-lasting pain, erythema, localized edema, and blisters after 24 hours. Partial-thickness burns (previously second degree) involve skin loss, blisters within minutes of injury, pain throughout the healing process, and scarring (Fig. 40-6A); they are classified as either superficial partial-thickness skin loss (involving the epidermis and upper dermis) or deep partial-thickness skin loss (involving the epidermis and deep dermis). Full-thickness burns (previously third degree) involve a waxy white appearance, surrounding partial-thickness involvement, diffuse edema, epithelialization from the hair follicles after 7 to 10 days, loss of epidermis and dermis, involvement of underlying subcutaneous tissue, muscle, or bone, dry leathery appearance, black or white eschar, visible thrombosed veins, and loss of pain and sensation (Fig. 40-6B).

Background Information
Burns may be caused by exposure to thermal heat, chemicals, electric current, or radiation. Activation of the emergency medical services at the time of onset is indicated if the burn is due to chemicals, if the burns are full thickness or extensive partial thickness, or if they are on the face, hands, or perineum. Subsequent management of these burns is best provided at a burn center.[13] Because superficial and partial-thickness burns usually heal in a timely sequence with standard wound care, individuals with nonhealing burn wounds being treated in an outpatient setting should be referred to an emergency department or primary care physician to determine the reason for poor healing. The most frequent complications of burn injuries are infection, hypovolemic shock, hypoproteinemia, and loss of range of motion due to adhesions.

■ Calciphylaxis

Chief Clinical Characteristics
This presentation commonly involves painful, indurated, purplish skin lesions that progress rapidly to skin necrosis and gangrene (Fig. 40-7). The lesions usually occur on the trunk and lower

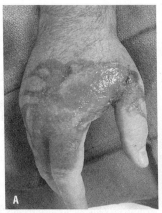 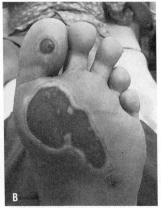

FIGURE 40-6 (A) Partial-thickness burns involve the epidermis and part of the dermis. (B) Full-thickness burns involve all of the dermis and extend into the subcutaneous tissue.

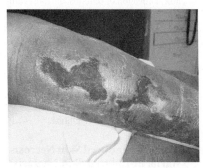

FIGURE 40-7 Wounds caused by calciphylaxis usually occur in individuals receiving long-term hemodialysis.

extremities and are frequently bilateral and symmetrical. Individuals with this condition will have palpable pulses distal to the lesions, unlike patients with peripheral arterial disease.

Background Information
The pathology involves microvascular calcification with superimposed intimal fibroblastic hyperplasia. This condition, often associated with hypercalcemia, hyperphosphatemia, and hyperparathyroidism, occurs in patients with end-stage renal disease. Individuals suspected of having this condition should be referred immediately to a renal specialist or endocrinologist. Interventions include parathyroidectomy, treatment to normalize calcium and phosphorus levels, and pain management.[14]

Usual wound management involves aggressive sharp or surgical debridement of all necrotic tissue, topical antibiotics, and moist wound dressings using sterile technique. Complications are secondary skin infection, sepsis, and death, with mortality rates as high as 60%. Individuals with lesions on the distal extremities and who receive early diagnosis and treatment have better survival rates.[15]

■ Cellulitis

Chief Clinical Characteristics
This presentation commonly includes erythema, edema, pain, drainage, warm to touch, induration, skin discoloration, and flaky or scaling skin. Periwound skin of a preexisting wound may be unresponsive to or exacerbated by standard wound care. In addition, there may or may not be systemic signs of infection, including fever, elevated white blood count, or erythematous streaking.

Background Information
This condition is caused by a bacterial infection of the dermis and subcutaneous tissue; most commonly the infective agents are *Staphylococcus aureus* and *Streptococcus*. Individuals with skin lesions, venous insufficiency, lymphedema, diabetes mellitus, and immunosuppression are at higher risk for developing cellulitis. Medical interventions include oral or intravenous antibiotics, depending on the severity and the cultured

bacteria, and prophylactic antibiotics for patients with frequent episodes.[16] Immediate referral to a primary care physician is advised. Standard wound management, including edema management with elevation and compression, is recommended for both acute and chronic conditions. Prophylactic compression hosiery is advised for patients with venous insufficiency or lymphedema. If not already present, cellulitis may cause open lesions in the affected area.

■ Chronic Venous Insufficiency

Chief Clinical Characteristics

This presentation typically involves wounds that occur proximal to the malleoli on the lower one-third of the leg (gaiter area), and are characterized by uneven edges, copious serous drainage, and shallow depth with a red granulated base (Fig. 40-8). In addition, the surrounding skin will have hyperpigmentation caused by the deposition of hemosiderin in the skin when red blood cells trapped in the interstitial tissue are lysed; lipodermatosclerosis, defined as the scaly or bark appearance of the skin; a dilated long saphenous vein; atrophie blanche, defined as ivory white atrophic plaques in the skin; unilateral or bilateral edema; dermatitis or eczema with or without exudate; or thickened skin that is warm to the touch due to the inflammatory process. The venous wound is usually less painful than the arterial one, and the pain is alleviated by elevation.

Background Information

This condition occurs when there is obstruction, reflux, or both that inhibits the return of fluid through the veins to the heart. Incompetent valves are usually the cause of fluid reflux. The buildup of chronic interstitial fluid in the distal leg causes venous hypertension and triggers cellular and chemical changes in the tissue, typical of a systemic inflammatory response, which result in skin breakdown. Comorbid pathologies that increase the risk for developing this condition include varicose veins, deep venous thrombosis, previous vein surgery, multiple pregnancies, obesity, congestive heart failure, coronary artery bypass surgery with saphenous vein harvesting, hip trauma, ankle immobility, and prolonged standing. Screening tests to determine the cause of venous insufficiency include approximation of central venous pressure, augmented venous flow, valve competency, percussion test, and ankle-brachial index. Medical intervention for antibiotic therapy is indicated if there are signs of clinical infection or cellulitis, the most common complication of venous ulcers. Standard wound care, compression therapy, and exercise to activate the venous pump can be initiated if there are no signs of infection. If infection is suspected, referral to a primary care physician or vascular surgeon is indicated. Individuals with this condition also should be advised to avoid prolonged sitting or standing. The most common complication is cellulitis.

■ Coumadin-Induced Skin Necrosis (Warfarin-Induced Skin Necrosis)

Chief Clinical Characteristics

This presentation is characterized by severely painful full-thickness skin necrosis on the trunk or lower extremities where significant subcutaneous fat is present. Initial complaints include paresthesias, sensations of pressure, and extreme pain. Progression of the disease, which is fairly rapid, is characterized by edema and erythema, followed by petechiae, hemorrhagic bullae, and finally necrotic eschar.[17]

Background Information

The exact etiology of this condition is unknown; however, toxic vasculitis, acquired coagulopathy, and hypersensitivity are suggested causes. Symptoms usually occur within the first 10 days after initiating Coumadin therapy, but may occur later. This condition is associated with either serious medical diagnoses or chronic illnesses such as deep venous thrombosis,

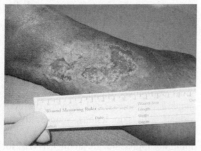

FIGURE 40-8 Chronic venous insufficiency wound. Note the dark hemosiderin staining in the skin around the wound.

stroke, and coronary artery disease. Immediate referral to a primary care physician is indicated to achieve reversal of the disease process and prevent progression of the necrosis. Aggressive wound care is indicated to prevent infection and facilitate closure.

■ Cryoglobulinemia

Chief Clinical Characteristics
This presentation typically involves palpable purpura, Raynaud's phenomenon, skin rash, supramalleolar ulcers, distal ischemia, gangrene, livedo reticularis (purplish mottling of the skin), and acrocyanosis. Ulcerations are severely painful. Systemic manifestations may include renal involvement, peripheral neuropathy (mixed or purely sensory), and central nervous system involvement.[18]

Background Information
Cryoglobulins are circulating immunoglobulins or immunoglobulin complexes that, under certain pathological conditions, precipitate from serum at cold temperatures (<37°C) causing thrombi within the microvascular system, which results in ulceration.[19] This condition is associated with autoimmune, chronic inflammatory, immunoproliferative, and infectious diseases. The most common types of this condition are associated with hepatitis C and chronic liver failure. Ulcerations occur as a result of either small vessel obstruction or inflammation of the vessel walls induced by the deposition of the cryoglobulins. Individuals suspected of having this condition should be referred to a physician or emergency department for treatment of the underlying disease in conjunction with receiving standard wound care and compression therapy. Most common complications include infection (including osteomyelitis), arthralgia, loss of joint range of motion, and gait impairments.

■ Cutaneous Lymphoma

Chief Clinical Characteristics
This presentation involves firm, erythematous, violaceous, and/or brown lesions that usually occur on the trunk, face, or extremities accompanied by pruritus.

Background Information
This condition refers to a whole host of malignancies affecting B and T cells. Broadly, this condition is divided among Hodgkin's and

non-Hodgkin's lymphomas. Hodgkin's lymphomas are a group of five separate conditions that arise from a specific B-cell abnormality, whereas non-Hodgkin's lymphomas number approximately 30. A combination of genetic and environmental factors has been implicated in the development of this condition. Environmental factors include exposure to solvents and organic chemicals, pesticides and herbicides, wood preservatives, and radiation. In addition, states of immunocompromise, including autoimmune conditions and acquired immunodeficiency virus, have been implicated in this condition's development. Interventions range from phototherapy, topical chemotherapy, local electron beam or x-ray therapy, and/or interferon alpha for local lesions to systemic chemotherapy, corticosteroids, antibiotics, and various combinations of treatment for extracutaneous involvement. Individuals suspected of having this condition should be referred to an oncologist; no physical therapy interventions are indicated.

■ Dermal Viral Infections

Chief Clinical Characteristics
This presentation commonly includes a rash or a cluster of inflamed vesicles that usually erupt and become crusty. Pain, paresthesias, burning, or itching may precede the appearance of skin lesions.

Background Information
This condition is caused by minute intracellular parasites that depend on the enzymes of the host cells for survival, causing the host to produce neutralizing antibodies that result in the viral activity.[20] The most common dermal viral infections are:

1. Herpes simplex virus, most commonly manifested as oral, perioral, or nasal cold sores or fever blisters
2. Herpes varicella or chickenpox manifested by diffuse macules, papules, and vesicles during childhood
3. Herpes zoster or shingles manifested by vesicular eruptions that follow a specific dermatome
4. Warts, a benign round rough gray lesion that can occur anywhere on the skin as a result of the human papillomavirus.

If detected early, individuals suspected of having this condition should be referred to the primary physician or dermatologist for medical management. No topical treatment is indicated for herpes simplex or herpes varicella.

■ Factitious Disorder

Chief Clinical Characteristics
This presentation is characterized by wounds with a consistent appearance of healing, including a good granulation base.

Background Information
The wounds are caused by self-inflicted injuries such as compulsive scratching; individuals with this condition usually have associated psychiatric disorders. Associated signs to observe are prematurely removed bandages, scratching of the periwound skin, and other suspicious behaviors such as self-mutilation. Both medical and psychiatric referrals are indicated and standard wound care should be provided in conjunction with medical and psychiatric intervention. The most common complication is infection.

■ Foreign Body Reaction

Chief Clinical Characteristics
This presentation typically involves drainage, edema, erythema, skin necrosis, and pain that increases with weight-bearing activities (when the foot or hand are involved).

Background Information
Common examples of foreign bodies include splinters, needles, or other sharp objects in the plantar foot; suture remnants or staples in or around surgical incisions; bone chips or debris in traumatic injuries; or metal slivers in high-risk occupations. A foreign body embedded in subcutaneous or deep wound tissue may be undetectable until an inflammatory response is initiated and superficial signs are noted. If the foreign body cannot be easily located and removed with sterile instruments, individuals with this condition should be immediately referred to an emergency room or primary care physician for surgical removal. Complications of foreign bodies are infection and further soft tissue damage with delayed or prolonged healing times.

■ Fungal Infection

Chief Clinical Characteristics
This presentation involves dry, scaly, erythematous, pruritic patches on the skin.

Background Information
This condition is caused by fungi, called tinea, that thrive on keratin in the stratum corneum, hair, and nails. These fungi are classified by the affected location. For example, tinea pedis is on the foot, tinea capitis on the scalp, tinea cruris on the groin, and tinea manus on the hand. Onychomycosis is a fungal infection of the nails, seen commonly in patients with diabetes mellitus or peripheral vascular disease. Fungal infections commonly occur in individuals with systemic administration of antibiotics, diabetes mellitus, pregnancy, immunosuppression, Cushing's disease, certain blood neoplasms, debilitated states, or infants under 6 months of age with decreased immune reactivity.[3] Individuals with tinea capitis, onychomycosis, or severe fungal infections should be referred to a primary care physician; no physical therapy treatment is indicated.

■ Kaposi's Sarcoma

Chief Clinical Characteristics
This presentation usually includes multifocal purplish brown macules that develop into plaques and nodules, usually on the lower extremities or upper body. The lesions can be painful and pruritic.

Background Information
This condition is classified as a vascular malignancy.[21] It most frequently occurs in individuals who are immune deficient (such as secondary to human immunodeficiency virus and acquired immunodeficiency syndrome) or in individuals who take immunosuppressive medications (such as following organ transplantation). Lesions are usually treated medically or surgically.[22] Local treatment of the sarcoma is not indicated; however, wounds may occur in tissue irradiated for treatment of this condition. These wounds may or may not respond to standard wound care and are often recalcitrant due to the inhibitory effects of the radiation on the cellular mitotic activity.

LYMPHEDEMAS

■ Primary Lymphedema (Milroy's Disease, Meige Disease)

Chief Clinical Characteristics
This presentation can involve a distal to proximal progression of unilateral or bilateral extremity edema in an individual with possible

hypoparathyroidism, yellow nails, ptosis, and webbing at the neck.[23] There may or may not be open chronic wounds with weeping of clear lymphatic drainage and surrounding low-grade inflammation. Most commonly, the lower extremities are involved; however, all four extremities may be affected. Initially the edema is soft and pitting, but over time the edema will progress to become hard, indurated, and fibrotic with little or no pitting. The limb can become quite large with abnormal deposition of fat cells, which leads to loss of joint spaces and a columnar-like appearance. Skin changes (such as papillomatosis and hyperkeratosis) and development of lymphocytes can occur.

Background Information

This condition develops as a result of a malformation of the lymph vessels or lymph nodes that occurred as the embryo was developing *in utero*. The limb is at risk for developing cellulitis, erysipelas, and fungal infections. The infections increase the lymphatic load and further increase the edema. In severe cases, elephantiasis may develop. Hypoplasia is the most common cause of this condition. Several ages of onset are possible including at or around the time of birth (congenital lymphedema; Milroy's disease); at puberty, when it is called lymphedema praecox (Meige disease); and during adulthood (lymphedema tarde). This condition remains a diagnosis of exclusion from all other causes of edema. Lymphoscintigraphy, bioelectrical impedance, magnetic resonance imaging, and computed tomography can assist in determining the appropriate diagnosis. The individual with lymphedema will require lifelong self-treatment, compression therapy, and physical therapy intervention if the individual experiences repeated infections or has difficulty in controlling acute exacerbations.[24]

■ Secondary Lymphedema

Chief Clinical Characteristics

This presentation typically includes heaviness, achiness, tightness, tingling and numbness of the involved extremity, and painless swelling of a limb that initially fluctuates with rest or elevation but with time does not dissipate. There may or may not be open chronic wounds

with weeping of clear lymphatic drainage and surrounding low-grade inflammation. If the hand or foot is involved, the individual will have difficulty making a fist or curling the toes. These concerns may worsen with activity, increased heat and humidity, or during changes in elevation. The distal aspect of the limb (foot or hand) may be affected initially; however, in some cases the proximal part of the limb may swell first. The edema usually spreads distally to proximally if left untreated. Initially, pitting edema is present and palpation of the limb is soft. Chronic edema causes fibrosis to develop within the subcutaneous tissues, which may lead to a loss of skin mobility and decrease range of motion. As fibrosis develops, the edema becomes harder to pit and palpation of the limb becomes hard and firm.

Background Information

As the edema becomes indurated, the skin can develop a "peau d'orange" appearance. Over time hyperkeratosis and papillomatosis may develop. The skin may begin to break down and infections such as cellulitis and erysipelas may occur. In lower extremity lymphedema, inability to pinch the skin at the base of the metatarsal heads (positive Stemmer sign) is present.[25] If the condition is untreated, repeated infections may occur and the combination of obstruction and infection can lead to elephantiasis. The limb becomes grossly enlarged; hyperkeratosis, papillomatosis, and the development of a lymphocele may occur and result in severe disfigurement and disability. This condition occurs as a result of abnormal accumulation of protein molecules and fluid in the interstitial spaces of the body from an acquired impairment of the lymphatic system that affects reabsorption of the interstitial fluid and transportation of lymph (lymphatic drainage). Cancer surgery and radiation therapy are considered the most frequent causes of secondary lymphedema. Diagnosis of lymphedema is primarily a diagnosis of exclusion. All other causes of edema are ruled out before this diagnosis is reached. Lymphoscintigraphy, bioelectrical impedance, magnetic resonance imaging, and computed tomography can be used to assist in the diagnosis. Treatment of this condition begins first with treating any infections that might be present. Treatment may include manual lymphatic drainage mobilization followed by compression bandages with short-stretch materials, joint range of motion, proper skin care, and exercise. Patient education regarding skin care, independent bandaging techniques, and lymph drainage massage techniques are critical in order for the individual to control the lymphedema. The individual with this condition will require lifelong self-treatment and physical therapy intervention if the individual experiences repeated infections or has difficulty in controlling acute exacerbations.

■ Marjolin's Ulcer

Chief Clinical Characteristics
This presentation involves history of repeated trauma, unusual location and no obvious etiology, and active and abnormal cellular proliferation that continues indefinitely if untreated. It is characterized by a vague irregular outline.

Background Information
Marjolin's ulcer wounds usually occur secondary to squamous cell carcinoma or basal cell carcinoma.[26] Any chronic wound of 2 to 3 months' duration that is nonresponsive to standard care for a patient without identifiable comorbidities should be suspected of being malignant. Characteristics to alert the clinician to the possibility of malignancy within a wound include the following: nonencapsulated with invasive fingers of abnormal tissue, systemically detrimental wounds, inflamed edges, a process that limits the growth into adjacent tissue and sometimes causes a bulbous or cauliflower appearance, or it may be vascular or necrotic, depending on the blood supply in the tissue connecting the neoplasm to the host.[27,28] Individuals with nonhealing wounds that are suspected of being malignant should be referred to a primary care physician. Debridement, modalities, and negative pressure therapy are contraindicated until malignancy has been excluded.

■ Martorell's Ulcer

Chief Clinical Characteristics
This presentation can be characterized by wounds on the anterolateral or posterior aspect of the lower third of the leg and cause moderate to severe pain, more than is usually expected

with ulcers in this location. The wound edges are irregular and satellite ulcers are often present.

Background Information
This condition is more prevalent in females and rarely seen in African Americans. These ulcers occur in individuals who have uncontrolled hypertension, particularly diastolic hypertension, and do not respond to standard wound care until the hypertension is adequately managed. In addition, there may be a history of minor trauma. Pathophysiology is characterized by classic hyalinization and thickening of the arteriole media (without atheroma and calcification) and a decrease in skin perfusion.[29] Referral to a medical specialist is imperative for management underlying hypertension in conjunction with nonsurgical wound management. Aggressive wound management (eg, surgical debridement and closure with flaps) may cause wound exacerbation.

■ Melanoma

Chief Clinical Characteristics
This presentation is defined by the ABCDE rule (Fig. 40-9):
Asymmetry,
Border irregularity,
Color variegation,
Diameter more than 5 mm, and
Evolution, indicating that the lesion changes in size, color, and shape.[30]

Background Information
This condition occurs when normal cutaneous melanocytes (the cells responsible for skin pigmentation) become malignant. The abnormal

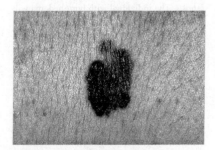

FIGURE 40-9 Melanoma has the following characteristics: **A**symmetry, **B**order irregularity, **C**olor variegation, **D**iameter more than 5 mm, and **E**volution, indicating that the lesion changes in size, color, and shape.

transformation of cells can occur in the basal layer of the epidermis where the melanocytes are located or in a preexisting nevus. Similar to other skin cancers, risk factors for melanoma include intense sun exposure with a history of childhood sunburns. Other risk factors include fair skin, family history of melanoma, multiple nevi, ethnicity (white vs. black), regular use of tanning beds before age 30, and immunosuppressive therapy.[17] Because this condition is highly curable by surgical excision during the early stages and is usually fatal if undetected until the later stages when the abnormal cells penetrate the dermis and potentially metastasize, early detection and expeditious treatment are necessary for optimal chances of survival. Therefore, individuals with any dermatological changes suspicious of this condition should be immediately referred to a primary care physician or dermatologist. Physical therapy intervention for wound management is not indicated.

■ Necrotizing Fasciitis

Chief Clinical Characteristics
This presentation involves a wound that is characterized by erythema and edema without demarcated borders; severe pain; tense shiny skin progressing to ischemic skin as tissue necrosis advances; clear or hemorrhagic blisters, progressing to bullae filled with gray odiferous fluid (dishwater pus); separation of necrotic tissue along fascial planes with myonecrosis; high fever and chills; decreased urinary output; change in mental status; weakness and fatigue; and dry black eschar in advanced disease.

Background Information
Necrotizing fasciitis usually occurs on the extremities, especially the lower ones. The abdominal wall, groin, perianal area, and postoperative wounds are also common sites of occurrence. If the affected area is the male genitalia, the disease is referred to as Fournier's gangrene.[31] This condition is a life-threatening infection of the fascia underlying the skin and subcutaneous tissue that is characterized by acute onset and rapid progression. It occurs when bacteria enter the skin (from, eg, minor trauma, skin disorders, needlesticks, or any existing ulceration) and elicit an intense inflammatory response. The bacteria spread throughout the underlying tissue, causing release of

bacterial toxins and enzymes and damage to the endothelial lining. This leads to fluid leakage into extravascular spaces, diminished blood flow, tissue hypoxemia, and necrosis, as well as production of oxygen-free radicals and nitrous oxide. Shock, immunosuppression, depression of myocardial function, and failure of multiple organs leading to death are consequences of the fascial inflammatory process. This condition is classified into two types. Type 1 is a polymicrobial infection caused by aerobic and anaerobic microbes (eg, *Clostridium* and *Bacteroides* species). Type 2 necrotizing fasciitis is caused by group A *Streptococcus*, with or without *Staphylococcus*.[20] Individuals with diabetes mellitus, immunosuppression (eg, related to acquired immunodeficiency syndrome, malignancy, and chronic corticosteroid use), perirectal abscess, obesity, malnutrition, hypertension, or smoking history are predisposed to developing this condition.[32,33] Survival depends on immediate diagnosis and treatment, consisting of widespectrum intravenous antibiotics and thorough, immediate debridement of all infected tissue. Any individual suspected of having this condition should be referred immediately to an emergency department or transported by emergency medical services if needed.[34] Standard wound care is indicated only after surgical debridement and medical management have been initiated.

■ Neuropathic Wounds

Chief Clinical Characteristics
This presentation may involve blisters, calluses, punctures, skin tears, or cracks, usually on the plantar surface of the foot, over the first and fifth metatarsal heads, on the distal digits, or in the interdigital spaces (Fig. 40-10).

Background Information
This condition occurs as a result of abnormal mechanical forces or minor trauma to the insensate foot. Bony abnormalities, diminished or absent protective sensation, decreased tissue oxygen saturation, and anhidrosis caused by autonomic neuropathy in combination with poorly fitting shoes increase the risk of calluses and blisters that become nonhealing wounds. The most frequently associated medical comorbidity is type 2 diabetes mellitus; however, neuropathic wounds also occur in individuals with Hansen's disease, spinal cord injury, spina

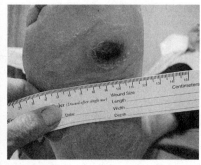

FIGURE 40-10 Neuropathic wound. Wound caused by mechanical trauma on a foot with sensory neuropathy, most commonly seen in patients with diabetes.

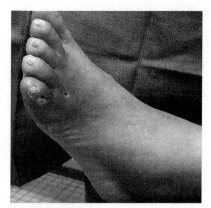

FIGURE 40-11 Any wound that can be probed to bone is suspicious of having osteomyelitis.

bifida, and other neuropathic conditions that may be associated with vascular pathology. This condition is best treated by redistribution of the foot pressures to eliminate the mechanical forces causing the wound and with standard wound care. The most common complication is infection, at which time the patient should be referred to a primary care physician.

■ Osteomyelitis

Chief Clinical Characteristics

This presentation includes pain, edema, erythema, and drainage; limited range of motion; pain or tenderness during palpation or weight bearing; or draining sinus under superficial granulation tissue (Fig. 40-11). Other symptoms and signs include fever, fatigue and malaise, and reluctance to use the involved extremity.

Background Information

This condition begins as an inflammatory response in the bone secondary to the presence of pyogenic organisms, such as bacteria, fungi, or viruses. Subsequently, edema and leukocytic activity result in abscess formation; small terminal vessels in the bones thrombose; exudates seal the canaliculi and extend into the metaphysis, marrow cavity, and cortex; and infection weakens the cortex, predisposing the bone to fracture.[6] When this condition is associated with chronic wounds, it usually occurs in conjunction with neuropathic ulcers where the soft tissue between the skin and bone is less dense. This condition should be suspected in any chronic wound that can be probed to the bone.[33] The diagnosis is confirmed by radiographs, magnetic resonance imaging, radionuclide bone scan, or computed tomography. Therefore, immediate referral to the primary care physician or orthopedist is advised. Local wound management, including irrigation, debridement, and absorbent antimicrobial dressings, is indicated for immediate care. The use of occlusive dressings is not recommended while the infection is active. Offloading of the involved area with accommodative dressings, adaptive shoes, and assistive devices will facilitate wound closure.

■ Pemphigus

Chief Clinical Characteristics

This presentation typically includes intraepidermal bullae of the skin and mucous membranes, which present as flaccid bullae and crusted erosions of the skin and mucosal membranes, accompanied by skin or oral pain and pruritus. The blisters are flaccid and can be transient (differentiating this condition from bullous pemphigoid) and result in diffuse crusts or scabs.

Background Information

This condition refers to a group of autoimmune diseases. The blisters that characterize this condition are caused by binding of the antibodies to adhesion proteins in the epidermis and/or mucosal membranes.[35] Two prototypical pemphigus diseases are pemphigus vulgaris and pemphigus foliaceus, both of which are chronic disorders requiring long-term treatment. Individuals suspected of having this condition should be referred to a dermatologist for medical management. The primary complication is infection of the open wounds.

■ Pressure Ulcers

Chief Clinical Characteristics

This presentation varies based on the extent of tissue involvement, including the following six stages:

- *Stage I: Intact skin with nonblanchable redness of a localized area usually over a bony prominence. Darkly pigmented skin may not have visible blanching; its color may differ from the surrounding area. Further description: The area may be painful, firm, soft, warmer or cooler as compared to adjacent tissue. Stage I may be difficult to detect in individuals with dark skin tones. May indicate "at-risk" persons (Fig. 40-12A).*

- *Stage II: Partial-thickness loss of dermis presenting as a shiny or dry shallow open ulcer with a red-pink wound bed, without slough or bruising. Also may present as an intact or open/ruptured serum-filled blister. This stage should not be used to describe skin tears, tape burns, perineal dermatitis, maceration, or excoriation (Fig. 40-12B).*

- *Stage III: Full-thickness tissue loss. Subcutaneous fat may be visible but bone, tendon, or muscle is not exposed. Slough may include undermining and tunneling. Further description: The depth of a Stage III pressure ulcer varies by anatomical location and subcutaneous tissue. Stage III ulcers can be shallow. In contrast, areas of significant adiposity can develop extremely deep Stage III pressure ulcers. Bone/tendon is not visible or directly palpable (Fig. 40-12C).*

- *Stage IV: Full-thickness loss with exposed bone, tendon, or muscle. Slough or eschar may be present on some parts of the wound bed. Often includes undermining and tunneling. Further description: The depth of Stage IV pressure ulcers varies by anatomical location. The bridge of the nose, ear, occiput, and malleolus do not have subcutaneous tissue and these ulcers can be shallow. Stage IV ulcers can extend into muscle and/or supporting structures (eg, fascia, tendon, or joint capsule), making osteomyelitis possible. Exposed bone/tendon is visible or directly palpable (Fig. 40-12D).*

- *Stage V: Purple or maroon localized area of discolored intact skin or blood-filled blister due to damage of underlying soft tissue from pressure and/or shear. The area may be preceded by tissue that is painful, firm, mushy, boggy, warmer or cooler as compared to adjacent tissue. Further description: Deep tissue injury may be difficult to detect in individuals with dark skin tones. Evolution may include a thin blister over a dark wound bed. The wound may further evolve and become covered by thin eschar. Evolution may be rapid, exposing additional layers of tissue even with optimal treatment (Fig. 40-12E).*

- *Stage VI: Full-thickness tissue loss in which the base of the ulcer is covered by slough (yellow, tan, gray, green, or brown) and/or eschar (tan, brown, or black) in the wound bed. Further description: Until enough slough and/or eschar is removed to expose the base of the wound, the true depth and, therefore, stage cannot be determined. Stable (dry, adherent, intact without erythema or fluctuance) eschar on the heels serves as "the body's natural (biological) cover" and should not be removed (Fig. 40-12F).[36]*

Background Information

Lesions occur over bony prominences where there is minimal soft tissue to absorb the external forces that are applied to the skin, such as the sacrum, ischial tuberosities, greater trochanters, heels, malleoli, medial femoral condyles, elbows, scapular spine, and vertebrae. This condition results primarily from four causative factors: shear forces on subcutaneous tissue, friction of the skin against a support surface, external pressure that is greater than the capillary closing pressure, and excessive moisture resulting in skin maceration. Because subcutaneous tissue damage can occur before any external skin necrosis is visible, this condition is usually more extensive than initially visible with skin inspection. Risk factors include immobility, joint contractures, decreased or absent sensation, age, poor nutrition, incontinence, and psychosocial factors (eg, altered mental status, depression, stress, polypharmacy, drug and alcohol abuse, and poor social support systems). Standard care begins with offloading or reducing the pressure to the affected area using specialty

FAILURE OF WOUNDS TO HEAL

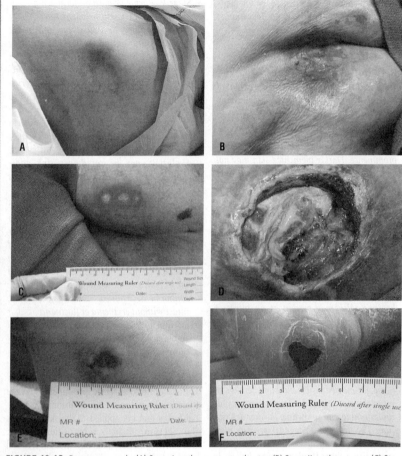

FIGURE 40-12 Pressure wounds: (A) Stage I on the greater trochanter; (B) Stage II on the sacrum; (C) Stage III on the gluteal region; the dark purple area on the sacrum is a suspected deep tissue injury; (D) Stage IV on the greater trochanter extends to the fascia and muscle; (E) suspected deep tissue injury on the lateral malleolus; (F) wound on the heel that is considered an unstageable wound because the wound bed cannot be visualized.

support surfaces and periodic repositioning, along with debridement of necrotic tissue and moist wound dressings. If this condition is extensive, medical referral is indicated. Complications include soft tissue infection, osteomyelitis, and impaired mobility.

■ Pyoderma Gangrenosum

Chief Clinical Characteristics

This presentation includes sterile pustules and rapidly progresses to painful, purplish, suppurative, undermined ulcers. Smaller pustules will often coalesce to become a larger ulceration. The initial wounds may develop spontaneously or in response to minor trauma or to an operative procedure (pathergy) (Fig. 40-13).[37]

Background Information

Usually occurring on the trunk or lower extremities, this condition occurs in conjunction with several systemic diseases, including irritable bowel syndrome, rheumatoid arthritis, hematologic diseases, or malignancies.[38] The exact pathogenesis is unknown; therefore,

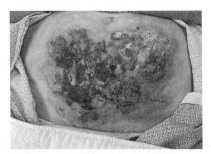

FIGURE 40-13 Pyoderma gangrenosum usually occurs in immunocompromised patients.

this condition is a diagnosis of exclusion. Biopsy results may include an interstitial neutrophilic infiltrate expanding into the subcutaneous tissue.[39] Immediate medical referral is advised for treatment of any underlying systemic disease, immunosuppressive therapy, anti-inflammatory medications such as corticosteroids, cytotoxic therapy, and pain management. Unlike the majority of wounds with necrotic tissue, debridement is contraindicated because it causes further pathergy.[40] Local wound management includes topical antibiotic creams, topical steroids, and moisture-retentive dressings. Use of sterile technique with dressing changes is recommended to prevent infection, the most common complication.

■ Raynaud's Disease

Chief Clinical Characteristics

This presentation may involve pallor, numbness, and cold sensations of the fingers and, less commonly, of the toes. As this condition progresses, symptoms may include rubor, throbbing, and paresthesias.

Background Information

The cause of this condition is vasospasm of the small arteries and arterioles, causing hypoxia of the digits, beginning with the tips and advancing to the proximal phalanges. Attacks are triggered by cold exposure or by emotional stress. This condition is more prevalent in women, and it also can be a manifestation of collagen vascular diseases (eg, scleroderma and systemic lupus erythematosus), pulmonary hypertension, thoracic outlet syndrome, myxedema trauma, serum sickness, or long-term exposure to cold or vibrating machinery during work.[41] There is no indication for local wound care.

Referral to a physician is indicated if there are complications, including ulceration and gangrene, in which case amputation may be necessary.

■ Sickle Cell Disease

Chief Clinical Characteristics

This presentation typically includes lower extremity wounds on the malleolar sites, hemosiderosis, prominent superficial veins, and lower extremity edema. This condition may cause complications in multiple organ systems, including stroke, skin ulcers, and blindness.

Background Information

This condition involves abnormal red blood cell morphology that causes them to become rigid and sticky, disrupting blood flow to bones, and resulting in painful bone infarcts. Wounds are most common in individuals who are homozygous for this condition. The pathophysiology of wounds includes venous hypertension and vaso-occlusion that leads to skin infarct.[38] This condition may be complicated by lower oxygen saturation levels due to fewer red blood cells being oxygenated. There is no cure for this condition; treatment is palliative and preventive. Local wound care includes debridement, moist wound dressings, and compression therapy.[42] Individuals with this condition who have nonhealing wounds are advised to see a hematologist for treatment including blood transfusions and chelation of high iron levels as a result of the transfusions.[43]

■ Squamous Cell Carcinoma

Chief Clinical Characteristics

This presentation commonly involves gray to yellow-brown hyperkeratosis and may progress to crusty wart-like lesions that sometimes bleed, irregular red scaly patches, persistent open wounds that crust or bleed, or raised lesions with indented centers.[44] This condition is a malignant proliferation of the keratinocytes in the epidermis (Fig. 40-14).[45]

Background Information

Squamous cell carcinoma most commonly occurs in areas that are exposed to the sun or in areas where the skin has been previously injured by burns, trauma, radiation, diabetes, chronic osteomyelitis, or chronic venous insufficiency. Individuals suspected of having this condition should be referred to a primary care physician or

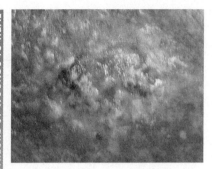

FIGURE 40-14 Squamous cell carcinoma.

dermatologist. Physical therapy intervention for wound management is not indicated.

■ Traumatic Injury

Chief Clinical Characteristics

This presentation may take on many different appearances depending on the mechanism of injury and will follow a normal healing sequence unless untreated comorbidities exist (eg, diabetes, immunosuppressive conditions, protein energy malnutrition, or infection). An embolic or thrombotic arterial occlusion after a traumatic event will cause absent pulses, pain, paresthesias, loss of skin color, and possible paralysis distal to the occlusion.

Background Information

The occlusion may result from an embolus that breaks away from a proximal hematoma and lodges in a peripheral artery or from a thrombus that forms at the site of injury, leading to peripheral tissue ischemia that must be treated emergently to avoid tissue necrosis and possible loss of limb. Immediate referral to an emergency department is indicated if hemostasis is not achieved within 30 minutes, or if the individual demonstrates symptoms and signs of acute thrombosis. Referral to a primary care physician is also recommended if a post-traumatic wound fails to heal in a timely sequence. Physical therapy intervention is indicated after normal circulation has been restored.

■ Vasculitis

Chief Clinical Characteristics

This presentation typically includes palpable purpura, petechiae, urticaria, painful or tender nodules, patches of skin necrosis (cutaneous necrotizing vasculitis), or small black necrotic dots on the fingers and toes (Fig. 40-15).[46]

Background Information

This condition is caused by an inflammation of blood vessels, usually as a result of an immune reaction in the vessel wall. This condition may be cutaneous, involving the post-capillary venules, or systemic, involving any of the organs. Symptoms vary according to the type of tissue involved and the extent of the tissue involvement. Wounds related to this condition frequently occur in conjunction with other autoimmune connective tissue diseases (eg, systemic lupus erythematosus, scleroderma, rheumatoid arthritis, Wegener's granulomatosis, temporal arteritis, and cryoglobulinemia) or with some malignancies (eg, leukemia or lymphoma).[43] This condition also can occur without any obvious associated infection or other illness. Referral to a medical specialist is recommended for diagnosis and interventions that may include immunosuppressants, systemic corticosteroids, cytotoxic drugs if corticosteroids are ineffective, and identification and treatment of any underlying infection.[47] Wound management includes standard care and compression therapy if the wounds are on the lower extremity.

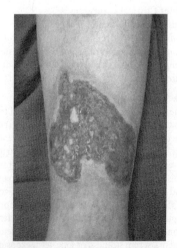

FIGURE 40-15 Vasculitis on the lower extremity of a patient with polyarteritis nodosa.

References

1. Lazarus GS, Cooper DM, Knighton DR, et al. Definitions and guidelines for assessment of wounds and evaluation of healing. *Arch Dermatol.* Apr 1994; 130(4):489–493.
2. Enoch S, Harding K. Wound bed preparation: the science behind the removal of barriers to healing. *Wounds.* 2003;15(7):213–229.
3. Huether SE, Kravitz M. Structure, function, and disorders of the integument. In: Huether SE, McCance KL, eds. *Understanding Pathophysiology.* St. Louis, MO: Mosby; 1996:1084–1121.
4. Hagood CO, Wilson JR. Necrotic wounds produced by spider bites. In: Sheffield PJ, Smith APS, Fife CE, eds. *Wound Care Practice.* Flagstaff, AZ: Best Publishing; 2004:389–403.
5. Wilson JR, Hagood CO Jr, Prather ID. Brown recluse spider bites: a complex problem wound. A brief review and case study. *Ostomy Wound Manage.* Mar 2005; 51(3):59–66.
6. Mourad LA, McCance KL. Alterations of musculoskeletal function. In: Huether SE, McCance KL, eds. *Understanding Pathophysiology.* St. Louis, MO: Mosby; 1996:1036–1070.
7. Gordon RM. Skin cancer: more than skin deep. *Adv Skin Wound Care.* Dec 2009;22(12):574–580; quiz 581–582.
8. Foundation TSC. About basal cell carcinoma. http://www.skincancer.org/basal/index.php. Accessed April 7, 2003.
9. Garcia EJ. Infections of the leg that mimic malignancy. *Infect Med.* 1998;15(8):557–567.
10. Hanley EJ. Buerger disease (thromboangiitis obliterans). http://www.medscape.com. Accessed August 27, 2005.
11. Lin MD, Phillips TJ. Bullous pemphigoid. *Wounds.* 2002;14(5):36–41.
12. Chan L. Bullous pemphigoid. http://emedicine.medscape.com/article/1062391-overview, 2002. Accessed October 12, 2008.
13. Barillo DJ, Paulsen SM. Management of burns to the hand. *Wounds.* 2003;15(1):4–9.
14. Polizzotto MN, Bryan T, Ashby MA, Martin P. Symptomatic management of calciphylaxis: a case series and review of the literature. *J Pain Symptom Manage.* Aug 2006;32(2):186–190.
15. Burkhart CG, Mian A. Calciphylaxis: a case report and review of literature. *Wounds.* 1999;11(2):58–61.
16. Hirschmann JV. Fungal, bacterial, and viral infections of the skin. http://www.medscape.com Accessed March 9, 2003.
17. Beitz JM. Coumadin-induced skin necrosis. *Wounds.* 2002;14(6):217–220.
18. Lin MD, Phillips TJ. Type II cryoglobulinemia. *Wounds.* 2002;14(5):85–91.
19. Shah JB. Approach to commonly misdiagnosed wound and unusual leg ulcers. In: Sheffield PJ, Smith APS, Fife CE, eds. *Wound Care Pract.* Flagstaff, AZ: Best Publishing; 2004:405–422.
20. Trent JT, Kirsner RS. Necrotizing fasciitis. *Wounds.* 2002;14(8):282–292.
21. Sakakibara S, Tosato G. Regulation of angiogenesis in malignancies associated with Epstein-Barr virus and Kaposi's sarcoma-associated herpes virus. *Future Microbiol.* Sep 2009;4:903–917.
22. Lin P, Phillips TJ. Kaposi's sarcoma. *Wounds.* 2001; 13(6):237–240.
23. Levinson KL, Feingold E, Ferrell RE, Glover TW, Traboulsi EI, Finegold DN. Age of onset in hereditary lymphedema. *J Pediatr.* Jun 2003;142(6):704–708.
24. Rockson SG. Diagnosis and management of lymphatic vascular disease. *J Am Coll Cardiol.* Sep 2 2008;52(10):799–806.
25. Cheville AL. Current and future trends in lymphedema management: implications for women's health. *Phys Med Rehabil Clin N Am.* Aug 2007; 18(3):539–553, x.
26. Snyder RJ, Stillman RM, Weiss SD. Epidermoid cancers that masquerade as venous ulcer disease. *Ostomy Wound Manage.* Apr 2003;49(4):63–64, 65–66.
27. Fallis BD. Neoplasia. In: Robbins SL, ed. *Textbook of Pathology.* 2nd ed. Philadelphia, PA: W. B. Saunders; 1964:103–133.
28. Trent JT, Kirsner RS. Herpesvirus infections and herpetic wounds. *Adv Skin Wound Care.* Sep–Oct 2003;16(5):236–243.
29. Davison S, Lee E, Newton ED. Martorell's ulcer revisited. *Wounds.* 2003;15(6):208–212.
30. Friedman RJ, Rigel DS, Kopf AW. Early detection of malignant melanoma: the role of physician examination and self-examination of the skin. *CA Cancer J Clin.* May–Jun 1985;35(3):130–151.
31. Ribo JC, Boucher B, Merwath D, Olive J. Case report: implications for a patient diagnosed with Fournier's gangrene. *Wounds.* 2002;14(9):340–347.
32. Norton KS, Johnson LW, Perry T, Perry KH, Sehon JK, Zibari GB. Management of Fournier's gangrene: an eleven year retrospective analysis of early recognition, diagnosis, and treatment. *Am Surg.* Aug 2002; 68(8):709–713.
33. Armstong DG, Boulton AJM, Jospeh WS, Lipsky BL. Diagnosing and treating osteomyelitis. *Podiatry Today.* 2003:8–12.
34. Yuen JC, Feng Z. Salvage of limb and function in necrotizing fasciitis of the hand: role of hyperbaric oxygen treatment and free muscle flap coverage. *South Med J.* Feb 2002;95(2):255–257.
35. Woldegiorgis S, Swerlick RA. Pemphigus in the southeastern United States. *South Med J.* Jul 2001;94(7):694–698.
36. National Pressure Ulcer Advisory Panel. Pressure ulcer stages revised by NPUAP. http://www.npuap.org/pr2.htm. Accessed 15 December, 2009.
37. Walusimbi M, Mannari RJ, Payne WG, Ochs D, Blue ML, Robson MC. Pyoderma gangrenosum: case report of novel treatment with topical steroid and silver sulfadiazine. *Wounds.* 2002;14(6):227–229.
38. Wollina U. Clinical management of pyoderma gangrenosum. *Am J Clin Dermatol.* 2002;3(3):149–158.
39. Chakrabaarty A, Phillips TJ. Pyoderma gangrenosum. *Wounds.* 2002;14(8):302–305.
40. Paparone PP, Paparone PW, Paparone P. Post-traumatic pyoderma gangrenosum. *Wounds.* 2009;21(4):89–94.
41. National Institutes of Health. Questions and answers about Reynaud's phenomenon. http://www.niams.nih.gov. Accessed August 28, 2005.
42. Hamm RL, Rodrigues J, Weitz IC. Pathophysiology and multidisciplinary management of leg wounds in sickle cell disease: a case discussion and literature review. *Wounds.* 2006;18(10):277–285.

43. Hahn BH. Lupus and vasculitis. http://www.lupus.org. Accessed August 24, 2005.
44. Foundation TSC. About squamous cell carcinoma. http://www.skincancer.org/squamous/index.php. Accessed April 7, 2003.
45. Dasgeb B, Ghosn S, Phillips T. Well differentiated squamous cell carcinoma with verrucous clinical presentation. *Wounds*. 2005;17(3):67–72.

46. Lee J, Phillips TJ. Livedoid vasculitis. *Wounds*. 2001;13(4):132–134.
47. de Araujo TS, Kirsner RS. Vasculitis. *Wounds*. 2001;13(3):99–112.

CHAPTER 41

Case Demonstration: Fatigue

■ *Kim Levenhagen, PT, DPT, WCC* ■ *Chris A. Sebelski, PT, DPT, OCS, CSCS*

NOTE: This case demonstration was developed using the diagnostic process described in Chapter 4 and demonstrated in Chapter 5. The reader is encouraged to use this diagnostic process in order to ensure thorough clinical reasoning. If additional elaboration is required on the information presented in this chapter, please consult Chapters 4 and 5.

THE DIAGNOSTIC PROCESS

Step 1 Identify the patient's chief concern.

Step 2 Identify *barriers to communication*.

Step 3 Identify *special concerns*.

Step 4 Create a symptom timeline and sketch the anatomy (if needed).

Step 5 Create a diagnostic hypothesis list considering all possible forms of *remote* and *local* pathology that could cause the patient's chief concern.

Step 6 Sort the diagnostic hypothesis list by epidemiology and specific case characteristics.

Step 7 Ask specific questions to rule specific conditions or pathological categories less likely.

Step 8 Re-sort the diagnostic hypothesis list based on the patient's responses to specific questioning.

Step 9 Perform tests to differentiate among the remaining diagnostic hypotheses.

Step 10 Re-sort the diagnostic hypothesis list based on the patient's responses to specific tests.

Step 11 Decide on a diagnostic impression.

Step 12 Determine the appropriate patient disposition.

Case Description

Alex is a frail 42-year-old male presenting with concerns of fatigue and generalized weakness. He attributes his symptoms to being inactive and losing 20 lbs recently during his illness. He has noted excessive sweating especially at night. Past medical history includes human immunodeficiency virus (HIV; 8 years) and hospitalization for Pneumocystis carinii pneumonia 1 month ago. Prior to this recent bout of pneumonia, Alex was active as a self-employed business owner and participated in triathlons. He has been off work for the past month following a hospitalization for pneumonia. Since that episode of care, he has been too tired and short of breath to ride his bike or run. His goals are to return to work and eventually return to triathlon training. The employees at his business and his family have not been informed of his diagnosis of HIV. His most recent blood testing indicates CD4+ T lymphocytes 450 cells/mm^3. Alex's medication includes the highly active antiviral reactive therapy (HAART) regimen (for the past 8 months), which includes tenofovir, emtricitabine, ritonavir, and a daily multivitamin.

Teaching comments: The U.S. Department of Health and Human Services Panel on Clinical Practices for Treatment of HIV Infection sets guidelines for the treatment of HIV including initialization of HAART regimen. In the question of "when to start" this therapy, the panel has been unable to reach a two-thirds consensus for their recommendations. The 2009 guidelines stated: "Based on cumulative observational cohort data demonstrating benefits of antiretroviral therapy in reducing [acquired immune deficiency syndrome] AIDS- and non-AIDS-associated morbidity and mortality, the Panel now recommends antiretroviral therapy for patients with CD4 count between 350 and 500 cells/mm^3. This recommendation is made with 50% of the Panel in agreement."[1]

STEP #1: Identify the patient's chief concern.

- Fatigue/generalized weakness. *Note:* This symptom is his primary concern; however, the diagnostic category list below includes pathologies that involve the symptoms of shortness of breath due to his comment regarding his perceived limitation in daily activities.

STEP #2: Identify *barriers to communication*.

- Inability to collect information due to the patient's eagerness to return to work. Alex may be less likely to share information that will lead to a diagnostic impression with a prognosis that is inconsistent with his goals.
- Social stigma related to the diagnosis of HIV. The therapist may require additional sensitivity to Alex's perception of how his condition is received socially, particularly because of the documented nondisclosure to family and coworkers regarding the underlying diagnosis of HIV. In addition, therapists should examine their own perceptions and beliefs about HIV in order to minimize the potential impact on the ability of the therapist to fully engage in the diagnostic process.
- Medication adherence. Adherence to the HAART medications is necessary for long-term viral suppression, yet it is known that adherence to HAART medications over a long period of time is often compromised. Financial burden, psychosocial stigma, side effects, and the recent change in health status indicate that reconfirmation of adherence to the medication regimen is necessary at this time. With inconsistent adherence, there is an increased threat of development of a strain of the virus that is resistant to known agents. Due to the importance of compliance with the regimen of medications, it is strongly recommended that this topic be explored. Provision of support via open dialogue can make a small but significant effect on adherence. Questions regarding the medication, its side effects, and the prescription dosage should be referred to Alex's pharmacist.[2]

- Gender issues with communication. Therapists of a different gender than Alex may feel less comfortable asking sensitive questions. Conversely, Alex also may feel less comfortable divulging sensitive information to a therapist of another gender.

> **Teaching comments:** Alex is a "nondiscloser." He has not informed his family, friends, and/or colleagues of his diagnosis. There is conflicting evidence in the literature regarding the overall effect of disclosing HIV status to select people and the reasoning behind disclosing versus nondisclosing. In a meta-analysis of the literature, a small but statistical relationship was shown between social support and disclosing. Additionally, the authors of the meta-analysis postulated that the act of nondisclosure was driven by the stigma surrounding the disease.[3]

STEP #3: Identify *special concerns*.

- Recent profound weight loss. The weight loss, in combination with fatigue and reports of excessive sweating, suggests an underlying systemic disease process that must be investigated.
- Presence of HIV. The presence of HIV is a caution secondary to the complicated medical course and medication regimen.

STEP #4: Create a symptom timeline and sketch the anatomy (if needed).

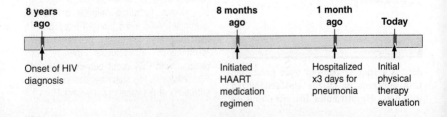

8 years ago	8 months ago	1 month ago	Today
Onset of HIV diagnosis	Initiated HAART medication regimen	Hospitalized x3 days for pneumonia	Initial physical therapy evaluation

STEP #5: Create a diagnostic hypothesis list considering all possible forms of *remote* and *local* pathology that could cause the patient's chief concern.

T   Trauma

Exercise
Pneumothorax

I   Inflammation

Aseptic
Cardiomyopathy

Chronic inflammatory demyelinating polyneuropathy

Inflammatory myopathies:
- Dermatomyositis

- Inclusion body myositis

- Multifocal motor neuropathy
- Polymyositis

Pleural effusion
Pleurisy
Systemic lupus erythematosus

Septic
Cardiomyopathy
Idiopathic pulmonary fibrosis
Pleurisy
Pleural effusion
Pneumonia

M   Metabolic

Diabetes mellitus polyneuropathy
Diabetic myopathy
Medication toxicity/toxic myopathy
Myasthenia gravis

Va   Vascular

Anemia
Arteriovenous malformation within the spine

Atherosclerosis
Cardiomyopathy
Transient ischemic attack/stroke

STEP #6: Sort the diagnostic hypothesis list by epidemiology and specific case characteristics.

T   Trauma

Exercise
~~Pneumothorax~~ (unassociated with night sweats and extreme weight loss)

I   Inflammation

Aseptic
~~Cardiomyopathy~~ (unassociated with night sweats and extreme weight loss)
~~Chronic inflammatory demyelinating polyneuropathy~~ (unassociated with night sweats and extreme weight loss)
~~Inflammatory myopathies:~~
- ~~Dermatomyositis~~ (unassociated with night sweats and extreme weight loss)
- ~~Inclusion body myositis~~ (age; unassociated with night sweats and extreme weight loss)
- ~~Multifocal motor neuropathy~~ (time course)
- ~~Polymyositis~~ (unassociated with night sweats and extreme weight loss)

Pleural effusion
Pleurisy
~~Systemic lupus erythematosus~~ (gender, presentation)

Septic
Cardiomyopathy
Idiopathic pulmonary fibrosis
Pleurisy
Pleural effusion
Pneumonia

M   Metabolic

Diabetes mellitus polyneuropathy
Diabetic myopathy
Medication toxicity/toxic myopathy
~~Myasthenia gravis~~ (unassociated with night sweats and extreme weight loss)

Va   Vascular

Anemia
~~Arteriovenous malformation within the spine~~ (unassociated with night sweats and extreme weight loss)
Atherosclerosis
Cardiomyopathy
~~Transient ischemic attack/stroke~~ (time course)

De Degenerative

Deconditioning

Tu Tumor

Malignant Primary, such as:
- AIDS- and non-AIDS-related malignancy
- Colon
- Hematologic
- Kidney
- Lung
- Pancreas
- Prostate
- Spinal tumor

Teaching comments: This listing of malignant primary tumors is due to the multiple comments of the patient including recent weight loss, night sweats, and generalized weakness or fatigue. Complicating the picture is that these same symptoms are common in the presentation of HIV secondary to both the disease course and the medications used to treat the disease course.

Malignant Metastatic, such as:
- AIDS- and non-AIDS-related malignancy
- Colon metastases
- Kidney metastases
- Pancreas metastases
- Prostate metastases
- Spinal metastases

De Degenerative

Deconditioning

Tu Tumor

Malignant Primary, such as:
- AIDS- and non-AIDS-related malignancy
- Colon
- Hematologic
- Kidney
- Lung
- Pancreas
- Prostate
- Spinal tumor

Malignant Metastatic, such as:
- AIDS- and non-AIDS-related malignancy
- Colon metastases
- Kidney metastases
- Pancreas metastases
- Prostate metastases
- Spinal metastases

Teaching comments: Per the Panel on Clinical Practices for Treatment of HIV Infection, "The incidence of non-AIDS malignancy in HIV-infected subjects is higher than in matched HIV-uninfected controls. Large cohort studies of mostly patients receiving antiretroviral treatment have reported a consistent link between low CD4 counts (<350–500 cells/mm^3) and the risk of AIDS- and/or non-AIDS-defining malignancy. The ANRS C04 demonstrated a statistically significant relative risk of all cancers evaluated (except for anal carcinoma) in patients with CD4 counts <500 cells/mm^3 compared with patients with current CD4 counts >500 cells/mm^3 and a protective effect of antiretroviral therapy for HIV-associated malignancies."[1]

Benign:
Not applicable

Co Congenital

Not applicable

Ne Neurogenic/Psychogenic

Depression
Neurological compromise due to acquired
  immunodeficiency virus

Peripheral /myopathy due to HIV

Benign:
Not applicable

Co Congenital

Not applicable

Ne Neurogenic/Psychogenic

Depression
~~Neurological compromise due to
acquired immunodeficiency virus~~
  (unassociated with night sweats and
  extreme weight loss)
Peripheral neuropathy/myopathy due
  to HIV

> **Teaching comments:** Severity of depression and anxiety in patients with a diagnosis of HIV are more related to the magnitude of symptomatology rather than to the degree of immunodeficiency or the number of opportunistic infections.[4]

STEP #7: Ask specific questions to rule specific conditions or pathological categories less likely.

- **Do you have shortness of breath at rest?** "No, I become short of breath and exhausted with any activities that requires a lot of effort such as climbing the stairs. I can catch my breath after sitting down for a few minutes." This response makes less likely primary cardiopulmonary pathology and pulmonary disorders such as pneumonia-related pleurisy, pulmonary embolism, and pulmonary fibrosis.

- **Do you have back pain?** "No." This response makes less likely conditions affecting the lumbar region, kidney pathology, and pneumonia.

- **Have you noticed a change in frequency, color, or urgency with urination or bowel function?** "No." This response makes less likely conditions affecting the kidney, diabetes mellitus, the colon, the pancreas, or the prostate.

- **Do you experience numbness or tingling?** "Yes, my toes and the bottoms of my feet tingle; at times, so do my hands. I have noticed in the past couple of years that I do not like to walk barefoot due to the sensitivity of my feet." This response makes more likely sources of symptoms that are associated with sensory changes.

> **Teaching comments:** This is not in a dermatome pattern. The clinician should consider pathologies with dermatome-type sensory changes as less likely than others. Oftentimes the initial presentation of diabetes mellitus or peripheral neuropathy due to disease progression is a change of sensation at the most distal aspects of the extremity. The clinician should be suspicious of protective sensation loss as assessed by Semmes-Weinstein monofilament testing.

STEP #8: Re-sort the diagnostic hypothesis list based on the patient's responses to specific questioning.

T Trauma

Not applicable

I Inflammation

Aseptic
~~Pleural effusion~~ (no shortness of breath or back pain)
~~Pleurisy~~ (no shortness of breath)

Septic
~~Cardiomyopathy~~ (no shortness of breath)
~~Idiopathic pulmonary fibrosis~~ (no shortness of breath)
~~Pleural effusion~~ (no shortness of breath)

~~Pleurisy~~ (no shortness of breath or back pain)
~~Pneumonia~~ (no shortness of breath or back pain)

M Metabolic

Diabetes mellitus polyneuropathy
Diabetic myopathy
Medication toxicity/toxic myopathy

Va Vascular

Anemia
Atherosclerosis
~~Cardiomyopathy~~ (no shortness of breath)

De Degenerative

Deconditioning

Tu Tumor

Malignant Primary, such as:
- AIDS- and non-AIDS-related malignancy
- ~~Colon~~ (no change in bowel function)
- Hematologic
- ~~Kidney~~ (no signs of blood in urine)
- ~~Lung~~ (no shortness of breath, no back pain)
- ~~Pancreas~~ (no change in bowel function, no back pain)
- ~~Prostate~~ (no back pain, no change in frequency/urgency in urination)
- ~~Spinal tumor~~ (no back pain)

Malignant Metastatic, such as:
- AIDS- and non-AIDS-related malignancy
- ~~Colon metastases~~ (no change in bowel function)
- ~~Kidney metastases~~ (no change in color of urine)
- ~~Pancreas metastases~~ (no back pain, no change in bowel function)
- ~~Prostate metastases~~ (no change in frequency/urgency in urination)
- ~~Spinal metastases~~ (no back pain)

Benign:
Not applicable

Co Congenital

Not applicable

Ne Neurogenic/Psychogenic

Depression
Peripheral neuropathy/myopathy due to HIV

STEP #9: Perform tests to differentiate among the remaining diagnostic hypotheses.

- **Observation.** Patient is not in apparent distress sitting at rest in the clinic, making less likely conditions associated with anxiety.

The patient answers questions with appropriate affect, making less likely conditions associated with depressed mood. There are bruises throughout the upper and lower extremities, but none appear on the trunk. Upon specific questioning, Alex acknowledges that recently he has been bruising more easily. This finding, although nonspecific, may increase the index of suspicion for AIDS-associated lymphoma. Palpation of painless, swollen lymph nodes in the neck, chest, axillary, or groin regions can further increase the index of suspicion. There are signs of lipodystrophy, including thinning of the face and arms and increased bulk at the back of the neck, which is a nonspecific finding associated with HAART adherence of greater than 6 months.[5]

- **Auscultation.** Lungs: No crackles or wheezing noted, confirming the suspicion based on history that acute restrictive or obstructive pulmonary pathologies are less likely. Heart sounds: No murmur or S_4 noted, confirming the initial impression that primary pathology of the myocardium is less likely.

- **Vitals.** Heart rate: 88 beats per minute at rest. Respiratory rate: 15 breaths/min at rest. Body temperature: 99.8°. Blood pressure: 136/88 SpO$_2$: 95% at rest on room air.

STEP #10: Re-sort the diagnostic hypothesis list based on the patient's responses to specific tests.

T Trauma

Not applicable

I Inflammation

Aseptic
Not applicable

Septic
Not applicable

M Metabolic

Diabetic myopathy
Medication toxicity/toxic myopathy

Va Vascular

Anemia
Atherosclerosis

De Degenerative

Deconditioning

Tu Tumor

AIDS- and non-AIDS-related malignancy

C   Congenital

Not applicable

Ne Neurogenic/Psychogenic

Depression

Peripheral neuropathy/myopathy due to HIV

STEP #11: Decide on a diagnostic impression.

- AIDS and non-AIDS malignancy vs. medication toxicity.

Teaching comment: Although certain conditions could not be ruled less likely, this should not preclude the clinician from using this process for differential diagnosis with a complex patient case. The conditions of atherosclerosis, anemia, and depression are common secondary conditions associated with a diagnosis of HIV. The clinician should attempt to fit all of the patient's concerns to the pathological condition. Though one or two of Alex's concerns may meet the patient presentation of atherosclerosis, anemia, or depression, not all do. Although deconditioning secondary to recent bed rest and illness with pneumonia could not be completely excluded based on the history findings, the patient's report of extreme weight loss (20 lbs over 1 month), fatigue with daily activities, and excessive sweating at night, in combination with the physical findings of low-grade temperature and bruising on the extremities, indicates the need for referral to exclude tumors and metabolic issues associated with the patient's underlying HIV infection and treatment.[6]

Teaching comment: Lipodystrophy is a collection of symptoms seen since the advent of HAART. Symptoms include metabolic changes, insulin resistance, glucose intolerance, diabetes, and hyperlipidemia. Physical signs may occur due to the redistribution of adipose tissue such as increased visceral fat in the abdomen, breasts, and neck; a "buffalo hump" at the back of the neck; and a decrease of fat on the extremities. These metabolic and fat changes increase the risk in this population of atherosclerosis and cardiac conditions such as myocardial infarction affirming the importance for vital sign monitoring for safe exercise prescription.[6,7]

STEP #12: Determine the appropriate patient disposition.

- Initiate physical therapy treatment with consult to address diagnostic impression.

Teaching comment: Physical therapy interventions are seldom prescribed in isolation for patients receiving HAART. The complexity of the disease process coupled with the side effects of the medications results in the need for a multidisciplinary approach including physicians, psychologists, nutritionists, and therapies.

Case Outcome

The consultation with the referring physician included a discussion on the results of Alex's recently completed blood tests, the results of which demonstrated anemia and an elevated white blood count. These results, in combination with Alex's symptoms, necessitated putting a hold on therapy services for 4 weeks for further investigation of his health status. The patient was diagnosed with AIDS-related lymphoma.

After confirmation of the diagnosis, initiation of chemotherapy and completion of an exercise stress test, Alex resumed physical therapy.[6] An aerobic training program was initiated that involved intermittent bouts of short-duration exercise and rest to accommodate the "down days" that are often associated with chemotherapy treatment.[8] Alex's goals were reevaluated based on the results of the exercise stress test. Several studies have documented improvements in both the physical and psychosocial status of patients with a diagnosis of lymphoma or HIV/AIDS and the interventions of aerobic and progressive resistance training. Outcome expectations from this episode of physical therapy care for Alex will include an increased rate of completing the planned chemotherapy treatment session,[8] an improvement in patient self-report of quality-of-life measures, and physical improvements such as improved peak oxygen consumption.[8] An outline of suggested training regimens is given here:

	DIAGNOSIS	PRESCRIPTION	OUTCOME
Progressive resistance exercise	HIV/AIDS	Up to four sets of eight repetitions at 70%–80% of 1 repetition maximum (RM) were utilized. Large and small muscle groups were involved.[9]	Improved strength and psychological status.
Aerobic training	HIV/AIDS	20-minute sessions three times per week for 4 weeks.	Improved cardiorespiratory fitness and psychological status.[10]
Progressive resistance exercise	Lymphoma	8–10 exercises of major muscle groups involving 10–15 repetitions of from one to three sets, 2 to 3 days per week at 60%–70% of 1 RM.[6,11]	Improved quality of life reported.[11]
Aerobic training	Lymphoma	Upright or recumbent cycle ergometer three times per week for 12 weeks. Duration was up to 20 minutes at 60% peak power output until week 4; 45 minutes by week 9 at 75% of peak power output.	Improved cardiorespiratory fitness and psychological status. Did not interfere with chemotherapy or completion rate.[8]

References

1. U.S. Department of Health and Human Services, Panel on Clinical Practices for Treatment of HIV Infection. Guidelines for the use of antiretroviral agents in HIV-1-infected adults and adolescents. http://aidsinfo.nih.gov/ContentFiles/AdultandAdolescentGL.pdf. Accessed May 17, 2010.
2. Simoni JM, Amico KR, Smith L, Nelson K. Antiretroviral adherence interventions: translating research findings to the real world clinic. Curr HIV/AIDS Rep. Feb 2010;7(1): 44–51.
3. Smith R, Rossetto K, Peterson BL. A meta-analysis of disclosure of one's HIV-positive status, stigma and social support. AIDS Care. Nov 2008;20(10):1266–1275.
4. Perdices M, Dunbar N, Grunseit A, Hall W, Cooper DA. Anxiety, depression and HIV related symptomatology across the spectrum of HIV disease. Aust N Z J Psychiatry. Dec 1992;26(4):560–566.
5. Anuurad E, Bremer A, Berglund L. HIV protease inhibitors and obesity. Curr Opin Endocrinol Diabetes Obes. Oct 2010;17(5):478–485.
6. American College of Sports Medicine, ed. ACSM's Resource for Clinical Exercise Physiology: Musculoskeletal, Neuromuscular, Neoplastic, Immunologic, and Hematologic Conditions. 2nd ed. ed. Philadelphia, PA: Lippincott Williams & Wilkins; 2010.
7. Gopal M, Bhaskaran A, Khalife WI, Barbagelata A. Heart disease in patients with HIV/AIDS—an emerging clinical problem. Curr Cardiol Rev. May 2009;5(2): 149–154.
8. Courneya KS, Sellar CM, Stevinson C, et al. Randomized controlled trial of the effects of aerobic exercise on physical functioning and quality of life in lymphoma patients. J Clin Oncol. Sep 20 2009;27(27):4605–4612.
9. Dolan SE, Frontera W, Librizzi J, et al. Effects of a supervised home-based aerobic and progressive resistance training regimen in women infected with human immunodeficiency virus: a randomized trial. Arch Intern Med. Jun 12, 2006;166(11):1225–1231.
10. Lucia A, Earnest C, Perez M. Cancer-related fatigue: can exercise physiology assist oncologists? Lancet Oncol. Oct 2003;4(10):616–625.
11. Cramp F, James A, Lambert J. The effects of resistance training on quality of life in cancer: a systematic literature review and meta-analysis. Support Care Cancer. Nov 2010;18(11):1367–1376.

CHAPTER **42**

Special Diagnostic Issues in Children

■ *Sharon K. DeMuth, PT, DPT, MS* ■ *Hugh G. Watts, MD*

IN THIS CHAPTER:
- Special features of history taking in children
- Special features of the physical examination in children
- Unique features of bone growth and injury

OUTLINE

Introduction

"Children are not small adults."

This is a well-known, but often overlooked maxim. When pointed out, it is so obvious that writing about it may seem unnecessary, but it bears emphasis and should be kept in mind throughout the various discussions in this chapter.

Pediatric practice like all physical therapy practice is constantly evolving. With the adoption of *Vision 2020* by the American Physical Therapy Association, physical therapists are expected to practice as doctors of physical therapy.[1] Pediatric physical therapists serve children and their families in many environments where they may be the initial health care provider evaluating a child's or infant's ability to move. Because pediatric physical therapy practice is the only physical therapy practice that is federally mandated (IDEA),[2] the expectation that pediatric physical therapists will recognize signs and symptoms and accurately diagnose patients as part of providing those services is crucial.

Special Features of History Taking in Children

The Age of a Child is the Defining Feature in Differential Diagnosis

Many diseases only occur at specific ages or are extremely rare at other ages. For example, Legg-Calvé-Perthes disease more commonly occurs in the hip of boys ages 4 to 6, while a slipped capital femoral epiphysis would be more commonly expected in a boy ages 12 to 15. If a boy presents with increasing weakness at age 7 or 8, Duchenne muscular dystrophy is a more likely diagnosis than spinal muscular atrophy III.

Exact age is important to establish. In some cultures, for example, in Saudi Arabia where birthdays are not celebrated, a child's exact age is not well documented. The ages of children adopted from another country are often only estimates. This has been the case in children from orphanages in Romania, Russia, and some parts of China. A healthy skepticism is needed if such a child does not fit within the expected range of norms. Bone age radiographs and standardized developmental testing may help to determine an approximate age. Additionally, infants who are born prematurely (more than 3 weeks early) are evaluated based on "adjusted age" until they are 2 years old. This means that a child born 2 months early, who has now lived 4 months since delivery, would be regarded as a 2-month-old in terms of developmental performance, not as a 4-month-old.[3]

The History is Generally Obtained Secondhand Through the Parent

Especially when children are young, parents provide all the information. It is easy to overlook the fact that the information provided by a parent may be misinterpreted by the health care provider.

PARENTS (OR THEIR SURROGATES) MAY BRING ASSUMPTIONS TO THE CLINICIAN

"My child hurts when she...." This may be true, but it may not be true. Such a statement may well set you on the wrong track when developing your list of possible diagnoses. Cultural background may pose additional challenges, related to assumptions about disease etiology, privacy customs, and language barriers.[4]

The clinician should search for the original problem that concerned the parent. For example, if parents state that they want their child evaluated for a leg-length difference, the clinician may focus on that particular issue when in reality the problem the parent initially was concerned about was a limp that a friend or grandparent might have suggested was due to the unequal leg length.

The clinician should try to get as much history as possible from the child. Even a 2-year-old can provide valuable information

if the question is asked in simple language and the answer interpreted with wisdom. If the child states that she has a "tummy ache" and when asked to point to where it hurts she points to her head, this information can be helpful.

Asking a child questions may also give you important information about how the family interacts. Does the parent constantly interrupt or insist on interpreting? If so, it is important to give the child a chance to speak for herself and reassure the parent that he will get his chance to give information in a minute. If the child always looks at the parent first as if looking for permission to speak, this can also provide an indication about the family dynamics.

Obtaining Information About a Child's Development

A physical therapist may be the first health care provider to interact with some children especially in settings such as "early intervention" programs (serving children from birth to 3 years of age) or the school system. The child may not have received a formal assessment from a primary care physician or pediatrician and the family may not have access to any health care services. Again the age of the child and the setting direct the evaluation.

For an infant, activities such as feeding and sleeping should be assessed as well as the infant's gross- and fine-motor abilities. It is also important to screen the infant's vision and hearing. An infant with torticollis may keep the head turned to one side because of a visual loss as well as a tight sternocleidomastoid muscle. Infants with hypotonia or hypertonia may have difficulty feeding. All infants go through periods in their development when they cry more than other periods, and an infant who has a central nervous system injury may be hard to console or get to sleep, increasing strain on the family and the risk for child abuse. Older children with known diagnoses such as cerebral palsy or myelodysplasia may be underweight or overweight and may need a referral to a pediatrician and or a registered dietician in order to help the family provide better care for the child.

In the early intervention setting, the focus is on the family[5] and the use of open-ended questions such as "Tell me about your baby's typical schedule," "What types of activities does the baby enjoy?" and "Does the baby sleep through the night?" may elicit more information than a question requiring only a yes or no answer. Open-ended questions also work well with older children in the preschool or school setting because they allow the physical therapist to begin to assess the child's cognitive ability and interests while getting acquainted with the child and the family and developing a mental list of potential diagnoses.

Knowing when the child accomplished certain motor skills such as rolling over (4 to 5 months), moving alone from lying to sitting up (6 to 7 months), walking (12 to 15 months), and reaching for objects (3 to 4 months) is important.[5] However, some parents will be better historians than others. Often with a first child the family may be able to tell you exactly what happened but they may not be able to give the same details for the fourth child.

In addition, certain cultures place value on certain motor activities, for example, independence in dressing, and will encourage those activities. For this reason, the timeline for accomplishment of certain tasks will be different for different infants. For example, in some African countries children are not allowed or encouraged to crawl but are carried until they can walk alone, a task often achieved at 8 or 9 months of age.[5]

The "back to sleep movement," which has been endorsed by the American Academy of Pediatrics and others since 1966, encourages parents to place babies face up to sleep to reduce the incidence of sudden infant death syndrome. This has altered the expected age for accomplishment of crawling and walking by decreasing prone experiences.[6,7]

The clinician uses this knowledge about whether a child accomplished motor skills within a range of expected norms to assess if the child is behaving appropriately for his or her age. If not, the clinician determines whether the child needs to be referred to a specialist such as a physical therapist who is a pediatric certified specialist (PCS), developmental pediatrician, pediatric neurologist, or pediatric orthopedist. If the family has no access to health care services, should they be referred to a social worker or to a state system such as Medicaid? The family may be unwilling to accept that there is anything really wrong with the infant or child and it may take a number of visits by the physical therapist and/or referral to another health care provider to help the family accept and begin to cope with their child's diagnosis.

Some Pitfalls

A HISTORY OF A FALL IS ALWAYS SUSPECT

Children fall frequently so it is easy to ascribe the cause of some problem to a fall. If a mother notes a swollen knee when her 3-year-old is being given a bath, she may well think that it is due to the fall off of the sofa she witnessed 2 days ago. On the other hand, the swollen knee could be due to juvenile rheumatoid arthritis. If there is a history of a fall, it is important to get the details. Was the child able to get up and walk or run right away? Was the crying inordinately prolonged? Was there a wound or scrape? These details will give a better understanding of the seriousness of the fall.

A HISTORY OF FEVER ALWAYS NEEDS FULL DETAILS

Children in their initial school years frequently bring upper respiratory infections home with them. These fevers can easily confuse the diagnostic problem. A parent may, for example, inadvertently overlook an important fever that heralds osteomyelitis by ascribing the fever to a "cold." Did the child have a runny nose or a cough?

"TICKET OF EXIT" ISSUES

Children often develop a strong wish to avoid unpleasant social situations by inventing illnesses. Gym class at school is commonly an activity a child wants to avoid. A preteen girl who is embarrassed about her delayed physical development in comparison to her classmates may not want to participate in gym class if she is required to change clothes in a locker room where she has to expose herself. A teenage boy with gynecomastia may feel the same way. Unwilling to discuss the real issues with their parents, a backache or foot pain may become the means of getting an excuse from gym class. Similarly, a child who is being pushed into competing in an activity such as skating or gymnastics may feel overwhelmed and look for a way to get out of the competition by developing a malady. It may take particularly sensitive questioning to get to the root of such matters.

THE "BY THE WAY" CONSULTATIONS
Parents often bring siblings along when one of their other children is being seen in the clinic. It is not unusual for the parent to take the opportunity to have one of the sibs evaluated at the same time with the common "Oh, by the way, what about my other child's flat feet?" As with any informal consultation (see Chapter 3), such interactions are fraught with potential problems. Time is limited since the appointment has been scheduled for only one child; the history is frequently hurried and superficial; and often no record of the visit is made. While it is a nuisance for the mother to make a separate appointment for the additional child, your reasons for this need to be carefully explained to the parent if disgruntlement is to be avoided.

Never Forget the Possibility of Child Abuse[2]

Child abuse can happen in what appear to be "the best" of families. Overlooking the possibility may mean that the next time it happens, the child may be badly maimed or, even worse, killed. Question the details of any story that involves trauma, a fall off of a changing table, or a fall down the stairs. One does not need to sound accusatory while doing so. Look for bruises that appear to have different dates of occurrence—that is, some that are blue-black while others are yellowish or greenish. Do the bruises suggest finger or hand marks left behind by a vigorous slap? Does the child raise his arm as if to protect himself from a blow when you approach? For the school-age child has there been a change in behavior at school, a change in academic performance, or frequent absences that are unexplained?

Physical therapists, like all health care providers, are mandated reporters if child abuse is suspected. All local and state departments of health have systems in place for reporting. It is incumbent on the physical therapist to know the procedures for the state in which he or she is licensed to practice.

Special Features of the Physical Examination of a Child

Get to the Child's Level

Imagine yourself lying on an examining table in your underwear when a 10-foot-tall person comes in to examine you. That's not unlike the situation for a child. Lower yourself to the child's level by sitting down or squatting.

Watch While the Child is Waiting to Be Seen

Often the parent will bring a child in for evaluation of a limp or in-toeing only to be frustrated when the child walks absolutely normally in front of the clinician. If possible, keep an eye on the waiting area and watch the children before you see them—that is, when they are not putting on a studied gait for your eyes. Other tricks such as asking a child to rub his tummy with one hand while patting the top of his head with the other hand, then asking him to walk, may fool the child into walking with his more usual gait.

Potential Problems with Disrobing

An adequate examination requires the child to disrobe. Feet and lower extremity problems cannot be appropriately evaluated by just pulling up the child's trouser legs. Spinal deformities cannot be evaluated properly without being able to see the child's entire trunk and pelvis. Many children are unhappy about undressing for an examination. They may be shy or afraid that this is the first step to getting an injection. If this occurs, being arbitrary and insisting may lead to a totally unsatisfactory examination. Some techniques that can work are to avoid eye contact with the child and simply state to the parent which clothes you want to have removed. It may also help to step out of room saying you'll return when the child is ready for examination.

Examine the Painful Area Last

This seems obvious, but it is frequently forgotten. Evaluate all the normal areas first. This may require a prior explanation to the parent who may think you are inept or forgetful if they see you examining the left leg when it is the right leg that is the problem. When finally coming to the painful extremity, log rolling the extremity gently should be done first before going to a range-of-motion (ROM) evaluation.

Confirmation of Discrepancies

If in doubt about the extent or intensity of a pain, a child can be asked to roll prone. Examine the opposite side as if it was the alleged painful side and ask the child if it hurts.

Examining the Child to Obtain Information About the Child's Development

As stated earlier, the physical therapist may be the first health care provider a child has seen, so there may not be a prior physician evaluation or history to review. In this situation it is important to try to estimate the child's cognitive, language, emotional, and self-help capabilities as well as her motor skills. Is the child able to talk to you? Can you understand what she is saying and does the vocabulary seem appropriate for her age? You can expect that by 2 years of age children will have a vocabulary of around 100 words.[5]

If the child is shy and will not talk to you, listen while he talks to the family or be prepared to try again later in the evaluation after he has gotten used to you. If the child is old enough, ask him to take off his clothing. Children ages 3 to 4 years usually can manage most of this.[8] This gives you a chance to see how they problem solve and it allows you to start to generate ideas about areas to focus on during your physical exam. If the child cannot remove her shoes or socks, if she cannot unbutton buttons, or sit alone to even attempt these activities you are gaining a lot of valuable information. This may be another area where cultural expectations of independence differ. If the child appears very frightened, it might be helpful to allow her to play with a toy or use a piece of equipment such as a ride-on-toy or slide in order to begin to "make friends" so you can perform your assessment.

To evaluate children successfully, you need to be familiar with the timing of typical developmental activities. That information is beyond the scope of this book but resources can be found in other excellent references.[5,9–11]

The physical therapist is also expected to provide accurate information about a child's ROM, muscle strength, and functional abilities. A child of 4 years can usually cooperate with ROM testing and may even be able to understand the concept of pushing against the therapist, allowing an active assessment of muscle strength by manual muscle testing (MMT). By 6 years of age children who are cognitively at their appropriate age level should be able to follow directions for ROM and MMT. Therapists should be familiar with changes in ROM at different ages[5] and may need to be prepared to estimate muscle strength based on observation of various functional activities if the child is unable to cooperate with a traditional examination.

It is critical to be able to provide accurate records of strength and mobility for many childhood illnesses in order to determine if the child is getting better or worse. The physical therapist usually has more time and more toys than other medical practitioners who only see the child in an office and is thus able to gain a better understanding of a child's capabilities. Providing care in the home or school settings also allows the physical therapist to understand how the child and family function most of the time. This information can be extremely important in making an accurate diagnosis and will need to be shared with the child's other health care providers.

We cannot stress enough the importance of the physical therapist in assessing for signs of child abuse. Look for the signs described above: bruises that appear to have different dates of occurrence; bruises that suggest finger or hand marks left behind by a vigorous slap; does the child raise his arm as if to protect himself from a blow when you approach. Look for additional signs of the loss of previously accomplished skills such as toilet training or problems with nightmares and excessive weight gain or loss.

Issues Related to Growth of Bones in Children

Growth of the Long Bones

This growth takes place at the *physis*, known in the past more commonly as the *epiphyseal growth plate*. Abnormalities in longitudinal growth in children most frequently result from trauma, infection, or loss of vascular supply. On the other hand, growth can be stimulated, presumably due to increased blood supply, as a result of fracture healing and/or chronic inflammation as seen in juvenile rheumatoid arthritis.

Differential inhibition of longitudinal growth (eg, medial versus lateral) may result in angular deformity. This is commonly seen after fractures of the physis medially at the ankle. Inhibition of growth of the physeal cells due to excessive asymmetric longitudinal loading is presumed to be the cause of the progressive genu varum seen in Blount's disease.

Growth Disturbances Due to Abnormal Muscle Activity

Bone growth responds to the muscle forces applied to the bones. What is often overlooked is that the shape of the bones may be modified by the growth of the apophyses, for example, the greater trochanter of the femur. In the past, when poliomyelitis was much more common, the effects of lack of muscle pull on the growth in length and shape of the bones was seen frequently by medical personnel caring for these children. Ewald and others[12,13] showed that the shape of the upper end of the femur, and especially the neck-shaft angle, was markedly decreased in experimental animals when the hip abductor muscles were removed or defunctioned. This effect is presumed to be the etiology of the increased proximal femoral valgus seen in children with cerebral palsy where their hip abductor muscles may be reciprocally inhibited by the spasticity of the hip adductor muscles.

Leg-Length Discrepancy

Causes for leg-length discrepancy are numerous.[14] Probably the commonest are due to the results of a fracture, either shortening due to healing with overlap or lengthening due to the stimulation of the healing fracture causing longitudinal overgrowth. Other causes are dislocation of the hip, osteomyelitis, traumatic physeal injury, Legg-Calvé-Perthes disease, and congenital conditions.

The concern about leg-length discrepancy varies with the specialty of the person evaluating the child—the more specialized a clinician, the less concerned he or she is about the lesser degrees of leg-length difference. Pediatric orthopedic surgeons are not concerned with a leg-length difference if, at maturity, the difference will be less than 2 cm.

The main issue with leg-length differences in children is not the current difference, but what the difference will be at maturity. A difference of 2 cm at the current time may be of little concern if the difference is stable in absolute terms. However, if the difference is due to a congenital decrease in longitudinal growth of the femur, for example, a 10% difference in a 1-year-old boy, the ultimate difference at maturity could be an additional 4 cm.

The management of leg-length discrepancy requires an adequate series of measurement data, usually at yearly intervals. Simple tape-measure evaluations are not adequate. Radiographs taken so that magnification is eliminated are important (either scanograms or orthoroentgenograms). Because bone length norms have been established based on bone age rather than calendar age, a simultaneous x-ray of the left hand is also taken and compared to norms. Because of the importance of having baseline measurements and appropriate serial measurements, a child with this problem should be given an early referral to an orthopedic surgeon who is familiar with leg-length discrepancies.

Differences in Fractures Between Children and Adults

Fractures in children are different from those seen in adults in a number of ways.

Epiphyseal Fractures

The most obvious anatomical difference is the presence of the physes (epiphyseal growth plates) responsible for longitudinal growth that are susceptible to injury. Furthermore, the subarticular physis, which allows for the growth in width and in shape of the ends of the bones, is also vulnerable to injury.

Nomenclature for fractures is not firmly agreed on. Fractures that take place at the ends of the bones in children where the physis, the secondary center of ossification, and the subarticular physis may be involved have generally been classified as *epiphyseal fractures*. Although a number of different classification schemes are available, the most commonly used is the Salter and Harris system (Fig. 42-1).[15]

- *Salter-Harris I:* In these fractures, the break takes place across the zone of provisional mineralization. Although the line of separation is not always exclusively at that level, the proliferating cells are usually not involved; hence, growth disturbance is not a common feature. The issue with these fractures is recognition. There is no break in the osseous tissue so there is nothing to be seen on the bones on a plain radiograph. Deep soft tissue swelling seen on the x-ray may be the only clue. Recognition comes from the knowledge that such a lesion could take place and an understanding of the mechanism of injury.
- *Salter-Harris II:* In these fractures, the break takes place across the zone of provisional mineralization, but as the fracture reaches the far side of the bone, the line of the break turns toward the metaphysis and leaves a telltale small triangle of bone attached to the physis. Because of this small fragment of bone attached to the physis, the lesion is usually readily recognized on an x-ray.

As with Salter-Harris I fractures, the line of separation along the physis is not always exclusively at that level; however, the proliferating cells are usually not injured, so growth disturbance is not a common feature of this fracture.

- *Salter-Harris III:* In these fractures, the line of the break goes across the zone of provisional mineralization, then turns toward the joint and breaks the secondary center of ossification. It may, or may not continue across the subarticular physis and articular cartilage into the joint itself. If the fracture extends totally into the joint, the loose fragment can easily dislodge and result in an incongruous joint surface with long-term dire consequences for joint function and growth. Although the fracture extends along the zone of provisional mineralization initially, the turn toward the joint crosses the layer of proliferating cells in the physis with a considerable probability of causing a growth disturbance. Such fractures often require accurate replacement of the fragments and fixation by surgery.
- *Salter-Harris IV:* In this fracture, the break takes place at approximately right angles to the physis, and extends from the metaphysis into the joint. The free fragment contains a piece of metaphysis, a segment of the physis and of the bony secondary center of ossification.

  Usually, the free fragment moves toward the joint, not only causing joint incongruity, but the bone of the metaphysis may heal across to the bone of the secondary center of ossification, which prevents the physis from growing. Such fractures, seen most commonly at the ankle and elbow, result in an

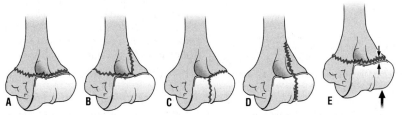

FIGURE 42-1 Salter-Harris fracture classification: (A) Salter-Harris I; (B) Salter-Harris II; (C) Salter-Harris III; (D) Salter-Harris IV; (E) Salter-Harris V.

asymmetrical growth arrest that requires treatment.

- *Salter-Harris V:* In this fracture, the mechanism of injury is presumed to be excessive axial loading that damages the proliferating cells of the physis. Injury to the blood supply may play a part. There is nothing to see on the x-ray, and the injury is recognized after the fact when the bone is discovered to have stopped growing.

Physiological Differences

Children's fractures also differ physiologically from those in adults. They heal more rapidly, which leads to both good and bad results. Rapid healing, with less likelihood of delayed union or nonunion, makes children's fractures easier to treat. However, if the bones are malpositioned, rapid healing may require that the bones be refractured in order to gain appropriate alignment if the malunited fracture is not treated early enough.

GROWTH IN LENGTH
Growth in length may be partially or totally inhibited by the trauma or by the injury to the vessels that supply nutrition to the multiplying cells of the physis. However, as noted above, a healing fracture may stimulate a rapidly growing bone to grow longer. This is particularly common with fractured femurs, especially where the fracture is close to the rapidly growing physis at the distal femur. Recognition of this phenomenon may lead the treating orthopedic surgeon to leave the ends of the fracture intentionally overlapped by 1 to 2 cm in anticipation of the overgrowth. It is important for all health care providers working with children to understand these treatment principles because they may be questioned about issues like this by parents and patients.

EFFECTS OF REMODELING
Periosteal growth controls the increase in bone diameter. This growth can result in remarkable remodeling of a child's bone following fractures. Judgment of this effect allows the orthopedic surgeon to accept considerable angulation in a long bone fracture alignment in anticipation of the straightening. Although angular remodeling readily takes place, the angulation between the line of the shaft and the line parallel to the physis does not necessarily remodel. If the angulation of the physis is in the plane of the joint motion (eg, flexion or extension of the knee in a proximal tibial fracture), remodeling is more likely. However, there is much less likely to be remodeling in the varus, valgus plane. At best, malrotation should be expected to show only minimal correction.

Mechanical Differences

Children's bones differ from those of adults in three important mechanical ways, as discussed next.

PERIOSTEUM
The periosteum is more of a structure in children's bones than in adults'. The tissue is much stronger and may not tear when the bone shaft breaks, thus leaving the broken bone more stable within an intact sleeve of the soft tissue periosteum. This can help the orthopedic surgeon because it can make the job of aligning the bone fragments easier through simple traction. The tough periosteum may allow a small child to continue walking after a spiral fracture of the shaft of the tibia. This can present a diagnostic dilemma because it may lead to health care workers assuming that a fracture could not be the cause of a limp because the child would ordinarily not be able to walk.

THE MECHANICAL PROPERTIES OF BONE IN CHILDREN ARE DIFFERENT
Bones can bend without breaking, a phenomenon that is sometimes called *plastic deformation*.[16,17] Bones can crush longitudinally, creating a stable break that shows in an x-ray as a bulging ring around the bone at about the junction of the metaphysis and diaphysis. This is called a *buckle* or *torus fracture* because its appearance on x-ray is similar to the ring at the top of a Greek Doric column (Fig. 42-2).

LIGAMENTS ARE STRONGER THAN THE ATTACHMENT OF THE PHYSES TO THE METAPHYSIS
Ligamentous structures in adults are less strong than the bones to which they are

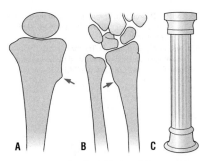

FIGURE 42-2 (A, B) Buckle (torus) fractures share a resemblance to (C) the top of a Doric column.

attached. Hence, they are the structures most likely to be torn with a varus or valgus stress at the knee. However, in children, the opposite is true. The ligaments are stronger than the bones. Hence, a valgus stress at the knee is much more likely to result in a fracture at the physeal-metaphyseal junction (the zone of provisional mineralization) than a torn ligament. This difference becomes less noticeable as the child grows toward the mid-teen years, at which time torn ligaments may be seen more frequently.

Other Considerations

ACTIVITY AND CAUTION

Children are usually more active and less cautious than adults, making them more vulnerable to fractures. However, this increased activity and devil-may-care attitude makes it less likely that their joints will stiffen during the immobilization needed for fracture healing.

FREQUENT FRACTURES

Some children will be seen who seem to have an inordinate number of fractures. Two potential causes come to mind: osteogenesis imperfecta and child abuse. It is often difficult to differentiate between these, *but they must always be kept in mind and a proper diagnosis is critical.*

Conclusion

Making a diagnosis for a child requires special techniques in history taking that are different

from those used with adults. The history is generally obtained secondhand through the parent and it is easy to overlook the fact that the parent's information may be misinterpreted by the clinician. For example, a history of a fall is always suspect (because children fall so frequently), because it is easy to ascribe a traumatic cause related to the fall when another form of pathology may be responsible. Cultural differences in childrearing may pose additional challenges. The physical therapist needs to be aware of the ages at which particular conditions affect a child, and the unique features of growth and injury that should alter how one assesses the likelihood of a diagnosis. Similarly, approaching children to examine them requires special techniques: get to the child's level; watch while the child is in the waiting area (and not afraid); and examine the painful area last.

References

1. American Physical Therapy Association. *Vision 2020.* http://www.apta.org/vision2020. Accessed June 28, 2011.
2. Phillips WE, Spotts ML. Medico-legal issues in the United States. In: Campbell SK, Vander Linden DW, Palisano RJ, eds. *Physical Therapy for Children.* 3rd ed. Philadelphia, PA: Elsevier; 2006:1123–1139.
3. Carter S. Neonatology: frequently asked questions: calculating corrected age. Emory University Department of Pediatrics. http://www.pediatrics.emory.edu/divisions/neonatology/dpc/faq.html. Accessed September 14, 2009.
4. Fadiman A. *The Spirit Catches You and You Fall Down.* New York: Farrar, Straus and Giroux; 1998.
5. Long T, Toscano K. *Handbook of Pediatric Physical Therapy.* 2nd ed. Philadelphia, PA: Lippincott Williams & Wilkins; 2002.
6. Dewey C, Fleming P, Golding J, Team AS. Does the supine sleeping position have any adverse effects on the child? II. Development in the first 18 months. *Pediatrics.* 1998;101(1, E5).
7. Davis BE, Moon RY, Sachs HC, Ottolini MC. Effects of sleep position on infant motor development. *Pediatrics.* 1998;102:1135–1140.
8. Ratliffe KT. The typically developing child. In *Clinical Pediatric Physical Therapy: A Guide for the Physical Therapy Team.* Philadelphia, PA: Mosby; 1998:45–51.
9. Adolph KE. Learning in the development of infant locomotion. *Monogr Soc Res Child Dev.* 1997;62(3):1–140.
10. Adolph KE, Berger SE. Motor development. In: Damon W, Lerner RM, eds. *Handbook of Child Psychology.* Vol II. 6th ed. New York: Wiley; 2006.
11. Campbell SK. Understanding motor performance in children. In Campbell SK, Vander Linden DW, Palisano RJ, eds. *Physical Therapy for Children.* 3rd ed. Philadelphia, PA: Elsevier; 2006:3–190.
12. Hoyt WA, Troyer ML, Reef T. The proximal femoral epiphysis. *JBJS.* 1966;48–A:1026.

13. Ewald FC, Hirohashi K. Effect of distal transfer of the greater trochanter in growing animals. *JBJS*. 1973;55(4): 1064–1067.

14. Moseley CF. Leg-length discrepancy. In: Morrissy RT, Weinstein SL, eds. *Lovell and Winter's Pediatric Orthopaedics*. Vol 2. 6th ed. Philadelphia, PA: Lippincott Williams & Wilkins; 2006:1213–1256.

15. Salter R, Harris WR. Injuries involving the epiphyseal plate. *JBJS*. 1963;45–A:587.

16. Vorlat P, DeBroeck H. Bowing fractures of the forearm in children: a long term followup. *Clin Orthop*. 2003;413:233–237.

17. Sanders WE, Heckman JD. Traumatic plastic deformation of the radius and ulna. A closed method of correction of deformity. *Clin Orthop*. 1984;188:58–67.

CHAPTER **43**

Elbow Pain in a Child

▨ *Julia L. Burlette, PT, DPT, OCS* ▨ *Jill S. Masutomi, PT, DPT, PCS*

Description of the Symptom

This chapter describes possible causes of elbow pain in a child. **Local causes** of elbow pain are defined as occurring in the region bounded by the distal one-third of the humerus, proximal one-third of the radius and ulna, and corresponding articular and periarticular structures.

Remote causes are defined as occurring outside this region.

Special Concerns

■ Decreased pulses
■ Recent change of status from previous
■ Skin breakdown and wound problems
■ Warmth and swelling associated with a fever

CHAPTER PREVIEW: Conditions That May Lead to Elbow Pain in a Child

T Trauma

REMOTE	LOCAL GENERALIZED	LOCAL ANTERIOR
COMMON		
Acute brachial plexus injury 859	Dislocations: • Elbow dislocation 861 Fractures: • Supracondylar fracture of the humerus 863	Not applicable
UNCOMMON		
Obstetric brachial plexus injury 860	Fractures: • Monteggia fracture-dislocation 863 • Transphyseal fracture 864	Nerve injury: • Median nerve injury 865
RARE		
Cervical radiculopathy 860	Not applicable	Fractures: • Coronoid process 862

I Inflammation

REMOTE	LOCAL GENERALIZED	LOCAL ANTERIOR
COMMON		
Not applicable	Not applicable	Not applicable

LOCAL LATERAL	LOCAL POSTERIOR	LOCAL MEDIAL
Fractures: • Lateral condyle 862 Osteochondritis/osteochondrosis: • Osteochondritis of the capitellum (Little Leaguer's elbow) 866 • Osteochondrosis of the capitellum (Panner's disease) 867 Pulled elbow (nursemaid's elbow, acute radial head subluxation) 867	Not applicable	Fractures: • Medial epicondyle 862
Muscle strains: • Extensor muscle strain 865 Nerve injury: • Radial nerve injury 866	Fractures: • Olecranon 863	Medial collateral ligament sprain/disruption or insufficiency 865 Muscle strains: • Flexor/pronator muscle strain 865 Nerve injury: • Ulnar nerve injury 866
Dislocations: • Radial head dislocation, traumatic 861 Fractures: • Capitellar fracture 862	Not applicable	Not applicable

LOCAL LATERAL	LOCAL POSTERIOR	LOCAL MEDIAL
Aseptic Tendinopathies (tendinitis): • Lateral epicondylitis (tennis elbow) 868 **Septic** Not applicable	**Aseptic** Apophysitis: • Olecranon 860 **Septic** Not applicable	**Aseptic** Apophysitis: • Medial epicondyle (Little Leaguer's elbow) 860 Tendinopathies (tendinitis): • Medial epicondylitis (golfer's elbow) 868 **Septic** Not applicable

(continued)

Inflammation (*continued*)

REMOTE	LOCAL GENERALIZED	LOCAL ANTERIOR
UNCOMMON		
Not applicable	**Aseptic** Juvenile idiopathic arthritis 864 **Septic** Septic arthritis (pyogenic arthritis) 867	Not applicable
RARE		
Not applicable	**Aseptic** Not applicable **Septic** Osteomyelitis 867 Systemic fungal infection 868 Tuberculosis 869	**Aseptic** Tendinopathies (tendinitis): • Distal biceps tendinitis 868 **Septic** Not applicable

M   Metabolic

REMOTE	LOCAL GENERALIZED	LOCAL ANTERIOR
COMMON		
Not applicable	Not applicable	Not applicable
UNCOMMON		
Not applicable	Myositis ossificans 865	Not applicable
RARE		
Not applicable	Gout 864	Not applicable

Va   Vascular

REMOTE	LOCAL GENERALIZED	LOCAL ANTERIOR
COMMON		
Not applicable	Not applicable	Not applicable
UNCOMMON		
Not applicable	Arterial injury 861 Compartment syndrome 861	Not applicable
RARE		
Not applicable	Hemophilia 864	Not applicable

De   Degenerative

REMOTE	LOCAL GENERALIZED	LOCAL ANTERIOR
COMMON		
Not applicable	Not applicable	Not applicable
UNCOMMON		
Not applicable	Not applicable	Not applicable

LOCAL LATERAL	LOCAL POSTERIOR	LOCAL MEDIAL
Not applicable	**Aseptic** Tendinopathies (tendinitis): • Triceps tendinitis 868 **Septic** Not applicable	Not applicable
Not applicable	Not applicable	Not applicable

LOCAL LATERAL	LOCAL POSTERIOR	LOCAL MEDIAL
Not applicable	Not applicable	Not applicable
Not applicable	Not applicable	Not applicable
Not applicable	Not applicable	Not applicable

LOCAL LATERAL	LOCAL POSTERIOR	LOCAL MEDIAL
Not applicable	Not applicable	Not applicable
Not applicable	Not applicable	Not applicable
Not applicable	Not applicable	Not applicable

LOCAL LATERAL	LOCAL POSTERIOR	LOCAL MEDIAL
Not applicable	Not applicable	Not applicable
Not applicable	Not applicable	Not applicable

(continued)

Degenerative *(continued)*

REMOTE	LOCAL GENERALIZED	LOCAL ANTERIOR
RARE		
Not applicable	Not applicable	Not applicable

Tu Tumor

REMOTE	LOCAL GENERALIZED	LOCAL ANTERIOR
COMMON		
Not applicable	Not applicable	Not applicable
UNCOMMON		
Not applicable	Not applicable	Not applicable
RARE		
Not applicable	*Malignant Primary, such as:* • Ewing's sarcoma 869 • Osteosarcoma 870 • Rhabdomyosarcoma 870 *Malignant Metastatic:* Not applicable *Benign, such as:* • Aneurysmal bone cyst 869 • Fibromatosis 869 • Lipoma 869 • Osteoblastoma 870 • Osteochondroma 870 • Osteoid osteoma 870	Not applicable

Co Congenital

REMOTE	LOCAL GENERALIZED	LOCAL ANTERIOR
COMMON		
Not applicable	Not applicable	Not applicable
UNCOMMON		
Not applicable	Radioulnar synostosis 867	Not applicable
RARE		
Not applicable	Not applicable	Not applicable

Ne Neurogenic/Psychogenic

REMOTE	LOCAL GENERALIZED	LOCAL ANTERIOR
COMMON		
Not applicable	Not applicable	Not applicable

LOCAL LATERAL	LOCAL POSTERIOR	LOCAL MEDIAL
Not applicable	Not applicable	Not applicable

LOCAL LATERAL	LOCAL POSTERIOR	LOCAL MEDIAL
Not applicable	Not applicable	Not applicable
Not applicable	Not applicable	Not applicable
Not applicable	Not applicable	Not applicable

LOCAL LATERAL	LOCAL POSTERIOR	LOCAL MEDIAL
Not applicable	Not applicable	Not applicable
Dislocations: • Radial head dislocation, congenital 861	Not applicable	Not applicable
Not applicable	Not applicable	Not applicable

LOCAL LATERAL	LOCAL POSTERIOR	LOCAL MEDIAL
Not applicable	Not applicable	Not applicable

(continued)

Neurogenic/Psychogenic *(continued)*

REMOTE	LOCAL GENERALIZED	LOCAL ANTERIOR
UNCOMMON		
Not applicable	Not applicable	Not applicable
RARE		
Not applicable	Not applicable	Not applicable

Note: These are estimates of relative incidence because few data are available for the less common conditions.

Common Ages at Which Elbow Pain Presents in a Child

APPROXIMATE AGE	CONDITION
Birth to 3 Years	Juvenile idiopathic arthritis Obstetric brachial plexus injury Osteomyelitis Pulled elbow Septic arthritis Transphyseal fracture
Preschool (3–5 Years)	Juvenile idiopathic arthritis Monteggia fracture-dislocation Osteomyelitis Pulled elbow Radial head or neck fracture Supracondylar humerus fracture Transphyseal fracture Traumatic radial head dislocation
Elementary School (6–11 Years)	Aneurysmal bone cyst Juvenile idiopathic arthritis Lateral condyle fracture Medial collateral ligament sprain/disruption Medial epicondyle apophysitis Medial epicondyle fracture Monteggia fracture-dislocation Olecranon apophysitis Osteoblastoma Osteochondrosis of the capitellum Osteoid osteoma Radial head or neck fracture Supracondylar humerus fracture Traumatic radial head dislocation
Middle School (12–14 Years)	Aneurysmal bone cyst Capitellar fracture Elbow dislocation Extensor muscle strain Flexor/pronator muscle strain Juvenile idiopathic arthritis Lateral epicondylitis Medial condyle fracture Medial epicondyle fracture Medial epicondylitis Olecranon fracture Osteoblastoma

LOCAL LATERAL	LOCAL POSTERIOR	LOCAL MEDIAL
Not applicable	Not applicable	Not applicable
Not applicable	Not applicable	Not applicable

Common Ages at Which Elbow Pain Presents in a Child—cont'd

APPROXIMATE AGE	CONDITION
	Osteochondritis of the capitellum
	Osteochondrosis of the capitellum
	Osteoid osteoma
	Radial head or neck fracture
High School (15–18 Years)	Acute brachial plexus injury
	Aneurysmal bone cyst
	Capitellar fracture
	Elbow dislocation
	Extensor muscle strain
	Flexor/pronator muscle strain
	Lateral epicondylitis
	Medial collateral ligament sprain/disruption
	Medial epicondylitis
	Olecranon fracture
	Osteoblastoma
	Osteochondritis of the capitellum
	Osteoid osteoma
	Triceps tendinitis

Overview of Elbow Pain in a Child

The elbow is the most common joint injured in childhood. Elbow injuries in the skeletally immature child have increased as participation in organized athletics has expanded for this age group. Juvenile and adolescent athletes are participating at earlier ages—and at higher intensities of competition—in year-round sports, placing excessive amounts of stress on immature structures. There are several conditions unique to the pediatric elbow that can be attributed to the presence of the growth plates or physes that distinguish these injuries from their adult counterpart. The high prevalence of convoluted physes in the distal humerus, proximal radius, and proximal ulna make the recognition of fractures difficult on plain radiographs. The strength of the musculoskeletal tissue is age dependent, and injury patterns are commonly observed in association with the skeletal developmental stage of the growing child's elbow. Tumors, infections, and arthritides are less likely to occur in the pediatric elbow, given that much less longitudinal growth occurs at the distal humerus and proximal radius and ulna in relation to their opposite ends.

Description of Conditions That May Lead to Elbow Pain in a Child

Remote

■ Acute Brachial Plexus Injury

Chief Clinical Characteristics

This presentation includes burning pain down the arm, numbness, weakness, and dysesthesia.

Background Information

Also known as a *burner*, the mechanism of injury involves collision sports and typically includes traction to the brachial plexus from a blow that depresses the shoulder. The upper trunks (C5–C6) are most commonly involved, resulting in more numbness and pain in the C5 and C6 dermatomes and weakness in the deltoid and biceps. Assessment includes screening for osseous injury and a thorough neurological examination. Most acute brachial plexus injuries from collision sports will resolve with complete recovery within minutes to hours. The athlete may return to sports when neurological function is normal. The athlete with a severe injury resulting in weakness lasting longer than 6 months should not return to collision sports.[1]

■ Cervical Radiculopathy

Chief Clinical Characteristics

This presentation can be characterized by pain in the cervical region and the corresponding dermatome for the involved nerve root. Pain is typically increased with cervical movement, use of the involved upper extremity, and coughing or sneezing. This presentation may also include motor loss, sensory disturbances, and diminished or absent reflexes corresponding to the involved nerve root.

Background Information

Cervical radiculopathy may be caused by trauma or other lesions (ie, space-occupying lesion, infection, or hemorrhage). The diagnosis is confirmed with magnetic resonance imaging. Progressive neurological deficits indicate surgical intervention.

■ Obstetric Brachial Plexus Injury

Chief Clinical Characteristics

This presentation can be characterized by weakness of the muscles innervated by the involved brachial plexus trunk.

Background Information

The mechanism of injury is traction of the brachial plexus during delivery when the head is pulled laterally away from the shoulder. The injury is classified by the level of trunk involvement. The upper trunk (C5 and C6) is most commonly involved.[2] It is also known as upper plexus palsy or Erb's palsy. Complete recovery by 3 months of age is observed in up to 92% of injured infants.[3] Additional involvement of the C7 nerve will result in the classic "waiter tip deformity" with the shoulder adducted and internally rotated, elbow extended, forearm pronated, and wrist and fingers flexed. Risk factors for obstetric brachial plexus injury include high birth weight, prolonged labor, and breech presentation.[3] Treatment includes stretching and splinting to prevent further contracture. Microsurgery may be beneficial if no recovery occurs by 3 to 6 months. Tendon transfers and osteotomies may be indicated to increase function.

Local

APOPHYSITIS

■ Medial Epicondyle (Little Leaguer's Elbow)

Chief Clinical Characteristics

This presentation may include pain, swelling, and localized tenderness over the medial epicondyle. Reproduction of symptoms will occur with resisted wrist flexion, resisted forearm pronation, and passive wrist extension with the elbow extended. Application of a valgus stress to an elbow flexed 20 degrees increases pain and may also demonstrate laxity.[4]

Background Information

Medial epicondyle apophysitis is a repetitive stress injury typically found in the skeletally immature child and adolescent thrower, ages 8 to 12.[1,5] Its cause is excessive distractive force produced on the medial side of the elbow with repetitive valgus stress leading to a series of microavulsions at the bone–cartilage junction.[6] It is seen most commonly in throwers during the acceleration phases of throwing, but can occur in gymnasts, tennis players, golfers, or with any repetitive valgus stress to the elbow.[6,7] Treatment includes rest until the child is asymptomatic, followed by gradual stretching and strengthening, with a slow progression of throwing or return to sports.[8]

■ Olecranon

Chief Clinical Characteristics

This presentation may involve pain, mild swelling, and tenderness at the insertion of the triceps at the tip of the olecranon. Pain is exacerbated by resisted elbow extension, and a decrease in elbow range of motion may be present.[8]

Background Information
Traction apophysitis at the distal triceps insertion is the most common posterior elbow injury in skeletally immature pitchers, 8 to 12 years of age. The olecranon is subject to minor stress fractures in throwing secondary to the excessive triceps pull in the early acceleration phase, coupled with the impaction of the olecranon into the humeral fossa in the late follow-through phase.[4,5,8,9] This condition is associated with overuse[4] in any movement or task that involves repeated maximal extension of the elbow in a skeletally immature child.[7] Treatment includes rest and ice in the acute stage followed by stretching and strengthening.

■ **Arterial Injury**

Chief Clinical Characteristics
This presentation typically involves pain out of proportion to the injury that increases with passive stretch of the involved muscles. Pulses are decreased or absent, skin temperature is decreased, and skin color is poor. This presentation may also include weakness and hypoesthesia.

Background Information
The mechanism of injury is usually traumatic and may include fracture or laceration. Surgical repair is required.

■ **Compartment Syndrome**

Chief Clinical Characteristics
This presentation involves pain, feelings of increased pressure, tense compartment, weakness, numbness, and swelling. Pain is out of proportion than expected for injury and increases with passive stretching of the muscles. Pain related to this condition is not relieved with immobilization. Peripheral pulses are usually intact unless an arterial injury has occurred.

Background Information
The mechanisms of injury are numerous and include fracture, crush injury, burns, and vascular injury. Prolonged external pressure from a compressive cast or bandage may also cause compartment syndrome. Immediate identification of compartment syndrome is critical

to prevent muscle ischemia. A decompressive fasciotomy is required to alleviate the pressure. The major complication of compartment syndrome is a Volkmann contracture.[10]

DISLOCATIONS

■ **Elbow Dislocation**

Chief Clinical Characteristics
This presentation includes severe pain, swelling, deformity, and inability to flex or extend the elbow.

Background Information
The mechanism of injury is typically a fall. Dislocations account for 5% of elbow injuries in children.[11] The most frequent pattern of dislocation is posterior. Associated fractures are common. Other associated injuries include disruption of the anterior capsule, ulnar collateral ligament injury, and brachialis muscle tear. Arterial and nerve injuries are uncommon. Peak incidence occurs in the second decade, usually between 12 and 14 years of age.[5,11] Spontaneous reduction is common.[12] Closed reduction with splinting for simple dislocations usually results in good outcomes although loss of elbow motion may occur. Dislocation with associated injury may require surgical intervention.

■ **Radial Head Dislocation, Congenital**

Chief Clinical Characteristics
This presentation may involve restricted pronation or supination and bony prominence at the location of the dislocation, usually posteriorly or laterally.[13]

Background Information
This condition is uncommon and typically occurs unilaterally. The radial head has a rounded shape and the capitellum is underdeveloped.[14] It is usually not detected until later in childhood. Treatment consists of observation unless pain develops. Surgical intervention may be indicated once skeletal maturation has been achieved.

■ **Radial Head Dislocation, Traumatic**

Chief Clinical Characteristics
This presentation may be characterized by lateral elbow pain and restricted range of

motion. The radial head may be palpable in the dislocated position.

Background Information
The mechanism of injury is typically a fall onto the hyperextended elbow or outstretched, pronated hand. Isolated radial head dislocation is rare and often associated with plastic deformation of the ulna.[3] It is considered a variant of the Monteggia lesion. This injury is frequently missed and may result in future problems if left untreated. It may be treated with closed reduction and immobilization. Open reduction is indicated if closed reduction is unsuccessful, with delayed reduction greater than 3 weeks postinjury,[12] and with persistent dislocation.[3] Complications are uncommon; they include posterior interosseous nerve lesion and decreased elbow range of motion.

FRACTURES
■ Capitellar Fracture
Chief Clinical Characteristics
This presentation can involve pain and swelling at the lateral elbow and antecubital fossa. Range of motion is restricted, especially with flexion. The lateral elbow may be tender.

Background Information
The mechanism of injury is typically a fall, with the elbow extended, onto an outstretched arm. The fracture may also occur with a fall onto a flexed elbow.[12] Capitellar fractures are rare and usually occur in children older than 12 years.[15] Cubitus recurvatum and cubitus valgus may facilitate this injury. One-third of these injuries are associated with a radial head fracture.[15] Capitellar fractures usually require internal fixation; however, minimally displaced fractures may be managed with closed reduction.

■ Coronoid Process
Chief Clinical Characteristics
This presentation includes pain and swelling at the antecubital fossa. Crepitus may occur with end-range elbow extension. Isolated injury is rare.

Background Information
This fracture may occur with elbow dislocation or severe trauma. This condition is commonly unrecognized and may contribute to continued instability following elbow trauma.

■ Lateral Condyle
Chief Clinical Characteristics
This presentation is characterized by lateral elbow pain and swelling.

Background Information
The mechanism of injury is typically a varus stress with the elbow in extension. The fracture can also occur with an elbow dislocation or a fall onto a flexed elbow. Lateral condyle fractures occur between the ages of 2 and 14 years, but are more common between the ages of 6 and 10 years.[16] These fractures are relatively common, accounting for 15% to 20% of distal humerus fractures in children,[17] and they occur more frequently in boys. This fracture usually requires internal fixation. An undisplaced and stable fracture may be treated with external immobilization or percutaneous pinning. Complications of lateral condyle fracture include nonunion, avascular necrosis, ulnar nerve palsy, cubitus valgus deformity, and physeal arrest.[5,11]

■ Medial Condyle
Chief Clinical Characteristics
This presentation may include medial elbow pain and swelling.

Background Information
The mechanism of injury is typically a fall onto the point of a flexed elbow or a valgus stress on an extended elbow causing an avulsion fracture.[16] Isolated medial condyle fractures are rare. Surgical intervention is indicated for displaced fractures. Nondisplaced fractures may be managed with immobilization only.

■ Medial Epicondyle
Chief Clinical Characteristics
This presentation can be characterized by medial elbow pain, tenderness, and valgus instability. Mild to moderate swelling may occur. The fracture may result in mild to severe ulnar nerve injury.

Background Information
The mechanism of injury is typically a fall on an outstretched hand, but may also occur

with a direct blow to the medial elbow. Fifty percent of cases are associated with elbow dislocation.[5,18] Dislocation with spontaneous reduction may occur. Medial epicondyle fractures typically occur between the ages of 10 and 14 years.[5,17] It is a relatively common fracture, comprising 12% of elbow fractures.[19] Indications for surgical intervention include valgus instability, ulnar neuropathy, entrapped fragment in the elbow joint, and displacement greater than 5 mm. Athletes will usually require surgical fixation.

■ Monteggia Fracture-Dislocation

Chief Clinical Characteristics
This presentation may involve pain, tenderness, swelling, and angulation of the ulna. Elbow range of motion is restricted. The dislocation of the radial head may be visualized on the lateral aspect of the elbow.

Background Information
The mechanism of injury is typically a fall onto the hyperextended elbow but less commonly may occur from a direct blow or a hyperpronation injury. This condition refers to dislocation of the radial head associated with ulnar fracture or bowing. The Monteggia lesion is classified according to the direction of the radial head dislocation and the trauma to the ulna. It is an uncommon injury in children accounting for less than 1% of all pediatric forearm fractures.[20] It occurs most often in children younger than 10 years of age.[20] The posterior interosseous nerve may be injured with an anterior dislocation; however, associated nerve injuries are less common than in adults. Additional complications include failure or loss of reduction, elbow stiffness, avascular necrosis of the radial head, and radioulnar synostosis.[20] The injury is usually treated by closed methods but may require surgical intervention if the elbow is unstable. The prognosis is good.

■ Olecranon

Chief Clinical Characteristics
This presentation includes posterior elbow pain, tenderness, swelling, and decreased elbow range.

Background Information
The mechanism of injury is typically a fall on an outstretched hand, but may also occur

with a direct blow or twisting injury.[11,21] The fracture is uncommon, accounting for 4% to 6% of elbow fractures in children.[11,22] Thirty-two percent of olecranon fractures have associated elbow injuries including radial neck fracture, medial epicondyle fracture, coronoid fracture, and osteochondral fracture.[11] Treatment is determined by the fracture site and pattern, amount of displacement, stability, and associated injuries. Most of these injuries are nondisplaced or minimally displaced requiring immobilization only. Complications are uncommon and outcomes are good with the majority of children regaining functional elbow range. Between 10% and 20% olecranon fractures require open reduction.[11]

■ Radial Head or Neck

Chief Clinical Characteristics
This presentation may involve pain, swelling, and tenderness along the lateral aspect of the elbow over the proximal radius. Pronation and supination are limited and painful with pain often referred to the wrist.

Background Information
The mechanism of injury is typically a fall on the outstretched extremity with a valgus moment at the elbow, resulting in a fracture just distal to, or at the epiphyseal plate, or a fracture of the neck of the radius.[21] These fractures may be associated with a rupture of the medial collateral ligament, avulsion of the medial epicondylar apophysis, olecranon fracture, and rarely with dislocation. A stress fracture of the radial neck with angular deformity may occur in pediatric athletes. This injury typically occurs in children ages 4 to 14 years.[11,17] Fracture management is determined by the degree of angulation, translation, elbow motion, and any concomitant injuries.[23] Treatment options include immobilization without reduction, closed reduction, or open reduction with or without internal fixation.

■ Supracondylar Fracture of the Humerus

Chief Clinical Characteristics
This presentation typically includes pain, tenderness, and swelling medially and laterally in the supracondylar area. Swelling

may be present posteriorly and anteriorly following high-energy injuries with greater displacement.

Background Information

This fracture is the most common elbow fracture in children, and accounts for 60% of elbow injuries.[11] The mechanism of injury is typically a fall on the outstretched arm or with the elbow positioned a little flexed with the forearm pronated. The incidence of this injury is greatest in the first decade of life with a peak between the ages of 5 and 10 years.[5] Injuries to the anterior interosseus nerve, radial nerve, median nerve, and brachial artery can occur in up to 18% of displaced fractures.[5] Treatment of these fractures is guided by the amount of displacement. Nondisplaced to mildly displaced fractures are treated by cast immobilization or through closed reduction followed by cast immobilization.[17] With greater degrees of displacement, these injuries necessitate surgical intervention with either closed reduction and percutaneous pin fixation or open reduction.[5,11]

■ Transphyseal Fracture

Chief Clinical Characteristics

This presentation involves swelling, deformation, muffled crepitus, and instability.[17]

Background Information

This injury is a fracture-separation of the distal humeral epiphysis that is observed in children from birth to 7 years of age, with a peak occurring before the child is 2½ years of age.[11] Multiple mechanisms of injury have been reported, with the most common a rotatory shear force, either at birth secondary to traumatic delivery, child abuse, or from a fall onto an extended arm.[17] Closed reduction is performed under anesthesia followed by cast immobilization if necessary. Percutaneous pin stabilization is used to prevent loss of reduction and malunion with postsurgical cast immobilization for 3 weeks. Damage to the physis is rare and cubitus varus is an uncommon complication.[11,17]

■ Gout

Chief Clinical Characteristics

This presentation involves a sudden onset of pain, swelling, redness of the superficial tissues,

and tenderness of the joint or bursal cavity. Advanced cases may have palpable firm tophi.

Background Information

Gout commonly manifests as acute olecranon bursitis. The olecranon bursa is a common location for tophi. The toes should also be assessed for metatarsal joint involvement. Gout is usually associated with elevated uric acid levels. Gout is rare in children, although it may be associated with inherited conditions that are, in turn, associated with hyperuricemia. Polarized microscopic examination of aspirated synovial fluid confirms the diagnosis. Treatment includes inflammation control, medication, and diet modification.

■ Hemophilia

Chief Clinical Characteristics

This presentation can be characterized by swelling, pain, warmth, stiffness, and the child holding the elbow in a flexed position.

Background Information

This condition is an inherited, recessive, sex-linked disorder that affects blood clotting predominantly in males. Hemorrhages may occur anywhere in the body, but are most often found in joints; typically the knee, elbow, and ankle.[24] Muscles are the second most common site of bleeding, with the iliopsoas, gastrocnemius, and forearm flexor muscle compartment most frequently involved.[25] Depending on the severity of the disorder, bleeding may occur spontaneously, or more commonly, secondary to a minor trauma such as a sprain or muscle pull. Infants or toddlers may develop subcutaneous ecchymosis over bony prominences or large hematomas after receiving intramuscular vaccinations. Factor replacement therapy, given intravenously, is the mainstay of treatment for an acute bleeding episode.[25] In addition to factor replacement, management of an acute bleed includes rest, ice, compression, and elevation, pain-free movement, splinting, and pain medication as needed (aspirin is contraindicated in this patient population).[24]

■ Juvenile Idiopathic Arthritis

Chief Clinical Characteristics

This presentation typically includes insidious onset of multiple peripheral joint swelling, heat, decreased extension greater than flex-ion range of motion, and pain and tender-ness with joint motion. Joint stiffness is most marked in the morning or after a period of inactivity and improves with movement. The muscles surrounding the elbow may show marked wasting, especially when the more acute painful stage of the disease is subsiding. With chronic conditions, the pain may subside; however, the joint is left with limited move-ment and possibly long-term deformity.

Background Information
This condition is one of the most common rheumatic diseases of childhood, and is one of the more frequent chronic illnesses of chil-dren.[26] There is a peak age of onset between 1 and 3 years of age and a secondary peak just before puberty.[26,27] Treatment includes med-ications, activity modification, general condi-tioning, splinting, and casting. Surgical inter-vention may be necessary to improve long-term joint function.

■ Medial Collateral Ligament Sprain/Disruption or Insufficiency

Chief Clinical Characteristics
This presentation can involve medial elbow pain, tenderness, and laxity with valgus stress testing.

Background Information
The mechanism of injury typically includes a history of repetitive overhead throwing activities but may also occur from a fall on the outstretched hand. Valgus force at the elbow may cause complete or partial tearing of the medial collateral ligament. Ligamentous injury in children occurs more commonly before the growth spurt and after growth plate closure in adolescents.[6] Medial collat-eral ligament disruption usually requires surgical repair to allow a full return to sports.

MUSCLE STRAINS
■ Extensor Muscle Strain

Chief Clinical Characteristics
This presentation may be characterized by muscle soreness and tenderness of the wrist extensor musculature. Symptoms are repro-duced with active wrist extension and increased when resistance is applied. Reproduction of

symptoms may occur with passive wrist flexion.

Background Information
The mechanism of injury is typically in-creased wrist extensor use 1 to 2 days prior to the onset of symptoms. Resolution of symp-toms will usually occur in 1 to 3 days with avoidance of aggravating activities.

■ Flexor/Pronator Muscle Strain

Chief Clinical Characteristics
This presentation may include muscle soreness and tenderness of the wrist flexor/pronator musculature. Reproduction of symptoms will occur with active wrist flexion and forearm pronation with increased symptoms when resistance is applied. Symptoms may be re-produced with passive wrist extension and forearm supination.

Background Information
The mechanism of injury is typically in-creased forearm use 1 to 2 days prior to the onset of symptoms. Symptoms will typically resolve in 1 to 3 days with rest.

■ Myositis Ossificans

Chief Clinical Characteristics
This presentation can involve swelling, tender-ness, and warmth over the involved muscle.

Background Information
The mechanism of injury is typically a direct blow to the muscle mass that causes a signifi-cant contusion. The etiology of this condition is theorized to be due to a hematoma organi-zation involving a progressive transformation of fibrous tissue to cartilage and then bone; hematoma calcification; intramuscular bone formation after detachment of periosteal flaps, periosteal rupture, metaplasia of intramuscu-lar connective tissue into cartilage and bone, and an individual predisposition to myosi-tis.[28,29] Radiographic changes may occur 3 to 4 weeks following the injury. Surgical resection is rarely indicated unless function is impaired.

NERVE INJURY
■ Median Nerve Injury

Chief Clinical Characteristics
This presentation may include aching pain in the anterior forearm and palpable pain

along the course of the nerve. Reproduction of symptoms may occur with resisted forearm, elbow, or finger motions. The patient may present with weakness in the muscles innervated by the median nerve and numbness in the hand, primarily the first and second digits.

Background Information
The mechanism of injury may be acute trauma or chronic, repetitive microtrauma. Repetitive, resisted pronation and supination of the forearm may contribute to microtrauma of the median nerve. Median nerve compression should initially be managed conservatively with inflammation control and activity modification. Traumatic median nerve injuries from fractures usually resolve spontaneously.[30]

■ Radial Nerve Injury

Chief Clinical Characteristics
This presentation involves minimal to severe aching pain in the lateral forearm and tenderness in the supinator region. Resisted wrist extension with the elbow extended or resisted supination of the forearm may reproduce symptoms. The child suspected of this condition may present with partial or complete paralysis of the muscles innervated by the radial nerve.

Background Information
Radial nerve injury may occur from trauma, space-occupying lesions, inflammation, excessive muscular activity, and is associated with extension type supracondylar fracture.[30]

■ Ulnar Nerve Injury

Chief Clinical Characteristics
This presentation may involve aching pain in the medial elbow and forearm and paresthesias in the sensory dermatome of the ulnar nerve. Weakness and atrophy of the muscles innervated by the ulnar nerve may be found depending on the extent of the injury.

Background Information
The mechanism of injury may be traumatic or secondary to microtrauma to the nerve.

Microtrauma may be caused by chronic subluxation, valgus stress, and flexor carpi ulnaris muscle compression.[4] Ulnar nerve injury is associated with medial condyle fracture and flexion type supracondylar fracture.[30] Ulnar neuritis may occur in young athletes from repeated throwing and may be associated with medial instability.[9] Treatment for this condition includes rest and inflammation control. Strengthening is initiated when the acute phase resolves. Traumatic nerve injuries from fractures or following surgery usually resolve spontaneously.[31]

OSTEOCHONDRITIS/ OSTEOCHONDROSIS

■ Osteochondritis of the Capitellum (Little Leaguer's Elbow)

Chief Clinical Characteristics
This presentation can involve dull pain, tenderness over the lateral elbow, effusion, and loss of elbow range, most commonly extension. Catching, locking, and crepitus may also occur with elbow motion.[32] Symptoms are aggravated with use of the involved extremity and relieved with rest.

Background Information
Osteochondritis of the capitellum is associated with frequent repetitive overuse of the elbow and is most common in young throwing athletes between the ages of 13 and 16 years. It is also associated with loose body formation. Treatment is guided by clinical findings and radiographs. Magnetic resonance imaging may aid in early detection of this condition.[33] Nonsurgical intervention includes rest and activity modification. Surgical intervention may be indicated to remove loose bodies. Prognosis depends on the size and extent of the lesion and the patient's age. Younger patients have a better prognosis but functional limitations are common and a return to sports is not always achieved. A poor outcome has been correlated with advanced lesions, a large osteochondral defect, and development of osteoarthritis.[34]

■ Osteochondrosis of the Capitellum (Panner's Disease)

Chief Clinical Characteristics
This presentation includes aching pain, tenderness over the lateral side of the elbow, local swelling, and decreased range, typically a loss of 5 to 20 degrees of extension. Symptoms are aggravated with activity and relieved with rest.

Background Information
Osteochondrosis of the capitellum is associated with repetitive microtrauma to the lateral elbow from valgus stress or increased axial load as observed with throwing athletes and gymnasts. It occurs more commonly in boys, in the dominant extremity, and usually between the ages of 7 and 12 years.[35] Radiographs demonstrate abnormalities of the capitellum. Treatment includes inflammation control, rest, and activity modification. The prognosis is good but healing may require a prolonged period. Residual deformity is rare.

■ Osteomyelitis

Chief Clinical Characteristics
This presentation typically involves a rapid onset of symptoms including general malaise, high fever, chills, severe constant pain, swelling, and tenderness over the metaphysis of the involved bone. The limb is painful with any movement, which leads to an appearance of paralysis in infants. The older child with this condition may refuse to use the affected limb.[26,27]

Background Information
Osteomyelitis occurs most frequently from birth to 5 years old and is rarely found in the elbow. The disease occurs 2.5 times more commonly in males than in females.[36] In some cases the infection starts in the bony metaphysis and spreads to an adjacent joint, creating a septic arthritis. It is caused by an infection in the bone secondary to a minor injury with the most common causative bacterium being *Staphylococcus aureus*.[27,36] Treatment includes aspiration, antibiotics, immobilization of the affected area, and surgical drainage if necessary.

■ Pulled Elbow (Nursemaid's Elbow, Acute Radial Head Subluxation)

Chief Clinical Characteristics
This presentation can be characterized by pain, local tenderness, and the forearm positioned in pronation. The child is typically unwilling to move the elbow and rotation of the forearm will provoke pain.

Background Information
The mechanism of injury is typically axial traction to the extended elbow but less commonly occurs secondary to a fall. Pulled elbow is common in children less than 5 years of age, but occurs most frequently between the ages of 6 months to 3 years. The injury is observed more frequently in girls. Treatment consists of a simple reduction maneuver and immobilization is typically not indicated unless the child has persistent pain.[12] The rate of recurrence ranges around 5%.[37]

■ Radioulnar Synostosis

Chief Clinical Characteristics
This presentation involves restricted forearm pronation and supination. The elbow is typically positioned in midpronation or hyperpronation. Pain is usually not a feature of this condition.

Background Information
This condition occurs equally in males and females and over half of cases are bilateral. Congenital radioulnar synostosis is an uncommon condition with a hereditary predisposition.[13] Unilateral cases present with minimal functional disability. Bilateral cases may require surgical intervention to improve pronation/supination position to enhance function. Although rare, synostosis can also occur between the humerus, radius, and ulna.

■ Septic Arthritis (Pyogenic Arthritis)

Chief Clinical Characteristics
This presentation can be characterized by acute onset and by symptoms that include a high-grade fever, malaise, and pain, with joint involvement including swelling, intra-articular effusion, and warmth. The child will typically hold the elbow in approximately 30 to 60 degrees of flexion with reports of severe pain and muscle spasm on attempting any slight movement.[26,27]

Background Information
Septic arthritis is an infection of the joint usually caused by a cocci bacterial organism, most commonly *Staphylococcus aureus*.[27] Septic arthritis can occur at any age but is most frequently seen in children younger than 3 years of age and is two to three times more frequent in boys than girls.[26,27] The elbow is the third most commonly affected joint and is treated by immediate aspiration and drainage and intravenous administration of antibiotics.[27,36]

■ Systemic Fungal Infection

Chief Clinical Characteristics
This presentation can include pain, tenderness, and swelling over the elbow or the surrounding soft tissues.

Background Information
Exposure and subsequent infection may be insidious in nature, with the majority of those infected asymptomatic. Musculoskeletal involvement is rare; however, lesions of bones and joints result in diffuse soft tissue swelling, bone destruction, and sinus formation. Systemic fungal infections occur most frequently in the young, old, and immunocompromised populations.[27] Treatment includes long-term antibiotics, irrigation, and debridement of the affected area.

TENDINOPATHIES (TENDINITIS)

■ Distal Biceps Tendinitis

Chief Clinical Characteristics
This presentation includes pain and tenderness in the anterior elbow. Reproduction of symptoms will occur with resisted elbow flexion and forearm supination.

Background Information
This is a rare injury in adolescents that may present secondary to weight lifting or carrying heavy loads with flexed elbows. Treatment includes activity modification and inflammation control.

■ Lateral Epicondylitis (Tennis Elbow)

Chief Clinical Characteristics
This presentation includes pain, inflammation, and localized tenderness at the lateral epicondyle. Tenderness may also be present just anterior and distal to the lateral epicondyle at the origin of the extensor carpi radialis brevis. Reproduction of symptoms will occur with resisted wrist extension and passive wrist flexion.

Background Information
This condition is found frequently in adolescent tennis players secondary to the repetitive loading to the extensor carpi radialis brevis tendon, but can also be found in young throwers and swimmers.[4,38] Lateral epicondylitis occurs after skeletal maturation, which happens at approximately fourteen years of age in males and thirteen years of age in females.[9] Treatment includes activity modification, inflammation control, stretching, bracing, and strengthening when inflammation has resolved.

■ Medial Epicondylitis (Golfer's Elbow)

Chief Clinical Characteristics
This presentation involves medial elbow pain and localized tenderness at the common flexor origin. Tenderness may also occur at the proximal flexor and pronator teres muscle bellies. Reproduction of symptoms will occur with resisted wrist flexion, resisted forearm pronation, and passive wrist extension.

Background Information
This condition typically occurs in adolescent throwers and pitchers secondary to overuse and repetitive valgus stress to the elbow during the acceleration phase of their delivery, however it is also found in golfers, tennis players, and gymnasts.[7,9] Epicondylitis versus apophysitis is more likely to occur after closure of the medial epicondyle physis, which occurs at approximately 17 years of age in males and 14 years of age in females.[4] Treatment includes activity modification, inflammation control, and stretching and strengthening when the acute symptoms have subsided.

■ Triceps Tendinitis

Chief Clinical Characteristics
This presentation involves pain, inflammation, and localized tenderness at the insertion of the distal triceps tendon. Reproduction of

symptoms will occur with resisted elbow extension and passive elbow flexion.

Background Information
Triceps tendinitis is more common in older throwers but can present with any repetitive elbow extension in adolescents after skeletal maturation.[4,9] Triceps tendinitis is often associated with other injuries such as loose bodies and osteochondral defects and is typically a result of overuse rather than poor throwing mechanics.[4] Treatment includes activity modification and inflammation control in the acute stage followed by strengthening.

▪ Tuberculosis

Chief Clinical Characteristics
This presentation includes a period of general malaise, poor appetite, loss of weight, and low-grade fever prior to any local symptoms. The initial local symptoms include swelling or interference with function rather than pain. Pain develops gradually in the affected joint and is aggravated by movement and later becomes severe at night.[27]

Background Information
The infecting organism is usually *Mycobacterium tuberculosis* and the primary infection takes place through the lungs, tonsils, or alimentary tract.[27] Unlike acute osteomyelitis, infection is more likely to affect a synovial joint than the shaft of the bone.[27] Tuberculosis of the elbow usually responds to antibiotic treatment; however, sometimes clearance of the disease by surgical excision involving the humerus or the ulna may be needed.

TUMORS

▪ Aneurysmal Bone Cyst

Chief Clinical Characteristics
This presentation typically involves dull pain and swelling.

Background Information
An aneurysmal bone is a benign, vascular lesion. It is frequently seen in individuals during the second decade of life.[39] In 30% of cases, aneurysmal bone cysts occur in association with other benign and malignant tumors.[40] Surgical excision is usually required

and 25% may require additional surgery secondary to recurrence.[41]

▪ Ewing's Sarcoma

Chief Clinical Characteristics
This presentation includes pain and local swelling at the site of the tumor. Constitutional symptoms such as fever and malaise may be present specifically when metastatic disease is present.[42]

Background Information
Ewing's sarcoma is the second most common malignant bone tumor in children and adolescents. These tumors most commonly develop in the axial skeleton, but may arise in any bone, particularly the diaphyses of the humerus and femur. Approximately 25% of patients with this condition may present with overt metastasis, typically in the lungs, bone marrow, or bone.[43] Ewing's tumors are typically sensitive to both chemotherapy and radiotherapy; surgical excision is utilized as well.[44]

▪ Fibromatosis

Chief Clinical Characteristics
This presentation, although highly variable, typically includes an enlarging soft tissue mass associated with localized pain.[45]

Background Information
Fibromatoses represent a group of rare fibroproliferative disorders comprising 12% of soft tissue tumors identified in childhood.[46] Although benign, they are locally invasive and prone to recurrence.[47] Loss of function has been frequently observed in the affected extremity.[45] Surgical excision with a wide margin of resection remains the primary treatment for this condition.

▪ Lipoma

Chief Clinical Characteristics
This presentation involves a small, asymptomatic soft tissue mass.

Background Information
A lipoma is a benign soft tissue neoplasm comprised of adipose tissue. Surgical intervention is indicated in cases where the lipoma interferes with function or becomes symptomatic.

■ Osteoblastoma

Chief Clinical Characteristics
This presentation may include pain that is not significantly relieved by aspirin.

Background Information
Osteoblastoma is an uncommon, benign tumor and usually occurs between the ages of 10 and 25 years.[37] It is more likely to occur in males. The tumor is locally aggressive and requires surgical excision. Recurrence is common.

■ Osteochondroma

Chief Clinical Characteristics
This presentation commonly includes hard swelling adjacent to the involved joint.[37] Elbow motion may be impaired and irritation of the involved tissues may cause pain.

Background Information
Osteochondroma is a very common benign tumor, but is uncommon in the elbow. It can occur at any age but is usually diagnosed in patients younger than 21 years of age.[48] Growth of the tumor usually ceases after the patient has reached skeletal maturity. Surgical excision is indicated for lesions that cause pain or impair motion.

■ Osteoid Osteoma

Chief Clinical Characteristics
This presentation can involve sharp pain that is worse at night and relieved significantly with aspirin.

Background Information
Osteoid osteoma is a relatively common, benign tumor and usually occurs between the ages of 5 and 24 years.[48] It is two times more likely to occur in males. It is a small (1 cm or less) tumor commonly located in long bones. Plain radiographs may fail to reveal the tumor. Treatment consists of surgical excision.

■ Osteosarcoma

Chief Clinical Characteristics
This presentation may be characterized by deep achy pain that is usually mechanical in nature (exacerbated by activity of the extremity),[42] local swelling, and decreased range of motion.[49] Symptoms are often caused by microfractures through the involved area, and in severe cases secondary to stretching and compression of the surrounding structures.[50]

Background Information
Osteosarcoma is the most common primary malignancy of bone in children, but it is rare in the elbow. It typically occurs between 10 and 20 years of age, with the peak age incidence during the adolescent growth spurt.[51] The onset of symptoms is insidious in nature and often related to a minor trauma such as a sports-related injury.[50] Treatment of the tumor requires surgical ablation and adjuvant chemotherapy.

■ Rhabdomyosarcoma

Chief Clinical Characteristics
This presentation includes a mass in an extremity that may or may not be painful. Pain or tenderness may be present if the tumor is displacing a peripheral nerve.

Background Information
Rhabdomyosarcoma is the most common pediatric soft tissue sarcoma, and two-thirds of patients are less than 10 years of age.[50,52] They can develop anywhere in the body but are often found in the extremities. Approximately half the tumors of the limbs are alveolar in nature and are therefore highly metastatic.[53] Treatment typically includes presurgical neoadjuvant chemotherapy, surgical excision, and postsurgical chemotherapy; radiation therapy is used if needed.

References

1. Gomez JE. Upper extremity injuries in youth sports. *Pediatr Clin North Am.* Jun 2002;49(3):593–626, vi–vii.
2. Waters PM. Update on management of pediatric brachial plexus palsy. *J Pediatr Orthop.* Jan–Feb 2005; 25(1):116–126.
3. Cramer KE, Scherl SA, Tornetta P, Einhorn TA. *Pediatrics.* Philadelphia, PA: Lippincott Williams & Wilkins; 2003.
4. Gerbino PG. Elbow disorders in throwing athletes. *Orthop Clin North Am.* Jul 2003;34(3):417–426.
5. Kocher MS, Waters PM, Micheli LJ. Upper extremity injuries in the paediatric athlete. *Sports Med.* Aug 2000;30(2):117–135.
6. Saperstein AL, Nicholas SJ. Pediatric and adolescent sports medicine. *Pediatr Clin North Am.* Oct 1996;43(5): 1013–1033.
7. Zetaruk MN. The young gymnast. *Clin Sports Med.* Oct 2000;19(4):757–780.

8. Rudzki JR, Paletta GA, Jr. Juvenile and adolescent elbow injuries in sports. *Clin Sports Med.* Oct 2004;23(4): 581–608, ix.

9. Reider B. *Sports Medicine: The School-Age Athlete.* 2nd ed. Philadelphia, PA: W. B. Saunders; 1996.

10. Mubarak SJ, Wallace CD. Complications of supracondylar fractures of the elbow. In: Morrey BF, ed. *The Elbow and Its Disorders.* 3rd ed. Philadelphia, PA: W. B. Saunders; 2000.

11. Lins RE, Simovitch RW, Waters PM. Pediatric elbow trauma. *Orthop Clin North Am.* Jan 1999;30(1):119–132.

12. Letts M, Fox J. Elbow and forearm. In: Anderson SJ, Sullivan JA, eds. *Care of the Young Athlete.* Rosemont, IL: American Academy of Orthopaedic Surgeons; 2000: 309–332.

13. Weiner DS, Jones K. *Pediatric Orthopedics for Primary Care Physicians.* 2nd ed. Cambridge: Cambridge University Press; 2004.

14. Letts RM. Dislocations of the child's elbow. In: Morrey BF, ed. *The Elbow and Its Disorders.* 3rd ed. Philadelphia, PA: W. B. Saunders; 2000:261–286.

15. Abraham E. Fractures and dislocations elbow. In: Cramer KE, Scherl SA, Tornetta P, Einhorn TA, ed. *Pediatrics.* Philadelphia, PA: Lippincott Williams & Wilkins; 2003:110–125.

16. Peterson HA. Physeal fractures of the elbow. In: Morrey BF, ed. *The Elbow and Its Disorders.* 3rd ed. Philadelphia, PA: W. B. Saunders; 2000.

17. Early SD, Tolo VT. Pediatric elbow fractures. In: Mirzayan R, Itamura JM, eds. *Shoulder and Elbow Trauma.* New York, NY: Thieme Medical Publishers; 2004:115–131.

18. Case SL, Hennrikus WL. Surgical treatment of displaced medial epicondyle fractures in adolescent athletes. *Am J Sports Med.* Sep–Oct 1997;25(5):682–686.

19. Farsetti P, Potenza V, Caterini R, Ippolito E. Long-term results of treatment of fractures of the medial humeral epicondyle in children. *J Bone Joint Surg Am.* Sep 2001;83-A(9):1299–1305.

20. Flynn JM, Nagda S. Upper extremity injuries. In: Dormans JP, ed. *Pediatric Orthopaedics and Sports Medicine: The Requisites in Pediatrics.* St. Louis, MO: Mosby; 2004.

21. Evans MC, Graham HK. Radial neck fractures in children: a management algorithm. *J Pediatr Orthop B.* Apr 1999;8(2):93–99.

22. Graves SC, Canale ST. Fractures of the olecranon in children: long-term follow-up. *J Pediatr Orthop.* Mar–Apr 1993;13(2):239–241.

23. D'Souza S, Vaishya R, Klenerman L. Management of radial neck fractures in children: a retrospective analysis of one hundred patients. *J Pediatr Orthop.* Mar–Apr 1993;13(2):232–238.

24. McFarland EG, Gill HS, Laporte DM, Streiff M. Miscellaneous conditions about the elbow in athletes. *Clin Sports Med.* Oct 2004;23(4):743–763, xi–xii.

25. Lane H, Audet M, Herman-Hilker S, Houghton S. *Physical Therapy in Bleeding Disorders.* New York, NY: National Hemophilia Foundation; 2004.

26. Cassidy JT, Petty RE. *Textbook of Pediatric Rheumatology.* 4th ed. Philadelphia, PA: W. B. Saunders; 2001.

27. Sharrard SJW. *Paediatric Orthopaedics and Fractures.* 3rd ed. New York, NY: Blackwell Science; 1993.

28. Booth DW, Westers BM. The management of athletes with myositis ossificans traumatica. *Can J Sport Sci.* Mar 1989;14(1):10–16.

29. Beiner JM, Jokl P. Muscle contusion injury and myositis ossificans traumatica. *Clin Orthop Relat Res.* Oct 2002(403 suppl):S110–119.

30. Amillo S, Mora G. Surgical management of neural injuries associated with elbow fractures in children. *J Pediatr Orthop.* Sep–Oct 1999;19(5):573–577.

31. Lyons JP, Ashley E, Hoffer MM. Ulnar nerve palsies after percutaneous cross-pinning of supracondylar fractures in children's elbows. *J Pediatr Orthop.* Jan–Feb 1998;18(1):43–45.

32. Kobayashi K, Burton KJ, Rodner C, Smith B, Caputo AE. Lateral compression injuries in the pediatric elbow: Panner's disease and osteochondritis dissecans of the capitellum. *J Am Acad Orthop Surg.* Jul–Aug 2004;12(4): 246–254.

33. Takahara M, Shundo M, Kondo M, Suzuki K, Nambu T, Ogino T. Early detection of osteochondritis dissecans of the capitellum in young baseball players. Report of three cases. *J Bone Joint Surg Am.* Jun 1998;80(6):892–897.

34. Takahara M, Ogino T, Sasaki I, Kato H, Minami A, Kaneda K. Long term outcome of osteochondritis dissecans of the humeral capitellum. *Clin Orthop Relat Res.* Jun 1999(363):108–115.

35. Shaughnessy WJ. Osteochondritis dissecans. In: Morrey BF, ed. *The Elbow and Its Disorders.* 3rd ed. Philadelphia, PA: W. B. Saunders; 2000.

36. Sonnen GM, Henry NK. Pediatric bone and joint infections. Diagnosis and antimicrobial management. *Pediatr Clin North Am.* Aug 1996;43(4):933–947.

37. Choung W, Heinrich SD. Acute annular ligament interposition into the radiocapitellar joint in children (nursemaid's elbow). *J Pediatr Orthop.* Jul–Aug 1995;15 (4):454–456.

38. Kibler WB, Safran MR. Musculoskeletal injuries in the yound tennis player. *Clin Sports Med.* Oct 2000;19(4): 781–792.

39. Erol B, States, L. Musculoskeletal tumors in children. In: Dormans JP, ed. *Pediatric Orthopaedics and Sports Medicine: The Requisites in Pediatrics.* St. Louis, MO: Mosby; 2004.

40. Erol B, Dormans JP. Tumors. In: Cramer KE, Scherl SA, Tornetta P, Einhorn TA, eds. *Pediatrics.* Philadelphia, PA: Lippincott Williams & Wilkins; 2004:250–270.

41. Pritchard DJ, Unni KK. Neoplasms of the elbow. In: Morrey BF, ed. *The Elbow and Its Disorders.* 3rd ed. Philadelphia, PA: W. B. Saunders; 2000.

42. Gibbs CP, Jr., Weber K, Scarborough MT. Malignant bone tumors. *Instr Course Lect.* 2002;51:413–428.

43. Vlasak R, Sim FH. Ewing's sarcoma. *Orthop Clin North Am.* Jul 1996;27(3):591–603.

44. Himelstein BP, Dormans JP. Malignant bone tumors of childhood. *Pediatr Clin North Am.* Aug 1996;43(4): 967–984.

45. Spiegel DA, Dormans JP, Meyer JS, et al. Aggressive fibromatosis from infancy to adolescent. *J Pediatr Orthop.* Nov–Dec 1999;19(6):776–784.

46. Baerg J, Murphy JJ, Magee JF. Fibromatoses: clinical and pathological features suggestive of recurrence. *J Pediatr Surg.* Jul 1999;34(7):1112–1114.

47. Dormans JP, Spiegel D, Meyer J, et al. Fibromatoses in childhood: the desmoid/fibromatosis complex. *Med Pediatr Oncol.* Aug 2001;37(2):126–131.

48. Copley L, Dormans JP. Benign pediatric bone tumors. Evaluation and treatment. *Pediatr Clin North Am.* Aug 1996;43(4):949–966.

ELBOW PAIN IN A CHILD

49. Widhe B, Widhe T. Initial symptoms and clinical features in osteosarcoma and Ewing sarcoma. *J Bone Joint Surg Am.* May 2000;82(5):667–674.

50. Arndt CA, Crist WM. Common musculoskeletal tumors of childhood and adolescence. *N Engl J Med.* Jul 29 1999;341(5):342–352.

51. Meyers PA, Gorlick R. Osteosarcoma. *Pediatr Clin North Am.* Aug 1997;44(4):973–989.

52. Conrad EU 3rd, Bradford L, Chansky HA. Pediatric soft-tissue sarcomas. *Orthop Clin North Am.* Jul 1996;27(3):655–664.

53. Pappo AS, Shapiro DN, Crist WM. Rhabdomyosarcoma. Biology and treatment. *Pediatr Clin North Am.* Aug 1997;44(4):953–972.

CHAPTER 44

Back Pain in a Child

■ *Munesha Ramsinghani Lona, PT, DPT, PCS* ■ *Josiane Stickles, PT, DPT*

Description of the Symptom

This chapter describes possible causes of back pain in a child, including the region of the posterior body between the eighth rib and posterior superior iliac spines.

Special Concerns
- Changes in functional mobility
- Fever

- Night pain, pain at rest, or unremitting pain
- Unexplained weight loss
- New or evolving neurological symptoms:
  - Abnormal reflexes/posturing
  - Loss of bowel and/or bladder function
  - Sensory changes
  - Radiating pain
- Abdominal tenderness
- Skin rash, tenderness on palpation
- Postural changes

CHAPTER PREVIEW: Conditions That May Lead to Back Pain in a Child

☐ T ☐ Trauma

REMOTE	LOCAL
COMMON	
Not applicable	Muscle strain/overuse syndrome 885 Scheuermann's disease (idiopathic/structural kyphosis) 888 Spondylolisthesis 890 Spondylolysis 890
UNCOMMON	
Not applicable	Fractures: • Burst 881 • Compression 881 • Flexion-distraction 882 • Fracture-dislocations 882 Lumbar radiculopathy 884
RARE	
Not applicable	Slipped vertebral apophysis 889

☐ I ☐ Inflammation

REMOTE	LOCAL
COMMON	
Not applicable	**Aseptic** Juvenile rheumatoid arthritis 883 **Septic** Not applicable

(continued)

Inflammation *(continued)*

REMOTE	LOCAL
UNCOMMON	
Not applicable	**Aseptic** Rheumatoid arthritis–like conditions of the spine: • Juvenile ankylosing spondylitis 886 **Septic** Discitis 880 Tuberculous spondylitis (spinal tuberculosis) 891
RARE	
Aseptic Not applicable **Septic** Acute pelvic inflammatory disease 878 Appendicitis 879 Cholecystitis 879 Pancreatitis 879 Pleuritis (pleurisy) 879 Pyelonephritis 880	**Aseptic** Rheumatoid arthritis–like conditions of the spine: • Arthritis with inflammatory bowel disease 886 • Juvenile dermatomyositis 887 • Psoriatic arthritis 887 • Systemic lupus erythematosus 888 Transverse myelitis 891 **Septic** Meningitis 884 Spinal epidural abscess 889 Vertebral osteomyelitis 895

M   Metabolic

REMOTE	LOCAL
COMMON	
Not applicable	Not applicable
UNCOMMON	
Not applicable	Not applicable
RARE	
Not applicable	Idiopathic juvenile osteoporosis 883 Metabolic bone disease 885 Osteogenesis imperfecta (brittle bone disease) 885

Va   Vascular

REMOTE	LOCAL
COMMON	
Not applicable	Not applicable
UNCOMMON	
Not applicable	Not applicable
RARE	
Not applicable	Hemophilia 882 Sickle cell anemia (crisis) 889

De Degenerative

REMOTE	LOCAL
COMMON	
Not applicable	Not applicable
UNCOMMON	
Not applicable	Not applicable
RARE	
Not applicable	Not applicable

Tu Tumor

REMOTE	LOCAL
COMMON	
Not applicable	Not applicable
UNCOMMON	
Not applicable	*Malignant Primary, such as:* • Ewing's sarcoma 892 • Leukemia 893 • Lymphoma 893 • Osteosarcoma (osteogenic sarcoma) 895 *Malignant Metastatic:* Not applicable *Benign:* Not applicable
RARE	
Malignant Primary, such as: • Nephroblastoma (Wilms' tumor) 880 *Malignant Metastatic:* Not applicable *Benign:* Not applicable	*Malignant Primary:* Not applicable *Malignant Metastatic, such as:* • Astrocytoma 892 • Neuroblastoma 894 • Rhabdomyosarcoma 895 *Benign, such as:* • Aneurysmal bone cyst 891 • Langerhans' cell histiocytosis 892 • Osteoblastoma 894 • Osteoid osteoma 894

Co Congenital

REMOTE	LOCAL
COMMON	
Not applicable	Not applicable
UNCOMMON	
Not applicable	Not applicable
RARE	
Not applicable	Joint hypermobility syndrome 883

Ne Neurogenic/Psychogenic

REMOTE	LOCAL
COMMON	
Not applicable	Not applicable
UNCOMMON	
Not applicable	Psychosomatic back pain 886
RARE	
Not applicable	Not applicable

Note: These are estimates of relative incidence because few data are available for the less common conditions.

Common Ages at Which Back Pain Presents in a Child

APPROXIMATE AGE	CONDITION
Birth to 3 Years	Discitis
	Hemophilia
	Langerhans' cell histiocytosis
	Meningitis
	Metabolic bone disease
	Neuroblastoma
	Pleuritis
	Pyelonephritis
	Spinal epidural abscess
	Transverse myelitis
	Tuberculous spondylitis
	Vertebral osteomyelitis
	Wilms' tumor
Preschool (3–5 Years)	Appendicitis
	Astrocytoma
	Discitis
	Joint hypermobility syndrome
	Langerhans' cell histiocytosis
	Leukemia
	Lymphoma
	Meningitis
	Neuroblastoma
	Pleuritis
	Pyelonephritis
	Rhabdomyosarcoma
	Vertebral osteomyelitis
	Wilms' tumor
Elementary School (6–11 Years)	Aneurysmal bone cyst
	Appendicitis
	Astrocytoma
	Discitis
	Ewing's sarcoma
	Fractures
	Hemophilia
	Idiopathic juvenile osteoporosis
	Joint hypermobility syndrome
	Juvenile dermatomyositis
	Langerhans' cell histiocytosis

Common Ages at Which Back Pain Presents in a Child—cont'd

APPROXIMATE AGE	CONDITION
	Leukemia
	Lymphoma
	Meningitis
	Osteoblastoma
	Osteogenesis imperfecta
	Osteoid osteoma
	Osteosarcoma
	Pleuritis
	Rhabdomyosarcoma
	Sickle cell anemia
	Spondylolisthesis
	Spondylolysis
	Systemic lupus erythematosus
Middle School (12–14 Years)	Aneurysmal bone cyst
	Appendicitis
	Ewing's sarcoma
	Fractures
	Hemophilia
	Lumbar radiculopathy
	Idiopathic juvenile osteomyelitis
	Joint hypermobility syndrome
	Juvenile dermatomyositis
	Juvenile rheumatoid arthritis
	Langerhans' cell histiocytosis
	Leukemia
	Lymphoma
	Muscle strain/overuse syndrome
	Osteoblastoma
	Osteogenesis imperfecta
	Osteoid osteoma
	Osteosarcoma
	Pancreatitis
	Psychosomatic back pain
	Scheuermann kyphosis
	Sickle cell anemia
	Slipped vertebral apophysis
	Spondylolisthesis
	Spondylolysis
	Transverse myelitis
High School (15–18 Years)	Acute pelvic inflammatory disease
	Aneurysmal bone cyst
	Appendicitis
	Cholecystitis
	Ewing's sarcoma
	Fractures
	Hemophilia
	Lumbar radiculopathy
	Idiopathic juvenile osteomyelitis
	Joint hypermobility syndrome
	Juvenile ankylosing spondylitis
	Juvenile dermatomyositis
	Juvenile rheumatoid arthritis
	Leukemia
	Lymphoma

Continued

Common Ages at Which Back Pain Presents in a Child—cont'd

APPROXIMATE AGE	CONDITION
	Meningitis
	Muscle strain/overuse syndrome
	Psoriatic arthritis
	Osteoblastoma
	Osteogenesis imperfecta
	Osteoid osteoma
	Osteosarcoma
	Pancreatitis
	Psychosomatic back pain
	Scheuermann's kyphosis
	Sickle cell anemia
	Slipped vertebral apophysis
	Spondylolisthesis
	Spondylolysis
	Transverse myelitis

Overview of Back Pain in a Child

There are differing points of view on whether reports of back pain in children should be taken seriously. Studies have shown that back pain is common in about 34% to 60% of children.[1,2] Some research has shown that at least 50% of children with back pain have a significant spinal disease,[3] while other research[4] has found that less than 30% are diagnosed with spinal disease. Reports of back pain are generally not as serious as previously thought; however, they still require careful consideration. The patient's history and pain pattern are extremely important.

The spine and related structures of a child differ significantly from those of an adult and this should affect how the physical therapist evaluates and treats the child with back pain. Unlike in adults, vascular channels are present in children that connect the cartilaginous growth plate to the nucleus pulposus, allowing direct invasion of infectious organisms.[5] The pediatric spine has increased hydration of the intervertebral disks, incomplete ossification of vertebrae, the presence of ring apophyses, and increased elasticity and ligamentous laxity resulting in greater flexibility. Younger children also tend to be relatively weaker than adults, especially in the abdominal region, resulting in increased lordosis. In trauma the increased elasticity of the ligaments and muscles may allow for neurological damage even in the presence of normal radiographs.[6]

Description of Conditions That May Lead to Back Pain in a Child

Remote

■ Acute Pelvic Inflammatory Disease

Chief Clinical Characteristics
This presentation commonly includes lower abdominal pain in adolescents, associated with dull, constant, and poorly localized pain. Many adolescents will also demonstrate emotional distress because of the unknown source or cause of pain.[7] Other symptoms such as abnormal vaginal discharge, fever, pain in the right upper quadrant, painful intercourse, and irregular menstrual bleeding can occur as well.

Background Information
The U.S. Centers for Disease Control and Prevention now recommends that only one of the following criteria be identified to confirm the diagnosis: adnexal (pertaining to the uterus appendages), cervical motion, or uterine tenderness.[8] This condition is caused by a bacterial infection in the upper genital tract, most commonly associated with sexually transmitted infections such as gonorrhea and chlamydia. Each year 1 million adolescents in the United States will become infected, with the most prevalence in women between 15 and 23 years of age.[9] Treatment typically includes aggressive antibiotics and hospitalization. If left untreated, this condition often leads to

more serious problems such as infertility, ectopic pregnancy, and chronic pelvic pain.

■ Appendicitis

Chief Clinical Characteristics

This presentation typically involves pain in the middle of the abdomen, near the navel, that gradually moves to the lower right area of the abdomen. Pain is often accompanied by nausea with vomiting and fever. Tenderness in the right lower quadrant, specifically rebound tenderness, is a component for diagnosis confirmation.

Background Information

Diagnosis is difficult in young children, a factor contributing to perforation rates of 30% to 60% in this population. Approximately 80,000 children experience this condition in the United States annually, a rate of 4 per 1,000 children younger than 14 years of age. The incidence of this condition increases with age, peaking in adolescence and rarely occurring in children younger than 1 year old. Diagnosis is confirmed by detailed abdominal examination. Laboratory evaluation may include complete blood cell count and urinalysis. Ultrasound and computed tomography will reveal an enlarged appendix. Treatment requires immediate surgical removal of the appendix.[10]

■ Cholecystitis

Chief Clinical Characteristics

This presentation typically involves right upper quadrant or epigastric pain, nausea, vomiting, fever, and jaundice. Right upper quadrant guarding and tenderness are present. Pain may radiate to an area just below the right scapula.

Background Information

This condition refers to inflammation or infection of the gallbladder. In children, it is usually caused by an underlying infection. It can also be a result of gallstones causing an obstruction of the gallbladder ducts. This condition is rare in otherwise healthy children. It occurs more commonly in children with various other predisposing conditions such as chronic hemolytic disease (ie, sickle cell anemia), obesity, ileac disease, cystic fibrosis, chronic liver disease, Crohn's disease, prolonged parenteral nutrition, premature birth with complicated medical or surgical course,

prolonged fasting or rapid weight reduction, treatment for childhood cancer, abdominal surgery, and pregnancy. Laparoscopic cholecystectomy is commonly performed in symptomatic infants and children. In cases of obstructive jaundice and pancreatitis, endoscopic retrograde cholangiography with stone extractions is also performed.[11]

■ Pancreatitis

Chief Clinical Characteristics

This presentation can include back pain in combination with abdominal pain, persistent vomiting, and fever. Thoracolumbar pain is more commonly reported in older children and adolescents with this condition, and younger children commonly report primary symptoms of abdominal pain and vomiting. The pain is epigastric and steady, often resulting in the child assuming an antalgic position with hip and knees flexed, sitting upright, or lying on the side to alleviate pain. Lying supine and extension of the spine aggravate the symptoms of pain. Children with this condition will also be very uncomfortable and irritable. The abdomen may be distended and tender; a mass may be palpable.

Background Information

This condition is the most common pancreatic disorder in children. Blunt abdominal injuries, mumps and other viral illnesses, multisystem disease, congenital anomalies, and biliary microlithiasis account for most known etiologies. Many cases are of unknown etiology or are secondary to a systemic disease process. Diagnosis can be established by measuring the serum amylase and amylase isozyme levels. Treatment is focused on alleviating pain and restoring metabolic homeostasis. Pain medication is prescribed and fluid electrolyte and mineral balance should be maintained.[12]

■ Pleuritis (Pleurisy)

Chief Clinical Characteristics

This presentation typically involves a dull ache localized over the chest wall and is referred to the shoulder or the back. If pleuritis is caused by pleural effusion, the primary symptom is pain, which is exaggerated by deep breathing, coughing, and straining. Pain with breathing accounts for grunting and guarding of respiration, and children with this condition will often lie on the affected side in an attempt to decrease respiratory excursions.

Background Information
The most common causes of this condition in children are bacterial pneumonia, heart failure, rheumatological causes, and metastatic intrathoracic malignancy. A variety of other diseases account for the remaining cases, including tuberculosis, lupus erythematosus, aspiration pneumonitis, uremia, pancreatitis, subdiaphragmatic abscess, and rheumatoid arthritis. Boys and girls are affected equally. Diagnosis is confirmed upon radiographic examination, and often a pleural tap is performed to examine the exudates of pleural effusion. Treatment is dependent on the underlying disease. Antibiotics are often prescribed when the underlying pleural effusion is caused by bacterial pneumonia. When large amounts of fluid are present, the fluid can be drained to make the patient more comfortable.[13]

■ Pyelonephritis

Chief Clinical Characteristics
This presentation commonly includes chills, fever, pain in the lower part of the back on either side, malaise, nausea, vomiting, and occasionally diarrhea. Some newborns and infants may show nonspecific symptoms such as jaundice, poor feeding, irritability, and weight loss. About one-third of individuals with this condition also have symptoms of cystitis, including frequent, painful urination. One or both kidneys may be enlarged and tender, with tenderness felt in the flank on the affected side.

Background Information
This condition is a form of urinary tract infection occurring in the upper urinary tract. Involvement of the renal parenchyma is called acute pyelonephritis, whereas if there is no parenchymal involvement, the condition may be called pyelitis. The term *cystitis* is used when there is bladder involvement. Urinary tract infections occur in 3% to 5% of girls and 1% of boys. In girls, the first urinary tract infection usually occurs by the age of 5 years, with peaks during infancy and toilet training. After the first urinary tract infection, 60% to 80% of girls will develop a second urinary tract infection within 18 months. In boys, most urinary tract infections occur during the

first year of life. The prevalence of urinary tract infections varies with age. Diagnosis is confirmed usually by urine culture and common course of treatment is with a wide spectrum of antibiotics.[14]

TUMORS

■ Nephroblastoma (Wilms' Tumor)

Chief Clinical Characteristics
This presentation typically includes an asymptomatic, nontender mass in the abdomen. Associated symptoms may be abdominal pain, fever, nausea, and vomiting. Hematuria, anemia, and hypertension can occur, since the kidneys are instrumental in controlling blood pressure. Shortness of breath may be present if metastases to the lungs are present.[15,16]

Background Information
This condition involves a tumor that originates from renal precursor cells. It is the second most common abdominal tumor in infants and children up to 5 years old and is the most common primary malignant tumor of the kidney. Multiple laboratory tests, including complete blood count, ultrasound, magnetic resonance imaging, or computed tomography, are indicated. Treatment includes removal of the kidney containing the tumor followed by chemotherapy and/or radiation. The survival rate is typically 70% to 95%, especially in young children, or those with stage I, II, or III tumors.[15] Recurrences are usually seen within 3 years. Postradiation scoliosis may follow in the second decade.

Local

■ Discitis

Chief Clinical Characteristics
This presentation consists of back pain as a presenting symptom in approximately 50% of children with discitis. Children under 3 years of age often will refuse to bear weight on lower extremities or will limp during ambulation. Infants may refuse to crawl or sit up. Children ages 3 to 8 years of age may also avoid other activities and report having vague abdominal and back pain. Older children and adolescents may report abdominal pain that is usually

localized to the thoracolumbar region of the lumbar spine (although discitis is rare in this particular age group).[17] They may also report leg and buttock pain due to nerve root irritation. In all age groups, a low-grade fever may be present. Commonly there are spasms of the paravertebral musculature, decreased range of motion of the spine, and tightness of the hamstrings. Children will tend to keep their back stiff and rigid during walking and squatting activities, avoiding fluid motion of the spine. Children will often maintain a flexed position. If left untreated, the pain can progress such that the only position of relief is supine.[5]

Background Information

This condition is an inflammation, irritation, and swelling of the intervertebral disk space or vertebral end plate. This is an uncommon condition usually seen in children younger than 10 years of age. It can be caused by a bacterial or viral infection or other inflammatory process, such as autoimmune diseases. The lumbar disks are most commonly affected, followed by the thoracic spine.[18] Laboratory studies include a complete blood workup; however, children with discitis will often have normal white blood cell counts and be afebrile, demonstrating no systemic symptoms.[19] *Staphylococcus aureus* is the most common source of infection for children with discitis. X-rays will reveal changes in the disk space and end plates of vertebral bodies. Magnetic resonance imaging will assist with early diagnosis and assist in differentiating discitis from other infectious disease processes. Nonsurgical treatment includes immobilization with a thoracolumbar orthosis and rest. Antibiotic treatment is often added to ensure eradication of the infection. If the child continues to have symptoms and is not showing signs of improvement, surgical drainage may be necessary. If left untreated, the infection can spread to adjacent vertebral bodies, progressing to vertebral osteomyelitis. Children presenting with symptoms of septic discitis should be referred to a physician for evaluation and treatment. Treatment includes an intensive course of antibiotics, immobilization of the affected spine, and rest. Immobilization with a brace, cervicothoracic orthosis, or halo may help prevent deformity and aid in pain relief. Surgery is indicated to drain abscesses

causing sepsis and to stabilize structures at risk for deformity causing neurological damage.[5]

FRACTURES

■ Burst

Chief Clinical Characteristics

This presentation includes acute back pain in the region of injury that will depend on the severity of the injury, limitations in movement, and tenderness on palpation. With severe injury neurological signs may be present as a result of spinal cord compression.

Background Information

These fractures are rare in children, accounting for approximately 10% of thoracolumbar fractures with a mean age of 14 years.[20] Burst fractures are a result of axial compression combined with flexion and involve the anterior and middle column structures. With severe injury the posterior longitudinal ligament can be damaged, resulting in instability and potential neurological injury.[21,22] Radiographs will show less than 50% of anterior vertebral body collapse and less than 35-degree kyphosis with a stable injury.[22] There may also be bone fragment in the spinal canal from the middle column and a vertical laminar fracture. A computed tomography scan will show disruption of the anterior and posterior vertebral ring. For stable fractures treatment includes immobilization with hyperextension casting or bracing. Unstable injuries and the presence of neurological symptoms may require surgical intervention including internal fixation and decompression.

■ Compression

Chief Clinical Characteristics

This presentation includes acute back pain in the region of injury that will depend on the severity of the injury, limitations in movement, and tenderness on palpation. With severe injury neurological signs may be present as a result of spinal cord compression.

Background Information

These fractures are uncommon injuries in children and adolescents, but child abuse results in about 3% of spinal fractures in children, typically at the thoracolumbar junction.[20,23] An axial compression fracture can occur at any age and is typically a result of severe trauma such as a fall on the buttocks. In the absence of trauma, vertebral compression fractures may also be found in children with osteopenia and hepatoblastoma.[14] Radiographs will show decreased anterior vertebral height and computed tomography scan may show anterior end-plate fracture with intact posterior wall. Symptoms may be relieved with casting or bracing in extension to allow healing.

■ Flexion-Distraction

Chief Clinical Characteristics
This presentation includes acute back pain in the region of injury that will depend on the severity of the injury, limitations in movement, and tenderness on palpation. With severe injury neurological signs may be present as a result of spinal cord compression.

Background Information
Flexion-distortion fractures are more common in children than burst and compression fractures, and result in tension failure of the middle and posterior columns with intact anterior longitudinal ligament.[21] A variant of this injury is a Chance fracture, which is a transverse fracture through the posterior and middle vertebral body. Flexion-distraction injuries typically occur as a result of motor vehicle accidents secondary to seat-belt restraints that are designed for adults. In a child the lap restraint tends to rest across the abdomen, creating a fulcrum for distraction when the child is thrown forward into flexion during a head-on collision.[20,22] Incidence of this injury is unknown; however, occurrences are increasing with mandatory use of restraints. If the child presents with the classic lap-belt sign across the abdomen, flexion-distraction should be suspected. Posterior element injury may not be appreciated in plain radiographs and therefore the child may be diagnosed only with a compression fracture.[20] A high incidence of intra-abdominal trauma is associated with a flexion-distraction injury and should be assessed and treated accordingly. Treatment includes hyperextension casting or bracing. Surgical intervention is reserved for vertebral body involvement and typically involves posterior fusion with compression instrumentation for stability. For those without surgical intervention, progressive kyphosis can occur.[20]

■ Fracture-Dislocations

Chief Clinical Characteristics
This presentation includes acute back pain in the region of injury that will depend on the severity of the injury, limitations in movement, and tenderness on palpation. With severe injury neurological signs may be present as a result of spinal cord compression. Fracture-dislocations are highly unstable injuries that involve failure of all three columns of the spine, which are disrupted by any combination of compression, tension, rotation, or shear.[21,22]

Background Information
The most common method of injury is flexion with axial compression. The child may present with neurological signs if there is cord compression following severe fracture-dislocation. The child should undergo a complete neurological examination and a computed tomography or magnetic resonance imaging scan to determine the extent of central cord involvement if any due to the malalignment of the vertebral bodies. Life-threatening intra-abdominal injuries and rib fractures are typically present with fracture-dislocation and should be assessed and treated appropriately. Treatment can include immobilization, traction, internal fixation into hyperextension, or vertebral fusion if the fracture-dislocation is unstable. If there is injury to the spinal cord, the child should be managed with an intensive multidisciplinary rehabilitation approach.[20–22,24]

■ Hemophilia

Chief Clinical Characteristics
This presentation commonly involves pain and restricted movement in the lumbar spine in combination with symptoms in the hinge joints of the elbow, knee, and ankle; muscle pain in the gastrocnemius, iliopsoas, or forearm; and an absence of fever. Neurological deficits may occur several hours to days after hemorrhage depending on the severity of the hemorrhage.

Background Information
Usually a known diagnosis of hemophilia will prompt clinicians to investigate this condition as

a diagnostic possibility. However, in cases of a mild form of the disease process or in younger children who have not yet been diagnosed, a careful history that may lead a clinician to believe the child may have a blood clotting disorder should also make the clinician suspicious of the possibility of spontaneous spinal epidural hematoma (SSEH) when a child presents with back pain. This term is used to collectively identify several X-linked disorders of blood coagulation. The most common of these are Factor VIII deficiency, or hemophilia A, comprising 80% to 90% of the population with hemophilia. The next most common is Factor IX deficiency, also known as hemophilia B.[25] These factors are necessary precursors for the blood clotting process to occur to stop bleeding. Uncontrolled bleeding can occur in organ systems, the central nervous system, muscle tissue, and most frequently in joint spaces. The most common hemorrhage is spinal epidural hematoma. Spontaneous spinal epidural hematoma is rare in children; the cervicothoracic region is the most common site.[26] The diagnosis of SSEH is confirmed by magnetic resonance imaging. Treatment includes administration of factor replacement and rest. Generally, children have good neurological outcome and the hematoma resolves after factor therapy is administered. Surgical treatment is reserved for severe cases and is considered for intractable or progressive cases.[27]

■ Idiopathic Juvenile Osteoporosis

Chief Clinical Characteristics
This presentation may be characterized by low back pain in combination with long bone and joint pain due to spontaneous vertebral fractures and to spinal deformities, primarily kyphosis.

Background Information
This condition is very rare, with multiple causes related to consequences of primary endocrine, gastrointestinal, bone marrow, connective tissue, or developmental diseases. Onset is typically before puberty.[28] This condition is a diagnosis of exclusion, and it is made when no obvious underlying cause can be detected.

■ Joint Hypermobility Syndrome

Chief Clinical Characteristics
This presentation commonly includes arthralgia, abnormal gait, joint deformity, and back pain. Developmental history may reveal delayed walking (~15 months of age). Children may be considered "clumsy" or having poor coordination.[29] Examination of joints may reveal hypermobility, most commonly in knees, elbows, wrist, hand metacarpophalangeal joints, and ankles.

Background Information
This condition may result from ligamentous laxity, which is inherent and determined by genes that encode for collagen, elastin, fibrillin, and tenascin. Most people who present with only joint hypermobility have no symptoms or ill effects. Children are diagnosed with this condition when the musculoskeletal symptoms of pain persist greater than 12 weeks and when there is exercise-induced pain and exercise intolerance with joint hypermobility. Benign joint hypermobility syndrome is said to exist provided that patients do not have signs of any other rheumatic, neurological, skeletal, or metabolic disease, such as Ehlers-Danlos syndrome or Marfan's syndrome. Physical therapy is indicated, including strengthening of musculature surrounding hypermobile joints, education about joint protection, and pain management techniques.[30]

■ Juvenile Rheumatoid Arthritis

Chief Clinical Characteristics
This presentation may include generalized back pain, accompanied by peripheral joint pain of affected joints: knees, ankles, elbows, wrist, and hands. Initial symptoms often include morning stiffness of affected joints; easy fatigability, particularly after school in the early afternoon; joint pain later in the day; and joint swelling. Arthritis is evidenced by joint swelling or effusion and the presence of two or more of the following signs: heat, limitation of range of motion, and tenderness or pain on motion. Symptoms must persist for a minimum of 6 weeks. Typically, joints of the extremities are affected; however, the spine may also be affected. Back pain associated with this condition may be the result of spinal involvement or habitual posture secondary to pain.

Background Information
This condition is one of the most common rheumatic diseases of children and a major

cause of chronic disability. The etiology of juvenile rheumatoid arthritis (JRA) is unknown; however, it is believed to be an autoimmune response against cells in the joint fluid. The end result of the autoimmune response can include adhesions and osteophyte proliferation in the joint space, fibrosis of surrounding tissue (tendons and ligaments) resulting in contracture, and scarring of the underlying bone, causing the joint shape to be irregular.[31] It affects the cervical spine more often than it affects the joints of the thoracic and lumbar spine.[32] The age of onset is set younger than 16 years to distinguish this condition from adult-onset disease. Complications of major concern are acute iritis and uveitis leading to blindness. These complications are seen most often in those children with the pauciarticular form of this condition. Because no definitive laboratory tests are available to identify JRA, the diagnosis is made by exclusion of other rheumatic diseases or diagnoses such as joint infections, trauma, malignancies, or systemic illnesses, depending on the presenting symptoms. Medical management includes a variety of oral medications used to control joint inflammation such as nonsteroidal antiinflammatory drugs, antirheumatic drugs, and glucocorticoids. Intra-articular injections of glucocorticoids may be used to target single joints. In some severe cases, surgical intervention may be indicated for soft tissue releases, synovectomies, osteotomies, and arthroplasty.

■ Lumbar Radiculopathy

Chief Clinical Characteristics

This presentation includes back pain with radiation to the lower extremity, positive Lasègue's sign,[33] decreased lumbar range of motion, lumbar muscle spasm, gait abnormalities, scoliosis, hyperlordosis, and lower extremity sensory changes.[33,34] Unlike adults, children do not typically present with abnormal reflexes or lower extremity weakness.

Background Information

Lumbar radiculopathy varies in severity with the severity of disk herniation. The direction of herniation is usually posterolateral or posterior. In adolescents, the protruding disk material is more fibrous and secured to the cartilaginous plate and, therefore, appears more like a fracture of fibrocartilage.[33] Lumbar radiculopathies rarely occur in children and adolescents, and are usually the result of cumulative trauma rather than a single episode as in adults. Adolescents account for only 1% to 4% of reported herniations.[1,35] Often there is a family history of lumbar disk disease. Sacralization of the fifth lumbar vertebrae is frequently accompanied by low back pain and disk herniation proximal to the transitional vertebra. Radiographs rarely show loss of intervertebral disk height and, therefore, a magnetic resonance imaging or computed tomography scan should be obtained. The most common levels are L4–L5 and L5–S1.[1,36] Most patients respond well to conservative treatment that includes rest, nonsteroidal anti-inflammatory drugs, and gradual return to activities. Surgical treatment is usually reserved for those with positive nerve tension signs, persistent abnormal sensation and reflexes, lower extremity weakness, and sciatic pain. Excision of the intervertebral disk may be necessary, and in rare cases of spinal instability, fusion may be indicated.[34]

■ Meningitis

Chief Clinical Characteristics

This presentation can be characterized by back pain associated with systemic infection and meningeal irritation including fever, nausea, altered level of consciousness, irritability, lethargy, anorexia, poor appetite, symptoms of upper respiratory tract infection, myalgias, arthralgias, tachycardia, hypotension, and various cutaneous signs. Most commonly, this condition is preceded by several days of fever accompanied by upper respiratory tract or gastrointestinal symptoms, followed by the previously mentioned, nonspecific symptoms.[37] Other possible signs include nuchal rigidity (stiff neck), positive Kernig's sign (flexion of the hip to 90 degrees with subsequent pain upon passive extension of the hip), and positive Brudzinski sign (involuntary flexion of the knees and hips after passive flexion of the neck in supine). Positive Brudzinski and Kernig's signs are not consistently present in all children, especially children younger than 12 to 18 months old. Acute forms of this condition can present in a dramatic fashion with sudden onset and rapid progression, frequently leading to death within 24 hours. Rarely, the presentation involves decreased level of consciousness, seizure activity, and purpura (unblanchable lesion caused by bleeding in the skin).

Background Information
This condition is an infection of the meninges, the outer covering of the spinal cord and brain. The infection can be due to bacteria, virus, or protozoa. In 1986, there was a significant decrease in meningitis caused by certain strains due to the implementation of universal immunization against these certain bacterium. Major risk factors are lack of immunity to specific pathogens associated with young age, nonimmunization, and being in close contact with infected people (household, day care centers, and schools). Transmission of the disease is via person-to-person contact with respiratory tract secretions or droplets. Fifty-five percent of those diagnosed with meningitis are younger than 19 years of age and incidence is higher among children younger than 2 years of age.[38,39] Diagnosis is confirmed by blood culture analysis and cerebrospinal fluid collected by lumbar puncture. Electroencephalography, magnetic resonance imaging, and computed tomography give valuable information regarding brain function and swelling. Antibiotics are most commonly used as treatment for meningitis originating from bacteria. Corticosteroids may also be used in conjunction to reduce the resulting edema that may produce additional neurological injury. A large portion of the treatment will focus on supportive care of the secondary problems resulting from the infection (pain, cardiovascular insufficiency, and decreased kidney function). Children and adolescents presenting with back pain and other symptoms of this condition should immediately be referred to their primary care physician.

■ Metabolic Bone Disease

Chief Clinical Characteristics
This presentation commonly includes radial metaphysic, femoral neck, and lumbar vertebrae fractures in an infant.

Background Information
The risk for fracture is high; however, very few infants present with these fractures due to decreased amounts of movement at this age. This condition is also known as osteopenia of prematurity; it occurs in very low birth weight infants (<1,500 g) and in infants born preterm (<32 weeks gestation). The rate of osteopenia is inversely related to birth weight and gestational age and correlates to rate of fractures.[40] Infants suspected of having this condition are administered nutritional supplements in the neonatal intensive care units to improve bone strength, which further decreases incidence of fractures. Decreased bone mineral density in the lumbar vertebrae usually resolves by age 3 to 4 years.[41]

■ Muscle Strain/Overuse Syndrome

Chief Clinical Characteristics
This presentation includes pain, muscle spasms, and tenderness. Pain may increase with excessive flexion or extension and rarely radiates.

Background Information
Muscle strains can occur as acute injuries, often from improper technique or from chronic overuse. Injuries occur frequently in children who carry heavy backpacks or wear them improperly, participate in sports requiring excessive motion such as gymnastics, or practice improper body mechanics. Diagnostic tests will be negative and x-rays will be normal. Both resisted contraction and stretching of the affected muscle may reproduce characteristic pain. Treatment includes rest, nonsteroidal anti-inflammatory and muscle relaxant medications, gradual return to activities, and physical therapy.

■ Osteogenesis Imperfecta (Brittle Bone Disease)

Chief Clinical Characteristics
This presentation commonly involves a spectrum of disablement ranging from mild to lethal. Children with milder forms (osteogenesis imperfecta [OI] type I) sustain vertebral fractures usually after mild to moderate trauma, such as falls when learning to walk. This risk of fracture decreases after puberty. Children with moderate to severe forms (OI types III and IV) may be born with vertebral fractures or will sustain several vertebral fractures over their lifetime. Children with this condition commonly have blue sclera, which distinguishes it from other metabolic disease processes.

Background Information
This condition is the most common cause of genetically mediated osteoporosis. Treatment

is aimed at fracture and deformity management. Individuals with this condition are also treated with bisphosphonate agents and intravenous pamidronate to enhance bone mineralization.[42]

■ Psychosomatic Back Pain

Chief Clinical Characteristics
This presentation includes back pain in the absence of a definitive diagnosis of inclusion or exclusion. In children and adolescents whose symptoms seem to exceed the findings and who may be subject to other home or school factors, psychosomatic reactions must be considered. These patients generally report severe symptoms but rarely have positive physical findings. They may report a relatively minor preceding trauma. The patients often report other nonspecific symptoms including headaches, neck pain, shoulder pain, chest pain, fatigue, abdominal pain, limb pain, and difficulty breathing.[26]

Background Information
Of children and adolescents reporting symptoms, 10% to 25% can be of psychosomatic origin.[26,43] The prevalence of this disorder tends to increase with age; adolescents ages 16 to 18 years are more likely to have psychosomatic symptoms. Some studies have also shown a higher prevalence in girls than in boys.[44] The symptoms of neck, shoulder, and back pain were earlier thought to be the result of carrying weight and the frequency of use of backpacks and school bags; however, psychosomatic factors appear to be more strongly related to the occurrence of neck, shoulder, and/or back pain complaints than weight and type of school bag.[45] Diagnostic studies often include administering standardized tests such as the Family Environmental Scale, Brief Symptom Inventory, and Children's Depression Inventory to obtain objective measures and establish a diagnosis. It is also not uncommon to find that another family member has similar problems and that the child has subconsciously taken on those symptoms.[46] A detailed medical evaluation must be completed to rule out organic causes of back pain before the consideration of psychosocial problems as the cause of symptoms. Treatment of these patients includes aggressive psychological treatment and physical therapy.[47]

RHEUMATOID ARTHRITIS–LIKE CONDITIONS OF THE SPINE

■ Arthritis with Inflammatory Bowel Disease

Chief Clinical Characteristics
This presentation involves sacroiliac joint or low back pain and stiffness associated with an acute episode of gastrointestinal upset.

Background Information
Children with this disease are likely to be HLA-B27 positive, suggesting an underlying genetic predisposition. In some cases, when the inflammatory bowel disease is latent, the course of arthritis may be similar to the course of juvenile ankylosing spondylitis.[48,49]

■ Juvenile Ankylosing Spondylitis

Chief Clinical Characteristics
This presentation includes an insidious onset of sacroiliac and/or low back pain and stiffness that may be unilateral or bilateral and difficult to localize initially. Sacroiliitis is the hallmark sign, however, along with spinal pain and stiffness, usually does not manifest until 2 to 5 years after onset. The pain will become more persistent over time, along with gradual loss of spinal mobility and a reduction in normal lumbar lordosis. Symptoms are typically worse at night or in the morning and last at least 30 minutes. In ankylosing spondylitis pain may be relieved with rest or only mild activity. During active disease, systemic symptoms such as fever and weight loss may be present, and the child may refuse to walk. Associated complications may include atlantoaxial subluxation, uveitis leading to blindness, acute iritis, aortic valve insufficiency, decreased vital capacity, neurological complications, and, rarely, gastrointestinal and renal problems.

Background Information
This condition is the most prevalent spondyloarthropathy in children, found primarily in adolescent boys and young men. Onset is usually in the second or third decade of life, but 10% to 20% of those affected will have onset prior to age 16. Only about 25% of children with this disease will present initially with sacroiliac or spinal symptoms.

Peripheral joints are involved in 30% to 50% of patients, usually within the first 10 years of disease. Ankylosing spondylitis is a chronic disease with intermittent periods of remission; it is rarely active persistently. There is no specific laboratory test for ankylosing spondylitis; however, most patients have the presence of HLA-B27 (human leukocyte antigen), elevated erythrocyte sedimentation rate and C-reactive protein level, and absence of rheumatoid factor. Radiographic changes include erosion, sclerosis, and eventually fusion of the sacroiliac joint and vertebrae. Magnetic resonance imaging and computed tomography of the sacroiliac joint may assist with early diagnosis. Enthesitis distinguishes this condition from juvenile rheumatoid arthritis. Individuals with this condition typically begin a course of nonsteroidal anti-inflammatory medications upon diagnosis for pain control. Corticosteroids are used only short term due to associated problems including osteoporosis. Research indicates that treatment with tumor necrosis factor can significantly improve symptoms.[50]

■ Juvenile Dermatomyositis

Chief Clinical Characteristics
This presentation is characterized by a skin rash that may be located on the torso, low back, and buttocks area early on in the disease process. The characteristic skin rash may also be found around the shoulder girdle, extensor surfaces of the arms and legs, medial malleoli of the ankles, and face. Disease onset is often insidious and may include fatigue, low-grade fever, weight loss, irritability, arthralgia, and abdominal pain. Proximal muscle weakness is usually recognized after a median of 2 months.[51] Back pain, although an uncommon symptom of this condition, is often reproduced with palpation of the low back. Although this condition is rare in children, it is the most common of its type.

Background Information
The disease process is triggered by an antigen-driven response, which manifests as a skin rash. In the absence of prompt diagnosis and treatment, the development of myositis with subsequent calcinosis occurs, causing severe limitation of range of motion of involved joints. The onset of proximal weakness is insidious and difficult to recognize. It is often detected by difficulty in everyday activities such as climbing stairs, reaching overhead, going from sitting to standing, and going from the floor to standing.[52] This condition occurs in approximately 1 to 3 children per million every year. The average age of onset is between 6 and 7 years of age with a higher prevalence in girls. Laboratory investigations include blood tests, muscle biopsy, and specific antibody tests. Treatment includes protection from the sun and a possible course of corticosteroids. Physical therapy is indicated with close supervision from the child's rheumatologist and pediatrician. Physical therapy should include passive range of motion and stretching during the disease course. Once active inflammation has resolved, treatment should focus on strengthening deconditioned muscle, regaining range of motion, and performing weight-bearing activities to ensure adequate bone mineralization. Bed rest and immobilization are contraindicated.

■ Psoriatic Arthritis

Chief Clinical Characteristics
This presentation involves psoriatic rash, arthritis, nail pitting, dactylitis (or "sausage digit"), and occasional fatigue. As the disease progresses sacroiliitis is present, resulting in hip and low back pain. In children arthritis may manifest prior to psoriasis, or onset of arthritis and psoriasis is concurrent.

Background Information
Chronic iridocyclitis is seen in approximately 15% of children.[48,49] This condition typically occurs in young girls, usually manifesting between 7 and 13 years of age, but always occurring prior to age 16 years. There is almost always a family history of psoriasis. Radiographs and computed tomography scan will determine extent of involvement of the spine, hips, and sacroiliac joint. Treatment includes nonsteroidal anti-inflammatory medications, corticosteroids, and topical or systemic medications for psoriasis.

Modalities can also be used to control inflammation and pain.

■ Systemic Lupus Erythematosus

Chief Clinical Characteristics

This presentation may initially include musculoskeletal pain in any or all regions of the body including the back in 74% of children,[53] in the presence of fever, fatigue, arthralgia, malar rash, anorexia, lymphadenopathy, pleuritic pain, and seizures.

Background Information

This condition is a rheumatic disease of unknown cause characterized by autoantibodies directed against self-antigens and resulting in inflammatory damage to target organs including kidneys, blood-forming cells, and the central nervous system. The incidence varies by ethnicity and location. Prevalence rates vary from 4 to 250 in 100,000 children. The median age at diagnosis is approximately 10 years, and onset before age 8 is uncommon.[54] Diagnosis is confirmed by the combination of clinical and laboratory manifestations revealing multisystem disease. Treatment regimen depends on the affected target organs. Nonsteroidal anti-inflammatory agents are used to treat arthralgia and arthritic symptoms. Corticosteroids have been demonstrated to control symptoms and autoantibody production in systemic lupus erythematosus. Patients with severe disease may require cytotoxic therapy. When the child is cleared for activity, physical therapy should focus on stretching, joint protection, and relaxation techniques to manage joint and muscle pain. During periods of remission, an exercise program of strengthening and cardiovascular exercise may be implemented to maintain the strength of surrounding musculature and to prevent the detrimental effects of bone demineralization due to prolonged use of corticosteroids.[54] Physical therapy treatment should be provided under supervision of the child's physician. The natural history is unpredictable; patients may present with a history of many years of symptoms or with acute, life-threatening disease. Left untreated, this condition may result in spontaneous remission, years of disease, or rapid death.

■ Scheuermann's Disease (Idiopathic/Structural Kyphosis)

Chief Clinical Characteristics

This presentation includes pain and mild to severe rigid thoracic kyphosis with inability to actively correct the deformity.[34] There is often point tenderness over the apex of deformity, which is usually localized between T_7 and T_9. Neurological complications are rare.

Background Information

This condition results in an increase in the normal kyphotic curvature of the thoracic spine that is rigid. It results in wedge-shaped vertebrae with loss of anterior height.[6,15,34] The problem is typically cosmetic, with mild pain that is localized to the area of the deformity during forward flexion.[1] In many cases of this condition, there is compensatory lumbar lordosis that can be painful. Due to increased lordosis there is a high incidence of spondylolysis due to increased strain on the L_5 pars interarticularis.[1,22] Etiology is unknown; theories include heredity, increased anterior pressure on the vertebrae impairing anterior growth, mechanical weakening, and collagen defects.[34,36] Incidence is approximately 8%, and is most common in adolescent males. Diagnosis is confirmed with lateral standing radiographs that show the vertebral deformities of decreased anterior height, reduced disk space, end-plate irregularities, and Schmorl's nodes, which are thought to be disk herniation into the vertebral body. A consistent criterion is wedging of 5 degrees in three or more adjacent vertebra.[6,55] Radiographs will differentiate Scheuermann kyphosis from postural round back, in which there are no structural changes and which is correctable with hyperextension.[6,34,55] Treatment will vary depending on the degree of deformity and the age of the child. Skeletally mature asymptomatic individuals do not require treatment. Younger children with mild deformity may respond favorably to activity modification and an exercise program emphasizing hyperextension activities to relieve pain and increase flexibility. Physical therapy will not change the structural deformities. Extension bracing may be beneficial in those who are skeletally immature. Surgical correction is reserved for individuals who are skeletally mature and who are symptomatic and have not responded to conservative treatment. This may include anterior and/or posterior spinal fusion with instrumentation.[34,56]

■ Sickle Cell Anemia (Crisis)

Chief Clinical Characteristics

This presentation includes joint pain with possible physical signs in the spine including local tenderness over the spinous process and decreased range of back motion.[57] *Bone changes cause pain due to marrow hyperplasia, tissue ischemia, and infarction due to vaso-occlusion.*

Background Information

This condition results from a point mutation in the genetic code that causes structural changes to the hemoglobin molecule. This structural change decreases the affinity of oxygen to red blood cells, thereby decreasing delivery of oxygen to structures of the body. There are different strains of the disease, depending on the component of genetic code affected, which causes various levels of severity and involvement expressed in the disease process. Newborn infants seldom exhibit features of sickle cell disease; however, it can be diagnosed by blood tests. Clinical manifestations are uncommon prior to age 5 to 6 months. Infants with sickle cell anemia have abnormal immune function, making bacterial sepsis the greatest risk for morbidity and mortality. By age 5, most children will have a painful episode of the small bones of the hands and feet that is believed to be caused by choking off of blood supply as a result of rapidly expanding bone marrow. Depending on the type of sickle cell disease, children may have symptoms ranging from never experiencing any painful episodes to experiencing some pain on nearly a daily basis. Episodes of severe pain requiring hospitalization occur on average one time per year. Young children usually experience pain of the extremities and older children/adolescents are more likely to experience pain in the head, chest, abdomen, and back. Sickle cell anemia affects most of the other organ systems of the body, leading to a variety of complications.[58] Avascular necrosis leading to collapse of vertebral bodies and infective spondylitis are some of the more serious complications of the spine, the majority of which require anterolateral decompression and bone grafting.[59] Treatment of pain caused by sickle cell disease focuses on pain management using nonsteroidal anti-inflammatory drugs and limited use of opiate medication. Other treatments targeting the disease process are aimed at decreasing red blood cell adhesions, increasing cellular hydration, lowering blood viscosity, and elevating hemoglobin levels. Bone marrow transplantation is the only cure for sickle cell disease, but is only an option for children younger than 16 years of age.

■ Slipped Vertebral Apophysis

Chief Clinical Characteristics

This presentation involves low back pain, a positive Lasègue's sign, and motor and sensory signs that correspond with a spinal root distribution.[20,36] *This injury is most common in adolescent boys participating in sports that require repeated heavy lifting.*

Background Information

Injury is usually the result of repetitive axial loading causing the ring apophysis to slip, or even separate, and move into the spinal canal. The majority of these injuries occur at L4–L5 or L5–S1. In young adolescents the ring apophysis is not yet fully ossified and adhered to the vertebral body. Radiographs may show the apophysis fragment within the spinal canal, but this is best viewed with computed tomography or magnetic resonance imaging. Treatment typically requires surgical excision of the fragment, and most patients respond well.[34]

■ Spinal Epidural Abscess

Chief Clinical Characteristics

This presentation commonly includes fever, back pain, and radiculopathy.[60] *The radicular symptoms can progress to weakness and paralysis.*

Background Information

Staphylococcus aureus is the bacteria most commonly responsible for this condition. Children at higher risk include those with diabetes mellitus, and those who have suffered a recent trauma or have recently had a lumbar puncture. This condition most commonly occurs in adults, but also can occur in young infants who have suppressed immune systems.

The main challenge with this condition is achieving early diagnosis before these neurological symptoms occur. Diagnosis in infants can be difficult due to the inconsistent presentation. Older infants and toddlers who are ambulatory may limp or refuse to bear weight on an extremity because of weakness, paraplegia, or paraparesis, indicative of neurological deficits. Magnetic resonance imaging displays the greatest diagnostic accuracy. Lumbar puncture to determine cerebrospinal fluid protein concentration is not indicated for diagnosis because it could lead to bacteria spreading into the subarachnoid space, placing the child at risk for meningitis.[61] Nonsurgical management involves treatment with antibiotics, and this approach often is effective in children diagnosed early in the disease process. In the later stages of the disease process, children with neurological deficits may require surgical intervention in conjunction with local antibiotics. Laminectomy is the most common surgical procedure used to decompress the lesion on the spinal cord. Children suspected of having this condition should immediately be referred for medical evaluation and treatment by a physician.

■ Spondylolisthesis

Chief Clinical Characteristics

This presentation includes low back pain that may radiate to the lower extremities, limitations in range of motion, a positive Lasègue's sign, and tenderness over the lumbar spinous processes with or without a palpable step. Significant hamstring tightness or spasm may result in an abnormal gait pattern with short stride length, flexed knees, and pelvic waddle. Decreased lumbar lordosis, scoliosis, and flattened buttocks may also be present. Neurological signs are rare, but may be present even in low-grade slips secondary to nerve root compression.[6,22,36,62] As with spondylolysis (see next entry), symptoms are usually aggravated by activities that require repetitive flexion and extension such as gymnastics.

Background Information

This condition involves the forward displacement of a proximal vertebra on the one below it, typically as a result of bilateral pars interarticularis defect. The pars defect is not present in congenital spondylolisthesis. The most common site for slippage is the fifth lumbar vertebra on the sacrum. Standing anteroposterior and lateral radiographs are needed to determine the grade of slippage, and an oblique view is necessary to appreciate the pars defect. In high-grade slips with neurological deficits, a complete neurological exam is indicated. Treatment is determined by symptoms, clinical signs, and the grade of slip. Asymptomatic patients do not require intervention. Those with low-grade slips and pain tend to do well with conservative treatment of activity restriction, bracing, and exercises. Fusion is recommended for grade II slips or greater even if they are asymptomatic because they are at risk for further slippage during growth spurts.[22,36] Reduction of the slip is not recommended because of the high risk of neurological injury.[6,22,36] Patients are more prone to recurrent symptoms and clinical deformity if forward slipping is allowed to progress. Progression of slip, delayed union, neuropathy of the fifth nerve root, and cauda equina syndrome have all been reported as postsurgical complications.[22,36]

■ Spondylolysis

Chief Clinical Characteristics

This presentation can include low back pain with hyperextension that rarely radiates, scoliosis, decreased lumbar lordosis, and increased lumbosacral kyphosis.[34] The child will often have hamstring tightness that can affect gait.[1,6] Adolescents participating in sports that require repetitive hyperextension, such as gymnastics, wrestling, and football, appear to be at increased risk.[6] Most children with spondylolysis are asymptomatic or may have symptoms that are mild and therefore often overlooked.

Background Information

This condition is a congenital or acquired defect of the pars interarticularis, the bone between the superior and inferior facets of the vertebrae. An acquired defect would arise as a stress or fatigue fracture of the pars.[1,36] The pars interarticularis defect can occur at any level, most commonly at L5, and can occur unilaterally or bilaterally. A bilateral defect no longer provides posterior stability and may result in forward slippage, especially of L5 over S1, known as spondylolisthesis. Spondylolysis can occur at any age, but is rarely seen before age 10; it appears to be more prevalent in boys. An oblique standing view is the best view to show the pars defect that can easily be overlooked if only anteroposterior and lateral views are taken.[1,22,63] Computed tomography or bone scan is used if radiographs are inconclusive, and single-photon emitted computed tomography will determine if the lesion is acute or chronic.[36] Treatment depends on the degree of the defect and whether the patient is symptomatic. If pain is present in the absence of spondylolisthesis, immobilization with a thoracic-lumbar-sacral orthosis for 3 to 6 months may be most beneficial. Physical therapy should focus on hamstring and lumbar musculature stretching, abdominal strengthening, and monitoring of gradual return to activity. With persistent pain unrelieved by nonsteroidal anti-inflammatory medication, rest, and physical therapy, surgical stabilization can be achieved through posterior spinal fusion.[6,34] Any child with this condition should be followed closely, because they are at risk for progression to spondylolisthesis. Girls tend to have a higher rate of progression.

■ Transverse Myelitis

Chief Clinical Characteristics
This presentation involves sudden onset of severe back pain and progressive symmetric lower extremity numbness and weakness that begins distally. Progression to complete paralysis may take several hours to several days depending on the severity and location of the inflammation. There may also be loss of deep tendon reflexes and bowel and bladder control. Patients often experience tightness in a belt-like fashion around the stomach at the level affected.

Background Information
Onset of symptoms typically follows fever, malaise, and a viral infection, often Lyme disease, or influenza, rubella, mumps, varicella, herpes, or Epstein-Barr viruses. Computed tomography or magnetic resonance imaging is indicated to rule out cord compression, abscess, or neoplasm, and cerebrospinal fluid exam will differentiate transverse myelitis from Guillain-Barré syndrome, meningitis, poliomyelitis, and other infectious diseases. Partial or full spontaneous recovery occurs in most patients, but can take up to several months. High doses of corticosteroids have also been used, however, there is no evidence that they significantly affect outcome.[15,24]

■ Tuberculous Spondylitis (Spinal Tuberculosis)

Chief Clinical Characteristics
This presentation may include pain, tenderness, and weakness in the presence of possible systemic signs including fever, night sweats, anorexia, weight loss, and sensory changes. Neurological deficits are uncommon in children, but if present, may be due to pressure from paravertebral abscess.

Background Information
This condition originates and affects the anterior vertebral bodies in the lower thoracic and upper lumbar spine at onset and may affect the disks in later stages of the disease. In some cases vertebral collapse occurs, resulting in kyphosis. Diagnostic testing includes skin tests, erythrocyte sedimentation rate, histology, and computed tomography. Treatment includes antibiotics, antituberculosis therapy such as pyrazinamide, isoniazid, and rifampin, and in some cases, chemotherapy. Bracing may be necessary to prevent progression of kyphosis. Surgical treatment is usually indicated for abscesses resulting in cord compression, children younger than 15 years of age with kyphosis of at least 30 degrees, and children younger than 10 years with destruction of the vertebral bodies.[22]

TUMORS

■ Aneurysmal Bone Cyst

Chief Clinical Characteristics
This presentation may include chronic back pain and neurological signs due to cord compression; however, these tumors are typically asymptomatic and are usually discovered when a pathological fracture or hemorrhage occurs.

Background Information
This condition involves a highly vascularized mass with fibrous connective tissue.[64] Locally, the lesion can be aggressive and destructive. Rarely, it is found in the sacrum.[65] Peak age of diagnosis is typically between 10 and 20 years of age with a slight female predominance.[64,65] Radiographs

suggestive of this condition will show an expansile, lytic lesion that can involve the entire bone, extending into the vertebral body. There may also be involvement of adjacent vertebral bodies, the intervertebral disks, posterior ribs, and paravertebral soft tissue.[65] Differential diagnosis includes unicameral bone cyst, giant cell tumor, and malignancy. Treatment can include excision or curettage with bone graft, and possible fusion with care to preserve nerve roots.[1,66] Complete resection is not always achieved due to proximity to neurovascular structures. Radiation may also be necessary, but this poses a risk for future radiation-induced sarcomas. Recurrence is generally 20% to 30% and this increases with incomplete resection.[65,67]

■ Astrocytoma

Chief Clinical Characteristics

This presentation includes localized pain, motor weakness, gait abnormalities, stiffness, scoliosis, and sphincter dysfunction. Paresthesia may occur with disease progression. Pain may be exacerbated with coughing or sneezing.

Background Information

This condition refers to a neoplasm of astrocytal origin, which is a type of glial cell. Astrocytomas account for about half of all childhood brain tumors with peak age around 5 to 9 years. These tumors become widespread, infiltrating via cerebrospinal fluid pathways, and therefore are difficult to cure. They are rarely found outside of the central nervous system.[68,69] Approximately 15% of individuals with this condition become hydrocephalic.[36,70] A biopsy is necessary to grade an infiltrating astrocytoma so growth rate can be determined.[68] Spinal lesions are best viewed with magnetic resonance imaging. Low-grade forms of this condition can be surgically excised, although complete resection is difficult. The 5-year survival rate is approximately 65% to 70%. High-grade lesions are best treated with radiation and chemotherapy.[26]

■ Ewing's Sarcoma

Chief Clinical Characteristics

This presentation typically manifests as severe, persistent pain especially at night, localized swelling, palpable mass, tenderness, and decreased range of motion. Other symptoms can include fever, malaise, and weight loss when there are metastases.[71]

Background Information

This condition is the most common malignant primary tumor found in the pediatric spine[56] and the second most common pediatric malignancy overall.[72] Approximately 2.1 children per million are diagnosed with this condition each year with predominance in males. Diagnosis is usually between the ages of 10 and 20 years, and is uncommon before age 5.[72] Treatment includes a combination of multiagent chemotherapy, followed by radiation and resection for local control. Prognosis for cure is approximately 75% in those who present without metastasis, and less than 30% for those with metastasis.

■ Langerhans' Cell Histiocytosis

Chief Clinical Characteristics

This presentation commonly consists of pain that is usually relieved with nonsteroidal anti-inflammatory medications, rest, and, if necessary, bracing. Associated symptoms may be hepatosplenomegaly, anemia, leukopenia, and thrombocytopenia. Neurological symptoms may manifest if there is cord compression.

Background Information

This condition is commonly found in the anterior elements of the spine as a single lesion or is multifocal. A single, localized lesion is also known as eosinophilic granuloma. This condition is generally found in children 3 to 15 years of age with a predominance for white males, but can manifest at any age.[34,64,73] Radiographs will show a well-defined lesion, with focal bone destruction and possible vertebral collapse, or vertebral plana. This condition appears to be the most common cause of vertebral plana.[73] The intervertebral disks are not affected.[73] Treatment is usually reserved for those with organ dysfunction, unrelieved symptoms, or osseous deformity, because this condition is usually self-limiting.[73] Treatment can include a combination of any or all of radiation, chemotherapy, steroid therapy and curettage, and bracing.[64,66]

■ Leukemia

Chief Clinical Characteristics

This presentation commonly involves reports of aches and pains in the back, extremities, and joints; fatigue; and anorexia. There may also be intermittent low-grade fever, enlarged lymph nodes, weight loss, petechiae, lethargy, shortness of breath, bruises, and excessive bleeding.

Background Information

Leukemia is the most common malignancy in children and adolescents, with a higher incidence in males.[16,74] It is typically diagnosed within the first decade of life and accounts for about 40% of all childhood malignancies. The two most common types account for approximately 90% of all leukemias: acute lymphoblastic leukemia (ALL), 77% to 80%, and acute myelogenous leukemia (AML), 10% to 13%. Some symptoms may be consistent with a viral infection, but the symptoms persist longer. Other symptoms are a result of progressive disease and bone marrow failure as a result of bone marrow infiltration by malignant cells, leading to anemia and decreased production of clotting factors.[74] Diagnostic evaluation of patients with leukemia includes complete blood count and bone marrow biopsy. Examination of bone marrow aspirate is necessary for confirmation, and a spinal tap determines if leukemia is present in the central nervous system.[75] Infiltration of bone and bone marrow may also be viewed on magnetic resonance imaging.[64] Rarely radiographs may show osteopenia and compression fractures. Analysis of chromosome abnormalities in the leukemia cells is very important to assess prognosis and formulate treatment. Treatment is specific to the type of leukemia present and typically has several phases. It involves multiple courses of chemotherapy and antibiotics to prevent infection, and often a child will require blood transfusions. Side effects of chemotherapy and steroid treatment include neutropenia, thrombocytopenia, and risk for infection. Long-term complications can include osteoporosis, and avascular necrosis. Bone marrow or stem cell transplant is reserved for situations where standard chemotherapy has failed and has a better success rate if performed in remission.[76] With current advances in treatment the 5-year survival rate, without relapse is reaching 80% to 90%.[77]

■ Lymphoma

Chief Clinical Characteristics

This presentation initially involves asymptomatic, chronically swollen lymph nodes, most commonly in the neck, axillae, or groin. Other symptoms may include neurological symptoms due to cord compression, fever, itching or irritation of the skin, weight loss, night sweats, cough, or shortness of breath.[75] Symptoms depend on the type of lymphoma present and the proximity to other structures and organs.

Background Information

Lymphoma is one of the most prevalent malignant tumors of childhood, and can manifest quickly. The two general types of lymphoma are Hodgkin's lymphoma and non-Hodgkin's lymphoma (NHL), and each has its own subtypes. Hodgkin's disease is distinguished from non-Hodgkin's by the presence of specific cancer cells in the biopsy material, termed Reed-Sternberg cells.[75,78] Approximately 40% of pediatric cases are of the Hodgkin's type, and 60% are non-Hodgkins.[16] Approximately 10% to 15% of all cases of Hodgkin's disease, and about 5% of all NHL cases, are children under age 19, both with a higher prevalence in boys. NHL is more common in children under age 5.[78,79] Biopsy, radiographs, computed tomography, and blood tests are performed for definitive diagnosis and to assess the stage of disease. Bone marrow biopsy is done to evaluate bone marrow involvement. Radiographs and computed tomography typically show enlarged lymph nodes in the affected areas and can show extensive, destructive lesions in patients with osseous involvement. Magnetic resonance imaging is indicated to evaluate soft tissue involvement.[71] Laboratory tests may show anemia and elevated sedimentation rate. Treatment includes chemotherapy and radiation, the course of which depends on the type of lymphoma, the stage of disease, and if there is bone marrow metastasis. Bone marrow transplant may be indicated if there is failure to respond to standard chemotherapy and radiation. Survival rates are 90 to 95% for those with local lesions, and 75 to 80% for those with more diffuse disease.[16]

■ Neuroblastoma

Chief Clinical Characteristic

This presentation may include severe localized back pain, weakness, scoliosis, and neurological signs secondary to spinal cord compression. Other symptoms may include a palpable mass, hepatomegaly, constipation, abdominal pain, bladder dysfunction, and ecchymoses. It is one of the few cancers that cause diarrhea.[16,68,71,80]

Background Information

This condition is a solid tumor that develops in neural crest tissue, most commonly in the abdomen, chest, or adrenal glands.[16] It rarely originates in the brain or spinal cord. If the primary lesion originates somewhere other than the spinal cord, metastases is hematogenic in nature, and can spread to bone, bone marrow, skin, lungs, and the brain. This is the most common extracranial cancer of childhood and the third most common pediatric neoplasm overall. Approximately 500 new cases are diagnosed each year. It is usually diagnosed in infancy, almost always by 5 years of age, and is rarely seen in children over 10 years of age.[16,68,71,80] Low-risk tumors (stage I) in infants treated with surgical excision and observation have an approximately 90% survival rate without relapse. Children over 3 years of age with stage IV tumors only have a 10% to 15% survival rate.[16] In infants the tumor may regress completely with spontaneous cell death or mature to normal ganglion cells and become benign. In children over 1 year of age, the disease progression may be rapidly metastatic and often fatal.[16,68]

■ Osteoblastoma

Chief Clinical Characteristics

This presentation produces night pain that demonstrates limited responsiveness to nonsteroidal anti-inflammatory medications or aspirin.[1,71] *The pain is dull and localized to the affected region of the lumbar spine.*[65] *In addition neurological signs such as paraparesis and paresthesia may be present,*

suggesting cord compression. Scoliosis is rare, but when present, it is typically convex toward the site of the tumor.

Background Information

Although rare, this condition is one of the more common lesions found in the spine, typically in the posterior elements of the lumbar and thoracic vertebrae. They tend to be large, destructive tumors, and may extend into the vertebral bodies and infiltrate soft tissue.[71] Diagnosis is usually between 10 and 20 years of age and there is a 2:1 male predominance.[65] Radiographs show a lucent area with a sclerotic border, and may include multifocal calcifications. Computed tomography will more clearly define the sclerotic borders, while magnetic resonance imaging is optimal for showing central cord compression. Treatment consists of surgical resection with an approximately 10% to 15% recurrence rate.

■ Osteoid Osteoma

Chief Clinical Characteristics

This presentation involves predominantly intense nocturnal pain that may be relieved with nonsteroidal anti-inflammatory medications or aspirin.[1,64] *The pain may be referred or localized. Gait deviations and muscle atrophy are often present. About 50% of children present with nonstructural, painful scoliosis,*[56] *which should be a red flag because idiopathic scoliosis is not painful.*

Background Information

This condition includes highly vascularized connective tissue bundles, usually sclerotic, surrounding an osteoid nidus or growth center. They are small round or ovate tumors that are usually less than 1 cm in diameter.[71,81] Spinal osteoid lesions are found primarily in the posterior elements of the lumbar vertebra.[34,56,64,71,81] Soft tissue changes are rare. This condition is typically found in children between the ages of 5 and 20, with an approximate 2:1 male-to-female ratio.[65,71] Erythrocyte sedimentation rate, leukocyte count, and protein electrophoresis should be normal. Radiographs and computed tomography will also differentiate osteoid osteomas from osteoblastomas, infection, lymphoma, and facet abnormalities such as spondylolysis.[65] Spinal lesions typically require open surgical excision. In most cases, the scoliosis will resolve and pain will subside completely.[62]

■ Osteosarcoma (Osteogenic Sarcoma)

Chief Clinical Characteristics
This presentation may be characterized by persistent night pain.

Background Information
This condition is related to highly malignant and locally aggressive lesions.[82] It rarely originates in the axial skeleton, but when it does it is usually found in the vertebral bodies.[66,67,82] Vertebral sarcomas comprise about 10% of all cases.[56] These tumors are typically found in the metaphyses of long bones and may metastasize to the spine. Diagnosis usually occurs between 10 and 20 years of age, and adolescent growth spurts appear to be the greatest risk periods for development.[64,83] Children with certain hereditary conditions such as retinoblastoma have a significant predisposition for developing this condition. Treatment includes local control with surgical excision and radiation or chemotherapy for metastatic lesions. If neurological signs are present, surgical decompression and laminectomy may be necessary.[22] Without metastasis approximately 70% of cases are cured with surgery and chemotherapy. If metastases are present upon diagnosis, the survival rate is less than 20%.

■ Rhabdomyosarcoma

Chief Clinical Characteristics
This presentation may include back pain associated with neurological signs due to cord compression when present in the lumbar spine.[67,75]

Background Information
This condition is thought to originate from striated skeletal muscle cells.[67] Alveolar rhabdomyosarcoma is typically found in the extremities and in paravertebral soft tissue. Although it is rare, this condition is the most common solid soft tissue tumor in children under 10 years of age, accounting for 5% to 8% of pediatric neoplasms. It is usually diagnosed prior to age 6 and is most prevalent in male infants.[67,71,75] Diagnostic tests include biopsy, computed tomography, and magnetic resonance imaging.[71,75] Treatment includes chemotherapy, radiation, and, if necessary, complete resection. For those diagnosed and treated in the early stages, the survival rate is approximately 80% to 90%.[67,75] Prognosis is poor for those with the alveolar subtype, larger tumors, or who are over 10 years of age.[67,71,75]

■ Vertebral Osteomyelitis

Chief Clinical Characteristics
This presentation commonly includes back pain as a presenting symptom. Children with this condition will tend to keep their back stiff and rigid during walking and squatting activities, avoiding fluid motion of the spine. Children with this condition will often maintain a flexed position. If left untreated, the pain can progress such that the only position of relief is supine.[5] Neurological abnormalities may be present due to cord compression after vertebral collapse. When cervical spine is involved, the child may have symptoms of torticollis or dysphagia.

Background Information
Although this condition and discitis can occur at any age, this condition is more likely to occur in adolescents, and discitis is more commonly seen in children <3 years of age. The final diagnosis is made by radiographic evaluation of the spine and blood work.[17] Also, children who have history of immunocompromise after organ transplant or chemotherapy may be at higher risk for infections such as this.

References
1. Payne WK 3rd, Ogilvie JW. Back pain in children and adolescents. *Pediatr Clin North Am.* Aug 1996;43(4):899–917.
2. Troussier B, Davoine P, de Gaudemaris R, Fauconnier J, Phelip X. Back pain in school children. A study among 1178 pupils. *Scand J Rehabil Med.* Sep 1994;26(3):143–146.
3. Turner PG, Green JH, Galasko CS. Back pain in childhood. *Spine (Phila Pa 1976).* Aug 1989;14(8):812–814.
4. Feldman DS, Hedden DM, Wright JG. The use of bone scan to investigate back pain in children and adolescents. *J Pediatr Orthop.* Nov–Dec 2000;20(6):790–795.
5. Tay BK, Deckey J, Hu SS. Spinal infections. *J Am Acad Orthop Surg.* May–Jun 2002;10(3):188–197.
6. Pierz K, Dormans J. Spinal disorders. In: Dormans JP, ed. *Pediatric Orthopedics and Sports Medicine: The Requisites in Pediatrics.* St. Louis, MO: Mosby; 2004:155, 168.

7. Sacchetti A. Pelvic infections. In: Harwood-Nuss A, ed. *The Clinical Practice of Emergency Medicine*. Philadelphia, PA: Lippincott Williams & Wilkins; 1991.

8. Risser WL, Cromwell PF, Bortot AT, Risser JM. Impact of new diagnostic criteria on the prevalence and incidence of pelvic inflammatory disease. *J Pediatr Adolesc Gynecol*. Feb 2004;17(1):39–44.

9. Igra V. Pelvic inflammatory disease in adolescents. *AIDS Patient Care STDS*. Feb 1998;12(2):109–124.

10. Hartman G. Acute appendicitis. In: Behrman RE, Kliegman RM, Jenson HB, eds. *Nelson Textbook of Pediatrics*. 17th ed. Philadelphia, PA: W. B. Saunders; 2004.

11. Suchy F. Diseases of the gallbladder. In: Behrman RE, Kliegman RM, Jenson HB, eds. *Nelson Textbook of Pediatrics*. 17th ed. Philadelphia, PA: W. B. Saunders; 2004.

12. Werlin S. Exocrine pancreas. In: Behrman RE, Kliegman RM, Jenson HB, eds. *Nelson Textbook of Pediatrics*. 17th ed. Philadelphia, PA: W. B. Saunders; 2004.

13. Winnie G. Pleurisy. In: Behrman RE, Kliegman RM, Jenson HB, eds. *Nelson Textbook of Pediatrics*. 17th ed. Philadelphia, PA: W. B. Saunders; 2004.

14. Elder K. Urologic disorders in infants and children. In: Behrman RE, Kliegman RM, Jenson HB, eds. *Nelson Textbook of Pediatrics*. 17th ed. Philadelphia, PA: W. B. Saunders; 2004.

15. Beers MH. *The Merck Manual of Medical Information*. 2nd ed. Whitehouse Station, NJ: Merck; 2003.

16. Golden CB, Feusner JH. Malignant abdominal masses in children: quick guide to evaluation and diagnosis. *Pediatr Clin North Am*. Dec 2002;49(6):1369–1392, viii.

17. Fernandez M, Carrol CL, Baker CJ. Discitis and vertebral osteomyelitis in children: an 18-year review. *Pediatrics*. Jun 2000;105(6):1299–1304.

18. Early SD, Kay RM, Tolo VT. Childhood diskitis. *J Am Acad Orthop Surg*. Nov–Dec 2003;11(6):413–420.

19. Crawford AH, Kucharzyk DW, Ruda R, Smitherman HC Jr. Diskitis in children. *Clin Orthop Relat Res*. May 1991(266):70–79.

20. Segal L. Spine and pelvis trauma. In: Dormans JP, ed. *Pediatric Orthopedics and Sports Medicine: The Requisites in Pediatrics*. St. Louis, MO: Mosby; 2004:2.

21. Denis F. Spinal instability as defined by the three-column spine concept in acute spinal trauma. *Clin Orthop Relat Res*. Oct 1984(189):65–76.

22. Wheeless CR. *Wheeless' Textbook of Orthopedics*. Durham, NC: Duke University Medical Center; 2005.

23. King J, Diefendorf D, Apthorp J, Negrete VF, Carlson M. Analysis of 429 fractures in 189 battered children. *J Pediatr Orthop*. Sep–Oct 1988;8(5):585–589.

24. Haslam R. Spinal cord disorders. In: Behrman RE, Kliegman RM, Jenson HB, eds. *Nelson Textbook of Pediatrics*. 17th ed. Philadelphia, PA: W. B. Saunders; 2004.

25. McGee SM. Hemophilia. In: Campbell SK, Palisano RJ, Vander Linden DW, eds. *Physical Therapy for Children*. Philadelphia, PA: W. B. Saunders; 1994:247–259.

26. Brill SR, Patel DR, MacDonald E. Psychosomatic disorders in pediatrics. *Indian J Pediatr*. Jul 2001;68(7): 597–603.

27. Hamre MR, Haller JS. Intraspinal hematomas in hemophilia. *Am J Pediatr Hematol Oncol*. May 1992;14(2): 166–169.

28. Chesney R. Metabolic bone disease. In: Behrman RE, Kliegman RM, Jenson HB, eds. *Nelson Textbook of Pediatrics*. 17th ed. Philadelphia, PA: W. B. Saunders; 2004.

29. Adib N, Davies K, Grahame R, Woo P, Murray KJ. Joint hypermobility syndrome in childhood. A not so benign multisystem disorder? *Rheumatology (Oxford)*. Jun 2005;44(6):744–750.

30. Engelbert RH, Kooijmans FT, van Riet AM, Feitsma TM, Uiterwaal CS, Helders PJ. The relationship between generalized joint hypermobility and motor development. *Pediatr Phys Ther*. Winter 2005;17(4):258–263.

31. Miller M, Cassidy J. Juvenile rheumatoid arthritis. In: Behrman RE, Kliegman RM, Jenson HB, eds. *Nelson Textbook of Pediatrics*. 17th ed. Philadelphia, PA: W. B. Saunders; 2004.

32. Scull S. Juvenile rheumatoid arthritis. In: Campbell SK, Palisano RJ, Vander Linden DW, eds. *Physical Therapy for Children*. Philadelphia, PA: W. B. Saunders; 1995.

33. Epstein JA, Epstein NE, Marc J, Rosenthal AD, Lavine LS. Lumbar intervertebral disk herniation in teenage children: recognition and management of associated anomalies. *Spine (Phila Pa 1976)*. May–Jun 1984; 9(4):427–432.

34. Thompson G. The spine. In: Behrman RE, Kliegman RM, Jenson HB, eds. *Nelson Textbook of Pediatrics*. 17th ed. Philadelphia, PA: W. B. Saunders; 2004:2287.

35. Durham SR, Sun PP, Sutton LN. Surgically treated lumbar disc disease in the pediatric population: an outcome study. *J Neurosurg*. Jan 2000;92(1 suppl):1–6.

36. Thompson G. Back pain in children. In: Heckman JD, ed. *Instructional Course Lectures*. Rosemont, IL: American Academy of Orthopaedic Surgeons; 1993.

37. Prober CG. Central nervous system infections. In: Behrman RE, Kliegman RM, Jenson HB, eds. *Nelson Textbook of Pediatrics*. 17th ed. Philadelphia, PA: W. B. Saunders; 2004:2038–2047.

38. Shepard CW, Rosenstein NE, Fischer M. Neonatal meningococcal disease in the United States, 1990 to 1999. *Pediatr Infect Dis J*. May 2003;22(5):418–422.

39. Sotir MJ, Ahrabi-Fard S, Croft DR, et al. Meningococcal disease incidence and mortality in Wisconsin, 1993–2002. *WMJ*. Apr 2005;104(3):38–44.

40. Litmanovitz I, Dolfin T, Friedland O, et al. Early physical activity intervention prevents decrease of bone strength in very low birth weight infants. *Pediatrics*. Jul 2003;112(1 pt 1):15–19.

41. Fewtrell MS, Cole TJ, Bishop NJ, Lucas A. Neonatal factors predicting childhood height in preterm infants: evidence for a persisting effect of early metabolic bone disease? *J Pediatr*. Nov 2000;137(5):668–673.

42. Marini J. Osteogenesis imperfecta. In: Behrman RE, Kliegman RM, Jenson HB, eds. *Nelson Textbook of Pediatrics*. 17th ed. Philadelphia, PA: W. B. Saunders; 2004.

43. Alfven G. One hundred cases of recurrent abdominal pain in children: diagnostic procedures and criteria for a psychosomatic diagnosis. *Acta Paediatr*. 2003;92(1): 43–49.

44. Vikat A, Rimpela M, Salminen JJ, Rimpela A, Savolainen A, Virtanen SM. Neck or shoulder pain and low back pain in Finnish adolescents. *Scand J Public Health*. Sep 2000;28(3):164–173.

45. van Gent C, Dols JJ, de Rover CM, Hira Sing RA, de Vet HC. The weight of schoolbags and the occurrence of neck, shoulder, and back pain in young adolescents. *Spine (Phila Pa 1976)*. May 1, 2003;28(9):916–921.

46. King H. Back pain in children. In: Weinstein SL, ed. *The Pediatric Spine: Principles and Practice*. New York, NY: Raven Press; 1993:182.

47. Broocks A. [Physical training in the treatment of psychological disorders]. *Bundesgesundheitsblatt Gesundheitsforschung Gesundheitsschutz.* Aug 2005;48(8):914–921.

48. Miller M, Petty R. Ankylosing spondylitis and other spondyloarthropathies. In: Behrman RE, Kliegman RM, Jenson HB, eds. *Nelson Textbook of Pediatrics.* 17th ed. Philadelphia, PA: W. B. Saunders; 2004.

49. Scalzi L, Lou J. Synovial disorders. In: Dormans JP, ed. *Pediatric Orthopedics and Sports Medicine: The Requisites in Pediatrics.* St. Louis, MO: Mosby; 2004:349.

50. Gorman JD, Sack KE, Davis JC, Jr. Treatment of ankylosing spondylitis by inhibition of tumor necrosis factor alpha. *N Engl J Med.* May 2, 2002;346(18):1349–1356.

51. Pachman L. Juvenile dermatomyositis. In: Behrman RE, Kliegman RM, Jenson HB, eds. *Nelson Textbook of Pediatrics.* 17th ed. Philadelphia, PA: W. B. Saunders; 2004.

52. Pilkington CA, Wedderburn LR. Paediatric idiopathic inflammatory muscle disease: recognition and management. *Drugs.* 2005;65(10):1355–1365.

53. Iqbal S, Sher MR, Good RA, Cawkwell GD. Diversity in presenting manifestations of systemic lupus erythematosus in children. *J Pediatr.* Oct 1999;135(4):500–505.

54. Miettunen PM, Ortiz-Alvarez O, Petty RE, et al. Gender and ethnic origin have no effect on long-term outcome of childhood-onset systemic lupus erythematosus. *J Rheumatol.* Aug 2004;31(8):1650–1654.

55. King HA. Back pain in children. *Pediatr Clin North Am.* Oct 1984;31(5):1083–1095.

56. Luedtke LM, Flynn JM, Ganley TJ, Hosalkar HS, Pill SG, Dormans JP. The orthopedists' perspective: bone tumors, scoliosis, and trauma. *Radiol Clin North Am.* Jul 2001;39(4):803–821.

57. Roger E, Letts M. Sickle cell disease of the spine in children. *Can J Surg.* Aug 1999;42(4):289–292.

58. Quirolo K, Vichinsky E. Hemoglobin disorders. In: Behrman RE, Kliegman RM, Jenson HB, eds. *Nelson Textbook of Pediatrics.* 17th ed. Philadelphia, PA: W. B. Saunders; 2004.

59. Sadat-Ali M, Ammar A, Corea JR, Ibrahim AW. The spine in sickle cell disease. *Int Orthop.* Jun 1994;18(3):154–156.

60. Alvarez M. Spinal epidural abscess—from onset to rehabilitation: case study. *J Neurosci Nurs.* Apr 2005;37(2):72–78.

61. Reihsaus E, Waldbaur H, Seeling W. Spinal epidural abscess: a meta-analysis of 915 patients. *Neurosurg Rev.* Dec 2000;23(4):175–204; discussion 205.

62. Hosalkar H, Dormans JP. Back pain in children requires extensive workup. *Biomechanics.* Jun 2003;10(6):51–58.

63. Luedtke L. Back pain in children and adolescents: Understanding and diagnosing spondylolysis and spondylolisthesis. In: *A Pediatric Perspective.* Vol 1. St. Paul, MN: Gillette Children's Specialty Healthcare; 2002.

64. Miller SL, Hoffer FA. Malignant and benign bone tumors. *Radiol Clin North Am.* Jul 2001;39(4):673–699.

65. Murphey MD, Andrews CL, Flemming DJ, Temple HT, Smith WS, Smirniotopoulos JG. From the archives of the AFIP. Primary tumors of the spine: radiologic pathologic correlation. *Radiographics.* Sep 1996;16(5):1131–1158.

66. Hosalkar J, Dormans J. Back pain in children requires extensive workup. *Biomechanics.* 2003(June):51–58.

67. Arndt C. Soft tissue sarcomas. In: Behrman RE, Kliegman RM, Jenson HB, eds. *Nelson Textbook of Pediatrics.* 17th ed. Philadelphia, PA: W. B. Saunders; 2004:1714.

68. *Detailed Guide: Brain/CNS Tumors in Children: What Are Children's Brain and Spinal Cord Cancers?* American Cancer Society; 2005.

69. Kuttesch J, Ater J. Brain tumors in childhood. In: Behrman RE, Kliegman RM, Jenson HB, eds. *Nelson Textbook of Pediatrics.* 17th ed. Philadelphia, PA: W. B. Saunders; 2004:1704.

70. MacDonald T. Astrocytoma. http://emedicine.medscape.com/article/985927-overview. Accessed August 27, 2005.

71. Erol B, States L. Musculoskeletal tumors in children. In: Dormans JP, ed. *Pediatric Orthopedics and Sports Medicine: The Requisites in Pediatrics.* St. Louis. MO: Mosby; 2004:325.

72. Horowitz ME, Neff JR, Kun LE. Ewing's sarcoma. Radiotherapy versus surgery for local control. *Pediatr Clin North Am.* Apr 1991;38(2):365–380.

73. Levine SE, Dormans JP, Meyer JS, Corcoran TA. Langerhans' cell histiocytosis of the spine in children. *Clin Orthop Relat Res.* Feb 1996(323):288–293.

74. Tubergen D, Bleyer A. Cancer and benign tumors. In: Behrman RE, Kliegman RM, Jenson HB, eds. *Nelson Textbook of Pediatrics.* 17th ed. Philadelphia, PA: W. B. Saunders; 2004:1694–1698.

75. Johns Hopkins University. Types of childhood cancers. http://www.jhscout.org//types/index.cfm. Accessed August 27, 2005.

76. Johns Hopkins University. Types of childhood cancers. In: *The Scout:* Sidney Kimmel Comprehensive Cancer Center, Johns Hopkins University; 2005.

77. Miller S, Hoffer F. Malignant and benign bone tumors. *Radiol Clin North Am Pediatr Musculoskel Radiol.* 2001;39(4):673–699.

78. Gilchrist G. Lymphoma. In: Behrman RE, Kliegman RM, Jenson HB, eds. *Nelson Textbook of Pediatrics.* 17th ed. Philadelphia, PA: W. B. Saunders; 2004.

79. Kurtzberg J, Graham ML. Non-Hodgkin's lymphoma. Biologic classification and implication for therapy. *Pediatr Clin North Am.* Apr 1991;38(2):443–456.

80. Ater J. Neuroblastoma. In: Behrman RE, Kliegman RM, Jenson HB, eds. *Nelson Textbook of Pediatrics.* 17th ed. Philadelphia, PA: W. B. Saunders; 2004:1709.

81. Guzey FK, Seyithanoglu MH, Sencer A, Emei E, Alatas I, Izgi AN. Vertebral osteoid osteoma associated with paravertebral soft-tissue changes on magnetic resonance imaging. Report of two cases. *J Neurosurg.* May 2004;100(5 suppl Pediatrics):532–536.

82. Meyer WH, Malawer MM. Osteosarcoma. Clinical features and evolving surgical and chemotherapeutic strategies. *Pediatr Clin North Am.* Apr 1991;38(2):317–348.

83. Kay RM, Eckardt JJ, Mirra JM. Osteosarcoma and Ewing's sarcoma in a retinoblastoma patient. *Clin Orthop Relat Res.* Feb 1996(323):284–287.

CHAPTER 45

Hip Pain in a Child

Stephanie A. Jones, PT, DPT, OCS, NCS

Description of the Symptom

This chapter describes possible causes of hip pain in a child between the proximal one-third of the thigh, inguinal region, and buttock.

Special Concerns

- Any hip pain associated with rapidly ascending symmetrical weakness and hyporeflexia
- Severe hip pain with an acute onset associated with an inability to bear weight, decreased range of motion, and stiffness
- Any post-traumatic hip pain
- Hip pain associated with local swelling, fever, and chills

CHAPTER PREVIEW: Conditions That May Lead to Hip Pain in a Child

T Trauma

REMOTE	LOCAL
COMMON	
Spondylolisthesis 905	Muscle strain 911
	Slipped femoral capital epiphyses 917
	Tendinitis 918
UNCOMMON	
Spondylolysis 906	Chondral injury 908
	Contusion 908
	Snapping hip syndrome 917
RARE	
Lumbar disk herniation/radiculopathy 905	Avulsion injuries:
	• Psoas off lesser trochanter 907
	• Rectus femoris off the anterior inferior iliac spine 907
	• Sartorius or tensor fascia lata off the anterior superior iliac spine 907
	Fracture 908
	Labral tear 910
	Meralgia paresthetica 911
	Traumatic dislocation 918

I Inflammation

REMOTE	LOCAL
COMMON	
Not applicable	**Aseptic**
	Transient synovitis 918

Inflammation *(continued)*

REMOTE	LOCAL
COMMON	
	Septic Osteomyelitis (pyogenic or granulomatous) 912 Septic arthritis 916
UNCOMMON	
Not applicable	**Aseptic** Bursitis 907 Osteochondritis dissecans 912
	Septic Lyme disease (tick paralysis) 911
RARE	
Aseptic Not applicable **Septic** Appendicitis 904 Chronic granulomatous disease 905 Discitis 905	**Aseptic** Apophysitis 907 Demyelinating polyneuropathies: • Acute demyelinating polyradiculoneuropathy (Guillain-Barré syndrome) 908 • Chronic demyelinating polyradiculoneuropathy 908 Juvenile dermatomyositis 909 Juvenile rheumatoid arthritis 909 Osteitis pubis 912 Rheumatic fever 913 Rheumatoid arthritis–like diseases of the hip: • Arthritis with inflammatory bowel disease 913 • Juvenile ankylosing spondylitis 914 • Juvenile dermatomyositis 914 • Psoriatic arthritis 915 • Reactive arthritis (Reiter's syndrome) 915 • Systemic lupus erythematosus 915 Scleroderma (focal or systemic sclerosis) 916 **Septic** Poliomyelitis 913 Pyomyositis 913 Tuberculosis arthritis 918

M Metabolic

REMOTE	LOCAL
COMMON	
Not applicable	Not applicable
UNCOMMON	
Not applicable	Osteogenesis imperfecta 912 Rickets, vitamin D–resistant (hypophosphatasia) 916
RARE	
Metabolic myopathy 905	Ehlers-Danlos syndrome 908 Gaucher's disease 909

(continued)

Metabolic (*continued*)

REMOTE	LOCAL
RARE	
	Lesch-Nyhan syndrome 910
	Myositis ossificans (heterotopic ossification) 912
	Osteopetrosis 913
	Rickets, vitamin D–dependent (nutritional) 916

Va Vascular

REMOTE	LOCAL
COMMON	
Not applicable	Avascular necrosis of the hip 907
	Legg-Calvé-Perthes disease 910
	Sickle cell anemia 917
UNCOMMON	
Not applicable	Not applicable
RARE	
Not applicable	Hemophilic arthropathy 909
	Henoch-Schönlein purpura (small-vessel vasculitis) 909
	Polyarteritis nodosa (medium- and large-vessel vasculitis) 913

De Degenerative

REMOTE	LOCAL
COMMON	
Not applicable	Not applicable
UNCOMMON	
Not applicable	Not applicable
RARE	
Not applicable	Not applicable

Tu Tumor

REMOTE	LOCAL
COMMON	
Not applicable	Not applicable
UNCOMMON	
Not applicable	*Malignant Primary, such as:*
	• Nephroblastoma (Wilms' tumor) 920
	Malignant Metastatic:
	Not applicable
	Benign, such as:
	• Osteoid osteoma 921

Tumor *(continued)*

REMOTE	LOCAL
RARE	
Not applicable	*Malignant Primary, such as:*
	• Ewing's sarcoma 919
	• Leukemia 919
	• Lymphoma 920
	• Neuroblastoma 920
	• Osteosarcoma (osteogenic sarcoma) 921
	• Rhabdomyosarcoma 922
	• Synovial sarcoma 922
	Malignant Metastatic:
	Not applicable
	Benign, such as:
	• Langerhans' cell histiocytosis 919
	• Osteochondroma 921

Co Congenital

REMOTE	LOCAL
COMMON	
Not applicable	Not applicable
UNCOMMON	
Not applicable	Acetabular dysplasia 906
RARE	
Not applicable	Metaphyseal chondrodysplasia 911
	Multiple epiphyseal dysplasia 911
	Myelodysplasia (spina bifida) 911

Ne Neurogenic/Psychogenic

REMOTE	LOCAL
COMMON	
Not applicable	Not applicable
UNCOMMON	
Not applicable	Not applicable
RARE	
Not applicable	Meralgia paresthetica 911
	Spastic cerebral palsy 918

Note: These are estimates of relative incidence because few data are available for the less common conditions.

Common Ages at Which Hip Pain Presents in a Child

APPROXIMATE AGE	CONDITION
Birth to 3 Years	Chronic inflammatory demyelinating polyneuropathy
	Discitis
	Juvenile rheumatoid arthritis (polyarticular)

(continued)

Common Ages at Which Hip Pain Presents in a Child—cont'd	
APPROXIMATE AGE	**CONDITION**
	Lesch-Nyhan syndrome
	Leukemia
	Lyme disease (tick paralysis)
	Metabolic myopathy
	Myelodysplasia (spina bifida)
	Nephroblastoma
	Neuroblastoma
	Osteochondroma
	Osteogenesis imperfecta
	Osteomyelitis
	Osteopetrosis
	Poliomyelitis
	Polyarteritis nodosa
	Rhabdomyosarcoma
	Rickets
	Scleroderma
	Septic arthritis
	Transient synovitis
	Tuberculosis arthritis
Preschool (3–5 Years)	Acute transient synovitis
	Discitis
	Gaucher's disease
	Henoch-Schönlein purpura
	Legg-Calvé-Perthes disease
	Leukemia
	Lyme disease (tick paralysis)
	Metabolic myopathy
	Nephroblastoma
	Neuroblastoma
	Osteochondroma
	Osteomyelitis
	Rhabdomyosarcoma
	Scleroderma
	Septic arthritis
	Tuberculosis arthritis
Elementary School (6–11 Years)	Chronic granulomatous disease
	Ewing's sarcoma
	Guillain-Barré syndrome
	Hemophilic arthropathy
	Henoch-Schönlein purpura
	Hip dislocation (traumatic)
	Juvenile dermatomyositis
	Juvenile rheumatoid arthritis (pauciarticular)
	Legg-Calvé-Perthes disease
	Leukemia
	Lyme disease (tick paralysis)
	Lymphoma
	Metaphyseal chondrodysplasia
	Multiple epiphyseal dysplasia
	Osteochondritis dissecans
	Osteochondroma
	Osteoid osteoma
	Osteomyelitis

Common Ages at Which Hip Pain Presents in a Child—cont'd

APPROXIMATE AGE	CONDITION
	Osteosarcoma
	Psoriatic arthritis
	Pyomyositis
	Rhabdomyosarcoma
	Scleroderma
	Sickle cell anemia
	Spondylolysis
Middle School (12–14 Years)	Acetabular dysplasia
	Avascular necrosis
	Epiphyseal dysplasias
	Ewing's sarcoma
	Hip bursitis
	Hip contusion
	Hip fractures
	Juvenile ankylosing spondylitis
	Juvenile chronic arthritis
	Juvenile dermatomyositis
	Juvenile rheumatoid arthritis (polyarticular)
	Leukemia
	Lyme disease (tick paralysis)
	Lymphoma
	Metabolic myopathy
	Muscle strain
	Myelodysplasia (spina bifida)
	Myositis ossificans
	Osteochondritis dissecans
	Osteoid osteoma
	Osteosarcoma
	Psoriatic arthritis
	Reactive arthritis (Reiter's syndrome)
	Rhabdomyosarcoma
	Rheumatic fever
	Scleroderma
	Slipped femoral capital epiphysis
	Snapping hip syndrome
	Spondylolysis
	Tendinitis
High School (15–18 Years)	Apophysitis
	Appendicitis
	Avulsion injury
	Cerebral palsy (spastic)
	Chondral injury
	Ehlers-Danlos syndrome
	Ewing's sarcoma
	Heterotopic ossification
	Hip bursitis
	Hip contusion
	Hip fractures
	Juvenile ankylosing spondylitis
	Labral tears
	Lumbar disk herniation/radiculopathy
	Lyme disease (tick paralysis)

(continued)

Common Ages at Which Hip Pain Presents in a Child—cont'd

APPROXIMATE AGE	CONDITION
	Meralgia paresthetica
	Metaphyseal chondrodysplasia
	Muscle strain
	Myelodysplasia (spinal bifida)
	Myositis ossificans
	Osteitis pubis
	Osteochondritis dissecans
	Osteochondroma
	Osteoid osteoma
	Osteosarcoma
	Rhabdomyosarcoma
	Rheumatic fever
	Scleroderma
	Septic arthritis
	Sickle cell anemia
	Slipped capital femoral epiphysis
	Snapping hip syndrome
	Spondylolisthesis
	Spondylolysis
	Synovial sarcoma
	Systemic lupus erythematosus
	Tendinitis
	Tuberculosis arthritis

Overview of Hip Pain in a Child

Hip pain is common in children. A child with a painful hip will commonly present with difficulty weight bearing, a limp if at an age old enough to walk, and pain-limited range of motion. Young children in particular might have difficulty describing their symptoms or cooperating with the examination. This same clinical presentation occurs in a wide variety of underlying pathologies. The correct diagnosis is important due to the potential for long-term dysfunction from hip disease if proper treatment is delayed or absent. This is particularly relevant in diseases such as septic arthritis and slipped capital femoral epiphysis, which can lead to severe joint destruction if not treated expeditiously. Since the presenting symptoms for fairly benign disorders such as transient synovitis are similar to those that require urgent medical attention such as septic arthritis, prompt evaluation of any acute onset of hip pain in a child is critical. Referred pain to the medial knee joint results in the frequent misdiagnosis of primary hip disease.

The most common childhood diseases resulting in hip pain include slipped capital femoral epiphysis, Legg-Calvé-Perthes disease, acetabular dysplasia, septic arthritis, transient synovitis, and muscular injuries.[1-3] For infants and toddlers transient synovitis of the hip and septic arthritis are the most common causes of hip pain.[4] In children under the age of 10 years, Legg-Calvé-Perthes disease, septic arthritis, transient synovitis, and various cancers are the most likely sources of hip pain. In adolescence, as sports participation increases, traumatic injuries such as slipped capital femoral epiphysis, muscle strains, tendinitis, and spondylolisthesis are more frequent.

Description of Conditions That May Lead to Hip Pain in a Child

Remote

■ Appendicitis

Chief Clinical Characteristics

This presentation can include tenderness or pain in the right anterior pelvis or psoas region.[5]

Background Information

Retrocecal appendicitis typically presents with right lower abdominal or lumbar pain with tenderness of the right ilium or lumbar areas.[6] If appendiceal rupture occurs there may also be an ilial abscess causing right flank or costovertebral pain.[6] These symptoms might also be accompanied by anorexia, low-grade fever, and leukocytosis.[6] Treatment includes surgery and antibiotic medications.

■ Chronic Granulomatous Disease

Chief Clinical Characteristics

This presentation commonly involves thigh or hip pain, painful limp, limited hip range of motion, and recurrent abscesses.[7]

Background Information

This disorder includes recurrent purulent bacterial and fungal infections, which are the most common underlying condition in extracranial osteomyelitis.[7] It may present as an osseous infection.[7] Imaging tests or biopsy is used to differentiate the disease.[7] Treatment includes antibiotic medications and chemotherapy.[7]

■ Discitis

Chief Clinical Characteristics

This presentation for infants or toddlers may include a limp, avoidance of ambulation, or abdominal pain.[8]

Background Information

Pain or spasm may be present when the hip is placed in extension (log-roll test).[8] This infection of the disk space is common in children. Moderately elevated erythrocyte sedimentation rate, disk space narrowing with irregular vertebral end plates on imaging studies, and local tenderness to palpation can be used to confirm the diagnosis.[2,8] Treatment is with antibiotic medication.[8]

■ Lumbar Disk Herniation/ Radiculopathy

Chief Clinical Characteristics

This presentation includes local or referred pain from the disk injury as well as radicular symptoms due to encroachment on a nerve root that can refer to the buttocks, groin, or elsewhere in the lower extremity in a dermatomal pattern.

Background Information

Onset can be insidious or related to mechanical trauma. Bending, lifting, and prolonged sitting often increase symptoms. Damage of the intervertebral disk due to a disruption in the annulus fibrosus or vertebral end plate is an uncommon phenomenon in adolescents.[9] Most cases are managed nonsurgically. Related saddle numbness or bowel and bladder dysfunction indicate a need for referral to a spine surgeon in order to consider urgent surgical decompression.

■ Metabolic Myopathy

Chief Clinical Characteristics

The classic presentation can include pain, cramping, stiffness, and fatigue during intense exercise.[10]

Background Information

Myophosphorylase deficiency (McArdle's syndrome) is the most common of these nine glycogen defect related disorders.[10] The onset is in childhood to early adolescence.[10] Diagnosis is made with muscle biopsy and the forearm ischemic exercise test.[10] Another presentation of this disease includes progressive weakness similar to that in the dystrophies. This presentation most commonly occurs in infancy to early childhood.[11] Treatment may include diet modification and exercise.[12,13]

■ Spondylolisthesis

Chief Clinical Characteristics

This presentation includes hip and low back pain that may radiate to the lower extremities, limitations in range of motion, a positive Lasègue's sign, and tenderness over the lumbar spinous processes with or without a palpable step. Significant hamstring tightness or spasm may result in an abnormal gait pattern with short stride length, flexed knees, and pelvic waddle. Decreased lumbar lordosis, scoliosis, and flattened buttocks may also be present. Neurological signs are rare, but may be present even in low-grade slips secondary to nerve root compression.[14–17] As with spondylolysis (see next entry), symptoms are usually aggravated by activities that require repetitive flexion and extension such as gymnastics.

Background Information

This condition involves the forward displacement of a proximal vertebra on the one below it, typically as a result of bilateral pars interarticularis defect. The pars defect is not present in congenital spondylolisthesis. The most common site for slippage is the fifth lumbar vertebra on the sacrum. Standing anteroposterior and lateral radiographs are needed to determine the grade of slippage, and an oblique view is necessary to appreciate the pars defect. In high-grade slips with neurological deficits a complete neurological exam is indicated. Treatment is determined by symptoms, clinical signs, and the grade of slip. Asymptomatic patients do not require intervention. Those with low-grade slips and pain tend to do well with conservative treatment of activity restriction, bracing, and exercises. Fusion is recommended for grade II slips or greater even if they are asymptomatic because they are at risk for further slippage during growth spurts.[16,17] Reduction of the slip is not recommended because of the high risk of neurological injury.[15–17] Patients are more prone to recurrent symptoms and clinical deformity if forward slipping is allowed to progress. Progression of slip, delayed union, neuropathy of the fifth nerve root, and cauda equina syndrome have all been reported as postsurgical complications.[16,17]

■ Spondylolysis

Chief Clinical Characteristics

This presentation can include hip and low back pain with hyperextension that rarely radiates, scoliosis, decreased lumbar lordosis and increased lumbosacral kyphosis.[18] The child will often have hamstring tightness that can affect gait.[15,19] Adolescents participating in sports that require repetitive hyperextension, such as gymnastics, wrestling, and football appear to be at increased risk.[15] Most children with spondylolysis are asymptomatic or may have symptoms that are mild and therefore often overlooked.

Background Information

This condition is a congenital or acquired defect of the pars interarticularis, the bone between the superior and inferior facets of the vertebrae. An acquired defect would arise as a stress or fatigue fracture of the pars.[16,19] The pars interarticularis defect can occur at any level, most commonly at L5, and can occur unilaterally or bilaterally. A bilateral defect no longer provides posterior stability and may result in forward slippage, especially of L5 over S1, known as spondylolisthesis. Spondylolysis can occur at any age, but is rarely seen before age ten; it appears to be more prevalent in boys. An oblique standing view is the best view to show the pars defect that can easily be overlooked if only anteroposterior and lateral views are taken.[17,19,20] Computed tomography or bone scan is used if radiographs are inconclusive, and single-photon emitted computed tomography will determine if the lesion is acute or chronic.[16] Treatment depends on the degree of the defect and whether the patient is symptomatic. If pain is present in the absence of spondylolisthesis, immobilization with a thoracic-lumbar-sacral orthosis for 3 to 6 months may be most beneficial. Physical therapy should focus on hamstring and lumbar musculature stretching, abdominal strengthening, and monitoring of gradual return to activity. With persistent pain unrelieved by nonsteroidal anti-inflammatory medication, rest, and physical therapy, surgical stabilization can be achieved through posterior spinal fusion.[15,18] Any child with this condition should be followed closely, because they are at risk for progression to spondylolisthesis. Girls tend to have a higher rate of progression.

Local

■ Acetabular Dysplasia

Chief Clinical Characteristics

This presentation involves pain in the hip that may be associated with a limp. Usually the range of motion is unchanged. While dysplasia of the acetabulum is seen as an infant, it is not a cause of pain until the early to middle teenage years.

Background Information

This condition is characterized by a shallow acetabulum or slanted acetabular roof (Fig. 45-1).[21] Overall developmental dysplasia is far more common in females with a ratio of 6:1.[21] Acetabular dysplasia has also been associated with labral tears due to the hypertrophy of the labrum from impingement by the acetabulum, resulting in pain as well as osteoarthritis later in adulthood.[22]

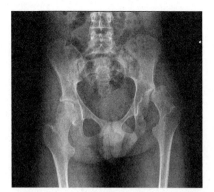

FIGURE 45-1 Developmental dysplasia of the left hip with dislocation (anteroposterior view). (Image courtesy of Nishant Verma, MD, diagnostic radiology resident, Indiana University School of Medicine.)

The diagnosis is confirmed with x-rays. Treatment in infants may include bracing such as with a Pavlik harness. Other interventions include physical therapy for strengthening and positioning or in more severe cases surgery such as an osteotomy.[23]

■ Apophysitis

Chief Clinical Characteristics
This presentation involves the gradual onset of mild pain at the muscle attachment sites.[24]

Background Information
Pain and inflammation are due to excessive traction to the apophysis, attachment site, or insertion of muscle into bone.[24] This condition is managed with rest and progressive rehabilitation.[25]

■ Avascular Necrosis of the Hip

Chief Clinical Characteristics
This presentation involves groin pain, difficulty weight bearing, limited hip extension, and internal rotation.[26]

Background Information
The vascular supply to the femoral head can be disturbed by trauma, treatments requiring very high-dose steroids (such as in post–kidney allograft rejection), and disorders including endocrine dysfunction, human immunodeficiency virus, and sickle cell disease.[27] This is a

separate disorder from Legg-Calvé-Perthes disease. It may require surgical management.[26]

AVULSION INJURIES
Chief Clinical Characteristics
This presentation includes a variable clinical picture that depends on the affected muscle group.

Background Information
Sprinting or sports activities are the most common mechanism of injury for avulsion injuries.[24,25] The force of the muscle contraction is beyond of the strength of the apophyseal muscle attachment, resulting in an avulsion fracture.[28] Recovery is expected in 4 to 6 weeks with rehabilitation.[24]

■ Psoas Off Lesser Trochanter
Chief Clinical Characteristics
This presentation may include anterior hip pain.[28]

■ Rectus Femoris Off the Anterior Inferior Iliac Spine
Chief Clinical Characteristics
This presentation can be characterized by groin pain, weakness with active hip flexion and knee extension, limited hip extension motion, and difficulty weight bearing.[24]

■ Sartorius or Tensor Fascia Lata Off the Anterior Superior Iliac Spine
Chief Clinical Characteristics
This presentation includes anterior hip pain, weakness with hip flexion, external rotation and abduction, limited hip extension, and internal rotation motion as well as difficulty weight bearing.[24]

■ Bursitis
Chief Clinical Characteristics
This presentation commonly includes pain localized over the bursa that might radiate distally.[24]

Background Information
This condition involves inflammation and swelling of the synovial fluid-filled sacs called bursas.[24] The most common location is the trochanteric bursa followed by the ischial, iliopsoas, and iliopectineal bursae.[24]

This disorder can be caused by a direct blow to the bursae, prolonged pressure to the area, friction over the bursae from muscle imbalances, bony alignment, and/or environmental factors in sports activity.[24] Treatment includes rest, anti-inflammatory medications, ultrasound, and therapeutic exercise to restore muscle balance.[25] Sometimes corticosteroid injections are used for the inflammation, as well.

■ Chondral Injury

Chief Clinical Characteristics
This presentation includes reports of hip joint locking.[22,29]

Background Information
This condition is frequently associated with a jumping or twisting mechanism.[29] Surgery may be indicated if nonsurgical management does not alleviate symptoms.[29]

■ Contusion

Chief Clinical Characteristics
This presentation includes pain, spasm, and transient weakness of affected muscles.[24,25]

Background Information
This injury results in hematoma formation from a blow to the musculature surrounding the hip.[25] *Hip pointer* is the term used to indicate a contusion to the musculature that attaches to the iliac crest.[24] In severe cases this can lead to the development of myositis ossificans.[24] Treatment includes ice, ultrasound, anti-inflammatory medications, or steroid injection.[25]

DEMYELINATING POLYNEUROPATHIES

■ Acute Demyelinating Polyradiculoneuropathy (Guillain-Barré Syndrome)

Chief Clinical Characteristics
This presentation commonly involves ascending weakness and muscle pain.[30] *Leg pain often precedes symptoms of weakness.*[3] *Prodromal symptoms or events such as gastroenteritis, upper respiratory infection, surgery, or immunization 1 to 4 weeks prior to weakness may be reported.*[30,31]

Background Information
This condition is a rapidly progressive lower motor neuron disease that affects boys more commonly than girls.[31] It can rapidly lead to respiratory failure in acute stages if not treated. Intravenous immunoglobulin has been shown to be the most effective medical therapy but plasma exchange and corticosteroids are also utilized.[31] Most patients undergo extensive rehabilitation to regain strength and restore function.

■ Chronic Demyelinating Polyradiculoneuropathy

Chief Clinical Characteristics
This presentation involves ascending weakness and muscle pain with a subacute onset over at least 2 months.[32]

Background Information
The course of disease may include chronic progression or periodic relapses. Intravenous immunoglobulin has been shown to be the most effective medical therapy but plasma exchange and corticosteroids are also utilized.[31] Most patients undergo extensive rehabilitation to regain strength and restore function.

■ Ehlers-Danlos Syndrome

Chief Clinical Characteristics
This presentation includes joint hypermobility that can lead to recurrent hip dislocations and joint effusion in these children.[10,33] *Individuals with this condition are also prone to experiencing dislocations at the knee, shoulder, elbow, and clavicle and typically have cardiac defects.*

Background Information
This is an inherited connective tissue disorder with 10 distinct variations.[33] Management may include bracing or physical therapy for strengthening.

■ Fracture

Chief Clinical Characteristics
This presentation involves an acute onset of activity-limiting hip pain and swelling.[24]

Background Information
This would include any fracture to the pelvis or proximal femur of the following types: traumatic or stress.[24] Traumatic fractures due to compression or a blow in children are most

commonly a result of a motor vehicle accident, fall from height, or sports activity.[24] Traumatic avulsion fractures result from traction to a muscle origin or attachment, usually in ballistic sport activities.[24] This is the most common fracture type in children and typically occurs at the anterior superior iliac spine, anterior inferior iliac spine, ischial tuberosity, or lesser trochanter.[24] Stress fractures are of insidious onset and typically related to overuse from sports activities such as running. Overall the incidence of pediatric hip fractures is rare.[24] Management ranges from surgical fixation of fracture segments to rehabilitation.

■ Gaucher's Disease

Chief Clinical Characteristics
This presentation typically involves musculoskeletal symptoms such as a recurrent ache in the hip, knee, or shoulder joint and bone crisis of the femur or tibia, which can include severe pain, swelling, and erythema.[10]

Background Information
This disorder is deficiency of a fat metabolizing enzyme that results in fatty infiltration of tissues including bone marrow. Osteonecrosis of the femoral head and pathological long bone fractures may also occur.[10] The juvenile form of this disease (type 3) has an onset in early childhood.[10] Treatment includes enzyme replacement therapy and in some cases bone marrow transplantation.[34]

■ Hemophilic Arthropathy

Chief Clinical Characteristics
This presentation includes physical signs of inflammation due to only minor joint trauma that results in hemarthrosis.[10]

Background Information
Synovium proliferation or pannus usually occurs in the knee, ankle, and elbow joints of children with this blood clotting disorder.[35] Hip osteonecrosis may develop from vascular occlusion due to bleeding or synovial hyperplasia.[35] Hemophilia is almost exclusive to males.[10] Treatment of the hemophilia may include infusion of treated plasma-derived factor or recombinant factor. The joint damage may necessitate joint arthroplasty surgery.[36]

■ Henoch-Schönlein Purpura (Small-Vessel Vasculitis)

Chief Clinical Characteristics
This presentation often includes abdominal pain after an upper respiratory infection followed by a rash (petechiae) and edema in dependent areas of the extremities.[10]

Background Information
Arthritis and nephritis can develop.[10] The course of the disease usually resolves in 2 weeks without intervention.[10] Nonsteroidal antiinflammatory medication may be used to manage symptoms.

■ Juvenile Dermatomyositis

Chief Clinical Characteristics
This presentation includes a vasculitic rash on the face, elbows, and knees and the slow onset of signs of proximal weakness such as difficulty walking and clumsiness.[10]

Background Information
Muscle pain due to the inflammation of the blood vessels may also occur.[10] This condition should be excluded in cases of chronic arthritis and muscle inflammation. Muscle enzyme testing, electromyography, and muscle biopsy are used to confirm the diagnosis.[10] Corticosteroid therapy will reverse the disease in 6 months for most cases.[10] Complications include dysphagia, chronic abdominal pain leading to perforation, cerebritis, and diffuse calcification of muscle or subcutaneous tissues.[10]

■ Juvenile Rheumatoid Arthritis

Chief Clinical Characteristics
This presentation commonly involves the consistent presence for 6 or more weeks of joint swelling, or the presence of two or more of the following: limited joint range of motion, palpable tenderness, painful movement, or joint warmth.[10]

Background Information
Hip involvement may present 1 to 6 years after initial disease onset in 30% to 50% of affected children and typically is bilateral.[37] Other associated problems include osteoporosis, growth disturbance due to epiphyseal plate damage, coxa magna, and less commonly hip subluxations, avascular necrosis, and, rarely, fusion.[37] Hip involvement is usually also associated with

the more severe forms requiring aggressive medical management with long-term remission-inducing drugs such as methotrexate and intensive physical therapy for contracture management, bracing, strengthening, and gait training.[37] Functional problems include altered gait possibly with a limp and difficulty with stair climbing and rising from a seated position.[37] The three subtypes of this condition are systemic, polyarticular, and pauciarticular. Pauciarticular or oligoarticular must affect five or fewer joints.[21] Late-onset pauciarthritis occurs mostly in boys after age 8.[21] It involves concomitant enthesitis or tendinitis and arthritis that asymmetrically affects the knees, shoulders, spine, or hips.[10] The polyarticular type involves more than five joints symmetrically and usually occurs in small joints but can involve the hips.[23] This type is more common in females. Systemic arthritis is characterized by fever and rash but may also include thrombocytosis, leukocytosis, anemia, pleuritis, pericarditis, osteopenia, delayed growth, hepatosplenomegaly, and lymphadenopathy.[10,23] Patients with monoarticular disease report morning stiffness, joint pain, and swelling in the initial stages.[10] The joints are warm and limited in range of motion.

■ Labral Tear

Chief Clinical Characteristics
This presentation includes catching, clicking, giving way, pain, and decreased range of motion of the hip.[22,29]

Background Information
These tears are associated with sports activities that involve running, pivoting, jumping, and kicking such as in tennis, soccer, martial arts, dance, and football.[29] Children may describe the mechanism of injury as twisting or an axial load on a flexed hip if they recall an acute event.[29] Hip dysplasia can also result in labral tears most commonly occurring anteriorly.[22] Such tears can sometimes be managed nonsurgically; otherwise surgery might be indicated.

■ Legg-Calvé-Perthes Disease

Chief Clinical Characteristics
This presentation involves groin, thigh, and/or knee pain, a limp (typically with the femur externally rotated), limited hip abduction, and internal rotation.[23]

Background Information
This disease can have an acute traumatic or insidious onset over months. The femoral head ceases to grow due to a disturbance in blood supply. The secondary center of ossification becomes fragmented as revascularization occurs and then reossification follows (Fig. 45-2).[21] It is more common in males by a 4:1 ratio.[21] Smaller, highly active boys with delayed skeletal maturity may be predisposed to developing this disorder.[21] Between 8% and 24% of cases are bilateral.[25] Most cases are self-limiting but need monitoring with radiographs and periodic clinical assessments.[25] More severe cases might require strengthening, splinting, weight-bearing limitations, and even surgery.[21] It is important to avoid weight bearing for a period to allow for revascularization and prevent permanent bony deformity.[25]

■ Lesch-Nyhan Syndrome

Chief Clinical Characteristics
This presentation includes gouty arthritis, mental retardation, hypertonicity resulting in hip dislocation, movement disorders, and self-mutilating behaviors.[21,38]

Background Information
This is a rare genetic disorder characterized by an enzyme deficiency that results in uric acid accumulation.[38] This disorder only occurs in boys.[21] Death due to renal failure typically occurs in the first two decades. Medical management may include allopurinol to address the excess uric acid and various medications to manage the neurological symptoms.[38]

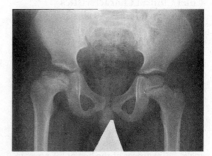

FIGURE 45-2 Legg-Calvé-Perthes disease of the right hip (anteroposterior view). (Image courtesy of Nishant Verma, MD, diagnostic radiology resident, Indiana University School of Medicine.)

■ Lyme Disease (Tick Paralysis)

Chief Clinical Characteristics

This presentation involves a rash commonly with central clearing, fever, fatigue, malaise, headache, myalgias, and polyarthritis in the early stage.[10]

Background Information

This condition involves infection by a tick-borne spirochete *Borrelia burgdorferi*. The joint pain is secondary to an autoimmune reaction rather than a septic arthritis due to the organism. Ninety percent of cases in the United States have been in the states of Connecticut, Massachusetts, Minnesota, New Jersey, New York, Pennsylvania, Rhode Island, and Wisconsin.[10] It is treated with antibiotic medication.[39]

■ Meralgia Paresthetica

Chief Clinical Characteristics

This presentation includes numbness, burning, tingling, and/or pain of the anterolateral thigh.[24] This condition results from an entrapment or compression of the superficial branch of the lateral femoral cutaneous nerve.[24]

Background Information

This condition is typically due to obesity, a direct blow, or the wearing of tight garments or heavy accessories (such as a tool belt) over the anterior hip. It can also follow prolonged operations done in the prone position, such as in posterior spine fusions in children.[24] Management is nonsurgical, consisting of measures to provide relief from mechanical compression of the nerve.

■ Metaphyseal Chondrodysplasia

Chief Clinical Characteristics

This presentation of this metaphyseal pathology can produce hip pain, short/bowed legs, and a waddling gait with the Schmid type.[10]

Background Information

This autosomal dominant group of disorders may present in infancy or childhood. Radiologic examination will demonstrate metaphyseal abnormalities with limb shortening or deformity.[40] Treatment may include surgery for correction of deformity.

■ Multiple Epiphyseal Dysplasia

Chief Clinical Characteristics

This presentation is characterized by abnormal ossification of multiple physes, resulting in lower limb stiffness and pain, usually symmetrically and most often in the hips and knees. Irregular epiphyseal and physeal development may also result in skeletal deformities such as coxa vara.[41]

Background Information

The Fairbank and Ribbing types have been further differentiated. Fairbank-type dysplasia is more severe and includes short extremities, waddling gait, and joint pain.[10] The Ribbing type may be difficult to distinguish from symmetrical Legg-Calvé-Perthes with its proximal femur involvement.[10] This is a predominantly autosomal dominant inherited disorder. Treatment may include activity modification or surgery.[41]

■ Muscle Strain

Chief Clinical Characteristics

This presentation includes an acute onset of local pain, spasm, swelling, weakness, and/or echymosis.[24,25]

Background Information

This injury is common in the hip adductor, iliopsoas, and hamstring muscle groups.[24,25] It results from an overstretching or tearing of the muscle.[24] Strains commonly occur in sports such as soccer, basketball, and sprinting.[24] Management includes ice, compression, rest, anti-inflammatory medications, ultrasound, and gradual return to exercise and sport.[25]

■ Myelodysplasia (Spina Bifida)

Chief Clinical Characteristics

This presentation includes muscle imbalances that result from weakness due to spinal cord injury and can result in hip dislocation.[21]

Background Information

In rare cases children with this condition might also develop neuropathic arthropathy of their hips or a monoarthritis resulting in pain and swelling.[10,42] This is a group of congenital disorders that results in neural tube defects that alter the development of the spinal cord, spine, or brain. It includes meningocele, myelomeningocele, and spina bifida occulta.

Surgical intervention is typically indicated to close the spinal canal defect. Other interventions may include bracing and rehabilitation to address the weakness that results from the spinal cord injury.[43]

■ Myositis Ossificans (Heterotopic Ossification)

Chief Clinical Characteristics

This presentation may include localized pain and limited joint range of motion following the resolution of a soft tissue trauma.[24]

Background Information

Heterotopic ossification is the laying down of bone at an abnormal site.[44] Hip fractures especially those followed by surgery are associated with the development of this disorder in the periarticular space.[44] In the pediatric population such fractures are most likely associated with high-velocity injuries such as motor vehicle accidents or a fall from a height.[44] The incidence for this disorder is approximately 20% in patients with brain or spinal cord injury with the hip being the most common site.[44] Children with cerebral palsy undergoing hip surgery are at higher risk for this complication. The three primary sites of involvement in this region are inferomedial to the hip, between the anterosuperior iliac spine and the proximolateral femur, and the posterior hip.[44] Treatment is controversial and may include therapy to maintain ROM, diphosphonate treatment, manipulation, and surgical excision.[44] When the formation of heterotopic bone follows direct trauma to a muscle, especially in the quadriceps or adductors, the term *myositis ossificans* is often used, but the biological process is the same. Early return to activity, soft tissue mobilization, ultrasound, or use of heat soon after a contusion may increase the risk for developing this disorder.[25] Surgical excision is performed if the pain and range-of-motion restriction limit function, but surgery is not recommended until at least 1 year postinjury to prevent recurrence.[25]

■ Osteitis Pubis

Chief Clinical Characteristics

This presentation is characterized by an insidious onset of pain over the pubic symphysis sometimes radiating to the groin.[24]

Background Information

This overuse disorder is associated with sports such as running, soccer, and football.[25] It is treated with rest, anti-inflammatory medications, and progressive return to sport.[25]

■ Osteochondritis Dissecans

Chief Clinical Characteristics

This presentation includes hip pain and difficulty weight bearing.[21]

Background Information

This is a subchondral bone defect that is rarely seen in the proximal femur except in children with healed Legg-Calvé-Perthes disease.[21] It may be caused by minor trauma or ischemia and often resolves without intervention.[21]

■ Osteogenesis Imperfecta

Chief Clinical Characteristics

This presentation includes fracture due to brittle bones as a potential cause of hip pain in these patients.[10] This is an autosomal dominant disorder resulting in poor collagen synthesis and brittle bones that develop abnormally, resulting in short stature and bowing of long bones. Many children with this condition have bone pain relating to old fractures as well as muscle weakness and ligamentous laxity.[21]

Background Information

Management may include bracing, rehabilitation, and possibly surgery for stabilization of the joints.

■ Osteomyelitis (Pyogenic or Granulomatous)

Chief Clinical Characteristics

This presentation may include a sudden onset of throbbing pain and swelling over the site of infection, along with fever, chills, and malaise.[5,21,45]

Background Information

This is an inflammatory disease of bone and bone marrow, most commonly due to a bacterial infection from a preceding trauma, systemic illness, or surgery.[5,8,21] In children the lesions are most common in the metaphyses of long, tubular bones and less often at the greater trochanter, femoral neck, or innominate of the pelvis.[21,46] Osteomyelitis is more common in boys and can be misdiagnosed as septic arthritis.[45,47] Delay in treatment of osteomyelitis with antibiotic medications can result in destruction of the involved bone.[21] Lack of response to antibiotic medications may necessitate surgical debridement.[8]

■ Osteopetrosis

Chief Clinical Characteristics
This presentation commonly results in epiphyseal separations and femur fractures.[48]

Background Information
Osteoclast dysfunction results in excessive bone density in this rare congenital disorder.[48] The goal of medical management is osteoclast stimulation through calcium restriction, steroids, parathyroid hormone, and interferon.[49] Children may also undergo a bone marrow transplant in certain forms of this condition.[49]

■ Poliomyelitis

Chief Clinical Characteristics
This presentation includes muscle tenderness and pain especially hamstring muscle spasm or tightness that may precede the onset of weakness.

Background Information
This is a viral infection involving the motor neurons of the central nervous system, especially in the spinal cord.[50] While the incidence has been reduced dramatically during the past decade, the disease is still an important one in India and parts of Africa. Treatment includes supportive care and rehabilitation.[50]

■ Polyarteritis Nodosa (Medium- and Large-Vessel Vasculitis)

Chief Clinical Characteristics
This presentation at onset is variable, but may include abdominal or extremity pain, rash, hypertension, hematuria, and/or fever.[10]

Background Information
It can be difficult to distinguish from Kawasaki disease, systemic-onset juvenile rheumatoid arthritis, small-vessel vasculitis, infection, neoplasm, and inflammatory bowel disease.[10] This disease is rare in children. Treatment includes steroid therapy.[10]

■ Pyomyositis

Chief Clinical Characteristics
This presentation may include limited, painful hip movements with an inability to bear weight.[51,52]

Background Information
This can be difficult to differentiate from septic arthritis.[51] It is more common in tropical climates or warm North American climates during summer.[52] An abscess is a subcategory of pyomyositis that has been described in the psoas, obturator externus or internus muscles, and retroperitoneal space in children.[52,53] A primary psoas abscess is formed without any detectable underlying infection and is more common in children.[53] A secondary abscess relates to an underlying infection such as tuberculosis, appendicitis, or osteomyelitis.[53] This condition may also be related to a history of trauma or strenuous exercise.[53] Treatment may include surgical drainage, aspiration, and/or a course of antibiotic medications.[52]

■ Rheumatic Fever

Chief Clinical Characteristics
This presentation may be characterized by rapid onset of migrating pain and inflammation.[10]

Background Information
This is an inflammatory disease that results from a *Streptococcus* bacterial infection. Incidence is higher in non-Western countries.[54] It is associated with a transient form of polyarthritis with lower extremity involvement preceding upper extremity early in the course of the illness.[10] Treatment is with anti-inflammatory medications.[10]

RHEUMATOID ARTHRITIS–LIKE DISEASES OF THE HIP

■ Arthritis with Inflammatory Bowel Disease

Chief Clinical Characteristics
This presentation involves hip, sacroiliac joint, or low back pain and stiffness associated with an acute episode of gastrointestinal upset. There are two forms of peripheral arthropathy associated with inflammatory bowel disease that occur in about 25% of patients.[55] The type I arthropathy associated with inflammatory bowel disease presents in a

pauciarticular distribution and it is considered self-limiting.[55]

Background Information

Inflammatory bowel disease is an idiopathic immune disorder affecting the intestinal tract. The most common types are Crohn's disease and ulcerative colitis.[56] Children with this disease are likely to be HLA-B27 positive, suggesting an underlying genetic predisposition. In some cases, when the inflammatory bowel disease is latent, the course of arthritis may be similar to the course of juvenile ankylosing spondylitis.[57,58] Treatment may include aminosalicylate or steroid medications and bowel resection depending on the severity of the disorder.[56]

■ Juvenile Ankylosing Spondylitis

Chief Clinical Characteristics

This presentation includes an insidious onset of hip, sacroiliac, and/or low back pain and stiffness that may be unilateral or bilateral and difficult to localize initially. Sacroiliitis is the hallmark sign, however, along with spinal pain and stiffness, it usually does not manifest until 2 to 5 years after onset. The pain will become more persistent over time along with gradual loss of spinal mobility and a reduction in normal lumbar lordosis. Symptoms are typically worse at night or in the morning and lasting at least 30 minutes. In ankylosing spondylitis pain may be relieved with rest or only mild activity. During active disease, systemic symptoms such as fever and weight loss may be present, and the child may refuse to walk. Associated complications may include atlantoaxial subluxation, uveitis leading to blindness, acute iritis, aortic valve insufficiency, decreased vital capacity, neurological complications, and, rarely, gastrointestinal and renal problems.

Background Information

This condition is the most prevalent spondyloarthropathy in children, found primarily in adolescent boys and young men. Onset is usually in the second or third decade of life, but 10% to 20% will have onset prior to age 16. Only about 25% of children with this disease will present initially with sacroiliac or spinal symptoms. Peripheral joints are involved in 30% to 50% of patients, usually within the first 10 years of disease. Ankylosing spondylitis is a chronic disease with intermittent periods of remission; it is rarely active persistently. There is no specific laboratory test for ankylosing spondylitis, however, most patients have the presence of HLA-B27 (human leukocyte antigen), elevated erythrocyte sedimentation rate and C-reactive protein level, and absence of rheumatoid factor. Radiographic changes include erosion, sclerosis, and eventually fusion of the sacroiliac joint and vertebrae. Magnetic resonance imaging and computed tomography of the sacroiliac joint may assist with early diagnosis. Enthesitis distinguishes this condition from juvenile rheumatoid arthritis. Individuals with this condition typically begin a course of nonsteroidal anti-inflammatory medications upon diagnosis for pain control. Corticosteroids are used only short term due to associated problems including osteoporosis. Research indicates that treatment with tumor necrosis factor can significantly improve symptoms.[59]

■ Juvenile Dermatomyositis

Chief Clinical Characteristics

This presentation is characterized by a skin rash that may be located on the torso, low back, and buttocks area early on in the disease process. The characteristic skin rash may also be found around the shoulder girdle, extensor surfaces of the arms and legs, medial malleoli of the ankles, and face. Disease onset is often insidious and may include fatigue, low-grade fever, weight loss, irritability, arthralgia, and abdominal pain. Proximal muscle weakness is usually recognized after a median of 2 months.[60] *Hip pain, although an uncommon symptom of this condition, is often reproduced with palpation of the affected region. Although this condition is rare in children, it is the most common of its type.*

Background Information

The disease process is triggered by an antigen-driven response, which manifests as a skin rash. In the absence of prompt diagnosis and treatment, the development of myositis with subsequent calcinosis occurs, causing severe limitation of range of motion of involved joints. The onset of proximal weakness is insidious and difficult to recognize. It is often detected by difficulty in everyday activities such as climbing stairs, reaching overhead, going from sitting to standing, and going from the floor to standing.[61] This condition occurs in approximately 1 to 3 children per million every year. The average age of onset is between 6 and 7 years of age with a higher prevalence in girls. Laboratory investigations include blood tests, muscle biopsy, and specific antibody tests. Treatment should include passive range-of-motion exercises and stretching during the disease course. Once active inflammation has resolved, treatment should focus on strengthening deconditioned muscle, regaining range of motion, and performing weight-bearing activities to ensure adequate bone mineralization. Bed rest and immobilization are contraindicated.

■ Psoriatic Arthritis

Chief Clinical Characteristics
This presentation involves psoriatic rash, arthritis, nail pitting, dactylitis (or "sausage digit"), and occasional fatigue. As the disease progresses sacroiliitis is present, resulting in hip and low back pain. In children arthritis may manifest prior to psoriasis, or onset of arthritis and psoriasis is concurrent.

Background Information
Chronic iridocyclitis is seen in approximately 15% of children.[57,58] This condition typically occurs in young girls, usually manifesting between 7 and 13 years of age, but always occurring prior to age 16 years. There is almost always a family history of psoriasis. Radiographs and computed tomography scan will determine extent of involvement of the spine, hips, and sacroiliac joint. Treatment includes nonsteroidal anti-inflammatory medications, corticosteroids, and topical or systemic medications for psoriasis. Modalities can also be used to control inflammation and pain.

■ Reactive Arthritis (Reiter's Syndrome)

Chief Clinical Characteristics
This presentation of reactive arthritis or Reiter's syndrome can be characterized by pain with passive and active movement that accompanies discoloration (dusky blue or redness), enthesitis, swelling, warmth, and tenderness to palpation of the involved joints.[11]

Background Information
It is asymmetrical, affecting an average of four joints and predominantly the lower extremities.[10] Hip involvement occurs uncommonly. It is most common in Caucasian males.[10] The onset of symptoms is usually preceded by a genitourinary or gastrointestinal infection.[10] While the underlying cause is an infection, the condition itself is a reactive arthritis to the bacterial proteins, not an infection. It has also been associated with human immunodeficiency virus. In children a genitourinary infection may be an indication of sexual abuse.[10] This condition is medically managed with anti-inflammatory medications or in severe cases with low-dose corticosteroids.[10]

■ Systemic Lupus Erythematosus

Chief Clinical Characteristics
This presentation may initially include musculoskeletal pain in any or all regions of the body including the back in 74% of children.[62] This may be accompained by the presence of fever, fatigue, arthralgia, malar (butterfly) rash, anorexia, lymphadenopathy, pleuritic pain, and seizures.

Background Information
This condition is a rheumatic disease of unknown cause characterized by autoantibodies directed against self-antigens and resulting in inflammatory damage to target organs including kidneys, blood-forming cells, and the central nervous system. The incidence varies by ethnicity and location. Prevalence rates vary from 4 to 250 per 100,000 children. The median age at diagnosis is approximately 10 years, and onset before age 8 is uncommon.[63] Diagnosis is confirmed by the combination of clinical and laboratory manifestations revealing multisystem disease. Treatment regimen depends on the affected target organs. Nonsteroidal anti-inflammatory agents are used to treat arthralgia and arthritic symptoms. Corticosteroids have been demonstrated to control symptoms and autoantibody production in systemic lupus erythematosus. Patients with severe disease may

require cytotoxic therapy. When the child is cleared for activity, physical therapy should focus on stretching, joint protection, and relaxation techniques to manage joint and muscle pain. During periods of remission, an exercise program of strengthening and cardiovascular exercise may be implemented to maintain the strength of surrounding musculature and to prevent the detrimental effects of bone demineralization due to prolonged use of corticosteroids.[63] Physical therapy treatment should be provided under supervision of the child's physician. The natural history is unpredictable; patients may present with a history of many years of symptoms or with acute, life-threatening disease. Left untreated, this condition may result in spontaneous remission, years of disease, or rapid death.

■ Rickets, Vitamin D–Dependent (Nutritional)

Chief Clinical Characteristics
This presentation includes profound weakness, skeletal deformity such as bowing of long bones, and an inability to ambulate.[64]

Background Information
In the underdeveloped world, children who are undernourished may have a vitamin D deficiency resulting in osteomalacia that can lead to hip pain due to stress fracture or slipped capital femoral epiphysis.[64] Lack of exposure to sunlight can also be a precipitating factor.[5] Vitamin D supplements to address the specific deficiency can resolve this disorder.

■ Rickets, Vitamin D–Resistant (Hypophosphatasia)

Chief Clinical Characteristics
This presentation involves spine, pelvic, and long bone deformity due to poor bone mineralization and overgrowth of unmineralized bone matrix.[5]

Background Information
In the industrialized world vitamin D–resistant rickets or hypophosphatasia is the most common form of rickets. This form is not related to dietary deficiency but instead due to vitamin D metabolism derangement or malabsorption, or homeostasis of calcium or phosphorus due to kidney or liver disease,

uremia, and prolonged treatment with certain anticonvulsants.[5] This condition is an autosomal dominant inherited disorder. It can be associated with renal osteodystrophy, another metabolic disease found in children with renal disease.[64] Supplements and medications are not indicated for this form of rickets. Surgery, bracing and rehabilitation may be necessary to address orthopedic complications.

■ Scleroderma (Focal or Systemic Sclerosis)

Chief Clinical Characteristics
This presentation includes fatigue, arthralgias or myalgias, and Raynaud's syndrome (vasospasm of arteries in response to cold).[10] It also can result in arthritis, tendinitis, weakness, and joint contractures.[10]

Background Information
This rare, chronic multisystem connective tissue disease results in fibrosis, small-vessel vasculitis, and an autoimmune response.[10] Pharmacologic therapy is the primary means of management with therapy involved for management of contractures and systemic effects.[10]

■ Septic Arthritis

Chief Clinical Characteristics
This presentation commonly includes severe pain and spasm with all hip movements, limp or inability to bear weight, fever, tenderness to palpation, local warmth, and edema.[10,51]

Background Information
Children often maintain their hip in a position of flexion, abduction, and external rotation.[10] The majority of cases in children are monoarticular, affect the knee or hip, and result from a bacterial infection.[10] It occurs less commonly due to tuberculosis or fungal infections such as coccidioidomycosis.[10] An elevated erythrocyte sedimentation rate helps to confirm the diagnosis.[10] In neonates or infants anorexia, irritability, and failure to thrive may be the only indications of pathology.[10] In sexually active adolescents the infection may be due to gonococcus and presents as a migratory mono- or polyarticular arthritis with accompanying hemorrhagic or pustular skin lesions.[10] Complications of the disease include osteomyelitis and osteonecrosis of the hip.[10] Treatment includes antibiotic therapy, surgical drainage, and debridement.[10]

■ Sickle Cell Anemia

Chief Clinical Characteristics

This presentation is characterized by painful vaso-occlusive crisis triggered by infection, dehydration, or acidosis that results in diffuse joint pain.[10]

Background Information

Complications of the vaso-occlusion that occurs in this disease include osteonecrosis of the femoral head, osteomyelitis, and septic and reactive arthritis.[5,10] Slipped capital femoral epiphysis should be excluded in these children due to similar age and presentation.[65] Management includes folic acid supplements and pain management during acute crises.

■ Slipped Femoral Capital Epiphyses

Chief Clinical Characteristics

This presentation involves acute or insidious onset of groin pain, which may radiate into the anteromedial thigh or knee, increased pain with weight bearing, and a passive limitation of abduction, flexion, and internal rotation.[25]

Background Information

The pathology is due to a disruption of the capital epiphyseal plate resulting in a slipping of the head on the neck of the femur (Fig. 45-3).[66,67] This disorder occurs bilaterally in 18% to 50% of children with higher frequency in the African American population.[67] Overall this disorder is most common in males, and is more common in Pacific Islanders and African Americans than other ethnic groups.[67] It is also associated with an obese, hypogonadal, or tall and thin body type.[25,68] Prevalence is higher in children with hypothyroidism on growth hormone therapy and is associated in rare cases with radiation therapy.[68] Complications of this disorder include avascular necrosis and chondrolysis.[67] Intervention options include immobilization with a hip-spica cast and various types of surgical fixation.[67]

■ Snapping Hip Syndrome

Chief Clinical Characteristics

This presentation includes clicking and pain located over the greater trochanter or the groin depending on the structure involved.[24]

Background Information

This phenomenon of clicking of the hip is typically due to the iliotibial band snapping over the greater trochanter, but it also can occur from the iliopsoas over the iliopectineal eminence, biceps femoris long head over the

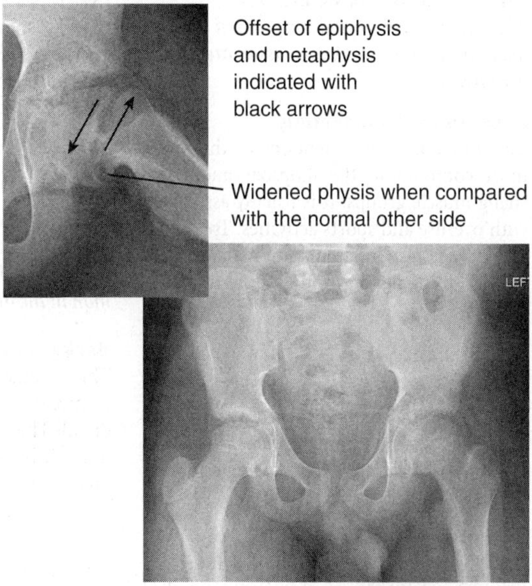

Offset of epiphysis and metaphysis indicated with black arrows

Widened physis when compared with the normal other side

FIGURE 45-3 Slipped capital femoral epiphysis of the leg hip, anteroposterior view. *Inset:* frog leg view. (Images courtesy of Keven Preston, MD, diagnostic radiology resident, Indiana University School of Medicine.)

ischial tuberosity, and the iliofemoral ligaments over the femoral head.[24] These extraarticular disorders can progress into bursitis.[24] Intra-articular problems such as loose bodies can also cause the same symptoms.[24] Snapping hip is typically associated with activities such as dancing and running.[25] Management includes inflammation management and restoring of muscle balance.[24,25]

■ Spastic Cerebral Palsy

Chief Clinical Characteristics
This presentation may include hip subluxation or dislocation as a result of the muscle imbalance between spastic hip adductors and other weak hip musculature.[69]

Background Information
A child with this condition may also have increased femoral anteversion and femoral neck-to-shaft angle, decreasing the stability of the hip articulation.[70] Subluxations or dislocations are more common in nonambulatory children with cerebral palsy and may be more likely during growth spurts and do not tend to be a problem until their second decade of age.[21] Nonsurgical management may include positioning and stretching.

■ Tendinitis

Chief Clinical Characteristics
This presentation includes a gradual onset of local pain and weakness associated with activity.[24]

Background Information
This inflammation of tendons of the hip is most common in the iliopsoas and hamstring muscle groups. It is usually associated with overuse and sports activities. Treatment can include rest, inflammation management, taping, strengthening, and gradual return to activity.

■ Transient Synovitis

Chief Clinical Characteristics
This presentation commonly involves unilateral hip joint pain and a limp.[71] Often, hip motion is limited and children maintain a position of hip flexion and external rotation.[71]

Background Information
Boys are more commonly affected between the ages of 3 and 8.[71] This condition may be linked to a prior viral infection, microtrauma, or allergic reaction but is largely a diagnosis of exclusion with diseases such as bacterial synovitis, septic arthritis, osteomyelitis, and pyarthrosis being ruled out.[71] This is usually a self-limiting disorder treated with rest and anti-inflammatory medications.[71]

■ Traumatic Dislocation

Chief Clinical Characteristics
This presentation is characterized by a range of presentations that correspond with the direction of dislocation. A child with a posterior dislocation will present with a flexed, adducted, and internally rotated limb that appears shortened. The posturing is the opposite for an anterior dislocation without shortening. An inferiorly dislocated hip will present in hyperflexion.[72]

Background Information
Hip dislocation due to trauma is rare in the pediatric population with most cases due to a motor vehicle accident, a fall from height, or a sports activity.[73] The hip is dislocated in the posterior direction in the majority of cases with a few being anterior or inferior.[24] The dislocation is sometimes associated with a concomitant hip fracture (17%).[73] Complications after this injury include avascular necrosis (3% to 15%), heterotopic ossification, coxa magna, and instability.[72,73] There is a significant association between the time from dislocation to reduction and the incidence of avascular necrosis.[72] Management includes reduction of dislocation and rehabilitation.

■ Tuberculosis Arthritis

Chief Clinical Characteristics
This presentation includes joint pain and swelling.[10] This form of arthritis is most common in the hips and knees.[10]

Background Information
This condition can be related to an adjacent osteomyelitis involving the hands or feet in children.[10] This is a chronic, slowly progressive disorder. It is confirmed by a tissue and synovial fluid culture that is positive for *Mycobacterium tuberculosis* due to joint invasion.[74] Treatment may include combination chemotherapy and surgery for debridement, stabilization, or synovectomy.[10]

TUMORS

◼ Ewing's Sarcoma

Chief Clinical Characteristics

This presentation typically manifests as severe, persistent pain especially at night, localized swelling, palpable mass, tenderness, and decreased range of motion. Other symptoms can include fever, malaise, and weight loss when there are metastases.[75]

Background Information

This condition is the most common malignant primary tumor found in the pediatric spine[76] and the second most common pediatric malignancy overall.[77] Approximately 2.1 children per million are diagnosed with this condition each year with predominance in males. Diagnosis is usually between the ages of 10 and 20 years, and is uncommon before age 5.[77] Treatment includes a combination of multiagent chemotherapy, followed by radiation and resection for local control. Prognosis for cure is approximately 75% in those who present without metastasis, and less than 30% for those with metastasis.

◼ Langerhans' Cell Histiocytosis

Chief Clinical Characteristics

This presentation commonly consists of pain that is usually relieved with nonsteroidal anti-inflammatory medications, rest, and, if necessary, bracing. Associated symptoms may be hepatosplenomegaly, anemia, leukopenia, and thrombocytopenia. Neurological symptoms may manifest if there is cord compression.

Background Information

This condition is commonly found in the anterior elements of the spine as a single lesion or is multifocal. A single, localized lesion is also known as eosinophilic granuloma. This condition is generally found in children 3 to 15 years of age with a predominance for white males, but can manifest at any age.[18,78,79] Radiographs will show a well-defined lesion, with focal bone destruction and possible vertebral collapse, or vertebral plana. This condition appears to be the most common cause of vertebral plana.[78] The intervertebral disks are not affected.[78] Treatment is usually reserved for those with organ dysfunction, unrelieved symptoms, or osseous deformity, because this condition is usually self-limiting.[78] Treatment can include a combination of any or all of radiation, chemotherapy, steroid therapy and curettage, and bracing.[79,80]

◼ Leukemia

Chief Clinical Characteristics

This presentation commonly involves reports of aches and pains in the extremities, back, and joints; fatigue; and anorexia. There may also be intermittent low-grade fever, enlarged lymph nodes, weight loss, petechiae, lethargy, shortness of breath, bruises, and excessive bleeding.

Background Information

Leukemia is the most common malignancy in children and adolescents, with a higher incidence in males.[81,82] It is typically diagnosed within the first decade of life and accounts for about 40% of all childhood malignancies. The two most common types account for approximately 90% of all leukemias: acute lymphoblastic leukemia (ALL), 77% to 80%, and acute myelogenous leukemia (AML), 10% to 13%. Some symptoms may be consistent with a viral infection, but the symptoms persist longer. Other symptoms are a result of progressive disease and bone marrow failure as a result of bone marrow infiltration by malignant cells, leading to anemia and decreased production of clotting factors.[82] Diagnostic evaluation of patients with leukemia includes complete blood count and bone marrow biopsy. Examination of bone marrow aspirate is necessary for confirmation, and a spinal tap determines if leukemia is present in the central nervous system.[83] Infiltration of bone and bone marrow may also be viewed on magnetic resonance imaging.[79] Rarely radiographs may show osteopenia and compression fractures. Analysis of chromosome abnormalities in the leukemia cells is very important to assess prognosis and formulate treatment. Treatment is specific to the type of leukemia present and typically has several phases. It involves multiple courses of chemotherapy and antibiotics to prevent infection, and often a child will require blood transfusions. Side effects of chemotherapy and steroid treatment include neutropenia, thrombocytopenia, and risk for infection. Long-term complications can include osteoporosis, and avascular necrosis. Bone marrow or stem cell transplant is reserved for situations where standard chemotherapy has failed and has a better success rate if performed in remission.[83] With current advances in treatment the 5-year survival rate, without relapse is reaching 80% to 90%.[84]

■ Lymphoma

Chief Clinical Characteristics

This presentation initially involves asymptomatic, chronically swollen lymph nodes, most commonly in the neck, axillae, or groin. Other symptoms may include neurological symptoms due to cord compression, fever, itching or irritation of the skin, weight loss, night sweats, cough, or shortness of breath.[83] Symptoms depend on the type of lymphoma present and the proximity to other structures and organs.

Background Information

Lymphoma is one of the most prevalent malignant tumors of childhood, and can manifest quickly. The two general types of lymphoma are Hodgkin's lymphoma and non-Hodgkin's lymphoma (NHL), and each has its own subtypes. Hodgkin's disease is distinguished from non-Hodgkin's by the presence of specific cancer cells in the biopsy material, termed Reed-Sternberg cells.[83,85] Approximately 40% of pediatric cases are of the Hodgkin's type, and 60% are non-Hodgkin's.[81] Approximately 10% to 15% of all cases of Hodgkin's disease, and about 5% of all NHL cases, are children under age 19, both with a higher prevalence in boys. NHL is more common in children under age 5.[85,86] Biopsy, radiographs, computed tomography, and blood tests are performed for definitive diagnosis and to assess the stage of disease. Bone marrow biopsy is done to evaluate bone marrow involvement. Radiographs and computed tomography typically show enlarged lymph nodes in the affected areas and can show extensive, destructive lesions in patients with osseous involvement. Magnetic resonance imaging is indicated to evaluate soft tissue involvement.[75] Laboratory tests may show anemia and elevated sedimentation rate. Treatment includes chemotherapy and radiation, the course of which depends on the type of lymphoma, the stage of disease, and if there is bone marrow metastasis. Bone marrow transplant may be indicated if there is failure to respond to standard chemotherapy and radiation. Survival rates are 90 to 95% for those with local lesions, and 75 to 80% for those with more diffuse disease.[81]

■ Nephroblastoma (Wilms' Tumor)

Chief Clinical Characteristics

This presentation typically includes an asymptomatic, nontender mass in the abdomen. Associated symptoms may be abdominal pain, fever, nausea, and vomiting. Hematuria, anemia, and hypertension can occur, since the kidneys are instrumental in controlling blood pressure. Shortness of breath may be present if metastases to the lungs are present.[81,87]

Background Information

This condition involves a tumor that originates from renal precursor cells. It is the second most common abdominal tumor in infants and children up to 5 years old and is the most common primary malignant tumor of the kidney. Multiple laboratory tests, including complete blood count, ultrasound, magnetic resonance imaging, or computed tomography, are indicated. Treatment includes removal of the kidney containing the tumor followed by chemotherapy and or radiation. The survival rate is typically 70% to 95%, especially in young children, or those with stage I, II, or III tumors.[87] Recurrences are usually seen within 3 years. Postradiation scoliosis may follow in the second decade.

■ Neuroblastoma

Chief Clinical Characteristics

This presentation may include severe localized back pain, weakness, scoliosis, and neurological signs secondary to spinal cord compression. Other symptoms may include a palpable mass, hepatomegaly, constipation, abdominal pain, bladder dysfunction, and ecchymoses. It is one of the few cancers that cause diarrhea.[75,81,88,89]

Background Information

This condition is a solid tumor that develops in neural crest tissue, most commonly in the abdomen, chest, or adrenal glands.[81] It rarely originates in the brain or spinal cord. If the primary lesion originates somewhere other than the spinal cord, metastases is hematogenic in nature, and can spread to bone, bone marrow, live, skin, lungs, and the brain. This is the most common extracranial cancer of childhood and the third most common pediatric neoplasm overall. Approximately 500 new cases are diagnosed each year. It is usually diagnosed in infancy, almost always by 5 years of age, and is rarely seen in children over 10 years of age.[75,81,88,89] Low-risk tumors (stage I) in infants treated with surgical excision and observation have an approximately 90% survival rate without relapse. Children over 3 years of age with stage IV tumors only have a 10% to 15% survival rate.[81] In infants the tumor may regress completely with spontaneous cell death, or mature to normal ganglion cells and become benign. In children over 1 year of age, the disease progression may be rapidly metastatic and often fatal.[81,88]

■ Osteochondroma

Chief Clinical Characteristics

This presentation involves hip pain that can result from compression of a nerve by or fracture of the exostosis.[5]

Background Information

This cartilaginous exostosis is more common in males and sometimes occurs in the pelvis.[5] It is more common in late adolescence to young adulthood.[5] Familial osteochondromatosis or multiple hereditary exostosis is an autosomal dominant inherited variant in which more than two osteochondromas are present.[5] This form is more common in males during childhood and is more likely to involve the hip region.[5]

■ Osteoid Osteoma

Chief Clinical Characteristics

This presentation involves predominantly intense nocturnal pain that may be relieved with nonsteroidal anti-inflammatory medications or aspirin.[19,79] The pain may be referred or localized. Gait deviations and muscle atrophy are

often present. About 50% of children present with nonstructural, painful scoliosis,[76] which should be a red flag because idiopathic scoliosis is not painful.

Background Information

This condition includes highly vascularized connective tissue bundles, usually sclerotic, surrounding an osteoid nidus or growth center. They are small round or ovate tumors that are usually less than 1 cm in diameter.[75,90] Spinal osteoid lesions are found primarily in the posterior elements of the lumbar vertebra.[18,75,76,79,90] Soft tissue changes are rare. This condition is typically found in children between the ages of 5 and 20, with an approximate 2:1 male-to-female ratio.[75,91] Erythrocyte sedimentation rate, leukocyte count and protein electrophoresis should be normal. Radiographs and computed tomography will also differentiate osteoid osteomas from osteoblastomas, infection, lymphoma, and facet abnormalities such as spondylolysis.[91] Spinal lesions typically require open surgical excision. In most cases, the scoliosis will resolve and pain will subside completely.[14]

■ Osteosarcoma (Osteogenic Sarcoma)

Chief Clinical Characteristics

This presentation may be characterized by persistent night pain.

Background Information

This condition is related to highly malignant and locally aggressive lesions.[92] It rarely originates in the axial skeleton, but when it does it is usually found in the vertebral bodies.[80,92,93] Vertebral sarcomas comprise about 10% of all cases.[76] These tumors are typically found in the metaphyses of long bones and may metastasize to the spine. Diagnosis usually occurs between 10 and 20 years of age, and adolescent growth spurts appear to be the greatest risk periods for development.[79,94] Children with certain hereditary conditions such as retinoblastoma have a significant predisposition for developing this condition. Treatment includes local control with surgical excision and radiation or chemotherapy for metastatic lesions. If neurological signs are present, surgical decompression and laminectomy may be necessary.[17] Without metastasis approximately 70% of cases are cured with surgery and chemotherapy. If metastases are present on diagnosis, the survival rate is less than 20%.

■ Rhabdomyosarcoma

Chief Clinical Characteristics

This presentation may include back pain associated with neurological signs due to cord compression when present in the lumbar spine.[83,93]

Background Information

This condition is thought to originate from striated skeletal muscle cells.[93] Alveolar rhabdomyosarcoma is typically found in the extremities and in paravertebral soft tissue. Although it is rare, this condition is the most common solid soft tissue tumor in children under 10 years of age, accounting for 5% to 8% of pediatric neoplasms. It is usually diagnosed prior to age 6 and is most prevalent in male infants.[75,83,93] Diagnostic tests include biopsy, and computed tomography and magnetic resonance imaging.[75,83] Treatment includes chemotherapy, radiation, and if necessary, complete resection. For those diagnosed and treated in the early stages, the survival rate is approximately 80% to 90%.[83,93] Prognosis is poor for those with the alveolar subtype, larger tumors, or who are over 10 years of age.[75,83,93]

■ Synovial Sarcoma

Chief Clinical Characteristics

This presentation includes a painful mass in approximately half of patients.[10]

Background Information

Synovial sarcoma is a slow-growing, malignant tumor that is typically found proximal to tendons or fascia but sometimes also near or inside of a joint.[10] It is more common in the lower extremity than in other regions of the body.[10] The tissue origin for this tumor has not been determined but resembles nerve sheath tumor cells.[95] It makes up 9% of soft tissue sarcomas and typically occurs in young adults.[96] Treatment with surgical excision and radiation results in good local outcomes.[96,97] Chemotherapy may be used in larger tumors or with distal metastases.[96]

References

1. Fischer SU, Beattie TF. The limping child: epidemiology, assessment and outcome. *J Bone Joint Surg Br.* Nov 1999;81(6):1029–1034.
2. Malleson PN, Beauchamp RD. Rheumatology: 16. Diagnosing musculoskeletal pain in children. *CMAJ.* Jul 24 2001;165(2):183–188.
3. Tang T, Noble-Jamieson C. Lesson of the week: A painful hip as a presentation of Guillain-Barré syndrome in children. *BMJ.* Jan 20 2001;322(7279): 149–150.
4. Hesse B, Kohler G. Does it always have to be Perthes' disease? What is epiphyseal dysplasia? *Clin Orthop Relat Res.* Sep 2003(414):219–227.
5. Cotran RS, Kumar V, Robbins SL, Schoen FJ. *Pathologic Basis of Disease.* 5th ed. Philadelphia, PA: W. B. Saunders; 1994.
6. Wiener SL. *Differential Diagnosis of Acute Pain: By Body Region.* New York: McGraw-Hill; 1993.
7. Hosalkar HS, Gill IP, Monsell F, Sau I, Ramsay A. Hip pain in a 12-year-old boy. *Clin Orthop Relat Res.* Nov 2003(416):325–332.
8. McCarthy JJ, Dormans JP, Kozin SH, Pizzutillo PD. Musculoskeletal infections in children: basic treatment principles and recent advancements. *Instr Course Lect.* 2005;54:515–528.
9. Lundon K, Bolton K. Structure and function of the lumbar intervertebral disk in health, aging, and pathologic conditions. *J Orthop Sports Phys Ther.* Jun 2001;31(6): 291–303; discussion 304–306.
10. Klippel JH. *Primer on the Rheumatic Diseases.* 12th ed. Atlanta, GA: Arthritis Foundation; 2002.
11. Gilbert-Barness E. Review: Metabolic cardiomyopathy and conduction system defects in children. *Ann Clin Lab Sci.* Winter 2004;34(1):15–34.
12. Haller RG, Wyrick P, Taivassalo T, Vissing J. Aerobic conditioning: an effective therapy in McArdle's disease. *Ann Neurol.* Jun 2006;59(6):922–928.
13. Quinlivan R, Beynon RJ, Martinuzzi A. Pharmacological and nutritional treatment for McArdle disease (glycogen storage disease type V). *Cochrane Database Syst Rev.* 2008(2):CD003458.
14. Hosalkar H, Dormans JP. Back pain in children requires extensive workup; *Biomechanics.* Jun 2003;10(6):51–58.
15. Pierz K, Dormans, J. Spinal disorders. In: Dormans JP, ed. *Pediatric Orthopedics and Sports Medicine: The Requisites in Pediatrics.* St. Louis, MO: Mosby; 2004.
16. Thompson G. Back pain in children. In: Heckman JD, ed. *Instructional Course Lectures.* Rosemont, IL: American Academy of Orthopaedic Surgeons; 1993.
17. Wheeless CR. *Wheeless' Textbook of Orthopedics.* Durham, NC: Duke University Medical Center; 2005.
18. Thompson G. The spine. In: Behrman RE, Kliegman RM, Jenson HB, eds. *Nelson Textbook of Pediatrics.* 17th ed. Philadelphia, PA: W. B. Saunders; 2004:2287.
19. Payne WK 3rd, Ogilvie JW. Back pain in children and adolescents. *Pediatr Clin North Am.* Aug 1996;43(4): 899–917.
20. Luedtke L. Back pain in children and adolescents: Understanding and diagnosing spondylolysis and spondylolisthesis. In: *A Pediatric Perspective.* Vol 1. St. Paul, MN: Gillette Children's Specialty Healthcare; 2002.
21. Ratliffe KT. *Clinical Pediatric Physical Therapy: A Guide for the Physical Therapy Team.* St. Louis, MO: Mosby; 1997.

22. McCarthy J, Noble P, Aluisio FV, Schuck M, Wright J, Lee JA. Anatomy, pathologic features, and treatment of acetabular labral tears. *Clin Orthop Relat Res.* Jan 2003(406):38–47.

23. Clohisy JC, Nunley RM, Curry MC, Schoenecker PL. Periacetabular osteotomy for the treatment of acetabular dysplasia associated with major aspherical femoral head deformities. *J Bone Joint Surg Am.* Jul 2007;89(7): 1417–1423.

24. Zachazewski JE, Magee DJ, Quillen WS. *Athletic Injuries and Rehabilitation.* Philadelphia, PA: W. B. Saunders; 1996.

25. Arnheim DD, Prentice WE. *Principles of Athletic Training.* 8th ed. St. Louis, MO: Mosby; 1992.

26. Loth TS, Wadsworth CT. *Orthopedic review for physical therapists.* St. Louis, MO: Mosby; 1997.

27. Gaughan DM, Mofenson LM, Hughes MD, Seage GR 3rd, Ciupak GL, Oleske JM. Osteonecrosis of the hip (Legg-Calvé-Perthes disease) in human immunodeficiency virus-infected children. *Pediatrics.* May 2002; 109(5):E74.

28. Behrman RE, Kliegman RM, Jenson HB. *Nelson Textbook of Pediatrics.* 17th ed. Philadelphia, PA: W. B. Saunders; 2004.

29. Berend KR, Vail TP. Hip arthroscopy in the adolescent and pediatric athlete. *Clin Sports Med.* Oct 2001;20(4): 763–778.

30. Korinthenberg R, Monting JS. Natural history and treatment effects in Guillain-Barré syndrome: a multicentre study. *Arch Dis Child.* Apr 1996;74(4):281–287.

31. Govoni V, Granieri E. Epidemiology of the Guillain-Barré syndrome. *Curr Opin Neurol.* Oct 2001;14(5): 605–613.

32. Connolly AM. Chronic inflammatory demyelinating polyneuropathy in childhood. *Pediatr Neurol.* Mar 2001;24(3):177–182.

33. Giunta C, Superti-Furga A, Spranger S, Cole WG, Steinmann B. Ehlers-Danlos syndrome type VII: clinical features and molecular defects. *J Bone Joint Surg Am.* Feb 1999;81(2):225–238.

34. Martins AM, Valadares ER, Porta G, et al. Recommendations of diagnosis treatment and monitoring for Gaucher's disease. *J Pediatr.* 2009;155(4 Suppl):S10-18.

35. Kilcoyne RF, Nuss R. Femoral head osteonecrosis in a child with hemophilia. *Arthritis Rheum.* Jul 1999;42(7): 1550–1551.

36. Hilgartner MW. Current treatment of hemophilic arthropathy. *Curr Opin Pediatr.* Feb 2002;14(1):46–49.

37. Spencer CH, Bernstein BH. Hip disease in juvenile rheumatoid arthritis. *Curr Opin Rheumatol.* Sep 2002;14(5):536–541.

38. Jinnah HA. Lesch-Nyhan disease: from mechanism to model and back again. *Dis Model Mech.* Mar–Apr 2009;2(3–4):116–121.

39. Halperin JJ. Nervous system lyme disease: diagnosis and treatment. *Rev Neurol Dis* 2009;6(1):4–12.

40. Savarirayan R, Cormier-Daire V, Lachman RS, Rimoin DL. Schmid type metaphyseal chondrodysplasia: a spondylometaphyseal dysplasia identical to the "Japanese" type. *Pediatr Radiol.* Jul 2000;30(7):460–463.

41. Treble NJ, Jensen FO, Bankier A, Rogers JG, Cole WG. Development of the hip in multiple epiphyseal dysplasia. Natural history and susceptibility to premature osteoarthritis. *J Bone Joint Surg Br.* Nov 1990;72(6): 1061–1064.

42. Nagarkatti DG, Banta JV, Thomson JD. Charcot arthropathy in spina bifida. *J Pediatr Orthop.* 2000; 20(1):82.

43. Botto LD, Moore CA, Khoury MJ, Erickson JD. Neural-tube defects. *N Engl J Med.* Nov 11 1999;341(20): 1509–1519.

44. Garland DE. Clinical observations on fractures and heterotopic ossification in the spinal cord and traumatic brain injured populations. *Clin Orthop Relat Res.* Aug 1988(233):86–101.

45. Davidson D, Letts M, Khoshhal K. Pelvic osteomyelitis in children: a comparison of decades from 1980–1989 with 1990–2001. *J Pediatr Orthop.* Jul–Aug 2003;23(4): 514–521.

46. Zvulunov A, Gal N, Segev Z. Acute hematogenous osteomyelitis of the pelvis in childhood: Diagnostic clues and pitfalls. *Pediatr Emerg Care.* Feb 2003;19(1):29–31.

47. Auh JS, Binns HJ, Katz BZ. Retrospective assessment of subacute or chronic osteomyelitis in children and young adults. *Clin Pediatr (Phila).* Jul–Aug 2004;43(6): 549–555.

48. Armstrong DG, Newfield JT, Gillespie R. Orthopedic management of osteopetrosis: results of a survey and review of the literature. *J Pediatr Orthop.* Jan–Feb 1999; 19(1):122–132.

49. Kocher MS, Kasser JR. Osteopetrosis. *Am J Orthop.* May 2003;32(5):222–228.

50. Victor M, Ropper AH. *Adams and Victor's Principles of Neurology.* 7th ed. New York, NY: McGraw-Hill; 2001.

51. Hosalkar HS, Chatoo MB, Jones S, McHugh K, Monsell F, Jones DH. Hip pain in a 6-year-old girl. *Clin Orthop Relat Res.* Feb 2004(419):311–315.

52. Orlicek SL, Abramson JS, Woods CR, Givner LB. Obturator internus muscle abscess in children. *J Pediatr Orthop.* Nov–Dec 2001;21(6):744–748.

53. Song J, Letts M, Monson R. Differentiation of psoas muscle abscess from septic arthritis of the hip in children. *Clin Orthop Relat Res.* Oct 2001(391):258–265.

54. Tibazarwa KB, Volmink JA, Mayosi BM. Incidence of acute rheumatic fever in the world: a systematic review of population-based studies. *Heart.* Dec 2008;94 (12):1534–1540.

55. Wordsworth P. Arthritis and inflammatory bowel disease. *Curr Rheumatol Rep.* Apr 2000;2(2):87–88.

56. Andres PG, Friedman LS. Epidemiology and the natural course of inflammatory bowel disease. *Gastroenterol Clin North Am.* Jun 1999;28(2):255–281, vii.

57. Miller M, Petty R. Ankylosing spondylitis and other spondyloarthropathies. In: Behrman RE, Kliegman RM, Jenson HB, eds. *Nelson Textbook of Pediatrics.* 17th ed. Philadelphia, PA: W. B. Saunders; 2004.

58. Scalzi L, Lou J. Synovial disorders. In: Dormans JP, ed. *Pediatric Orthopedics and Sports Medicine: The Requisites in Pediatrics.* St. Louis, MO: Mosby; 2004:349.

59. Gorman JD, Sack KE, Davis JC, Jr. Treatment of ankylosing spondylitis by inhibition of tumor necrosis factor alpha. *N Engl J Med.* May 2, 2002;346(18): 1349–1356.

60. Pachman L. Juvenile dermatomyositis. In: Behrman RE, Kliegman RM, Jenson HB, eds. *Nelson Textbook of Pediatrics.* 17th ed. Philadelphia, PA: W. B. Saunders; 2004.

61. Pilkington CA, Wedderburn LR. Paediatric idiopathic inflammatory muscle disease: recognition and management. *Drugs.* 2005;65(10):1355–1365.

62. Iqbal S, Sher MR, Good RA, Cawkwell GD. Diversity in presenting manifestations of systemic lupus erythematosus in children. *J Pediatr.* Oct 1999;135(4): 500–505.

63. Miettunen PM, Ortiz-Alvarez O, Petty RE, et al. Gender and ethnic origin have no effect on long-term outcome of childhood-onset systemic lupus erythematosus. *J Rheumatol.* Aug 2004;31(8):1650–1654.

64. Mankin PN, Beauchamp RD. Metabolic bone disease. In: Heckman JD, ed. *Instructional Course Lectures.* Rosemont, IL: American Academy of Orthopaedic Surgeons; 1993.

65. Segal LS, Wallach DM. Slipped capital femoral epiphysis in a child with sickle cell disease. *Clin Orthop Relat Res.* Feb 2004(419):198–201.

66. Castriota-Scanderbeg A, Orsi E. Slipped capital femoral epiphysis: ultrasonographic findings. *Skeletal Radiol.* 1993;22(3):191–193.

67. Loder RT, Aronsson DD, Dobbs MB, Weinstein SL. Slipped capital femoral epiphysis. *J Bone Joint Surg Am.* 2000;82-A(8):1170–1188.

68. Loder RT, Hensinger RN, Alburger PD, et al. Slipped capital femoral epiphysis associated with radiation therapy. *J Pediatr Orthop.* Sep–Oct 1998;18(5): 630–636.

69. McHale KA, Bagg M, Nason SS. Treatment of the chronically dislocated hip in adolescents with cerebral palsy with femoral head resection and subtrochanteric valgus osteotomy. *J Pediatr Orthop.* Jul–Aug 1990;10(4): 504–509.

70. Jozwiak M, Marciniak W, Piontek T, Pietrzak S. Dega's transiliac osteotomy in the treatment of spastic hip subluxation and dislocation in cerebral palsy. *J Pediatr Orthop B.* Oct 2000;9(4):257–264.

71. Do TT. Transient synovitis as a cause of painful limps in children. *Curr Opin Pediatr.* Feb 2000;12(1):48–51.

72. Salisbury RD, Eastwood DM. Traumatic dislocation of the hip in children. *Clin Orthop Relat Res.* Aug 2000(377):106–111.

73. Mehlman CT, Hubbard GW, Crawford AH, Roy DR, Wall EJ. Traumatic hip dislocation in children. Long-term followup of 42 patients. *Clin Orthop Relat Res.* Jul 2000(376):68–79.

74. Bodur H, Erbay A, Yilmaz O, Kulacoglu S. Multifocal tuberculosis presenting with osteoarticular and breast involvement. *Ann Clin Microbiol Antimicrob.* Mar 19 2003;2:6.

75. Erol B, States L. Musculoskeletal tumors in children. In: Dormans JP, ed. *Pediatric Orthopedics and Sports Medicine: The Requisites in Pediatrics.* St. Louis, MO: Mosby; 2004:325.

76. Luedtke LM, Flynn JM, Ganley TJ, Hosalkar HS, Pill SG, Dormans JP. The orthopedists' perspective: bone tumors, scoliosis, and trauma. *Radiol Clin North Am.* Jul 2001;39(4):803–821.

77. Horowitz ME, Neff JR, Kun LE. Ewing's sarcoma. Radiotherapy versus surgery for local control. *Pediatr Clin North Am.* Apr 1991;38(2):365–380.

78. Levine SE, Dormans JP, Meyer JS, Corcoran TA. Langerhans' cell histiocytosis of the spine in children. *Clin Orthop Relat Res.* Feb 1996(323):288–293.

79. Miller SL, Hoffer FA. Malignant and benign bone tumors. *Radiol Clin North Am.* Jul 2001;39(4):673–699.

80. Hosalkar J, Dormans J. Back pain in children requires extensive workup. *Biomechanics.* 2003(June):51–58.

81. Golden CB, Feusner JH. Malignant abdominal masses in children: quick guide to evaluation and diagnosis. *Pediatr Clin North Am.* Dec 2002;49(6):1369–1392, viii.

82. Tubergen D, Bleyer A. Cancer and benign tumors. In: Behrman RE, Kliegman RM, Jenson HB, eds. *Nelson Textbook of Pediatrics.* 17th ed. Philadelphia, PA: W. B. Saunders; 2004:1694–1698.

83. Johns Hopkins University. Types of childhood cancers. http://www.jhscout.org//types/index.cfm. Accessed August 27, 2005.

84. Miller S, Hoffer F. Malignant and benign bone tumors. *Radiol Clin North Am Pediatr Musculoskel Radiol.* 2001;39(4):673–699.

85. Gilchrist G. Lymphoma. In: Behrman RE, Kliegman RM, Jenson HB, eds. *Nelson Textbook of Pediatrics.* 17th ed. Philadelphia, PA: W. B. Saunders; 2004.

86. Kurtzberg J, Graham ML. Non-Hodgkin's lymphoma. Biologic classification and implication for therapy. *Pediatr Clin North Am.* Apr 1991;38(2):443–456.

87. Beers MH. *The Merck Manual of Medical Information.* 2nd ed. Whitehouse Station, NJ: Merck; 2003.

88. *Detailed Guide: Brain/CNS Tumors in Children: What Are Children's Brain and Spinal Cord Cancers?* American Cancer Society; 2005.

89. Ater J. Neuroblastoma. In: Behrman RE, Kliegman RM, Jenson HB, eds. *Nelson Textbook of Pediatrics.* 17th ed. Philadelphia, PA: W. B. Saunders; 2004:1709.

90. Guzey FK, Seyithanoglu MH, Sencer A, Emei E, Alatas I, Izgi AN. Vertebral osteoid osteoma associated with paravertebral soft-tissue changes on magnetic resonance imaging. Report of two cases. *J Neurosurg.* May 2004;100(5 suppl Pediatrics):532–536.

91. Murphey MD, Andrews CL, Flemming DJ, Temple HT, Smith WS, Smirniotopoulos JG. From the archives of the AFIP. Primary tumors of the spine: radiologic pathologic correlation. *Radiographics.* Sep 1996;16(5): 1131–1158.

92. Meyer WH, Malawer MM. Osteosarcoma. Clinical features and evolving surgical and chemotherapeutic strategies. *Pediatr Clin North Am.* Apr 1991;38(2):317–348.

93. Arndt C. Soft tissue sarcomas. In: Behrman RE, Kliegman RM, Jenson HB, eds. *Nelson Textbook of Pediatrics.* 17th ed. Philadelphia, PA: W. B. Saunders; 2004:1714.

94. Kay RM, Eckardt JJ, Mirra JM. Osteosarcoma and Ewing's sarcoma in a retinoblastoma patient. *Clin Orthop Relat Res.* Feb 1996(323):284–287.

95. Ladanyi M, Antonescu CR, Leung DH, et al. Impact of SYT-SSX fusion type on the clinical behavior of synovial sarcoma: a multi-institutional retrospective study of 243 patients. *Cancer Res.* Jan 1 2002;62(1):135–140.

96. Eilber FC, Dry SM. Diagnosis and management of synovial sarcoma. *J Surg Oncol.* Mar 15, 2008;97 (4):314–320.

97. Ladenstein R, Treuner J, Koscielniak E, et al. Synovial sarcoma of childhood and adolescence. Report of the German CWS-81 study. *Cancer.* Jun 1, 1993;71(11): 3647–3655.

CHAPTER 46

Case Demonstration: Hip Pain in a Child

■ *Hugh G. Watts, MD* ■ *Chris A. Sebelski, PT, DPT, OCS, CSCS*

NOTE: This case demonstration was developed using the diagnostic process described in Chapter 4 and demonstrated in Chapter 5. The reader is encouraged to use this diagnostic process in order to ensure thorough clinical reasoning. If additional elaboration is required on the information presented in this chapter, please consult Chapters 4 and 5.

THE DIAGNOSTIC PROCESS

Step 1 Identify the patient's chief concern.
Step 2 Identify *barriers to communication*.
Step 3 Identify *special concerns*.
Step 4 Create a symptom timeline and sketch the anatomy (if needed).
Step 5 Create a diagnostic hypothesis list considering all possible forms of *remote* and *local* pathology that could cause the patient's chief concern.
Step 6 Sort the diagnostic hypothesis list by epidemiology and specific case characteristics.
Step 7 Ask specific questions to rule specific conditions or pathological categories less likely.
Step 8 Re-sort the diagnostic hypothesis list based on the patient's responses to specific questioning.
Step 9 Perform tests to differentiate among the remaining diagnostic hypotheses.
Step 10 Re-sort the diagnostic hypothesis list based on the patient's responses to specific tests.
Step 11 Decide on a diagnostic impression.
Step 12 Determine the appropriate patient disposition.

Case Description

You receive a phone call from a good friend of yours who is a graduate student at the University of Southern California. Her son has mentioned that he has pain in his right hip. Your friend is unsure of exactly where the pain is. She's hoping that you will check out her child to see if an expensive journey through the medical system can be avoided.

Billy is 7 years old and is a good student in the second grade. Questions directed to your friend indicate that Billy's pain came on gradually about 2 months ago, a few days after he fell off his bicycle. He is a healthy boy overall and has had all of his immunizations. She admits that he has had several intermittent low-grade fevers, but there have been a lot of "bugs" going around his school. Billy has a 5-year-old sister who is developing typically.

You agree to see him. Billy walks into the clinic with a right antalgic gait pattern. When asked, Billy points vaguely to his right hip above the greater trochanter and in front of his upper thigh.

STEP #1: Identify the patient's chief concern.

- Right anterolateral hip pain

STEP #2: Identify *barriers to communication*.

- This is a personal referral from a friend.
- Patient is a 7-year-old male, which suggests associated issues with communication.

STEP #3: Identify *special concerns*.

- **Family history.** Though no details are known, the mother has identified a possible family history of a bleeding disorder.
- **Recent illness.** This may raise the index of clinical suspicion for causes of pain that are associated with illness.

STEP #4: Create a symptom timeline and sketch the anatomy (if needed).

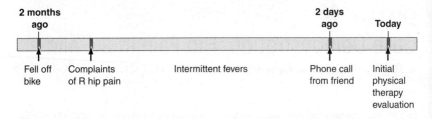

2 months ago		Intermittent fevers	2 days ago	Today
Fell off bike	Complaints of R hip pain		Phone call from friend	Initial physical therapy evaluation

STEP #5: Create a diagnostic hypothesis list considering all possible forms of *remote* and *local* pathology that could cause the patient's chief concern.

Remote

T   Trauma

Lumbar disk herniation/radiculopathy

Spondylolisthesis

Spondylolysis

I   Inflammation

Aseptic
Not applicable

Septic
Appendicitis (especially retrocecal)

Chronic granulomatous disease
Discitis
Osteomyelitis of the lumbar vertebra
Septic arthritis of sacroiliac joint

M   Metabolic

Metabolic myopathy

Va   Vascular

Polyarteritis nodosa

De   Degenerative

Not applicable

Tu   Tumor

Lymphoma
Neuroblastoma

Co   Congenital

Not applicable

Ne   Neurogenic/Psychogenic

Not applicable

STEP #6: Sort the diagnostic hypothesis list by epidemiology and specific case characteristics.

Remote

T   Trauma

~~Lumbar disc herniation/radiculopathy~~ (would require major trauma)
~~Spondylolisthesis~~ (too young; congenital type is painless)
~~Spondylolysis~~ (too young)

I   Inflammation

Aseptic
Not applicable

Septic
~~Appendicitis (especially retrocecal)~~ (timeline too long)
Chronic granulomatous disease
Discitis
Osteomyelitis of the lumbar vertebra
Septic arthritis of sacroiliac joint

M   Metabolic

~~Metabolic myopathy~~ (not associated with fever)

Va   Vascular

~~Polyarteritis nodosa~~ (rare in children)

De   Degenerative

Not applicable

Tu   Tumor

Lymphoma
~~Neuroblastoma~~ (too old)

Co   Congenital

Not applicable

Ne   Neurogenic/Psychogenic

Not applicable

Local

T Trauma

Avulsion injuries:
- Psoas off the lesser trochanter
- Rectus off the AIIS
- Sartorius off the ASIS

Chondral injury

Delayed-onset muscle soreness

Heterotopic ossification due to trauma

Hip contusion
Hip dislocation

Hip fracture
Labral tear
Meralgia paresthetica

Muscle strain
Myositis ossificans
Slipped capital femoral epiphyses

Snapping hip syndrome

I Inflammation

Aseptic

Apophysitis of greater trochanter
Chronic inflammatory demyelinating
  polyneuropathy
Guillain-Barré syndrome
Hip bursitis
Juvenile rheumatoid arthritis (and related
  diseases):
- Juvenile dermatomyositis
- Juvenile spondyloarthropathies
- Scleroderma
- Systemic lupus erythematosus

Osteitis pubis
Reactive arthritis
Rheumatic fever
Tendinitis
Transient synovitis

Septic

Acute:
Lyme disease (tick paralysis)
Osteomyelitis of femoral neck
Poliomyelitis
Pyomyositis
Septic arthritis of the hip

Local

T Trauma

~~Avulsion injuries:~~
- ~~Psoas off the lesser trochanter~~ (too young)
- ~~Rectus off the AIIS~~ (too young)
- ~~Sartorius off the ASIS~~ (too young)

~~Chondral injury~~ (not associated with fever)

~~Delayed-onset muscle soreness~~ (not
  associated with fever)

~~Heterotopic ossification due to trauma~~ (not
  associated with fever)

~~Hip contusion~~ (not associated with fever)
~~Hip dislocation~~ (can walk; not associated
  with fever)

~~Hip fracture~~ (can walk)
~~Labral tear~~ (too young)
~~Meralgia paresthetica~~ (not associated with
  fever)

~~Muscle strain~~ (not associated with fever)
~~Myositis ossificans~~ (too young)
~~Slipped capital femoral epiphyses~~ (too
  young, unless major metabolic,
  endocrine, renal problem)

~~Snapping hip syndrome~~ (not associated
  with fever)

I Inflammation

Aseptic

~~Apophysitis~~ (not associated with fever)
Chronic inflammatory demyelinating
  polyneuropathy
Guillain-Barré syndrome
~~Hip bursitis~~ (not associated with fever)
Juvenile rheumatoid arthritis (and related
  diseases):
- Juvenile dermatomyositis
- Juvenile spondyloarthropathies
- Scleroderma
- Systemic lupus erythematosus

~~Osteitis pubis~~ (not associated with fever)
~~Reactive arthritis~~ (too young)
~~Rheumatic fever~~ (timeline too long)
~~Tendinitis~~ (not associated with fever)
~~Transient synovitis~~ (too old)

Septic

Acute:
Lyme disease (tick paralysis)
Osteomyelitis of femoral neck
~~Poliomyelitis~~ (would be known by this time)
~~Pyomyositis~~ (not sick enough)
~~Septic arthritis of the hip joint~~ (timeline too
  long)

Chronic:
Brucellosis of the proximal femur or pelvis

Fungal infection of the proximal femur or pelvis (such as actinomycosis, coccidioidomycosis, or histoplasmosis)

Tuberculosis of the proximal femur or pelvis

M Metabolic

Ehlers-Danlos syndrome

Gaucher's disease

Gout
Lesch-Nyhan syndrome

Osteogenesis imperfecta

Osteopetrosis

Rickets:
* Vitamin D–dependent (nutritional)

* Vitamin D–resistant (hypophosphatasia)

Va Vascular

Hemophilic arthropathy

Legg-Calvé-Perthes/osteonecrosis

Henoch-Schönlein purpura

Osteochondritis dissecans

Sickle cell anemia

De Degenerative

Not applicable

Tu Tumor

Malignant Primary, such as:
* Ewing's sarcoma
* Leukemia
* Osteosarcoma
* Rhabdomyosarcoma
* Synovial sarcoma

Chronic:
~~Brucellosis of the proximal femur or pelvis~~ (wrong country)

~~Fungal infection of the proximal femur or pelvis (such as actinomycosis coccidioidomycosis, or histoplasmosis)~~ (wrong geography)

Tuberculosis of the proximal femur or pelvis

M Metabolic

~~Ehlers-Danlos syndrome~~ (not associated with fever)

~~Gaucher's disease~~ (not specifically associated with fever, otherwise normal growth, development, and appearance to date)

~~Gout~~ (possible but unlikely at this age)
~~Lesch-Nyhan syndrome~~ (would be known by this time)

~~Osteogenesis imperfecta~~ (would be known by this time; not associated with fever)

~~Osteopetrosis~~ (would be known by this time; not associated with fever)

~~Rickets:~~
* ~~Vitamin D–dependent (nutritional)~~ (not associated with fever)

* ~~Vitamin D–resistant (hypophosphatasia)~~ (not associated with fever)

Va Vascular

~~Hemophilic arthropathy~~ (would be known by this time)

~~Legg-Calvé-Perthes/osteonecrosis~~ (not associated with fever)

~~Henoch-Schönlein purpura~~ (would be known by this time)

~~Osteochondritis dissecans~~ (not associated with fever)

~~Sickle cell anemia~~ (would be known by this time)

De Degenerative

Not applicable

Tu Tumor

Malignant Primary, such as:
* Ewing's sarcoma
* Leukemia
* Osteosarcoma
* Rhabdomyosarcoma
* Synovial sarcoma

Malignant Metastatic

Benign, such as:
* Langerhans' cell histiocytosis (eosinophilic granuloma)
* Osteochondroma

* Osteoid osteoma

Co Congenital

Acetabular dysplasia

Epiphyseal dysplasias

Myelodysplasia (spina bifida/ myelomeningocele)

Ne Neurogenic/Psychogenic

School phobia
Spastic cerebral palsy

~~Malignant Metastatic~~ (unlikely at this age)

Benign, such as:
* Langerhans' cell histiocytosis (eosinophilic granuloma)
* ~~Osteoid osteoma~~ (not associated with fever)
* ~~Osteochondroma~~ (not associated with fever)

Co Congenital

~~Acetabular dysplasia~~ (not associated with fever)

~~Epiphyseal dysplasias~~ (not associated with fever)

~~Myelodysplasia (spina bifida/ myelomeningocele)~~ (would be known by this time)

Ne Neurogenic/Psychogenic

~~School phobia~~ (not associated with fever)
~~Spastic cerebral palsy~~ (not associated with fever)

STEP #7: Ask specific questions to rule specific conditions or pathological categories less likely.

* **Have you had any weakness in your legs or arms?** No, the patient denies any symptoms of weakness. This would exclude diagnostic categories associated with weakness such as Guillain-Barré and chronic demyelinating polyradiculoneuropathy.

* **Have you been more tired than usual?** No, making forms of cancer, such as lymphoma and metastatic disease, less likely.

* **Have you had any back pain?** No, making osteomyelitis of lumbar vertebrae and discitis unlikely.

* **Have you been hiking in the woods (or otherwise exposed to ticks)?** No, making Lyme disease less likely.

STEP #8: Re-sort the diagnostic hypothesis list based on the patient's responses to specific questioning.

Remote

T Trauma

Not applicable

I Inflammation

Aseptic
Not applicable

Septic
Chronic granulomatous disease
~~Discitis~~ (no back pain)
~~Osteomyelitis of the lumbar vertebra~~ (no back pain)
Septic arthritis of sacroiliac joint

M Metabolic
Not applicable

Va Vascular
Not applicable

De Degenerative
Not applicable

Tu Tumor
~~Lymphoma~~ (absence of fatigue)

Co Congenital
Not applicable

Ne Neurogenic/Psychogenic
Not applicable

Local

T **Trauma**

Not applicable

I **Inflammation**

Aseptic

~~Chronic inflammatory demyelinating polyneuropathy~~ (no symptoms of weakness)

~~Guillain-Barré syndrome~~ (no symptoms of weakness)

Juvenile rheumatoid arthritis (and related diseases):

- Juvenile dermatomyositis
- Juvenile spondyloarthropathies
- Scleroderma
- Systemic lupus erythematosus

Septic

Acute:

~~Lyme disease (tick paralysis)~~ (no chance for exposure to ticks)

Osteomyelitis of femoral neck

Chronic:

Fungi (such as actinomycosis or coccidioidomycosis)

Tuberculosis of the proximal femur or pelvis

M **Metabolic**

Not applicable

Va **Vascular**

Not applicable

De **Degenerative**

Not applicable

Tu **Tumor**

Malignant Primary, such as:

- Ewing's sarcoma
- ~~Leukemia~~ (absence of fatigue)
- Osteosarcoma
- Rhabdomyosarcoma
- Synovial sarcoma

Malignant Metastatic:

Not applicable

Benign, such as:

- Langerhans' cell histiocytosis (eosinophilic granuloma)

Co **Congenital**

Not applicable

Ne **Neurogenic/Psychogenic**

Not applicable

STEP #9: Perform tests to differentiate among the remaining diagnostic hypotheses.

- **Oral temperature:** 100°F.

Teaching Comments: Body temperature is the most discriminating test at this point for further differentiation of the remaining diagnostic categories. A positive finding allows the clinician to be more efficient with the remaining physical exam measures. Additionally, a positive finding with the temperature narrows the diagnostic categories, demonstrating that Billy will require referral to a physician because the remaining categories are not appropriate for direct access care by a physical therapist.

- **Palpation/percussion of the lumbar spine:** There was no pain or limitation in segmental mobility found during this exam, making chronic granulomatous disease and discitis less likely.
- **Active range of motion of the hip:** Normal and pain free, making primary hip pathologies less likely.
- **Compression of the sacroiliac joint via the ilial wings:** Acute pain, making septic arthritis of the sacroiliac joint more likely.

Teaching Comments: Many physical therapists would continue the physical exam in order to collect further data to share with the patient and with the health care practitioner to whom they will refer the patient. Interpretation of test results should be based on the keys of evidence-based practice: patient viewpoint, clinician's experience, and research. The sacroiliac compression test has been studied extensively with mixed reviews on reliability.[1] However, with consideration of all three components of evidence-based practice, the information received from the physical exam techniques in combination with that of the temperature strengthens the diagnostic impression.

STEP #10: Re-sort the diagnostic hypothesis list based on patient's responses to specific tests.

Remote

T Trauma

Not applicable

I Inflammation

Aseptic

Not applicable

Septic

~~Chronic granulomatous disease~~ (no pain with palpation)

~~Discitis~~ (no pain with palpation and percussion)

Septic arthritis of sacroiliac joint

M Metabolic

Not applicable

Va Vascular

Not applicable

De Degenerative

Not applicable

Tu Tumor

Not applicable

Co Congenital

Not applicable

Ne Neurogenic/Psychogenic

Not applicable

Local

T Trauma

Not applicable

I Inflammation

Aseptic

~~Juvenile rheumatoid arthritis (and related diseases):~~

- ~~Juvenile dermatomyositis~~ (pain is not reproduced with ileal wing compression)
- ~~Juvenile spondyloarthropathies~~ (pain is not reproduced with ileal wing compression)
- ~~Scleroderma~~ (pain is not reproduced with ileal wing compression)
- ~~Systemic lupus erythematosus~~ (pain is not reproduced with ileal wing compression)

Septic

Acute:

~~Osteomyelitis of femoral neck~~ (no pain with hip active range of motion)

Chronic:

~~Fungi (such as actinomycosis or coccidioidomycosis)~~ (no pain with hip active range of motion)

~~Tuberculosis of the proximal femur or pelvis~~ (no pain with hip active range of motion)

M Metabolic

Not applicable

Va Vascular

Not applicable

De Degenerative

Not applicable

Tu Tumor

Malignant Primary, such as:

- ~~Ewing's sarcoma~~ (no pain with hip active range of motion)
- ~~Leukemia~~ (no pain with hip active range of motion)
- ~~Osteosarcoma~~ (no pain with hip active range of motion)
- ~~Rhabdomyosarcoma~~ (no pain with hip active range of motion)
- ~~Synovial sarcoma~~ (no pain with hip active range of motion)

Malignant Metastatic:

Not applicable

Benign, such as:

- ~~Langerhans' cell histiocytosis (eosinophilic granuloma)~~ (no pain with hip active range of motion)

Co Congenital

Not applicable

Ne Neurogenic/Psychogenic

Not applicable

STEP #11: Decide on a diagnostic impression.

- Septic arthritis of the sacroiliac joint

STEP #12: Determine the appropriate patient disposition.

- Refer Billy to physician urgently for additional evaluation.

Case Outcome

Billy was referred to a pediatric orthopedic surgeon, who confirmed the diagnosis of septic arthritis of the sacroiliac joint. Billy was treated with a course of antibiotic therapy that began with high-dose intravenous agents administered on an inpatient basis followed by high-dose oral agents on an outpatient basis. As a result of this intervention, Billy's condition resolved.

Reference

1. van der Wurff P, Hagmeijer RH, Meyne W. Clinical tests of the sacroiliac joint. A systematic methodological review. Part 1: reliability. *Man Ther.* 2000;5(1):30–36.

CHAPTER 47

Knee Pain in a Child

■ *Jennifer Lundberg, PT, DPT* ■ *Cassandra Sanders-Holly, PT, DPT, PCS*

Description of the Symptom

This chapter describes possible causes of knee pain in a child. Local causes are defined as occurring between the distal one-third of the thigh and proximal one-third of the lower leg in a child. Remote causes are defined as occurring outside this region.

Special Concerns
■ Sudden onset of knee pain in the absence of trauma

■ Knee pain associated with fever, flu-like symptoms, skin changes in appearance and temperature
■ Knee pain that is worse at night, unrelenting pain, pain associated with night sweats, rapid unexplained weight changes
■ Pain that persists for several weeks with no known mechanical etiology

CHAPTER PREVIEW: Conditions That May Lead to Knee Pain in a Child

T Trauma	
REMOTE	**LOCAL**
COMMON	
Slipped capital femoral epiphysis 941	Contusion (bone/muscle) 943
	Fat pad impingement 944
	Fractures:
	• Avulsion, supracondylar (Segond fracture) 944
	• Epiphyseal injuries 944
	• Stress fracture 944
	Growing pains 945
	Iliotibial band friction syndrome 945
	Ligament sprains/tears:
	• Anterior cruciate ligament sprain/rupture 946
	• Lateral collateral ligament sprain/rupture 946
	• Medial collateral ligament sprain/rupture 947
	• Posterior cruciate ligament sprain/rupture 947
	Muscle strain (eg, quadriceps, hamstrings, adductors) 948
	Osgood-Schlatter disease 949
	Patellar dislocation 950
	Patellofemoral pain syndrome (chondromalacia patella) 951
	Sinding-Larsen-Johansson disease 952
UNCOMMON	
Not applicable	Blount's disease 942
	Meniscus tears:
	• Lateral meniscus tear 947
	• Medial meniscus tear 948

(continued)

Trauma *(continued)*

REMOTE	LOCAL
RARE	
Lumbar radiculopathies: • L4 radiculopathy 940 • L5 radiculopathy 941 • S1 radiculopathy 941	Nerve entrapments: • Common peroneal nerve at the fibular head 948 • Saphenous nerve 949 Plica syndrome 951

I Inflammation

REMOTE	LOCAL
COMMON	
Not applicable	**Aseptic** Bursitis: • Infrapatellar 942 • Pes anserine (Voshell's bursitis) 942 • Prepatellar 943 Patellar tendonitis 951 Transient synovitis 953 **Septic** Lyme disease (Lyme arthritis) 947 Osteomyelitis of the distal femur, proximal tibia, or fibula 950 Pyogenic arthritis (septic arthritis) 952
UNCOMMON	
Aseptic Ankylosing spondylitis 939 **Septic** Epidural abscess 940 Septic hip 941	**Aseptic** Erythema nodosum 944 Juvenile rheumatoid arthritis 946 Rheumatic fever 952 Systemic lupus erythematosus 953 **Septic** Not applicable
RARE	
Not applicable	Not applicable

M Metabolic

REMOTE	LOCAL
COMMON	
Not applicable	Not applicable
UNCOMMON	
Not applicable	Osteogenesis imperfecta 949
RARE	
Not applicable	Gout 944 Myositis ossificans 948

Va Vascular

REMOTE	LOCAL
COMMON	
Avascular necrosis of the femoral head (Legg-Calvé-Perthes disease) 940	Osteochondritis desiccans 949
UNCOMMON	
Not applicable	Hemophilia 945 Sickle cell disease 952
RARE	
Not applicable	Henoch-Schönlein purpura 945 Thrombus (venous or arterial) 953 Vascular malformation 956

De Degenerative

REMOTE	LOCAL
COMMON	
Not applicable	Not applicable
UNCOMMON	
Not applicable	Not applicable
RARE	
Not applicable	Popliteal cyst 951

Tu Tumor

REMOTE	LOCAL
COMMON	
Not applicable	*Malignant Primary, such as:* • Leukemia 954 *Malignant Metastatic:* Not applicable *Benign, such as:* • Osteochondroma 954
UNCOMMON	
Not applicable	Not applicable
RARE	
Not applicable	*Malignant Primary, such as:* • Ewing's sarcoma 953 • Lymphoma 954 • Osteosarcoma (osteogenic sarcoma) 955 • Synovial sarcoma 956 *Malignant Metastatic, such as:* • Neuroblastoma 954 *Benign, such as:* • Ganglion cysts 954

(continued)

Tumor *(continued)*

REMOTE	LOCAL
RARE	
	• Osteoblastoma 954
	• Osteoid osteoma 955
	• Pigmented villonodular synovitis 955
	• Synovial chondromatosis 955

Co Congenital

REMOTE	LOCAL
COMMON	
Not applicable	Patella alta 950
	Patellar subluxation 950
UNCOMMON	
Not applicable	Discoid meniscus 943
RARE	
Not applicable	Bipartite patella 942
	Congenital dislocated patella 943

Ne Neurogenic/Psychogenic

REMOTE	LOCAL
COMMON	
Not applicable	Not applicable
UNCOMMON	
Not applicable	Not applicable
RARE	
Conversion syndrome 940 Somatization (psychogenic rheumatism) 941	Complex regional pain syndrome (reflex sympathetic dystrophy) 943

Note: These are estimates of relative incidence because few data are available for the less common conditions.

Common Ages at Which Knee Pain Presents in a Child

APPROXIMATE AGE	CONDITION
Birth to 3 Years	Hematogenous septic arthritis
	Hemophilia
	Neuroblastoma
	Osteogenesis imperfecta
	Osteomyelitis
	Pyogenic arthritis
	Septic hip
	Sickle cell anemia
	Thrombus
	Transient synovitis
	Venous malformation

Common Ages at Which Knee Pain Presents in a Child—cont'd

APPROXIMATE AGE	CONDITION
Preschool (3–5 Years)	Avascular necrosis of the proximal femur
	Contusion
	Discoid meniscus
	Epiphyseal injuries
	Ewing's sarcoma
	Fracture
	Hemophilia
	Henoch-Schönlein purpura
	Juvenile rheumatoid arthritis
	Leukemia
	Muscle strain
	Myositis ossificans
	Neuroblastoma (metastasis)
	Osteogenesis imperfecta
	Osteomyelitis
	Patellar subluxation
	Popliteal cyst
	Pyogenic arthritis
	Septic hip
	Sickle cell
	Stress fracture
	Transient synovitis
	Venous malformation
Elementary School (6–11 Years)	Avascular necrosis of the proximal femur
	Bursitis
	Congenital dislocated patella
	Contusion
	Discoid meniscus
	Epiphyseal injuries
	Ewing's sarcoma
	Hemophilia
	Henoch-Schönlein purpura
	Juvenile rheumatoid arthritis
	Ligamentous sprain/tear
	Muscle strain
	Osgood-Schlatter disease
	Osteochondritis desiccans
	Osteomyelitis
	Popliteal cyst
	Rheumatic fever
	Septic hip
	Sickle cell anemia
	Sinding-Larsen-Johannson disease
	Slipped capital femoral epiphysis
	Stress fracture
	Synovitis
	Tendonitis
	Thrombus
	Transient synovitis
	Venous malformation

(continued)

Common Ages at Which Knee Pain Presents in a Child—cont'd

APPROXIMATE AGE	CONDITION
Middle School (12–14 Years)	Ankylosing spondylitis
	Bursitis
	Contusion
	Conversion syndrome
	Discoid meniscus
	Embolism (venous or arterial)
	Epiphyseal injuries
	Ewing's sarcoma
	Fat pad impingement
	Fracture
	Gout
	Hemophilia
	Henoch-Schönlein purpura
	Juvenile rheumatoid arthritis
	Ligamentous sprain/tear
	Lyme disease
	Meniscus tear
	Muscle strain
	Myositis ossificans
	Osgood-Schlatter disease
	Osteoblastoma
	Osteochondritis desiccans
	Osteoid osteoma
	Osteomyelitis
	Osteosarcoma
	Patellar dislocation
	Popliteal cyst
	Rheumatic fever
	Saphenous nerve entrapments
	Septic hip
	Sickle cell anemia
	Sinding-Larsen-Johansson disease
	Slipped capital femoral epiphysis
	Stress fracture
	Supracondylar cortical avulsion
	Systemic lupus erythematosus
	Tendonitis
	Thrombus
	Venous malformation
High school (15–18 Years)	Ankylosing spondylitis
	Bursitis
	Contusion
	Conversion syndrome
	Epiphyseal injuries
	Ewing's sarcoma
	Fat pad impingement
	Hemophilia
	Juvenile rheumatoid arthritis
	Ligamentous sprain/tear
	Lyme disease
	Meniscus tear
	Muscle strain
	Myositis ossificans
	Osgood-Schlatter disease

Common Ages at Which Knee Pain Presents in a Child—cont'd

APPROXIMATE AGE	CONDITION
	Osteoblastoma
	Osteochondritis desiccans
	Osteoid osteoma
	Osteomyelitis
	Osteosarcoma
	Patellar dislocation
	Rheumatic fever
	Saphenous nerve entrapment
	Sickle cell anemia
	Slipped capital femoral epiphysis
	Stress fracture
	Supracondylar cortical avulsion
	Synovitis
	Systemic lupus erythematosus
	Tendonitis
	Thrombus

Overview of Knee Pain in a Child

In 1998, de Inocencio analyzed 1,000 consecutive pediatric clinic visits made by children at least 3 years of age and less than 15 years of age.[1] The study found that 61 of those 1,000 visits were related to musculoskeletal pain. Furthermore, the study found that the greatest number of these reports (33%) were due to knee pain. In the physical therapy setting, the patients present with the primary complaint of musculoskeletal dysfunction, and reports due to knee pain are common. This makes differential diagnosis of the pediatric knee of critical importance.

Knee pain in children can be difficult to diagnose. An infant or a young child cannot often describe, quantify, or localize the pain he or she feels. The clinician must be skilled in observation and palpation of the child, as well as adept at interviewing the child's parent(s). Physiological pain signs are important to recognize in nonverbal children. Often parents will cite a change in the child's gait, or a "limp," as their chief complaint. Parents may note that their infant or toddler is refusing to move a leg or bear weight. Parents may also be concerned that the infant is delayed in walking. Children often will not mention pain for various reasons such as difficulty describing it, or fear of losing the ability to participate in play, sports, and/or fear of painful treatments, such as an injection in young children.

When the cause of the knee pain is traumatic, there would likely be a known mechanism of injury and the patient has typically sought intervention from a medical doctor. It is not uncommon, however, for a physical therapist to receive a diagnosis from a physician that is general, such as "knee pain," and requires further evaluation. Many of these diagnoses need to be confirmed by radiographic evidence or other special tests that are outside of the scope of physical therapy, and if suspected should be referred back to a physician. Another fact to be aware of is that prepubescent or skeletally immature children who participate in sports are more prone to injury involving the growth plates of the tibia and femur.

Description of Conditions That May Lead to Knee Pain in a Child

Remote

■ Ankylosing Spondylitis

Chief Clinical Characteristics

This presentation includes dull and diffuse pain or stiffness in the lumbar spine and buttock region that persists for several months. The pain and stiffness is usually described as worse in the morning and at night and can be alleviated by a warm shower and light activity.

Background Information

Symptoms can begin in a peripheral joint such as the hip or knee caused by an inflammation of the site of bony attachment of tendons and ligaments in the joint. Chronic inflammation in the vertebral joints can lead to bony overgrowth with fusion and immobilization of these joints. Inflammation of the eye can accompany this diagnosis. This condition is often referred to as "bamboo spine" because of the characteristic appearance on x-ray. Physical therapy intervention is directed at impairments such as pain, limited range of motion, weakness, and gait deviations. Gentle aerobic activity or aquatherapy may also be indicated.

■ Avascular Necrosis of the Femoral Head (Legg-Calvé-Perthes Disease)

Chief Clinical Characteristics

This presentation typically includes pain of an insidious onset that radiates to the anteromedial aspect of the knee. Often a Trendelenburg limp is the first sign with no known history of injury. Common reports also include muscle stiffness that may increase with activity. Clinical findings include mild limitation of hip range of motion, especially extension, abduction, and internal rotation.

Background Information

This condition most commonly presents in boys ages 5 to 7 years, though it can range from 2 years old to adolescence. It is a self-limiting disease characterized by avascular necrosis of the femoral head. Revascularization occurs almost invariably without treatment. Complications such as femoral head deformation have been identified.[2,3] Physical therapy intervention is directed at impairments such as pain, limited range of motion, weakness, and gait deviations.

■ Conversion Syndrome

Chief Clinical Characteristics

This presentation consists of knee pain in which history and examination data are inconsistent with any predictable pattern of underlying anatomy and physiology. Adolescents suspected of having this condition are often emotionally labile, dramatic, sexually provocative, and ego-centric, and demonstrate attention-seeking behaviors.[4] The child may also appear indifferent to the symptoms described.

Background Information

This psychosomatic pain condition is usually related to secondary gain for the child with family and/or friends. It is also likely to help him or her deal with the environment. It may be related to stress in the child's life as well. This syndrome may assist the child in dealing with stress in his or her life and thus decrease anxiety.[5] In a study by Fritz and colleagues, at least two of the following factors must be present in a child for the diagnosis of conversion syndrome:

1. History of symptoms varied significantly in the telling.
2. Pain was out of proportion to exam findings.
3. Only vague adjectives used to describe the pain.
4. Evidence of emotional difficulties in other areas.[6]

Children suspected of having this condition should be referred to a psychiatrist or other mental health diagnostician for additional evaluation and management.

■ Epidural Abscess

Chief Clinical Characteristics

The child presents with motor and/or sensory signs and symptoms in a dermatomal/myotomal distribution. Orbital inflammation with forehead edema and headache are clinical signs of an infection in the cranium.

Background Information

This type of abscess is an infection of the epidural space that can encroach on the spinal cord and compromise the vascular supply of the region. Epidural abscess can be a complication of severe or chronic sinus infections in children. Medical management includes antibiotic therapy and surgical drainage. Physical therapy management is important for any resultant impairments.[7]

LUMBAR RADICULOPATHIES

■ L4 Radiculopathy

Chief Clinical Characteristics

This presentation can be characterized by pain in the lumbar spine and paresthesias radiating from the anterior aspect of the hip, thigh, and knee, sometimes ending antero-medially from the knee to the foot. Depending on the severity, this presentation may also include a decreased or absent patellar tendon reflex and motor loss in the muscles innervated by the L4 nerve. Prone knee bend may reproduce symptoms.

Background Information
A lumbar disk herniation is the most common cause for this condition. The diagnosis is confirmed with magnetic resonance imaging. Surgical intervention may be indicated in severe cases of lower extremity pain accompanied by neurological signs.

■ L5 Radiculopathy

Chief Clinical Characteristics
This presentation includes pain in the lumbar spine and paresthesias radiating from the lateral aspect of the hip and buttock to the lateral aspect of the knee, extending anterolaterally down to the foot. Depending on the severity, this presentation may also include motor loss in the muscles innervated by the L5 nerve root.

Background Information
A lumbar disk herniation is the most common cause for this condition. The diagnosis is confirmed with magnetic resonance imaging. Surgical intervention may be indicated in severe cases of lower extremity pain accompanied by neurological signs.

■ S1 Radiculopathy

Chief Clinical Characteristics
This presentation typically includes pain in the lumbar spine and paresthesias radiating from the buttock to the posterior aspect of the knee and extending posterolaterally from the knee to the foot. Depending on the severity, this presentation may also include a decreased or absent Achilles tendon reflex and motor loss in the muscles innervated by the S1 nerve.

Background Information
A lumbar disk herniation is a common cause for this condition. The diagnosis is confirmed with magnetic resonance imaging. Surgical intervention may be indicated in severe cases of lower extremity pain accompanied by neurological signs.

■ Septic Hip

Chief Clinical Characteristics
This presentation includes painful, restricted active and passive motion of the hip, but may present as anteromedial knee pain. Difficulty with weight bearing and a limp with gait are common. Typically this condition is accompanied by fever.[8]

Background Information
Such a problem requires immediate referral to an orthopedic surgeon. This may also be referred to as septic arthritis or infectious arthritis. Surgical or medical intervention is typically indicated. Following medical management, physical therapy intervention is directed at impairments such as pain, limited range of motion, weakness, and gait deviations.

■ Slipped Capital Femoral Epiphysis

Chief Clinical Characteristics
This presentation involves hip, knee, and medial thigh pain that occurs insidiously or suddenly, and can be unilateral or bilateral. Clinical signs include a slight limp with foot in external rotation and limited hip abduction, internal rotation, and flexion. There may or may not be a history of trauma. Pain is aggravated with activity and is alleviated with rest.

Background Information
This condition most commonly occurs between the ages of 10 and 15 years with a greater incidence in obese male children. This condition requires immediate surgical attention.[9,10] The physical therapy intervention that follows is directed at impairments such as pain, limited range of motion, weakness, and gait deviations.

■ Somatization (Psychogenic Rheumatism)

Chief Clinical Characteristics
This presentation consists of history and examination data that are inconsistent with anatomy and physiology. Adolescents suspected of having this condition are often emotionally labile, dramatic, sexually provocative, and egocentric and demonstrate attention-seeking behaviors.[4] *The child may also appear indifferent to the symptoms described.*

Background Information

In contrast to conversion syndrome, children with this condition may demonstrate symptoms of psychosis and severe mental illness such as hallucinations, strange symptom explanations, and an inability to relate to his or her peers.[4]

Local

■ Bipartite Patella

Chief Clinical Characteristics

This presentation involves tenderness at the superior pole of the patella. Children suspected of having this condition may report activity-related aching.[11] There may be a palpable ridge on the patella. Pain is felt on the patella and range of motion may be uncomfortable.

Background Information

This condition is seen most commonly in adolescents, and boys are affected more often than girls. It is usually found incidentally in very active children. History of a single event causing the pain is not usual as there is often a minor trauma to the area, which then reveals the bipartite patella. It occurs when the secondary ossification centers do not fuse to the primary ossification centers, causing bipartite patella. Treatment is nonsurgical with modification of activity, aspirin, and splinting if necessary.[11]

■ Blount's Disease

Chief Clinical Characteristics

This presentation consists of bowing of the lower extremities in the infantile form. The bowing is asymmetrical, though usually bilateral, and the child is frequently obese and has internal tibial torsion and leg-length discrepancy. In-toeing is commonly seen along with the tibial torsion. In children 4 years of age and older, the primary complaint is often pain and then bowing of the lower extremity. The child is frequently obese.[12]

Background Information

This condition is an abnormal growth of the medial proximal tibial epiphysis where it begins to wedge and cause increased varus. It is thought to be due to growth suppression at the medial proximal tibia caused by compressive trauma. It is the most common pathology that causes tibial varus.[12] It can occur at any age,

but is classified based on ages: infantile (0 to 3 years), juvenile (4 to 10 years), and adolescent (11 years and older). The infantile form is the most common and is seen more in females, early walkers (<1 year), and African Americans, and it presents with bilateral involvement in 80% of cases and a prominent medial metaphyseal "beak."[12,13] The late-onset groups also show obesity, and African American predominance, but in contrast to the infantile form, males are affected more frequently and only 50% have bilateral involvement.[13] Treatment in the infantile group begins with nonsurgical bracing utilizing knee-ankle-foot orthoses. Treatment in the late-onset groups is surgical with a proximal tibial valgus osteotomy and a fibular diaphyseal osteotomy.

BURSITIS

■ Infrapatellar

Chief Clinical Characteristics

This presentation commonly includes localized edema over the inferior aspect of the patellofemoral joint and pain in the infrapatellar region with palpation.

Background Information

With malalignment of the extensor mechanism or irritation to the infrapatellar fat pad, the infrapatellar bursa may become enlarged, inflamed, and painful. Pain is often associated with hyperextension or extension overpressure. Treatment includes rest and inflammation control.

■ Pes Anserine (Voshell's Bursitis)

Chief Clinical Characteristics

This presentation includes pain, tenderness, and localized edema at the anteromedial aspect of the knee. Patients may report pain with ascending stairs and tenderness to palpation at the insertion site of the three tendons that comprise the pes anserine group (semitendinosus, gracilis, and sartorius). Pain is typically located approximately 4 cm below the joint line at the anteromedial aspect of the knee.[14]

Background Information

Activities that involve repetitive cutting or side-to-side stepping may also result in pes anserine bursitis. Chronic bursitis has been associated with degenerative joint disease of the knee or rheumatoid arthritis.[15,16] Treatment includes rest, control of inflammation, orthotic therapy, and strengthening to reduce stress on the medial structures of the knee.

■ Prepatellar

Chief Clinical Characteristics
This presentation is characterized by superficial edema and diffuse pain over the anterior aspect of the knee with palpation.

Background Information
The mechanism of injury typically involves repeated minor trauma or kneeling, inciting inflammation of the subcutaneous bursa over the patella. Treatment includes avoidance of kneeling and inflammation control. Inflamed bursae need to be monitored for infection.

■ Complex Regional Pain Syndrome (Reflex Sympathetic Dystrophy)

Chief Clinical Characteristics
This presentation typically includes pain that is disproportionate to any causative or traumatic event (allodynia) and excessive sensitivity (hyperalgesia), edema, skin temperature changes, trophic changes, and impaired motor function.

Background Information
Diagnosis is by exclusion of other conditions. In children, complex regional pain syndrome is seen in the adolescent population. This condition is usually treated nonsurgically with desensitization and restoration of normal use of the lower extremity.

■ Congenital Dislocated Patella

Chief Clinical Characteristics
This presentation is characterized by quadriceps weakness. Pain may or may not be a significant feature. The child will often present with a knee flexion contracture and/or a patella that is held laterally.[17]

Background Information
Infants may demonstrate a delay in gait.[17] This condition is commonly found bilaterally. This condition is quite distinct from a subluxating or dislocating patella. The patella is firmly fixed laterally, making knee extension difficult. The lateral pull of the quadriceps mechanism usually results in a rotary subluxation of the tibia on the femur. The child will also likely have a positive apprehension test. This condition requires surgical correction.

■ Contusion (Bone/Muscle)

Chief Clinical Characteristics
This presentation typically involves swelling, pain, and limited joint range of motion near the injury. Bruising is noted and pain and stiffness with muscle activation can also occur.

Background Information
Contusions occur from direct or repeated blows from a blunt object that damage the muscle fibers or bone without breaking the skin. Bone marrow contusions can frequently be identified on magnetic resonance imaging and result from a direct blow to the bone, compressive forces from adjacent bones, or traction forces as in an avulsion injury. Common contusions in the knee joint include dashboard injuries, pivot shift injury (valgus load applied to the knee in flexion combined with external rotation of the tibia or internal rotation of the femur), hyperextension injury, and lateral patellar dislocation.[18] Physical therapy intervention is directed at impairments such as pain, limited range of motion, weakness, and gait deviations.

■ Discoid Meniscus

Chief Clinical Characteristics
This presentation typically includes symptoms indicative of a torn meniscus: dull, aching pain, edema, and locking.[19] It may cause a palpable and audible click and tenderness over the joint line on the side of meniscus. "Snapping" at the knee is also common. Many children are asymptomatic.

Background Information
This condition is an abnormally shaped meniscus that is thicker and rounder and covers more of the tibial plateau than does the normal semilunar-shaped meniscus. A positive McMurray's test and joint line tenderness help with diagnosis. However, the symptoms of a torn discoid meniscus may not present with the typical mechanism of injury and, in fact, the child may not have a recent history of trauma. The lateral meniscus is most commonly affected. Treatment

usually includes saucerization (debridement) of the meniscus.[19]

■ Erythema Nodosum

Chief Clinical Characteristics

This presentation involves sudden onset of swollen, red, and painful nodules on the anterior aspect of the bilateral lower extremities. The child may also demonstrate fever and malaise.

Background Information

The etiology is unknown but precipitating factors include streptococcal infection, tuberculosis, and drug reactions. The inflammation is of the fat cells under the skin. The treatment is medical and attends to the precipitating factors. This condition usually lasts approximately 2 weeks.[13] However, it may take up to 6 weeks to alleviate.

■ Fat Pad Impingement

Chief Clinical Characteristics

This presentation includes anterior knee pain that is typically localized near the inferior pole of the patella. It often occurs in the absence of eccentric loading, may be sudden onset following a hyperextension injury, and is aggravated by prolonged standing or stairs and passive overpressure with extension.[20]

Background Information

This condition may be caused by a direct blow or can be due to chronic irritation. Pain with palpation is primarily along either side of the patellar tendon and at the inferior pole. Physical therapy intervention may be indicated to address muscle imbalances and symptoms such as pain. Taping the superior patella may also be used to decrease the angle of the inferior pole of the patella into the fat pad.

FRACTURES

■ Avulsion, Supracondylar (Segond Fracture)

Chief Clinical Characteristics

This presentation typically involves pain with adduction located at the posterior lateral knee, proximal to the joint line.

Background Information

This condition is an avulsion of the tibia at the insertion of the lateral capsular ligament. It results from excessive internal rotation and varus stress of the knee and is frequently comorbid with anterior cruciate ligament or meniscal tears.[21] It is typically diagnosed by x-ray examination. Stabilization through bracing, casting, or surgical intervention is typically indicated by a physician. Growth disturbances are a potential complication of fractures in children. Physical therapy intervention is directed at impairments such as pain, limited range of motion, weakness, and gait deviations.

■ Epiphyseal Injuries

Chief Clinical Characteristics

This presentation can be characterized by localized tenderness to palpation over the plate that is often aggravated by contraction of the hip adductors. Pain may also be over the posteromedial aspect of knee proximal to the joint line.

Background Information

These injuries typically occur at the epiphyseal plate of children and adolescents and have been classified by type by Salter and Harris. Type I is a fracture along the plate, type II extends into the metaphysis on one side, type III extends into the epiphysis on one side, and type IV extends through the epiphyseal plate into the metaphysis.

■ Stress Fracture

Chief Clinical Characteristics

This presentation involves pain at and surrounding the fracture site with impaired ability to bear weight. Children with this condition will demonstrate a limp with attempts to weight bear.

Background Information

This condition is frequently seen in the pediatric athletic population, because they are skeletally immature and susceptible to the stress and strain of high-intensity muscle activity. This condition is common at the epiphyseal growth plates of the long bones and the shaft of the proximal tibia. Treatment includes rest and splinting.

■ Gout

Chief Clinical Characteristics

This presentation includes acute, recurrent episodes of severely painful arthritis with inflammation of the joints.

Background Information

This condition is primarily a disease of adults and is rare in children. Children with Type I glycogen storage disorder can have gouty arthritis, typically during the adolescent years. If gout occurs in a child, it is almost always secondary to another condition. At least 95% of gout happens in postpubertal men. It is a condition of purine metabolism characterized by elevation of levels of uric acid in serum. Surgical intervention may be indicated including amputation of the toes, partial resection of tendons or joints, and arthroplasty or arthrodesis of symptomatic joints.[12,22]

■ Growing Pains

Chief Clinical Characteristics

This presentation typically involves diffuse pain that is deep, intermittent, and poorly localized. It is most frequently felt bilaterally and at night.[8,17] The pain is not articular, nor is the joint tender.

Background Information

The child may report a "cramping" sensation. It is theorized to be the result of fatigue of the muscles in the thighs and calves, usually bilateral. The theory is that the longitudinal growth of the bones is greater than the longitudinal muscle-tendon unit growth and this leads to tightness around the joints, causing an overuse-type injury and subsequent pain.[5] Growing pains are most common in 4- to 12-year-old children.[17] Treatment includes massage and stretching.

■ Hemophilia

Chief Clinical Characteristics

This presentation typically includes pain in the knee with a red, swollen, and warm joint that has decreased range of motion.

Background Information

This condition is a genetic condition caused by a sex-linked recessive gene (seen in boys) that results in impaired blood clotting abilities where the child bleeds into the joint. The knee is one of the most frequently affected joints. The child may also have deep soft tissue hemorrhages that occur most frequently in the calf, thigh, iliopsoas, and upper extremities. Additionally, muscle weakness and atrophy may be present due to the child's decreased mobility.[23] Medical treatment is necessary and typically includes clotting factor replacement therapy. Physical therapy consists of range and strength restoration after a joint bleed. Family and patient education on joint protection precautions is imperative to help minimize bleeds.

■ Henoch-Schönlein Purpura

Chief Clinical Characteristics

This presentation can be characterized by joint swelling, redness, tenderness, pain, periarticular swelling, and warmth. The child develops a skin rash and abdominal pain, in addition to the arthritic pain. The rash is palpable and purpuric and is noted on the legs and buttocks; however, it may occur days to weeks after the first symptoms are noted. According to Hoekelman, the most common feature is the rash, followed by arthritis.[4] The child may also exhibit a low-grade fever, malaise, headache, nosebleeds, and/or scrotal and scalp swelling.

Background Information

This condition is a hypersensitivity vasculitis syndrome, which is an inflammatory process of the blood vessels. This inflammation can cause damage to the parts of the body supplied by the affected vessels. It is often seen after a respiratory viral illness. A definitive etiology is not known. The knee and the ankle are the two most common sites where arthritic pain is experienced. The physician needs to be involved to monitor renal function and the arthritis. The physical therapist will determine impairments and limitations once the child is cleared by the physician.

■ Iliotibial Band Friction Syndrome

Chief Clinical Characteristics

This presentation involves localized pain over the lateral femoral epicondyle that occurs during activity. Symptoms are aggravated by knee flexion and ambulation, typically alleviated with rest and a position of full knee extension.

Background Information

This condition is an overuse syndrome in which friction of the iliotibial band causes inflammation of the underlying structures. Physical therapy intervention includes addressing muscle imbalances surrounding the knee and hip joints.

■ Juvenile Rheumatoid Arthritis

Chief Clinical Characteristics

This presentation includes fever, abdominal pain, and joint swelling and heat with decreased range of motion. Local pain presents with a gradual onset. Occasionally, a rash may also develop; this is evident only in the systemic type of juvenile rheumatoid arthritis (JRA). Stiffness is usually worse in the morning and after rest. In addition to the above-mentioned signs/symptoms, the child will also demonstrate muscle atrophy due to the chronic inflammation of the joints, causing immobility and thus loss of muscle.

Background Information

The cause of JRA is unknown. It is thought to be autoimmune in response to an unknown infectious agent with a possible genetic predisposition. Criteria for diagnosis include greater than 6 weeks of inflammation of joints (synovial), less than or equal to 16 years of age, and a determination of the onset type and number of joints involved. Traditionally, three types were described; now several additional patterns have been described.[23] The three traditional types include pauciarticular, polyarticular, and systemic. The pauciarticular type demonstrates involvement in less than or equal to four joints and is the most common of the three types. The knee joint is the most frequently involved in the pauciarticular subtype.[24] Here the findings are usually a swollen knee without redness and may be accompanied by a small leg-length discrepancy due to overgrowth from the inflammatory stimulation of the physes. The polyarticular type demonstrates involvement in greater than or equal to five joints, and is usually symmetric. Both the pauciarticular and polyarticular types are seen more frequently in females and children who are 1 to 4 years of age at onset. The systemic type of JRA is characterized by spiking fevers that peak in the night and return to normal by the morning. This group demonstrates a rash and has fevers one to two times daily for greater than/equal to 2 weeks.[24] Males and females are affected equally. Chronic inflammation at the knee joint may lead to an overgrowth of the distal femoral and proximal tibial physes, resulting in a leg-length difference of up to 2 to 3 cm. All patients with this condition need to see a physician for medical management of the inflammation and its symptoms. Treatment includes aerobic activity to help decrease the frequency and severity of the joint flares as well as modalities to control symptoms during a flare. Consistent stretching and strengthening are beneficial as well as patient and family education on management techniques and joint protection precautions.

LIGAMENT SPRAINS/TEARS

■ Anterior Cruciate Ligament Sprain/Rupture

Chief Clinical Characteristics

This presentation includes hypermobility of the accessory motions at the knee joints, which is clinically tested with special tests such as the anterior drawer test, Lachman test, and others. Typically edema is observed and tenderness to palpation is present.

Background Information

Patients may note an audible pop or click during the injurious event that is typically a "plant and twist" or cut-and-pivot type of motion, or sudden deceleration. In children, the ligaments are usually stronger than the bone at the physis, so Salter I and II fractures are more likely to occur than ligament tears. As children reach their teen-aged years, the likelihood of ligament tears becomes more like that of adults.[25] Nonsurgical management of this condition in children has not demonstrated good outcomes; hence, surgical treatment is recommended. Physical therapy intervention is directed at impairments such as pain, limited range of motion, weakness, and gait deviations.

■ Lateral Collateral Ligament Sprain/Rupture

Chief Clinical Characteristics

This presentation involves pain, localized edema along the lateral aspect of the knee, and lateral joint line tenderness. Pain and/or laxity is present with varus stress testing at 30 degrees of knee flexion. This injury generally results in minimal effusion and pain with walking; however, the patient may report difficulty with running and cutting activities.

Background Information

The mechanism of injury is typically from a varus stress applied to the knee, such as a direct blow to the medial aspect of the knee. During varus stress testing, pain with no joint laxity is a Grade I (stretch) injury. Laxity with a firm end-feel is a Grade II (partial tear) injury, and no firm end-feel is a Grade III (complete tear) injury.[26] Clinical examination and magnetic resonance imaging confirm the diagnosis. Grade I, II, and III injuries are managed nonsurgically.[26,27] Surgical repair may be necessary to address associated meniscal or combined ligament tears.

■ Medial Collateral Ligament Sprain/Rupture

Chief Clinical Characteristics
This presentation includes pain, localized edema along the medial aspect of the knee, and medial joint line tenderness. Pain and/or laxity is present with valgus stress testing at 30 degrees of knee flexion. This injury generally results in minimal effusion and pain with walking; however, it also may cause difficulty with running and cutting activities.

Background Information
The mechanism of injury involves a valgus stress applied to the knee, such as a direct blow to the lateral aspect of the knee. The incidence of medial meniscus tears increases with increased severity of the sprain because of its attachment to the medial collateral ligament. With valgus stress testing, pain with no joint laxity is a Grade I injury (stretch). Laxity with a firm end-feel is a Grade II injury (partial tear), and no firm end-feel is a Grade III injury (complete tear).[26] Clinical examination and magnetic resonance imaging confirm the diagnosis.

■ Posterior Cruciate Ligament Sprain/Rupture

Chief Clinical Characteristics
This presentation typically includes pain, edema, and tenderness in the region of the popliteal fossa. Positive posterior sag sign of the tibia with the hip and knee flexed to 90 degrees and a positive posterior drawer test may be present.

Background Information
The mechanism of injury is typically from a hyperextension force or a direct anterior blow to the knee in a flexed position. This condition occurs with falls onto a flexed knee with the foot in plantarflexion, causing the tibial tubercle to contact the ground first, and in motor vehicle accidents resulting from contact with the dashboard. Magnetic resonance imaging confirms the diagnosis. Most tears are treated conservatively, but may be surgically repaired in an adolescent who is skeletally mature.

■ Lyme Disease (Lyme Arthritis)

Chief Clinical Characteristics
This presentation may be characterized by an achiness in the joints, and joint stiffness in addition to malaise and fever. Children with this condition may have edema, pain, and warmth, but frequently the child is without erythema about the knee.[28] The pattern has remissions and recurrences. If a rash is present, it typically shows "central clearing."

Background Information
This condition involves a history of tick bite months or up to 2 years prior to symptoms. The tick bite may have demonstrated the circular-type rash around the bite. In comparison to children with other causes of arthritis, patients with Lyme arthritis had a higher frequency of episodic arthritis and initial knee joint arthritis, reported tick bites more frequently, were older, had a lower frequency of initial arthralgias, and fewer large joints were involved.[29] According to Hoekelman, 85% of cases involve the knee and the arthritis lasts 1 to 2 weeks.[4] Medical treatment is necessary. Physical therapy treatment is based on the child's impairments and functional limitations that result from the disease.

MENISCUS TEARS

■ Lateral Meniscus Tear

Chief Clinical Characteristics
This presentation may involve pain, lateral joint line tenderness, and reports of catching, clicking, and locking. Mild joint line effusion is present, and pain or a palpable click may be provoked with McMurray's and Apley's compression tests.

Background Information
Mechanism of injury involves an acute, non-contact rotatory force with the knee flexed and the foot planted. Meniscal compromise

leads to increased stress on the articular cartilage and early degenerative changes. Magnetic resonance imaging confirms this diagnosis.[30–32] Tears located in the peripheral one-third of the meniscus respond well to surgical intervention. Some researchers advocate that tears in the middle one-third zone also be repaired.[33,34]

■ Medial Meniscus Tear

Chief Clinical Characteristics
This presentation can be characterized by pain, medial joint line tenderness, and reports of catching, clicking, and locking. Mild joint line effusion is present, and pain or a palpable click may be provoked with McMurray's and Apley's compression tests.

Background Information
Mechanism of injury involves an acute, noncontact rotatory force with the knee flexed and the foot planted. The medial meniscus is more commonly injured than the lateral meniscus because it is less mobile.[33] This condition often is associated with medial collateral ligament injuries because of its rigid attachment to the ligament and the joint capsule. Meniscal compromise leads to increased stress on the articular cartilage and early degenerative changes. Magnetic resonance imaging confirms the diagnosis.[30–32] Typically, tears located in the peripheral one-third of the meniscus heal well with surgical intervention, and some researchers also advocate repair of tears in the middle one-third zone.[33,34]

■ Muscle Strain (eg, Quadriceps, Hamstrings, Adductors)

Chief Clinical Characteristics
This presentation includes pain or tenderness with localized edema over the muscle belly or tendon that is aggravated by contraction or stretching of the muscle.

Background Information
Children with this condition often cite an audible "pop" with a tear of the muscle. A strain occurs when a muscle or tendon is overstretched or torn. Physical therapy intervention such as gentle stretching and strengthening of the surrounding musculature may be indicated as well as edema management and pain control.

■ Myositis Ossificans

Chief Clinical Characteristics
This presentation involves pain, focal swelling, and limited joint range of motion, commonly occurring in the arm or thigh. In the progressive form, the patient presents with painful lumps in the muscle and stiffness in adjacent joints.

Background Information
Symptoms progress from proximal to distal. This condition is an aberrant reparative process that causes benign heterotopic ossification of the soft tissue. There are two forms; one can develop in response to a soft tissue injury or in the absence of injury, the other is a progressive form that is an autosomal dominant genetic condition.

NERVE ENTRAPMENTS

■ Common Peroneal Nerve at the Fibular Head

Chief Clinical Characteristics
This presentation may be characterized by a partial or total loss of sensation in the distribution of the peroneal nerve. Weakness with ankle dorsiflexion and extension of the toes and a positive Tinel's sign at the fibular head may also be present.

Background Information
Pain is an uncommon feature unless it is related to the specific cause of the nerve entrapment, such as entrapment secondary to soft tissue swelling and inflammation from direct trauma. Causes include sitting crossed-legged, prolonged immobility in bed against bedrails or firm mattresses, trauma, squatting, crouching, kneeling, and idiopathic origins. Dynamic entrapments also may occur during activities such as running. The common peroneal nerve may be injured at any location along the nerve; however, entrapment most frequently occurs at the fibular head. The nerve may become compressed under the fibrous arch in the region where the bifurcation of the nerve into its deep and superficial branches occurs.[35,36] An electrodiagnostic evaluation, including nerve conduction velocity and needle electromyography may confirm the diagnosis. Treatment is generally conservative; however, surgical decompression may be indicated in recalcitrant

cases in which the anatomical site of entrapment is well characterized.

■ Saphenous Nerve

Chief Clinical Characteristics

This presentation involves pain and/or paresthesias in the medial thigh and knee, tenderness to palpation over the adductor canal, and normal motor function of the affected extremity. Symptoms include a deep ache that may radiate into the foot along the saphenous nerve distribution. Symptoms are exacerbated by prolonged walking or standing.

Background Information

Entrapment typically occurs where the saphenous nerve pierces the fascia of the adductor canal, resulting in inflammation. Mechanisms for saphenous nerve entrapment may be traumatic, nontraumatic, or iatrogenic (eg, following knee surgery or saphenous vein harvest). Diagnosis may be confirmed with injection of local anesthetic. Symptoms typically improve following an injection with a local anesthetic and steroids and avoiding aggravating activities. Neurolysis or neurectomy may be performed if nonsurgical treatment fails in recalcitrant cases in which the anatomical site of entrapment is well characterized.[37]

■ Osgood-Schlatter Disease

Chief Clinical Characteristics

This presentation includes swelling of the tibial tubercle with tenderness and sometimes warmth; the pain may increase with activity.

Background Information

This condition is caused by stress on the patellar ligament at its insertion on the tibia, with microfractures of the apophysis of the tibial tubercle causing pain.[17] Children with this condition often demonstrate a slight limp. Pain can be elicited with resisted quadriceps contraction. This condition is more commonly seen in boys.[38] Physical therapy intervention may include stretching and strengthening of the surrounding musculature, especially the quadriceps and antagonists.

■ Osteochondritis Desiccans

Chief Clinical Characteristics

This presentation involves pain, edema, and a limp in gait. The clinician usually appreciates an increase in pain with activity and a decrease in pain with rest. Onset is usually insidious and eventually quad atrophy is present.[21]

Background Information

This condition is necrosis of bone and cartilage with an unknown cause. Theories include abnormal vascular anatomy causing necrosis, the failure of an ossification center to fuse, trauma, or constitutional factors.[5] The most common site is the lateral middle-to-posterior portion of the medial femoral condyle, but the lateral femoral condyle can be affected as well. A positive Wilson's test is indicative of this condition. Williams and colleagues advocate non–weight-bearing activities in a knee immobilizer and range of motion during the nonsurgical management of this process.[39] The pain is gone in 6 to 18 months usually with full return to previous activity.[40] If a loose body is present, surgical resection of the loose body may be indicated.

■ Osteogenesis Imperfecta

Chief Clinical Characteristics

This presentation commonly involves deformities of the long bones and ligamentous laxity. The child may have a history of a few fractures to many fractures, depending on the severity of the disease. The child often has short stature, blue sclerae, and thin dentin.

Background Information

Osteogenesis imperfecta is a genetic condition and most forms of this condition result from a defect in Type I collagen. This defect makes the child's bones osteoporotic and fragile. This disease is often called *brittle bone disease* because the children frequently sustain multiple fractures from seemingly mild trauma. There are four major types of this condition varying from death in the prenatal/perinatal period to mild bone fragility.[28] However, in 2003, Zeitlin and colleagues described three additional types of this condition that are noncollagenous types.[41] Hearing may also be impaired due to problems with the bones of the middle ear. It is critical to rule out child abuse on children who present with multiple fractures. The multiple deformities and ligamentous laxity can be a clue for the clinician. The current treatment is frequently medical intravenous treatments along with surgical rodding of the lower extremities as well as physical therapy for pregait and gait once fixation is stable.[41]

Osteomyelitis of the Distal Femur, Proximal Tibia, or Fibula

Chief Clinical Characteristics

This presentation is acute with extreme bone pain and includes a limp and/or refusal to walk on affected leg. Additionally, warmth, edema, and redness will likely be present near the knee joint. An infant may demonstrate lack of movement of the involved leg (pseudoparalysis) and may refuse feeding. A fever is usually present. The pain is constant and progressively more severe and is aggravated by movement.

Background Information

This condition is an inflammation of bone that is primarily due to infection. It is most frequently a response to infection of the bone and of the medullary canal that may follow trauma to that area or result from remote seeding. However, it is most commonly due to a hematogenous source in children due to slow blood flow near the metaphysis. Up to 70% of hematogenous osteomyelitis is found in the femur or tibia.[23] A history of recent illness, inoculations, and so on may indicate an infectious agent that traveled via the blood to the long bones adjacent to the knee (ie, metaphyseal region). This condition requires immediate referral to medical care for antibiotics and likely surgical excision.

Patella Alta

Chief Clinical Characteristics

This presentation commonly includes a high-riding and usually small patella. The patella does not glide in the patellar groove.

Background Information

This condition is seen most commonly in kids with cerebral palsy due to the continuous muscle forces on the patella.[42] Children with this condition typically demonstrate a crouch position in gait. It can also be found during rapid growth spurts in the adolescent population or after trauma.[42] Treatment may consist of quadriceps stretching and bracing.

Patellar Dislocation

Chief Clinical Characteristics

This presentation includes a displaced patella. The direction of displacement is almost always lateral. Effusion is usually present.

Background Information

Ligamentous laxity is often found in patients who have recurrences. Malalignments such as genu valgum and external tibial torsional deformities can additionally contribute to disruption of the quadriceps mechanism and recurrent dislocation. Patella alta with elongation of the patellar tendon can predispose an individual to patellar dislocation because the normal support within the trochlear groove is gone. This condition usually occurs with a blow to the medial side of the leg, or more frequently to an indirect blow, such as a fall.[17] It is the most common musculoskeletal dislocation in the young athlete.[4] In a study by Neitosvaara and colleagues, 9 to 15 years of age was the most common age group to experience dislocations of the patella.[43] With knee flexion and extension, recurrent patellar dislocation can cause patellar arthritis and other degenerative patellofemoral joint changes.[22] Additionally, fracture incidence after patellar dislocation was 39%. Treatment consists of rest and edema/pain control, patellar taping, transcutaneous electrical nerve stimulation, and quadriceps and gluteal strengthening.

Patellar Subluxation

Chief Clinical Characteristics

This presentation involves tenderness on the anterior knee at the medial side of the patella and edema. Children with this condition may report a "going out" sensation.[5] Often, medial knee pain is present due to the stretch/tear of medial retinaculum.

Background Information

The patella usually dislocates laterally. The positive apprehension test is an indicator of this issue. This condition may be associated with an avulsion fracture of the lateral femoral condyle or the medial portion of the patella. Physical therapy treatment includes rest and edema/pain control, patellar taping, transcutaneous electrical nerve stimulation, and quadriceps and gluteal strengthening.

■ Patellar Tendonitis

Chief Clinical Characteristics

This presentation may involve anterior knee pain with flexion and extension of the knee; it is often worse at night. Children with this condition may have swelling, pain with activity, and restricted motion at the knee. The tenderness is usually at the lower pole of the patella and on the patellar tendon.[21]

Background Information

This condition is an inflammation of the patellar tendon caused by overuse or repetitive activities such as jumping or running. It is common in the active adolescent age group. Treatment includes stretching and strengthening the surrounding musculature and controlling the symptoms of inflammation.

■ Patellofemoral Pain Syndrome (Chondromalacia Patella)

Chief Clinical Characteristics

This presentation is such that pain begins insidiously, most commonly in adolescent females, with feelings of grinding, clicking, popping, or buckling. The pain may follow trauma as well, but this is not the most common presentation. Pain is anterior and may be described as aching around the patella. The pain is usually exacerbated by activities requiring flexion and extension of the knee, such as the stairs. The child may also indicate that he or she feels the pain with kneeling, squatting, running, and/or sitting as well. The physical therapist may be able to palpate crepitus as the child flexes/extends knee, though point pain with palpation is not usually present. Muscle atrophy and patellar hypermobility may be seen upon examination. Pain is activity related and relieved by rest. One does not usually palpate edema, warmth, or redness with patellofemoral pain syndrome, and most patients have full range of motion at the knee. The pain is often felt bilaterally. An additional finding may be that the child has a painful or unstable single limb stance on the involved leg and a limp with gait when symptomatic.

Background Information

The patella does not track in the femoral groove as it should and may be related to increased stress and pain. It can be congenital or acquired and has been thought to be due to malalignment of the patellofemoral mechanism where,

most often, the patella deviates laterally with quadriceps contractions. Patella alta, joint hypermobility, increased quadriceps angle, increased femoral anteversion, increased external tibial torsion, abnormal iliotibial band attachment, genu valgum, and genu recurvatum may all lead to this malalignment.[42,44,45] Pronated feet are another finding seen with patellofemoral pain syndrome. It is most commonly seen after an adolescent growth spurt. It may also be due to overuse leading to an inflammatory response that causes pain.[28] Treatment includes rest, elevation, and ice followed by restoration of range of motion, strengthening of gluteals and quadriceps, patellofemoral taping, and orthotics.

■ Plica Syndrome

Chief Clinical Characteristics

This presentation typically involves anterior or anteromedial pain that is intermittent and often reported with clicking, snapping, catching, or buckling sensations.

Background Information

It is typically aggravated by squatting, stair climbing, and prolonged sitting and standing. Tenderness along the inferior and medial patella can be elicited, and often hypertrophied tissue can be palpated. This condition is an overuse injury in which inflammation leads to a hypertrophied synovial membrane in the knee that loses elasticity. The medial plica is a band of tissue originating medially at the undersurface of the quadriceps tendon and attaches distally to the synovium, covering the infrapatellar fat pad. Plica syndrome is a rare cause of knee pain, but more common in adolescents.[46,47]

■ Popliteal Cyst

Chief Clinical Characteristics

This presentation involves a cyst behind the knee between the semimembranosus and the medial head of the gastrocnemius muscle. The swelling is not midline or lateral in position. The mass transluminates and is not tender. It does not limit motion. Pain does not typically increase with activity.

Background Information

A popliteal cyst is a form of bursitis. The cyst is caused by distention of the gastrocnemius and semimembranosus bursa that is fed by the muscle tenosynovium.[12] It is thought to be from chronic irritation and is seen more in boys than girls.[28] It is often misnamed a Baker cyst; however, this condition should not be confused with the "Baker's cyst" that is found in adults. This condition is a connection of the popliteal mass with the knee joint and follows an effusion into the joint.[5] It is usually self-limiting.

■ Pyogenic Arthritis (Septic Arthritis)

Chief Clinical Characteristics

This presentation includes a child who is acutely ill with fever, chills, irritability, and malaise. Children with this condition will report pain and local tenderness over the affected joint. The child will limp with weight bearing or refuse to use the leg. Redness, warmth, edema, muscle spasm, and limited range of motion are also signs of this infection. Additionally, slight flexion of the knee may be preferred as pain increases with motion. More so than other causes of knee pain, severe pain on attempted movement of the joint is possible. The joint is extremely painful, hot, and very red in its presentation.[28]

Background Information

This condition is an infection of the joint space caused by transient bacteremia, or a direct wound. The bacteria then colonizes the vascular synovium of the knee.[17] This infection can cause destruction of the articular cartilage and long-term bony growth problems. The knee is the second-most common joint involved, just after the hip.[48] This condition requires immediate referral to medical care for antibiotics and surgical drainage. According to Hamer, urgent surgical draining is critical.[49]

■ Rheumatic Fever

Chief Clinical Characteristics

This presentation may be characterized by an acute onset of a very painful knee joint that may not be edematous. The pain usually becomes migratory after 2 to 3 days, and responds well to aspirin. Joint involvement is sequential and this fact, along with the extreme pain that appears out of proportion to what is found physically, can help differentiate rheumatic fever from other conditions.[28] Finberg notes that the pain is so great that at times the child may not be able to tolerate a sheet or blanket covering the knee.[23] Children with this condition

may also have a rash on his or her upper arms, thighs, and trunk (though this is not common).

Background Information

This condition is due to an abnormal immune response to a streptococcal infection. It causes an arthritic joint that is painful. This condition may not often show symptoms for 10 to 20 days after the previous streptococcal infection (strep throat and/or tonsillitis). This condition is seen most commonly in the 5- to 15-year-old range.[12,23] Medical treatment is required. Physical therapy follows to address the child's impairments and functional limitations.

■ Sickle Cell Disease

Chief Clinical Characteristics

This presentation commonly includes edema, fever, erythema, warmth, and severe pain in the long bones and surrounding muscles that lasts 3 to 5 days. There may be mild swelling and limited range of motion as well as a low-grade fever. Initial crisis typically occurs around ages 3 to 4 years of age, The child is often smaller and weighs less than his or her peers when under 2 years of age. Symptoms may be migratory and are recurrent.[50]

Background Information

This condition contains a subset of vascular conditions that are more prevalent in children of African American descent. Pain due to sickle cell disease is caused by excessive clustering of the sickled red blood cells, which lead to bone infarcts and a secondary inflammatory response. It can also cause avascular necrosis, septic and reactive arthritis, and leg ulcers, all of which can cause pain. Roger found the knee to be the most common site of bony involvement in sickle cell anemia, whereas Hanissian and Silverman showed the elbow to be the most common site, and the knee the second most common.[50,51] Treatment is multifactorial, though the pain crises are treated with fluids, pain medication, and oxygen. Medical management is required and cardiorespiratory challenges should be avoided.[47,52]

■ Sinding-Larsen-Johansson Disease

Chief Clinical Characteristics

This presentation involves tenderness at the inferior pole of the patella, peripatellar swelling, and pain that increases with activity-related pain.

Background Information
This condition is common in the pediatric/adolescent athletic population. It occurs due to microfractures at the inferior pole of the patella at the patellar tendon.[17] Often the quadriceps muscle is shortened and weak. Radiographic evidence may include fragmentation of the distal patellar pole.[38]

■ Systemic Lupus Erythematosus

Chief Clinical Characteristics
This presentation typically is characterized by transient and migratory pain, redness, swelling, and stiffness, as well as a malar (butterfly) rash and symmetric joint inflammation. Fever, weight loss, and decreased energy are also reported. Joint movements are more painful, but have an intermittent pattern as compared to children with juvenile rheumatoid arthritis.[28] Additionally, edema is slight compared to the pain the children experience.[28]

Background Information
The cause is unknown. Theories include an autoimmune disease process and/or B-lymphocyte hyperactivity with genetic and environmental relationships. This condition may recur with exacerbations.[23] Girls are five times more likely than boys to have the disease, and children of African American descent are more frequently affected than Caucasian children. Children suspected of having this condition must be evaluated by their physician for treatment to control organ and joint inflammation. Physical therapy focuses on the patient's impairments and limitations.

■ Thrombus (Venous or Arterial)

Chief Clinical Characteristics
This presentation includes swelling of the leg, warmth and redness, and pain worse with standing or walking.

Background Information
This condition develops typically following prolonged immobility, trauma to the area, and most frequently after a vascular access device was used. A clot in the vessel obstructs blood flow and causes pain. This condition is rare in children. Most cases are found in neonates who

have used vascular access devices. Greenway and colleagues indicated that 90% of all neonatal thromboses were seen in neonates that had such devices.[53] If the child is in the age range of 10 to 17 years, another risk has been noted in the literature. In these ages, girls are affected 2:1 over boys. Nguyen et al. studied 10 children diagnosed in this age range and found 7/10 females were taking oral contraception.[54] The deep venous thromboses were most commonly found on the left iliofemoral vein (11/15).[54,55] Treatment for this condition is medical, involving the administration of anticoagulant medications.

■ Transient Synovitis

Chief Clinical Characteristics
This presentation can involve unilateral hip, groin, medial thigh, or anteromedial knee pain. Clinically, the child is able to move the joint, but stiffness is present. Often the complaint of pain follows a recent respiratory infection.

Background Information
The condition causes arthralgia and arthritis secondary to transient inflammation of the synovium of the hip joint that typically resolves. It is the most common cause of acute hip pain in children ages 3 to 10 years and it occurs twice as often in boys than girls.[8] Physical therapy intervention is directed at impairments such as pain, limited range of motion, weakness, and gait deviations.

TUMORS

■ Ewing's Sarcoma

Chief Clinical Characteristics
This presentation typically includes an insidious onset with night and rest pain. Children with this condition may have a fever. A soft tissue mass is common as is severe pain and edema. Erythema and decreased energy are also symptoms noted with this disease.[56]

Background Information
This condition is a cancerous lesion that can start anywhere in the body but develops in the bone. It tends to locate in weight-bearing bones and typically affects boys in the teenage years. It is found most frequently in the femur, then the tibia, then the humerus, then

the fibula (diaphysis of long bones).[56] It is the second most common primary malignant bone tumor seen in children.[28] Treatment includes surgical resection and chemotherapy; with this regimen, survival rates are now 65% to 70% with localized disease.[57] Physical therapy focuses on the child's postoperative impairments.

■ Ganglion Cysts

Chief Clinical Characteristics
This presentation involves a nonpainful or minimally painful soft tissue mass.

Background Information
Patients may report pain, clicking, or locking with range of motion. This condition is frequently found at the insertion sites of ligaments, near the region of the epiphysis. Intra-articular cysts typically present with greater losses of range of motion compared to intraosseous cysts.[58] Ganglion cysts are more common in women and 70% occur in people between the ages of 20 and 40 years, but they are not frequently located in the knee. Treatment typically involves aspiration or surgical excision; however, most cysts do not require any intervention.

■ Leukemia

Chief Clinical Characteristics
This presentation typically includes fever, weight loss, malaise, fatigue, swollen lymph nodes, and joint swelling. Limping is frequently an early sign. The child has diffuse, nonspecific pain that is asymmetric. Children with this condition appear systemically ill with fever, pallor, bruises, and excessive bleeding.

Background Information
This condition is a cancer of the white blood cells and is the most common type of childhood cancer. The two major types include acute lymphoblastic leukemia (ALL) and acute myeloid or (nonlymphoblastic) lymphoma. Although ALL predominantly affects children ages 1 to 4 years, the peak age of incidence is 2 to 3 years.[23,59] Medical management with chemotherapy is the primary treatment course at this time.

■ Lymphoma

Chief Clinical Characteristics
This presentation at the knee can involve pain caused by the lymph nodes in the popliteal fossa or inguinal area, which causes knee pain. However, the most common presentation is cervical or supraclavicular lymphadenopathy that is progressive. Additional findings include fever, night sweats, and weight loss.

Background Information
This condition is a cancer of the lymph system and is present in boys 3:1 over girls.[12] Medical management is necessary for chemotherapy and radiation.

■ Neuroblastoma

Chief Clinical Characteristics
This presentation can involve pain; infants present with refusal to walk, irritability, and limping in ambulatory children.[13]

Background Information
At the knee, this condition is a malignant, metastatic tumor that consists mainly of immature nerve cells. It is most common in children under the age of 4 to 5 years.

■ Osteoblastoma

Chief Clinical Characteristics
This presentation typically includes mild pain that is not well defined. Pain is usually worse at night and may be relieved by aspirin. Osteoblastoma is more common in older male teens. Pain is progressive though mild.

Background Information
Treatment is surgical excision if symptomatic.[60]

■ Osteochondroma

Chief Clinical Characteristics
This presentation can involve a visible and/or palpable firm, bony mass that is typically painless. Pain can occur in the presence of a fracture at the lesion site.[12] Children with this condition are generally asymptomatic, but a decrease in range of motion may present depending on the location of the lesion.

Background Information
This condition is the most common benign tumor of bone. It originates near the ends of

long bones and typically grows away from the joint. Growth of these lesions is typically during childhood and ceases with epiphyseal closure. They typically occur as single lesions, with most occurring at the knee at the ends of the femur and tibia.[12] This condition is typically asymptomatic, and it is often incidentally discovered on plain radiographs obtained for some other reason. Treatment generally only involves surgical resection of the lesion.

■ Osteoid Osteoma

Chief Clinical Characteristics
This presentation typically includes bone pain that is often worse at night. Pain is frequently relieved with aspirin and does not typically increase with activity. The onset is usually insidious and described as diffuse, aching, or throbbing. May also see joint effusion and a flexion contracture.[61]

Background Information
In a study by Torg and colleagues, the major physical finding was quadriceps atrophy.[62] None of their subjects demonstrated effusion, decreased range of motion, tenderness at the knee, signs of internal derangement, or neurological deficits. Surgical excision may be performed if symptomatic.

■ Osteosarcoma (Osteogenic Sarcoma)

Chief Clinical Characteristics
This presentation includes deep pain, especially at night, that is not related to activity. Children with this condition may have a palpable mass that is firm and tender.

Background Information
This condition is a cancerous lesion near the epiphyseal plates of the long bones (eg, distal femur, proximal tibia). There is no known cause. Pain usually is present for more than 6 weeks. It is a rare disease that is more common in males between the ages of 10 and 25 years during rapid growth spurts. This condition is the most common primary bone malignancy in children. Fifty percent are located in the distal femur, proximal tibia, or metaphysis of fibula.[61] Treatment includes chemotherapy and surgical excision.

■ Pigmented Villonodular Synovitis

Chief Clinical Characteristics
This presentation can involve diffuse, recurrent edema that is initially pain free, repeated hemarthrosis in the absence of trauma, progressive and insidious onset of pain, palpable nodules, and decreased range of motion. Symptoms may include locking and catching.

Background Information
This condition is a benign, proliferative pathology of unknown etiology that affects synovial tissue. The condition results in various degrees of villous and/or nodular changes in the joints, with the knee being the most commonly involved.[19,63–65] The two forms of the condition are diffuse and focal. The diffuse form typically involves large joints and involves the entire synovial lining, resulting in destructive changes in the joint. In contrast, the focal form involves small joints, such as the hands and feet, and results in mechanical symptoms like locking and catching. Surgical intervention is the optimal choice of treatment and the best results are most often observed with the focal form.[30] For the focal form, resection of the localized synovium often results in success. For the diffuse form, partial or complete removal of the entire synovial lining is required, however, the recurrence rate is high.

■ Synovial Chondromatosis

Chief Clinical Characteristics
This presentation can involve a chronic history of pain, swelling, stiffness, progressive loss of range of motion, and joint locking. Palpable nodules may also be present.

Background Information
This condition is a benign condition of unknown etiology that is characterized by synovial membrane proliferation and metaplasia. Nodular proliferation of the synovial lining occurs and fragments may break off into the joint to calcify and grow, resulting in gradual joint degeneration and secondary osteoarthritis. Almost any joint can be affected, however the knee is affected in more than half of all reported cases. The condition

most commonly presents at 30 to 50 years of age, is observed more often in males than females, and most often occurs on the right side of the body (4:1 ratio).[15,66] Treatment requires surgical excision of the proliferating synovium. To minimize risk of recurrence, total synovectomies are preferred.

■ Synovial Sarcoma

Chief Clinical Characteristics

This presentation usually includes pain and tenderness accompanied by swelling or mass. Children with this condition may also have decreased range at the knee. Synovial sarcoma is a rare cancer usually found in joints of the legs and arms.

Background Information

This condition typically presents at ages 20 to 40 years and is rare in children. The malignancy most commonly affects the lower extremities around the knees. Patients most commonly cite a slowly enlarging, deep-seated mass that is often painful. Children with this condition need medical management.

■ Vascular Malformation

Chief Clinical Characteristics

This presentation can be characterized by pain that is worse with exertion, diffuse muscular edema, and dependent pain. Other findings included pain in the morning and intermittent swelling.[67]

Background Information

This condition is frequently found intramuscularly. Roughly two-thirds of the malformations are seen at birth and the rest are not found until childhood and adolescence.[67] This condition is more common in females than in males, and in a study by Hein et al., 21 of the 46 lower extremity venous malformations were found in the quadriceps muscle.[67] The most common finding in a study by Theruvil and colleagues was diffuse edema in the involved muscle, followed by tenderness of that muscle.[68] The majority of the venous malformations in that study were located in the vastus medialis. Current treatments include compression stockings, radiotherapy, sclerotherapy, embolization, and excision.[68]

References

1. de Inocencio J. Musculoskeletal pain in primary pediatric care: analysis of 1000 consecutive general pediatric clinic visits. *Pediatrics*. Dec 1998;102(6):E63.
2. Dolman CL, Bell HM. The pathology of Legg-Calve-Perthes disease. A case report. *J Bone Joint Surg Am*. Jan 1973;55(1):184–188.
3. Herring JA, Kim HT, Browne R. Legg-Calve-Perthes disease. Part II: Prospective multicenter study of the effect of treatment on outcome. *J Bone Joint Surg Am*. Oct 2004;86-A(10):2121–2134.
4. Hoekelman RA, Adam HM, Nelson NM, Weitzman ML, Wilson MH. *Primary Pediatric Care*. St. Louis, MO: Mosby; 2001.
5. Davids JR. Pediatric knee. Clinical assessment and common disorders. *Pediatr Clin North Am*. Oct 1996;43 (5):1067–1090.
6. Fritz GK, Bleck EE, Dahl IS. Functional versus organic knee pain in adolescents. A pilot study. *Am J Sports Med*. Jul–Aug 1981;9(4):247–249.
7. Kuczkowski J, Narozny W, Mikaszewski B, Stankiewicz C. Suppurative complications of frontal sinusitis in children. *Clin Pediatr (Phila)*. Oct 2005;44(8):675–682.
8. Campbell SK, Vander Linden DW, Palisano RJ. *Physical Therapy for Children*. 2nd ed. Philadelphia, PA: W. B. Saunders; 2000.
9. Ankarath S, Ng AB, Giannoudis PV, Scott BW. Delay in diagnosis of slipped upper femoral epiphysis. *J R Soc Med*. Jul 2002;95(7):356–358.
10. Causey AL, Smith ER, Donaldson JJ, Kendig RJ, Fisher LC 3rd. Missed slipped capital femoral epiphysis: illustrative cases and a review. *J Emerg Med*. Mar–Apr 1995;13(2):175–189.
11. Singer KM, Henry J. Knee problems in children and adolescents. *Clin Sports Med*. Apr 1985;4(2):385–397.
12. Behrman RE, Kliegman RM, Jenson HB. *Nelson Textbook of Pediatrics*. 17th ed. Philadelphia, PA: W. B. Saunders; 2004.
13. Shah BR, Laude TA. *Atlas of Pediatric Clinical Diagnosis*. Philadelphia, PA: W. B. Saunders; 2000.
14. Johansson JE, Ajjoub S, Coughlin LP, Wener JA, Cruess RL. Pigmented villonodular synovitis of joints. *Clin Orthop Relat Res*. Mar 1982(163):159–166.
15. Larsson LG, Baum J. The syndrome of anserina bursitis: an overlooked diagnosis. *Arthritis Rheum*. Sep 1985;28(9):1062–1065.
16. Zeiss J, Coombs RJ, Booth RL Jr, Saddemi SR. Chronic bursitis presenting as a mass in the pes anserine bursa: MR diagnosis. *J Comput Assist Tomogr*. Jan–Feb 1993;17(1):137–140.
17. Staheli LT. *Pediatric Orthopedic Secrets*. Philadelphia, PA: Hanley and Belfus; 1998.
18. Sanders TG, Medynski MA, Feller JF, Lawhorn KW. Bone contusion patterns of the knee at MR imaging: footprint of the mechanism of injury. *Radiographics*. Oct 2000;20 Spec No:S135–151.
19. Kocher MS, Klingele K, Rassman SO. Meniscal disorders: normal, discoid, and cysts. *Orthop Clin North Am*. Jul 2003;34(3):329–340.
20. Brukner P, Khan K. *Clinical Sports Medicine*. 2nd ed. New York, NY: McGraw-Hill; 2000.
21. Speer DP. Differential diagnosis of knee pain in children. *Ariz Med*. May 1977;34(5):330–332.

22. Tachdjian MO. *Pediatric Orthopaedics*. 2nd ed. Philadelphia, PA: Elsevier Health Sciences; 1972.

23. Finberg L, Kleinman RE. *Saunders Manual of Pediatric Practice*. Philadelphia, PA: W. B. Saunders; 2002.

24. Cassidy JT, Levinson JE, Bass JC, et al. A study of classification criteria for a diagnosis of juvenile rheumatoid arthritis. *Arthritis Rheum*. Feb 1986;29(2): 274–281.

25. Calmbach WL, Hutchens M. Evaluation of patients presenting with knee pain: Part II. Differential diagnosis. *Am Fam Physician*. Sep 1, 2003;68(5):917–922.

26. Kruse RW. Evaluation of knee injuries. In: Lilliegard WA, Rucker KS, eds. *Handbook of Sports Medicine. A Symptom-Oriented Approach*. Newton, MA: Andover Medical Publishers; 1993:135–149.

27. Indelicato PA. Non-operative treatment of complete tears of the medial collateral ligament of the knee. *J Bone Joint Surg Am*. Mar 1983;65(3):323–329.

28. Zitelli BJ, Davis HW. *Atlas of Pediatric Physical Diagnosis*. 4th ed. Philadelphia, PA: Mosby; 2002.

29. Huppertz HI, Bentas W, Haubitz I, et al. Diagnosis of paediatric Lyme arthritis using a clinical score. *Eur J Pediatr*. Apr 1998;157(4):304–308.

30. Ekstrom JE. Arthrography. Where does it fit in? *Clin Sports Med*. Jul 1990;9(3):561–566.

31. Mink JH, Levy T, Crues JV 3rd. Tears of the anterior cruciate ligament and menisci of the knee: MR imaging evaluation. *Radiology*. Jun 1988;167(3):769–774.

32. Reicher MA, Hartzman S, Duckwiler GR, Bassett LW, Anderson LJ, Gold RH. Meniscal injuries: detection using MR imaging. *Radiology*. Jun 1986;159(3):753–757.

33. McCarty EC, Marx RG, DeHaven KE. Meniscus repair: considerations in treatment and update of clinical results. *Clin Orthop Relat Res*. Sep 2002;(402):122–134.

34. van Trommel MF, Simonian PT, Potter HG, Wickiewicz TL. Arthroscopic meniscal repair with fibrin clot of complete radial tears of the lateral meniscus in the avascular zone. *Arthroscopy*. May–Jun 1998;14 (4):360–365.

35. Kopell HP, Thompson WAL. Peripheral entrapment neuropathies. Baltimore, MD: Williams and Wilkins; 1963:34–47.

36. Maudsley RH. Fibular tunnel syndrome. In proceedings of the North-West Metropolitan Othopaedic Club. *J Bone Joint Surg*. 1967;49–B:384.

37. Deese MJ, Baxter DE. Compressive neuropathies of the lower extremity. *J Musculoskel Med*. 1988;5(11):68–91.

38. Hogan KA, Gross RH. Overuse injuries in pediatric athletes. *Orthop Clin North Am*. Jul 2003;34(3):405–415.

39. Williams JS Jr, Bush-Joseph CA, Bach BR Jr. Osteochondritis dissecans of the knee. *Am J Knee Surg*. Fall 1998;11(4):221–232.

40. Sales de Gauzy J, Mansat C, Darodes PH, Cahuzac JP. Natural course of osteochondritis dissecans in children. *J Pediatr Orthop B*. Jan 1999;8(1):26–28.

41. Zeitlin L, Fassier F, Glorieux FH. Modern approach to children with osteogenesis imperfecta. *J Pediatr Orthop B*. Mar 2003;12(2):77–87.

42. Stanitski CL, DeLee JC, Drez D Jr. *Pediatric and Adolescent Sports Medicine*. Philadelphia, PA: W. B. Saunders; 1994.

43. Nietosvaara Y, Aalto K, Kallio PE. Acute patellar dislocation in children: incidence and associated osteochondral fractures. *J Pediatr Orthop*. Jul–Aug 1994;14(4):513–515.

44. Adirim TA, Cheng TL. Overview of injuries in the young athlete. *Sports Med*. 2003;33(1):75–81.

45. Shea KG, Pfeiffer R, Curtin M. Idiopathic anterior knee pain in adolescents. *Orthop Clin North Am*. Jul 2003;34(3):377–383, vi.

46. Boles CA, Butler J, Lee JA, Reedy ML, Martin DF. Magnetic resonance characteristics of medial plica of the knee: correlation with arthroscopic resection. *J Comput Assist Tomogr*. May–Jun 2004;28(3):397–401.

47. Irha E, Vrdoljak J. Medial synovial plica syndrome of the knee: a diagnostic pitfall in adolescent athletes. *J Pediatr Orthop B*. Jan 2003;12(1):44–48.

48. Wang CL, Wang SM, Yang YJ, Tsai CH, Liu CC. Septic arthritis in children: relationship of causative pathogens, complications, and outcome. *J Microbiol Immunol Infect*. Mar 2003;36(1):41–46.

49. Hamer AJ. Pain in the hip and knee. *BMJ*. May 1 2004;328(7447):1067–1069.

50. Hanissian AS, Silverman A. Arthritis of sickle cell anemia. *South Med J*. Jan 1974;67(1):28–32.

51. Roger E, Letts M. Sickle cell disease of the spine in children. *Can J Surg*. Aug 1999;42(4):289–292.

52. Meremikwu M. Sickle cell disease. *Clin Evid*. Dec 2003(10):21–36.

53. Greenway A, Massicotte MP, Monagle P. Neonatal thrombosis and its treatment. *Blood Rev*. Jun 2004;18 (2):75–84.

54. Nguyen LT, Laberge JM, Guttman FM, Albert D. Spontaneous deep vein thrombosis in childhood and adolescence. *J Pediatr Surg*. 1986;21(7):640–643.

55. DeAngelis GA, McIlhenny J, Willson DF, et al. Prevalence of deep venous thrombosis in the lower extremities of children in the intensive care unit. *Pediatr Radiol*. Nov 1996;26(11):821–824.

56. Kennedy JG, Frelinghuysen P, Hoang BH. Ewing's sarcoma: current concepts in diagnosis and treatment. *Curr Opin Pediatr*. Feb 2003;15(1):53–57.

57. Marec-Berard P, Philip T. Ewing's sarcoma: the pediatrician's point of view. *Pediatr Blood Cancer*. May 2004;42(5):477–480.

58. Gunter P, Schwellnus MP. Local corticosteroid injection in iliotibial band friction syndrome in runners: a randomised controlled trial. *Br J Sports Med*. Jun 2004;38(3):269–272; discussion 272.

59. Brower V. New initiatives aim to test more cancer drugs for children. *J Natl Cancer Inst*. Dec 15 2004;96(24):1808–1810.

60. Papagelopoulos PJ, Galanis EC, Sim FH, Unni KK. Clinicopathologic features, diagnosis, and treatment of osteoblastoma. *Orthopedics*. Feb 1999;22(2):244–247; quiz 248–249.

61. Gebhardt MC, Ready JE, Mankin HJ. Tumors about the knee in children. *Clin Orthop Relat Res*. Jun 1990(255): 86–110.

62. Torg JS, Loughran T, Pavlov H, et al. Osteoid osteoma. Distant, periarticular, and subarticular lesions as a cause of knee pain. *Sports Med*. Jul–Aug 1985;2(4):296–304.

63. Handy JR. Popliteal cysts in adults: a review. *Semin Arthritis Rheum*. Oct 2001;31(2):108–118.

64. Holman PJ, Suki D, McCutcheon I, Wolinsky JP, Rhines LD, Gokaslan ZL. Surgical management of metastatic disease of the lumbar spine: experience with 139 patients. *J Neurosurg Spine*. May 2005;2(5): 550–563.

65. Nishihara RM, Helmstedter CS. Chondroblastoma: an unusual cause of knee pain in the adolescent. *J Adolesc Health.* Jan 2000;26(1):49–52.

66. Mann HA, Goddard NJ, Lee CA, Brown SA. Periarticular aneurysm following total knee replacement in hemophilic arthropathy. A case report. *J Bone Joint Surg Am.* Dec 2003;85-A(12):2437–2440.

67. Hein KD, Mulliken JB, Kozakewich HP, Upton J, Burrows PE. Venous malformations of skeletal muscle. *Plast Reconstr Surg.* Dec 2002;110(7):1625–1635.

68. Theruvil B, Kapoor V, Thalava R, Nag HL, Kotwal PP. Vascular malformations in muscles around the knee presenting as knee pain. *Knee.* Apr 2004;11 (2):155–158.

CHAPTER 48

Case Demonstration: Knee Pain and Limping in a Child

■ *Todd E. Davenport, PT, DPT, OCS* ■ *Sharon K. DeMuth, PT, DPT, MS*

NOTE: This case demonstration was developed using the diagnostic process described in Chapter 4 and demonstrated in Chapter 5. The reader is encouraged to use this diagnostic process in order to ensure thorough clinical reasoning. If additional elaboration is required on the information presented in this chapter, please consult Chapters 4 and 5.

THE DIAGNOSTIC PROCESS

Step 1 Identify the patient's chief concern.
Step 2 Identify *barriers to communication*.
Step 3 Identify *special concerns*.
Step 4 Create a symptom timeline and sketch the anatomy (if needed).
Step 5 Create a diagnostic hypothesis list considering all possible forms of *remote* and *local* pathology that could cause the patient's chief concern.
Step 6 Sort the diagnostic hypothesis list by epidemiology and specific case characteristics.
Step 7 Ask specific questions to rule specific conditions or pathological categories less likely.
Step 8 Re-sort the diagnostic hypothesis list based on the patient's responses to specific questioning.
Step 9 Perform tests to differentiate among the remaining diagnostic hypotheses.
Step 10 Re-sort the diagnostic hypothesis list based on the patient's responses to specific tests.
Step 11 Decide on a diagnostic impression.
Step 12 Determine the appropriate patient disposition.

Case Description

Sophie is a 6-year-old female who presents to your clinic with her mother, a current patient and friend of yours that you have been treating for a while. Sophie's mother is at the clinic for her usual appointment, but she also would like your quick advice about Sophie. Sophie's mother was unable to schedule an appointment with Sophie's pediatrician, so no physician referral is available for consultation. Sophie has not been playing outside and her teachers have told Sophie's mother that Sophie has preferred to stay inside at her desk at recess for the past 3 months. Your daughter, who is a classmate and friend of Sophie's, also has talked about the fact that Sophie has not been playing as much lately. Sophie's mother reports that Sophie has reported pain in her left knee and feeling tired. This keeps her from playing games outside with her friends. Sophie's mother thought a physical therapist's advice would be especially useful. Sophie's mother reports she cannot recall Sophie talking about specifically injuring her knee, but Sophie's mother knows that at Sophie's age falls are common on the playground.

STEP #1: Identify the patient's chief concern.
- Left knee pain and fatigue that precludes usual play

STEP #2: Identify *barriers to communication*.
- **Informal referral.** This route of referral often requires that rapid assessments be made without the routine documentation. The clinician should be careful to take the time necessary to be thorough and generate follow-up documentation for the patient and patient's family, clinic, and the pediatrician as needed. Legal issues also may exist given the request to evaluate this patient without physician referral.

- **Patient and patient's mother are acquaintances.** The clinician should be careful to collect all necessary information in order to arrive at a diagnostic conclusion, since some information unconsciously might be considered "too personal" to be collected. Acquaintance with the patient and her mother also might bias the clinician away from collecting information that could be useful to exclude or confirm the presence of pathology that is serious or carries social stigma.

- **Patient is a child.** Obtaining history and physical examination information from children requires special consideration.

STEP #3: Identify *special concerns.*

- **Knee pain without specific mechanism of injury.** Potentially raises the index of clinical suspicion for nontraumatic etiology.

STEP #4: Create a symptom timeline and sketch the anatomy (if needed).

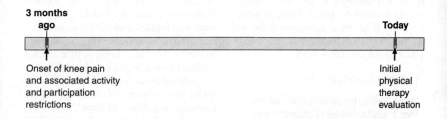

3 months ago

Today

Onset of knee pain and associated activity and participation restrictions

Initial physical therapy evaluation

STEP #5: Create a diagnostic hypothesis list considering all possible forms of *remote* and *local* pathology that could cause the patient's chief concern.

Remote

T Trauma

Lumbar radiculopathies:
- L3 radiculopathy
- L4 radiculopathy
- L5 radiculopathy

Slipped capital femoral epiphysis

I Inflammation

Aseptic
Transient synovitis of the hip

Septic
Epidural abscess
Septic hip

M Metabolic
Not applicable

Va Vascular
Avascular necrosis of the proximal femur

Legg-Calvé-Perthes disease

STEP #6: Sort the diagnostic hypothesis list by epidemiology and specific case characteristics.

Remote

T Trauma

Lumbar radiculopathies:
- L3 radiculopathy
- L4 radiculopathy
- L5 radiculopathy

~~Slipped capital femoral epiphysis~~ (patient age)

I Inflammation

Aseptic
Transient synovitis of the hip

Septic
Epidural abscess
Septic hip

M Metabolic
Not applicable

Va Vascular
~~Avascular necrosis of the proximal femur~~ (absence of significant trauma; patient age)

Legg-Calvé-Perthes disease

De Degenerative

Not applicable

Tu Tumor

Not applicable

Co Congenital

Not applicable

Ne Neurogenic/Psychogenic

Not applicable

Local

T Trauma

Blount's disease
Contusion
Fat pad impingement
Foreign body in the knee
Fractures:
- Avulsion
- Epiphyseal
- Standard
- Stress

Growing pains
Iliotibial band syndrome

Ligament sprain/tear

Meniscus tear

Muscle strain

Osgood-Schlatter disease
Patellar dislocation

Patellofemoral pain syndrome

Plica syndrome
Saphenous nerve entrapment

Sinding-Larsen-Johansson disease

I Inflammation

Aseptic
Bursitis:
- Infrapatellar
- Pes anserinus
- Prepatellar

Dermatomyositis
Erythema nodosum

De Degenerative

Not applicable

Tu Tumor

Not applicable

Co Congenital

Not applicable

Ne Neurogenic/Psychogenic

Not applicable

Local

T Trauma

Blount's disease
~~Contusion~~ (absence of significant trauma)
Fat pad impingement
Foreign body in the knee
~~Fractures:~~
- ~~Avulsion~~ (absence of significant trauma)
- ~~Epiphyseal~~ (absence of significant trauma)
- ~~Standard~~ (absence of significant trauma)
- ~~Stress~~ (absence of significant trauma)

Growing pains
~~Iliotibial band syndrome~~ (absence of significant trauma; not associated with fatigue)
~~Ligament sprain/tear~~ (absence of significant trauma; not associated with fatigue)
~~Meniscus tear~~ (absence of significant trauma; not associated with fatigue)
~~Muscle strain~~ (absence of significant trauma; not associated with fatigue)
~~Osgood-Schlatter disease~~ (patient age)
~~Patellar dislocation~~ (absence of significant trauma)
~~Patellofemoral pain syndrome~~ (not associated with fatigue)
~~Plica syndrome~~ (not associated with fatigue)
~~Saphenous nerve entrapment~~ (not associated with fatigue)
~~Sinding-Larsen-Johansson disease~~ (patient age)

I Inflammation

Aseptic
Bursitis:
- Infrapatellar
- Pes anserinus
- Prepatellar

Dermatomyositis
~~Erythema nodosum~~ (unilateral involvement; duration of symptoms)

Juvenile ankylosing spondylitis

Juvenile psoriatic arthritis
Juvenile rheumatoid arthritis
Juvenile scleroderma
Patellar tendonitis

Rheumatic fever

Systemic lupus erythematosus
Septic
Lyme disease
Osteomyelitis
Pyogenic arthritis
Systemic fungal infection (eg,
   actinomycosis, blastomycosis,
   coccidiomycosis, histoplasmosis)
Tuberculosis

M Metabolic

Gout

Myositis ossificans

Va Vascular

Hemophilia
Henoch-Schönlein purpura
Osteochondritis desiccans

Sickle cell anemia
Thrombus (venous or arterial)

Vascular malformation

De Degenerative

Not applicable

Tu Tumor

Malignant Primary, such as:
- Ewing's sarcoma
- Leukemia
- Lymphoma
- Osteosarcoma
- Synovial sarcoma
Malignant Metastatic, such as:
- Neuroblastoma
Benign, such as:
- Ganglion cyst
- Osteoblastoma
- Osteochondroma
- Osteoid osteoma
- Pigmented villonodular synovitis

~~Juvenile ankylosing spondylitis~~ (patient age
   and sex, uncommon initial presentation
   in the knee)
Juvenile psoriatic arthritis
Juvenile rheumatoid arthritis
Juvenile scleroderma
~~Patellar tendonitis~~ (not associated with
   fatigue)
~~Rheumatic fever~~ (duration of symptoms;
   lack of migratory pains)
Systemic lupus erythematosus
Septic
Lyme disease
Osteomyelitis
Pyogenic arthritis
Systemic fungal infection (eg,
   actinomycosis, blastomycosis,
   coccidiomycosis, histoplasmosis)
Tuberculosis

M Metabolic

~~Gout~~ (patient age, uncommon first
   presentation in the knee)
~~Myositis ossificans~~ (absence of significant
   trauma)

Va Vascular

~~Hemophilia~~ (patient sex)
Henoch-Schönlein purpura
~~Osteochondritis desiccans~~ (not associated
   with fatigue)
~~Sickle cell anemia~~ (duration of symptoms)
~~Thrombus (venous or arterial)~~ (symptom
   location)
Vascular malformation

De Degenerative

Not applicable

Tu Tumor

Malignant Primary, such as:
- Ewing's sarcoma
- Leukemia
- Lymphoma
- Osteosarcoma
- Synovial sarcoma
Malignant Metastatic, such as:
- ~~Neuroblastoma~~ (patient age)
Benign, such as:
- Ganglion cyst
- Osteoblastoma
- Osteochondroma
- Osteoid osteoma
- Pigmented villonodular synovitis

- Popliteal cyst
- Synovial chondromatosis

Co Congenital

Bipartite patella

Congenital dislocated patella
Discoid meniscus
Osteogenesis imperfecta

Patella alta
Patellar subluxation

Ne Neurogenic/Psychogenic

Conversion syndrome
Complex regional pain syndrome

Somatization

- Popliteal cyst
- ~~Synovial chondromatosis~~ (patient age)

Co Congenital

~~Bipartite patella~~ (not associated with
fatigue)
Congenital dislocated patella
Discoid meniscus
~~Osteogenesis imperfecta~~ (patient age at
presentation; depends on OI type)
Patella alta
Patellar subluxation

Ne Neurogenic/Psychogenic

Conversion syndrome
~~Complex regional pain syndrome~~
(absence of significant trauma)
Somatization

STEP #7: Ask specific questions to rule specific conditions or pathological categories less likely.

> **Teaching Comment:** Sophie's mother may be more helpful in providing many aspects of the history, but it is important for the clinician to address Sophie as much as possible to solicit her perspectives and gain rapport for the physical examination.

Questions for Sophie:

- **Where does it hurt?** Sophie rubs her left leg vaguely between her thigh and her shin anteriorly. (This shows you that Sophie is willing to provide information but needs help to be specific enough for your evaluation.) Makes less likely popliteal cyst due to the location of the pain since Sophie has indicated anteriorly not posteriorly.

- **Can you show me with one finger where it hurts?** Sophie points to left knee. (This localizes the pain to the left knee.) Makes less likely bilateral conditions.

- **Does your leg ever feel funny, like it is going to sleep or does it tingle?** Sophie shakes her head no. Makes less likely spinal pathology.

- **Does your leg ever feel numb or dead so you can't feel things that touch the skin of your legs or feet?** Sophie shakes her head no. Makes less likely spinal pathology.

> **Teaching Comment:** Sophie provides nonverbal answers to the questions about pain and sensation. This is common for children until they become comfortable with the examiner; if a child is very shy, this may be all they are able to do. It is safer to ask similar questions in different ways to be more certain of the answers.

Questions for Sophie's Mother:

- **Has Sophie gained or lost weight recently?** No, making less likely primary and malignant metastatic disease.

- **Is Sophie's pain worse at night?** No, making less likely osteoid osteoma.

STEP #8: Re-sort the diagnostic hypothesis list based on the patient's responses to specific questioning.

Remote

T Trauma

~~Lumbar radiculopathies:~~
- ~~L3 radiculopathy~~ (no numbness and
tingling)
- ~~L4 radiculopathy~~ (no numbness and
tingling)
- ~~L5 radiculopathy~~ (no numbness and tingling)

I Inflammation

Aseptic
Transient synovitis of the hip

Septic

~~Epidural abscess~~ (no numbness and tingling)

Septic hip

M Metabolic

Not applicable

Va Vascular

Legg-Calvé-Perthes disease

De Degenerative

Not applicable

Tu Tumor

Not applicable

Co Congenital

Not applicable

Ne Neurogenic/Psychogenic

Not applicable

Local

T Trauma

Blount's disease

Fat pad impingement

Foreign body in the knee

~~Growing pains~~ (unilateral pain; no pain at night)

I Inflammation

Aseptic

Bursitis:

● Infrapatellar

● Pes anserinus

● Prepatellar

Dermatomyositis

Juvenile psoriatic arthritis

Juvenile rheumatoid arthritis

Juvenile scleroderma

Systemic lupus erythematosus

Septic

Lyme disease

Osteomyelitis

Pyogenic arthritis

Systemic fungal infection (eg, actinomycosis, blastomycosis, coccidiomycosis, histoplasmosis)

Tuberculosis

M Metabolic

Not applicable

Va Vascular

Henoch-Schönlein purpura

De Degenerative

Not applicable

Tu Tumor

Malignant Primary, such as:

● ~~Ewing's sarcoma~~ (no weight changes)

● ~~Leukemia~~ (no weight changes)

● ~~Lymphoma~~ (no weight changes)

● ~~Osteosarcoma~~ (no weight changes)

● ~~Synovial sarcoma~~ (no weight changes)

Malignant Metastatic:

Not applicable

Benign, such as:

● Ganglion cyst

● Osteoblastoma

● Osteochondroma

● ~~Osteoid osteoma~~ (no increase in pain at night)

● Pigmented villonodular synovitis

● ~~Popliteal cyst~~ (pain location anterior not posterior)

Co Congenital

Congenital dislocated patella

Discoid meniscus

Patella alta

Patellar subluxation

Ne Neurogenic/Psychogenic

Conversion syndrome

Somatization

STEP #9: Perform tests to differentiate among the remaining diagnostic hypotheses.

● **Inspection and palpation.** The affected knee is edematous with increased surface temperature. Makes less likely benign tumors.

There are no rashes or skin lesions present on the lower extremities or face. Makes less likely dermatomyositis, Henoch-Schönlein purpura, juvenile psoriatic arthritis, juvenile scleroderma, systemic lupus erythematosus.

There are no local masses or areas of focal tenderness in the knee. Makes less likely bursitis, discoid meniscus, fat pad impingement, ganglion cyst, osteochondroma, pigmented villonodular synovitis.

The knee and patella have normal alignment and tracking. Makes less likely congenital dislocated patella, patella alta, patellar subluxation, and Blount's disease.

- **Log rolling of the hips.** Unremarkable for pain, guarding, and reproduction of pain. Makes less likely transient synovitis of the hip, septic hip, Legg-Calvé-Perthes disease.

- **Oral temperature.** Normal, ruling less likely pyrogenic conditions. Makes less likely osteomyelitis, pyogenic arthritis, systemic fungal infections, tuberculosis.

STEP #10: Re-sort the diagnostic hypothesis list based on the patient's responses to specific tests.

Remote

T   Trauma

Not applicable

I   Inflammation

Aseptic

Transient synovitis of the hip (no reproduction with hip provocation tests)

Septic

Septic hip (no reproduction with hip provocation tests; no fever)

M   Metabolic

Not applicable

Va   Vascular

Legg-Calvé-Perthes disease (no reproduction with hip provocation tests)

De   Degenerative

Not applicable

Tu   Tumor

Not applicable

Co   Congenital

Not applicable

Ne   Neurogenic/Psychogenic

Not applicable

Local

T   Trauma

Blount's disease (normal knee alignment)

Fat pad impingement (no local masses; no focal tenderness)

Foreign body in the knee (no local masses; no focal tenderness)

I   Inflammation

Aseptic

Bursitis:
- Infrapatellar (no focal tenderness)
- Pes anserinus (no focal tenderness)
- Prepatellar (no focal tenderness)

Dermatomyositis (no skin lesions)

Juvenile psoriatic arthritis (no skin lesions)

Juvenile rheumatoid arthritis

Juvenile scleroderma (no skin lesions)

Systemic lupus erythematosus (no skin lesions; no facial rash)

Septic

Lyme disease

Osteomyelitis (no fever)

Pyogenic arthritis (no fever)

Systemic fungal infection (eg, actinomycosis, blastomycosis, coccidiomycosis, histoplasmosis) (no fever)

Tuberculosis (no fever)

M   Metabolic

Not applicable

Va   Vascular

Henoch-Schönlein purpura (no skin lesions)

De   Degenerative

Not applicable

Tu   Tumor

Malignant Primary:
Not applicable
Malignant Metastatic:
Not applicable
Benign, such as:
- Ganglion cyst (no masses; no focal tenderness)
- Osteoblastoma (no masses; no focal tenderness)
- Osteochondroma (no masses; no focal tenderness)
- Pigmented villonodular synovitis (no masses; no focal tenderness)

Co   Congenital

Congenital dislocated patella (normal position)

Discoid meniscus (no focal tenderness)

~~Patella alta~~ (normal position)
~~Patellar subluxation~~ (normal position)

Ne Neurogenic/Psychogenic

~~Conversion syndrome~~ (not associated with objective signs of apparent knee inflammation)

~~Somatization~~ (not associated with objective signs of apparent knee inflammation)

STEP #11: Decide on a diagnostic impression.

- Rule out pauciarticular juvenile rheumatoid arthritis versus Lyme disease.

STEP #12: Determine the appropriate patient disposition.

- Refer the patient to the pediatrician by telephone for additional evaluation and treatment.

- Educate Sophie and Sophie's mother that the appointment should take place urgently.

Case Outcome

Sophie was referred to a pediatric rheumatology clinic where x-rays of her knees confirmed the absence of a primary malignant or benign tumor. A blood test was taken that was negative for Lyme disease and positive for an elevated sedimentation rate. A diagnosis of pauciarticular juvenile rheumatoid arthritis was made. Sophie was referred to an ophthalmologist for a slit-lamp examination to rule out the anterior uveitis that is often associated with pauciarticular juvenile rheumatoid arthritis. The slit-lamp examination was negative.

CHAPTER 49

Shin Pain in a Child

■ *Covey J. Lazouras, PT, DPT, NCS*

Description of the Symptom

This chapter describes possible causes of shin pain in a child. **Local causes** are defined as occurring distal to the knee and proximal to the ankle along the anterior portion of the lower leg. **Remote causes** are defined as occurring outside this region.

Special Concerns

■ Sudden onset of pain after mechanical injury particularly with weight bearing and/or palpation
■ Complaint of bone pain without mechanical injury that has persisted for longer than 2 weeks

■ Muscle pain that has persisted for longer than 2 weeks
■ Pain with repetitive activities, such as running
■ Any neurological signs suggesting increased compartmental pressure (ie, paresthesia or weakness of muscles below the knee)
■ Pain, edema, and redness over soft tissue of the calf or anterior compartment
■ Any of the above with fever, nausea, malaise, or fatigue

CHAPTER PREVIEW: Conditions That May Lead to Shin Pain in a Child

T Trauma	
REMOTE	**LOCAL**
COMMON	
Not applicable	Bone bruise 972
	Fracture of the tibia or fibula 974
	Muscle contusion 974
	Muscle strain/tear 975
	Stress fracture of the tibia or fibula 977
	Toddler's fracture of the tibia 977
UNCOMMON	
Lumbar radiculopathies:	Epiphyseal fractures 973
• L4 radiculopathy 971	Nerve entrapments:
• L5 radiculopathy 971	• Common peroneal nerve 975
• S1 radiculopathy 971	• Superficial peroneal nerve 975
RARE	
Not applicable	Not applicable

(continued)

I Inflammation

REMOTE	LOCAL
COMMON	
Not applicable	**Aseptic** Medial tibial stress syndrome (shin splints) 974
	Septic Not applicable
UNCOMMON	
Not applicable	Not applicable
RARE	
Aseptic Not applicable	**Aseptic** Not applicable
Septic Osteomyelitis of the lumbar vertebra 972	**Septic** Cellulitis 972 Dengue fever (break bone fever) 973 Osteomyelitis of the tibia or fibula 976

M Metabolic

REMOTE	LOCAL
COMMON	
Not applicable	Not applicable
UNCOMMON	
Not applicable	Not applicable
RARE	
Not applicable	Not applicable

Va Vascular

REMOTE	LOCAL
COMMON	
Not applicable	Not applicable
UNCOMMON	
Not applicable	Anterior compartment syndrome 972
RARE	
Not applicable	Sickle cell anemia/crisis 976

De Degenerative

REMOTE	LOCAL
COMMON	
Not applicable	Not applicable
UNCOMMON	
Not applicable	Not applicable

Degenerative *(continued)*

REMOTE	LOCAL
RARE	
Not applicable	Not applicable

Tu Tumor

REMOTE	LOCAL
COMMON	
Not applicable	Not applicable
UNCOMMON	
Not applicable	Not applicable
RARE	
Not applicable	*Malignant Primary, such as:* • Ewing's sarcoma 978 • Leukemia 978 • Osteosarcoma 979 • Rhabdomyosarcoma 979 *Malignant Metastatic, such as:* • Metastatic disease 978 *Benign, such as:* • Aneurysmal bone cyst 977 • Osteochondroma 978 • Osteoid osteoma 978 • Unicameral bone cyst 979

Co Congenital

REMOTE	LOCAL
COMMON	
Not applicable	Not applicable
UNCOMMON	
Not applicable	Not applicable
RARE	
Not applicable	Not applicable

Ne Neurogenic/Psychogenic

REMOTE	LOCAL
COMMON	
Not applicable	Idiopathic leg pain (growing pains) 974
UNCOMMON	
Not applicable	Not applicable
RARE	
Not applicable	Not applicable

Note: These are estimates of relative incidence because few data are available for the less common conditions.

SHIN PAIN IN A CHILD

Common Ages at Which Shin Pain Presents in a Child

APPROXIMATE AGE	CONDITION
Birth to 3 Years	Bone bruise
	Cellulitis
	Dengue fever
	Leukemia
	Muscle contusion
	Osteomyelitis
	Sickle cell anemia/crisis
	Toddler's fracture
Preschool (3–5 Years)	Bone bruise
	Cellulitis
	Dengue fever
	Idiopathic leg pain (growing pains)
	Muscle contusion
	Osteomyelitis
	Sickle cell anemia/crisis
	Toddler's fracture
Elementary School (6–11 Years)	Bone bruise
	Cellulitis
	Dengue fever
	Epiphyseal fractures
	Fracture
	Idiopathic leg pain (growing pains)
	Malignant tumors
	Muscle contusion
	Osteoid osteoma
	Sickle cell anemia/crisis
	Unicameral bone cyst
Middle School (12–14 Years)	Aneurysmal bone cyst
	Bone bruise
	Cellulitis
	Dengue fever
	Epiphyseal fractures
	Fracture
	Idiopathic leg pain (growing pains)
	Malignant tumors
	Medial tibial stress syndrome
	Muscle contusion
	Muscle strain/tear
	Osteochondroma
	Osteoid osteoma
	Sickle cell anemia/crisis
	Unicameral bone cyst
High School (15–18 Years)	Aneurysmal bone cyst
	Anterior compartment syndrome
	Bone bruise
	Cellulitis
	Common peroneal nerve entrapment
	Contusion
	Fracture
	Malignant tumors
	Medial tibial stress syndrome

Common Ages at Which Shin Pain Presents in a Child—cont'd

APPROXIMATE AGE	CONDITION
	Muscle contusion
	Muscle strain/tear
	Osteoid osteoma
	Sickle cell anemia/crisis
	Stress fracture
	Superficial peroneal nerve entrapment

Overview of Shin Pain in a Child

Shin pain is a common symptom reported in the pediatric population. Shin pain can occur as a result of a clearly defined mechanical event or be a sign and symptom of the normal growing process, that is, "growing pains." The former usually occurs at night. Shin pain from a nonmechanical event should be explored further. Remote causes of shin pain are rare but the theoretical possibility exists. One must consider pathology at L4, such as an epidural abscess, osteomyelitis, or a tumor, as a potential source of nerve root compression or central canal stenosis at the L4–L5 level. Impingement on the roots of L4–L5 of the lumbar plexus as they traverse the pelvis could theoretically be caused by an intrapelvic tumor or infection.

Description of Conditions That May Lead to Shin Pain in a Child

Remote

LUMBAR RADICULOPATHIES

■ L4 Radiculopathy

Chief Clinical Characteristics
This presentation can be characterized by pain in the lumbar spine and paresthesias radiating from the anterior aspect of the hip, thigh, and knee, sometimes ending anteromedially from the knee to the foot. Depending on the severity, this presentation may also include a decreased or absent patellar tendon reflex and motor loss in the muscles innervated by the L4 nerve. Prone knee bend may reproduce symptoms.

Background Information
A lumbar disk herniation is the most common cause for this condition. The diagnosis is confirmed with magnetic resonance imaging. Surgical intervention may be indicated in severe cases of lower extremity pain accompanied by neurological signs.

■ L5 Radiculopathy

Chief Clinical Characteristics
This presentation includes pain in the lumbar spine and paresthesias radiating from the lateral aspect of the hip and buttock to the lateral aspect of the knee, extending anterolaterally down to the foot. Depending on the severity, the presentation may also include motor loss in the muscles innervated by the L5 nerve root.

Background Information
A lumbar disk herniation is the most common cause for this condition. The diagnosis is confirmed with magnetic resonance imaging. Surgical intervention may be indicated in severe cases of lower extremity pain accompanied by neurological signs.

■ S1 Radiculopathy

Chief Clinical Characteristics
This presentation typically includes pain in the lumbar spine and paresthesias radiating from the buttock to the posterior aspect of the knee and extending posterolaterally from the knee to the foot. Depending on the severity, the presentation may also include a decreased or absent Achilles tendon reflex and motor loss in the muscles innervated by the S1 nerve.

Background Information
A lumbar disk herniation is a common cause for this condition. The diagnosis is confirmed with magnetic resonance imaging. Surgical intervention may be indicated in severe cases of lower extremity pain accompanied by neurological signs.

■ Osteomyelitis of the Lumbar Vertebra

Chief Clinical Characteristics

This presentation may include an insidious onset of localized pain over the infected vertebral body, fever, chills, and malaise.[1]

Background Information

As the infection progresses pain can refer in a dermatomal pattern and neurological compromise may occur.[1] Treatment is with antibiotic medications.[1]

Local

■ Anterior Compartment Syndrome

Chief Clinical Characteristics

This presentation includes pain out of proportion to the injury or increasing pain over time.

Background Information

Compartment syndrome is due primarily to increased intracompartmental pressure. The mechanism involved in the development of increased pressure depends on the precipitating event.[2] Two distinct types of compartment syndrome have been recognized. The first type is associated trauma to the affected compartment, as seen in fractures or muscle injuries contained in a compartment of the limb. The second type is associated with repetitive loading or microtrauma associated with physical activity. This second type is what is described as exertional compartment syndrome. Thus, this syndrome may be acute or chronic in nature. The most serious complication of a contusion is compartment syndrome. Contused tissue within a confined compartment can rapidly reach elevated or critical pressure levels.[2] Clinicians should have a low threshold for testing compartments for increased pressure if compartment syndrome is suspected. Surgical intervention to release compartment pressure may be indicated because irreversible damage such as nerve entrapment, vascular compromise, and tissue necrosis may occur with prolonged elevated pressures. In general, however, early diagnosis, with institution of the appropriate treatment, results in a good outcome.[3]

■ Bone Bruise

Chief Clinical Characteristics

This presentation includes swelling, skin discoloration, and pain to touch and possibly with weight-bearing activity (eg, during peak anterior tibialis muscle activity during gait). Stretching or contraction of affected muscle also reproduces the symptom of pain. The mechanism of injury is typically blunt trauma via a fall or projectile.

Background Information

Conventional radiographic techniques are limited in providing accurate bone marrow characterization and therefore the diagnosis of bone bruising is essentially based on magnetic resonance imaging findings.[4] Radiographs, however, are able to identify a fracture that may have occurred as a result of trauma. A complication of bruising of the shin bone includes compartment syndrome and the possibility of a fracture.[4] Treatment typically involves relative rest, nonsteroidal anti-inflammatory medications, and rehabilitation interventions intended to reduce pain.

■ Cellulitis

Chief Clinical Characteristics

This presentation includes redness of the skin, red streaking of the skin or broad areas of redness, swelling, warmth, pain or tenderness, and drainage or leaking of yellow clear fluid or pus from the skin. If the condition spreads to the body via the blood, then fevers and chills can result.

Background Information

This condition can occur in almost any part of the body. Most commonly it occurs in areas that have been damaged or are inflamed for other reasons, such as inflamed lesions, contaminated cuts or abrasions, foreign objects in the skin, and areas with poor circulation.[5] This condition has no predilection for any racial or ethnic group or gender. For the vast majority of cases, there is no age-group predilection. Perianal cellulitis usually occurs in children younger than 3 years. Group B *Streptococcus* cellulitis occurs in infants younger than 6 months.[6] Pain disproportional to the physical examination or severe pain on passive movement of the extremities requires prompt evaluation by a surgeon. Uncomplicated forms of this condition have an excellent prognosis with standard antibiotic treatment.[6]

■ Dengue Fever (Break Bone Fever)

Chief Clinical Characteristics

This presentation includes shin pain, headache, retro-orbital pain, myalgia, arthralgia, rash, and hemorrhagic manifestations. Fever and other symptoms may subside after 3 to 4 days. An individual with this condition may recover completely, or the fever may return with a rash within 1 to 3 days. The clinical symptoms are often persisting fatigue and exhaustion, even after the fever has subsided.

Background Information

This condition is an acute benign febrile syndrome that occurs in tropical regions. It is caused by a virus transmitted to humans through the bite of an infected *Aedes aegypti* mosquito. Most cases in the United States occur in returning travelers, but the incidence of dengue is increasing along the Texas–Mexico border and in other parts of the southern United States. A serious complication of this condition is dengue hemorrhagic fever, which can result in internal bleeding and death. Ninety percent of cases of dengue hemorrhagic fever occur in individuals less than 15 years of age.[7] Course of treatment for dengue fever without complications includes analgesics, fluid replacement, and bed rest.[8]

■ Epiphyseal Fractures

Chief Clinical Characteristics

This presentation typically includes complaints of localized joint pain, usually following a traumatic event (eg, fall, collision). Swelling near a joint with focal tenderness over the physis is usually present. Injuries to the physes are more likely to occur in an active pediatric population, especially boys, in part due to the greater structural strength and integrity of the ligaments and joint capsules than of the growth plates. These binding filamentous structures are two to five times stronger than the growth plates at either end of a long bone and, therefore, are less often injured in children sustaining excessive external loads to the joints.[9] Plain radiographs may depict physeal widening as the only sign of displacement. Radiographic stress views (varus and valgus) may be indicated in certain patients. Magnetic resonance imaging has proved to be the most accurate evaluation tool for the fracture anatomy when performed in the acute phase of injury. Magnetic resonance imaging can depict altered arrest lines and transphyseal bridging abnormalities prior to their being evident on plain radiographs.

Background Information

The age of the patient at the time of injury is of paramount importance in helping predict clinical outcomes because more correction, or loss of growth, can be anticipated in younger patients. Injuries to the physes of 14- to 15-year-old girls or 17- to 18-year-old boys are of little consequence due to their limited growth potential.[10] As a result, any growth plate injury is unlikely to be clinically significant. However, injuries in younger children with full growth potential can cause significant problems and a wide range of clinical effects. Long-term follow-up is essential to determine whether or not complications will occur. Most physeal injuries should be reevaluated in the short term to ensure maintenance of reduction and proper anatomical relationships. After initial fracture healing has occurred, physeal fractures require additional follow-up radiographs 6 months and 12 months following injury to assess for growth disturbance. Management of such physeal fractures can thus be divided into two phases. The first phase involves ensuring bone healing, and the second phase is monitoring growth.[11] Ligamentous laxity tests of the joints of the injured side may elicit pain and positive findings similar to those indicative of joint injury. Do not dismiss positive joint laxity test findings as only involving the related joint. Complete growth retardation or partial growth arrest may result in progressive limb-length discrepancies. Complete growth arrest is uncommon and depends on when the injury to the physis occurs in relation to the remaining skeletal growth potential.[11] The younger the patient, the greater the potential for problems associated with growth. While fractures involving the tibia and fibula are the most common lower extremity pediatric fractures, those involving the proximal tibial epiphysis are among the most uncommon but have the highest rate of complications. When displacement occurs, the popliteal artery is vulnerable. At the tibial metaphysis, the artery is just posterior to the popliteus muscle. Complications of these injuries may include vascular insufficiency, peroneal nerve palsy, and anterior physis closure, which may cause significant genu recurvatum.[12]

■ Fracture of the Tibia or Fibula

Chief Clinical Characteristics

This presentation includes pain, swelling, and possible lower leg angulation from either direct trauma or indirect trauma (rotational forces). Fractures of the legs, especially the lower legs, often come from simple falls during active play. There is an inability to ambulate with tibia fracture; however, ambulation is possible with isolated fibula fracture.

Background Information

Fractures of the tibia generally are associated with fibula fracture, because the force is transmitted along the interosseous membrane to the fibula. Significant numbers of these injuries are open, because the skin and subcutaneous tissue are very thin over the anterior tibia.[13] Open fractures require immediate orthopedic referral for irrigation, debridement, and possible open reduction and internal fixation. These variations require long leg posterior splints. Isolated midshaft or proximal fibula fractures do not require immobilization in a long leg cast. A few days without weight-bearing activity until swelling resolves, followed by weight-bearing activity as tolerated, is recommended.[14] Prognosis is generally good yet is dependent on degree of soft tissue injury and bony comminution.[15] Complications of this injury may include neurovascular compromise, compartment syndrome, peroneal nerve injury, infection, gangrene, osteomyelitis, delayed union, nonunion, or malunion.[14]

■ Idiopathic Leg Pain (Growing Pains)

Chief Clinical Characteristics

This presentation includes pain late in the day or that awakens a child at night. The pain is not specifically related to joints. Pain is intermittent with symptom-free intervals of days, weeks, or months. The specific etiology of growing pains is unknown and it is often a diagnosis of exclusion.[16] The most likely causes are the aches and discomforts resulting from the jumping, climbing, and running that active children do during the day.

Background Information

This condition is a common pediatric disorder with an incidence of about 15%. Two peak incidences exist from 3 to 5 years of age, and later on, in 8- to 12-year-olds. There is a greater incidence in girls.[17] Physical examination is normal without any evidence of trauma, joint swelling, erythema, decreased range of motion, limp, or tenderness. Evaluations, including radiographs and erythrocyte sedimentation rate, are normal.[16] Typical treatment involves watchful waiting.

■ Medial Tibial Stress Syndrome (Shin Splints)

Chief Clinical Characteristics

This presentation includes pain and swelling located at the anteromedial aspect of the lower leg (ie, insertion of the posterior tibialis tendon in the leg). Overuse is the most common etiology including repetitive, sustained exertion or insufficient recovery time between activities.[18]

Background Information

Runners running on hard surfaces without proper footwear are predisposed to this condition. Improper stretching and neglecting to warm up before exercising also may contribute to shin injury. Conservative treatment includes nonsteroidal anti-inflammatory medications, splinting, and/or immobilization. A change in training routine and/or equipment may be indicated.[19] Corticosteroid injections are considered for individuals with this condition in whom rest, immobilization, and anti-inflammatory medications have failed. In general, the prognosis is very good with rest and conservative management. Possibility of full tendon rupture or stress fracture exists if condition is ignored.[3]

■ Muscle Contusion

Chief Clinical Characteristics

This presentation is characterized by direct trauma to the muscle group with subsequent swelling, tenderness to palpation, and pain with passive and active range of motion resulting from bleeding within the muscle.

Background Information

This condition accounts for one-third of all sports injuries.[20] This condition is caused by blunt trauma to the outer aspect of the muscle, resulting in tissue and cellular damage and bleeding deep within the muscle and between the muscle planes. The resultant tissue necrosis and hematoma lead to inflammation. A contusion usually can be distinguished from a muscle rupture because residual function remains after a contusion.[20] Depending on the size of the lesion, a hematoma also may be appreciated. A complete examination of the injured area and surrounding areas must be emphasized to identify other possible injuries. Typical treatment involves relative rest and rehabilitative interventions. The most serious complication is compartment syndrome. Signs and symptoms of compartment syndrome include pain out of proportion to the injury or increasing pain over time. Contused tissue within a confined compartment can rapidly reach elevated or critical pressure levels. Surgical intervention should not be necessary unless the diagnosis of compartment syndrome is considered and confirmed. Heterotopic ossification may also be a complication of muscle contusions.[21]

■ Muscle Strain/Tear

Chief Clinical Characteristics
This presentation includes swelling, bruising or redness, muscle spasm, pain at rest, pain when the specific muscle or the joint in relation to that muscle is used, and weakness of the muscle or tendons and inability to use the muscle.[22] Symptoms can vary, depending on how severe the strain.

Background Information
The mechanism of injury is typically caused by twisting or pulling a muscle or tendon. This condition can be acute or chronic. An acute strain is caused by trauma or an injury such as a blow to the body; it can also be caused by improperly lifting heavy objects or overstressing the muscle tissue.[23] Chronic strains are usually the result of overuse—prolonged, repetitive movement of the muscles and tendons. Minor or moderate strain often heals well with home treatment and rehabilitation. Severe strains may require surgery to repair the torn muscles or tendons. Complications of an acute severe muscle strain if left untreated include long-term pain, limited movement, and deformity resulting from muscle imbalances and chronic compensation.[24]

NERVE ENTRAPMENTS

■ Common Peroneal Nerve

Chief Clinical Characteristics
This presentation can be characterized by exercise-related leg pain with or without associated dermatomal numbness. Pain is not universal, and if present, it is often related to the specific cause of the nerve compromise.[25] For example, a nerve compromise secondary to traumatic injury from blunt trauma will likely result in pain secondary to soft tissue swelling and inflammation.

Background Information
Traumatic causes can include wounds and contusions, direct fractures involving the lateral knee, and direct lacerations.[26] This condition may be caused by ankle sprains with associated proximal fibula fractures, knee dislocations, or compression from intraneural or extraneural tumors. Compression of the nerve against the fibrous or fascial layers of the well-developed muscles of the legs of athletes has also been seen as a causal factor.[27] Treatment for this condition is typically nonsurgical, with surgical intervention reserved for cases in which the anatomical site of entrapment is well characterized.

■ Superficial Peroneal Nerve

Chief Clinical Characteristics
This presentation includes numbness or paresthesia in the distribution of the nerve, and occasionally vague pain about the lateral leg extending to the dorsum of the foot. The pain can be chronic and present for several years and may be associated with other foot and ankle symptoms, or the pain can be acute and associated with recent trauma or surgery about the ankle.[28] Infrequently, weakness of the dorsiflexors and everters of the foot may be seen with associated foot drop in more proximal entrapments of the superficial peroneal nerve. Typically, symptoms increase with activity such as running, walking, and squatting.[29] Rest or avoiding the precipitating activity often relieves the symptoms.

Background Information
Percussion along the superficial course of the nerve over the proximal fibula, lateral leg, or the anterior ankle may cause a positive result on Tinel test, with reproduction of radiating

pain.[30] Direct palpation with pressure on the site of entrapment may also induce or exacerbate symptoms. Repeating the examination after a particular activity that exacerbates symptoms may produce findings not present on the initial examination at rest. In some cases of superficial peroneal nerve entrapment associated with direct or indirect trauma, patients may present with symptoms of complex regional pain syndrome, which creates a diagnostic and therapeutic challenge.[31] Although rare, plain radiographs of the leg may reveal bony abnormalities that may contribute or be the cause of entrapment. In cases of suspected proximal entrapment, knee radiographs may show abnormalities of the proximal fibula, such as exostoses, osteochondromas, and fracture callus.[28] If necessary, computed tomography or sonography can provide more detailed information on the bony anatomy of the area, and a sonogram can help localize cystic masses that cause impingement of the nerve. Surgical decompression may be indicated in cases when symptoms are not relieved by nonoperative options. This can include release of the superficial peroneal nerve at the lateral leg for surgical decompression with partial or full fasciotomy.[31]

■ Osteomyelitis of the Tibia or Fibula

Chief Clinical Characteristics

This presentation includes a rapid onset of symptoms including general malaise, high fever, chills, severe constant pain, swelling, and tenderness over the metaphysis of the involved bone. The limb is painful with any movement, which leads to an appearance of paralysis in infants.[32]

Background Information

Approximately 50% of cases occur in preschool-aged children. Preponderance in males is observed in all age groups. In some cases the infection starts in the bony metaphysis and spreads to an adjacent joint, creating a septic arthritis. It is caused by an infection in the bone secondary to a minor injury with the most common causative bacterium being *Staphylococcus aureus* followed by *Streptococcus pneumoniae* and *Streptococcus pyogenes*.[33] To confirm the diagnosis, adequate radiologic

and laboratory data are necessary. Three-phase technetium radionuclide bone scanning is used for imaging studies; however, magnetic resonance imaging is increasingly being used to define bone involvement in patients with a negative bone scan.[34] Blood, bone, and joint aspirate cultures are obtained before any antibiotics are given to identify the pathogen. Treatment includes aspiration, antibiotics, immobilization of the affected area, and surgical drainage if necessary.[33]

■ Sickle Cell Anemia/Crisis

Chief Clinical Characteristics

This presentation involves four patterns of acute presentation: sudden acute chest pain where coughing up of blood can occur, abdominal crisis, joint crisis, and bone crisis. Bone crisis is an acute or sudden pain in a bone usually in an arm or leg. The affected area may be tender to palpation. Common bones involved include the large bones in the arm or leg: the humerus, tibia, and femur. The same bone may be affected repeatedly in future episodes of bone crisis.[35] This presentation includes severe pain, which is the most common sign of sickle cell disease emergencies (acute sickle cell crises).[36] Commonly no mechanical event precedes a crisis, but one or more of the following situations may have contributed to the start of the painful sickle crisis: dehydration, infection, fever, hypoxia (decrease in oxygen to body tissue), bleeding, cold exposure, drug and alcohol use, pregnancy, or stress.[35]

Background Information

This condition is a hereditary condition of the blood where the red blood cells become distorted (into a sickle shape) under conditions of hypoxia and clog the vessels, resulting in vascular occlusion. This disease is present mostly in individuals of African descent. It also is found, with much less frequency, in eastern Mediterranean and Middle Eastern populations. The male-to-female ratio is 1:1. This disease process is a lifelong condition. It first manifests in the second half of the first year of life and persists for the entire life span.[37] Further complicating this presentation is that children with sickle cell disease have weakened immune systems and are at increased risk for developing secondary infection, especially in the lungs, kidneys, bones, and central nervous system. There is a frequent occurrence of *Salmonella* osteomyelitis in areas of bone weakened by infarction. Repeated infarction of joints, bones, and growth plates leads to aseptic necrosis, especially in weight-bearing areas such as the femur. This complication is associated with chronic pain and disability and may require changes in employment and lifestyle.[38] A sickle cell crisis can often be managed efficiently and quickly in a hospital's emergency department with intravenous fluids and pain medicines. A person suspected of having this condition should not delay going to the hospital for emergent medical evaluation and treatment.[35–37]

■ Stress Fracture of the Tibia or Fibula

Chief Clinical Characteristics
This presentation is characterized by insidious onset of activity-related pain. Pain is reproduced with palpation or percussion of the affected area. Inspection of the site may reveal localized swelling and possible erythema. Loading the affected bone using specific maneuvers may reproduce pain.[39] Early on, the pain typically is mild and occurs toward the end of the inciting activity. The proximal tibial shaft is the most common site of stress fractures.

Background Information
Stress fractures are overuse injuries of bone. Girls have a higher incidence of stress fractures than boys. Muscle fatigue and structural malalignments may contribute to stress fractures.[40] Treatment consists of activity restriction to minimize symptoms (ie, a period of non–weight-bearing ambulation may be necessary) before engaging in a program of increasingly demanding strengthening and conditioning exercise leading to eventual return to play in 8 to 12 weeks.[39] Treat cortical stress fractures of the anterior tibial midshaft with care since they tend to heal more slowly (average of 6 months) and are prone to delayed union or nonunion. In most cases, stress fractures can be managed successfully with conservative measures. High-risk displaced stress fractures, however, require surgical intervention to ensure proper healing.

■ Toddler's Fracture of the Tibia

Chief Clinical Characteristics
This presentation may include pain, limping, or refusal to bear weight on the affected side.

Tenderness, swelling, warmth, and pain with palpation of the lower third of the tibia also may be noted.[41]

Background Information
This is a common fracture of toddlers and preschoolers. The term refers to an undisplaced oblique or spiral fracture of the tibial diaphysis with an intact fibula.[42] Because the periosteum in the toddler is sufficiently tough, the child may be able to walk on the leg, even though fractured, albeit with pain and a limp. Typically there is an acute onset without known history of trauma. It occurs when the child is learning to walk, running, or steps on something and loses his or her footing. A sudden twisting of the tibia (shin bone), perhaps from getting the foot caught in a crib slat, causes a fracture in a spiral pattern. The fracture may be very subtle on the initial radiograph and may only be recognized on a follow-up film when callus is evident. Treatment consists of a below-knee walking cast for approximately 3 weeks. A long-leg cast is applied to relieve the symptoms. Healing is rapid, within 3 or 4 weeks.[43]

TUMORS

■ Aneurysmal Bone Cyst

Chief Clinical Characteristics
This presentation may include pain of relatively acute onset that rapidly increases in severity over 6 to 12 weeks. Local skin temperature may increase and a palpable bony swelling may be present.

Background Information
This condition is a benign tumor; therefore it is not the type of disease that will spread to other areas. However, a bone cyst can cause destruction of bone and isolated symptoms at the site of the bone cyst.[44] Compared with males, females have an increased incidence. This condition may occur in patients ages 10 to 30 years, with a peak incidence in those 16 years of age. About 75% of patients are younger than 20 years. The most common site is the metaphyseal region of the knee; however, any bone may be affected with the lower leg being affected in 24% of the cases.[45] The most common problem caused by this condition is weakening of the bone. This may lead to increased susceptibility to

fracture at that location. Because of this, the bone cyst may need to be treated in the operating room to prevent a fracture. Sometimes the bone cyst will not be found until after a fracture has happened. In this case, treatment of the fracture will also include treatment of the bone cyst to prevent a recurrence of this problem.[44] Documented cases of malignant conversion exist; however, this scenario is rare.[46]

■ Ewing's Sarcoma

Chief Clinical Characteristics

This presentation includes pain and local swelling at the site of the tumor. Constitutional symptoms such as fever and malaise may be present specifically when metastatic disease is present.[47]

Background Information

Ewing's sarcoma is the second most common malignant bone tumor in children and adolescents. These tumors most commonly develop in the axial skeleton, but may arise in any bone; particularly the diaphyses of the humerus and femur. Approximately 25% of patients with this condition may present with overt metastasis, typically in the lungs, bone marrow, or bone.[48] Ewing's tumors are typically sensitive to both chemotherapy and radiotherapy; surgical excision is utilized as well.[49]

■ Leukemia

Chief Clinical Characteristics

This presentation typically includes diffuse, nonspecific bone pain with fever and elevated white blood cell and sedimentation rates. Lesions to the mouth are also often seen later.[50]

Background Information

This condition is a cancer of the white blood cells and is the most common form of childhood cancer.[51] Changes on x-ray may show focal lesions of bone resorption seen in the long bones of the body. Occasionally, children with this condition can have pathological fractures associated with osteopenia/osteoporosis of the bones, such as the tibia.[51] Treatment consists of the primary interventions of chemotherapy, radiation, and bone marrow transplant.

■ Metastatic Disease

Chief Clinical Characteristics

This presentation typically involves bone or soft tissue pain in combination with pallor, fatigue, tachycardia, and headache and fever. Pain may be the only local presenting symptom.

Background Information

If a mechanical source of injury is not easily identified or if the child presents with the above systemic symptoms, the diagnosis of malignancy of the blood (leukemia), bone (osteosarcoma), or soft tissue (rhabdomyosarcoma) should be considered. Immediate referral to a primary care physician is indicated. Treatment options range from surgical resection and reconstruction of host tissues to chemotherapy and radiation treatment.

■ Osteochondroma

Chief Clinical Characteristics

This presentation can include pain around the area of the bony protrusion and may cause secondary nerve and tendon inflammation.

Background Information

This condition involves cartilage-covered bony excrescence (exostosis) that arises from the surface of a bone. This condition is the most common bone tumor in children, accounting for 50% of all benign bone tumors in children. Its peak incidence is in the second decade of life with a male-to-female ratio of approximately 2:1.[52] This condition can occur at any time from birth to the cessation of growth. Complications of osteochondromas include fractures, bony deformities, neurological and vascular injuries, bursa formation, and malignant transformation.[53] The treatment of symptomatic osteochondromas is surgical excision. Hereditary multiple exostosis is a hereditary autosomal dominant disorder where many exostoses are noted. Growth disturbances may occur as one result of this complication.[54]

■ Osteoid Osteoma

Chief Clinical Characteristics

This presentation consists of focal bone pain at the site of the tumor. The condition worsens at night and increases with activity, and it is dramatically relieved with small doses of aspirin.

Background Information

The most common skeletal sites are the metaphysis or diaphysis of long bones, which are affected in 73% of patients. This condition more commonly affects males than females. The male-to-female ratio is 2:1. The age range in patients is 5 to 56 years. The lesion initially appears as a small sclerotic bone island within a circular lucent defect. The tumors may regress spontaneously. This condition is classified as cortical, cancellous, or subperiosteal.[55,56] The tumor usually does not grow, and it occasionally regresses spontaneously or becomes dormant, leaving residual sclerosis. The tumor has no malignant potential.[57] Complications include pathological fractures secondary to decreased structural integrity of the affected bone.[58] Several techniques are available for ablation of osteoid osteoma. The tumor can be percutaneously ablated by using radiofrequency, ethanol, laser, or thermocoagulation therapy under computed tomographic guidance.[59]

■ Osteosarcoma

Chief Clinical Characteristics

This presentation may be characterized by deep achy pain that is usually mechanical in nature (exacerbated by activity of the extremity),[47] local swelling, and decreased range of motion.[60] Symptoms are often caused by microfractures through the involved area, and in severe cases secondary to stretching and compression of the surrounding structures.[61]

Background Information

Osteosarcoma is the most common primary malignancy of bone in children. It typically occurs between 10 and 20 years of age, with the peak age incidence during the adolescent growth spurt.[62] The onset of symptoms is insidious in nature, often related to a minor trauma such as a sports-related injury.[61] Treatment of the tumor requires surgical ablation and adjuvant chemotherapy.

■ Rhabdomyosarcoma

Chief Clinical Characteristics

This presentation includes a mass in an extremity that may or may not be painful. Pain or tenderness may be present if the tumor is displacing a peripheral nerve.

Background Information

Rhabdomyosarcoma is the most common pediatric soft tissue sarcoma, and two-thirds of affected patients are less than 10 years of age.[61,63] They can develop anywhere in the body but are often found in the extremities. Approximately half the tumors of the limbs are alveolar in nature and are therefore highly metastatic.[64] Treatment typically includes presurgical neoadjuvant chemotherapy, surgical excision, and postsurgical chemotherapy; radiation therapy is used if needed.

■ Unicameral Bone Cyst

Chief Clinical Characteristics

This presentation usually includes local pain over one bone in an individual who is skeletally immature. Most individuals with this condition present with symptoms and signs of a pathological fracture.

Background Information

This condition is a common benign fluid-filled lesion found almost exclusively in children. It occurs most frequently in children ages 5 to 15 years, with an average age of approximately 9 years.[65,66] Much has been written about the diagnosis and management of these lesions, and evidence of a variety of successful treatment strategies can be found in the literature. In general, treatment may be summarized as watchful waiting more than trying to promote natural healing. When such cysts are immediately adjacent to a growth plate, they are referred to as active cysts; when they have achieved some distance from the growth plate, they are considered to be latent cysts. This distinction has been used in the past, because it was believed to have prognostic significance. Injury to the growth plate (physis) may occur secondary to direct cyst expansion, pathological fracture, or unintended mechanical disturbance during surgical intervention. Growth arrest secondary to unicameral bone cysts is related to direct cyst expansion across the growth plate and into the epiphysis of the proximal humerus.[67] Growth arrest also has been reported following treatment of the cyst either by local injection of steroids or by curettage and bone grating.[68] Growth disturbance leading to angular deformity or disturbed longitudinal growth has been estimated to possibly occur in approximately 14% of cases.[66] Steroid injection has been a successful treatment, even in the setting of cyst extension into the epiphysis.[69] The overall outcome and prognosis is good. The lesion is believed to resolve spontaneously in most cases if given enough time.

References

1. Jevtic V. Vertebral infection. *Eur Radiol.* Mar 2004;14 (suppl 3):E43–52.
2. Hutchinson MR, Ireland ML. Common compartment syndromes in athletes. Treatment and rehabilitation. *Sports Med.* Mar 1994;17(3):200–208.
3. Detmer DE, Sharpe K, Sufit RL, Girdley FM. Chronic compartment syndrome: diagnosis, management, and outcomes. *Am J Sports Med.* May–Jun 1985;13(3): 162–170.
4. Miller MD, Osborne JR, Gordon WT, Hinkin DT, Brinker MR. The natural history of bone bruises. A prospective study of magnetic resonance imaging-detected trabecular microfractures in patients with isolated medial collateral ligament injuries. *Am J Sports Med.* Jan–Feb 1998;26(1):15–19.
5. Sadow KB, Chamberlain JM. Blood cultures in the evaluation of children with cellulitis. *Pediatrics.* Mar 1998; 101(3):E4.
6. Darmstadt GL. Oral antibiotic therapy for uncomplicated bacterial skin infections in children. *Pediatr Infect Dis J.* Feb 1997;16(2):227–240.
7. Anderson LJ. Human parvoviruses. *J Infect Dis.* Apr 1990; 161(4):603–608.
8. Schwartz GR. *Principles and Practice of Emergency Medicine.* 3rd ed. Philadelphia, PA: Lippincott Williams & Wilkins; 1992.
9. Brighton CT. Structure and function of the growth plate. *Clin Orthop Relat Res.* Oct 1978(136):22–32.
10. Peterson HA. Physeal & apophyseal injuries. In: Rockwood CA, Wilkins KE, Beaty JH, eds. *Fractures in Children.* 4th ed. Philadelphia, PA: Lippincott Williams & Wilkins; 1996.
11. Bright RW. Physeal injuries. In: Wilkins KE, Rockwood CA, eds. *Fractures in Children.* 3rd ed. Philadelphia, PA: Lippincott Williams & Wilkins; 1991:87–186.
12. Salter RB, Harris WR. Injuries involving the epiphyseal plate. *J Bone Joint Surg Am.* 1963;4(A):587–622.
13. Russell TA. Fractures of the tibia and fibula. In: Rockwood CA, Green DP, eds. *Fractures in Adults.* 4th ed. Philadelphia, PA: Lippincott Williams & Wilkins; 1996:2127–2201.
14. Roberts DM, Stallard TC. Emergency department evaluation and treatment of knee and leg injuries. *Emerg Med Clin North Am.* Feb 2000;18(1):67–84, v–vi.
15. Haller PR, Harris CR. The tibia and fibula. In: *Emergent Management of Skeletal Injuries.* St. Louis, MO: Mosby; 1995:499–517.
16. Peterson H. Growing pains. *Pediatr Clin North Am.* Dec 1986;33(6):1365–1372.
17. Weiner SR. Growing pains. *Am Fam Physician.* Jan 1983; 27(1):189–191.
18. Lord J, Winell JJ. Overuse injuries in pediatric athletes. *Curr Opin Pediatr.* Feb 2004;16(1):47–50.
19. Kortebein PM, Kaufman KR, Basford JR, Stuart MJ. Medial tibial stress syndrome. *Med Sci Sports Exerc.* Mar 2000;32(3 suppl):S27–33.
20. Best TM. Soft-tissue injuries and muscle tears. *Clin Sports Med.* Jul 1997;16(3):419–434.
21. Jackson DW, Feagin JA. Quadriceps contusions in young athletes. Relation of severity of injury to treatment and prognosis. *J Bone Joint Surg Am.* Jan 1973;55 (1):95–105.
22. Garrett WE Jr. Muscle strain injuries. *Am J Sports Med.* 1996;24(6 suppl):S2–8.
23. Kirkendall DT, Garrett WE Jr. Clinical perspectives regarding eccentric muscle injury. *Clin Orthop Relat Res.* Oct 2002(403 suppl):S81–89.
24. Garrett WE Jr. Muscle strain injuries: clinical and basic aspects. *Med Sci Sports Exerc.* Aug 1990;22(4):436–443.
25. Katirji MB, Wilbourn AJ. Common peroneal mononeuropathy: a clinical and electrophysiologic study of 116 lesions. *Neurology.* Nov 1988;38(11):1723–1728.
26. Fabre T, Piton C, Andre D, Lasseur E, Durandeau A. Peroneal nerve entrapment. *J Bone Joint Surg Am.* Jan 1998; 80(1):47–53.
27. Mitra A, Stern JD, Perrotta VJ, Moyer RA. Peroneal nerve entrapment in athletes. *Ann Plast Surg.* Oct 1995; 35(4):366–368.
28. Kim DH, Kline DG. Management and results of peroneal nerve lesions. *Neurosurgery.* Aug 1996;39(2): 312–319; discussion 319–320.
29. Lorei MP, Hershman EB. Peripheral nerve injuries in athletes. Treatment and prevention. *Sports Med.* Aug 1993;16(2):130–147.
30. McAuliffe TB, Fiddian NJ, Browett JP. Entrapment neuropathy of the superficial peroneal nerve. A bilateral case. *J Bone Joint Surg Br.* Jan 1985;67(1):62–63.
31. Johnston EC, Howell SJ. Tension neuropathy of the superficial peroneal nerve: associated conditions and results of release. *Foot Ankle Int.* Sep 1999;20(9):576–582.
32. Scott RJ, Christofersen MR, Robertson WW Jr, Davidson RS, Rankin L, Drummond DS. Acute osteomyelitis in children: a review of 116 cases. *J Pediatr Orthop.* Sep–Oct 1990;10(5):649–652.
33. Bradley JS, Kaplan SL, Tan TQ, et al. Pediatric pneumococcal bone and joint infections. The Pediatric Multicenter Pneumococcal Surveillance Study Group (PMPSSG). *Pediatrics.* Dec 1998;102(6):1376–1382.
34. Schauwecker DS, Braunstein EM, Wheat LJ. Diagnostic imaging of osteomyelitis. *Infect Dis Clin North Am.* Sep 1990;4(3):441–463.
35. Ballas SK. Complications of sickle cell anemia in adults: guidelines for effective management. *Cleve Clin J Med.* Jan 1999;66(1):48–58.
36. Bookchin RM, Lew VL. Pathophysiology of sickle cell anemia. *Hematol Oncol Clin North Am.* Dec 1996;10(6): 1241–1253.
37. Platt OS, Brambilla DJ, Rosse WF, et al. Mortality in sickle cell disease. Life expectancy and risk factors for early death. *N Engl J Med.* Jun 9, 1994;330(23):1639–1644.
38. Quinn CT, Buchanan GR. Sickle-cell anemia with unusual bone changes. *J Pediatr.* 2003;143(3):350.
39. Orava S, Karpakka J, Hulkko A, et al. Diagnosis and treatment of stress fractures located at the mid-tibial shaft in athletes. *Int J Sports Med.* Aug 1991;12(4): 419–422.
40. Arendt EA. Stress fractures and the female athlete. *Clin Orthop Relat Res.* Mar 2000(372):131–138.

41. Mellick LB, Reesor K, Demers D, Reinker KA. Tibial fractures of young children. *Pediatr Emerg Care.* Jun 1988; 4(2):97–101.

42. Oudjhane K, Newman B, Oh KS, Young LW, Girdany BR. Occult fractures in preschool children. *J Trauma.* Jun 1988;28(6):858–860.

43. Halsey MF, Finzel KC, Carrion WV, Haralabatos SS, Gruber MA, Meinhard BP. Toddler's fracture: presumptive diagnosis and treatment. *J Pediatr Orthop.* Mar–Apr 2001;21(2):152–156.

44. Clough JR, Price CH. Aneurysmal bone cyst: pathogenesis and long term results of treatment. *Clin Orthop Relat Res.* Nov–Dec 1973(97):52–63.

45. Cottalorda J, Kohler R, Sales de Gauzy J, et al. Epidemiology of aneurysmal bone cyst in children: a multicenter study and literature review. *J Pediatr Orthop B.* Nov 2004;13(6):389–394.

46. Brindley GW, Greene JF Jr, Frankel LS. Case reports: malignant transformation of aneurysmal bone cysts. *Clin Orthop Relat Res.* Sep 2005;438:282–287.

47. Gibbs CP Jr, Weber K, Scarborough MT. Malignant bone tumors. *Instr Course Lect.* 2002;51:413–428.

48. Vlasak R, Sim FH. Ewing's sarcoma. *Orthop Clin North Am.* Jul 1996;27(3):591–603.

49. Himelstein BP, Dormans JP. Malignant bone tumors of childhood. *Pediatr Clin North Am.* Aug 1996;43(4): 967–984.

50. Kling T. The sick child. In: Staheli LT, ed. *Pediatric Orthopedic Secrets.* 2nd ed. Philadelphia, PA: Hanley & Belfus; 2002.

51. Goodwin R. Hematologic disorders. In: Staheli LT, Song K, eds. *Pediatric Orthopedic Secrets.* 3rd ed. Philadelphia, PA: Hanley & Belfus; 2007.

52. Schmale GA, Conrad EU 3rd, Raskind WH. The natural history of hereditary multiple exostoses. *J Bone Joint Surg Am.* Jul 1994;76(7):986–992.

53. Wicklund CL, Pauli RM, Johnston D, Hecht JT. Natural history study of hereditary multiple exostoses. *Am J Med Genet.* Jan 2 1995;55(1):43–46.

54. Nawata K, Teshima R, Minamizaki T, Yamamoto K. Knee deformities in multiple hereditary exostoses. A longitudinal radiographic study. *Clin Orthop Relat Res.* Apr 1995(313):194–199.

55. Adam G, Neuerburg J, Vorwerk D, Forst J, Gunther RW. Percutaneous treatment of osteoid osteomas: combination of drill biopsy and subsequent ethanol injection. *Semin Musculoskelet Radiol.* 1997;1(2):281–284.

56. Cove JA, Taminiau AH, Obermann WR, Vanderschueren GM. Osteoid osteoma of the spine treated with percutaneous computed tomography-guided thermocoagulation. *Spine (Phila Pa 1976).* May 15, 2000; 25(10):1283–1286.

57. Hosalkar HS, Garg S, Moroz L, Pollack A, Dormans JP. The diagnostic accuracy of MRI versus CT imaging for osteoid osteoma in children. *Clin Orthop Relat Res.* Apr 2005(433):171–177.

58. Ortiz EJ, Isler MH, Navia JE, Canosa R. Pathologic fractures in children. *Clin Orthop Relat Res.* Mar 2005(432): 116–126.

59. Donley BG, Philbin T, Rosenberg GA, Schils JP, Recht M. Percutaneous CT guided resection of osteoid osteoma of the tibial plafond. *Foot Ankle Int.* Jul 2000; 21(7):596–598.

60. Widhe B, Widhe T. Initial symptoms and clinical features in osteosarcoma and Ewing sarcoma. *J Bone Joint Surg Am.* May 2000;82(5):667–674.

61. Arndt CA, Crist WM. Common musculoskeletal tumors of childhood and adolescence. *N Engl J Med.* Jul 29, 1999;341(5):342–352.

62. Meyers PA, Gorlick R. Osteosarcoma. *Pediatr Clin North Am.* Aug 1997;44(4):973–989.

63. Conrad EU 3rd, Bradford L, Chansky HA. Pediatric soft-tissue sarcomas. *Orthop Clin North Am.* Jul 1996; 27(3):655–664.

64. Pappo AS, Shapiro DN, Crist WM. Rhabdomyosarcoma. Biology and treatment. *Pediatr Clin North Am.* Aug 1997;44(4):953–972.

65. Capanna R, Campanacci DA, Manfrini M. Unicameral and aneurysmal bone cysts. *Orthop Clin North Am.* Jul 1996;27(3):605–614.

66. Lokiec F, Ezra E, Khermosh O, Wientroub S. Simple bone cysts treated by percutaneous autologous marrow grafting. A preliminary report. *J Bone Joint Surg Br.* Nov 1996;78(6):934–937.

67. Gupta AK, Crawford AH. Solitary bone cyst with epiphyseal involvement: confirmation with magnetic resonance imaging. A case report and review of the literature. *J Bone Joint Surg Am.* Jun 1996;78(6):911–915.

68. Stanton RP, Abdel-Mota'al MM. Growth arrest resulting from unicameral bone cyst. *J Pediatr Orthop.* Mar–Apr 1998;18(2):198–201.

69. Malawer MM, Markle B. Unicameral bone cyst with epiphyseal involvement: clinicoanatomic analysis. *J Pediatr Orthop.* Mar 1982;2(1):71–79.

CHAPTER 50

Ankle and Foot Pain in a Child

■ *Robert C. Sieh, PT, DPT*

Description of the Symptom

This chapter describes possible causes of ankle and foot pain in a child. **Local causes** are defined as occurring between the distal one-third of the tibia and the toes, inclusive of musculoskeletal and neurovascular structures that cross the ankle joint, rearfoot, midfoot, forefoot, and toes. **Remote causes** are defined as occurring outside this region.

Special Concerns
■ Pain of sudden onset without known cause
■ Pain that continues with rest or elevation of the feet

■ Skin breakdown, rash, or infection of any area around the foot
■ Unexplained mass(es)
■ Swelling of one limb for longer than 24 hours
■ Pain that increases with exercise
■ Any numbness, tingling, or other loss of sensation
■ Sudden inability to walk or loss of muscle strength

CHAPTER PREVIEW: Conditions That May Lead to Ankle and Foot Pain in a Child

T Trauma	
REMOTE	**LOCAL**
COMMON	
Not applicable	Fractures:
	• Calcaneal 993
	• Epiphyseal 993
	• Pathological 994
	• Stress 994
	• Talar 994
	• Toddler's fracture of the tibia 994
	Ill-fitting shoes 996
	Ligament sprains:
	• Anterior talofibular ligament 997
	• Calcaneofibular ligament 997
	• Metatarsophalangeal joint (turf toe) 998
	Muscle strain 998
	Puncture wounds 1000

Trauma *(continued)*

REMOTE	LOCAL
UNCOMMON	
Not applicable	Ankle impingement syndromes:
	• Anterior 989
	• Posterior 990
	Apophysitis:
	• Achilles tendon insertion (Sever's disease) 990
	• Fifth metatarsal (Iselin's disease) 990
	Nerve entrapments:
	• Common peroneal nerve entrapment 998
	• Lateral plantar nerve 999
	• Tarsal tunnel syndrome 999
RARE	
Lumbar radiculopathies:	Not applicable
• L5 radiculopathy 988	
• S1 radiculopathy 988	
Popliteal entrapment syndrome 988	

ⓘ Inflammation

REMOTE	LOCAL
COMMON	
Not applicable	**Aseptic**
	Bursitis:
	• Retrocalcaneal bursitis 991
	• Subcutaneous Achilles bursitis 991
	Tendinitis:
	• Achilles tendinitis 1001
	• Flexor hallucis longus tenosynovitis 1001
	• Tibialis posterior tendinitis 1002
	Septic
	Ingrown toenails 996
UNCOMMON	
Not applicable	**Aseptic**
	Juvenile rheumatoid arthritis 997
	Plantar fasciitis 1000
	Retrocalcaneal bursitis 1000
	Septic
	Cellulitis 991
	Fungal disease 995
	Hand-foot-mouth disease 996
	Joint sepsis 996
	Osteomyelitis 999

(continued)

Inflammation *(continued)*

REMOTE	LOCAL
RARE	
Not applicable	**Aseptic** Rheumatic fever 1000 Seronegative spondyloarthropathies 1000 **Septic** Necrotizing fasciitis 998 Tuberculosis 1002

M Metabolic

REMOTE	LOCAL
COMMON	
Not applicable	Not applicable
UNCOMMON	
Not applicable	Gout 995
RARE	
Not applicable	Ehlers-Danlos syndrome 992 Fabry's disease 992 Gaucher's disease 995 Myositis ossificans 998

Va Vascular

REMOTE	LOCAL
COMMON	
Not applicable	Hemophilia 996
UNCOMMON	
Not applicable	Osteochondritis dissecans of the talus 999 Sickle cell anemia 1001
RARE	
Not applicable	Avascular necrosis: • Navicular (Köhler's disease) 990 • Second metatarsal head (Freiberg's infarction) 990 Compartment syndrome 992 Peripheral arterial disease 999 Thalassemia (familial Mediterranean fever) 1002

De Degenerative

REMOTE	LOCAL
COMMON	
Not applicable	Bunions 991 Heel spurs 996
UNCOMMON	
Not applicable	Not applicable

Degenerative *(continued)*

REMOTE	LOCAL
RARE	
Not applicable	Hallux rigidus 995
	Peroneal tendon subluxation 999

Tu Tumor

REMOTE	LOCAL
COMMON	
Not applicable	Not applicable
UNCOMMON	
Not applicable	Not applicable
RARE	
Not applicable	*Malignant Primary, such as:*
	• Ewing's sarcoma 1003
	• Leukemia 1003
	• Osteosarcoma 1004
	• Rhabdomyosarcoma 1004
	• Synovial sarcoma 1004
	Malignant Metastatic:
	Not applicable
	Benign, such as:
	• Calcaneal cysts 1002
	• Ganglion cyst 1003
	• Giant cell tumor of the tendon sheath 1003
	• Glomangioma 1003
	• Osteoblastoma 1003
	• Osteochondroma 1004
	• Osteoid osteoma 1004

Co Congenital

REMOTE	LOCAL
COMMON	
Not applicable	Accessory navicular 989
	Flat-foot deformities:
	• Flexible 993
UNCOMMON	
Not applicable	Flat-foot deformities:
	• Rigid 993
	Tarsal coalitions:
	• Calcaneonavicular coalition 1001
	• Talocalcaneal coalition 1001

(continued)

Congenital *(continued)*

REMOTE	LOCAL
RARE	
Not applicable	Claw toes 991
	Congenital oblique talus 992
	Congenital vertical talus 992
	Hallux varus 995
	Hammer toes 995
	Polydactyly 1000
	Trevor's disease (dysplasia epiphysealis hemimelica) 1002

Ne   Neurogenic/Psychogenic

REMOTE	LOCAL
COMMON	
Not applicable	Not applicable
UNCOMMON	
Not applicable	Complex regional pain syndrome (reflex sympathetic dystrophy) 992
RARE	
Not applicable	Not applicable

Note: These are estimates of relative incidence because few data are available for the less common conditions.

Common Ages at Which Ankle/Foot Pain Presents in a Child

APPROXIMATE AGE	CONDITION
Birth to 3 Years	Congenital vertical and oblique talus
	Hand-foot-mouth disease
	Hemophilia
	Juvenile rheumatoid arthritis
	Leukemia
	Sickle cell anemia
Preschool (3–5 Years)	Cellulitis
	Ewing's sarcoma
	Fractures
	Hand-foot-mouth disease
	Hemophilia
	Ill-fitting shoes
	Juvenile rheumatoid arthritis
	Leukemia
	Osteoid osteoma
	Puncture wounds
	Rheumatic fever
	Sickle cell anemia
	Tuberculosis
Elementary School (6–11 Years)	Accessory navicular
	Avascular necrosis of the metatarsal head
	Avascular necrosis of the navicular

Common Ages at Which Ankle/Foot Pain Presents in a Child—cont'd

APPROXIMATE AGE	CONDITION
	Complex regional pain syndrome
	Ewing's sarcoma
	Fabry's disease
	Familial Mediterranean fever
	Fungal infection
	Gaucher's disease
	Giant cell tumor of the tendon sheath
	Hemophilia
	Juvenile rheumatoid arthritis
	Osteochondroma
	Osteoid osteoma
	Rheumatic fever
	Sickle cell anemia
	Tarsal coalitions
Middle School (12–14 Years)	Accessory navicular
	Ankle impingement syndromes
	Ankle sprain
	Avascular necrosis of the metatarsal head
	Avascular necrosis of the navicular
	Bursitis
	Calcaneal apophysitis
	Complex regional pain syndrome
	Dysplasia epiphysealis hemimelica
	Ewing's sarcoma
	Fabry's disease
	Familial Mediterranean fever
	Fracture (calcaneus)
	Fungal infection
	Gaucher's disease
	Giant cell tumor of the tendon sheath
	Glomangioma
	Hallux rigidus
	Heel spurs
	Hemophilia
	Ingrown toenails
	Juvenile rheumatoid arthritis
	Muscle strain
	Necrotizing fasciitis
	Osteochondritis dissecans of the talus
	Osteochondroma
	Osteoid osteoma
	Osteomyelitis
	Peroneal tendon subluxation
	Popliteal entrapment syndrome
	Puncture wounds
	Rheumatic fever
	Rigid flat foot
	Seronegative spondyloarthropathies
	Sickle cell anemia
	Tarsal coalitions
	Tendinitis

(continued)

Common Ages at Which Ankle/Foot Pain Presents in a Child—cont'd

APPROXIMATE AGE	CONDITION
High School (15–18 Years)	Avascular necrosis of the metatarsal head
	Compartment syndrome
	Ehlers-Danlos syndrome
	Fabry's disease
	Gout
	Hemophilia
	Myositis ossificans
	Necrotizing fasciitis
	Osteochondritis dissecans of the talus
	Osteomyelitis
	Popliteal entrapment syndrome
	Rheumatic fever
	Seronegative spondyloarthropathies
	Sickle cell anemia

Overview of Ankle and Foot Pain in a Child

Ankle and foot pain is relatively rare in young children. In many cases, the ankle or foot pain will have simple causes that can be treated easily by the therapist. However, it is very important to rule out other causes of the pain due to the harmful effects of some causes if overlooked. These include many forms of inflammation, vascular compromise, systemic diseases, and other such problems that would require a referral to the appropriate physician. The following section describes the thought process used when considering such a referral.

Description of Conditions That May Lead to Ankle and Foot Pain in a Child

Remote

LUMBAR RADICULOPATHIES

■ L5 Radiculopathy

Chief Clinical Characteristics

This presentation includes pain in the lumbar spine and paresthesias radiating from the lateral aspect of the hip and buttock to the lateral aspect of the knee, extending anterolaterally down to the foot. Depending on the severity, the presentation may also include motor loss in the muscles innervated by the L5 nerve root.

Background Information

A lumbar disk herniation is the most common cause for this condition. The diagnosis is confirmed with magnetic resonance imaging. Surgical intervention may be indicated in severe cases of lower extremity pain accompanied by neurological signs.

■ S1 Radiculopathy

Chief Clinical Characteristics

This presentation typically includes pain in the lumbar spine and paresthesias radiating from the buttock to the posterior aspect of the knee and extending posterolaterally from the knee to the foot. Depending on the severity, the presentation may also include a decreased or absent Achilles tendon reflex and motor loss in the muscles innervated by the S1 nerve.

Background Information

A lumbar disk herniation is a common cause for this condition. The diagnosis is confirmed with magnetic resonance imaging. Surgical intervention may be indicated in severe cases of lower extremity pain accompanied by neurological signs.

■ Popliteal Entrapment Syndrome

Chief Clinical Characteristics

This presentation may be characterized by symptoms and signs consistent with claudication and lower limb ischemia with exercise.[1]

Background Information

This is a rare condition in which the popliteal artery is compressed by various muscle tendons in the region. History, physical examination with auscultating and palpating the peripheral pulses, and use of Doppler sonography if available before and after exercise can help identify this condition.[1] Use of magnetic resonance imaging can also identify possible compression sites due to individual differences in anatomy. Treatment should be a referral for surgical treatment.[1]

Local

■ Accessory Navicular

Chief Clinical Characteristics

This presentation includes pain with weight bearing and palpation to the navicular region (Fig. 50-1).[2,3] Tight shoes may increase

symptoms due to increased pressure in the area.[4] This condition is more common in girls, with pain and tenderness medial to the navicular as the most common sign.[2,3]

Background Information

An external oblique x-ray is needed to properly visualize this condition.[2] Physical testing may include pain with testing the posterior tibialis tendon.[5] This is due to the tendon inserting on the accessory bone instead of the true navicular, causing too much stress to the area.[5] Treatment includes use of a walking cast, with occasional need for surgical resection if symptoms persist.[2–5]

ANKLE IMPINGEMENT SYNDROMES

■ Anterior

Chief Clinical Characteristics

This presentation involves restriction with pain when the foot is dorsiflexed, and palpation tenderness to the anterior ankle joint. Often osteophyte formation is present in the tibiotalar region and is the cause of the impingement and resulting pain (Fig. 50-2).[6]

Background Information

An oblique anteromedial impingement radiograph is usually the best method of looking for these osteophytes.[6] Treatment consists of

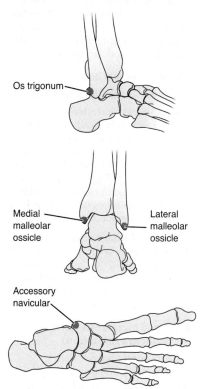

FIGURE 50-1 Common accessory ossification centers.

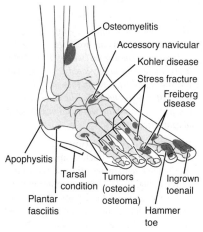

FIGURE 50-2 Pain localization points about the ankle and foot.

surgical removal of the osteophytes that are causing the trauma to the surrounding tissues.[6]

■ **Posterior**

Chief Clinical Characteristics

This presentation involves restriction with pain when the foot is plantarflexed, with palpation tenderness to the posterior ankle joint.

Background Information

This syndrome is very common in dancers and soccer players, especially those with a history of flexor hallucis tenosynovitis.[7,8] Many times an ankle sprain injury with a congenital abnormality such as large talus, os trigonum (see Fig. 50-2), or loose bodies will result in an impingement of the posterior capsule of the ankle.[9] This results in pain and limited plantarflexion. Physical testing including pain with passive plantarflexion reproducing the child's pain is positive for posterior impingement. Nonsurgical management consisting of antiinflammatory modalities, taping, stretching, and/or steroid injections is the treatment for this condition.[7] If unsuccessful, surgical intervention may be warranted.[7]

APOPHYSITIS

■ **Achilles Tendon Insertion (Sever's Disease)**

Chief Clinical Characteristics

This presentation commonly involves often bilateral focal pain and swelling near the insertion on the calcaneous (see Fig. 50-1), tight heel cords leading to decreased dorsiflexion of the ankle, and walking on toes secondary to pain with weight bearing. The child usually has just increased the workload or intensity of competitive sports.

Background Information

This condition is a traction apophysitis of the Achilles tendon insertion at the calcaneus (see Fig. 50-2). The most commonly affected age range is 8 to 12 years.[3,10,11] X-rays can be helpful to confirm the diagnosis by ruling out other causes of pain.[3,4,10] Treatment consists of stretching, strengthening, activity limitation, and use of heel cups/change in footwear. Most children respond

to nonsurgical treatment and return to full activity in 4 to 8 weeks.[3,4,10]

■ **Fifth Metatarsal (Iselin's Disease)**

Chief Clinical Characteristics

This presentation usually involves pain, swelling, and tenderness under the proximal region of the fifth metatarsal (especially with weight bearing near the attachment of the peroneus brevis; see Fig. 50-1).[3,12]

Background Information

This is an overuse injury to the region while performing running, jumping, and cutting type activities. The most common group affected is 10- to 12-year-olds.[12] Due to the ligaments and tendons being stronger than bone at this age, the bone can avulse or cause a traction apophysitis similar to that in the calcaneus in Sever's disease. Physical testing elicits pain with resisted eversion with end-range plantarflexion or dorsiflexion.[12] The usual course of treatment is immobilization and then strength and proprioceptive training.[3,12]

AVASCULAR NECROSIS

■ **Navicular (Köhler's Disease)**

Chief Clinical Characteristics

This presentation involves pain and limping with forefoot supination in young children (ie, 3 to 7 years old).[3] The pain is often localized to the medial border of the midfoot (see Fig. 50-1). Swelling in the talonavicular joint and pain with motion (supination/pronation) can help with diagnosis if the child is too young for conclusive x-rays.[3,5]

Background Information

This condition is avascular necrosis of the navicular (see Fig. 50-2).[3] The treatment consists of rest, a walking cast, and medial longitudinal arch supports until healing is complete, which can take up to a full year.[3,5]

■ **Second Metatarsal Head (Freiberg's Infarction)**

Chief Clinical Characteristics

This presentation commonly includes a female adolescent who reports pain on the ball of the foot with increased levels of lower extremity repetitive activities (see Fig. 50-1).[3,5]

Background Information
This is a condition of avascular necrosis of the second metatarsal head (see Fig. 50-2).[3,5,13] Physical examination demonstrates pain and stiffness near the region.[13] X-rays show an enlarged and flattened metatarsal head and decreased joint space.[13] Treatment consists of non–weight-bearing activities, and use of various orthoses to decrease stress in this region.[3,5] If symptoms persist, surgical intervention may be necessary.[13]

■ **Bunions**
Chief Clinical Characteristics
This presentation commonly includes pain or tightness with shoe wear. A bunion is an abnormality involving an increased angle between the first and second metatarsal with the big toe in a valgus position.[5,14]

Background Information
This condition is most commonly seen in young girls who are approximately 9 years old with pressure over the medial aspect of the foot near the first metatarsal head.[14] This condition is commonly found in children with neurological disorders and those with connective tissue disorders.[14] Treatment consists of wider width shoes and then surgery if necessary.[5]

BURSITIS
■ **Retrocalcaneal Bursitis**
Chief Clinical Characteristics
This presentation can involve pain, palpable warmth, tenderness to palpation, and some swelling at the medial and lateral aspects of the Achilles tendon. Pain is reproduced with firm palpation of the tissue anterior to the tendon, as well as with dorsiflexion of the ankle.

Background Information
This condition is the result of inflammation within the bursa that lies between the Achilles tendon and the calcaneus. Predisposing factors include trauma, systemic disease, and biomechanical or structural factors such as prominent posterosuperior calcaneal tuberosity (Haglund's deformity) and rearfoot varus. Clinical examination confirms the diagnosis. Treatment is nonsurgical and typically involves footwear modification.

■ **Subcutaneous Achilles Bursitis**
Chief Clinical Characteristics
This presentation includes local pain, tenderness to palpation, and swelling just posterior to the Achilles tendon insertion at the calcaneal tuberosity. Palpable warmth and observable redness may be present in the same area.

Background Information
Subcutaneous Achilles bursitis is a result of inflammation and swelling of the bursa between the Achilles tendon and the skin. This may occur from mechanical trauma to the tendon or it may be associated with insertional Achilles tendinopathy (tendinitis/tendinosis) or retrocalcaneal bursitis. Continued irritation of the inflamed and swollen bursa may lead to thickening of the bursal walls and fibrosis. Clinical examination confirms the diagnosis. Treatment is nonsurgical, and typically involves footwear modification.

■ **Cellulitis**
Chief Clinical Characteristics
This presentation typically involves warmth, tenderness to palpation, swelling, fever, malaise, and radiation of the symptoms toward the extremities can be seen.[15]

Background Information
This condition is an inflammation of the skin cells. It is usually differentiated from osteomyelitis based on appearance, with this condition demonstrating more swelling and redness.[16] Medical management is needed before treatment with physical therapy.[15] If not treated medically, the inflammation can spread rapidly.[15]

■ **Claw Toes**
Chief Clinical Characteristics
This presentation can be characterized by anatomical deformity and pain in the toes with weight bearing.[13]

Background Information
This condition is a deformity in which the metatarsophalangeal joint is in extension, while the proximal and distal interphalangeal joints are in flexion. It has been associated with some underlying neurological diseases such as hereditary sensory motor disorders or spinal

cord abnormalities.[13] If pain occurs, surgical intervention can be performed to correct the deformity.[13]

■ Compartment Syndrome

Chief Clinical Characteristics
This presentation typically involves decreased, painful dorsiflexion or plantarflexion of the foot and decreased circulation especially with increasing numbness or tingling.[2,17]

Background Information
Injuries that could cause this type of injury include trauma to the foot or lower leg, burns, poisonous agents, or compression from an ill-fitting garment or splint.[2,17] Children taking anticoagulant medication and long-distance runners are more at risk for this condition.[17] These factors can cause a building pressure when local venules collapse and have no place to drain.[17] In turn, increasing pressure leads to tissue ischemia and eventually necrosis.[17] Testing for this symptom includes plantar flexion of the foot and toes for the anterior and lateral aspects of the leg.[17] Congenital abnormalities such as an accessory soleus may also increase the mass effect on the posterior aspect of the ankle, creating ischemia.[18] If this syndrome is suspected, referral to a physician for probable surgical intervention is needed immediately to avoid amputation of the affected limb.[2,17,18]

■ Complex Regional Pain Syndrome (Reflex Sympathetic Dystrophy)

Chief Clinical Characteristics
This presentation usually includes pain that could be initiated from a minor trauma that has been forgotten. Typical symptoms include intense, poorly localized pain that is not relieved with rest, a hypersensitivity to touch, swelling, increased sweating, and changes in color and shininess of the skin.[2-4]

Background Information
If symptoms are recognized early, the least amount of treatment is needed. Mechanical stimulation to the foot, contrast baths, and other advanced medical management techniques are used to help break the pain cycle.[2-4]

■ Congenital Oblique Talus

Chief Clinical Characteristics
This presentation involves ankle and foot pain.

Background Information
This is an abnormality in which the navicular is dislocated dorsally, causing the talus to collapse into an equinus position. It contrasts from congenital vertical talus, however, in that the navicular is reducible on maximum plantarflexion x-rays. X-rays confirm the diagnosis. Surgical intervention involving Achilles tendon lengthening and use of orthoses is the best method of treatment.[19]

■ Congenital Vertical Talus

Chief Clinical Characteristics
This presentation involves ankle and foot pain.

Background Information
This is an abnormality in which the navicular is superiorly dislocated dorsally, causing the talus to collapse into an equinus position. It is important to differentiate this from calcaneovalgus (extreme dorsiflexion of the foot causing the valgus of the calcaneous) because calcaneovalgus responds to treatment more readily. X-rays are needed to differentiate these two conditions. Serial casting is the method of treatment for calcaneal valgus, but surgical intervention is the most common treatment for congenital vertical talus.[5,20]

■ Ehlers-Danlos Syndrome

Chief Clinical Characteristics
This presentation usually includes skin hyperextensibility, fragility of the connective tissue, joint hypermobility, and the increased ability to bruise.[21] On occasion it will present with small papules on the feet and heel that appear only with pressure. These papules will present with pain when they appear during weight-bearing activities.[21]

Background Information
This syndrome is a set of heritable connective tissue disorders. Treatment of ankle and foot consequences consists of decreasing pressure to the region.[21]

■ Fabry's Disease

Chief Clinical Characteristics
This presentation typically involves pain in the extremities, especially with limited movement in extension of the distal interphalangeal joints of the fingers. The other presenting symptoms can include a burning and tingling in the hands

and feet, fever, fatigue, and raised erythrocyte sedimentation rates.[22,23] Crises are induced by stress, temperature changes (especially cold), exercise, alcohol, and hot foods.[22,23]

Background Information
This condition is a genetic disorder involving the accumulation of ceramide trihexose, which is a neutral glycosphingolipid.[22,23] Diagnosis is made based on clinical observations of symptoms of crisis with previously mentioned stressors. In particular, differential diagnosis of Fabry's disease includes rheumatoid arthritis and rheumatic fever. Diagnosis is confirmed through a test of galactosidase A enzyme activity.[22,23] Treatment consists of medication, including diphenylhydantoin.[22,23]

FLAT-FOOT DEFORMITIES
■ Flexible
Chief Clinical Characteristics
This presentation commonly involves a depressed medial longitudinal arch and often has a genetic tendency. The two types of this disorder are flexible flat-foot deformity and flexible flat-foot deformity with short Achilles tendon.[24,25] Many children with this condition have ligamentous laxity, which can cause problems with activity.[24]

Background Information
With the increased ligamentous laxity, the muscles may have to work harder to maintain the stability of the ankle and foot. In this case, over-the-counter orthotics may help to reduce the need for stability.[24,25] The flexible flat-foot deformity with shortened Achilles tendon involves pain, redness, and callus formation under the head of the talus.[24,25] This condition is the same as the deformity without Achilles tendon shortening, but with less than 10 degrees of dorsiflexion with the knee extended. Stretching is the method of treatment with this form of flat feet.[24,25]

■ Rigid
Chief Clinical Characteristics
This presentation includes pain with activities or walking. This occurs with a shortening of the Achilles tendon, which then transfers dorsiflexion during stance phases to the regions of the midfoot, necessitating more pronation.[26] This is seen clinically by toe standing in which the heel elevates, but the subtalar joint does not change shape. The end result is an equinus foot with a flattened medial longitudinal arch and a painful callus beneath the talar head.[25]

Background Information
Common treatment for this condition is calf stretching. Other conditions such as a tarsal coalition, congenital vertical talus, juvenile rheumatoid arthritis, septic arthritis, and intra-articular fracture can also cause a rigid flatfoot.[25,26] If the rigid flatfoot persists, a referral to a surgeon is the appropriate course of treatment.[25,26]

FRACTURES
■ Calcaneal
Chief Clinical Characteristics
This presentation commonly involves foot pain, limping, and limited weight bearing on the affected lower extremity.

Background Information
These types of fractures, which are rare in children, occur in young patients (age 10 years and under) after jumping from a high surface. X-rays may help with diagnosis, with three views including the axial, anteroposterior, and lateral views.[10] A bone scan also may be needed to confirm the diagnosis.[10] Treatment consists of immobilization with non–weight bearing status for a span of 6 weeks.[10,27] In severe cases where the fracture is displaced or comminuted, surgical intervention is necessary.[10]

■ Epiphyseal
Chief Clinical Characteristics
This presentation commonly involves ankle and foot pain with limping.

Background Information
These types of fractures are commonly seen at the ankle in children and are classified by the Salter-Harris classification system (I through V). Type I involves a fracture across the growth plate, but it is not evident on x-ray. These usually occur around the distal fibula. The treatment is a short walking cast for 3 weeks and has an excellent prognosis.[27] Type II fractures occur with the fracture crossing the growth plate and part

of the metaphysis.[27] These are more common on the distal tibia. The treatment is reduction of the fracture, use of a long leg walking cast for 4 weeks and the prognosis is excellent. Type III fractures occur with a fracture crossing the growth plate and the epiphysis.[27] These will require surgical intervention of open reduction and internal fixation, a long leg walking cast with non–weight-bearing status for 4 weeks, then a short leg walking cast for 3 weeks. The prognosis for this fracture is poorer, especially fractures that were displaced. Type IV involves a complete fracture from the metaphysis to the epiphysis. These also will require surgical intervention with open reduction and internal fixation followed by casting for 6 weeks. With good surgical reduction, treatment of these fractures has a good success rate.[27] Type V involves a compression in the growth plate that often is not known about until later with the cessation of bone growth.

■ Pathological

Chief Clinical Characteristics
This presentation commonly involves ankle and foot pain with limping in response to trivial trauma.

Background Information
This condition occurs secondary to weakening of the bone from some other cause. In several disease processes, opportunistic osteomyelitis and/or osteonecrosis may decrease tensile strength in the long bones and cause a fracture.[16,28] Due to impaired healing, sites of bone crisis in Gaucher's disease are also at risk for pathological fractures, more typically in the hip and knee joint area.[28] Children with leukemia and other neoplasms with osteopenia, whether caused by chemotherapy or bone resorption by the tumor itself, are also prone to pathological fractures.[28] For the majority of fractures, the course of treatment is medical management and immobilization until healed.[16,28]

■ Stress

Chief Clinical Characteristics
This presentation typically involves reports of pain, swelling, limping, and/or tenderness usually around the proximal tibia or fifth metatarsal region (see Fig. 50-1).[4,10]

Background Information
This condition can occur with children due to stresses caused by overuse of an immature skeletal formation. Adolescents are most often affected by stress fractures in the foot. Usually a recent increase in activity such as marching in a band or sports participation is the cause of such fractures.[4,10,24] A bone scan or ultrasound can be useful for diagnosis.[3,4,10] Treatment usually consists of rest, casting/bracing with a walking boot for 2 to 3 weeks, and progressive training to resume the activity.[4,10]

■ Talar

Chief Clinical Characteristics
This presentation usually includes pain in the ankle and foot in response to forced dorsiflexion as a mechanism of injury.[27]

Background Information
X-rays confirm the diagnosis. If the fracture is nondisplaced, nonsurgical treatment usually consists of closed reduction in a long leg cast.[27] When there is evidence of healing, progressive weight bearing is resumed.[10,27] Displaced fractures require surgical intervention.[27]

■ Toddler's Fracture of the Tibia

Chief Clinical Characteristics
This presentation involves sudden onset of non–weight bearing, limping, and pain with palpation or percussion to the shaft of the tibia.[3]

Background Information
This is an undisplaced spiral fracture in the midshaft of the tibia with an intact fibula.[3] This condition primarily occurs in young children first learning to walk, hence the name.[3] The mechanism of injury is usually a sudden twisting motion. The child's ability to crawl may differentiate toddler's fracture of the tibia from hip pathology.[3] Follow-up x-rays can show a periosteal callus formation, indicating a previous fracture, to confirm diagnosis.[3] Treatment consists of a short leg walking cast for 3 to 4 weeks until healed.[3]

■ Fungal Disease

Chief Clinical Characteristics

This presentation involves nonspecific signs and symptoms of osteomyelitis or arthritis in children who are already immunodeficient or immunosuppressed due to long-term steroid or antibiotic treatment.[29,30]

Background Information

Different types of fungi create varying levels of concern with a patient. Some fungi remain in the superficial and subcutaneous layers of the skin such as those in "athlete's foot" and dermatophytes.[30] Yet other forms invade the body and spread systemically such as coccidioidomycosis, candidiasis, cryptococcosis, aspergillosis, sporotrichosis, blastomycosis, and actinomycosis.[29,30] Antifungal medications and surgical intervention are the treatment options, requiring a referral to a physician.[29]

■ Gaucher's Disease

Chief Clinical Characteristics

This presentation includes bone pain with or without crisis, enlarged liver and spleen, and bruising. Typical sites include the ribs, pelvis, hip, femur, tibia, and vertebrae.[31] Crisis can lead to severe pain as well as local warmth and tenderness with palpation.[31]

Background Information

This condition is a lipid storage disease in which an enzyme is not active to break down glucocerebroside in the reticuloendothelium.[31] There is a genetic link to those of Jewish descent.[31] Clinical and laboratory findings are very similar to osteomyelitis, but the use of magnetic resonance imaging and nuclear imaging is helping to differentiate the diagnosis.[31] This disease also has a high incidence of pathological fractures.[31] Medical enzyme replacement therapy is the course of treatment with this disease.[31]

■ Gout

Chief Clinical Characteristics

This presentation may include intense pain with weight bearing or palpation, commonly over the first metatarsophalangeal joint, but also may involve the ankle.[32]

Background Information

The pathophysiology, which primarily affects males, is the depositing of monosodium urate crystals in the joints.[32] Other risk factors include obesity, alcohol use, hypertension, renal disease, use of diuretics, and lead exposure. Treatment includes use of nonsteroidal anti-inflammatory or corticosteroid medication.[32]

■ Hallux Rigidus

Chief Clinical Characteristics

This presentation commonly involves pain and stiffness, which are the presenting signs especially in terminal stance in walking and running.[33]

Background Information

This is a disorder in which the first metatarsophalangeal joint becomes self-limiting in dorsiflexion. To differentiate this symptom from a tight flexor hallucis longus, compare the joint mobility with the foot plantarflexed and inverted to dorsiflexed and everted.[34] If the two conditions are the same, there is restriction in the joint. If the range is more with plantarflexion, then the problem is a short flexor hallucis longus muscle.[34] Use of mobilization and manipulation to the joint can help restore proper mechanics to the surrounding musculature to help with symptom relief.[34] Taping may also be a useful modality for treatment during the acute and subacute phases of treatment.[33,34]

■ Hallux Varus

Chief Clinical Characteristics

This presentation includes pain in the first ray, with a soft tissue band with palpation and possible partial or full duplication of the great toe on x-ray.

Background Information

As opposed to a bunion with a laterally deviated great toe, this condition is a fixed deformity in which the great toe is medially deviated.[13] Surgical intervention may be necessary if this condition interferes with shoe wear.[13]

■ Hammer Toes

Chief Clinical Characteristics

This presentation commonly involves toe pain and deformity concurrent with use of shoewear (see Fig. 50-1).[13]

Background Information

Hammer toe is a deformity of the metatarsophalangeal joint in extension, with the proximal interphalangeal joint plantar flexed, and the distal interphalangeal joint either normal or extended.[13] This is not very common in children. Unlike claw toes, this deformity is not usually caused from an underlying neurological disorder. Pain from pressure or shear stresses at the toe rubbing on the underside of the shoe is usually the only symptom. In these cases, surgical intervention is needed to fix the deformity.[13]

■ Hand-Foot-Mouth Disease

Chief Clinical Characteristics

This presentation is characterized by small vesicular lesions of the mouth as well as the hands and feet. The vesicles in the mouth are usually between 2 and 8 mm in size and 5 to 10 in number.[35] Other signs and symptoms may include sore throat, malaise, and fever, which usually are present 24 to 48 hours previously to the ulcers and are usually completed in 2 to 3 weeks.[35]

Background Information

This condition is a viral disease that is medically monitored.[35]

■ Heel Spurs

Chief Clinical Characteristics

This presentation typically involves pain around the calcaneous. In many instances, these spurs are asymptomatic.

Background Information

If the direction of the spur is in a downward direction, there may be some local impingement into soft tissues that causes pain. In many other instances, the pain may be a result of mechanical deformation of the plantar fascia.[11] Treatment consists of orthotic devices, steroid injections, and nonsteroidal anti-inflammatory medications. If these measures do not bring relief, surgical intervention may be pursued.[11]

■ Hemophilia

Chief Clinical Characteristics

This presentation includes a painful, warm, swollen joint.

Background Information

This is a sex-linked blood disorder that affects the body's ability to clot blood effectively. This affects mainly males. The most commonly affected joints are the knee, ankle, and elbow.[28] In younger children, the ankle is more involved due to more jumping. Treatment consists of splinting, range-of-motion exercises, monitoring of joint swelling due to influx of blood into the joint, nonsteroidal anti-inflammatory medications, and transfusions when needed to increase clotting factors.[28] If a muscle hemorrhage occurs with associated compartment syndrome, clotting factor is first added and then the appropriate surgical procedure is performed. Surgery may be needed during the course of the disease to address contractures at the ankle and knee.[28]

■ Ill-Fitting Shoes

Chief Clinical Characteristics

This presentation typically includes abnormal redness or reports of pain/pressure along the toes or either side of the foot.

Background Information

Such wear can cause related conditions, such as ingrown toenails and pressure sores to the sides or bottoms of the feet.[24] Treatment consists of obtaining properly fitting shoes.

■ Ingrown Toenails

Chief Clinical Characteristics

This presentation involves toe pain, most typically of the great toe (see Fig. 50-1).

Background Information

This condition is one in which the nail grows medially or laterally into the nearby soft tissue, causing inflammation and pain. The most common cause of this condition is improper nail trimming or shoes that are improperly fit, causing increased stresses to the soft tissues.[24,33,36] The most common age group for this condition is teenagers.[24] Children suspected of having this condition need further evaluation by a physician in these cases for warm water soaks, antibiotic treatment, or nail removal.[24,33,36]

■ Joint Sepsis

Chief Clinical Characteristics

This presentation commonly includes pain, increased temperature, tenderness to palpation, restriction of motion at the joint, and increased erythrocyte sedimentation rate.[26]

Background Information

Formal diagnosis is made by the use of aspiration of the joint.[26] Surgical intervention is the treatment.[26]

■ Juvenile Rheumatoid Arthritis

Chief Clinical Characteristics

This presentation includes a gradual increase in pain; joint stiffness (especially in the morning or after period of inactivity); swelling, heat, and diffuse tenderness to palpation, which remain for greater than 6 weeks; postural abnormalities; and gait deviations, including a decreased stride length and "stiff-legged" pattern leading to decreased velocity and cadence.[10,37,38] A high spiking fever, sore throat, stiff neck, and accompanying rash on the trunk and extremities that follows a daily pattern can also help with diagnosis of the systemic form of the disease.[38]

Background Information

This condition is a very common rheumatic disease in childhood, with three forms that include pauciarticular, polyarticular, and systemic. The pauciarticular type, in which four or fewer joints are involved, is the most common form and has a predominance in females 1 to 4 years of age. This form usually affects the knees, ankles, and wrists.[37] The polyarticular type, in which five or more joints are involved, also has a predominance in females, but with peaks in 1- to 4-year-olds and adolescents. This version tends to be symmetrical in nature, affecting the knees, ankles, wrist, spinal regions, and temporomandibular joints.[37] Systemic variation is equal in predominance and is diagnosed more with the symptoms of rash, high spiking fever at night, and other infections such as pericarditis and pleuritis.[37,38] Typical involvement at the foot and ankle include loss of subtalar and first metatarsophalangeal joint motion, overpronation, and possible hammertoe position.[37] Medical treatment consists of oral medications for decreasing inflammation and other features of the disease, injections of steroids to target individual joints, and possible surgical interventions to decrease contractures.[37] Physical therapy treatment may include strengthening and range-of-motion activities (often in an aquatic environment or limited weight-bearing manner), modalities such as heat to help decrease stiffness, gait training, and instruction on energy conservation.[37] Bracing/splinting techniques are also used to improve/maintain range of motion and help with walking.[10]

LIGAMENT SPRAINS

■ Anterior Talofibular Ligament

Chief Clinical Characteristics

This presentation involves lateral ankle pain following a mechanism of injury into plantarflexion and inversion.

Background Information

This condition involves the most frequently affected ligament. Physical examination using percussion to the bone 15 to 20 mm proximal to the tip of the fibula may differentiate this sprain from a fracture. If this percussion replicates the pain, the diagnosis is more indicative of a fracture.[39] X-ray examination also may be indicated to rule out a fracture. A common test for the integrity of this ligament is the anterior drawer test.[40] If acute, the child will need rest, ice, compression, elevation, and gait training with assistive devices. Strengthening and proprioceptive exercises with and without bracing can also help the child regain overall stability to the ankle region.[40] Final rehabilitation includes return to sports activities if the child is an athlete to prevent similar injuries in the future.[40]

■ Calcaneofibular Ligament

Chief Clinical Characteristics

This presentation involves lateral ankle pain following a mechanism of injury into plantarflexion and inversion, resulting in consensual injury with the anterior talofibular ligament.[40] Less commonly, this condition may result from inversion with the foot in a plantigrade position.

Background Information

The common test for the integrity of this ligament is the talar tilt test. If this test reveals excessive mobility compared to the unaffected ankle, the test is positive.[40] Treatment includes rest, ice, compression, elevation, progressive range-of-motion and strengthening exercises, and progression to simulation of regular activities.[40]

■ Metatarsophalangeal Joint (Turf Toe)

Chief Clinical Characteristics
This presentation typically includes tenderness to the joint, swelling, limited range of motion at joint, and limping during gait.

Background Information
A mechanism of injury of excessive forced dorsiflexion of the metatarsophalangeal joint is indicative of the diagnosis.[41] Initial treatment consists of rest, ice, compression, and elevation. After symptoms have lessened, gentle range-of-motion exercises, orthotics that limit dorsiflexion, and slow progression back to activity are the courses of action.[41]

■ Muscle Strain

Chief Clinical Characteristics
This presentation involves pain, swelling, and decreased strength in the affected muscle group.

Background Information
A variety of muscle strains can occur in the young athlete. Most of the injuries in the ankle/foot region occur to the calf or the tibialis anterior/posterior musculature. Pain, with resistance of the injured muscle group, or spasms can indicate a muscle strain. Treatment of an acute injury consists of using ice and nonsteroidal anti-inflammatory medications to reduce pain and inflammation. Activity modification, stretching, use of various modalities (ultrasound, electrical stimulation, heat, ice, soft tissue mobilization depending on age and site of injury), and use of medical intervention (anti-inflammatories or muscle relaxers) are used for treatment in the subacute phase of the injury. Progressive strengthening and return to sports/activity specific training (usually including open and closed chain exercises) are the final phases of rehabilitation.

■ Myositis Ossificans

Chief Clinical Characteristics
This presentation is characterized by a self-limiting decrease in motion in the region of the affected musculature.[42] Physical examination may include an unexplained mass. These lesions generally tend to form after a blunt trauma to the area in question.[42]

Background Information
Serial X-rays and computed tomography can help determine diagnosis. Mineralization is more dense peripherally in myositis ossificans, which differentiates this from osteosarcoma, which is the opposite formation.[42] Traditional treatment in the adult is immobilization of the area for 2 to 4 weeks then return to active range-of-motion and strengthening exercises, but movement of the affected region is self-limited by children requiring no immobilization.[42] Surgery may be needed in extreme cases.[42]

■ Necrotizing Fasciitis

Chief Clinical Characteristics
This presentation consists of symptoms and signs consistent with an aggressive infection that destroys the superficial fascia, with pain that is out of proportion for the injury as the most common symptom.[17] It can occur with even the most common skin wound.[17]

Background Information
Treatment is mostly medical, but the therapist may be utilized to help with debridement and wound care activities.[17]

NERVE ENTRAPMENTS

■ Common Peroneal Nerve Entrapment

Chief Clinical Characteristics
This presentation of a nerve entrapment near the neck of the fibula commonly involves weakness or eventually drop foot.[43]

Background Information
The cause of this entrapment can be blunt trauma to the area, or a variety of external and internal stresses located at the ankle with weight bearing.[43] Due to the peripheral location of the nerve, it is readily subject to injury.[43] A key to diagnosing this injury is the persistent pain or tingling after an inversion ankle sprain.[43] Consequently, many children with this type of nerve entrapment have weak ankle musculature and have a drop foot requiring surgical decompression of the area as the best means of treatment.[43]

■ Lateral Plantar Nerve

Chief Clinical Characteristics

This presentation usually involves palpation tenderness at the first branch of the lateral plantar nerve deep to the abductor hallucis on the medial aspect of the calcaneous. Typical symptoms in this entrapment often mimic overuse injury to the ankle.[44]

Background Information

Treatment consists of rest, nonsteroidal anti-inflammatory medication, taping or orthotics for overpronation, and use of iontophoresis. If necessary, a steroid injection or surgery will need to be performed.[44]

■ Tarsal Tunnel Syndrome

Chief Clinical Characteristics

This presentation may be characterized by burning pain on the bottom of the foot that increases with activity, a positive Tinel's sign (tapping the area of the posterior tibial nerve), and confirmation with electromyographic studies.[45]

Background Information

Tumors, an accessory flexor digitorum muscle, as well as os trigonum may contribute to the mass effect near the tarsal tunnel increasing pressure in these locations. Often excision of a space-occupying component can relieve symptoms.

■ Osteochondritis Dissecans of the Talus

Chief Clinical Characteristics

This presentation involves a painful, swollen ankle and a limp with walking.[2]

Background Information

The lesion can be confirmed on x-ray, usually appearing on the medial edge of the dome of the talus.[10] Treatment consists of casting for 6 to 12 weeks with serial x-rays to confirm healing. Surgical intervention may be needed if healing does not occur.[3,5]

■ Osteomyelitis

Chief Clinical Characteristics

This presentation involves fever, pain, general malaise, swelling in the hindfoot, and difficulty with walking.[10] Typical areas affected are the heel and the distal tibial epiphysis (see Fig. 50-1).[10,46]

Background Information

This condition is an infection of the bone. In infants, heel pricks for blood sampling are a common cause.[46,47] Puncture wounds from foreign objects are a more common reason in older children.[46] These puncture wounds, especially in rubber soled shoes, can quickly lead to infection from pseudomonas that can live in the shoe.[13] If suspected, medical referral is needed immediately due to the destructive nature of the infection. Treatment consists of antibiotics and possible surgical intervention.[16]

■ Peripheral Arterial Disease

Chief Clinical Characteristics

This presentation involves symptoms of intermittent claudication to the calf or buttock and thigh and/or decreased circulation to the foot.[48]

Background Information

This is a rare phenomenon in children, thus other causes such as muscle strain, arthritis, or back pain are more commonly diagnosed. The cause of this disease could be multifactorial including hyperlipidemia, family history, diabetes, smoking history, hypertension, or entrapments such as at the popliteal artery.[48] Palpation, listening to the pulses, and performing ankle/brachial index via Doppler scanning before and after exercise can help with the diagnosis. Neglected forms of this condition may lead to foot ulcers that can develop due to lack of blood flow to the area. If suspected as a diagnosis, the child needs referral to a physician for further testing.[48]

■ Peroneal Tendon Subluxation

Chief Clinical Characteristics

This presentation typically involves persistent pain, tenderness with palpation to the peroneals near the malleolus, and palpable mass with various positioning of the foot.[49]

Background Information

The mode of injury is typically a sudden dorsiflexion with eversion due to contraction of the peroneals.[49] Manual muscle testing of the peroneal tendons will usually elicit pain or the subluxation.[49] Nonsurgical management can be attempted, but surgical intervention is necessary if unsuccessful.[49]

■ Plantar Fasciitis

Chief Clinical Characteristics
This presentation involves a painful heel, tight calf musculature, plantarflexed first ray, and increased pain with first step or weight bearing in the morning (see Fig. 50-1).[33]

Background Information
This condition is caused by an inflammation of the plantar fascia. Children with this condition should not have any positive neurological signs that would differentiate it from a projected pain, such as a tarsal tunnel syndrome.[33] Use of modalities (eg, ice, ultrasound, iontophoresis), stretching and soft tissue mobilization of the calf and plantar fascia, orthotic intervention, and on occasion an injection of a steroid are utilized to treat the condition.[33]

■ Polydactyly

Chief Clinical Characteristics
This presentation involves an increase in the number of digits in the foot causing tightness or pain with shoe wear.

Background Information
The major problem with this condition is foot width, making appropriate shoes harder to find. Surgical removal can be performed on the extra digit to alleviate this problem.[20]

■ Puncture Wounds

Chief Clinical Characteristics
This presentation may involve pain, redness, and swelling in the surrounding area of the puncture. Children with this condition may exhibit limited weight bearing secondary to the pain.[46]

Background Information
Infections caused by pseudomonas may occur quite readily when wearing rubber-soled shoes (eg, tennis shoes, running shoes), very typical footwear for this population.[36] Consequently, if a child has a puncture wound it should be treated with added concern with referral to a physician to rule out osteomyelitis, cellulitis, tetanus, and other inflammatory conditions.[36] The course of treatment involves removal of the foreign body and surgical debridement of the surrounding tissues.[36]

■ Retrocalcaneal Bursitis

Chief Clinical Characteristics
This presentation involves pain in the posterior aspect of the heel/ankle. Often pain symptoms reduce if pressure is relieved such as when walking without shoes.[10]

Background Information
This condition is an inflammation of the bursa posterior to the calcaneus, which is common with sports-related activities. Treatment consists of rest and use of modalities as needed to decrease inflammation.[10]

■ Rheumatic Fever

Chief Clinical Characteristics
This presentation includes ankle and foot joint pain, but can have associated swelling, warmth, and tenderness to palpation, which migrates asymmetrically throughout the body as the process unfolds.[15,50]

Background Information
The most common age group is 5 to 15 years of age.[50] This is an inflammatory disease that affects many systems in the body. It is differentiated from leukemia in that it responds to anti-inflammatories and rest.[15,50] Treatment is either aspirin or nonsteroidal anti-inflammatory medication.[50]

■ Seronegative Spondyloarthropathies

Chief Clinical Characteristics
This presentation most commonly includes hip or foot pain in boys.[38,47] *If more systemic symptoms begin to emerge, refer to physician for further medical workup. These systemic pains include associated fatigue, fever, back pain, acute iritis, urethritis, oral lesions, conjunctivitis, and/or psoriasis.*[11]

Background Information
This group of diagnoses includes ankylosing spondylitis, psoriatic arthritis, inflammatory bowel disease, and Behçet's syndrome.[38,47] After positive identification of the cause, treatment consists of medical management of steroid injections and/or nonsteroidal anti-inflammatory medications for symptom relief.[38,47] Other treatments, including activity modification, orthotics, and stretching of the heel cord to decrease stress and strain

on the affected region, can be utilized as well.[10]

■ Sickle Cell Anemia

Chief Clinical Characteristics

This presentation involves episodic pain, swelling in the hands and feet, and fever. These symptoms can be initiated by cold weather or other situations associated with decreased oxygen use, such as a tourniquet. Symptoms in a crisis usually average about 14 days.[15,51]

Background Information

This disease affects primarily children of African descent in which the hemoglobin structure is altered. Decreased oxygen causes deformation of the red blood cells (into a crescentic shape, hence sickle cell disease) resulting in ischemia due to increased clotting of the deformed cells.[15,51] Medical lab testing is needed to confirm diagnosis. Treatment is medical in nature with steroids. Current experimental treatment involves bone marrow transplantation.[28]

TARSAL COALITIONS

■ Calcaneonavicular Coalition

Chief Clinical Characteristics

This presentation includes painful, flat feet with a significant reduction in subtalar joint motion. The symptoms are more localized to the region of interest in the calcaneonavicular coalition (see Fig. 50-1).[2,20]

Background Information

This is an abnormal failure of segmentation of two or three of the tarsal bones in adolescents.[2,10,20] There is a greater male-to-female ratio for this condition.[2,10,20] The most common tarsal coalition is the calcaneonavicular, usually seen in 8- to 12-year-olds.[2,10,20] X-ray examination (oblique views) and/or computed tomography may be necessary to see the appropriate union.[3,10,20] Surgical intervention is the best option for treatment for both of these conditions.[10,20]

■ Talocalcaneal Coalition

Chief Clinical Characteristics

This presentation includes painful, flat feet with a significant reduction in subtalar joint motion. The talocalcaneal version usually involves poorly localized pain in the hindfoot

(see Fig. 50-1).[2] The characteristic physical finding is sharp pain when the patient's foot is quickly inverted.[2]

Background Information

This is an abnormal failure of segmentation of two or three of the tarsal bones in adolescents.[2,10,20] There is a greater male-to-female ratio for this condition.[2,10,20] This condition commonly causes pain on inversion and leads to calcaneovalgus (peroneal spastic flat foot).[3,10,20] It is typical of 10- to 14-year-olds.[2] X-ray examination (oblique views) and/or computed tomography may be necessary to see the appropriate union.[3,10,20]

TENDINITIS

■ Achilles Tendinitis

Chief Clinical Characteristics

This presentation involves pain and tenderness to palpation near the insertion of the Achilles tendon into the calcaneous (see Fig. 50-1).[10]

Background Information

This is one of the most common overuse injuries. Due to its role of eccentrically controlling the heel lowering during jumping activities, the tendon can be damaged. This overuse in combination with decreased vascular compromise in this region leads to the injury. Chronic problems in this region could lead to degeneration and possible rupture later in life. The first course of treatment is to decrease inflammation with ice, rest, and/or use of orthotic inserts.[10] Range-of-motion and progressive eccentric strengthening exercises are the next stage of treatment.[10] The last stage of treatment is increasing the speed of activities, especially in sport-specific training. The child should be progressed cautiously before returning to sport due to the high risk of reinjury.

■ Flexor Hallucis Longus Tenosynovitis

Chief Clinical Characteristics

This presentation typically includes pain, tenderness, and swelling in the posterior portion of the ankle along the path of the tendon. This tenosynovitis is particularly common in dancers due to the majority of the time spent in extreme amounts of plantarflexion.[7]

Background Information
Common methods of testing include palpating the tendon with associated tenderness when moving the big toe. If symptoms mimic the pain with dancing, the diagnosis is made.[7] Nonsurgical methods—including modalities, taping, strengthening, and task analysis to improve the dancer's techniques—are typically utilized before surgical intervention.[7] If symptoms persist, referral to a physician for possible surgical intervention should be made.[7]

■ **Tibialis Posterior Tendinitis**

Chief Clinical Characteristics
This presentation commonly involves heel pain with weight bearing, especially with increased loading. Physical examination will reveal a swollen or tender posterior tibialis tendon area, a rearfoot that is neutral or slightly everted with a collapsed medial arch, and a single heel rise lack(s) calcaneal inversion.[52]

Background Information
During the gait cycle, children with this condition will lack an effective terminal stance and will overpronate throughout the stance phases of gait. Stretching tight myofascia, use of modalities, and orthotic intervention are warranted with treatment.[52] Later, active strengthening and muscular control activities may be utilized to restore the proper biomechanics for gait and other running activities.[52]

■ **Thalassemia (Familial Mediterranean Fever)**

Chief Clinical Characteristics
This presentation may involve symptoms of anemia, growth and developmental delays, and hepatosplenomegaly.[28] *In adolescence, physical examination can show evidence of scoliosis, and reports of arthralgias and low back pain are common.*[28]

Background Information
This is a multisystem genetic disorder of Mediterranean descent that affects multiple joints, as well as the chest wall and abdomen, and lasts 1 to 3 days.[28,53] Due to the symptoms,

infants who are not treated very early in life have a high mortality rate before the age of 5 years.[28] Due to the high level of skeletal involvement and associated osteoporosis, adolescents with this disease are at great risk for pathological fractures.[28] Treatment is medical including transfusions, chelation therapy, and bone marrow transplantation.[28,53]

■ **Trevor's Disease (Dysplasia Epiphysealis Hemimelica)**

Chief Clinical Characteristics
This presentation includes painless swelling and localized deformity with restricted motion.

Background Information
This is a condition of unusual overgrowth of one or more of the ossification centers at a joint.[54] It usually affects males. Usual sites in the foot and ankle are the talus and the distal tibia.[54] Typical treatment is surgery to limit the amount of deformity.[54]

■ **Tuberculosis**

Chief Clinical Characteristics
This presentation usually consists of pain as the only presenting symptom at the ankle and foot, but can be accompanied by low-grade fever, weight loss, or general malaise suggestive of the underlying systemic infection.[47]

Background Information
This is a condition in which signs and symptoms are not usually present years after initial infection. Immunosuppression due to anti-cancer medications, steroids, or acquired immunodeficiency syndrome can be an important precursor. The most common location in the skeletal system is the spine, followed by the long bones and joints including the talus and the distal fibula in children. An urgent referral to a physician is necessary for anyone who is suspected of having this diagnosis.[47]

TUMORS
■ **Calcaneal Cysts**

Chief Clinical Characteristics
This presentation is usually asymptomatic and located in the anterior/lateral aspect of the calcaneous.[10] *If there is microscopic*

damage to the cyst's cell wall, pain may occur in the region.[10]

Background Information
Treatment is usually nonsurgical with use of splinting and activity modification.[10]

■ **Ewing's Sarcoma**

Chief Clinical Characteristics
This presentation involves pain at night or with rest, and possible fever.

Background Information
The patient may have elevated erythrocyte sedimentation rates. Typical sites of this tumor are the long bones of the lower extremities and the pelvis.[50] Typical age for this type of tumor is 5 to 25 years old. Medical intervention involving chemotherapy, radiation, and limb salvage surgeries may be necessary.[55]

■ **Ganglion Cyst**

Chief Clinical Characteristics
This presentation commonly includes constant pain that increases with movement of the joint.

Background Information
This is a cystic tumor filled with a gel-like material that is adjacent to a joint or tendon. It may present in the ankle but more commonly in the subtalar joint in the sinus-tarsi. Many times cysts will disappear, but surgical removal maybe necessary.[56]

■ **Giant Cell Tumor of the Tendon Sheath**

Chief Clinical Characteristics
This presentation usually involves a long slow increase in painless swelling or slight pain with weight bearing or walking.[57]

Background Information
This condition is a tumor that develops out of the surrounding tendon sheath of the long tendons of the feet and hands. Surgical removal of the tumor is the best method of treatment.[57]

■ **Glomangioma**

Chief Clinical Characteristics
This presentation typically includes pain, tenderness to palpation, and a hallmark sign of difficulty with temperature changes.[58]

Background Information
A glomangioma is a type of benign tumor than consists of anastomoses containing unmyelinated neural cells.[58] These typically are found in the distal extremities. Many times these tumors mimic a musculoskeletal injury such as an injury to a long tendon. A bluish object may be seen underneath the nail as well.[58] Magnetic resonance imaging or computed tomography may be needed for further evaluation. Surgical excision of the tumor is the treatment of choice.[58]

■ **Leukemia**

Chief Clinical Characteristics
This presentation typically includes diffuse, nonspecific bone pain with fever and elevated white blood cell and sedimentation rates. Lesions to the mouth are also often seen later.[50]

Background Information
This condition is a cancer of the white blood cells and is the most common form of childhood cancer.[28] Changes on x-ray may show focal lesions of bone resorption seen in the long bones of the body. Occasionally, children with this condition can have pathological fractures associated with osteopenia/osteoporosis of the bones.[28] Treatment consists of the primary interventions of chemotherapy, radiation, and bone marrow transplants.

■ **Osteoblastoma**

Chief Clinical Characteristics
This presentation usually is characterized by pain in the ankle and foot region.

Background Information
These are rare tumors that usually are located in the foot and ankle.[59] This condition is very similar to osteoid osteoma upon histology reports, but the tumors are bigger in diameter and have the potential to turn malignant. These tumors also differ from osteoid osteoma in that night pain and relief from nonsteroidal anti-inflammatory medication is unpredictable.[59] These malignancies have the possibility to turn malignant in nature in rare cases.[59] Treatment consists of surgical removal of the tumor.[59]

ANKLE AND FOOT PAIN IN A CHILD

■ Osteochondroma

Chief Clinical Characteristics

This presentation can involve pain or a painless mass, but it may also exhibit a volume effect by compressing nerves and other vessels in the region.[60]

Background Information

This is the most common tumor in the skeletal system, usually affecting those in the first decades of life. The most common sites for this tumor in the lower extremity are the distal femur and proximal tibia, but tumors can occur in the bones of the foot.[60] It has a slightly greater prevalence in boys. The usual treatment is resection of the mass.[60]

■ Osteoid Osteoma

Chief Clinical Characteristics

This presentation involves localized night pain in the tarsal and foot bones with great relief from aspirin products.[3,10]

Background Information

This is a small benign bone tumor. The majority of these tumors are seen in the femur and the tibia, but there are some reported cases in the bones of the feet.[2] It can either be managed with nonsteroidal anti-inflammatory medications or surgical removal.[10]

■ Osteosarcoma

Chief Clinical Characteristics

This presentation typically includes pain, especially at night, and swelling.[61]

Background Information

This condition is the second most common malignant bone tumor, usually in the tarsal region of the foot if occurring in the ankle/foot in children 15 to 20 years of age.[61] Magnetic resonance imaging and computed tomography can be used to outline the extent of the tumor.[62] Treatment consists of chemotherapy and limb salvage surgeries.[55]

■ Rhabdomyosarcoma

Chief Clinical Characteristics

This presentation commonly involves a noticeable lump in muscle tissue.

Background Information

Histology is needed to confirm the diagnosis. This is the most common malignant soft tissue sarcoma in children. This is an aggressive tumor, so if suspected, referral to the appropriate physician is required.[56]

■ Synovial Sarcoma

Chief Clinical Characteristics

This presentation commonly occurs in the soft tissue of the mid and hindfoot and presents with pain, tenderness to palpation, swelling, and an enlarging mass.[2,63]

Background Information

Histology reports can confirm the diagnosis, with surgical removal as the treatment of choice.[2,63]

References

1. Schwarz T, Schellong SM, Neumann U, Traut H, Daniel WG. Popliteal entrapment syndrome: noninvasive diagnosis and complete recovery after surgery in an 11-year-old boy. *Pediatr Radiol.* Feb 1999;29(2):109–111.
2. Drennan JC. Foot pain. In: Staheli LT, ed. *Pediatric Orthopedic Secrets.* 2nd ed. Philadelphia, PA: Hanley & Belfus; 2002.
3. Wilkins KE. The painful foot in the child. *Instr Course Lect.* 1988;37:77–85.
4. Pattinson R, Bates E. Painful feet in childhood. *Aust Fam Physician.* Jun 1996;25(6):887–889; 892–883.
5. Trott AW. Children's foot problems. *Orthop Clin North Am.* Jul 1982;13(3):641–654.
6. Tol JL, Verhagen RA, Krips R, et al. The anterior ankle impingement syndrome: diagnostic value of oblique radiographs. *Foot Ankle Int.* Feb 2004;25(2):63–68.
7. Hamilton WG, Geppert MJ, Thompson FM. Pain in the posterior aspect of the ankle in dancers. Differential diagnosis and operative treatment. *J Bone Joint Surg Am.* Oct 1996;78(10):1491–1500.
8. Johnson RP, Collier BD, Carrera GF. The os trigonum syndrome: use of bone scan in the diagnosis. *J Trauma.* Aug 1984;24(8):761–764.
9. Jones DM, Saltzman CL, El-Khoury G. The diagnosis of the os trigonum syndrome with a fluoroscopically controlled injection of local anesthetic. *Iowa Orthop J.* 1999;19:122–126.
10. Kim CW, Shea K, Chambers HG. Heel pain in children. Diagnosis and treatment. *J Am Podiatr Med Assoc.* Feb 1999;89(2):67–74.
11. Scherer PR. Heel spur syndrome. Pathomechanics and nonsurgical treatment. Biomechanics Graduate Research Group for 1988. *J Am Podiatr Med Assoc.* Feb 1991; 81(2):68–72.
12. Canale ST, Williams KD. Iselin's disease. *J Pediatr Orthop.* Jan 1992;12(1):90–93.
13. Meehan AP. Toe deformities. In: Staheli LT, ed. *Pediatric Orthopedic Secrets.* 2nd ed. Philadelphia, PA: Hanley & Belfus; 2002.
14. Peterson H. Bunions. In: Staheli LT, ed. *Pediatric Orthopedic Secrets.* 2nd ed. Philadelphia, PA: Hanley & Belfus; 2002.
15. Gibson S, Kalinyak K. Pediatric management problems (hand-foot syndrome of sickle cell disease). *Pediatr Nurs.* Nov–Dec 1987;13(6):418–419.

16. Greene WB. Osteomyelitis. In: Staheli LT, ed. *Pediatric Orthopedic Secrets.* 2nd ed. Philadelphia, PA: Hanley & Belfus; 2002.

17. Johnson DE. When pain is out of proportion. *Emerg Med Serv.* Sep 2003;32(9):115–119.

18. Palaniappan M, Rajesh A, Rickett A, Kershaw CJ. Accessory soleus muscle: a case report and review of the literature. *Pediatr Radiol.* Aug 1999;29(8):610–612.

19. Katz MA, Davidson RS, Chan SH, Sullivan RJ. Plain radiographic evaluation of the pediatric foot and its deformities. *Univ Pennsylvania Orthoped J.* 2007;10:30–39.

20. Caselli MA, Sobel E, McHale KA. Pedal manifestations of musculoskeletal disease in children. *Clin Podiatr Med Surg.* Jul 1998;15(3):481–497, vi.

21. Kahana M, Levy A, Ronnen M, Cohen M, Schewach-Millet M. Painful piezogenic pedal papules on a child with Ehlers-Danlos syndrome. *Pediatr Dermatol.* Nov 1985;3(1):45–47.

22. Hilz MJ, Stemper B, Kolodny EH. Lower limb cold exposure induces pain and prolonged small fiber dysfunction in Fabry patients. *Pain.* Feb 2000;84(2–3):361–365.

23. Paira SO, Roverano S, Iribas JL, Barcelo HA. Joint manifestations of Fabry's disease. *Clin Rheumatol.* Dec 1992;11(4):562–565.

24. Gross RH. Foot pain in children. *Pediatr Clin North Am.* Dec 1986;33(6):1395–1409.

25. Mosca WS. Flatfoot. In: Staheli LT, ed. *Pediatric Orthopedic Secrets.* 2nd ed. Philadelphia, PA: Hanley & Belfus; 2002.

26. Luhmann SJ, Schoenecke PL. Septic arthritis. In: Staheli LT, ed. *Pediatric Orthopedic Secrets.* 2nd ed. Philadelphia, PA: Hanley & Belfus; 2002.

27. Sullivan A. Foot and ankle trauma in children. In: Staheli LT, ed. *Pediatric Orthopedic Secrets.* 2nd ed. Philadelphia, PA: Hanley & Belfus; 2002.

28. Keret D, Weintroub S. Hematologic disorders. In: Staheli LT, ed. *Pediatric Orthopedic Secrets.* 2nd ed. Philadelphia, PA: Hanley & Belfus; 2002.

29. Cheng Y, McNally DJ, Labbe C, Voyer N, Belzile F, Belanger RR. Insertional mutagenesis of a fungal biocontrol agent led to discovery of a rare cellobiose lipid with antifungal activity. *Appl Environ Microbiol.* May 2003;69(5):2595–2602.

30. Samuelson J. Infectious disease. In: Cotran RS, Kumar V, Collins T, eds. *Robbins Pathologic Basis of Disease.* 6th ed. Philadelphia, PA: W. B. Saunders; 1999.

31. Katz K, Kornreich L, Horev G, Ziv N, Soudry M, Cohen IJ. Involvement of the foot and ankle in patients with Gaucher disease. *Foot Ankle Int.* Feb 1999;20(2):104–107.

32. Mair SD, Coogan AC, Speer KP, Hall RL. Gout as a source of sesamoid pain. *Foot Ankle Int.* Oct 1995; 16(10):613–616.

33. Duckworth T. Painful conditions of the ankle and foot. *Practitioner.* Feb 1985;229(1400):153–154, 156, 158, passim.

34. Cibulka MT. Management of a patient with forefoot pain: a case report. *Phys Ther.* Jan 1990;70(1):41–44.

35. McKinney RV. Hand, foot, and mouth disease: a viral disease of importance to dentists. *J Am Dent Assoc.* Jul 1975;91(1):122–127.

36. Meehan AP. Nail puncture. In: Staheli LT, ed. *Pediatric Orthopedic Secrets.* 2nd ed. Philadelphia, PA: Hanley & Belfus; 2002.

37. Scull SA. Juvenile rheumatoid arthritis. In: Vander Lindin DW, Campbell SK, eds. *Physical Therapy for Children.* 2nd ed. Philadelphia, PA: W. B. Saunders; 2000.

38. Sherry D. Arthritis. In: Staheli LT, ed. *Pediatric Orthopedic Secrets.* 2nd ed. Philadelphia, PA: Hanley & Belfus; 2002.

39. Busch MT. Youth sports and related injuries. In: Staheli LT, ed. *Pediatric Orthopedic Secrets.* 2nd ed. Philadelphia, PA: Hanley & Belfus; 2002.

40. Anderson SJ. Soccer: a case-based approach to ankle and knee injuries. *Pediatr Ann.* Mar 2000;29(3):178–188.

41. Casillas MM, Jacobs, M. First metatarsophalangeal joint sprain (turf toe). In: Brontzman SB, Wilk KE, eds. *Clinical Orthopaedic Rehabilitation.* 2nd ed. Philadelphia, PA: Mosby; 2003.

42. Futani H, Itohara S, Maruo S, Tateishi H. A report on 2 cases of myositis ossificans in childhood. *Acta Orthop Scand.* Dec 1998;69(6):642–645.

43. Sidey JD. Weak ankles. A study of common peroneal entrapment neuropathy. *Br Med J.* Sep 13 1969; 3(5671):623–626.

44. Fredericson M, Standage S, Chou L, Matheson G. Lateral plantar nerve entrapment in a competitive gymnast. *Clin J Sport Med.* Apr 2001;11(2):111–114.

45. Cheung YY, Rosenberg ZS, Colon E, Jahss M. MR imaging of flexor digitorum accessorius longus. *Skeletal Radiol.* Mar 1999;28(3):130–137.

46. Rasool MN. Hematogenous osteomyelitis of the calcaneus in children. *J Pediatr Orthop.* Nov–Dec 2001; 21(6):738–743.

47. Kosinski M, Lilja E. Infectious causes of heel pain. *J Am Podiatr Med Assoc.* Jan 1999;89(1):20–23.

48. Hallett JW Jr, Greenwood LH, Robison JG. Lower extremity arterial disease in young adults. A systematic approach to early diagnosis. *Ann Surg.* Nov 1985;202(5): 647–652.

49. Forman ES, Micheli LJ, Backe LM. Chronic recurrent subluxation of the peroneal tendons in a pediatric patient. Surgical recommendations. *Foot Ankle Int.* Jan 2000;21(1):51–53.

50. Kling T. The sick child. In: Staheli LT, ed. *Pediatric Orthopedic Secrets.* 2nd ed. Philadelphia, PA: Hanley & Belfus; 2002.

51. Vanin E, Marcazzo L, Martini G, Mescoli G, Zulian F. Painful hand and foot swelling in a 6-month-old girl. *Eur J Pediatr.* Jan 2003;162(1):47–48.

52. Patla CE, Abbott JH. Tibialis posterior myofascial tightness as a source of heel pain: diagnosis and treatment. *J Orthop Sports Phys Ther.* Oct 2000;30(10):624–632.

53. Kubik NJ 3rd, Katz JD. Familial Mediterranean fever. *Am J Orthop.* Jul 2000;29(7):553–555.

54. Oates E, Cutler JB, Miyamoto EK, Hirose F, Lachman RS. Case report 305. Dysplasia epiphysealis hemimelica (Trevor disease) of left ankle with an associated osteochondral (post-traumatic) fracture fragment, probably arising from talus. *Skeletal Radiol.* 1985;13(2):174–178.

55. Bruckner JD. Bone tumors. In: Staheli LT, ed. *Pediatric Orthopedic Secrets.* 2nd ed. Philadelphia, PA: Hanley & Belfus; 2002.

56. Gebhardt MC. Soft tissue tumors. In: Staheli LT, ed. *Pediatric Orthopedic Secrets.* 2nd ed. Philadelphia, PA: Hanley & Belfus; 2002.

57. Gibbons CL, Khwaja HA, Cole AS, Cooke PH, Athanasou NA. Giant-cell tumour of the tendon sheath in the foot and ankle. *J Bone Joint Surg Br.* Sep 2002; 84(7):1000–1003.

ANKLE AND FOOT PAIN IN A CHILD

58. Miyano JA, Fitzgibbons TC. Glomangioma of the ankle simulating injury to the flexor hallucis longus: a case report. *Foot Ankle Int.* Dec 1996;17(12):768–770.

59. Temple HT, Mizel MS, Murphey MD, Sweet DE. Osteoblastoma of the foot and ankle. *Foot Ankle Int.* Oct 1998;19(10):698–704.

60. Erler K, Oguz E, Komurcu M, Atesalp S, Basbozkurt M. Ankle swelling in a 6-year-old boy with unusual presentation: report of a rare case. *J Foot Ankle Surg.* Jul–Aug 2003;42(4):235–239.

61. Biscaglia R, Gasbarrini A, Bohling T, Bacchini P, Bertoni F, Picci P. Osteosarcoma of the bones of the foot—an easily misdiagnosed malignant tumor. *Mayo Clin Proc.* Sep 1998;73(9):842–847.

62. Conrad III EU. Initial evaluation of musculoskeletal tumors in children. In: Staheli LT, ed. *Pediatric Orthopedic Secrets.* 2nd ed. Philadelphia, PA: Hanley & Belfus; 2002.

63. Scully SP, Temple HT, Harrelson JM. Synovial sarcoma of the foot and ankle. *Clin Orthop Relat Res.* Jul 1999 (364):220–226.

CHAPTER 51

Case Demonstration: Foot Pain in a Child

■ *Hugh G. Watts, MD*

NOTE: This case demonstration was developed using the diagnostic process described in Chapter 4 and demonstrated in Chapter 5. The reader is encouraged to use this diagnostic process in order to ensure thorough clinical reasoning. If additional elaboration is required on the information presented in this chapter, please consult Chapters 4 and 5.

THE DIAGNOSTIC PROCESS

Step 1 Identify the patient's chief concern.
Step 2 Identify *barriers to communication.*
Step 3 Identify *special concerns.*
Step 4 Create a symptom timeline and sketch the anatomy (if needed).
Step 5 Create a diagnostic hypothesis list considering all possible forms of *remote* and *local* pathology that could cause the patient's chief concern.
Step 6 Sort the diagnostic hypothesis list by epidemiology and specific case characteristics.
Step 7 Ask specific questions to rule specific conditions or pathological categories less likely.
Step 8 Re-sort the diagnostic hypothesis list based on the patient's responses to specific questioning.
Step 9 Perform tests to differentiate among the remaining diagnostic hypotheses.
Step 10 Re-sort the diagnostic hypothesis list based on the patient's responses to specific tests.
Step 11 Decide on a diagnostic impression.
Step 12 Determine the appropriate patient disposition.

Case Description

Oliver is a 14-year-old boy who presents with a chief concern of left dorsal midfoot pain. According to Oliver, the pain began more than a month ago. Oliver's mother is present to assist with giving the history. Oliver's primary concern is that kicking a soccer ball is particularly painful. The patient does not recall any particular incident 1 month ago. However, he does remember falling on his left leg during soccer about 6 months ago. Now his foot hurts with every step he takes, but it is better when he sits at school. The mother reports that Oliver "has always had flat feet" and she believes that is why he is currently having pain.

Oliver is healthy and does not take any medications. He is in the ninth grade at school and "likes it OK." No one in his family has similar problems. He has an older brother and a younger sister, both of whom have met normal developmental milestones without health issues.

Oliver is reticent in his responses to your questions. He is a little overweight. Gait observation as he walked into the interview revealed that he walks with his feet slightly externally rotated with a mild left antalgic gait pattern.

STEP #1: Identify the patient's chief concern.

- Left foot pain distal to the malleoli

STEP #2: Identify *barriers to communication.*

- **Fourteen-year-old male patient and its associated issues with communication.** History gathering from a child patient requires sensitivity to age-appropriate language and understanding of the body.

> **Teaching Comments:** The involvement of the child in health care consultations varies significantly from case to case.[1] The type of illness, parental and child preferences, and where within the disease course the consultation occurs all play roles in the level of involvement of the child.

STEP #3: Identify *special concerns.*
None identified at this time.

STEP #4: Create a symptom timeline and sketch the anatomy (if needed).

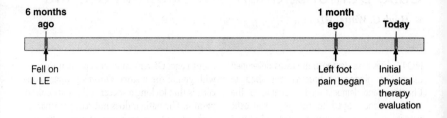

6 months
ago

1 month
ago

Today

Fell on
L LE

Left foot
pain began

Initial
physical
therapy
evaluation

STEP #5: Create a diagnostic hypothesis list considering all possible forms of *remote* and *local* pathology that could cause the patient's chief concern.

STEP #6: Sort the diagnostic hypothesis list by epidemiology and specific case characteristics.

Remote

T   Trauma

Lumbar radiculopathy

I   Inflammation

Aseptic
Seronegative spondylopathies

Septic
Not applicable

M   Metabolic

Not applicable

Va   Vascular

Popliteal artery entrapment syndrome

De   Degenerative

Not applicable

Tu   Tumor

Not applicable

Co   Congenital

Not applicable

Ne   Neurogenic/Psychogenic

Not applicable

Remote

T   Trauma

~~Lumbar radiculopathy~~ (worsens specifically with weight bearing over the affected foot)

I   Inflammation

Aseptic
Seronegative spondylopathies

Septic
Not applicable

M   Metabolic

Not applicable

Va   Vascular

~~Popliteal entrapment syndrome~~ (symptoms inconsistent with claudication)

De   Degenerative

Not applicable

Tu   Tumor

Not applicable

Co   Congenital

Not applicable

Ne   Neurogenic/Psychogenic

Not applicable

Local

T Trauma

Ankle impingement syndromes:
- Anterior
- Posterior

Calcaneal apophysitis (Sever's disease)

Fifth metatarsal apophysitis (Iselin's disease)

Fractures

Ill-fitting shoes

Ligament sprain

Muscle strain

Nerve entrapments:
- Common peroneal entrapment
- Lateral plantar nerve

- Tarsal tunnel syndrome

Puncture wounds

I Inflammation

Aseptic
Juvenile rheumatoid arthritis
Plantar fasciitis
Retrocalcaneal bursitis
Rheumatic fever
Tendinitis

Septic
Cellulitis
Fungal disease

Hand-foot-mouth disease
Ingrown toenail
Necrotizing fasciitis

Osteomyelitis
Sepsis of foot/ankle
Tuberculosis

M Metabolic

Ehlers-Danlos syndrome
Fabry's disease
Gaucher's disease

Gout

Myositis ossificans

Va Vascular

Avascular necrosis of the metatarsal head (Freiberg's infarction)

Local

T Trauma

Ankle impingement syndromes:
- Anterior
- ~~Posterior~~ (location of symptoms)

~~Calcaneal apophysitis (Sever's disease)~~ (location of symptoms)

~~Fifth metatarsal apophysitis (Iselin's disease)~~ (location of symptoms)

~~Fractures~~ (patient bearing weight with only mild gait deviation)

Ill-fitting shoes

Ligament sprain

Muscle strain

Nerve entrapments:
- Common peroneal entrapment
- ~~Lateral plantar nerve~~ (location of symptoms)

- ~~Tarsal tunnel syndrome~~ (location of symptoms)

Puncture wounds

I Inflammation

Aseptic
Juvenile rheumatoid arthritis
~~Plantar fasciitis~~ (location of symptoms)
~~Retrocalcaneal bursitis~~ (location of symptoms)
Rheumatic fever
Tendinitis

Septic
Cellulitis
~~Fungal disease~~ (unlikely due to absence of risk factors for immunocompromise)

Hand-foot-mouth disease
~~Ingrown toenail~~ (location of symptoms)
~~Necrotizing fasciitis~~ (lack of severe symptoms)

Osteomyelitis
Sepsis of foot/ankle
Tuberculosis

M Metabolic

Ehlers-Danlos syndrome
Fabry's disease
~~Gaucher disease~~ (less likely to cause isolated ankle and foot symptoms)

~~Gout~~ (rare in this age group and at this location)

~~Myositis ossificans~~ (location of symptoms)

Va Vascular

~~Avascular necrosis of the metatarsal head (Freiberg's infarction)~~ (location of symptoms)

Avascular necrosis of the navicular (Köhler's disease)

~~Avascular necrosis of the navicular (Köhler's disease)~~ (the anatomy of the area is sufficiently close together so the pain location is not at all specific)

Compartment syndrome

~~Compartment syndrome~~ (location of symptoms)

Familial Mediterranean fever

~~Familial Mediterranean fever~~ (age of onset is atypical of the norm for this condition)

Hemophilia

~~Hemophilia~~ (age of onset is atypical of the norm for this condition)

Osteochondritis dissecans of the talus

Osteochondritis dissecans of the talus

Peripheral arterial disease

~~Peripheral arterial disease~~ (symptoms not suggestive of claudication)

Sickle cell anemia

~~Sickle cell anemia~~ (age of onset is atypical of the norm for this condition)

De Degenerative

Bunion
Hallux rigidus
Heel spurs
Peroneal tendon subluxation

De Degenerative

~~Bunion~~ (location of symptoms)
~~Hallux rigidus~~ (location of symptoms)
~~Heel spurs~~ (location of symptoms)
~~Peroneal tendon subluxation~~ (location of symptoms)

Tu Tumor

Malignant Primary, such as:
- Ewing's sarcoma
- Leukemia
- Osteosarcoma
- Rhabdomyosarcoma
- Synovial sarcoma

Malignant Metastatic:
Not applicable

Benign, such as:
- Calcaneal cysts
- Ganglion
- Giant cell tumor of the tendon sheath
- Glomangioma
- Osteoblastoma
- Osteochondroma
- Osteoid osteoma

Tu Tumor

Malignant Primary, such as:
- Ewing's sarcoma
- Leukemia
- Osteosarcoma
- Rhabdomyosarcoma
- Synovial sarcoma

Malignant Metastatic:
Not applicable

Benign, such as:
- ~~Calcaneal cysts~~ (location of symptoms)
- Ganglion
- Giant cell tumor of the tendon sheath
- Glomangioma
- Osteoblastoma
- Osteochondroma
- Osteoid osteoma

Co Congenital

Accessory navicular
Claw toes
Congenital oblique talus
Congenital vertical talus
Flexible flat-foot deformity
Hallux varus
Hammer toes
Polydactyly
Rigid flat-foot deformity
Tarsal coalitions:
- Calcaneonavicular
- Talocalcaneal

Co Congenital

~~Accessory navicular~~ (location of symptoms)
~~Claw toes~~ (location of symptoms)
Congenital oblique talus
Congenital vertical talus
Flexible flat-foot deformity
~~Hallux varus~~ (location of symptoms)
~~Hammer toes~~ (location of symptoms)
~~Polydactyly~~ (location of symptoms)
Rigid flat-foot deformity
Tarsal coalitions:
- Calcaneonavicular
- Talocalcaneal

Trevor's disease (dysplasia epiphysealis
hemimelica)

Ne **Neurogenic/Psychogenic**

Complex regional pain syndrome

~~Trevor's disease (dysplasia epiphysealis
hemimelica)~~ (location of symptoms)

Ne **Neurogenic/Psychogenic**

~~Complex regional pain syndrome~~
(localization of symptoms atypical)

STEP #7: Ask specific questions to rule
specific conditions or pathological
categories less likely.

- Have you felt ill with a fever within
  the past several weeks? No. This response reduces the likelihood of pyrogenic forms of pathologies, such as in
  the septic inflammatory and tumor
  categories.

- Has there been any redness or swelling?
  No. This answer rules less likely the remaining pathologies in the septic inflammatory and vascular categories.

STEP #8: Re-sort the diagnostic
hypothesis list based on the patient's
responses to specific questioning.

Remote

T Trauma

   Not applicable

I **Inflammation**

   Aseptic

   ~~Seronegative spondylopathies~~ (no history of
   illness or swelling)

   Septic

   Not applicable

M **Metabolic**

   Not applicable

Va **Vascular**

   Not applicable

De **Degenerative**

   Not applicable

Tu **Tumor**

   Not applicable

Co **Congenital**

   Not applicable

Ne **Neurogenic/Psychogenic**

   Not applicable

Local

T **Trauma**

   Ankle impingement syndromes:
   - Anterior
   Ill-fitting shoes
   Ligament sprain
   Muscle strain
   Nerve entrapments:
   - Common peroneal entrapment
   Puncture wounds

I **Inflammation**

   Aseptic

   ~~Juvenile rheumatoid arthritis~~ (no history of
   illness or swelling)
   ~~Rheumatic fever~~ (no fever)
   Tendinitis

   Septic

   ~~Cellulitis~~ (no redness or swelling)
   ~~Hand-foot-mouth disease~~ (no redness or
   swelling)
   ~~Necrotizing fasciitis~~ (no redness or
   swelling)
   ~~Osteomyelitis~~ (no redness or swelling)
   ~~Tuberculosis~~ (no fever)
   ~~Sepsis of foot/ankle~~ (no redness or
   swelling)

M **Metabolic**

   Ehlers-Danlos syndrome
   ~~Fabry's disease~~ (no fever)

Va **Vascular**

   Osteochondritis dissecans of the talus

De **Degenerative**

   Not applicable

Tu **Tumor**

   Malignant Primary, such as:
   - ~~Ewing's sarcoma~~ (no illness or fever)
   - ~~Leukemia~~ (no illness or fever)
   - ~~Osteosarcoma~~ (no illness or fever, no
     swelling)

- ~~Rhabdomyosarcoma~~ (no illness or fever)
- ~~Synovial sarcoma~~ (no illness or fever)

Malignant Metastatic:
Not applicable

Benign, such as:
- Ganglion
- Giant cell tumor of the tendon sheath
- Glomangioma
- Osteoblastoma
- Osteochondroma
- Osteoid osteoma

Co Congenital

Congenital oblique talus
Congenital vertical talus
Flexible flat-foot deformity
Rigid flat-foot deformity
Tarsal coalitions:
- Calcaneonavicular
- Talocalcaneal

Ne Neurogenic/Psychogenic

Not applicable

STEP #9: Perform tests to differentiate among the remaining diagnostic hypotheses.

- **Examine the foot:** Foot has normal shape, making less likely congenital oblique or vertical talus.
- **Passive range of motion of the subtalar joint:** Limited and painful subtalar inversion and eversion on the affected side, but normal and pain free on the unaffected side.
- **Peroneal spasticity test:** Instant acute pain, making less likely a flexible flat-foot deformity.

Teaching Comments: The peroneal spasticity test is a quick inversion motion of the forefoot, which draws quick onset and reproduction of the patient's report of pain. It is only associated with talocalcaneal tarsal coalition. Do this test last because the child is unlikely to allow you to examine the foot any further.

STEP #10: Re-sort the diagnostic hypothesis list based on the patient's responses to specific tests.

- Talocalcaneal tarsal coalition

STEP #11: Decide on a diagnostic impression.

- Rule out talocalcaneal tarsal coalition.

STEP #12: Determine the appropriate patient disposition.

- Referral to a pediatric orthopedist prior to initiation of physical therapy. Plain-film x-rays may identify the nature of potential osseous pathology, but computed tomography may be needed.

Case Outcome

Subsequent plain film x-rays taken by the pediatric orthopedist confirmed the clinical diagnosis of talocalcaneal tarsal coalition. Oliver subsequently underwent successful excision. Subsequently, Oliver presented to physical therapy with chief concerns of inability to pursue premorbid activities secondary to postsurgical pain and swelling.

Reference
1. Taylor S, Haase-Casanovas S, Weaver T, Kidd J, Garralda EM. Child involvement in the paediatric consultation: a qualitative study of children and carers' views. *Child Care Health Dev.* 2010;36(5):678–685.

CHAPTER 52

Delayed Mobility (Crawling and Walking), Failure to Thrive, and Psychomotor Delay in a Child

■ *Phibun Ny, PT, DPT* ■ *Shelly Olivadoti-Santoro, PT, DPT*
■ *Cassandra Sanders-Holly, PT, DPT, PCS*

Description of the Symptom

Often, parents or caregivers present to the clinic with concerns that their child is not performing skills that other children his or her age are, or that perhaps a sibling did at the same age. The child may not be rolling, crawling, sitting, reaching, standing, or walking at the age that most children are able to perform those skills. This chapter discusses many of the causes that may contribute to delayed mobility, failure to thrive, and psychomotor delay.

Special Concerns

■ Neurological signs, such as rapid changes or loss of consciousness, sudden weakness/paralysis, sudden or new onset of uncontrolled seizures[1]
■ Rapid decline in function over short period of time, especially if associated with vomiting or lethargy
■ Evidence of abuse/neglect

CHAPTER PREVIEW: Conditions That May Lead to Delayed Mobility, Failure to Thrive, and Psychomotor Delay in a Child

T	Trauma

COMMON

Abuse/neglect 1017
Brachial plexus injury (Erb's palsy, Klumpke's palsy) 1018
Fractures 1024
Hypoxic-ischemic encephalopathy 1025
Limb deformities/bone and joint disorders:
• Amputation/agenesis of a limb 1026

UNCOMMON

Not applicable

RARE

Not applicable

(continued)

Inflammation

COMMON

Aseptic
Not applicable

Septic
Congenital infections 1022
Encephalitis 1024
Meningitis:
• Bacterial 1027
• Viral 1027

UNCOMMON

Aseptic
Acute inflammatory polyradiculopathy (Guillain-Barré syndrome) 1018
Inflammatory muscle diseases:
• Polymyositis 1025

Septic
Human immunodeficiency virus infection 1024

RARE

Aseptic
Chronic inflammatory demyelinating polyneuropathy 1022
Inflammatory muscle diseases:
• Dermatomyositis 1025
Poliomyelitis 1030

Septic
Not applicable

 Metabolic

COMMON

Intrauterine growth retardation or small for gestational age 1026
Maternal drug or alcohol exposure in utero/breast milk 1027
Mitochondrial disorders (eg, Leigh syndrome) 1028
Osteogenesis imperfecta 1029

UNCOMMON

Methylmalonic aciduria 1028
Peroxisomal disorders (Zellweger syndrome) 1030

RARE

Congenital hypothyroidism 1022
Metabolic brain disorders:
• Gray matter diseases:
  • Alpers disease 1027
  • Niemann-Pick disease 1027
• White matter diseases:
  • Phenylketonuria   1028
• Gray and white matter disease:
  • Mucopolysaccharidosis 1028
Myositis ossificans 1029

Va Vascular

COMMON

Hemophilia 1024
Intracranial hemorrhages:
- Epidural 1025
- Intracerebral (eg, shaken baby syndrome) 1025
- Subdural 1025

UNCOMMON

Not applicable

RARE

Klippel-Trenaunay-Weber syndrome 1026

De Degenerative

COMMON

Degenerative muscle diseases:
- Muscular dystrophies:
  - Duchenne muscular dystrophy 1023
  - Emery-Dreifuss muscular dystrophy 1023
  - Myotonic dystrophy (congenital myotonic dystrophy, Steinert disease) 1023
- Myasthenia gravis:
  - Congenital 1023
  - Transient neonatal 1023

UNCOMMON

Degenerative muscle diseases:
- Congenital myopathies:
  - Central core disease 1022
  - Congenital myopathies 1022
  - Nemaline body disease 1023
Spinal muscular atrophies:
- Acute Werdnig-Hoffmann disease (infantile, type I) 1032
- Chronic Werdnig-Hoffmann disease (intermediate, type II) 1032
- Kugelberg-Welander disease (juvenile, type III) 1032

RARE

Not applicable

Tu Tumor

COMMON

Not applicable

UNCOMMON

Malignant Primary, such as:
- Medulloblastoma 1033
Malignant Metastatic:
Not applicable
Benign, such as:
- Syringomyelia 1033

(continued)

Tumor (continued)

RARE

Malignant Primary, such as:
- Astrocytoma 1032
- Brainstem glioma 1032
- Craniopharyngioma 1033
- Ependymoma 1033
- Medulloblastoma 1033
- Neuroblastoma 1033

Malignant Metastatic:
Not applicable

Benign:
Not applicable

Co Congenital

COMMON

Auditory/visual impairments:
- Auditory impairment 1018
- Cortical visual impairment 1018

Central nervous system malformations:
- Agenesis of the corpus callosum (partial/complete) 1019
- Arnold-Chiari malformations (Chiari malformations):
  - Type I (adult onset) 1019
  - Type II (childhood onset) 1019
- Holoprosencephaly 1019
- Hydrocephalus 1019

Congenital heart defects (eg, tetralogy of Fallot) 1022
Developmental dysplasia of the hip 1024
Limb deformities/bone and joint disorders:
- Arthrogryposis multiplex congenita 1026
- Talipes equinovarus (clubfoot) 1026

Myelodysplasias:
- Meningocele (spina bifida occulta) 1029
- Myelomeningocele 1029

UNCOMMON

Chromosomal abnormalities:
- Angelman syndrome 1020
- Cockayne syndrome 1020
- Cystic fibrosis 1021
- Down syndrome (Trisomy 21) 1021
- Fragile X syndrome 1021
- Kabuki syndrome 1021
- Prader-Willi syndrome 1021
- Tay-Sachs disease 1022

Internal organ abnormalities/dysfunction 1025
Limb deformities/bone and joint disorders:
- Amputation/agenesis of a limb 1026
- Congenital constriction band syndrome (Streeter's dysplasia) 1026

Neurocutaneous disorders:
- Neurofibromatosis 1029
- Tuberous sclerosis 1029

Sex chromosomal or sex-linked syndromes:
- Rett syndrome 1031
- Turner syndrome (45XO) 1031

Congenital *(continued)*

RARE
Not applicable

Ne Neurogenic/Psychogenic

COMMON
Cerebral palsy 1020
Psychoses 1030
Seizure disorders:
• Infantile spasms 1031
• Lennox-Gastaut syndrome 1031
Sensory integrative dysfunction 1031

UNCOMMON
Peripheral neuropathies:
• Hereditary motor and sensory neuropathy Types I and II (Charcot-Marie-Tooth disease) 1030
• Hereditary motor and sensory neuropathy Type III (Dejerine-Sottas disease) 1030
Pervasive developmental disabilities 1030

RARE
Munchausen syndrome and Munchausen syndrome by proxy 1028

Note: These are estimates of relative incidence because few data are available for the less common conditions. Some information was extrapolated from the literature regarding the prevalence of developmental delay in general.

Overview of Delayed Mobility, Failure to Thrive, and Psychomotor Delay in a Child

Typical motor development follows a progression that can be measured by milestones that are generally accepted as being achieved by a certain age. Adequate developmental diagnosis requires that the clinician examine six domains of development or behavior: the adaptive/self-help, gross-motor, fine-motor, language, cognitive, and social-emotional domains.

The dynamic systems theory of motor control indicates that multiple variables drive the rate and variability of development.[1] Children learn functional motor skills through interactions with their environment. These motor skills then further drive cognitive changes by allowing exploration of their environment and self-directed play. The emergence of postural control and ability to adapt movement strategies is critical in motor development and the progression to mature gait. Typical motor development is dynamic in nature and is characterized by alternating advancement and regression in ability to perform skills.[2] It is normal for children to regress to simple, symmetrical patterns when learning a new skill. It takes practice to master complex, asymmetrical mobility as in a mature gait pattern. Also, typical motor development may vary across cultures, due to cultural practices and beliefs. The reader should take this into consideration when assessing children with possible developmental delays.

Description of Conditions That May Lead to Delayed Mobility, Failure to Thrive, and Psychomotor Delay in a Child

■ Abuse/Neglect

Chief Clinical Characteristics

This presentation commonly includes hematomas, frequent bony fractures, soft tissue injuries, welts, internal injuries, burns, excessive tenderness, excessively under- or overemotional, and behavioral alterations. Other issues may include soiled clothing or diapers, malnutrition, evidence of poor hygiene, skin breakdown, lack of compliance with medical/therapy appointments, and poor follow-through with administration of medication.[3]

Background Information

Abuse and neglect are common causes of mobility delay, failure to thrive, and psychomotor delay, and it is critical it be detected by physical therapists. Abuse and neglect are broadly defined as an act or failure to perform an act that results in physical, emotional, or sexual harm, abuse, or exploitation. Abuse and neglect may be perpetrated by parents, guardians, family members, or, less commonly, strangers. Abuse and neglect may be present in all socioeconomic and educational demographic groups. In addition to ethical obligations that require abuse and neglect reporting, legal mandatory reporting requirements similarly require physical therapists to communicate suspicions of this condition. Physical therapists should become familiar with accepted reporting mechanisms for abuse and neglect.

■ Acute Inflammatory Polyradiculopathy (Guillain-Barré Syndrome)

Chief Clinical Characteristics

This presentation includes weakness and loss of sensation that usually recovers completely after a few weeks or months. Typically this condition follows a throat/intestinal infection.

Background Information

There is a greater likelihood in male than female, and it is not hereditary. Some people experience recurrences of the condition throughout life.

AUDITORY/VISUAL IMPAIRMENTS

■ Auditory Impairment

Chief Clinical Characteristics

This presentation includes a failed newborn hearing screening, poor auditory responses, poor speech development, and/or an abnormal audiogram. Children with auditory impairments affecting the inner ear may have vestibular deficits, which cause balance disturbances, and this may affect early mobility. Children with multisensory impairments (visual and auditory) may avoid

or ignore stimuli that they have difficulty processing due to their visual and auditory deficits. These children may also demonstrate other less socially appropriate behaviors such as eye poking or pressing, rocking, head banging, hand waving in front of face, and teeth grinding.[4]

Background Information

Hearing loss may be the result of ototoxic drugs, infections, poor movement of the middle ear bones, or wax buildup. It is also common in conditions such as Down syndrome and neurofibromatosis.

■ Cortical Visual Impairment

Chief Clinical Characteristics

This presentation includes poor response to visual stimulation, shaking of the head, compulsive light gazing, difficulty with depth perception, and poor visual tracking. Children with multisensory impairments (visual and auditory) may avoid or ignore stimuli that they have difficulty processing due to their visual and auditory deficits.

Background Information

Cortical visual impairment may be permanent or transient and is typically a result of damage to the posterior visual pathways and/or cortical visual areas (occipital lobe primarily) due to ischemia. Vision is the driving force for a child acquiring early learning and developing typically. The origin of cortical visual impairment may be a tumor, other congenital anomalies, or central nervous system infections such as meningitis, trauma (eg, shaken baby syndrome), or perinatal asphyxia resulting in cerebral palsy.[5]

■ Brachial Plexus Injury (Erb's Palsy, Klumpke's Palsy)

Chief Clinical Characteristics

This presentation typically includes an inability to move an upper extremity throughout available range of motion; weakness or paralysis of the upper extremity musculature, particularly in the C5–C6 nerve root distribution; and posturing in shoulder extension, internal rotation, and adduction, elbow extension, forearm pronation, and wrist and finger flexion. Horner's syndrome is a group of signs indicating an injury to the sympathetic nerve tracts supplying the eye, which is exiting at the cervical level. Due to proximity of these sympathetic nerve tracts to the brachial plexus, they also may become injured along with the brachial plexus or as a result of a clavicular fracture during delivery.[6,7]

Background Information
Paralysis of the proximal shoulder musculature is not uncommon and grasp is typically intact with forearm support. This condition commonly follows a difficult vaginal delivery during which a traction force on the infant's shoulder can injure the cervical roots, fracture the clavicle or humerus, or sublux the shoulder.[3]

CENTRAL NERVOUS SYSTEM MALFORMATIONS

■ Agenesis of the Corpus Callosum (Partial/Complete)

Chief Clinical Characteristics
This presentation typically includes developmental delay in a child with dysmorphic features or other organ malformations or one who has an abnormal size or shape of the head. Children with this condition will typically have initial difficulty with midline orientation (in infants, bringing hands to midline), bilateral play, and tasks that require integration of both sides of the body. Motor development may be slow, age appropriate, or severely affected.

Background Information
This may occur independently, or along with other diagnoses such as myelodysplasia or cri du chat syndrome. The corpus callosum is responsible for coordinating bilateral limb and ocular movements, and contributes to learning and social understanding.[8–12]

ARNOLD-CHIARI MALFORMATIONS (CHIARI MALFORMATIONS)

■ Type I (Adult Onset)

Chief Clinical Characteristics
This presentation involves ataxic gait due to cerebellar involvement, headaches and vomiting due to obstructive hydrocephalus, vertigo, nystagmus, and lower cranial nerve palsies due to brainstem compression, and a cape-like distribution of decreased pain and temperature sensation due to syringomyelia.

Background Information
This condition is a congenital anomaly. It is the downward displacement of the cerebellar tonsils through the foramen magnum.[13] This interferes with the flow of cerebrospinal fluid to and from the brain. This condition is associated with meningomyelocele and hydrocephalus.

■ Type II (Childhood Onset)

Chief Clinical Characteristics
This presentation involves stridor and swallowing difficulties in infants. In older children, upper limb weakness and breathing difficulties are seen.

Background Information
Similar to Type I Arnold-Chiari malformation, this condition is also a congenital anomaly. It is the downward displacement of the cerebellar tonsils through the foramen magnum.[13] This interferes with the flow of cerebrospinal fluid to and from the brain. This condition is associated with meningomyelocele and hydrocephalus.

■ Holoprosencephaly

Chief Clinical Characteristics
This presentation includes varying degrees of deficit of midline facial development and incomplete morphogenesis of forebrain.

Background Information
If there is central nervous system involvement, prognosis is typically poor.[14]

■ Hydrocephalus

Chief Clinical Characteristics
This presentation includes changes in consciousness, muscle tone changes, visual changes, seizure activity, and cardiorespiratory consequences.

Background Information
May be initially diagnosed due to a visibly large cranium, with or without the presence of myelodysplasia. When suspected, children undergo imaging tests such as magnetic resonance imaging or head ultrasound to determine whether there are increased intracranial fluid levels with or without ventricular dilation. Children may undergo a ventriculoperitoneal shunt placement, or may go untreated under observation if hydrocephalus is showing signs of self-resolving.[15]

■ Cerebral Palsy

Chief Clinical Characteristics

This presentation includes a constellation of findings classified by topographic distribution of impairment (hemiplegia, diplegia, quadriplegia) and by types classified by clinical findings (spasticity, hypotonia, ataxia, dyskinesia/athetosis). In spastic cerebral palsy, muscles are perceived as stiff, especially during active movement. Muscle tone is increased; selective control is limited, resulting in the production of abnormal movement synergies; active range of motion is limited by coactivation of muscular activity; and the timing of the muscle activation and postural responses is abnormal.[16] Hypotonia is characterized by diminished resting muscle tone, hypermobility, decreased ability to produce voluntary force, and postural instability. Ataxia is a disorder of balance and control and in the timing of coordinated movement. Dyskinesia is associated with uncontrolled or purposeless movements that may present with both hypotonia and hypertonia.

Background Information

This condition includes clinical sequelae resulting from a nonprogressive encephalopathy in an immature brain. The cause may be pre-, peri-, or postnatal.[17] The primary impairments are typically impaired movement and posture. There are many possible causes of cerebral palsy, most common being a hypoxic event *in utero*, during delivery, or shortly after birth; drocephalus; intracerebral hemorrhage (any grade); prematurity; perinatal asphyxia; and head trauma. Some children may be diagnosed with cerebral palsy as a result of developmental delays that are unexplained by further testing when other metabolic or syndrome diagnoses have been ruled out. It is also typical for a child with a traumatic brain injury or infection (eg, encephalitis, meningitis) or abnormal magnetic resonance images (such as microcephaly) to be diagnosed with cerebral palsy as well. The diagnosis may be highly dependent on the classification provided by the diagnosing physician.

CHROMOSOMAL ABNORMALITIES

There are several hundred chromosomal abnormalities that may lead to delayed mobility.

The extent of these disorders is beyond the scope of this text. In this section, we describe a few of the more common disorders that a physical therapy practitioner is likely to encounter. Further information may be obtained by consulting other excellent textbooks on this subject.[14]

■ Angelman Syndrome

Chief Clinical Characteristics

This presentation includes marked mental retardation with accompanying minimal speech (receptive exceeding expressive language) and delayed gross-motor skills. Typically there is gait ataxia (puppet-like) and frequent inappropriate laughter/smiling.

Background Information

This condition is caused by loss of function of the *UBE3A* gene. The most common mechanism is deletion or inactivation of the segment containing the gene on chromosome 15, affecting up to 70% of individuals with this condition. In this instance, fair skin and blonde hair is also present secondary to a concomitant deletion or inactivation of the *OCA2* gene, which is also located on chromosome 15. Specific *UBE3A* gene mutations are responsible for 11% of cases. This condition affects 1 in 12,000 to 20,000 individuals. Affected people commonly have no family history, so this condition is considered to occur secondary to an inheritable random event during early embryonic development. Individuals with this condition have a life span that approximates normal.[18]

■ Cockayne Syndrome

Chief Clinical Characteristics

This presentation includes premature aging, severe growth retardation, ataxia, global delays in development, auditory and visual deficits, osteoporosis, and early death (average life span is 5 to 6 years of age).[14]

Background Information

This condition occurs secondary to mutations in either the *ERCC6* (CSB) or *ERCC8* (CSA) genes. When typically functioning, these genes provide for encoding appropriate responses to repairing deoxyribonucleic acid (DNA). Thus, this condition is characterized by deficient DNA repair, with consequent rapid aging and premature death. This condition occurs in 2 per 1 million live births. The pattern of heritability is autosomal dominant.[19]

■ Cystic Fibrosis

Chief Clinical Characteristics
This presentation may involve limited rib excursion, use of accessory muscles of respiration, and barrel-chest deformity. Advanced pulmonary complications can be manifested as digital clubbing. Nutritional status is usually compromised.[1]

Background Information
This is a progressive disorder of the exocrine glands. This disorder causes the obstruction of mucus-secreting exocrine glands by hyperviscous secretions. Blockage of the exocrine gland products prevents their delivery to target tissues and organs and thus creates abnormalities in multiple body systems. The etiology is related to the abnormal gene product, the cystic fibrosis transmembrane conductance regulator (CFTR) protein. Abnormal expression of this protein in airway epithelial cells results in abnormal amounts of fluid being removed from the airway lumen, leading to thick, dry mucus.[18] These thick secretions lead to progressive airway obstruction, secondary infection by opportunistic bacteria, inflammation, and subsequent bronchiectasis and irreversible airway damage.[3] The presentation of infants with failure to thrive and nutritional losses through steatorrhea accounts for up to 85% of the cases of this condition diagnosed in infancy.[18]

■ Down Syndrome (Trisomy 21)

Chief Clinical Characteristics
This presentation includes global hypotonia and hyperflexibility. Other characteristics include small stature, difficulty with feeding, heart defects, hearing loss, and atlanto-occipital instability. This diagnosis is also associated with moderate to severe cognitive delays.[1]

Background Information
This condition most commonly results from trisomy 21, in which three copies of chromosome 21 are present instead of the usual two copies. Typical development is consequently disrupted by the extra genetic material present in each cell. This condition is present in 1 in 740 live births. This condition is inheritable, and it occurs as a random error of nondisjunction early in fetal development. Women of advanced reproductive age are at higher risk for delivering a newborn with this condition.[20]

■ Fragile X Syndrome

Chief Clinical Characteristics
This presentation includes increased head circumference, prominent forehead, generalized hypotonia, torticollis, and scoliosis.

Background Information
This condition is the second most common known cause of mental retardation in males. A diagnosis of autism may coexist because findings such as poor eye contact, limited speech, and hand flapping are common.[1]

■ Kabuki Syndrome

Chief Clinical Characteristics
This presentation includes long palpebral fissures and eversion of the outer portions of the lower eyelid, with the result that the person appears to be wearing the makeup a Japanese Kabuki dancer. Children with this condition typically demonstrate joint hyperextensibility, hip abnormalities with possible recurrent surgeries, and low muscle tone. Cardiac defects are common and children with this condition may have seizures and visual and/or sensorimotor deficits.

Background Information
This condition is caused by a mutation of the *MLL2* gene on chromosome 12, which normally provides transcriptional control of estrogen receptor and beta globin. This condition is present in 1 per 32,000 Japanese individuals, but it is also present across various ethnic groups.[21]

■ Prader-Willi Syndrome

Chief Clinical Characteristics
This presentation includes cognitive delay, hypotonia, failure to thrive during infancy, as well as short stature and obsessive food disorder in childhood, which can result in severe obesity.[1]

Background Information

This condition occurs secondary to a dysfunction of the paternal copy of chromosome 15. The specific genes on chromosome 15 that are responsible for this condition are as yet unknown. However, this condition is known to occur with an OCA2 gene deletion, which causes blond hair and fair skin. This condition is present in 1 in 10,000 to 30,000 people worldwide. Most cases of this condition are not inherited.[22]

■ Tay-Sachs Disease

Chief Clinical Characteristics

This presentation includes listlessness and cognitive/motor regression.

Background Information

This condition is common in people of Jewish descent from the Mediterranean region. It is an autosomal recessive disorder that causes an enzyme deficiency that affects nerve cell metabolism. Without this enzyme, GM_2 ganglioside is not converted to a nontoxic substance and is allowed to build up in the nervous system, causing toxicity and the aforementioned clinical signs. Children with this condition develop typically until 5 to 10 months of age, when nervous system toxicity reaches a level at which it affects the child's development.[4]

■ Chronic Inflammatory Demyelinating Polyneuropathy

Chief Clinical Characteristics

This presentation includes weakness and loss of sensation that usually recovers completely after a few weeks or months. Typically this condition follows a throat/intestinal infection. This condition is progressive with frequent relapses. Clinical signs include upper and lower extremity weakness, hyporeflexia, decreased sensation, and pain.[19]

■ Congenital Heart Defects (eg, Tetralogy of Fallot)

Chief Clinical Characteristics

This presentation includes nailbed clubbing, muscle hypotonia, and changes in height/weight.

Background Information

This heart defect comprises four different cardiac anomalies that result in cyanosis, especially during exertion or when the child is upset. Surgical intervention is common in infants who are severely involved, and may also take place later on in early childhood years.

■ Congenital Hypothyroidism

Chief Clinical Characteristics

This presentation includes dry skin, constipation, lassitude, cold intolerance, bradycardia, and delayed relaxation phase of tendon reflexes, which usually appear in the first month or two after birth. Linear growth is impaired.[23]

Background Information

This condition is characterized by low serum thyroxine (T_4) and high thyroid-stimulating hormone (TSH) levels.

■ Congenital Infections

Chief Clinical Characteristics

This presentation may include microcephaly, hydrocephaly, blindness, deafness, mental retardation, and may also include a diagnosis of cerebral palsy.

Background Information

Underlying infections may include rubella virus, cytomegalovirus, herpes simplex virus, toxoplasmosis, and syphilis. Defects in limb, facial, and skeletal development; neurological abnormalities; opportunistic infections; failure to thrive; lymphoma; and heart defects can also result from these infections.[1]

DEGENERATIVE MUSCLE DISEASES

CONGENITAL MYOPATHIES

■ Central Core Disease

Chief Clinical Characteristics

This presentation includes hip displacement at birth and delayed motor development.

Background Information

Onset is in early infancy to childhood. This condition is variable in severity and progression and is autosomal dominant.[1]

■ Congenital Myopathies

Chief Clinical Characteristics

This presentation includes proximal muscle weakness, hypotonia, hyporeflexia, and normal creatine phosphokinase with onset in infancy or childhood.

Background Information

Relatively common congenital myopathies include central core disease, nemaline (rod) myopathy, and centronuclear (myotubular) myopathy. These conditions are inherited or caused by a spontaneous genetic mutation and cause nonprogressive problems with the muscles ranging from stiffness to weakness, with different degrees of severity.[13]

■ Nemaline Body Disease

Chief Clinical Characteristics

This presentation includes delayed motor development and weakness in the face and throat muscles. Onset is in early childhood with variable severity and progression.

Background Information

The pattern of heritability is autosomal dominant and autosomal recessive.[1]

MUSCULAR DYSTROPHIES

■ Duchenne Muscular Dystrophy

Chief Clinical Characteristics

This presentation includes symmetric weakness, especially proximally, that progresses over time. Typical gait is described as waddling and includes an increased lumbar lordosis and toe walking. Plantarflexion contractures occur over time. Calf muscles tend to enlarge, but muscle tissue is replaced by fat and connective tissue (pseudohypertrophy).

Background Information

This condition is an X-linked genetic disorder occurring in males, usually diagnosed when parents report noticing the child has lost motor skills or strength.[13]

■ Emery-Dreifuss Muscular Dystrophy

Chief Clinical Characteristics

This presentation involves weakness and muscle wasting of shoulder, upper arm, and chin muscles. Weakness of the elbow flexor and extensor musculature is usually seen first.

Background Information

Ankle equinus and elbow flexion contractures are common. Cardiac abnormalities are also common. Onset is in childhood to early teens, and progression is slow. This is an X-linked recessive disorder.[1]

■ Myotonic Dystrophy (Congenital Myotonic Dystrophy, Steinert Disease)

Chief Clinical Characteristics

This presentation includes marked temporalis muscle wasting and tenting of the upper lip, severe hypotonia at birth with impaired sucking and swallowing, and severe respiratory distress.

Background Information

Myotonic dystrophy is one of the most common causes of myopathic neonatal hypotonia. It is transmitted by an autosomal dominant pattern, most often from the mother. Muscle biopsy does not usually show any specific features and in most cases features consistent with myotonic dystrophy in the mother are used to confirm the diagnosis in the newborn. Overall, the severe weakness, which may require ventilatory support, is transient and gradually improves within days to weeks. However, severe weakness and hypotonia may continue and many infants with myotonic dystrophy also have mental retardation.

MYASTHENIA GRAVIS

■ Congenital

Chief Clinical Characteristics

This presentation involves ptosis and ophthalmoplegia when it presents rarely in the neonatal period. Hypotonia is common among most patients described with the disorder, as are intermittent episodes of generalized muscular weakness.

Background Information

This condition is caused by abnormalities of the neuromuscular junction structure and function, instead of the autoimmunity against nicotinic acetylcholine receptors that is common in the adult onset form of this condition. Thus, immunological medications are not used in treatment. Nevertheless, treatment is primarily pharmacologic. The specific medication used depends on the subtype of this condition.

■ Transient Neonatal

Chief Clinical Characteristics

This presentation includes floppiness, difficulty feeding, and fatigable bulbar weakness with defective respiration in a neonate.

DELAYED MOBILITY (CRAWLING AND WALKING), FAILURE TO THRIVE, AND PSYCHOMOTOR DELAY IN A CHILD

Background Information

This is a transient condition due to placental transfer of maternal acetylcholine receptor antibodies, which dissipate after several weeks. Diagnosis is made by these clinical signs, examination of the mother, a positive Tensilon test, and an electrophysiological study. Improvement usually occurs over the course of a few weeks as the antibodies clear the infant's system.

■ Developmental Dysplasia of the Hip

Chief Clinical Characteristics

This presentation includes waddling gait in a child between 18 and 24 months of age, if bilateral hip dislocation is present. Children with unilateral dislocation will limp, with a positive Trendelenburg sign on the involved side in the stance phase of gait.[3]

Background Information

This is an abnormal development of the hip joint in which the acetabulum and femoral head are not aligned normally. There are five types, defined by the alignment of the joint: (1) dysplasia, (2) subluxatable, (3) dislocatable, (4) dislocated, and (5) teratologic. Forms of this condition occur more often in girls and in the left hip. Associated problems include cervical torticollis, postural scoliosis, facial deformities, metatarsus adductus, and calcaneovalgus.[1]

■ Encephalitis

Chief Clinical Characteristics

This presentation includes acute confusion with fever, neck stiffness, photophobia, pain with eye movement, and mildly impaired consciousness.

Background Information

This condition is caused by childhood exanthems (ie, measles, mumps, varicella) or arthropod-borne (eg, tick, mosquito) viruses.

■ Fractures

Chief Clinical Characteristics

This presentation varies based on site and extent of fracture. Pain and warmth over fracture site are typically present.

Background Information

Fractures can be complicated by nerve injury or compression from swelling/bleeding that affects the bone's ability to heal. Example of fractures affecting children are supracondylar, greenstick (fracture of an immature skeleton, a break through one side of cortical bone), simple, comminuted, impaction, and avulsion fractures.

■ Hemophilia

Chief Clinical Characteristics

This presentation involves warm, swollen, and painful joints with limited range of motion during an acute hemarthrosis.

Background Information

This condition is related to a sex-linked recessive gene, so it is most commonly found in males. Typical microtrauma to joints and muscles that occur during daily activities can become acute episodes or "bleeds" that require immediate medical attention. With factor replacement injections, these bleeds are typically under control and occur with a traumatic event such as twisting an ankle or falling. Long-term effects of joint bleeds include hypertrophied synovium and degenerative changes to the cartilage in the joint, while muscle bleeds can cause atrophy, decreased range of motion, and nerve compression.[20]

■ Human Immunodeficiency Virus Infection

Chief Clinical Characteristics

This presentation includes distal symmetric sensorimotor polyneuropathy with pain, fatigue, weakness, and depressed lower extremity reflexes.[19]

Background Information

This condition is a bloodborne pathogen that may be transmitted to young children in several ways, including during delivery or via transfusion of infected blood products or transplantation of infected bone marrow. In developed countries, preventive technologies have made mother-to-child transmission less common than in developing countries. Older children may contract this condition from injectable drugs and sexual contact. This diagnosis is confirmed with a blood, saliva, or urine test for antibodies to human immunodeficiency virus. Treatment focuses on preventing the conversion of human immunodeficiency virus to acquired immunodeficiency syndrome, in which CD4+ T-lymphocyte counts are less than 200/µL, and opportunistic infections. Preventive efforts focus on a variety of antiretroviral medications administered in a cocktail.

■ Hypoxic-Ischemic Encephalopathy

Chief Clinical Characteristics
This presentation includes seizures, abnormal tone, posturing, reflexes, respiration, and autonomic dysfunction.

Background Information
Possible post-traumatic sequelae include motor deficits, mental retardation, and seizures. The principal cause in the newborn is perinatal asphyxia. Common causes in infants and children include upper airway obstruction (foreign body, physical trauma), pulmonary disease (near drowning, inhalation injury), cardiovascular disease (shock of any cause), neurological disorders (head trauma, status epilepticus, meningitis, encephalitis), intoxications (carbon monoxide), and metabolic disorders.

INFLAMMATORY MUSCLE DISEASES
■ Dermatomyositis

Chief Clinical Characteristics
This presentation includes progressive proximal symmetrical weakness.

Background Information
Diagnosis is confirmed by laboratory tests including muscle biopsy, elevated muscle enzymes, and an abnormal electromyogram. An associated cutaneous disease appears as a pruritic rash or dry scalp. In children, the onset of the dermatic symptoms is often insidious, and parents cite weakness with easy fatigability. Calcinosis is common in children, which presents as hard, painful nodules in the skin.

■ Polymyositis

Chief Clinical Characteristics
This presentation includes proximal limb and girdle weakness and wasting with pain, tenderness, dysphagia, and respiratory difficulty.

Background Information
Onset can occur at any age, and progression is variable.

■ Internal Organ Abnormalities/ Dysfunction

Chief Clinical Characteristics
This presentation includes hypotonia, poor endurance, frequent surgeries/hospitalization, and subsequent immobility.

Background Information
These factors mentioned above contribute to poor tolerance of physical activity, inadequate movement exploration, and possibly movement deprivation.

INTRACRANIAL HEMORRHAGES
■ Epidural

Chief Clinical Characteristics
This presentation involves loss of consciousness followed by a lucid interval for up to 2 days after a traumatic event that typically involves fracture of the lateral skull. Rapid evolution of headache, hemiparesis, and pupillary dilation follow and, if untreated, death.

Background Information
Hemorrhage typically occurs as a result of trauma as in a shaken baby, car accident, or other trauma that causes a shearing of the blood vessels in the brain.

■ Intracerebral (eg, Shaken Baby Syndrome)

Chief Clinical Characteristics
This presentation includes signs of meningeal irritation and hydrocephalus. Postinjury, behavioral problems are typically residual.[19]

Background Information
Hemorrhage typically occurs as a result of trauma as in a shaken baby, car accident, or other trauma that causes a shearing of the blood vessels in the brain. Intracerebral hemorrhage typically involves the frontal or temporal lobes.

■ Subdural

Chief Clinical Characteristics
This presentation involves headache and altered consciousness.

Background Information
The time between traumatic event and symptoms is typically longer in subdural hematomas. Hemorrhage typically occurs as a result of trauma as in a shaken baby, car accident, or other trauma that causes a shearing of the blood vessels in the brain.

■ Intrauterine Growth Retardation or Small for Gestational Age

Chief Clinical Characteristics
This presentation involves small fetal size that predisposes to various perinatal complications, such as asphyxia, polycythemia, hypoglycemia, and pulmonary hemorrhage.

Background Information
Each of these complications can further affect growth and development. The developmental outcomes of these children depend on the etiology of their small size and on any associated complications. Some fetuses develop this condition in response to maternal or unknown conditions that interfere with uteroplacental circulation, oxygenation, or nutrition, such as pregnancy-induced hypertension, maternal cyanotic congenital heart disease, and maternal chronic renal disease.[21] Poor growth may be an adaptive response of the fetus in order to maintain itself as efficiently as possible in constrained circumstances.[22]

■ Klippel-Trenaunay-Weber Syndrome

Chief Clinical Characteristics
This presentation includes disproportionate growth, hemangioma, joint discomfort, swelling, ulcers, or other chronic skin difficulties. Some children with this condition present with arteriovenous fistulas.

Background Information
This condition is an extremely rare congenital or early childhood hypertrophy of one or more limbs.[14]

LIMB DEFORMITIES/BONE AND JOINT DISORDERS

■ Amputation/Agenesis of a Limb

Chief Clinical Characteristics
This presentation often includes incomplete or malformation of an extremity, typically congenital, but may be traumatic.

Background Information
The child may have different levels of involvement depending on which limb(s) are involved and at what stage of development the child is in when the loss of limb took place. Children may often develop their own adaptive strategy to move or perform functional tasks. Whether or not the family chooses to pursue having the child fitted for a prosthesis and the child's aptitude at using it will have an effect on development as well.

■ Arthrogryposis Multiplex Congenita

Chief Clinical Characteristics
This presentation commonly includes contractures, fibrosis, and muscle weakness at the hip, knee, ankle, foot, shoulder, and elbow most severely in neonates. Children with this condition demonstrate abnormal joint creases and shape, and an imbalance of skeletal musculature, which contributes to worsening joint contractures with age.

Background Information
Prenatal viruses have been postulated to cause this condition; however, the etiology remains unknown because there are several forms, one of which is autosomal dominant.[3] Joint abnormalities will continue to progress if proper strengthening, positioning, and bracing are not initiated at birth.

■ Congenital Constriction Band Syndrome (Streeter's Dysplasia)

Chief Clinical Characteristics
This presentation includes malformed digits and/or limbs with visible ring-like concentric bands on the skin. Edema or enlargement of the limb may also be present.

Background Information
The etiology of this condition is unclear but it is hypothesized that tears in the amnion result in fibrous bands that entangle the fetal extremities and constrict or prevent proper formation *in utero*.[24]

■ Talipes Equinovarus (Clubfoot)

Chief Clinical Characteristics
This presentation typically includes a forefoot that is curved in medially (adducted),

the calcaneus is small, the hindfoot is in varus, and the ankle is in equinus. The calf and the foot are usually smaller on the involved side.

Background Information
This is a congenital deformity. It is often associated with myelomeningocele or arthrogryposis. Typical congenital clubfoot is probably due to abnormal intrauterine restriction in a genetically predisposed individual.[3]

■ **Maternal Drug or Alcohol Exposure In Utero/Breast Milk**

Chief Clinical Characteristics
This presentation involves growth retardation, cardiac anomalies, joint, and limb anomalies, visual impairments, behavioral/emotional disturbances, and learning disabilities.[1]

Background Information
Many substances can produce effects of delayed mobility and failure to thrive. Cocaine can produce cerebral hemorrhage, infarction, and genitourinary problems.[25] Narcotics such as heroin may cause gastrointestinal disturbances, sweating, and tremors. Excessive alcohol ingestion can lead to fetal alcohol syndrome. Legal drugs/medications taken by a mother can lead to congenital birth defects, dysmorphic features, and developmental sequelae. Frequently the number of anomalies correlates with the severity of cognitive impairment.[26] A variety of malformations are associated with the use of anticonvulsant medications. For example, one common anticonvulsant drug is associated with malformations in the neural tube, skeletal/limbs, head and neck, and skin/muscles.[1]

MENINGITIS
■ **Bacterial**

Chief Clinical Characteristics
This presentation includes headache, fever, sore throat, vomiting, seizures, confusion, and a stiff neck.

Background Information
This condition frequently follows a respiratory infection and is the leading cause of acute confusional states. Often cranial nerve palsies will be present.

■ **Viral**

Chief Clinical Characteristics
This presentation includes headache, fever, sore throat, vomiting, seizures, confusion, and a stiff neck.

Background Information
This condition is caused by enteric viruses found upon laboratory testing.

METABOLIC BRAIN DISORDERS
GRAY MATTER DISEASES

These diseases are characterized by seizures, failure of cognitive development, retinal disease, myoclonus, and spikes or sharp waves on the electroencephalogram.

■ **Alpers Disease**

Chief Clinical Characteristics
This presentation includes developmental delay, seizures, and failure to thrive. Neurological regression with impaired vision and hearing ensues.[23]

Background Information
This is an autosomal recessive disorder. A combination of gray matter neuronal degeneration and liver failure is characteristic of this disorder. Onset is during the first year of life.

■ **Niemann-Pick Disease**

Chief Clinical Characteristics
This presentation includes problems with feeding, failure to thrive, hepatosplenomegaly, and psychomotor regression. A cherry red macular spot is evident in about 50% of the cases.

Background Information
There are three types of this condition. Types A and B are caused by a deficiency in sphingomyelinase activity. In type A, sphingomyelin accumulates in all tissues, including the brain. The onset is in infancy. In type B, the presentation also includes hepatosplenomegaly without central nervous system involvement. Type C is caused by a defect in cholesterol esterification that leads to decreased sphingomyelinase activity. The early-onset form usually occurs after 2 years, with hepatosplenomegaly and developmental delay followed by ataxia and dementia. The delayed-onset form begins in

childhood with dystonia or cerebellar ataxia. Apraxia of vertical gaze, seizures, spasticity, and dementia then follow. The late-onset form begins in adolescence with similar characteristics as the delayed-onset form but the progression is slower.[23]

WHITE MATTER DISEASES

These diseases are metabolic brain disorders that primarily affect white matter and are characterized by marked motor deficits, including spasticity and slow encephalographic activity.

■ Phenylketonuria

Chief Clinical Characteristics
This presentation includes developmental delays and mental retardation, and other characteristics that include eczema, a musty odor, and seizures if left untreated.[23]

Background Information
This disorder is caused by the body's inability to convert phenylalanine to tyrosine.[23] It is believed that excess phenylalanine or its metabolites contribute to the brain damage in this condition.[27] If tested at birth and dietary treatment is adhered to, there are typically no developmental disabilities.[4]

GRAY AND WHITE MATTER DISEASES

These diseases are metabolic brain disorders that affect both gray and white matter.

■ Mucopolysaccharidosis

Chief Clinical Characteristics
This presentation includes coarse facial features, hepatosplenomegaly, and dysostosis multiplex. Intellectual dysfunction and neurological regression are also characteristic in the majority of these disorders.[23]

Background Information
These disorders are caused by a deficiency in activity of specific lysosomal enzymes responsible for the degradation of mucopolysaccharides. The majority are autosomal recessive.

■ Methylmalonic Aciduria

Chief Clinical Characteristics
This presentation includes acute neonatal ketoacidosis, with lethargy, vomiting, and

profound hypotonia. Additionally, the clinical picture includes mental retardation, seizures, failure to thrive, hypotonia, ataxia, and megaloblastic anemia.

Background Information
Infants with the classic form of the disease (absence of the apoenzyme methylmalonyl-CoA mutase) become symptomatic during the first week of life. This is usually after the onset of protein feedings. However, a large proportion of infants with the persistent (mild) form of this condition are asymptomatic and experience normal growth and mental development.[28]

■ Mitochondrial Disorders (eg, Leigh Syndrome)

Chief Clinical Characteristics
This presentation includes poor feeding, episodes of hypoventilation or apnea, seizures, hypotonia, weakness, cranial nerve dysfunction, disorders of movement such as dystonia, and developmental arrest followed by regression.

Background Information
Onset is usually in infancy or early childhood, but it can occur in the neonatal period. Diagnosis is based on the clinical and magnetic resonance imaging findings, and skin fibroblast culture or muscle biopsy finding.[23]

■ Munchausen Syndrome and Munchausen Syndrome by Proxy

Chief Clinical Characteristics
This presentation typically includes illness or impairment that is oddly difficult to treat, exceedingly rare, fails to follow the usual recovery, and has no organic cause or has an unknown/undetermined etiology. Additionally, caregivers who seem overly interested and involved in meetings with the medical team or completely disinterested are red flags. Clinicians should also be exceedingly cautious and astute at gathering evidence for this diagnosis and should refer patients and parents suspected of this condition to a psychologist for an assessment if suspected.[29]

Background Information
This condition is defined as overmedicalization, frequent and unnecessary medical care,

and caregiver actions or behavior that cause illness/impairment. The phrase *by proxy* identifies the psychopathology in the caregiver and is more likely than Munchausen syndrome (psychopathology in the patient) in the pediatric population.

MYELODYSPLASIAS

■ Meningocele (Spina Bifida Occulta)

Chief Clinical Characteristics
This presentation often includes a dimple or hairy patch on the skin overlying the lesion, which, along with unexplained weakness, may lead one to suspect this diagnosis.

Background Information
This condition is characterized by a lesion of the spinal cord involving membranes or nonfunctional nerves without a skin lesion.

■ Myelomeningocele

Chief Clinical Characteristics
This presentation includes, depending on location of cyst, symptoms ranging from mild weakness and limited bowel/bladder control to complete paraplegia with hydrocephalus.[1]

Background Information
There is a visible lesion involving inadequate skin closure about a cyst containing herniated cerebrospinal fluid and spinal cord. Surgery is indicated immediately within the first few days of life.

■ Myositis Ossificans

Chief Clinical Characteristics
This presentation includes pain, focal swelling, and limited joint range of motion, commonly occurring in the arm or thigh. In the progressive form, the patient presents with painful lumps in the muscle and stiffness in adjacent joints. Symptoms are progressive from proximal to distal.

Background Information
This condition is an aberrant reparative process that causes benign heterotopic ossification of the soft tissue. There are two forms: One can develop in response to a soft tissue injury or in the absence of injury, whereas the other is a progressive form that is an autosomal dominant genetic disorder.

NEUROCUTANEOUS DISORDERS

■ Neurofibromatosis

Chief Clinical Characteristics
This presentation includes existence of several café au lait spots, freckling, or lipoma on the skin by 1 to 3 years of age. Children with this condition may have difficulties with speech, coordination, and learning and may experience seizures.

Background Information
This condition is more likely in school-aged children but may be present at birth. In most affected individuals the course of these growths is benign.[4,14]

■ Tuberous Sclerosis

Chief Clinical Characteristics
This presentation includes delayed mobility with up to 90% of children with this condition demonstrating seizures. Skin abnormalities include depigmented white birthmarks and café au lait spots.

Background Information
This condition involves central nervous system abnormalities (tubers are large areas of disorganized cortex and white matter). Associated conditions include glial tumors, hydrocephalus, and retinal tumors.[1]

■ Osteogenesis Imperfecta

Chief Clinical Characteristics
This presentation involves short stature and growth retardation, blue sclerae, a triangular face shape, and osteopenia/osteoporosis, "brittle bones" that fracture easily with the first fractures occurring at birth or during early development (later in development for less severe forms). Children commonly have progressive bone/joint deformation with bowing of the long bones. Scoliosis may lead to cardiorespiratory compromise in later life.

Background Information
This condition is the most common cause of genetically mediated osteoporosis. Treatment is aimed at fracture and deformity management. Individuals with this condition are also treated with medications to enhance bone mineralization.

DELAYED MOBILITY (CRAWLING AND WALKING), FAILURE TO THRIVE, AND PSYCHOMOTOR DELAY IN A CHILD

PERIPHERAL NEUROPATHIES

■ Hereditary Motor and Sensory Neuropathy Types I and II (Charcot-Marie-Tooth Disease)

Chief Clinical Characteristics

This presentation includes weakness and atrophy of the muscles of the hands and lower leg, foot deformities, and loss of sensation in the feet. It has a slow but variable progression, and a normal life span.[1]

Background Information

This condition is one of the most common forms of peripheral neuropathy in children. It usually presents late in the first decade of life or early in the second decade. This disease causes a slowly progressive demyelination of peripheral Schwann cells. It occurs sporadically or with a dominant, X-linked, or recessive mode of inheritance.[13]

■ Hereditary Motor and Sensory Neuropathy Type III (Dejerine-Sottas Disease)

Chief Clinical Characteristics

This presentation includes delayed motor skills, such as walking. There is distal and truncal weakness. Areflexia may also be present. The presence of enlarged peripheral nerves is detectable by palpation.[27]

Background Information

This condition is a slowly progressive demyelinating disorder that usually has a recessive mode of inheritance. Onset is typically in infancy or childhood with severe disability by the third decade of life.[13]

■ Peroxisomal Disorders (Zellweger Syndrome)

Chief Clinical Characteristics

This presentation involves facial characteristics such as prominent forehead, epicanthal folds, low nasal bridge, anteverted nostrils, and narrow upper lip; also hepatomegaly, seizures, hypotonia, renal cysts, patellar stippled calcifications, visual problems (cataract, optic nerve hypoplasia, glaucoma), and lack of psychomotor development.[23]

Background Information

This condition is caused by mutations in genes involved in peroxisome biogenesis, leading to a decrease in the number or structure of peroxisomes.

■ Pervasive Developmental Disabilities

Chief Clinical Characteristics

This presentation includes delayed motor skills. Stereotypic body movements such as arm flapping, rocking, or hand wringing impede typical movement. Early play skills and social development are often affected and are atypical for the child's age.

Background Information

This condition encompasses a large spectrum of disabilities, including autism, that have an impact on social and cognitive development as well as speech/language skills and relating to people and objects. A referral to occupational therapy is typical for children with this condition because they will have impairments in social skills, self-help skills, activities of daily living, and hygiene maintenance.[4]

■ Poliomyelitis

Chief Clinical Characteristics

This presentation includes headache, nausea, vomiting, and soreness/stiffness in the posterior muscles of the neck, trunk, and limbs. Other signs and symptoms include muscle atrophy, joint pain, progressive weakness, and progressive skeletal deformity.

Background Information

Acute infection from the poliovirus causes a wide range of illness from none at all to severe paralysis and death. It is extremely rare in countries where a vaccination is available. Postpolio syndrome involves diffuse weakness or paralysis of the muscles that were affected in the initial poliovirus attack.

■ Psychoses

Chief Clinical Characteristics

This presentation includes inappropriate affect, poor behavioral control, a thought disorder, disturbed social relating ability, and auditory or visual hallucinations.

Background Information

This condition can lead to developmental delays and a decrease in cognitive function. It represents a severe disturbance in mental functioning that involves changes in cognition, perception, mood, impulse control, and reality testing.[23]

SEIZURE DISORDERS
▪ Infantile Spasms
Chief Clinical Characteristics
This presentation occurs in clusters of four or five and looks like jack-knifing jolts in which the trunk bends forward at the waist. Occurs primarily during periods of drowsiness or when arousing from sleep. This condition is characterized by abnormal electroencephalograms. Seizures cause a disturbance in development, causing difficulties with maintaining consciousness, and in cases with muscular involvement, interfere with the child's ability to attain motor skills.

Background Information
This condition begins around 4 to 8 months of age. Neurodevelopmental arrest or regression of skills is common. This condition is commonly treated with an intramuscular injection of adrenocorticotropic hormone.[1]

▪ Lennox-Gastaut Syndrome
Chief Clinical Characteristics
This presentation involves an atypical form of absence epilepsy characterized by diffuse slow spike waves often with atonic, tonic, or clonic seizures and mental retardation that persist into adulthood. It is characterized by abnormal electroencephalograms. Seizures cause a disturbance in development, causing difficulties with maintaining consciousness, and in cases with muscular involvement, interfere with the child's ability to attain motor skills.

Background Information
This condition often affects children with a history of infantile spasm. This condition begins between 1 and 8 years of age.[1]

▪ Sensory Integrative Dysfunction
Chief Clinical Characteristics
This presentation includes hyper- or hyposensitivity to movement (movement avoiders vs. movement seekers) or excessive falls that occur for no apparent reason, creating delays in walking. Children with this condition may have difficulty processing stimuli related to movement (ie, vestibular, tactile, and proprioceptive information), may have difficulty with coordination and body awareness, and may appear to have low muscle tone. Additionally, depending on their deficits in sensory processing, these children will develop compensatory behaviors. Children with this condition attempt to avoid movement, seek excessive movement, or, when they are not able to compensate, cry excessively.

Background Information
A major reason why children with this condition are referred to rehabilitation is that they are demonstrating adverse social behaviors such as self-injurious behaviors (eg, head banging, biting), or they may injure others for no apparent reason (eg, biting, hitting) or may have difficulty feeding or difficulty with activities of daily living and self-care (eg, sleeping, brushing teeth, brushing hair, bath time, dressing).[4]

SEX CHROMOSOMAL OR SEX-LINKED SYNDROMES
▪ Rett Syndrome
Chief Clinical Characteristics
This presentation includes apparent typical development in the first year or two of life, followed by a progressive decline in motor skills and the emergence of stereotypic hand movements (hand wringing/mouthing being most common), seen almost exclusively in females.

Background Information
Evidence has shown that the child with this condition may not be typically developing at birth.[30]

▪ Turner Syndrome (45XO)
Chief Clinical Characteristics
This presentation affects females and characteristics may include transient congenital lymphedema, short stature evident at birth, web-like appearance of the lateral neck, underdeveloped gonads, hearing impairments, learning disabilities, poor coordination, low muscle tone, deficits in visuospatial organization, and poor social awareness and nonverbal problem solving.[1]

Background Information

Turner syndrome is a sex-linked condition in females that involves a missing or partially missing X chromosome. This condition can be diagnosed at any time during the life span, but workup is common in childhood. Workup may include genetic testing and karyotyping. Additional blood tests and imaging may be necessary to characterize the extent of structural abnormalities of organs related to Turner syndrome, such as the heart and reproductive organs.

SPINAL MUSCULAR ATROPHIES

■ Acute Werdnig-Hoffmann Disease (Infantile, Type I)

Chief Clinical Characteristics

This presentation includes muscular weakness that occurs within the first 4 months of life. Primary impairments include contractures, talipes equinovarus, or other intrauterine deformities secondary to limited fetal movement. Also reported are muscle fasciculations.

Background Information

Secondary impairments include scoliosis and contractures, decreased respiratory capacity/respiratory distress and low endurance.[3] The pathology is an abnormality of the large anterior horn cells of the spinal cord. The number of cells is reduced, and there is progressive degeneration of the remaining cells leading to muscle weakness and loss of function.

■ Chronic Werdnig-Hoffmann Disease (Intermediate, Type II)

Chief Clinical Characteristics

This presentation includes onset of significant weakness that appears within the first year. Proximal muscles are affected most. Weakness is usually greatest in the hip and knee extensors and trunk musculature.

Background Information

Involvement of the distal musculature appears later in the course of the disease and is less severe than proximal involvement. The course of the disease is highly variable.[31] Contractures are not as common as in acute forms of this condition. Motor milestones are usually delayed due to

muscle weakness and reduced respiratory capacity.[3] The pathology is an abnormality of the large anterior horn cells of the spinal cord. The number of cells is reduced, and there is progressive degeneration of the remaining cells, leading to muscle weakness and loss of function.

■ Kugelberg-Welander Disease (Juvenile, Type III)

Chief Clinical Characteristics

This presentation includes muscle weakness that may appear within the first year of life in the proximal hip and shoulder girdle musculature. Typically, however, the onset of weakness occurs later in the first decade.[3] The most common impairment is proximal lower extremity weakness.

Background Information

Secondary impairments include postural compensations resulting from muscle weakness, contractures, and occasionally scoliosis.[32] The pathology is an abnormality of the large anterior horn cells of the spinal cord. The number of cells is reduced, and there is progressive degeneration of the remaining cells leading to muscle weakness and loss of function.

TUMORS

■ Astrocytoma

Chief Clinical Characteristics

This presentation includes visual disturbances, ataxia, and seizures. May also present with symptoms of increased intracranial pressure, such as the following in infants: bulging fontanelle, separated sutures, lethargy, and vomiting. In older children and adults, the presentation may involve vomiting, persistent headache, blurred vision, changes in behavior, progressive lethargy or decreased consciousness, neurological deficits, and seizures.

Background Information

This condition typically occurs in the cerebellar or supratentorial regions.[33]

■ Brainstem Glioma

Chief Clinical Characteristics

This presentation includes early signs and symptoms of progressive cranial nerve dysfunction and gait disorders.

Background Information
Typically prognosis for this condition is poor.

■ Craniopharyngioma

Chief Clinical Characteristics
This presentation includes visual disturbances, headaches, vomiting, and endocrine disturbances.

Background Information
Occurs primarily in the midline suprasellar region.[33]

■ Ependymoma

Chief Clinical Characteristics
This presentation includes seizures and focal cerebellar deficits. This condition may also present with symptoms of increased intracranial pressure, such as the following in infants: bulging fontanel, separated sutures, lethargy, and vomiting. In older children and adults, the presentation may involve vomiting, persistent headache, blurred vision, changes in behavior, progressive lethargy or decreased consciousness, neurological deficits, and seizures.

Background Information
This tumor occurs in the posterior fossa and cerebral hemispheres.[33]

■ Medulloblastoma

Chief Clinical Characteristics
This presentation includes ataxia and intracranial pressure as early signs. Symptoms of increased intracranial pressure include the following in infants: bulging fontanel, separated sutures, lethargy, and vomiting. In older children and adults, the presentation may involve vomiting, persistent headache, blurred vision, changes in behavior, progressive lethargy or decreased consciousness, neurological deficits, and seizures.

Background Information
This tumor occurs predominantly in the cerebellum. It can metastasize to the meninges and outside of the central nervous system.[33]

■ Neuroblastoma

Chief Clinical Characteristics
This presentation includes pain, abdominal mass, or persistent diarrhea.

Background Information
Some of these tumors regress spontaneously. This tumor develops in the neural crest cells anywhere in the sympathetic nervous system, but typically in the adrenal glands or paraspinal ganglion.[33]

■ Syringomyelia

Chief Clinical Characteristics
This presentation includes back pain; headaches; stiffness; weakness or pain in the back, shoulders, arms, or legs; and the loss of the ability to feel extremes of hot or cold. Neurological or cord signs may be present.

Background Information
This condition is caused by the formation of a cyst or syrinx that arises in the spinal cord and expands over time, damaging the cord. The condition may lie dormant for many years following a traumatic event to the spine. An Arnold-Chiari malformation may be associated with this condition.

References

1. Long T, Toscano K. *Handbook of Pediatric Physical Therapy.* 2nd ed. Philadelphia, PA: Lippincott Williams & Wilkins; 2001.
2. Shumway-Cook A, Woollacott MH. *Motor Control: Theory and Practical Applications.* Baltimore, MD: Williams & Wilkins; 1995.
3. Campbell S, Palisano RJ, Vander Linden DW. *Physical Therapy for Children.* 3rd ed. Philadelphia, PA: W. B. Saunders; 2000.
4. Case-Smith J, Allen A, Pratt PN. *Occupational Therapy for Children.* 3rd ed. St. Louis: Mosby-Year Book; 1996.
5. Good WV, Jan JE, DeSa L, Barkovich AJ, Groenveld M, Hoyt CS. Cortical visual impairment in children. *Surv Ophthalmol.* Jan–Feb 1994;38(4):351–364.
6. Shenaq SM, Kim JY, Armenta AH, Nath RK, Cheng E, Jedrysiak A. The surgical treatment of obstetric brachial plexus palsy. *Plast Reconstr Surg.* Apr 14, 2004; 113(4):54E–67E.
7. Vander Salm TJ, Cereda JM, Cutler BS. Brachial plexus injury following median sternotomy. *J Thorac Cardiovasc Surg.* Sep 1980;80(3):447–452.
8. Antshel KM, Conchelos J, Lanzetta G, Fremont W, Kates WR. Behavior and corpus callosum morphology relationships in velocardiofacial syndrome (22q11.2 deletion syndrome). *Psychiatry Res.* Apr 30 2005; 138(3):235–245.
9. Brown WS, Paul LK, Symington M, Dietrich R. Comprehension of humor in primary agenesis of the corpus callosum. *Neuropsychologia.* 2005;43(6):906–916.
10. Field M, Ashton R, White K. Agenesis of the corpus callosum: report of two pre-school children and review of the literature. *Dev Med Child Neurol.* Feb 1978; 20(1):47–61.
11. Huber-Okrainec J, Blaser SE, Dennis M. Idiom comprehension deficits in relation to corpus callosum agenesis

and hypoplasia in children with spina bifida meningomyelocele. *Brain Lang.* Jun 2005;93(3):349–368.

12. Saul RE, Biersner RJ. Spatial and visuomotor performance with agenesis of the corpus callosum. *Neurol Neurocir Psiquiatr.* 1977;18(2–3 suppl):105–113.

13. Simon RP, Aminoff MJ, Greenberg DA. *Clinical Neurology.* 4th ed. Stamford, CT: Appleton & Lange; 1999.

14. Smith DW, Jones KL. *Recognizable Patterns of Human Malformation: Genetic, Embryologic and Clinical Aspects.* 3rd ed. Philadelphia, PA: W. B. Saunders; 1982.

15. Saukkonen AL, Serlo W, von Wendt L. Epilepsy in hydrocephalic children. *Acta Paediatr Scand.* Feb 1990; 79(2):212–218.

16. Howie JM. Cerebral palsy. In: Campbell SK, ed. *Decision Making in Pediatric Neurologic Physical Therapy.* New York, NY: Churchill Livingston; 1999.

17. Bax MC. Terminology and classification of cerebral palsy. *Dev Med Child Neurol.* Jun 1964;6:295–297.

18. MacLusky IB, Levison H. Cystic fibrosis. In: Chernick V, Thomas F, Kendig BL, Kendig EL, eds. *Kendig's Disorders of the Respiratory Tract in Children.* 6th ed. Philadelphia, PA: W. B. Saunders; 1998:838–882.

19. Greenberg DA, Aminoff MJ, Simon RP. *Clinical Neurology.* 5th ed. New York, NY: McGraw-Hill/ Appleton & Lange; 2002.

20. Gilbert S, Wiedel J. *The Treatment of Hemophilia: Current Orthopedic Management.* New York, NY: National Hemophilia Foundation; 1995.

21. Allen MC. The high-risk infant. *Pediatr Clin North Am.* Jun 1993;40(3):479–490.

22. Warshaw JB. Intrauterine growth retardation: adaptation or pathology? *Pediatrics.* Dec 1985;76(6):998–999.

23. Bellet PS. *The Diagnostic Approach to Symptoms and Signs in Pediatrics.* 2nd ed. Philadelphia, PA: Lippincott Williams & Wilkins; 2002.

24. Tachdijan MO. *Pediatric Orthopaedics.* 2nd ed. Philadelphia, PA: Elsevier Health Sciences; 1972.

25. Merenstein GB, Kaplan DW, Rosenberg AA. *Handbook of Pediatrics.* 18th ed. New York, NY: McGraw-Hill; 1996.

26. Jones KL. *Smith's Recognizable Patterns of Human Malformations.* 4th ed. Philadelphia, PA: W. B. Saunders; 1988.

27. Cotran RS, Kumar V, Robbins SL, Schoen FJ. *Pathologic Basis of Disease.* 5th ed. Philadelphia, PA: W. B. Saunders; 1994.

28. Menkes JH, Sarnat HB. *Child Neurology.* 6th ed. Philadelphia, PA: Lippincott Williams & Wilkins; 2000.

29. Bursch B. Pediatric illness falsification: a new look at Munchausen by proxy. *Grand rounds presentation at Children's Hospital of Orange County;* 2005.

30. Leonard H, Bower C. Is the girl with Rett syndrome normal at birth? *Dev Med Child Neurol.* Feb 1998; 40(2):115–121.

31. Namba T, Aberfeld DC, Grob D. Chronic proximal spinal muscular atrophy. *J Neurol Sci.* Nov 1970; 11(5):401–423.

32. Dorsher PT, Sinaki M, Mulder DW, Litchy WJ, Ilstrup DM. Wohlfart-Kugelberg-Welander syndrome: serum creatine kinase and functional outcome. *Arch Phys Med Rehabil.* Jul 1991;72(8):587–591.

33. Tecklin JS. *Pediatric Physical Therapy.* 3rd ed. Philadelphia, PA: Lippincott Williams & Wilkins; 1998.

CHAPTER 53

The Child With a Painless Limp

■ *Hugh G. Watts, MD*

Description of the Symptom

A limp can be defined as any deviation, commonly asymmetric, from a normal gait pattern, and may be caused centrally, as a result of cerebral dysfunction, or peripherally, due to weakness or pain in the trunk or lower extremities.

This chapter describes possible causes of a limp in a child.

Special Concerns
■ Suspicion of child abuse
■ Associated with fever

CHAPTER PREVIEW: Conditions That May Lead to a Painless Limp in a Child

T Trauma

COMMON

Slipped femoral capital epiphyses 1051

UNCOMMON

Child abuse 1042
Chondral injury of the hip 1042
Tear of the acetabular labrum 1052
Toddler's fracture of the tibia 1052

RARE

Not applicable

I Inflammation

COMMON

Not applicable

UNCOMMON

Aseptic
Juvenile rheumatoid arthritis 1045
Juvenile rheumatoid arthritis–like diseases:
• Arthritis associated with inflammatory bowel disease 1046
• Dermatomyositis 1046
• Juvenile ankylosing spondylitis 1046
• Scleroderma 1047

Septic
Not applicable

(continued)

Inflammation (continued)

RARE

Aseptic
Ataxia telangiectasia 1042
Demyelinating polyradiculoneuropathies:
- Acute demyelinating polyradiculoneuropathy (Guillain-Barré syndrome) 1043
- Chronic demyelinating polyradiculoneuropathy 1043
Juvenile rheumatoid arthritis–like diseases:
- Polymyositis 1047
- Reactive arthritis (Reiter's syndrome) 1047
- Systemic lupus erythematosus 1047

Septic
Poliomyelitis 1050

M Metabolic

COMMON
Not applicable

UNCOMMON
Not applicable

RARE
Ehlers-Danlos syndrome 1045
Lesch-Nyhan syndrome 1048

Va Vascular

COMMON
Osteochondritis dissecans of the knee 1050

UNCOMMON
Legg-Calvé-Perthes disease 1048

RARE
Not applicable

De Degenerative

COMMON
Not applicable

UNCOMMON
Not applicable

RARE
Chondrolysis 1043
Friedreich's ataxia 1045
Muscular dystrophies:
- Becker muscular dystrophy 1049
- Duchenne muscular dystrophy 1049
Spinal muscular atrophies:
- Kugelberg-Welander disease (juvenile, type III) 1051

Tu Tumor

COMMON

Not applicable

UNCOMMON

Malignant Primary:
Not applicable
Malignant Metastatic:
Not applicable
Benign, such as:
• Syringomyelia 1054

RARE

Malignant Primary, such as:
• Leukemia 1053
Malignant Metastatic:
Not applicable
Benign, such as:
• Bone cysts of the lower extremity:
  • Aneurysmal 1052
  • Unicameral 1052
• Eosinophilic granuloma (Langerhans' cell histiocytosis) 1053
• Fibrous dysplasia 1053
• Osteochondroma 1053
• Trevor's disease (dysplasia epiphysealis hemimelica) 1054

Co Congenital

COMMON

Leg-length discrepancy 1047
Myelodysplasia 1049

UNCOMMON

Arthrogryposis:
• Amyoplasia (arthrogryposis multiplex congenita) 1041
• Distal arthrogryposis 1041
Limb deficiencies:
• Congenital deficiency of the tibia 1048
• Congenital short femur 1048
Myopathies, congenital 1049

RARE

Coxa vara, congenital 1043
Developmental dysplasia of the hip with dislocation 1043
Discoid lateral meniscus 1044
Dislocated patella, congenital 1044
Dysplasias of bone and cartilage:
• Epiphyseal dysplasia 1044
• Metabolic chondrodysplasia 1044
• Morquio's syndrome 1044
• Spondyloepiphyseal dysplasia 1044
Larsen's syndrome 1047

Ne Neurogenic/Psychogenic

COMMON

Cerebral palsy 1042
Encephalopathy (postencephalitis, postmeningitis, post-traumatic) 1045
Post–central nervous system vascular insufficiency or hemorrhage 1051

UNCOMMON

Spinal dysraphisms:
• Diastematomyelia 1051
• Tethered cord syndrome 1051

RARE

Malingering 1048
Myotonia congenita 1050
Peripheral neuropathies:
• Hereditary motor and sensory neuropathies Types I and II (Charcot-Marie-Tooth disease) 1050
• Hereditary motor and sensory neuropathy Type III (Dejerine-Sottas disease) 1050

Note: These are estimates of relative incidence because few data are available for the less common conditions.

Common Ages at Which Conditions Resulting in a Painless Limp Present in a Child

APPROXIMATE AGE	CONDITION
Birth to 3 Years	Cerebral palsy
	Child abuse
	Coxa vara, congenital
	Developmental dysplasia with hip dislocation
	Dysplasias of bone and cartilage
	Juvenile rheumatoid arthritis
	Leg-length discrepancy
	Lesch-Nyhan syndrome
	Spinal muscular atrophy
	Toddler's fracture
Preschool (3–5 Years)	Cerebral palsy
	Child abuse
	Coxa vara, congenital
	Developmental dysplasia with hip dislocation
	Dysraphisms
	Juvenile rheumatoid arthritis
	Leg-length discrepancy
	Lesch-Nyhan syndrome
	Leukemia
	Spinal muscular atrophy
	Syringomyelia
	Toddler's fracture
Elementary School (6–11 Years)	Cerebral palsy
	Child abuse
	Dysraphisms
	Ehlers-Danlos syndrome
	Juvenile rheumatoid arthritis
	Leg-length discrepancy

Common Ages at Which Conditions Resulting in a Painless Limp Present in a Child—cont'd

APPROXIMATE AGE	CONDITION
	Legg-Calvé-Perthes disease
	Leukemia
	Lupus
	Osteochondritis dissecans of the knee
	Spinal muscular atrophy
	Syringomyelia
Middle School (12–14 Years)	Cerebral palsy
	Chondral injury of the hip
	Chondrolysis of the hip
	Dysraphisms
	Ehlers-Danlos syndrome
	Juvenile rheumatoid arthritis
	Leg-length discrepancy
	Lupus
	Osteochondritis dissecans of the knee
	Slipped capital femoral epiphysis
	Spinal muscular atrophy
	Syringomyelia
High School (15–18 Years)	Cerebral palsy
	Chondrolysis
	Ehlers-Danlos syndrome
	Leg-length discrepancy
	Osteochondritis dissecans of the knee
	Slipped capital femoral epiphysis
	Spinal muscular atrophy
	Syringomyelia

Overview of a Painless Limp in a Child

Although pain is a major cause of limping, the presence of pain will usually lead to the source of the problem. However, there are a number of reasons why a child may limp without pain. A limp may alter the mechanics of walking sufficiently so that a child does not recognize the association with the limp. The painful event that precipitated the need for a limp may have been sufficiently distant in time so that the parents or child may not associate the two, as is common with Legg-Calvé-Perthes disease. The child may be afraid to report pain. Ordinarily one would expect that child abuse leading to a limp would be accompanied by pain. If, however, the child is sufficiently afraid of the abuser, the child may deny pain, which might, inappropriately, put to rest an examiner's suspicions.

When attempting to diagnose the cause of a painless limp in a child, the child must be sufficiently developed to be able to walk; furthermore, the child must not be bedridden.

The history, usually from a parent, is often uncertain. The history of prior trauma, especially in the young child under about 6 or 7 years of age, may often be a red herring since children of that age frequently fall, unrelated to the etiology of the limp.

To walk successfully, a child must achieve two important goals: stability during the stance phase (so that the child doesn't collapse and fall) and an efficiency of gait so as to expend as little energy as possible. An additional goal is to achieve the motion in as cosmetically appealing a manner as possible.

Causes of Limping

There are four primary reasons (or combinations of these reasons) for limping: to reduce pain; to compensate for muscle weakness; to accommodate deformity in the extremities or trunk; and as a result of central nervous system dysfunction.

Reduce Pain

Most commonly, pain reduction is achieved by decreasing the time that pain is felt. This is done by shortening the stance time—a gait pattern often called an *antalgic gait*. An antalgic gait is most readily seen in someone who has a stone in a shoe.

Another strategy to reduce pain is to decrease the need for the use of a painful muscle. A common example is the forward lean in midstance after quadriceps trauma. The forward lean brings the center of gravity anterior to the knee axis, which results in a stable knee in midstance without the use of the quadriceps (Fig. 53-1).

The use of the word *strategy* or *technique* implies conscious effort. However, these mechanisms are entirely unconscious.

Yet another technique for reduction of pain is to decrease the forces on a painful joint by decreasing the muscle pull across the joint. This is characteristically seen in the sideways lean during stance toward the affected side when the hip is painful, as seen in a child with Legg-Calvé-Perthes disease or with a slipped capital femoral epiphysis.

Compensate for Muscle Weakness

In the same way that a child might lean forward in stance to reduce the need to use a painful quadriceps, a weak quadriceps might require that a child lean forward in stance so that the knee will not collapse with weight bearing. This is a common observation in children who have had poliomyelitis.

Conversely, a child will lean backward during stance if the gluteus maximus is weak, as is usually seen in a child with myelodysplasia. Children with generalized weakness, as seen in

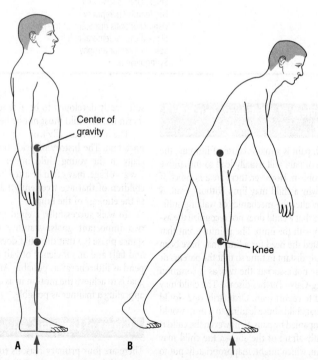

FIGURE 53-1 (A) Normal alignment of the knee in midstance. (B) If the quadriceps is painful for any reason, by leaning forward the floor reaction force falls anterior to the knee joint reducing the need for the quadriceps in midstance. This is the common limp seen in a "Charlie horse."

Duchenne muscular dystrophy, have to develop a complex balance pattern to compensate for both quadriceps and gluteus maximus weakness. To do that, the child must thrust the pelvis anteriorly so that the knees do not collapse into flexion, while at the same time extending the trunk posteriorly so that the hips do not collapse into flexion (Fig. 53-2).

Other strategies may be used to compensate for muscle weakness: A child may externally rotate the leg so that the knee axis is out of alignment with the line of progression, which will allow for stability in the knee in midstance with a weakened quadriceps muscle. With a weak gastrocnemius, a child may externally rotate the leg to permit a longer stride length to compensate for the lack of push-off at end-stance.

Accommodate a Deformity

A child may readily develop ankle equinus or an early heel-rise at end-stance to compensate for a short leg. A child with genu valgum, such as a child with Morquio's syndrome, will have to walk with the feet wide apart. This requires the child to adopt a waddling lean to the side in stance in order to get the weight over the foot that is in contact with the floor. Similarly, a child with very fat thighs may walk with the same bilateral sideways lean.

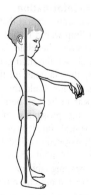

FIGURE 53-2 This child with Duchenne muscular dystrophy has developed a complex balance pattern to compensate for both quadriceps and gluteus maximus weakness; that is, the child thrusts the pelvis anteriorly so that the knees do not collapse into flexion, while at the same time extending the trunk posteriorly so that the hips do not collapse into flexion.

Central Nervous System Dysfunction

Efficient walking requires coordination and muscle control. Children with central nervous system disease such as cerebral palsy or post-traumatic encephalopathy commonly have an abnormal gait. Children who have disease of the cerebellum such as Friedreich's ataxia or a posterior fossa brain tumor will have trouble with their gait because of altered balance. Spinal cord pathology that is degenerative, as in spinal muscular atrophy, or post-traumatic paraplegia may also cause gait abnormalities.

Therefore, in assessing a child with a painless limp, it is important initially to examine the gait pattern carefully and reason out why the child walks the way he or she does.

Descriptions of Conditions That May Lead to a Painless Limp in a Child

ARTHROGRYPOSIS

■ Amyoplasia (Arthrogryposis Multiplex Congenita)

Chief Clinical Characteristics
This presentation is characterized by multiple joint contractures with muscle weakness or imbalance. The features of this condition are variable and while usually involving all four extremities, children with only upper extremity or only lower extremity involvement are not uncommon. The most common findings include rigid joints with significant contractures; featureless, cylindrical extremities that lack skin creases; atrophy or absence of muscle groups; diminished or absent deep tendon reflexes; and dislocations of joints with the hip being the most common. Sensation is intact.

Background Information
This is a nonprogressive disorder that is evident at birth and is not hereditary.

■ Distal Arthrogryposis

Chief Clinical Characteristics
This presentation is characterized by multiple joint contractures with muscle weakness or imbalance that involve the hands and feet.

Background Information
This condition is hereditary. Management is largely focused on enhancing the child's

functions through physical and occupational therapy.[1]

■ Ataxia Telangiectasia

Chief Clinical Characteristics

This presentation usually includes ataxia with an unsteady, clumsy gait. Dilated blood vessels (ie, telangiectasias) usually on the white portion of the conjunctiva of the eye usually occur after the onset of the ataxia, generally between 2 and 8 years of age. Telangiectasias may also be found on the ears, neck, and extremities.

Background Information

This condition is a progressive primary immune deficiency disease that involves loss of Purkinje cells in the cerebellar cortex; degeneration of neurons in the cerebral cortex, basal ganglia, brainstem, and anterior horns of the spinal cord; and later dilated blood vessels. Because of the immune deficiency the child has an increased susceptibility to infections and an increased risk for developing certain cancers, particularly cancers of the immune system, such as lymphoma and leukemia. It is inherited as an autosomal recessive trait. The treatment is largely supportive.[2]

■ Cerebral Palsy

Chief Clinical Characteristics

This presentation includes toe walking and an awkward gait. There may be a history of frequent tripping or falling. These features of mild spastic cerebral palsy can be exaggerated by asking the child to run. At that point, the awkwardness of gait becomes more evident, together with upper extremity posturing especially with scapular retraction and elbow flexion. Deep tendon reflexes are exaggerated, and the upper extremity "slap test" is positive. A history of prematurity or birth difficulties together with a history of poor performance at school can provide further clues.

Background Information

A child with a painless limp due to cerebral palsy is most likely to have a mild spastic variety of this condition, either hemiplegic or diplegic, because the other forms are usually very obvious by the age of walking. A number of other brain disorders in children are either included in many people's minds within the broad diagnostic category of cerebral palsy or

are sufficiently similar that the children are treated as if they had cerebral palsy. Such conditions are encephalopathies following meningitis or encephalitis or traumatic brain injuries and those due to an infantile central nervous system vascular insufficiency or hemorrhage. Some congenital conditions such as cerebellar ataxia or absent corpus callosum may fall into the same category. The presentation of these conditions will be the same as that seen in children with cerebral palsy, but a history of traumatic brain injury, meningitis or encephalitis, or high fever, especially with seizures during infancy or a history of seizures, may provide evidence for these other conditions that simulate cerebral palsy.

■ Child Abuse

Chief Clinical Characteristics

This presentation involves bruises that appear to have different dates of occurrence— some that are blue-black while others are yellowish or greenish. Do the bruises suggest finger or hand marks left behind by a vigorous slap? Does the child raise his arm as if to protect himself from a blow when you approach? For the school-age child, has there been a change in behavior at school, a change in academic performance, or frequent absences that are unexplained?

Background Information

Ordinarily one would expect that child abuse leading to a limp would be accompanied by pain. If, however, the child is sufficiently afraid of the abuser, the child may deny pain, easily putting the examiner off the appropriate track of suspicion. Child abuse can happen in what appear to be "the best" of families. Overlooking the possibility of abuse may mean that the next time it happens, the child may be badly maimed or killed. Question the details of any story that involves trauma—a fall off of a changing table or a fall down the stairs. One does not need to sound accusatory while doing so.

■ Chondral Injury of the Hip

Chief Clinical Characteristics

This presentation includes reports of intermittent locking with hip motion. There may or may not be pain.

Background Information

This presentation is frequently associated with a jumping or twisting mechanism. Surgery may be indicated if conservative management does not alleviate symptoms.[3]

■ Chondrolysis

Chief Clinical Characteristics

This presentation may include reports of intermittent locking with hip motion. There may or may not be pain.

Background Information

Surgery may be indicated if nonsurgical management does not alleviate symptoms.[3]

■ Coxa Vara, Congenital

Chief Clinical Characteristics

This presentation involves an abductor lurch (gluteus medius gait), some limb shortening, and proximal location of the greater trochanter of the femur. The physical findings may simulate a dislocated hip; however, the hip motion will be normal and there will be no laxity of the femoral head within the acetabulum.

Background Information

In congenital coxa vara, the neck of the femur makes less than the expected 135-degree angle with the shaft of the femur. The etiology is not known. It is usually not recognized until the child is 2 or 3 years of age. The varus results in a proximal location of the greater trochanter that puts the abductor muscle of the hip at a disadvantage, resulting in the abductor lurch. If left untreated, the condition usually worsens. Treatment is surgical—an osteotomy of the proximal femur to realign the normal neck shaft angle.

DEMYELINATING POLYRADICULONEUROPATHIES

■ Acute Demyelinating Polyradiculoneuropathy (Guillain-Barré Syndrome)

Chief Clinical Characteristics

This presentation involves a rapidly progressing lower motor neuron disease with ascending weakness and muscle pain.[4] Symptoms and signs are usually symmetrical, progressing over days or weeks. Severity may range from mild weakness to complete tetraplegia and

ventilatory failure. Peak deficits are usually reached by 4 weeks, and recovery usually begins 2 to 4 weeks after progression ceases. Leg pain often precedes symptoms of weakness.[5]

Background Information

Prodromal symptoms or events such as gastroenteritis, upper respiratory infection, surgery, or immunization 1 to 4 weeks prior to weakness may be reported.[6] This condition can rapidly progress to respiratory failure in acute stages if not treated. The condition is more common in males. Intravenous human immunoglobulin has been shown to be the most effective medical therapy but plasma exchange and corticosteroids are also utilized. Most children with this condition require extensive rehabilitation to regain strength and restore function.

■ Chronic Demyelinating Polyradiculoneuropathy

Chief Clinical Characteristics

This presentation involves a rapidly progressing lower motor neuron disease with ascending weakness and muscle pain,[4] similar to Guillain-Barré syndrome, but with a subacute onset over at least 2 months.[7]

Background Information

Treatment is also similar to that administered for Guillain-Barré syndrome. The course of disease is progressive in nature. The type of gait depends on the location of weakness and on the degree of proprioceptive loss. Children with this condition often have more profound gait abnormalities than adults.

■ Developmental Dysplasia of the Hip with Dislocation

Chief Clinical Characteristics

This presentation commonly involves a painless limp characterized by an abductor lurch (gluteus medius gait) and an increased lumbar lordosis. The range of motion of the affected hip is limited primarily in abduction. The greater trochanter is located proximal to Nélaton's line (ie, anterior superior iliac spine to ischial tuberosity). The femoral shortening that results from the dislocation may give a short leg component to the gait as well as asymmetry of the skinfolds of the medial thigh. When both hips are dislocated, these features are not evident.

Background Information
While the term *developmental dysplasia of the hip* spans a spectrum of conditions from mild subluxation of the hip in a newborn to the dislocation of one or both hips in a child, the nondislocated forms are not associated with a painless limp. Untreated hip dislocations may lead to permanent hip deformities or osteoarthritis.[8]

Discoid Lateral Meniscus

Chief Clinical Characteristics
This presentation may be asymptomatic; however, if torn, the child will present with symptoms indicative of a torn meniscus: pain, edema, and locking without any history of an injury. Commonly the patient reports an audible click or snapping, together with tenderness over the joint line together with a palpable "popping" over the joint line with knee flexion and extension. The child may report having a dull, aching pain, with the knee locking or giving way.

Background Information
A discoid meniscus is an abnormally shaped meniscus that is thicker and covers more of the tibial plateau than normal. The lateral meniscus is most commonly affected.[9]

Dislocated Patella, Congenital

Chief Clinical Characteristics
This presentation typically includes a fixed flexion contracture of the knee with the patella laterally placed and genu valgum, together with external rotation of the tibia.

Background Information
This condition is a rare condition that may occur in isolation or with syndromes such as nail-patella syndrome or Down syndrome. There are two groups of patients, one with a fixed dislocation at birth, and the other in whom the patella is normally located at birth, but progressively subluxates until it is in a fixed dislocated position. Diagnosis is generally not made until after walking age. There is increasing disability with age, especially weakness when climbing stairs, although the knee is painless. Treatment is surgical.[10]

DYSPLASIAS OF BONE AND CARTILAGE

Epiphyseal Dysplasia

Chief Clinical Characteristics
The presentation of this epiphyseal pathology commonly includes a waddling gait, short extremities, and joint pain. Joints are commonly affected symmetrically; the knee and hip are most commonly affected.

Background Information
The two types of epiphyseal dysplasia are the Fairbank and Ribbing types. The presentation in the Fairbank-type dysplasia involves more severe limb deformities, limping, and pain.[11] The Ribbing-type dysplasia is usually milder, though it may be difficult to distinguish from symmetrical Legg-Calvé-Perthes with its proximal femur involvement.

Metabolic Chondrodysplasia

Chief Clinical Characteristics
The presentation of this metaphysis pathology can produce hip pain, short/bowed legs, and waddling gait with the Schmid type.[11]

Background Information
This condition is caused by an X-linked chromosomal disorder. Structural abnormalities of the lower extremities and trunk are responsible for observed limping.

Morquio's Syndrome

Chief Clinical Characteristics
This presentation typically involves short stature with severe deformity of the spine and a characteristic prominence of the sternal manubrium, together with long bones with irregular epiphyses, enlarged joints, and flaccid ligaments. There is usually a marked genu valgum, giving a waddling gait.

Background Information
This condition is a genetic disorder of mucopolysaccharide metabolism with excessive urinary keratan sulfate and characterized by skeletal abnormalities, joint instability, and the gradual development of cervical myelopathy.[12]

Spondyloepiphyseal Dysplasia

Chief Clinical Characteristics
This presentation involves a short stature from birth, with a very short trunk and neck

and shortened limbs. The hands and feet are of average size. Kyphoscoliosis and lumbar lordosis progress during childhood. There may be decreased joint range of motion and signs of arthritis in those in their teens. There is a mild flattening of the midface.

Background Information

This condition is an inherited disorder of bone growth that results from a dysfunction of type II collagen synthesis. It is generally divided in the *congenita* and *tarda* forms. *Congenita* is identifiable in the newborn with short stature, disproportionate shortening of the limbs, flattening of the midface, a short neck, and barrel-shaped chest. It is inherited as an autosomal dominant condition. Affected individuals also have abnormalities affecting the eyes including myopia and retina detachment. Most individuals have hypotonia, kyphoscoliosis, excessive lumbar lordosis, and pectus carinatum. Adult height ranges from 3 to 4 feet. The *tarda* form is a much milder condition inherited as an X-linked disorder. There is usually disproportionate trunk shortening, but normal stature is possible. Spinal deformity is common, including scoliosis and increased lumbar lordosis. Hip pain and/or stiffness are common by the teenage years. Angular deformities of the limbs are not common. Radiographic findings include flattened, ovoid vertebral bodies and show a disorganized appearance of the epiphyses. The iliac bones are short. Myopia is common, as is hearing loss. The gravest problem is atlantoaxial instability and requires careful monitoring.[13]

■ Ehlers-Danlos Syndrome

Chief Clinical Characteristics

This presentation includes joint hypermobility that can lead to recurrent hip dislocations and joint effusion in children with this condition.[11]

Background Information

Treatment of ankle and foot consequences from this condition consists of decreasing pressure to the region.[14]

■ Encephalopathy (Postencephalitis, Postmeningitis, Post-Traumatic)

Chief Clinical Characteristics

This presentation is the same as that seen in children with cerebral palsy, but a history of

traumatic brain injury, meningitis or encephalitis, or high fever, especially with seizures during infancy or a history of seizures, may provide evidence for these other conditions that simulate cerebral palsy.

Background Information

Causes of this condition are multiple in children. The pattern of limping will depend on the area of the diencephalon that is affected, but will be caused by a combination of spasticity, sensorimotor, and cognitive deficits consistent with an upper motor neuron lesion.

■ Friedreich's Ataxia

Chief Clinical Characteristics

This presentation involves a child who shows the characteristics of ataxia with the classic signs of cerebellar dysfunction. Severe scoliosis is a frequent association.

Background Information

This condition is a hereditary disease resulting in atrophy and demyelination of the posterior columns of the spinocerebellar and corticospinal tracts of the spinal cord. It is inherited as an autosomal recessive trait with the responsible gene located on chromosome 9. Gait unsteadiness begins between the ages of 5 and 15 and is followed by upper extremity ataxia and dysarthria. Mental capacities often decline. Tremor, if present, is a minor feature. Children with this condition are areflexic and lose large-fiber sensory modalities (vibration and position sense). Progressive foot deformities and cardiomyopathy are common. Gait is wide based due to a combination of ataxia and spasticity.[15]

■ Juvenile Rheumatoid Arthritis

Chief Clinical Characteristics

This presentation may involve a painless limp. The knee is usually the most likely site affected, resulting in mild to moderate swelling. Frequently the parents think that their child's swollen knee is the result of a fall. The limp may be caused by a mild knee flexion contracture. If the problem has been going on for many months, a leg-length discrepancy may result from the overgrowth of the distal femoral physis due to the chronic inflammatory stimulus. To make the diagnosis of juvenile rheumatoid arthritis (JRA), the child must have the presence for 6 or more weeks of swelling of a joint or the presence of two or more of the following: limited joint range of motion, palpable tenderness, painful movement, or joint warmth. Joint stiffness is most marked in the mornings or after a period of inactivity and improves with movement.[11] Children with pauciarticular JRA and especially those with the monarticular variety are prone to develop iridocyclitis, which is diagnosed by slit-lamp examination. The presence of that complication helps to confirm the diagnosis.

Background Information

JRA is one of the most common rheumatic diseases of childhood, and is one of the more frequent chronic illnesses of children. There are three subtypes of JRA: systemic, polyarticular, and pauciarticular. The clinical signs during onset, defined as the first 6 months of the disease, are used to classify three distinct types of presentations: systemic in 10%, polyarticular in 40%, and pauciarticular (or oligoarthritis) in 50%.

Systemic JRA: Also known as Still's disease, systemic JRA can occur insidiously or acutely throughout childhood. It is characterized by high fever, rash (erythematous macules on the trunk and proximal extremities), hepatosplenomegaly, lymphadenopathy, and joint pains, which may lag behind the systemic symptoms by months to years. Additionally, leukocytosis, anemia, pleuritis, pericarditis, osteopenia, delayed growth, hepatosplenomegaly, and lymphadenopathy may be seen.

Polyarticular JRA: This type of JRA involves more than five joints symmetrically and commonly affects knees, ankles, elbows, wrists, cervical spine, and temporomandibular joint, typically with a symmetrical distribution. This type is more common in females.

Pauciarticular JRA: This is the most common subtype, with an insidious onset of swelling, stiffness, and sometimes local pain affecting one to four joints, typically large joints such as knees, hips, ankles, or elbows, often asymmetrically. Inflammation at a knee joint may, over many months, lead to overgrowth in length, giving a leg-length discrepancy of as much as 1 or 2 cm. *Monarticular JRA* is a subtype of the pauciarticular form in which only one joint is involved. These patients report morning stiffness, joint pain, and swelling in the initial stages. Pauciarticular

JRA occurs mostly in boys after 8 years of age.[16] It involves concomitant enthesitis or tendinitis and arthritis that asymmetrically affects the knees, shoulders, spine, or hips. Treatment of JRA includes medication, activity modification, general conditioning, splinting, and casting. Surgical intervention may occasionally be necessary to improve long-term function.

JUVENILE RHEUMATOID ARTHRITIS–LIKE DISEASES

■ Arthritis Associated with Inflammatory Bowel Disease

Chief Clinical Characteristics

This presentation includes abdominal pain, diarrhea, fever, and weight loss.

Background Information

This condition is episodic, corresponding to bowel symptom exacerbations, and involves large lower extremity joints. It can also lead to septic arthritis of the hip.

■ Dermatomyositis

Chief Clinical Characteristics

This presentation includes a vasculitic rash on the eyelids, cheeks, neck, chest, limbs, elbows, and knees and the slow onset of signs of proximal extremity weakness. Weakness manifests in difficulty walking and clumsiness.

Background Information

This condition is an inflammatory myopathy caused by an autoimmune attack on muscle capillaries and small arterioles. Muscle enzyme testing, electromyography, and muscle biopsy are used to confirm the clinical presentation. Corticosteroid therapy will usually control the disease until it resolves spontaneously. Complications include dysphagia, chronic abdominal pain leading to perforation, cerebritis, and diffuse calcification of muscle or subcutaneous tissues. The disease is generally active for 2 to 3 years.

■ Juvenile Ankylosing Spondylitis

Chief Clinical Characteristics

This presentation initially includes prolonged morning stiffness, asymmetrical hip pain or contractures, and knee, shoulder, or heel pain.[17–19]

Background Information
The course is usually episodic involving joints, especially the hip. It is the most common juvenile spondyloarthropathy and has a 6:1 male-to-female ratio. The disease causes fibrosis and ossification at the attachment sites of tendon, capsule, and ligaments to bone. It is associated with the presence of histocompatibility antigen HLA-B27.

■ Polymyositis

Chief Clinical Characteristics
This presentation is characterized by the acute onset of proximal, symmetric weakness and pain in the muscles and multiple joint stiffness.

Background Information
This condition is a systemic connective tissue disease. Corticosteroid therapy is the usual treatment.

■ Reactive Arthritis (Reiter's Syndrome)

Chief Clinical Characteristics
This presentation includes pain with passive and active movement. It is asymmetrical, affecting an average of four joints and predominantly the lower extremities. Hip involvement occurs uncommonly.

Background Information
This condition is most common in Caucasian males. The onset of symptoms is usually preceded by a genitourinary or gastrointestinal infection. Although the underlying cause is an infection, the condition itself is a reactive arthritis to the bacterial proteins, not an infection. In children a genitourinary infection may be an indication of sexual abuse.

■ Scleroderma

Chief Clinical Characteristics
This presentation includes fatigue, arthralgias, or myalgias and Raynaud's syndrome. Patchy areas of the skin become firm with a leathery quality, causing contractures if the involved skin is adjacent to a joint. Arthritis, tendinitis, and weakness may be seen.

Background Information
This rare, chronic multisystem disease results in fibrosis, small-vessel vasculitis, and autoimmune response. Drug therapy is the primary means of management with therapy involved for management of contractures and systemic effects.

■ Systemic Lupus Erythematosus

Chief Clinical Characteristics
This presentation involves a gradual onset of fatigue, malaise, pleural effusions, small joint synovitis, hemolytic anemia, proteinuria, and hematuria and frequently the characteristic malar rash in a "butterfly" shape is seen.

Background Information
The incidence varies by ethnicity and location. It is more common in adolescent females, African Americans, Asians, and Hispanics. Onset before age 8 is uncommon. The treatment regimen depends on the affected target organs. Nonsteroidal anti-inflammatory agents are used to treat arthralgia and arthritic symptoms.

■ Larsen's Syndrome

Chief Clinical Characteristics
This presentation involves multiple congenital dislocations, including hips, knees, and radial heads, together with a characteristic flattened facies with prominent forehead, brachydactyly, and clubfoot. Severe cervical spine kyphosis may present as weakness and ultimately quadriplegia.[20]

Background Information
This condition is caused by a disorder of the Filamin B gene, which creates a defect in growth hormone receptors in which they are resistant to growth hormone. The pattern of heritability for this condition is autosomal dominant.

■ Leg-Length Discrepancy

Chief Clinical Characteristics
This presentation typically includes a difference in the length of the legs present with nothing more than a painless short leg gait. Unilateral toe walking may be seen in cases of leg-length discrepancy as a compensatory strategy for limb advancement and toe clearance in gait.

Background Information
Causes for this condition are numerous, and are often associated with other syndromes or causes, such as proximal focal femoral deficiency, dislocation of the hip, or a physeal injury

due to infection or trauma. A leg-length discrepancy can also be idiopathic. While many leg-length discrepancies are not a major problem, it is important to remember that the leg-length difference may increase as growth progresses. Therefore, all such problems need to be seen initially by an orthopedic surgeon to determine the baseline measurements by x-ray together with x-ray evident of the child's skeletal age. These data are needed to calculate a prediction of the ultimate leg-length difference at maturity. This will allow for the necessary intervention to be planned for at an appropriate age.[21]

■ Legg-Calvé-Perthes Disease

Chief Clinical Characteristics
This presentation includes groin, thigh, and/or anteromedial knee pain, limited hip abduction and internal rotation, and a limp (typically with the femur externally rotated). Initially the limp may be painless.[16]

Background Information
This condition is an idiopathic osteonecrosis of the capital femoral epiphysis due to an interruption in its blood supply. This disease can have an acute traumatic or insidious onset over months. The femoral head ceases growth secondary to the disturbance in blood supply. The secondary center of ossification becomes fragmented after revascularization occurs and then reossification follows.[16] This condition is more common in males by a 4:1 ratio.[16] Smaller, highly active boys with delayed skeletal maturity may be predisposed to developing this disorder.[16] Between 8% and 24% of cases are bilateral.[22] The disease is self-limiting, but resultant deformation of the femoral head may lead to adulthood osteoarthrosis.[22] Those children with greater involvement may require weight-bearing limitations or bracing or surgery.[23]

■ Lesch-Nyhan Syndrome

Chief Clinical Characteristics
This presentation includes mental retardation, hypertonicity resulting in hip dislocation, movement disorders, and self-mutilating behaviors.

Background Information
This rare genetic disorder only occurs in boys.[16] It is characterized by an enzyme deficiency that results in uric acid accumulation.

Death due to renal failure typically occurs in the first two decades. Allopurinol may be used to address the excess uric acid, and various other medications are to manage the neurological symptoms.

LIMB DEFICIENCIES

■ Congenital Deficiency of the Tibia

Chief Clinical Characteristics
This presentation is characterized by a shortened limb, and often a deletion of one or more rays of the foot. Equinovalgus of the ankle is usual. There may be a dimple in the skin anteriorly over the midtibia accompanying a variable degree of anterior tibial bowing. This is the most likely limb deficiency.

Background Information
This condition may occur in syndromes involving other limb and hand malformations, congenital heart conditions, and learning disability. Common treatments involve surgical interventions ranging from transfers of the typically intact fibula to amputation.

■ Congenital Short Femur

Chief Clinical Characteristics
These children show a variable degree of lower limb shortening with little else to recognize. There may be a skin dimple laterally at the midfemur.

Background Information
This diagnosis is differentiated from proximal focal femoral deficiency (PFFD) by the absence of any ipsilateral tibial deformity and the absence of the abductor lurch characteristically seen in children with a PFFD due to abnormal muscles about the hip.[24] This is the second most likely limb deficiency.

■ Malingering

Chief Clinical Characteristics
This presentation involves limping without apparent organic cause.

Background Information
While malingering is a possibility, most children are not clever enough to be able to willfully sustain a consistent abnormal gait pattern. Asking a child to walk backwards is a way of confusing a child's ability to do so.

MUSCULAR DYSTROPHIES

■ Becker Muscular Dystrophy

Chief Clinical Characteristics

This presentation involves progressive symmetric weakness, especially proximally, which is later in onset than Duchenne muscular dystrophy. The gait is wide based, waddling, and includes an increased lumbar lordosis and slight toe walking. Calf muscles tend to enlarge, but muscle tissue is replaced by fat and connective tissue (pseudohypertrophy). An arbitrary means of distinguishing the two disorders depends on whether the affected person can still walk at age 16 years.

Background Information

Impairments are the same as those of Duchenne muscular dystrophy but less severe and much more variable. Life expectancy is more variable than for those with Duchenne muscular dystrophy and extends into the third and fourth decades. Occasionally, survival extends to middle age and older. A family history of older brothers with this condition makes the diagnosis easier. This condition is also an X-linked genetic disorder occurring in males.[25]

■ Duchenne Muscular Dystrophy

Chief Clinical Characteristics

This presentation includes frequent falling. Boys with this condition have progressive symmetric weakness, especially proximally. The gait is wide based, waddling, and includes an increased lumbar lordosis and slight toe walking. Calf muscles tend to enlarge, but muscle tissue is replaced by fat and connective tissue (pseudohypertrophy).

Background Information

The diagnosis usually comes to light when the child is about 5 years of age. A family history of older brothers with this condition makes the diagnosis easier and more likely to be discovered a year or two earlier. Children usually require full-time wheelchair use by about the age of 10 years, after which plantarflexion contractures and scoliosis usually develop. Life expectancy is limited to the later teenage years. This condition is an X-linked genetic disorder occurring in males.[26]

■ Myelodysplasia

Chief Clinical Characteristics

This presentation includes muscle weakness and loss of sensation with resulting foot sores.

Background Information

The term *myelodysplasia* includes spina bifida, myelomeningocele, lipomyelomeningocele, and neural tube defects. It is a condition resulting from the incomplete closure of the neural tube in prenatal development with its varying degrees of neurological involvement depending on the level of spinal lesion and the number of tissue layers exposed due to the neural tube defect. The resultant muscular weakness may cause a painless limp. While a myelomeningocele evident at birth would presumably be known to the parents as a cause of limping, a spina bifida occulta or a lipomyelomeningocele would not necessarily be recognized.

■ Myopathies, Congenital

Chief Clinical Characteristics

This presentation involves frequent falling as a common concern. Girls and boys may both be affected, usually starting in the first 3 to 5 years. They have progressive symmetric weakness, especially proximally. The gait is wide based and waddling. The increased lumbar lordosis and slight toe walking so characteristic of Duchenne muscular dystrophy is not as striking.

Background Information

Relatively common congenital myopathies include central core disease, nemaline (rod) myopathy, and centronuclear (myotubular) myopathy. Rare congenital myopathies include multicore (minicore) disease, fingerprint body myopathy, reducing body myopathy, sarcotubular myopathy, myopathies with tubular aggregates, hyaline body myopathy, trilaminar fiber myopathy, cap myopathy, zebra body myopathy, spheroid body myopathy, cytoplasmic body myopathy, desmin storage myopathies, X-linked myopathy with excessive autophagy, congenital myopathy with an excess of thin filaments, and congenital fiber type disproportion. These conditions are inherited or caused by a spontaneous genetic mutation and cause nonprogressive problems with the muscles ranging from stiffness to weakness, with different degrees of severity.[27]

■ Myotonia Congenita

Chief Clinical Characteristics

This presentation commonly involves symptoms that may include muscle stiffness, particularly in the leg muscles, and muscular hypertrophy. The muscle stiffness may be enhanced by cold and inactivity, and is often relieved by exercise. This condition often manifests in infancy as muscle stiffness and cramps and as abnormal muscle enlargement (a "body-builder–like" appearance). It may become apparent from infancy to approximately 2 to 3 years of age. In many cases, muscles of the eyelids, hands, and legs may be most affected, but other muscle groups may be involved as well. Individuals with Becker type (see Background Information section) may also experience pain and weakness in affected muscles. Becker type typically manifests between the ages of 4 and 12 years, but in rare cases, onset may occur as late as approximately 18 years of age.

Background Information

This condition is a rare genetic, neuromuscular disorder characterized by the slow relaxation of the muscles. There are two forms: a mild form called the Thomsen type that is autosomal dominant, and a more severe form, called Becker type, that is autosomal recessive. Most cases are relatively nonlimiting and not progressive so do not require treatment. Sometimes, however, symptoms of the disorder may be relieved with quinine, phenytoin, or other anticonvulsant drugs. Physical therapy and other rehabilitative measures may be used to help muscle function. Genetic counseling is advisable.[28]

■ Osteochondritis Dissecans of the Knee

Chief Clinical Characteristics

This presentation typically includes pain, edema, and a limp in gait. Typically the child has an increase in pain with activity and a decrease in pain with rest. If a loose body develops, the child may present with symptoms of locking in the knee.

Background Information

This condition is a necrosis of bone and cartilage in a small area of the knee joint surface of the distal femur. The cause is unknown but thought to be a result of a vessel occlusion. Trauma may play a role. The most common site is the lateral middle-to-posterior portion of the medial femoral condyle, but it can affect the lateral femoral condyle as well. The joint requires immobilization and occasionally surgery if a loose body is present.[29]

PERIPHERAL NEUROPATHIES

■ Hereditary Motor and Sensory Neuropathies Types I and II (Charcot-Marie-Tooth Disease)

Chief Clinical Characteristics

This presentation usually involves weakness and atrophy of muscles of the hands and lower leg and foot deformities, especially cavovarus. Typical age of onset occurs late in the first or early in the second decade of life. The gait is a typical "foot drop" pattern with compensating hyperflexion at the hips to clear the feet in swing phase. Loss of sensation in the feet is less evident in the childhood years.[30]

Background Information

This condition is one of the most common forms of hereditary motor and sensory neuropathy. This disease causes a slowly progressive demyelination of peripheral Schwann cells. It occurs sporadically or with a dominant, X-linked, or recessive mode of inheritance. The life span usually is normal.[31]

■ Hereditary Motor and Sensory Neuropathy Type III (Dejerine-Sottas Disease)

Chief Clinical Characteristics

This presentation involves a history of slowly progressive weakness, with muscle wasting. There may be slight loss of sensation in the feet and legs, as well as in the hands and the forearms. Scoliosis is common.

Background Information

This condition is a slowly progressive demyelinating disorder that is usually inherited by a recessive mode. The onset is in infancy or early childhood and results in severe disability by the third decade of life.[31]

■ Poliomyelitis

Chief Clinical Characteristics

This presentation may include a limp without the parents being aware that the child had poliomyelitis as an infant. The child may have had the acute episode at about 6 months of age while living in an undeveloped country. If the disease only mildly affected a few muscles of the lower extremity, the difficulty in walking may only be recognized several years later, at which time the parents are unable to relate the problem to the initial infection. The specific presentation will depend on which muscles are involved.

Background Information
This condition is a viral infection involving the motor neurons of the central nervous system, especially in the spinal cord.[32] While the incidence has been reduced dramatically during the past decade, the disease is still an important one in India and parts of Africa or in other regions where vaccination has been avoided for religious or social reasons. Other viruses, such as the coxsackie virus, may mimic poliomyelitis.

■ **Post–Central Nervous System Vascular Insufficiency or Hemorrhage**
Chief Clinical Characteristics
This presentation will be the same as that seen in children with cerebral palsy, but a history of traumatic brain injury, meningitis or encephalitis, or high fever, especially with seizures during infancy or a history of seizures, may provide evidence for these other conditions that simulate cerebral palsy.

Background Information
The pattern of limping will depend on the area of the diencephalon that is affected, but will be caused by a combination of spasticity, sensorimotor, and cognitive deficits consistent with an upper motor neuron lesion.

■ **Slipped Femoral Capital Epiphyses**
Chief Clinical Characteristics
This presentation involves either acute or insidious onset of groin pain that may radiate into the anteromedial thigh or knee and increased pain with weight bearing. However, a painless limp may be the only presenting symptom. Passive limitation of abduction, flexion, and internal rotation is usual.[23]

Background Information
The pathology is due to a disruption of the capital epiphyseal plate, resulting in a slipping of the head on the neck of the femur.[33,34] This disorder occurs bilaterally in 18% to 50% of children. The disorder is more common in males, Pacific-Islanders, and African Americans. It is also associated with an obese, hypogonadal, or tall and thin body type. The prevalence is higher in children with hypothyroidism on growth hormone therapy and is associated in rare cases with radiation therapy. Complications of this disorder include avascular necrosis and chondrolysis. Intervention usually involves surgical fixation of the femoral head to the neck.

SPINAL DYSRAPHISMS
■ **Diastematomyelia**
Chief Clinical Characteristics
This presentation varies with the level at which the cord is anomalous. Unilateral foot abnormalities, including talipes equinovarus, claw toes, gastrocnemius atrophy, and impaired pain/temperature sensation, may be apparent. A hairy patch on the skin or a dermal sinus may be seen on the back at the level of the anomaly.

Background Information
This condition is characterized by a spinal cord split into two longitudinally by a fibrous, cartilaginous, or bony band. It can occur as an isolated defect along with vertebral anomalies or in conjunction with myelomeningocele.[35]

■ **Tethered Cord Syndrome**
Chief Clinical Characteristics
This presentation involves a mixed upper and lower motor neuron pattern of deficits, bowel and bladder dysfunction, and progressive gait disturbances beginning at 2 to 3 years of age. This is seen commonly in children with myelodysplasia. A dermal sinus tract may be seen. Toe walking tends to increase in severity with age.

Background Information
The spinal cord is tethered to the spinal canal, and neurological deficits begin to present as the child grows and the cord is stretched.

SPINAL MUSCULAR ATROPHIES
■ **Kugelberg-Welander Disease (Juvenile, Type III)**
Chief Clinical Characteristics
This presentation includes muscle weakness that may appear within the first year of life

in the proximal hip and shoulder girdle musculature. Typically, however, the onset of weakness occurs later in the first decade.[35] Girls and boys are affected equally. The most common impairment is proximal lower extremity weakness resulting in difficulty climbing steps, or rising from a chair; there may be a slight tremor of the fingers.

Background Information
Secondary impairments include postural compensations resulting from muscle weakness, contractures, and occasionally scoliosis.[36] Contractures, however, are not common. Motor milestones are usually delayed due to muscle weakness and reduced respiratory capacity. The condition is transmitted as an autosomal recessive trait that causes lesions of the anterior horns of the spinal cord.

■ Tear of the Acetabular Labrum

Chief Clinical Characteristics
This presentation includes reports of intermittent locking with hip motion. There may or may not be pain.

Background Information
This presentation is frequently associated with a jumping or twisting mechanism. Surgery may be indicated if conservative management does not alleviate symptoms.[3]

■ Toddler's Fracture of the Tibia

Chief Clinical Characteristics
This presentation may include pain, limping, or refusal to bear weight on the affected side. Tenderness, swelling, warmth, and pain with palpation of the lower third of the tibia may be noted. Typically there is an acute onset without a known history of trauma.

Background Information
A toddler fracture of the tibia refers to an undisplaced oblique or spiral fracture of the tibial diaphysis without a concomitant fibular fracture. The fracture is common in toddlers and preschoolers. Because the periosteum in the toddler is sufficiently tough and the fibula is intact, the child may be able to walk on the leg, even though fractured, albeit with a limp and usually with pain. A sudden twisting of the tibia, perhaps from getting the foot caught in a crib slat, causes a spiral fracture. The fracture

may only be recognized on a follow-up film when callus becomes evident. Treatment consists of a below-knee walking cast for approximately 3 weeks. Healing is rapid, within 3 or 4 weeks.

TUMORS
BONE CYSTS OF THE LOWER EXTREMITY
■ Aneurysmal

Chief Clinical Characteristics
This presentation may include pain of relatively acute onset that rapidly increases in severity over 6 to 12 weeks. However, in the very early stages, pain may not be recognized as an issue and a painless limp may be the only symptom. Local skin temperature may increase and a palpable bony swelling may be present.

Background Information
This condition may occur in patients ages 10 to 30 years, with a peak incidence in those 16 years of age, with 75% of patients being younger than 20 years. The most common site is the metaphyseal region of the knee; however, any bone may be affected, with the lower leg being affected in 24% of the cases. The most common problem this condition will cause is weakening of the bone leading to increased susceptibility to fracture.

■ Unicameral

Chief Clinical Characteristics
This presentation may include pain of relatively acute onset that rapidly increases in severity over 6 to 12 weeks. However, in the very early stages, pain may not be recognized as an issue and a painless limp may be the only symptom.

Background Information
This condition is a common benign fluid-filled lesion found almost exclusively in children. When such cysts are immediately adjacent to a growth plate, they are referred to as active cysts. When they have achieved some distance from the growth plate, they are considered to be latent cysts. This condition occurs most frequently in children ages 5 to 15 years, with an average age of approximately 9 years.[37] Growth arrest may result

from the tumor or the surgical treatment of the tumor. The overall outcome and prognosis are good. The lesion is believed to resolve spontaneously in most cases if given enough time.[38]

■ Eosinophilic Granuloma (Langerhans' Cell Histiocytosis)

Chief Clinical Characteristics
This presentation will depend on the location of the tumor. Pain may be a feature.[39]

Background Information
This is a category of disorders that include a localized or generalized, reactive or neoplastic proliferation of cells, including histiocytes, eosinophils, plasma cells, and lymphocytes, due to the inflammatory response. This disease can present as a localized lesion or widespread disease affecting any organ. Bone lesions are most common in the skull, pelvis, and diaphyses of long bones.

■ Fibrous Dysplasia

Chief Clinical Characteristics
This presentation may include a painless abductor lurch (gluteus medius gait) if a shepherd's crook deformity of the proximal femurs has developed, but more likely the child will have had an earlier mild antalgic component. Cutaneous pigmentation occurs in more than 50% of cases of the polyostotic.

Background Information
The cutaneous pigmentation (also called café au lait spots) is confined to the side of the bony lesions and is different from the café au lait spots seen in neurofibromatosis. Pigmentation may occasionally precede the development of skeletal and endocrine abnormalities. In this condition, the medullary bone is replaced by fibrous tissue. The subsequent mechanically weakened bone is subject to fractures. On x-ray, the bones appear lucent. There are two forms: polyostotic and monostotic. The polyostotic form, while less common, is more severe and more likely to cause greater deformity. Approximately 90% of children will have involvement of the femur, most commonly proximal. The resulting deformity is a severe coxa vara with a neck-shaft angle of usually less than 90%,

hence the name "shepherd's crook" deformity. This puts the abductor muscles of the hip at a disadvantage, hence the abductor lurch. Onset of symptoms is usually after the age of 10 years. Sexual precocity in girls, with polyostotic fibrous dysplasia and cutaneous pigmentation, is called McCune-Albright syndrome. The monostotic form is more common (70% to 80% of fibrous dysplasia patients). This form involves the lower extremities in approximately one-third of children. This form may present with pain or a pathological fracture usually in older children to young adults.[40]

■ Leukemia

Chief Clinical Characteristics
This presentation may involve fatigue, fever, diminished appetite, large joint arthralgias, and arthritis. The limp may be painless and is characterized by decreased gastrocnemius push-off at end-stance or an external rotation of the entire leg so that end-stance push-off can be accomplished without stretching the gastrocnemius muscle. Joint involvement is usually asymmetric and polyarticular. Palpation of the joint may reveal bony tenderness. In some cases children may present with a chief complaint of an antalgic limp without a history of trauma.

Background Information
Severe pain results from infiltration of the bone periosteum and fractures may result from the weakened bones.[16,41] This bone marrow or lymph system cancer involves the hematopoietic cells and is the most common childhood cancer.[16] These children are also at risk for the development of multiple joint, symmetrical avascular necrosis associated with chemotherapy.[42]

■ Osteochondroma

Chief Clinical Characteristics
This presentation will depend on the location of the tumor. Pain may be a feature. Osteochondromata around the proximal femur may limit the hip range of motion, resulting in a painless limp.[43]

Background Information
This condition is a common childhood benign tumor that is more common in males and is more common in late adolescence to

young adulthood. *Familial osteochondromatosis,* also known as *multiple hereditary exostosis,* is an autosomal dominant inherited variant in which more than two osteochondromas are present. This form is more common in boys and is more likely to involve the hip region.

■ Syringomyelia

Chief Clinical Characteristics

This presentation usually involves loss of sensation, muscle wasting, and absent deep tendon reflexes. The presentation varies with the level and the extent of the lesion. A rapidly progressive scoliosis may be the initial manifestation of syringomyelia. Spastic paraplegia is a common finding.

Background Information

This condition is a cavitation of the spinal cord. In noncommunicating syringomyelia, there is a cystic dilation of the cord and the cerebrospinal fluid pathway is not affected. In communicating syringomyelia, cerebrospinal fluid flow communicates between the central canal of the spinal cord and the cavity. Communicating syringomyelia is often associated with the Arnold-Chiari malformation, which can lead to hydrocephalus, cerebellar ataxia, pyramidal signs, and impaired sensation. Progressive enlargement of the cavity impinges on the anterior horn cells and corticospinal tracts, resulting in the loss of lower level function.

■ Trevor's Disease (Dysplasia Epiphysealis Hemimelica)

Chief Clinical Characteristics

This presentation includes painless swelling about a joint that may result in an angular deformity with restricted joint motion.

Background Information

This is a condition of unusual overgrowth of one or more of the ossification centers within a joint. It usually affects males. Usual sites in the foot and ankle are the talus and the distal tibia. Typical treatment is surgery to limit the amount of deformity.[44]

References

1. Staheli L, Hall J, Paholke D, Jaffe K. *Arthrogryposis: A Text Atlas.* Cambridge, UK: Cambridge University Press; 1998.
2. Morrison P. Hereditary ataxias and paediatric neurology: new movers and shakers enter the field: a review. *Eur J Paediatr Neurol.* 2003;7(5):217–219.
3. Berend K, Vail T. Hip arthroscopy in the pediatric adolescent and pediatric athlete. *Clin Sports Med.* 2001;20 (4):763–778.
4. Korinthenberg R, Monting J. Natural history and treatment effects in Guillain Barre syndrome: a multicentre study. *Arch Dis Child.* 1996;74(4):281–287.
5. Tang T, Noble-Jamieson C. A painful hip as a presentation of Guillain-Barré syndrome in children. *Br Med J.* 2001;322:149–150.
6. Govoni V, Granieri E. Epidemiology of the Guillain-Barre syndrome. *Curr Opin Neurol.* 2001;14(5):605–613.
7. Connolly A. Chronic inflammatory demyelinating polyneuropathy in children. *Pediatr Neurol.* 2001;24(3): 177–182.
8. Weinstein S. Developmental hip dysplasia and dislocation. In: Morrissy R, Weinstein S, eds. *Pediatric Orthopedics.* Vol 2. 5th ed. Philadelphia, PA: Lippincott Williams & Wilkins; 2000:905–956.
9. Dickhaut S, DeLee J. The discoid lateral-meniscus syndrome. *J Bone Joint Surg.* 1982;64:1068.
10. Gordon J, Schoenecker P. Surgical treatment of congenital dislocation of the patella. *J Ped Orthop.* 1999;19(2): 260–264.
11. Klippel J, Crofford L, Stone J, Weyand C. *Primer on the Rheumatic Diseases.* 12th ed. Atlanta, GA: Arthritis Foundation; 2001.
12. Mikles M, Stanton R. A review of Morquio's syndrome. *Am J Orthop.* 1997;26:533.
13. Bassett G. The osteochondrodysplasia. In: Morrissy RT WS, ed. *Pediatric Orthopaedics.* Philadelphia, PA: Lippincott-Raven; 1996:203–249.
14. Kahana M, Levy A, Ronnen M, Cohen M, Schewach-Millet M. Painful piezogenic pedal papules on a child with Ehlers-Danlos syndrome. *Pediatr Dermatol.* Nov 1985;3(1):45–47.
15. Shapiro F, Spect J, Wiles D. The diagnosis and orthopedic treatment of spinal muscular atrophy, Friedreich's Ataxia and arthrogryposis. *J Bone Joint Surg.* 1993;75A: 1699.
16. Ratliffe KT. *Clinical Pediatric Physical Therapy.* St. Louis, MO: Mosby; 1998.
17. Bowyer S. Hip contracture as the presenting sign in children with HLA-B27 arthritis. *J Rheumatol.* 1995;22: 165–167.
18. Cate R, Hertzberger-ten, Dijkmans B, Breedveld F. Teenager with an irritable hip, anaemia and malaise. *Ann Rheum Dis.* 1995;54(9):701–705.
19. Law L, Haftel H. Shoulder, knee, and hip pain as initial symptoms of juvenile ankylosing spondylitis: a case report. *J Orthop Sports Phys Ther.* 1998;27(2): 167–172.
20. Laville J, Lakermance P, Limouzy F. Larsen's syndrome: review of the literature and analysis of thirty eight cases. *J Ped Orthop.* 1994;14:63.
21. Moseley C. Leg length discrepancy. In: Morrissy R, Weinstein S, eds. *Pediatric Orthopedics.* Vol 2. 5th ed. Philadelphia, PA: Lippincott Williams & Wilkins; 2000:1105–1150.
22. Arnheim DD, Prentice WE. *Principles of Athletic Training.* 8th ed. St. Louis, MO: Mosby-Year Book; 1993.
23. Herring J. Legg-Calve Perthes disease: a review of current knowledge. *Intsr Course Lect.* 1989;38:309.

24. Watts H, Clark MW. *Who Is Amelia*. Rosemont, IL: American Academy of Orthopedic Surgeons; 1998.

25. Hoffman E, Kunkel L, Angelini C, et al. Improved diagnosis of Becker muscular dystrophy by dystrophin testing. *Neurology*. 1989;39:1011.

26. Sutherland D, Olshen R, Cooper L, et al. The pathomechanics of gait in Duchenne muscular dystrophy. *Dev Med Child Neurol*. 1981;23:3.

27. Goebel H. Congenital myopathies. *Semin Pediatr Neurol*. 1996;3:152.

28. Chew K, Wong Y-S, Teoh H-L, Lim E. Myotonia congenita in a young active man. *Phys Sports Med*. 2004;32:7.

29. Twyman R, Desai K, Aichroth P. Osteochondritis dissecans of the knee: a long term study. *J Bone Joint Surg*. 1991;73B:461.

30. Long T, Toscano K. *Handbook of Pediatric Physical Therapy*. 2nd ed. Philadelphia, PA: Lippincott Williams & Wilkins; 2002.

31. Simon R, Aminoff M, Greenberg D. *Clinical Neurology*. 4th ed. New York, NY: Lange Medical Books/McGraw-Hill; 1999.

32. Victor M, Ropper A. *Adam and Victor's Principle's of Neurology*. 7th ed. New York, NY: McGraw-Hill; 2001.

33. Loder R, Aronsson D, Dobbs M, Weinstein S. Slipped capital femoral epiphysis. *J Bone Joint Surg*. 2000;82A:1170–1188.

34. Castriota-Scanderbeg A, Orsi E. Slipped capital femoral epiphysis: ultrasonographic findings. *Radiology*. 1993;22:191–193.

35. Campbell S. *Physical Therapy for Children*. 2nd ed. Philadelphia, PA: W. B. Saunders; 2000.

36. Dorscher P, Mehrsheed S, Mulder D, Litchy W, Ilstrup D. Wohlfart-Kugelberg-Welander syndrome: serum creatine kinase and functional outcome. *Arch Phys Med Rehabil*. 1991;72:587–591.

37. Capanna R, Campanacci D, Manfrini M. Unicameral and aneurysmal bone cysts. *Orthop Clin North Am*. 1996;27(3):605–614.

38. Gupta A, Crawford A. Solitary bone cyst with epiphyseal involvement: confirmation with magnetic resonance imaging. A case report and review of the literature. *J Bone Joint Surg*. 1996;78A(6):911–915.

39. Hosalkar H, Shaw B, Siongco A, Ceppi C. A 10-year-old boy with hip pain. *Clin Orthop Rel Res*. 2002; 397:434–441.

40. Guille J, Kumar S, MacEwen G. Fibrous dysplasia of the proximal part of the femur, Long term results of curettage and bone grafting and mechanical realignment. *J Bone Joint Surg*. 1998;80A:648.

41. Tuten H, Gabos P, Kumar S, Harter GD. The limping child: a manifestation of acute leukemia. *J Ped Orthop*. 1998;18(5):625–629.

42. Wei S, Esmail A, Bunin N, Dormans J. Avascular necrosis in children with acute lymphoblastic leukemia. *J Ped Orthop*. 2000;20(3):331–335.

43. Noonan KJ, Feinberg JR, Levenda A, Snead J, Wurtz LD. Natural history of multiple hereditary osteochondromatosis of the lower extremity and ankle. *J Ped Orthop*. 2002;22(1):120–124.

44. Oates E, Cutler J, Miyamoto E, Hirose F, Lachman R. Case report 305. *Skeletal Radiol*. 1985;13:174–178.

CHAPTER 54

Tripping and Falling in a Child

■ *Christy L. Skura, PT, DPT, PCS* ■ *Bach T. Ly, PT, DPT*

Description of the Symptom

Tripping and falling in the pediatric population are developmental traits that are normal but can be considered pathological if they (1) persist beyond a certain age, (2) present with a sudden onset, or (3) worsen over time. Tripping and falling may or may not be associated with changes in the gait pattern or with pain.

Special Concerns
■ Sudden onset
■ Signs of malfunctioning shunt (ie, ventricular-peritoneal shunt) and spinal cord tethering, such as nausea, vomiting, seizures, fever, decline in motor function, and change in affect
■ Proximal and worsening muscular weakness

CHAPTER PREVIEW: Conditions That May Lead to Tripping and Falling in a Child

T Trauma

COMMON

Peripheral nerve injury or entrapment 1066

UNCOMMON

Traumatic brain injury 1068

RARE

Traumatic spinal cord injury 1068

I Inflammation

COMMON

Not applicable

UNCOMMON

Aseptic
Juvenile rheumatoid arthritis 1064

Septic
Not applicable

RARE

Aseptic
Acute demyelinating polyradiculoneuropathy (Guillain-Barré syndrome) 1061
Secretory otitis media 1067

Septic
Poliomyelitis 1067

M   Metabolic

COMMON

Not applicable

UNCOMMON

Mitochondrial disease 1065

RARE

Hereditary motor and sensory neuropathy Type III (Dejerine-Sottas disease) 1064

Va   Vascular

COMMON

Not applicable

UNCOMMON

Stroke 1067

RARE

Ventriculoperitoneal shunt malfunction 1069

De   Degenerative

COMMON

Not applicable

UNCOMMON

Charcot-Marie-Tooth peripheral neuropathy 1062
Muscular dystrophies:
• Duchenne muscular dystrophy 1065

RARE

Adrenoleukodystrophy 1061
Cerebellar hypoplasia 1062
Kugelberg-Welander disease (juvenile, type III) 1065
Muscular dystrophies:
• Becker muscular dystrophy 1065
• Congenital myopathy 1065
• Emery-Dreifuss muscular dystrophy 1066
Neuronal ceroid lipofuscinosis (Batten disease) 1066

Tu   Tumor

COMMON

Not applicable

UNCOMMON

Not applicable

(continued)

TRIPPING AND FALLING IN A CHILD

Tumor *(continued)*

RARE

Malignant Primary, such as:
• Acute leukemia 1068
• Spinal cord tumor 1069
• Tumor in proximity to the fourth ventricle or vestibular nuclei 1069
Malignant Metastatic, such as:
• Pilocytic astrocytoma 1068
• Posterior fossa tumor 1068
Benign:
Not applicable

Co Congenital

COMMON

Angular variations of the knees (genu varum; bowlegs or genu valgum; knock knees) 1061
Clubfoot deformity (talipes equinovarus) 1062
Developmental dysplasia of the hip 1063
Down syndrome (Trisomy 21) 1063
Mental retardation 1065
Seizure disorder 1067

UNCOMMON

Attention deficit hyperactivity disorder 1061
Huntington's disease 1064
In-toeing (if severe) 1064
Out-toeing (if severe) 1066
Pes planus (flatfoot, if severe) 1067

RARE

Ehlers-Danlos syndrome 1063
Myelodysplasia 1066
Tethered cord syndrome 1067

Ne Neurogenic/Psychogenic

COMMON

Autism and pervasive developmental disorders 1062
Cerebral palsy (spastic or ataxic) 1062
Visual impairment 1069

UNCOMMON

Developmental coordination disorder 1063
Sensory processing disorder (including proprioceptive, tactile, and vestibular difficulties) 1067

RARE

Hereditary ataxias:
• Ataxia telangiectasia 1063
• Cerebellar ataxia 1064
• Friedreich's ataxia 1064

Note: These are estimates of relative incidence because few data are available for the less common conditions.

Common Ages at Which Tripping and Falling Present in a Child

APPROXIMATE AGE	CAUSES
Birth to 3 Years	Acute demyelinating polyradiculoneuropathy
	Acute leukemia
	Angular variations of the knees
	Ataxia telangiectasia
	Autism or pervasive developmental disorder
	Cerebellar hypoplasia
	Cerebral palsy
	Clubfoot deformity
	Congenital myopathy
	Developmental dysplasia of the hip
	Down syndrome (Trisomy 21)
	Ehlers-Danlos syndrome
	Emery-Dreifuss muscular dystrophy
	In-toeing, severe
	Juvenile rheumatoid arthritis
	Mental retardation
	Myelodysplasia
	Neuronal ceroid lipofuscinoses (Batten disease)
	Out-toeing, severe
	Pes planus, severe
	Secretory otitis media
	Seizure disorder
	Sensory processing disorder
	Stroke
	Tethered cord syndrome
	Traumatic brain injury (including shaken baby syndrome)
	Ventriculoperitoneal shunt malfunction
	Visual impairment
Preschool (3–5 Years)	Acute leukemia
	Adrenoleukodystrophy
	Attention deficit hyperactivity disorder
	Autism or pervasive developmental disorder
	Congenital myopathy
	Duchenne muscular dystrophy
	Ehlers-Danlos syndrome
	Emery-Dreifuss muscular dystrophy
	Juvenile rheumatoid arthritis
	Mitochondrial disease
	Neuronal ceroid lipofuscinoses (Batten disease)
	Secretory otitis media
	Sensory processing disorder
	Spinal cord tumor
	Ventriculoperitoneal shunt malfunction
	Visual impairment
Elementary School (6–11 Years)	Acute leukemia
	Attention deficit hyperactivity disorder
	Becker muscular dystrophy
	Charcot-Marie-Tooth peripheral neuropathy
	Developmental coordination disorder
	Duchenne muscular dystrophy
	Emery-Dreifuss muscular dystrophy
	Hereditary motor and sensory neuropathy Type III

(continued)

Common Ages at Which Tripping and Falling Present in a Child—cont'd	
APPROXIMATE AGE	**CAUSES**
	Juvenile rheumatoid arthritis
	Kugelberg-Welander disease
	Mitochondrial disease
	Neuronal ceroid lipofuscinoses (Batten disease)
	Pilocytic astrocytoma
	Poliomyelitis
	Posterior fossa tumor
	Spinal cord tumor
Middle School (12–14 Years)	Becker muscular dystrophy
	Friedreich's ataxia
	Kugelberg-Welander disease
	Pilocytic astrocytoma
	Seizure disorder
	Spinal cord tumor
High School (15–18 Years)	Acute demyelinating polyradiculoneuropathy (Guillain-Barré syndrome)
	Becker muscular dystrophy
	Cerebellar ataxia
	Friedreich's ataxia
	Huntington's disease
	Seizure disorder
	Spinal cord tumor
	Traumatic brain injury
	Traumatic spinal cord injury

Overview of Tripping and Falling in a Child

For typically developing children, the onset of ambulation usually occurs between 9 and 15 months of age. At first, the center of mass is high because the head is relatively large and the extremities are short. Because stability is inversely related to the distance of the center of mass from the base of support, children are very unsteady at this age, and tend to walk with a wide base of support. In addition, they are developing the strength, postural control, and balance reactions necessary to achieve a more mature gait pattern. Thus, frequent tripping and falling as children are learning to walk is considered normal. Heel strike tends to emerge around 18 months and becomes consistent by 24 months, or after 3 to 6 months after learning to walk. Around 3 years of age, joint angles during walking mature into an adult pattern, and electromyography demonstrates a mature pattern. Balance and postural control tend to have a period of disequilibrium at 4 to 6 years, but then renewed stability is seen at around 6 to 7 years of age.[1]

Tripping and falling may be associated with abnormal gait deviations, which may be symmetric or asymmetric, and should be noted for differential diagnosis. These gait deviations may be due to pain, weakness, structural abnormalities, decreased range of motion, or spasticity, all of which should be noted for differential diagnosis. Tripping and falling can occur with toe walking, as in cases of children with Duchenne muscular dystrophy, but occur in many other incidences without, as in the case of the child with an ataxic or in-toeing gait. The practitioner should note when tripping and falling began, the progression of symptoms (if any), and whether or not the child is reporting pain. Acute limping has a very broad differential diagnosis. For pain in a specific joint, the reader is referred to other appropriate chapters. In many incidences, tripping and falling are reported by parents but not observed in the clinic perhaps due to factors such as the physical environment, time of day, or the child's age-related hastiness and concentration level, fatigue level, or behavior.

When considering the differential diagnosis for tripping and falling, vestibular disturbances need to be ruled less likely. A child with recurrent falling that cannot be explained by the content of this chapter should be referred for vestibular testing. Certain impairments, such as spasticity, ankle contractures, muscular weakness, or ataxia, can stand on their own as causes of tripping and falling. However, because they are found as symptoms across numerous diseases, they are discussed within the description of diseases.

Description of Conditions That May Lead to Tripping and Falling in a Child

■ Acute Demyelinating Polyradiculoneuropathy (Guillain-Barré Syndrome)

Chief Clinical Characteristics
This presentation is usually associated with weakness that is ascending and symmetrical, progressing over days or weeks. Severity may range from mild weakness to complete tetraplegia and ventilatory failure. Peak deficits are usually reached by 4 weeks, and recovery usually begins 2 to 4 weeks after progression ceases.[2–5]

Background Information
Symptoms are thought to result from an immunologic reaction causing demyelination of peripheral nerves, and in severe cases, axonal degeneration as well. In addition to clinical presentation, differential diagnosis is established by the presence of only a few lymphocytes and an increase in protein in cerebrospinal fluid as well as electromyographic findings of reduction in amplitudes of muscle action potentials, slowed conduction velocity, conduction block in motor nerves, prolonged distal latencies, and prolonged or absent F responses. Standard treatment includes administration of intravenous immune globulin and plasma exchange. The majority of individuals recover completely or nearly so within a few weeks to a few months; however, the presence of axonal degeneration increases the regeneration time period.

■ Adrenoleukodystrophy

Chief Clinical Characteristics
This presentation includes hyperactivity, deterioration of handwriting, strabismus, and seizures. Other symptoms may include visual loss, learning disabilities, dysarthria, dysphagia, hearing loss, fatigue, and disturbances of gait and coordination. Further progression of the disease causes changes in muscle tone, stiffness, and contractures.

Background Information
This condition is a rare genetic disorder that involves progressive dysfunction of the adrenal gland and a breakdown of the myelin sheath surrounding nerve cells in the brain. The childhood form is the most severe and affects only boys. Death usually occurs within 1 to 10 years after onset of symptoms due to progressive neurological deterioration.[6,7]

■ Angular Variations of the Knees (Genu Varum; Bowlegs or Genu Valgum; Knock Knees)

Chief Clinical Characteristics
This presentation involves atypical variation in the frontal plane angle of the knees. Many children will look bowlegged when they start to walk and then knock-kneed between 3 and 7 years. The gradual change from varum to valgum may be caused by a widening pelvis. Unilateral deformity, progressive deformity, or lack of spontaneous resolution are reasons for referral to a physician.

Background Information
The severity of genu varum is measured by observing the distance between the medial femoral condyles when the lower extremities are positioned with the medial malleoli touching. The severity of genu valgum is measured by the distance between the medial malleoli with the medial femoral condyles touching. These are relative measurements that are affected by the child's size, thus measuring the femoral tibial angle with a goniometer is a more accurate way to quantify angulation. However, obtaining reliable goniometric measure on a child is often a challenge. If physiological genu varum or genu valgum persists beyond 7 to 8 years of age, orthopedic referral is indicated.[8,9]

■ Attention Deficit Hyperactivity Disorder

Chief Clinical Characteristics
This presentation involves children who appear to be clumsy or have motor deficits because they

are not able to focus on the task at hand. They may trip over obstacles in their environment because they do not attend to them.

Background Information

This condition is a behavioral disorder in which children have difficulty paying attention and focusing on tasks. The three symptoms are inattention, impulsivity, and hyperactivity.[10,11]

■ Autism and Pervasive Developmental Disorders

Chief Clinical Characteristics

This presentation is characterized by marked abnormalities in communication and social interactions and a restricted and socially atypical range of interests. Most individuals with this condition also exhibit some degree of mental retardation, and seizures are also commonly seen. Stereotypical behaviors and movements are often present, including hand flapping, spinning, and toe walking. Children with this condition often exhibit developmental delays, including difficulties with motor planning and coordination, and may appear clumsy.

Background Information

Pervasive developmental disorders encompass a broad range of diagnoses that are part of a grouping also known as autistic spectrum disorders. This includes autistic disorder, Asperger's syndrome, pervasive developmental disorder not otherwise specified, Rett's syndrome, and childhood disintegrative disorder. The etiology of autism continues to be studied, and current hypotheses include genetic abnormalities, exposure to toxins, and prenatal, perinatal, and postnatal infections.[11]

■ Cerebellar Hypoplasia

Chief Clinical Characteristics

This presentation may include developmental delay, hypotonia, ataxia, seizures, mental retardation, and nystagmus.

Background Information

This is a progressive developmental disorder characterized by underdevelopment of the cerebellum. It may be caused by thyroid abnormalities, drug exposure, viral infection, or stroke.[12]

■ Cerebral Palsy (Spastic or Ataxic)

Chief Clinical Characteristics

This presentation may be characterized by a child who demonstrates bilateral spasticity of the calf during gait and may toe walk and/or fall frequently. Asking the child to run often exaggerates the toe walking together with scapular retraction, making the diagnosis more evident.

Background Information

This condition is a nonprogressive chronic condition, noted at or about the time of birth, affecting muscle movement and coordination, caused by damage to the central nervous system before, during, or shortly after birth or in infancy. This condition is divided into four categories: spastic, athetoid (dyskinetic), ataxic, and mixed. Mixed forms of this condition include symptoms of more than one of the other three forms.[13–15] Very mild forms of spastic cerebral palsy are readily overlooked on routine examination so the cause of the gait disturbance is missed.

■ Charcot-Marie-Tooth Peripheral Neuropathy

Chief Clinical Characteristics

This presentation can be characterized by weakness of the peroneal and distal leg muscles, as well as the hand muscles. This condition also includes loss of proprioception at the feet and ankles in some cases.

Background Information

Also called peroneal muscular atrophy, this condition is usually of autosomal dominant inheritance. This neuropathy is chronic, symmetric, and involves demyelination of the peripheral nerve with axonal loss and loss of anterior horn cells and dorsal root ganglion neurons in the lumbar and sacral segments.[16,17]

■ Clubfoot Deformity (Talipes Equinovarus)

Chief Clinical Characteristics

This presentation involves a congenital structural abnormality of the foot apparent at birth and characterized by excessive ankle inversion, plantarflexion, and forefoot adduction. The affected foot and calf muscle are stiff and generally smaller than the other side, and children tend to walk on the toes and outer sole of the foot.[18–20]

Background Information

Depending on the extent of involvement and the child's age, both surgical and nonsurgical options are available to address this condition. This condition should be identified and treated early secondary to the detrimental effects of prolonged clubfoot positioning on the child's overall development and also to the affected foot's mechanical structure.

■ Developmental Coordination Disorder

Chief Clinical Characteristics

This presentation commonly involves a child who is described as clumsy and having poor strength, poor coordination, poor sequencing, poor spatial organization, and awkward gait.

Background Information

This condition is diagnosed when a child's poor motor coordination is not due to a medical condition, when the extent of incoordination is in excess of what is expected for the child's age and intelligence, and when it is interfering with academic achievement and activities of daily living. This condition can occur along with other diagnoses such as cerebral palsy and other neurological disorders, Down syndrome, brain tumors, loss of sensory functions such as vision and hearing, and mental retardation.[11,21–23]

■ Developmental Dysplasia of the Hip

Chief Clinical Characteristics

This presentation is often observed when the child begins to walk; at that time, the leg appears to be shorter on the affected side, and the child may walk up on the toes on that side to compensate for the discrepancy or may have a noticeable limp. If both hips are affected, the child may walk with a waddling gait and/or demonstrate excessive lumbar lordosis.

Background Information

This condition is caused when the femur does not fit securely into the acetabulum, usually because the socket is too shallow, which allows the femur to partially or completely slip out of the hip joint. Untreated, this condition may lead to permanent hip deformities or osteoarthritis.[8,24,25]

■ Down Syndrome (Trisomy 21)

Chief Clinical Characteristics

This presentation involves mental retardation as well as physical abnormalities, including musculoskeletal impairments such as low muscle tone and weakness. The characteristic appearance of a child with this condition includes a small head, flattening of the face and nose with a low nose bridge, epicanthal folds of skin at the inner eyes, and short broad hands with a single crease across the palm. Children with this condition present with global developmental delays, including delayed achievement of gross-motor milestones such as walking.

Background Information

This condition is a genetic disorder that is usually diagnosed at birth.[26–28]

■ Ehlers-Danlos Syndrome

Chief Clinical Characteristics

This presentation commonly includes abnormally flexible joints that may be unstable, loose and fragile skin, and fragile blood vessels that cause easy bruising. Children with this condition may appear clumsy, drop items, and trip or fall frequently.

Background Information

This condition is a group of hereditary disorders of connective tissue. Types include classical, hypermobility, vascular, kyphoscoliosis, arthrochalasia, dermatosparaxis, and tenascin-x–deficient types.[26]

HEREDITARY ATAXIAS

■ Ataxia Telangiectasia

Chief Clinical Characteristics

This presentation commonly involves parents of children with this condition describing their child as "clumsy" and their gait as "wobbly."

Background Information

Inherited as an autosomal recessive trait, this condition is a progressive disease that involves loss of Purkinje cells in the cerebellar cortex and degeneration of neurons in the cerebral cortex, basal ganglia, brainstem, and anterior horns of the spinal cord.[29,30]

■ Cerebellar Ataxia

Chief Clinical Characteristics

This presentation includes ataxic gait, dysarthria, and lack of limb coordination, with an eventual loss of ambulation.

Background Information

Also known as Marie's ataxia, cerebellar ataxia is an autosomal dominant disorder with symptoms that usually manifest in early adulthood.[31]

■ Friedreich's Ataxia

Chief Clinical Characteristics

This presentation commonly involves progressive involvement that begins in the lower extremities with eventual involvement of the upper extremities. Gait is wide based due to a combination of ataxia and spasticity.

Background Information

A degenerative disease with symptoms that appear in early adolescence, this condition is inherited as an autosomal recessive trait and involves the atrophy and demyelination of the posterior columns of the spinocerebellar and corticospinal tracts of the spinal cord.[31–34]

■ Hereditary Motor and Sensory Neuropathy Type III (Dejerine-Sottas Disease)

Chief Clinical Characteristics

This presentation includes intermittent attacks of ataxia of gait, numbness, weakness, and pain in the extremities. Deterioration is gradual and leads to an inability to walk by age 30 to 40 years.

Background Information

This condition is a peripheral neuropathy involving hypertrophy of peripheral nerves. It is slowly progressive, inherited as an autosomal recessive trait, and involves an abnormality of pyruvate metabolism, or poor conversion of lactate to pyruvate.[17,35]

■ Huntington's Disease

Chief Clinical Characteristics

This presentation involves progressive chorea and dementia. As the disease progresses, akinesia typically develops.

Background Information

This is an autosomal dominant condition. The onset of this condition is almost always in middle age; however, occasionally, the disease becomes evident in childhood.[36]

■ In-Toeing (If Severe)

Chief Clinical Characteristics

This presentation involves a child who appears to be "pigeon-toed" with the feet pointing medially. Tripping and falling may occur only in very severe cases.

Background Information

This condition is caused by structural abnormalities that can be observed, including femoral anteversion, internal tibial torsion, or metatarsus adductus. Although it is unclear how and even debatable if in-toeing actually causes falling and tripping, there appears to be an association between in-toeing gait and the frequency of falling and tripping episodes in children seen clinically. In-toeing in general is a very common reason why children are referred to the orthopedist. It may be due to developmental variation (ie, there is a wide range of normal bone development), family history, and intrauterine positioning. In addition to these congenital reasons, in-toeing may also have a neurogenic cause: a combination of spasticity-induced abnormal muscle forces and persistent physiological torsion due to delayed weight bearing.[8,9,37,38]

■ Juvenile Rheumatoid Arthritis

Chief Clinical Characteristics

This presentation includes the consistent presence for 6 or more weeks of swelling, or the presence of two or more of the following: limited joint range of motion, palpable tenderness, painful movement, or joint warmth. There are three subtypes: systemic, polyarticular, and pauciarticular.[39] This condition can be symmetric or asymmetric, and usually involves larger joints (knees, wrists, ankles). Children with this condition sometimes demonstrate compensatory gait patterns due to pain in a certain joint, including avoidance of hip extension, limited knee range of motion, and limited ankle dorsiflexion.

Background Information

The most common rheumatic disorder of childhood, this condition can affect multiple joints of the extremities and spine. Before a confirmed diagnosis or even a referral to a rheumatologist, a toddler, for example, has a typical onset of limping, pain, and falling. The child's parents may assume incorrectly that the swelling in her or his joint may be the result of a fall.[40,41]

■ Kugelberg-Welander Disease (Juvenile, Type III)

Chief Clinical Characteristics
This presentation commonly involves proximal lower extremity weakness, scoliosis, and ankle plantarflexion contractures.

Background Information
This condition is inherited as an autosomal recessive genetic defect on chromosome 5. This condition involves a reduced number of the large anterior horn cells of the spinal cord and the progressive degeneration of the remaining cells.[5,42,43]

■ Mental Retardation

Chief Clinical Characteristics
This presentation usually includes global developmental delay, including delayed achievement of gross-motor milestones.

Background Information
Many of the diagnoses that are listed here may be associated with some degree of mental retardation, including Down syndrome, cerebral palsy, and autism. However, mental retardation, defined as below-average intelligence with a deficit in adaptive behaviors, may have no known cause, which is estimated to occur in 75% to 85% of cases of mental retardation. It may be categorized by intelligence quotient scores into categories of mild, moderate, severe, and profound.[11,44,45]

■ Mitochondrial Disease

Chief Clinical Characteristics
This presentation may include loss of motor control and coordination, muscle weakness, and pain, which may lead to gait impairments, clumsiness, tripping, and falling.

Background Information
This is a large and varied group of disorders that results from failure of the mitochondria, the specialized compartment of the cell that is responsible for energy production. Organs most frequently affected include the brain, heart, liver, skeletal muscles, kidneys, and the endocrine and respiratory systems.[46,47]

MUSCULAR DYSTROPHIES

■ Becker Muscular Dystrophy

Chief Clinical Characteristics
This presentation involves proximal weakness, but progresses at a slow rate.

Background Information
Mild impairments and frequent falls and clumsiness may not appear until the mid- to late teenage years. Toe walking is uncommon in patients with this condition due to the lower incidence of ankle plantarflexor contractures than in other forms of this condition. When contractures are present, walking is no longer possible.[5,43]

■ Congenital Myopathy

Chief Clinical Characteristics
This presentation includes nonprogressive problems with the muscles ranging from stiffness to weakness, with different degrees of severity.

Background Information
Relatively common congenital myopathies include central core disease, nemaline (rod) myopathy, and centronuclear (myotubular) myopathy. Rare congenital myopathies include multicore (minicore) disease, fingerprint body myopathy, reducing body myopathy, sarcotubular myopathy, myopathies with tubular aggregates, hyaline body myopathy, trilaminar fiber myopathy, cap myopathy, zebra body myopathy, spheroid body myopathy, cytoplasmic body myopathy, desmin storage myopathies, X-linked myopathy with excessive autophagy, congenital myopathy with an excess of thin filaments, and congenital fiber type disproportion. Congenital myopathies are inherited or caused by a spontaneous genetic mutation.[5,48]

■ Duchenne Muscular Dystrophy

Chief Clinical Characteristics
This presentation typically includes symmetric weakness, especially proximally, that progresses over time. Typical gait is described as wide based and waddling and includes an increased lumbar lordosis and toe walking.

Parents report clumsiness, tripping, and falling. There is characteristic calf hypertrophy.

Background Information

This condition is an X-linked genetic disorder occurring in males, usually diagnosed when parents report noticing the child has lost motor skills or strength. Bilateral toe walking often begins at about the age of 4 or 5 and gradually becomes more pronounced. Plantarflexion contractures occur over time. Calf muscles tend to enlarge, as muscle tissue is replaced by fat and connective tissue (pseudohypertrophy).[5,27,43,49,50]

■ Emery-Dreifuss Muscular Dystrophy

Chief Clinical Characteristics

This presentation involves weakness predominantly in a humeroperoneal distribution. Independent walking is typically observed into adulthood, but ankle plantarflexion and elbow flexion are common.

Background Information

This condition is an X-linked recessive disorder.[33,43,51,52]

■ Myelodysplasia

Chief Clinical Characteristics

This presentation may include signs of a blood disorder, including paleness and bruising, or an associated syndrome such as neurofibromatosis, Down syndrome, Noonan syndrome, or ataxia telangiectasia. This results in muscular weakness that can cause falling and tripping. Clubfoot deformities can occur in children with this condition, and flaccidity is commonly found at their ankles.

Background Information

A rare condition resulting from the incomplete closure of the neural tube during prenatal development, this condition has varying degrees of neurological involvement depending on the level of spinal lesion and the number of tissue layers exposed due to the neural tube defect.[53,54]

■ Neuronal Ceroid Lipofuscinosis (Batten Disease)

Chief Clinical Characteristics

This presentation is characterized by progressive epilepsy, mental retardation, ataxia, and visual loss.

Background Information

This condition involves a group of recessively inherited neurodegenerative diseases. The subtypes are divided based on age of onset of symptoms, with the late infantile and juvenile forms also referred to as Batten disease.[55,56]

■ Out-Toeing (If Severe)

Chief Clinical Characteristics

This presentation involves feet that appear to be excessively turned out laterally. This condition is less common than in-toeing, and may be caused by femoral retroversion or external tibial torsion. Tripping and falling may occur only in very severe cases.

Background Information

Femoral retroversion is a common cause that is present in early infancy and is more common in obese children. It may gradually improve on its own in the first year of walking. Persistent femoral retroversion is associated with osteoarthritis, increased risk of stress fractures of the lower extremities, and slipped capital femoral epiphysis. External tibial torsion is often seen between 4 and 7 years of age, and is often unilateral. It usually worsens with age as the tibia rotates laterally with growth. It may be associated with patellofemoral instability and pain.[8,9,38]

■ Peripheral Nerve Injury or Entrapment

Chief Clinical Characteristics

This presentation may manifest as motor or sensory impairments, either of which may lead to an abnormal gait, and/or tripping or falling. This may include full or partial paralysis, weakness, tingling, or pain along the nerve distribution.

Background Information

Trauma to peripheral nerves is relatively common, and may be caused by a blunt trauma or associated with fractures/dislocations. Dysfunction results from damage to the neuron, the Schwann cells, or the myelin sheath, which causes the nerve to be unable to transmit impulses normally. Damage is classified into categories including neurapraxia, axonotmesis, or neurotmesis, depending on the severity and permanency of damage. Mechanisms of injury include mechanical, crush and percussion, laceration, penetrating trauma, stretch injury, high-velocity trauma, or cold injury.[17,57]

■ Pes Planus (Flatfoot, If Severe)

Chief Clinical Characteristics

This presence is characterized by the absence of the normal longitudinal arch of the foot. Associated tripping and falling may occur only in very severe cases.

Background Information

Congenital flexible flatfoot in infants is a normal developmental stage up through 2 years of age and does not require treatment, as it usually spontaneously corrects within a year of walking. A rigid flatfoot is usually caused by an osseous deformity. This condition is sometimes associated with tightness of the gastroc-soleus, which may cause toe walking or tripping.[8,9]

■ Poliomyelitis

Chief Clinical Characteristics

This presentation commonly involves initial fever and severe muscle pain, followed by asymmetric flaccid paralysis, which in turn can lead to tripping and falling.

Background Information

Commonly called polio, this condition involves paralysis resulting from a virus-induced loss of the motor neurons of the anterior horn cells of the spinal cord and of other parts of the central nervous system.[5,33]

■ Secretory Otitis Media

Chief Clinical Characteristics

This presentation commonly includes awkwardness, clumsiness, and a tendency of the child to fall.

Background Information

This condition is the most common cause of vestibular disturbances in young children. Effusion of the middle ear results from incomplete resolution of acute ear infections.[58,59]

■ Seizure Disorder

Chief Clinical Characteristics

This presentation may involve loss of consciousness or involuntary spasms, which may affect the gait pattern or cause tripping or falling.

Background Information

Also known as epilepsy, this is a condition characterized by recurrent seizures, which are a sudden disruption in the electrical activity of the brain. Although seizure disorders may be associated with head injuries, brain tumors, and certain genetic and infectious illnesses, sometimes there is no known cause. Seizures are classified according to whether they are generalized (diffuse) or focal (partial), which describes whether all or only part of the brain is involved. Types of seizures include generalized tonic-clonic (grand-mal), absence (petit-mal), myoclonic, simple partial, or complex partial.[4,60]

■ Sensory Processing Disorder (Including Proprioceptive, Tactile, and Vestibular Difficulties)

Chief Clinical Characteristics

This presentation commonly involves children who may appear disorganized or lacking purpose in their activities, may not explore their environment, may lack variety in their play, may appear clumsy or to have poor balance, may have difficulty calming themselves after becoming excited or upset, or may seek out excessive sensory input.

Background Information

This condition is the inability of the central nervous system to appropriately process sensory information in order to generate a meaningful response.[11,45,61]

■ Stroke

Chief Clinical Characteristics

This condition may result in muscle spasticity and a number of movement deviations. Symptoms are generally unilateral, opposite the side of the cortex that was affected, causing asymmetrical gait deviations.

Background Information

This condition also may occur in the cerebellum, causing an ataxic gait. Strokes occurring *in utero* or at birth cause hemiplegic cerebral palsy.[62–64]

■ Tethered Cord Syndrome

Chief Clinical Characteristics

This presentation may involve neurological deficits that begin to present as the child grows.

A mixed upper and lower motor neuron pattern of deficits involves bowel and bladder dysfunction and progressive gait disturbances beginning at 2 to 3 years of age.

Background Information
This condition occurs when the spinal cord is tethered and neurological symptoms increase positively with growth. Some of the more common causes of tethering include lipoma or lipomyelomeningocele, split cord malformation (diastematomyelia), dermal sinus tract, fatty or tight filum, or myelomeningocele (spina bifida or open spine).[53,62]

■ Traumatic Brain Injury

Chief Clinical Characteristics
This presentation may involve gait disturbances and ataxia with injury to the motor cortex or cerebellum. Motor deficits depend on the severity of the injury, and may include gait and balance problems, slowing, and visual motor deficits.

Background Information
Hematomas near the fourth ventricle or vestibular nuclei may cause unsteadiness or imbalance while standing and walking. This condition may be categorized as penetrating (if an object strikes the head with sufficient force to cause a depressed skull fracture), missile (if an object either lodges within brain tissue or exits the skull), or nonpenetrating (closed head injuries). Shaken baby syndrome is a collection of signs and symptoms caused by the violent shaking of an infant or small child (a form of child abuse). The severity and permanency of damage will depend on the extent of damage to the central nervous system.[58,63,64]

■ Traumatic Spinal Cord Injury

Chief Clinical Characteristics
This presentation depends on the level of the lesion within the pyramidal tract of the central nervous system. With a complete lesion at the level of L2, active hip flexion is preserved and reciprocal gait is possible with knee-ankle-foot orthoses (KAFOs). With an injury level of L3, ambulation with ankle-foot orthoses (AFOs) is possible; however, the hips remain unstable due to the lack of active hip abduction and extension.

Background Information
A child with this condition will need to use bilateral canes or crutches or a walker. This gait may be sufficient for community ambulation but still is laborious, and some patients may prefer a wheelchair. Children with spastic incomplete lesions tend to walk at a low velocity and have characteristic changes in gait pattern due in part to spasticity.[64,65]

TUMORS

■ Acute Leukemia

Chief Clinical Characteristics
This presentation may involve a sudden or a gradual onset, marked by fatigue, weakness, and bruising with joint pain.

Background Information
This disorder of white blood cells is the most common cancer of childhood. Two forms of leukemia include acute lymphoid leukemia (ALL), which originates in the lymph cells and accounts for about 80% to 90% of cases, and acute myelogenous leukemia (AML), which originates in the bone marrow and accounts for about 10% to 20%.[4,66]

■ Pilocytic Astrocytoma

Chief Clinical Characteristics
This presentation may include ataxia of gait, imbalance, and impulsiveness, which can be present postoperatively. This condition may include nausea, vomiting, headaches, drowsiness, ataxia (uncoordinated gait), and imbalance.

Background Information
This type of tumor is sometimes considered a posterior fossa tumor, but because astrocytomas usually begin in the cerebellar hemisphere, pilocytic astrocytoma has been reported as such and not as a posterior fossa tumor. These astrocytomas may also be located in the optic chiasm and hypothalamus.[67]

■ Posterior Fossa Tumor

Chief Clinical Characteristics
This presentation includes nausea, vomiting, headaches, drowsiness, ataxia (uncoordinated gait), and imbalance. Symptoms of cranial nerve damage may also be present, including hearing loss, visual field deficits, eye deviations,

unsteadiness when walking, facial muscle weakness, dilated pupils, taste disturbances, and loss of sensation of part of the face.

Background Information
This condition is an abnormal growth located in or near the posterior fossa, which is a depression on the interior, back portion of the base of the skull, near the cerebellum. The posterior fossa is a small, confined space and any growth there can block the flow of spinal fluid, causing increased pressure on the brain and spinal cord. Common types of posterior fossa tumors include cerebellar astrocytoma, primary neuroectodermal tumors, medulloblastoma, ependymoma and ependymoblastoma, choroid plexus papilloma and carcinoma, dermoid tumors, hemangioblastoma, metastatic tumors, and brainstem gliomas.[31,63]

■ **Spinal Cord Tumor**

Chief Clinical Characteristics
This presentation often includes nonspecific local pain or stiffness. Radicular (radiating) pain suggests nerve root impingement, which may be exacerbated with movement. The child may report weakness in one or both extremities. The onset of the pain symptoms is often insidious and followed by a gradually progressive course. However, once symptoms other than pain appear, symptom progression may be rapid.

Background Information
Direct compression of the spinal cord may be caused by tumors of the vertebral bodies, paravertebral spaces, or structures within the epidural space. Nerve tracts most vulnerable to mechanical pressure include the corticospinal and spinocerebellar tracts and the posterior spinal columns. Tumors of the spine may compromise the vascular supply, causing edema or ischemia.[5,68]

■ **Tumor in Proximity to the Fourth Ventricle or Vestibular Nuclei**

Chief Clinical Characteristics
This presentation may involve disequilibrium, or an imbalance or unsteadiness while standing and walking, as well as vertigo and nystagmus. Disequilibrium resolves in days to weeks.[58]

Background Information
This condition is caused by a tumor in the region of the cerebellum and midbrain. Mechanical compression and invasion of cerebellum and midbrain structures, in addition to restricted cerebrospinal fluid flow, may be responsible for presenting symptoms and signs. Optimal treatment varies based on tumor cell type and location.

■ **Ventriculoperitoneal Shunt Malfunction**

Chief Clinical Characteristics
This presentation may include fever, malaise, headache, onset of or increased strabismus, scoliosis, seizures, spasticity, and changes in activity level and quality of gait.

Background Information
This condition occurs when there is obstruction or infection of a shunt used to regulate the amount of cerebrospinal fluid in patients with hydrocephalus. Children with myelodysplasia may have shunted or nonshunted hydrocephalus.[69,70]

■ **Visual Impairment**

Chief Clinical Characteristics
This presentation may involve a child who rubs the eyes, shuts or covers one eye, leans forward to see better, uses a head tilt or turns the head to look at something, stumbles or trips over objects, or demonstrates clumsiness when reaching. Because vision is often a motivator for movement, motor milestones may be delayed, including walking.

Background Information
This condition may be congenital or acquired, and may be due to a peripheral or central nervous system defect. The list of eye conditions, syndromes, and diseases that may affect a child's vision is very extensive.[11,71]

References
1. Stout J. Gait: Development and analysis. In: Campbell S, Linden DV, Palisano R, eds. *Physical Therapy for Children.* 2nd ed. St. Louis, MO: W. B. Saunders; 2000: 88–116.
2. Hughes RA, Rees JH. Clinical and epidemiologic features of Guillain-Barré syndrome. *J Infect Dis.* Dec 1997; 176(suppl 2):S92–98.
3. Jones HR. Childhood Guillain-Barré syndrome: clinical presentation, diagnosis, and therapy. *J Child Neurol.* Jan 1996;11(1):4–12.

4. Ratliffe K. Medical disorders. In: Ratliffe K, ed. *Clinical Pediatric Physical Therapy*. St. Louis, MO: Mosby; 1998:385–428.

5. Simon R, Aminoff M, Greenberg D. Motor deficits. In: Simon R, Aminoff M, Greenberg D, eds. *Clinical Neurology*. 4th ed. Stamford, CT: Appleton & Lange; 1999:159–198.

6. Moser HW. Adrenoleukodystrophy: phenotype, genetics, pathogenesis and therapy. *Brain*. Aug 1997;120 (pt 8):1485–1508.

7. Moser HW, Moser AB, Naidu S, Bergin A. Clinical aspects of adrenoleukodystrophy and adrenomyeloneuropathy. *Dev Neurosci*. 1991;13(4–5):254–261.

8. Leach J. Orthopedic conditions. In: Campbell S, Linden DV, Palisano R, eds. *Physical Therapy for Children*. 2nd ed. St. Louis, MO: W. B. Saunders; 2000:398–428.

9. Sass P, Hassan G. Lower extremity abnormalities in children. *Am Fam Physician*. Aug 1, 2003;68(3):461–468.

10. Blondis TA. Motor disorders and attention-deficit/hyperactivity disorder. *Pediatr Clin North Am*. Oct 1999; 46(5):899–913, vi–vii.

11. Ratliffe K. Sensory, processing, and cognitive disorders. In: Ratliffe K, ed. *Clinical Pediatric Physical Therapy*. St. Louis, MO: Mosby; 1998:313–350.

12. Ramaekers VT, Heimann G, Reul J, Thron A, Jaeken J. Genetic disorders and cerebellar structural abnormalities in childhood. *Brain*. Oct 1997;120(pt 10):1739–1751.

13. Dabney KW, Lipton GE, Miller F. Cerebral palsy. *Curr Opin Pediatr*. Feb 1997;9(1):81–88.

14. Olney S, Wright M. Cerebral palsy. In: Campbell S, Linden DV, Palisano R, eds. *Physical Therapy for Children*. 2nd ed. St. Louis, MO: W. B. Saunders; 2000:533–570.

15. Ratliffe K. Cerebral palsy. In: Ratliffe K, ed. *Clinical Pediatric Physical Therapy*. St. Louis, MO: Mosby; 1998:163–218.

16. Holmes JR, Hansen ST Jr. Foot and ankle manifestations of Charcot-Marie-Tooth disease. *Foot Ankle*. Oct 1993; 14(8):476–486.

17. Simon R, Aminoff M, Greenberg D. Disorders of somatic sensation. In: Simon R, Aminoff M, Greenberg D, eds. *Clinical Neurology*. 4th ed. Stamford, CT: Appleton & Lange; 1999:199–227.

18. Faulks S, Luther B. Changing paradigm for the treatment of clubfeet. *Orthop Nurs*. Jan–Feb 2005;24(1): 25–30; quiz 31–32.

19. Miedzybrodzka Z. Congenital talipes equinovarus (clubfoot): a disorder of the foot but not the hand. *J Anat*. Jan 2003;202(1):37–42.

20. Roye DP Jr, Roye BD. Idiopathic congenital talipes equinovarus. *J Am Acad Orthop Surg*. Jul–Aug 2002; 10(4):239–248.

21. David K. Developmental coordination disorders. In: Campbell S, Linden DV, Palisano R, eds. *Physical Therapy for Children*. 2nd ed. St. Louis, MO: W. B. Saunders; 2000:471–501.

22. Hamilton SS. Evaluation of clumsiness in children. *Am Fam Physician*. Oct 15, 2002;66(8):1435–1440, 1379.

23. Willoughby C, Polatajko HJ. Motor problems in children with developmental coordination disorder: review of the literature. *Am J Occup Ther*. Sep 1995;49(8): 787–794.

24. Aronsson DD, Goldberg MJ, Kling TF Jr, Roy DR. Developmental dysplasia of the hip. *Pediatrics*. Aug 1994; 94(2 pt 1):201–208.

25. Ratliffe K. Disorders of the developing hip. In: Ratliffe K, ed. *Clinical Pediatric Physical Therapy*. St. Louis, MO: Mosby; 1998:71–98.

26. Cotran R, Kumar V, Robbins S, Schoen F. Genetic disorders. In: Cotran R, Kumar V, Robbins S, Schoen F, eds. *Robbins Pathologic Basis of Disease*. 5th ed. Philadelphia, PA: W. B. Saunders; 1994:123–170.

27. Ratliffe K. Genetic disorders. In: Ratliffe K, ed. *Clinical Pediatric Physical Therapy*. St. Louis, MO: Mosby; 1998:219–274.

28. Winders P. *Gross Motor Skills in Children with Down Syndrome*. Bethesda, MD: Woodbine House; 1997.

29. Chun HH, Gatti RA. Ataxia-telangiectasia, an evolving phenotype. *DNA Repair (Amst)*. Aug–Sep 2004;3(8–9): 1187–1196.

30. Gatti RA, Boder E, Vinters HV, Sparkes RS, Norman A, Lange K. Ataxia-telangiectasia: an interdisciplinary approach to pathogenesis. *Medicine (Baltimore)*. Mar 1991;70(2):99–117.

31. Simon R, Aminoff M, Greenberg D. Disorders of equilibrium. In: Simon R, Aminoff M, Greenberg D, eds. *Clinical Neurology*. 4th ed. Stamford, CT: Appleton & Lange; 1999:102–132.

32. Delatycki MB, Williamson R, Forrest SM. Friedreich ataxia: an overview. *J Med Genet*. Jan 2000;37(1):1–8.

33. Gilroy J. *Basic Neurology*. 2nd ed. New York, NY: McGraw-Hill; 1990.

34. Johnson WG. Friedreich ataxia. *Clin Neurosci*. 1995; 3(1):33–38.

35. Plante-Bordeneuve V, Said G. Dejerine-Sottas disease and hereditary demyelinating polyneuropathy of infancy. *Muscle Nerve*. Nov 2002;26(5):608–621.

36. Simon R, Aminoff M, Greenberg D. Movement disorders. In: Simon R, Aminoff M, Greenberg D, eds. *Clinical Neurology*. 4th ed. Stamford, CT: Appleton & Lange; 1999:228–252.

37. Karol LA. Rotational deformities in the lower extremities. *Curr Opin Pediatr*. Feb 1997;9(1):77–80.

38. Staheli LT. In-toeing and out-toeing in children. *J Fam Pract*. May 1983;16(5):1005–1011.

39. Klippel JH, Crofford LJ, Stone JH, Weyand CM. *Primer on the Rheumatic Diseases*. 12th ed. Atlanta, GA: Arthritis Foundation; 2001.

40. Reiff A. *Kids Get Arthritis Too!* El Monte, CA: Children's Medical Services; 2003.

41. Rhodes V. Physical therapy management of patients with juvenile rheumatoid arthritis. In *Pediatric Orthopedics*. Alexandria, VA: American Physical Therapy Association; 1992.

42. Carter GT, Wineinger MA, Walsh SA, Horasek SJ, Abresch RT, Fowler WM Jr. Effect of voluntary wheel-running exercise on muscles of the mdx mouse. *Neuromuscul Disord*. Jul 1995;5(4):323–332.

43. Stuberg W. Muscular dystrophy and spinal muscular atrophy. In: Campbell S, Linden DV, Palisano R, eds. *Physical Therapy for Children*. 2nd ed. St. Louis, MO: W. B. Saunders; 2000:339–369.

44. McEwen I. Children with cognitive impairments. In: Campbell S, Linden DV, Palisano R, eds. *Physical Therapy for Children*. 2nd ed. St. Louis, MO: W. B. Saunders; 2000:502–532.

45. Montgomery P, Gauger J. Sensory dysfunction in children who toe walk. *Phys Ther*. Oct 1978;58(10): 1195–1204.

46. Gropman AL. Diagnosis and treatment of childhood mitochondrial diseases. *Curr Neurol Neurosci Rep.* Mar 2001;1(2):185–194.

47. von Kleist-Retzow JC, Schauseil-Zipf U, Michalk DV, Kunz WS. Mitochondrial diseases—an expanding spectrum of disorders and affected genes. *Exp Physiol.* Jan 2003;88(1):155–166.

48. de Girolami U, Anthony D, Frosch M. Peripheral nerve and skeletal muscle. In: Cotran R, Kumar V, Robbins S, Schoen F, eds. *Robbins Pathologic Basis of Disease.* 5th ed. Philadelphia, PA: W. B. Saunders; 1994:1273–1294.

49. McDonald CM. Physical activity, health impairments, and disability in neuromuscular disease. *Am J Phys Med Rehabil.* Nov 2002;81(11 suppl):S108–120.

50. Williams EA, Read L, Ellis A, Morris P, Galasko CS. The management of equinus deformity in Duchenne muscular dystrophy. *J Bone Joint Surg Br.* Aug 1984;66(4): 546–550.

51. Dickey RP, Ziter FA, Smith RA. Emery-Dreifuss muscular dystrophy. *J Pediatr.* Apr 1984;104(4):555–559.

52. Merlini L, Granata C, Dominici P, Bonfiglioli S. Emery-Dreifuss muscular dystrophy: report of five cases in a family and review of the literature. *Muscle Nerve.* Jul–Aug 1986;9(6):481–485.

53. Anderson FM. Occult spinal dysraphism: a series of 73 cases. *Pediatrics.* Jun 1975;55(6):826–835.

54. Hinderer K, Hinderer S, Shurtleff DB. Myelodysplasia. In: Campbell S, Linden DV, Palisano R, eds. *Physical Therapy for Children.* 2nd ed. St. Louis, MO: W. B. Saunders; 2000:621–670.

55. Bennett MJ, Hofmann SL. The neuronal ceroid-lipofuscinoses (Batten disease): a new class of lysosomal storage diseases. *J Inherit Metab Dis.* Jun 1999;22(4): 535–544.

56. Goebel HH, Sharp JD. The neuronal ceroid-lipofuscinoses. Recent advances. *Brain Pathol.* Jan 1998;8(1):151–162.

57. Grant GA, Goodkin R, Kliot M. Evaluation and surgical management of peripheral nerve problems. *Neurosurgery.* Apr 1999;44(4):825–839; discussion 839–840.

58. Tusa R, Saada A, Niparko J. Dizziness in childhood. *J Child Neurol.* 1994;9:261–274.

59. Balkany T, Finkel R. The dizzy child. *Ear and Hearing.* 1986;7(3):138–141.

60. Simon R, Aminoff M, Greenberg D. Seizures & syncope. In: Simon R, Aminoff M, Greenberg D, eds. *Clinical Neurology.* 4th ed. Stamford, CT: Appleton & Lange; 1999:253–273.

61. Ayers J. *Sensory Integration and the Child.* Los Angeles, CA: Western Psychological Services; 1979.

62. Soonawala N, Overweg-Plandsoen WC, Brouwer OF. Early clinical signs and symptoms in occult spinal dysraphism: a retrospective case study of 47 patients. *Clin Neurol Neurosurg.* Mar 1999;101(1):11–14.

63. Kerkering G, Phillips W. Brain injuries: traumatic brain injuries, near-drowning, and brain tumors. In: Campbell S, Linden DV, Palisano R, eds. *Physical Therapy for Children.* 2nd ed. St. Louis, MO: W. B. Saunders; 2000:597–620.

64. Ratliffe K. Traumatic disorders. In: Ratliffe K, ed. *Clinical Pediatric Physical Therapy.* St. Louis, MO: Mosby; 1998:275–312.

65. Shakhazizian K, Massagli T, Southard T. Spinal cord injury. In: Campbell S, Linden DV, Palisano R, eds. *Physical Therapy for Children.* 2nd ed. St. Louis, MO: W. B. Saunders; 2000:571–596.

66. Tuten HR, Gabos PG, Kumar SJ, Harter GD. The limping child: a manifestation of acute leukemia. *J Pediatr Orthop.* Sep–Oct 1998;18(5):625–629.

67. Campbell JW, Pollack IF. Cerebellar astrocytomas in children. *J Neurooncol.* May–Jun 1996;28(2–3): 223–231.

68. Faerber EN, Roman NV. Central nervous system tumors of childhood. *Radiol Clin North Am.* Nov 1997;35(6): 1301–1328.

69. Dellorusso C, Crawford RW, Chamberlain JS, Brooks SV. Tibialis anterior muscles in mdx mice are highly susceptible to contraction-induced injury. *J Muscle Res Cell Motil.* 2001;22(5):467–475.

70. Hayes A, Williams DA. Beneficial effects of voluntary wheel running on the properties of dystrophic mouse muscle. *J Appl Physiol.* Feb 1996;80(2):670–679.

71. Simon R, Aminoff M, Greenberg D. Disturbances of vision. In: Simon R, Aminoff M, Greenberg D, eds. *Clinical Neurology.* 4th ed. Stamford, CT: Appleton & Lange; 1999:133–158.

CHAPTER 55

Toe Walking in a Child

■ *Christy L. Skura, PT, DPT, PCS* ■ *Bach T. Ly, PT, DPT*

Description of the Symptom

Toe walking in the pediatric population is a developmental trait that is normal but can be considered pathological if it (1) persists beyond a certain age, (2) presents with a sudden onset, or (3) worsens over time. Toe walking is common in new walkers, and a child who normally walks with a heel-toe pattern may regress to toe walking in order to find greater stability when faced with a more challenging task such as carrying a large object while walking. This chapter describes possible causes of toe walking in a child.

Special Concerns

■ Clumsiness and weakness, especially proximally
■ Sudden onset
■ Signs of shunt (ie, ventricular-peritoneal shunt) malfunction and spinal cord tethering, such as nausea, vomiting, seizures, fever, decline in motor function, and change in affect

CHAPTER PREVIEW: Conditions That May Lead to Toe Walking in a Child

T Trauma

COMMON

Post-traumatic weakness 1079

UNCOMMON

Traumatic brain injury 1080

RARE

Traumatic spinal cord injury 1080

I Inflammation

COMMON

Not applicable

UNCOMMON

Aseptic
Inflammatory muscle diseases:
• Dermatomyositis 1077
Juvenile rheumatoid arthritis 1077

Septic
Not applicable

Inflammation *(continued)*

RARE

Aseptic
Inflammatory muscle diseases:
• Polymyositis 1077

Septic
Poliomyelitis 1079

Metabolic

COMMON
Not applicable

UNCOMMON
Not applicable

RARE
Not applicable

Vascular

COMMON
Not applicable

UNCOMMON
Stroke 1079

RARE
Vascular malformation of the calf muscle 1084

De Degenerative

COMMON
Not applicable

UNCOMMON
Muscular dystrophies:
• Duchenne muscular dystrophy 1078

RARE
Kugelberg-Welander disease (juvenile, Type III) 1078
Muscular dystrophies:
• Becker muscular dystrophy 1078
• Congenital myopathy 1078
• Emery-Dreifuss muscular dystrophy 1078

Tu Tumor

COMMON
Not applicable

(continued)

Tumor *(continued)*

UNCOMMON

Malignant Primary:
Not applicable
Malignant Metastatic:
Not applicable
Benign, such as:
• Syringomyelia 1084

RARE

Malignant Primary, such as:
• Bone or soft tissue tumors of the lower extremity:
  • Ewing's sarcoma 1080
  • Langerhans' cell histiocytosis 1081
  • Leukemia 1081
  • Lymphoma 1081
  • Nephroblastoma (Wilms' tumor) 1082
  • Neuroblastoma 1082
  • Osteochondroma 1083
  • Osteoid osteoma 1083
  • Osteosarcoma (osteogenic sarcoma) 1083
  • Rhabdomyosarcoma 1083
  • Synovial sarcoma 1084
• Spinal cord tumor 1084
Malignant Metastatic:
Not applicable
Benign:
Not applicable

Co Congenital

COMMON

Clubfoot deformity (talipes equinovarus) 1076
Congenital tendo-Achilles contracture 1076
Idiopathic toe walking 1077

UNCOMMON

Tethered cord syndrome 1079

RARE

Hereditary motor and sensory neuropathy Type III (Dejerine-Sottas disease) 1077
Muscular dystrophies:
• Congenital myotonic muscular dystrophy 1078

Ne Neurogenic/Psychogenic

COMMON

Spastic cerebral palsy 1079

UNCOMMON

Sensory disturbance 1079

RARE

Not applicable

Note: These are estimates of relative incidence because few data are available for the less common conditions.

Common Ages at Which Toe Walking Presents in a Child

APPROXIMATE AGE	CAUSES
Birth to 3 Years	Bone or soft tissue tumor of the lower extremity Clubfoot deformity Congenital myopathy Congenital myotonic muscular dystrophy Congenital tendo-Achilles contracture Emery-Dreifuss muscular dystrophy Hereditary motor and sensory neuropathy Type III Idiopathic toe walking Juvenile rheumatoid arthritis Post-traumatic lower extremity pain/weakness with compensatory gait pattern Sensory disturbances Spastic cerebral palsy Stroke Tethered cord syndrome Traumatic brain injury
Preschool (3–5 Years)	Congenital myotonic muscular dystrophy Duchenne muscular dystrophy Emery-Dreifuss muscular dystrophy Juvenile rheumatoid arthritis Post-traumatic lower extremity pain/weakness with compensatory gait pattern Spastic cerebral palsy
Elementary School (6–11 Years)	Becker muscular dystrophy Dermatomyositis Duchenne muscular dystrophy Emery-Dreifuss muscular dystrophy Kugelberg-Welander disease Poliomyelitis Polymyositis Post-traumatic lower extremity pain/weakness with compensatory gait pattern
Middle School (12–14 Years)	Becker muscular dystrophy Bone or soft tissue tumor of the lower extremity Kugelberg-Welander disease Post-traumatic lower extremity pain/weakness with compensatory gait pattern Syringomyelia Vascular malformation of the calf
High School (15–18 Years)	Becker muscular dystrophy Post-traumatic lower extremity pain/weakness with compensatory gait pattern Spinal cord tumor Syringomyelia Traumatic brain injury Traumatic spinal cord injury Vascular malformation of the calf

Overview of Toe Walking in a Child

Toe walking is a part of normal development; children often walk up on their toes for the first few months after they have begun walking. Most children will change to a heel-to-toe pattern within 3 to 6 months of walking. However, some children will continue toe walking after this time. The main reasons for persistent toe walking include the following:

1. Spasticity (such as that seen in children with cerebral palsy, especially spastic diplegia, post-stroke or spinal lesion),
2. Lack of dorsiflexion range of motion (such as that seen in children with clubfoot or other tendo-Achilles shortening),
3. Weakness (such as that seen in children with Duchenne or other muscular dystrophies, and congenital myopathies),
4. Neurological immaturity (possibly related to impaired vestibular or proprioceptive processing), and
5. Idiopathic toe walking (where no known cause can be found).

When observing toe walking in children, the practitioner should note whether the gait deviation is symmetric or asymmetric, the age of the child, the rapidness/timing of onset, and whether or not spasticity is present. Achievement of gross-motor and other developmental milestones should be measured. It is also important to note the presence or absence of pain and its location. Be aware that asymmetric toe walking may be present due to pain in the hip, knee, ankle, or foot, and the reader is referred to the other chapters in this text for discussion of the appropriate differential diagnoses.

This section is prefaced with a note regarding leg-length discrepancy, because causes of leg-length discrepancy are numerous (eg, dislocation of the hip, osteomyelitis, traumatic physeal injury, and Legg-Calvé-Perthes disease), and can span several diagnostic groups such as trauma, inflammation, vascular, tumor, and congenital. Unilateral toe walking is seen in cases of leg-length discrepancy as a compensatory gait strategy for limb advancement and toe clearance.

The main issue with leg-length differences in children is not the current difference, but what the difference will be at maturity. A difference of 2 cm at the current time may be of little concern if the difference is stable in absolute terms. However, if the difference is due to a congenital decrease in longitudinal growth of the femur, for example, a 10% difference in a 1-year-old boy, the ultimate difference at maturity could be an additional 4 cm.

The management of leg-length discrepancy requires compiling an adequate series of measurement data, usually at yearly intervals. Simple tape-measure evaluations are not adequate. X-rays taken so that magnification is eliminated are important (either scanograms or orthoroentgenograms). Because bone length norms have been established based on bone age rather than calendar age, a simultaneous x-ray of the left hand is also taken and compared to norms. Because of the importance of having baseline measurements and appropriate serial measurements, early referral to an orthopedic surgeon is important.

Description of Conditions That May Lead to Toe Walking in a Child

■ Clubfoot Deformity (Talipes Equinovarus)

Chief Clinical Characteristics
This presentation involves a congenital structural abnormality of the foot apparent at birth and characterized by excessive ankle inversion, plantarflexion, and forefoot adduction. The affected foot and calf muscle are stiff and generally smaller than the other side, and children tend to walk on the toes and outer sole of the foot.[1–3]

Background Information
The etiology of this condition remains unknown, but risk factors such as male sex, family history, and exposure *in utero* to maternal smoking have been acknowledged. Treatment for this condition includes options ranging from surgical correction to serial casting and orthoses, depending on severity.

■ Congenital Tendo-Achilles Contracture

Chief Clinical Characteristics
This presentation involves toe walking when the child begins walking.[4]

Background Information
This condition involves a severe congenital shortening of the calf muscle.

■ Hereditary Motor and Sensory Neuropathy Type III (Dejerine-Sottas Disease)

Chief Clinical Characteristics
This presentation includes intermittent attacks of ataxia of gait, numbness, weakness, and pain in the extremities. Deterioration is gradual and leads to an inability to walk by age 30 to 40 years.

Background Information
This condition is a neuropathy involving hypertrophy of peripheral nerves. It is slowly progressive, inherited as an autosomal recessive trait, and involves an abnormality of pyruvate metabolism, or poor conversion of lactate to pyruvate.[5,6]

■ Idiopathic Toe Walking

Chief Clinical Characteristics
This presentation can be characterized by a child with normal birth weight and history who begins to walk on time, begins toe walking immediately, is able to walk on heels when cued, and toe walks intermittently. Children with this condition tend to lose range of motion over time, developing plantarflexor contractures.

Background Information
Authors of existing literature have used terms such as *hereditary*, *idiopathic*, and *habitual* to describe toe walking. In this chapter, the term *idiopathic toe walking* is used for presentations that cannot be otherwise explained. A positive family history may be reported. Hypersensitivity of the sole of the foot and a persistent primitive reflex (positive support reaction) will need to be ruled out in habitual toe walking. This condition has been shown to be associated with other developmental problems, especially language delays.[7-11]

INFLAMMATORY MUSCLE DISEASES

■ Dermatomyositis

Chief Clinical Characteristics
This presentation includes a rash on the eyelids, cheeks, neck, chest, and limbs, with weakness of neck and limb muscles. Children often begin toe walking due to ankle plantarflexion contractures.

Background Information
This is an inflammatory myopathy caused by an autoimmune attack on muscle capillaries and small arterioles. The disease is generally active for 2 to 3 years; approximately 20% of patients recover completely.[12-15]

■ Polymyositis

Chief Clinical Characteristics
This presentation includes an acute onset of proximal symmetric weakness, along with pain in the muscles and multiple joints. Muscle weakness can be the cause of falls and compensatory toe walking, because distal muscles are less affected than proximal muscles.

Background Information
Inflammatory and degenerative changes in the muscles are seen in this systemic connective tissue disease. The changes are caused by an autoimmune reaction. If these changes also occur in the skin and a rash is present, this condition is typically called dermatomyositis.[12,14,15]

■ Juvenile Rheumatoid Arthritis

Chief Clinical Characteristics
This presentation includes the consistent presence for 6 or more weeks of swelling, or the presence of two or more of the following: limited joint range of motion, palpable tenderness, painful movement, or joint warmth.[16] There are three subtypes: systemic, polyarticular, and pauciarticular.[16] Children with this condition will sometimes demonstrate compensatory gait patterns due to pain in a certain joint, including avoidance of hip extension, limited knee range of motion, and limited ankle dorsiflexion.

Background Information
When there is inflammation of a certain joint (especially the hip, knee, or ankle), a child with this condition may walk on his toes on one or both sides as a compensatory pattern to avoid weight bearing. This condition can be symmetric or asymmetric, and usually involves larger joints (knees, wrists, ankles).[17-21]

■ Kugelberg-Welander Disease (Juvenile, Type III)

Chief Clinical Characteristics

This presentation involves proximal lower extremity weakness, scoliosis, and ankle plantarflexion contractures.

Background Information

This condition, like the three other types, is inherited as an autosomal recessive genetic defect on chromosome 5. It involves a reduced number of the large anterior horn cells of the spinal cord and the progressive degeneration of the remaining cells.[15,22,23]

MUSCULAR DYSTROPHIES

■ Becker Muscular Dystrophy

Chief Clinical Characteristics

This presentation involves a slow and mild progression of proximal muscle weakness.

Background Information

Frequent falls and clumsiness may not appear until the mid- to late teenage years. Toe walking is less common due to a low incidence of ankle plantarflexor contractures, and these contractures usually do not occur until walking is no longer possible.[15,23]

■ Congenital Myopathy

Chief Clinical Characteristics

This presentation includes nonprogressive problems with the muscles ranging from stiffness to weakness, with different degrees of severity.

Background Information

Relatively common congenital myopathies include central core disease, nemaline (rod) myopathy, and centronuclear (myotubular) myopathy. Rare congenital myopathies include multicore (minicore) disease, fingerprint body myopathy, reducing body myopathy, sarcotubular myopathy, myopathies with tubular aggregates, hyaline body myopathy, trilaminar fiber myopathy, cap myopathy, zebra body myopathy, spheroid body myopathy, cytoplasmic body myopathy, desmin storage myopathies, X-linked myopathy with excessive autophagy, congenital myopathy with an excess of thin filaments, and congenital fiber type disproportion. Congenital myopathies

are inherited or caused by a spontaneous genetic mutation.[15,24]

■ Congenital Myotonic Muscular Dystrophy

Chief Clinical Characteristics

This presentation includes hypotonia and severe weakness. If the child survives the early weeks of life, he or she will show steady motor improvement up to age 10 years, with most developing independent walking. Fifty percent of children with this condition present with equinovarus contractures, and mental retardation is common.

Background Information

A rare form of myotonic muscular dystrophy, this condition is inherited as an autosomal dominant genetic defect of chromosome 19.[15,23–25]

■ Duchenne Muscular Dystrophy

Chief Clinical Characteristics

This presentation involves symmetric weakness, especially proximally, that progresses over time. Typical gait is described as waddling and includes an increased lumbar lordosis and toe walking.

Background Information

This condition is an X-linked genetic disorder occurring in males, usually diagnosed when parents report noticing the child has lost motor skills or strength. Bilateral toe walking often begins at about the age of 4 or 5 and gradually becomes more pronounced. Plantarflexion contractures occur over time. Calf muscles tend to enlarge, as muscle tissue is replaced by fat and connective tissue (pseudohypertrophy).[15,23,26–28]

■ Emery-Dreifuss Muscular Dystrophy

Chief Clinical Characteristics

This presentation involves weakness predominantly in a humeroperoneal distribution. Independent walking is typically observed into adulthood, but ankle plantarflexion and elbow flexion are common. Toe walking is possible but less commonly seen.

Background Information

This condition is an X-linked recessive disorder.[23,25,29,30]

▪ Poliomyelitis

Chief Clinical Characteristics
This presentation typically includes an initial fever and severe muscle pain, followed by asymmetric flaccid paralysis. It can be a cause of ipsilateral toe walking in the example of contralateral (unilateral) weakness of the anterior tibialis muscle resulting in a foot drop and excessive contralateral ankle plantarflexion and ipsilateral vaulting to allow for toe clearance in gait.

Background Information
Commonly called polio, this condition involves a viral infection of the motor neurons of the anterior horn cells of the spinal cord and of other parts of the central nervous system.[12–15,25]

▪ Post-Traumatic Weakness

Chief Clinical Characteristics
This presentation involves an acute or chronic injury to a structure in the lower extremities that can result in pain, muscle guarding, and weakness that leads to gait disturbances, including toe walking.

Background Information
Children presenting with pain in the lower extremity after a traumatic injury may exhibit an antalgic gait pattern (asymmetrical shortening of stance phase relative to swing phase) due to pain with weight bearing, and toe walking may be observed. After the initial injury has healed and pain is no longer present, toe walking may persist due to chronic weakness of the dorsiflexors (with the stronger plantarflexors contributing to an equinus contracture) or as a compensation for weak quadriceps (walking on the forefoot is used to generate an extension moment to stabilize the knee).

▪ Sensory Disturbance

Chief Clinical Characteristics
This presentation may be characterized by gait disturbances that vary with the affected sensory modality. For example, proprioceptive loss is sometimes associated with a stomping or slap-foot gait, and sometimes theorized to cause toe walking.

Background Information
Children with autism are often observed to walk up on their toes, which is theorized to be caused by an inability to adequately process vestibular information or visual-vestibular problems or to be a mechanism to provide increased proprioceptive feedback.[31–33]

▪ Spastic Cerebral Palsy

Chief Clinical Characteristics
This presentation may include spasticity of the calf during gait, and the child may toe walk, if ambulatory. Children with this condition may choose to toe walk due to weakness of the other antigravity extensor muscles; because the gluteal and quadriceps groups are weak, the compensatory approach is to excessively contract the ankle plantarflexors in order to stay upright. Asking the child to run often exaggerates the toe walking together with scapular retraction, making the diagnosis more evident.

Background Information
This is a nonprogressive chronic condition, noted at or about the time of birth, that affects muscle movement and coordination. It is caused by damage to the central nervous system before, during, or shortly after birth or in infancy. This condition is divided into four categories: spastic, athetoid (dyskinetic), ataxic, and mixed. Mixed forms of this condition include symptoms of more than one of the other three forms.[34–36] Very mild forms of spastic cerebral palsy are readily overlooked on routine examination so the cause of the toe walking is missed.

▪ Stroke

Chief Clinical Characteristics
This presentation consists of symptoms that are generally unilateral, opposite the side of the cortex that was affected, causing asymmetrical gait deviations, including toe walking due to muscle spasticity.

Background Information
A stroke may occur in the cerebellum, causing an ataxic gait. Strokes occurring *in utero* or at birth cause hemiplegic cerebral palsy.[37–39]

▪ Tethered Cord Syndrome

Chief Clinical Characteristics
This presentation may involve neurological deficits that begin to present as the child grows. A mixed upper and lower motor neuron pattern of deficits involves bowel and bladder

dysfunction and progressive gait disturbances beginning at 2 to 3 years of age.

Background Information

This condition occurs when the spinal cord is tethered and neurological symptoms increase positively with growth. Some of the more common causes of tethering include lipoma or lipomyelomeningocele, split cord malformation (diastematomyelia), dermal sinus tract, fatty or tight filum, or myelomeningocele (spina bifida or open spine).[40,41]

■ Traumatic Brain Injury

Chief Clinical Characteristics

This presentation, in the event of injury to the motor cortex or cerebellum, can be associated with gait disturbances and ataxia. Motor deficits depend on the severity of the injury, and may include gait and balance problems, slowing, and visual motor deficits.

Background Information

This condition may be categorized as penetrating (if an object strikes the head with sufficient force to cause a depressed skull fracture), missile (if an object either lodges within brain tissue or exits the skull), or nonpenetrating (closed head injuries).[42,43]

■ Traumatic Spinal Cord Injury

Chief Clinical Characteristics

This presentation includes weakness in a myotomal pattern below the level of the lesion, associated with loss of sensation in a dermatomal pattern, hypertonicity, spasticity, hyperreflexia, and sphincter dysfunction. Specific syndromes have characteristic presentations secondary to the location of the lesion. Incomplete forms of this condition may result in spasticity, which causes toe walking.

Background Information

Insult to the spinal cord results from fractured bone, displaced disk material, or a foreign object transecting or injuring the cord. Imaging is used to identify the cause of injury and direct surgical stabilization or intervention. Motor vehicle accidents and falls are the most common etiology of this condition.[44] Physical examination of strength and sensation is used to assign a score from the American Spinal Injury Association.[45] Injuries are classified in terms of neurological level (ie, most rostral segment where myotomal and dermatomal function is spared) and extent as either complete (total lack of sensory or motor function below level of injury) or incomplete (some motor or sensory function spared below the level of injury). Cervical spinal cord injury (SCI) results in tetraplegia and may cause paralysis or weakness of the respiratory musculature requiring mechanical ventilation and/or respiratory strengthening.[46] Thoracic or lumbar SCI results in paraplegia. Treatment consists of medical management, multidisciplinary rehabilitation, equipment prescription, and prevention of pressure ulcers, contractures, and further complications. Individuals with incomplete SCI may continue to recover strength and function, while individuals with complete SCI have a poor prognosis for recovery and instead use compensatory techniques and equipment. Individuals with SCI require adequate follow-up medical care to prevent secondary impairments.[47]

TUMORS

BONE OR SOFT TISSUE TUMORS OF THE LOWER EXTREMITY

■ Ewing's Sarcoma

Chief Clinical Characteristics

This presentation typically manifests as severe, persistent pain especially at night, localized swelling, palpable mass, tenderness, and decreased range of motion. Other symptoms can include fever, malaise, and weight loss when there are metastases.[48]

Background Information

This condition is the most common malignant primary tumor found in the pediatric spine[49] and the second most common pediatric malignancy overall.[50] Approximately 2.1 children per million are diagnosed with this condition each year with predominance in males. Diagnosis is usually between the ages of 10 and 20 years, and is uncommon before 5 years of age. Treatment includes a combination of multiagent chemotherapy, followed by radiation and resection for local control. Prognosis for cure is ~75% in those who present without metastasis, and less than 30% for those with metastasis.[50]

■ Langerhans' Cell Histiocytosis

Chief Clinical Characteristics

This presentation commonly consists of pain that is usually relieved with nonsteroidal anti-inflammatory medications and rest, and bracing if necessary. Associated symptoms may be hepatosplenomegaly, anemia, leukopenia, and thrombocytopenia. Neurological symptoms may manifest if there is cord compression.

Background Information

This condition is commonly found in the anterior elements of the spine as a single lesion or is multifocal. A single, localized lesion is also known as eosinophilic granuloma. This condition is generally found in children 3 to 15 years of age with a predominance in white males, but can manifest at any age.[51–53] Radiographs will show a well-defined lesion, with focal bone destruction and possible vertebral collapse, or vertebral plana. This condition appears to be the most common cause of vertebral plana. The intervertebral disks are not affected. Treatment is usually reserved for those with organ dysfunction, unrelieved symptoms, or osseous deformity, because this condition is usually self-limiting.[51] Treatment can include a combination of any or all of radiation, chemotherapy, steroid therapy, curettage, and bracing.[52,54]

■ Leukemia

Chief Clinical Characteristics

This presentation commonly involves reports of aches and pains in the extremities, back, and joints, fatigue, and anorexia. There may also be intermittent low-grade fever, enlarged lymph nodes, weight loss, petechiae, lethargy, shortness of breath, bruises, and excessive bleeding.

Background Information

Leukemia is the most common malignancy in children and adolescents, with a higher incidence in males.[55,56] It is typically diagnosed within the first decade of life and accounts for about 40% of all childhood malignancies. The two most common types account for ~90% of all leukemias: acute lymphoblastic leukemia (77% to 80%), and acute myelogenous leukemia (10% to 13%). Some symptoms may be consistent with a viral infection; however, they persist longer. Other symptoms are a result of progressive disease and bone marrow failure as a result of bone marrow infiltration by malignant cells, leading to anemia and decreased production of clotting factors.[56] Diagnostic evaluation of patients with leukemia includes complete blood count and bone marrow biopsy. Examination of bone marrow aspirate is necessary for confirmation, and a spinal tap determines if leukemia is present in the central nervous system.[57] Infiltration of bone and bone marrow may also be viewed on magnetic resonance imaging.[52] Rarely radiographs may show osteopenia and compression fractures. Analysis of chromosome abnormalities in the leukemia cells is very important to assess prognosis and formulate treatment. Treatment is specific to the type of leukemia present and typically has several phases. It involves multiple courses of chemotherapy and antibiotics to prevent infection, and often a child will require blood transfusions. Side effects of chemotherapy and steroid treatment include neutropenia, thrombocytopenia, and risk for infection. Long-term complications can include osteoporosis and avascular necrosis. Bone marrow or stem cell transplant is reserved for situations where standard chemotherapy has failed and has a better success rate if performed in remission. With current advances in treatment, the 5-year survival rate without relapse is 80% to 90%.[58]

■ Lymphoma

Chief Clinical Characteristics

This presentation initially involves asymptomatic, chronically swollen lymph nodes, most commonly in the neck, axillae, or groin. Other symptoms may include neurological symptoms due to cord compression, fever, itching or irritation of the skin, weight loss, night sweats, cough, or shortness of breath.[57] Symptoms will depend on the type of lymphoma present and the proximity to other structures and organs.

Background Information

Lymphoma is one of the most prevalent malignant tumors of childhood and can manifest quickly. The two general types of lymphoma are Hodgkin's lymphoma and non-Hodgkin's lymphoma, and each has its own subtypes. Hodgkin's disease is distinguished from non-Hodgkin's by the presence of specific cancer cells in the biopsy material, termed Reed-Sternberg cells.[57,59] Approximately 40% of pediatric cases are of the Hodgkin's type, and 60% are non-Hodgkins.[55] Approximately 10% to 15% of all cases of Hodgkin's disease and about 5% of all non-Hodgkin's lymphoma (NHL) cases are in children under age 19, both with a higher prevalence in boys. NHL is more common in children under 5 years of age.[59,60] Biopsy, radiographs, computed tomography, and blood tests are performed for definitive diagnosis and to assess the stage of disease. Bone marrow biopsy is done to evaluate bone marrow involvement. Radiographs and computed tomography typically show enlarged lymph nodes in the affected areas and can show extensive, destructive lesions in patients with osseous involvement. Magnetic resonance imaging is indicated to evaluate soft tissue involvement.[48] Laboratory tests may show anemia and an elevated sedimentation rate. Treatment includes chemotherapy and radiation, the course of which depends on the type of lymphoma, the stage of disease, and if there is bone marrow metastasis. Bone marrow transplant may be indicated if the patient fails to respond to standard chemotherapy and radiation. Survival rates are 90% to 95% for those with local lesions, and 75% to 80% for those with more diffuse disease.[55]

■ Nephroblastoma (Wilms' Tumor)

Chief Clinical Characteristics

This presentation typically includes an asymptomatic, nontender mass in the abdomen. Associated symptoms may be abdominal pain, fever, nausea, and vomiting. Hematuria, anemia, and hypertension can occur, since the kidneys are instrumental in controlling blood pressure. Shortness of breath may be present if there are metastases to the lungs.[55,61]

Background Information

This condition involves a tumor that originates from renal precursor cells. It is the second most common abdominal tumor in infants and children up to 5 years old and is the most common primary malignant tumor of the kidney. Multiple laboratory tests, including complete blood count, ultrasound, magnetic resonance imaging, or computed tomography, are indicated. Treatment includes removal of the kidney containing the tumor followed by chemotherapy and/or radiation. The survival rate is typically 70% to 95%, especially in young children, or those with stage I, II, or III tumors.[61] Recurrences are usually seen within 3 years. Postradiation scoliosis may follow in the second decade.

■ Neuroblastoma

Chief Clinical Characteristics

This presentation may include severe localized back pain, weakness, scoliosis, and neurological signs secondary to spinal cord compression. Other symptoms may include a palpable mass, hepatomegaly, constipation, abdominal pain, bladder dysfunction, and ecchymoses. It is one of the few cancers that cause diarrhea.[48,55,62,63]

Background Information

This condition is a solid tumor that develops in neural crest tissue, most commonly in the abdomen, chest, or adrenal glands.[55] It rarely originates in the brain or spinal cord. If the primary lesion originates somewhere other than the spinal cord, metastases is hematogenic in nature, and can spread to bone, bone marrow, liver, skin, lungs, and the brain. This is the most common extracranial cancer of childhood and the third most common pediatric neoplasm overall. Approximately 500 new cases are diagnosed each year. It is usually diagnosed in infancy, almost always by 5 years of age, and is rarely seen in children over 10 years of age.[48,55,62,63] Low-risk tumors (stage I) in infants treated with surgical excision and observation have an approximately 90% survival rate without relapse. Children over 3 years of age with stage IV tumors only have a 10% to 15% survival rate.[55] In infants the tumor may regress completely with spontaneous cell death, or mature to normal ganglion cells and become benign. In children over 1 year of age, the disease progression may be rapidly metastatic and often fatal.[55,62]

■ Osteochondroma

Chief Clinical Characteristics
This presentation involves pain that can alter gait pattern, resulting from compression of a nerve or fracture of the exostosis.[64]

Background Information
This cartilaginous exostosis is more common in males and sometimes occurs in the pelvis. It is more common in late adolescence to young adulthood. Familial osteochondromatosis or multiple hereditary exostosis is an autosomal dominant inherited variant in which more than two osteochondromas are present. This form is more common in males during childhood and is more likely to involve the hip region.[64]

■ Osteoid Osteoma

Chief Clinical Characteristics
This presentation involves predominantly intense nocturnal pain that may be relieved with nonsteroidal anti-inflammatory medications or aspirin.[52,65] The pain may be referred or localized. Gait deviations and muscle atrophy are often present. About 50% of children present with nonstructural, painful scoliosis,[49] which should be a red flag because idiopathic scoliosis is not painful.

Background Information
This condition includes highly vascularized connective tissue bundles, usually sclerotic, surrounding an osteoid nidus or growth center. They are small round or ovate tumors that are usually less than 1 cm in diameter.[48,66] Spinal osteoid lesions are found primarily in the posterior elements of the lumbar vertebra.[48,49,52,53,66] Soft tissue changes are rare. This condition is typically found in children between the ages of 5 and 20, with an approximate 2:1 male-to-female ratio.[48,67] Erythrocyte sedimentation rate, leukocyte count, and protein electrophoresis should be normal. Radiographs and computed tomography will also differentiate osteoid osteomas from osteoblastomas,

infection, lymphoma, and facet abnormalities such as spondylolysis.[67] Spinal lesions typically require open surgical excision. In most cases, the scoliosis will resolve and pain will subside completely.[54]

■ Osteosarcoma (Osteogenic Sarcoma)

Chief Clinical Characteristics
This presentation may be characterized by persistent night pain.

Background Information
This condition is related to highly malignant and locally aggressive lesions.[68] It rarely originates in the axial skeleton, but when it does it is usually found in the vertebral bodies.[54,68,69] Vertebral sarcomas comprise about 10% of all cases.[49] These tumors are typically found in the metaphyses of long bones and may metastasize to the spine. Diagnosis usually occurs between 10 and 20 years of age, and adolescent growth spurts appear to be the greatest risk periods for development.[52,70] Children with certain hereditary conditions such as retinoblastoma have a significant predisposition for developing this condition. Treatment includes local control with surgical excision and radiation or chemotherapy for metastatic lesions. If neurological signs are present, surgical decompression and laminectomy may be necessary.[71] Without metastasis approximately 70% of cases are cured with surgery and chemotherapy. If metastases are present on diagnosis, the survival rate is less than 20%.[69]

■ Rhabdomyosarcoma

Chief Clinical Characteristics
This presentation may include back pain associated with neurological signs due to cord compression when present in the lumbar spine.[57,69]

Background Information
This condition is thought to originate from striated skeletal muscle cells.[69] Alveolar rhabdomyosarcoma is typically found in the extremities and in paravertebral soft tissue. Although it is rare, this condition is the most common solid soft tissue tumor in children under 10 years of age, accounting for 5% to

8% of pediatric neoplasms. It is usually diagnosed prior to age 6 and is most prevalent in male infants.[48,57,69] Diagnostic tests include biopsy, and computed tomography and magnetic resonance imaging.[48,57] Treatment includes chemotherapy, radiation, and if necessary, complete resection. For those diagnosed and treated in the early stages, the survival rate is approximately 80% to 90%.[57,69] Prognosis is poor for those with the alveolar subtype, with larger tumors, or who are over 10 years of age.[48,57,69]

■ Synovial Sarcoma

Chief Clinical Characteristics

This presentation includes a painful mass in approximately half of patients.[72]

Background Information

A synovial sarcoma is a slow-growing, malignant tumor that is typically found proximal to tendons or fascia but sometimes also near or inside of a joint. It is more common in the lower extremity.[72]

■ Spinal Cord Tumor

Chief Clinical Characteristics

This presentation commonly involves nonspecific symptoms that include local pain or stiffness. Radicular (radiating) pain suggests nerve root impingement, which may be exacerbated with movement. The child may report weakness in one or both extremities. The onset of the pain symptoms is often insidious and followed by a gradually progressive course. However, once symptoms other than pain appear, symptom progression may be rapid.

Background Information

Direct compression of the spinal cord may be caused by tumors of the vertebral bodies, paravertebral spaces, or structures within the epidural space. Nerve tracts most vulnerable to mechanical pressure include the corticospinal and spinocerebellar tracts and the posterior spinal columns. Tumors of the spine may compromise the vascular supply, causing edema or ischemia.[15,73]

■ Syringomyelia

Chief Clinical Characteristics

This presentation includes lower motor neuron deficits above the level of the lesion, with

upper motor neuron signs below the lesion. There is dissociated sensory loss in the arms, with decreased response to pain or temperature, but with light touch preserved. Weakness and muscle wasting may be present at the level of the lesion, with increased tendon reflexes and spasticity in the lower extremities.

Background Information

This condition is a formation of a cavity in the inner part of the spinal cord, which may be congenital or acquired.[6]

■ Vascular Malformation of the Calf Muscle

Chief Clinical Characteristics

This presentation can be characterized by painful contracture of the calf muscle, resulting in equinus deformity and toe walking.[74] The affected limb may present with symptoms and signs ranging from dermatological features such as a soft blue mass and port wine stain to a hypertrophic limb. Mean age at diagnosis is 6 years. Other associated signs may include a limb-length discrepancy.

Background Information

This condition results from skeletal changes caused by a vascular malformation or tumor. The pain of this condition is related to either hemorrhage or hematoma. Treatment may involve nonsurgical options including analgesic medications and compression stockings. Surgical embolization also may be indicated if a specific location of vascular compromise is well characterized. Advanced forms of this condition can result in amputation of the affected limb.[75]

References

1. Faulks S, Luther B. Changing paradigm for the treatment of clubfeet. *Orthop Nurs*. Jan–Feb 2005;24(1):25–30; quiz 31–32.
2. Miedzybrodzka Z. Congenital talipes equinovarus (clubfoot): a disorder of the foot but not the hand. *J Anat*. Jan 2003;202(1):37–42.
3. Roye DP Jr, Roye BD. Idiopathic congenital talipes equinovarus. *J Am Acad Orthop Surg*. Jul–Aug 2002; 10(4):239–248.
4. Dupont-Versteegden EE, McCarter RJ, Katz MS. Voluntary exercise decreases progression of muscular dystrophy in diaphragm of mdx mice. *J Appl Physiol*. Oct 1994;77(4):1736–1741.
5. Plante-Bordeneuve V, Said G. Dejerine-Sottas disease and hereditary demyelinating polyneuropathy of infancy. *Muscle Nerve*. Nov 2002;26(5):608–621.

6. Simon R, Aminoff M, Greenberg D. Disorders of somatic sensation. In: Simon R, Aminoff M, Greenberg D, eds. *Clinical Neurology*. 4th ed. Stamford, CT: Appleton & Lange; 1999:199–227.

7. Caselli MA, Rzonca EC, Lue BY. Habitual toe walking: evaluation and approach to treatment. *Clin Podiatr Med Surg*. Jul 1988;5(3):547–559.

8. Hirsch G, Wagner B. The natural history of idiopathic toe walking: a long-term follow-up of fourteen conservatively treated children. *Acta Paediatr*. Feb 2004; 93(2):196–199.

9. Leach J. Orthopedic conditions. In: Campbell S, Linden DV, Palisano R, eds. *Physical Therapy for Children*. 2nd ed. St. Louis, MO: W. B. Saunders; 2000: 398–428.

10. Sala DA, Shulman LH, Kennedy RF, Grant AD, Chu ML. Idiopathic toe-walking: a review. *Dev Med Child Neurol*. Dec 1999;41(12):846–848.

11. Shulman LH, Sala DA, Chu ML, McCaul PR, Sandler BJ. Developmental implications of idiopathic toe walking. *J Pediatr*. Apr 1997;130(4):541–546.

12. Amato AA, Barohn RJ. Idiopathic inflammatory myopathies. *Neurol Clin*. Aug 1997;15(3):615–648.

13. Callen JP. Dermatomyositis. *Lancet*. Jan 1, 2000;355 (9197):53–57.

14. Dalakas MC, Hohlfeld R. Polymyositis and dermatomyositis. *Lancet*. Sep 20, 2003;362(9388):971–982.

15. Simon R, Aminoff M, Greenberg D. Motor deficits. In: Simon R, Aminoff M, Greenberg D, eds. *Clinical Neurology*. 4th ed. Stamford, CT: Appleton & Lange; 1999:159–198.

16. Klippel JH, Crofford LJ, Stone JH, Weyand CM. *Primer on the Rheumatic Diseases*. 12th ed. Atlanta, GA: Arthritis Foundation; 2001.

17. Reiff A. *Kids Get Arthritis Too!* El Monte, CA: Children's Medical Services; 2003.

18. Rhodes V. Physical therapy management of patients with juvenile rheumatoid arthritis. In *Pediatric Orthopedics*. Alexandria, VA: American Physical Therapy Association; 1992.

19. Ilowite NT. Current treatment of juvenile rheumatoid arthritis. *Pediatrics*. Jan 2002;109(1):109–115.

20. Ratliffe K. Developmental orthopedic disorders. In: Ratliffe K, ed. *Clinical Pediatric Physical Therapy*. St. Louis, MO: Mosby; 1998:99–130.

21. Scull S. Juvenile rheumatoid arthritis. In: Campbell S, Linden DV, Palisano R, eds. *Physical Therapy for Children*. 2nd ed. St. Louis, MO: W. B. Saunders; 2000: 227–246.

22. Carter GT, Wineinger MA, Walsh SA, Horasek SJ, Abresch RT, Fowler WM Jr. Effect of voluntary wheel-running exercise on muscles of the mdx mouse. *Neuromuscul Disord*. Jul 1995;5(4):323–332.

23. Stuberg W. Muscular dystrophy and spinal muscular atrophy. In: Campbell S, Linden DV, Palisano R, eds. *Physical Therapy for Children*. 2nd ed. St. Louis, MO: W. B. Saunders; 2000:339–369.

24. de Girolami U, Anthony D, Frosch M. Peripheral nerve and skeletal muscle. In: Cotran R, Kumar V, Robbins S, Schoen F, eds. *Robbins Pathologic Basis of Disease*. 5th ed. Philadelphia, PA: W. B. Saunders; 1994:1273–1294.

25. Gilroy J. *Basic Neurology*. 2nd ed. New York, NY: McGraw-Hill; 1990.

26. McDonald CM. Physical activity, health impairments, and disability in neuromuscular disease. *Am J Phys Med Rehabil*. Nov 2002;81(11 suppl):S108–120.

27. Ratliffe K. Genetic disorders. In: Ratliffe K, ed. *Clinical Pediatric Physical Therapy*. St. Louis, MO: Mosby; 1998:219–274.

28. Williams EA, Read L, Ellis A, Morris P, Galasko CS. The management of equinus deformity in Duchenne muscular dystrophy. *J Bone Joint Surg Br*. Aug 1984; 66(4):546–550.

29. Dickey RP, Ziter FA, Smith RA. Emery-Dreifuss muscular dystrophy. *J Pediatr*. Apr 1984;104(4):555–559.

30. Merlini L, Granata C, Dominici P, Bonfiglioli S. Emery-Dreifuss muscular dystrophy: report of five cases in a family and review of the literature. *Muscle Nerve*. Jul–Aug 1986;9(6):481–485.

31. Ayers J. *Sensory Integration and the Child*. Los Angeles, CA: Western Psychological Services; 1979.

32. Montgomery P, Gauger J. Sensory dysfunction in children who toe walk. *Phys Ther*. Oct 1978;58(10):1195–1204.

33. Ratliffe K. Sensory, processing, and cognitive disorders. In: Ratliffe K, ed. *Clinical Pediatric Physical Therapy*. St. Louis, MO: Mosby; 1998:313–350.

34. Dabney KW, Lipton GE, Miller F. Cerebral palsy. *Curr Opin Pediatr*. Feb 1997;9(1):81–88.

35. Olney S, Wright M. Cerebral palsy. In: Campbell S, Linden DV, Palisano R, eds. *Physical Therapy for Children*. 2nd ed. St. Louis, MO: W. B. Saunders; 2000:533–570.

36. Ratliffe K. Cerebral palsy. In: Ratliffe K, ed. *Clinical Pediatric Physical Therapy*. St. Louis, MO: Mosby; 1998: 163–218.

37. Gulati S, Kalra V. Stroke in children. *Indian J Pediatr*. Aug 2003;70(8):639–648.

38. Hutchison JS, Ichord R, Guerguerian AM, Deveber G. Cerebrovascular disorders. *Semin Pediatr Neurol*. Jun 2004;11(2):139–146.

39. Jain V, Sabharwal RK, Sachdeva A. Stroke in children. *Indian J Pediatr*. Mar 2003;70(suppl 1):S23–27.

40. Anderson FM. Occult spinal dysraphism: a series of 73 cases. *Pediatrics*. Jun 1975;55(6):826–835.

41. Soonawala N, Overweg-Plandsoen WC, Brouwer OF. Early clinical signs and symptoms in occult spinal dysraphism: a retrospective case study of 47 patients. *Clin Neurol Neurosurg*. Mar 1999;101(1):11–14.

42. Ratliffe K. Traumatic disorders. In: Ratliffe K, ed. *Clinical Pediatric Physical Therapy*. St. Louis, MO: Mosby; 1998: 275–312.

43. Kerkering G, Phillips W. Brain injuries: traumatic brain injuries, near-drowning, and brain tumors. In: Campbell S, Linden DV, Palisano R, eds. *Physical Therapy for Children*. 2nd ed. St. Louis, MO: W. B. Saunders; 2000:597–620.

44. Jackson AB, Dijkers M, Devivo MJ, Poczatek RB. A demographic profile of new traumatic spinal cord injuries: change and stability over 30 years. *Arch Phys Med Rehabil*. Nov 2004;85(11):1740–1748.

45. McDonald JW, Sadowsky C. Spinal-cord injury. *Lancet*. Feb 2, 2002;359(9304):417–425.

46. Gutierrez CJ, Harrow J, Haines F. Using an evidence-based protocol to guide rehabilitation and weaning of ventilator-dependent cervical spinal cord injury patients. *J Rehabil Res Dev*. Sep–Oct 2003;40(5 suppl 2):99–110.

47. Bloemen-Vrencken JH, de Witte LP, Post MW. Follow-up care for persons with spinal cord injury living in the community: a systematic review of interventions and their evaluation. *Spinal Cord*. Aug 2005;43 (8):462–475.

48. Erol B, States L. Musculoskeletal tumors in children. In: Dormans JP, ed. *Pediatric Orthopedics and Sports Medicine: The Requisites in Pediatrics*. St. Louis, MO: Mosby; 2004:325.

49. Luedtke LM, Flynn JM, Ganley TJ, Hosalkar HS, Pill SG, Dormans JP. The orthopedists' perspective: bone tumors, scoliosis, and trauma. *Radiol Clin North Am*. Jul 2001;39(4):803–821.

50. Horowitz ME, Neff JR, Kun LE. Ewing's sarcoma. Radiotherapy versus surgery for local control. *Pediatr Clin North Am*. Apr 1991;38(2):365–380.

51. Levine SE, Dormans JP, Meyer JS, Corcoran TA. Langerhans' cell histiocytosis of the spine in children. *Clin Orthop Relat Res*. Feb 1996(323):288–293.

52. Miller SL, Hoffer FA. Malignant and benign bone tumors. *Radiol Clin North Am*. Jul 2001;39(4):673–699.

53. Thompson G. The spine. In: Behrman RE, Kliegman RM, Jenson WS, eds. *Nelson Textbook of Pediatrics*. 17th ed. Philadelphia, PA: W. B. Saunders; 2004:2287.

54. Hosalkar HS, Dormans JP. Back pain in children requires extensive workup. *Biomechanics*. 2003(June):51–58.

55. Golden CB, Feusner JH. Malignant abdominal masses in children: quick guide to evaluation and diagnosis. *Pediatr Clin North Am*. Dec 2002;49(6):1369–1392, viii.

56. Tubergen D, Bleyer A. Cancer and benign tumors. In: Behrman RE, Kliegman RM, Jenson HB, eds. *Nelson Textbook of Pediatrics*. 17th ed. Philadelphia, PA: W. B. Saunders; 2004:1694–1698.

57. John Hopkins University. Types of childhood cancers. http://www.jhscout.org//types/index.cfm. Accessed August 27, 2005.

58. Miller S, Hoffer F. Malignant and benign bone tumors. *Radiol Clin North Am Pediatr Musculoskel Radiol*. 2001;39(4):673–699.

59. Gilchrist G. Lymphoma. In: Behrman RE, Kliegman RM, Jenson HB, eds. *Nelson Textbook of Pediatrics*. 17th ed. Philadelphia, PA: W. B. Saunders; 2004.

60. Kurtzberg J, Graham ML. Non-Hodgkin's lymphoma. Biologic classification and implication for therapy. *Pediatr Clin North Am*. Apr 1991;38(2):443–456.

61. Beers MH. *The Merck Manual of Medical Information*. 2nd ed. Whitehouse Station, NJ: Merck Research Laboratories 2003.

62. American Cancer Society. Detailed guide: Brain/CNS tumors in children: what are children's brain and spinal cord cancers? 2005.

63. Ater J. Neuroblastoma. In: Behrman RE, Kliegman RM, Jenson HB, eds. *Nelson Textbook of Pediatrics*. 17th ed. Philadelphia, PA: W. B. Saunders; 2004:1709.

64. Cotran RS, Kumar V, Robbins SL, Schoen FJ. *Pathologic Basis of Disease*. 5th ed. Philadelphia, PA: W. B. Saunders; 1994.

65. Payne WK 3rd, Ogilvie JW. Back pain in children and adolescents. *Pediatr Clin North Am*. Aug 1996;43(4):899–917.

66. Guzey FK, Seyithanoglu MH, Sencer A, Emei E, Alatas I, Izgi AN. Vertebral osteoid osteoma associated with paravertebral soft-tissue changes on magnetic resonance imaging. Report of two cases. *J Neurosurg*. May 2004;100(5 suppl Pediatrics):532–536.

67. Murphey MD, Andrews CL, Flemming DJ, Temple HT, Smith WS, Smirniotopoulos JG. From the archives of the AFIP. Primary tumors of the spine: radiologic pathologic correlation. *Radiographics*. Sep 1996;16(5):1131–1158.

68. Meyer WH, Malawer MM. Osteosarcoma. Clinical features and evolving surgical and chemotherapeutic strategies. *Pediatr Clin North Am*. Apr 1991;38(2):317–348.

69. Amdt C. Soft tissue sarcomas. In: Behrman RE, Kliegman RM, Jenson HB, eds. *Nelson Textbook of Pediatrics*. 17th ed. Philadelphia, PA: W. B. Saunders; 2004:1714.

70. Kay RM, Eckardt JJ, Mirra JM. Osteosarcoma and Ewing's sarcoma in a retinoblastoma patient. *Clin Orthop Relat Res*. Feb 1996(323):284–287.

71. Wheeless CR. *Wheeless' Textbook of Orthopedics*. Durham, NC: Duke University Medical Center; 2005.

72. Klippel JH. *Primer on the Rheumatic Diseases*. 12th ed. Atlanta, GA: Arthritis Foundation; 2002.

73. Faerber EN, Roman NV. Central nervous system tumors of childhood. *Radiol Clin North Am*. Nov 1997;35(6):1301–1328.

74. Domb BG, Khanna AJ, Mitchell SE, Frassica FJ. Toe walking attributable to venous malformation of the calf muscle. *Clin Orthop Relat Res*. Mar 2004(420):225–229.

75. Breugem CC, Maas M, Breugem SJ, Schaap GR, van der Horst CM. Vascular malformations of the lower limb with osseous involvement. *J Bone Joint Surg Br*. Apr 2003; 85(3):399–405.

CHAPTER 56

Joint Contractures in a Child

■ *Cassandra Sanders-Holly, PT, DPT, PCS* ■ *Cheri Kay Sessions, PT, DPT, ATC*

Description of the Symptom

Contracture has been defined as "a condition of fixed high resistance to passive stretch of a muscle, resulting from fibrosis of the tissues supporting the muscles or the joints, or from disorders of the muscle fibers." It is an abnormal, often permanent shortening of the muscle or scar tissue that results in distortion or deformity. This chapter describes possible causes of joint contractures in a child.

Special Concerns
■ Joint erythema
■ Joint warmth
■ Sudden onset of joint contracture
■ Increased pain within the joint
■ Changes in bony configuration

CHAPTER PREVIEW: Conditions That May Lead to Joint Contractures in a Child

 Trauma

COMMON

Brachial plexus injury (Erb's palsy, Klumpke's palsy) 1091
Third-degree burns 1097
Traumatic brain injury 1097

UNCOMMON

Surgical interventions (eg, limb lengthening) 1096

RARE

Not applicable

I **Inflammation**

COMMON

Aseptic
Juvenile rheumatoid arthritis 1094
Systemic lupus erythematosus 1097

Septic
Not applicable

UNCOMMON

Aseptic
Juvenile ankylosing spondylitis 1093
Psoriatic arthritis 1095
Reactive arthritis 1095
Scleroderma 1095

Septic
Human immunodeficiency virus encephalopathy 1092

(continued)

Inflammation *(continued)*

RARE

Aseptic
Juvenile dermatomyositis 1093

Septic
Poliomyelitis 1095

M   Metabolic

COMMON

Not applicable

UNCOMMON

Not applicable

RARE

Not applicable

Va   Vascular

COMMON

Not applicable

UNCOMMON

Not applicable

RARE

Not applicable

De   Degenerative

COMMON

Immobilization and prolonged bedrest 1093

UNCOMMON

Spinal muscular atrophy 1096

RARE

Not applicable

Tu   Tumor

COMMON

Not applicable

UNCOMMON

Malignant Primary:
Not applicable
Malignant Metastatic:
Not applicable
Benign, such as:
• Syringomyelia 1097

Tumor *(continued)*

RARE

Not applicable

Congenital

COMMON

Duchenne muscular dystrophy 1092
Talipes equinovarus (clubfoot) 1097

UNCOMMON

Arthrogryposis 1091

RARE

Epidermolysis bullosa 1092
Infantile spasms 1093
Lesch-Nyhan syndrome 1094
Sjögren-Larsson syndrome 1096

Ne Neurogenic/Psychogenic

COMMON

Cerebral palsy 1091
Hydrocephalus 1093
Immobilization and prolonged bedrest 1093
Myelodysplasia 1094
Seizure disorders 1096

UNCOMMON

Tethered cord syndrome 1097

RARE

Lennox-Gastaut syndrome 1094
Leukodystrophies 1094
Pelizaeus-Merzbacher disease 1095
Subacute sclerosing panencephalitis 1096

Note: These are estimates of relative incidence because few data are available for the less common conditions.

Common Ages at Which Joint Contractures Present in a Child

APPROXIMATE AGE	CONDITION
Birth to 3 Years	Brachial plexus injury
	Burns
	Cerebral palsy
	Hydrocephalus
	Immobilization
	Juvenile rheumatoid arthritis
	Lesch-Nyhan syndrome
	Leukodystrophies
	Myelodysplasia
	Pelizaeus-Merzbacher disease
	Poliomyelitis
	Seizure disorders

(continued)

Common Ages at Which Joint Contractures Present in a Child—cont'd

APPROXIMATE AGE	CONDITION
	Sjögren-Larsson syndrome
	Traumatic brain injury
Preschool (3–5 Years)	Burns
	Cerebral palsy
	Hydrocephalus
	Immobilization
	Juvenile rheumatoid arthritis
	Pelizaeus-Merzbacher disease
	Poliomyelitis
	Seizure disorders
	Traumatic brain injury
Elementary School (6–11 Years)	Burns
	Cerebral palsy
	Hydrocephalus
	Juvenile dermatomyositis
	Juvenile rheumatoid arthritis
	Immobilization
	Pelizaeus-Merzbacher disease
	Poliomyelitis
	Seizure disorders
	Systemic lupus erythematosus
	Traumatic brain injury
Middle School (12–14 Years)	Burns
	Cerebral palsy
	Duchenne muscular dystrophy
	Hydrocephalus
	Immobilization
	Juvenile dermatomyositis
	Juvenile rheumatoid arthritis
	Pelizaeus-Merzbacher disease
	Poliomyelitis
	Seizure disorders
	Systemic lupus erythematosus
	Traumatic brain injury
High School (15–18 Years)	Burns
	Cerebral palsy
	Duchenne muscular dystrophy
	Hydrocephalus
	Immobilization
	Juvenile rheumatoid arthritis
	Pelizaeus-Merzbacher disease
	Seizure disorders
	Systemic lupus erythematosus
	Traumatic brain injury

Overview of Joint Contractures in a Child

The etiology of a contracture may be dynamic or structural. A dynamic contracture is secondary to volitional muscle activity (ie, idiopathic toe walking) or caused by involuntary muscle activity (ie, spasticity). A structural contracture is an actual shortening of the musculotendinous unit or other joint structures. Clinically, physical therapists will find resistance perceived as stiffness while moving a joint through its range of motion or limited total available range of motion. Contractures typically develop in response to inadequate stretch stimulus, weakness/immobilization, and muscle imbalances. The primary factors in contracture formation are abnormal muscle structure, abnormal muscle tone, limb positioning, and activity level.

In diagnosing the cause of a child's contracture, it is important to consider the child's age, gender, and past medical history. The child may have a diagnosis for which contractures are considered a natural progression of the disease. The nature of the onset of contracture formation is important to consider, including whether the contracture was present at birth, developed in response to a sudden, traumatic event, or was insidious in nature. The physical therapist should note which joints are involved and potential symmetry to the involvement. The type and pattern of muscles also may be diagnostically significant.

During an assessment, the therapist needs to consider the etiology (dynamic vs. structural) of the contracture and the level of involvement at each joint by examining the child's functional mobility. Objective range-of-motion measurements should be taken, noting pain, stiffness, spasticity, or clonus during passive movement of the joint. Two measurements are typically taken clinically, the initial resistance and the final resistance. Measurements should be taken with slow movement of the joint to avoid resistance from spasticity. Major changes in mobility status are important to consider, as well as how the child is positioned throughout the course of a day. It is important to consider episodes of rapid growth because the rate of muscle elongation is slower than that of bone growth or elongation. These contractures may resolve over time or with minimal intervention.

> ## Description of Conditions That May Lead to Joint Contractures in a Child

■ Arthrogryposis

Chief Clinical Characteristics
This presentation—in its severe, generalized form (arthrogryposis multiplex congenita; amyoplasia)—is characterized by multiple joint contractures with muscle weakness or imbalance.

These features are variable and although all four extremities are often involved, children with only upper extremity or only lower extremity involvement are not uncommon. The most common findings include rigid joints with significant contractures; featureless, cylindrical extremities that lack skin creases; atrophy or absence of muscle groups; diminished or absent deep tendon reflexes; and dislocations of joints with the hip being the most common. Sensation is intact.

Background Information
This is a nonprogressive disorder that is evident at birth and is not hereditary. Another form of this condition, distal arthrogryposis, which primarily involves the hands and feet, however, is hereditary (autosomal dominant). Management is largely focused on enhancing the child's functions through physical and occupational therapy.[1]

■ Brachial Plexus Injury (Erb's Palsy, Klumpke's Palsy)

Chief Clinical Characteristics
This presentation typically involves an inability to move an upper extremity throughout available range of motion; weakness or paralysis of the upper extremity musculature, particularly in the C5–C6 nerve root distribution; and posturing in shoulder extension, internal rotation, and adduction, elbow extension, forearm pronation, and wrist and finger flexion. Contractures of the involved extremity (shoulder, elbow, wrist, and fingers) often develop over time due to imbalance of some musculature.

Background Information
Paralysis of the proximal shoulder musculature is not uncommon and grasp is typically intact with forearm support. This condition commonly follows a difficult vaginal delivery during which a traction force on the infant's shoulder can injure the cervical roots, fracture the clavicle or humerus, or sublux the shoulder.[2]

■ Cerebral Palsy

Chief Clinical Characteristics
This presentation typically ranges from very minimally affecting one extremity to severely affecting the entire body. Common manifestations include increased or decreased tone;

spasticity; developmental delay; visual, hearing, and speech abnormalities; and cognitive abnormalities.

Background Information

Cerebral palsy is a chronic nonprogressive disorder of posture and movement that results from a prepartum, peripartum, or shortly postpartum oxygen deprivation that affects the central nervous system. Joint contractures are common in the ankles, knees, hips, wrists, elbows, and shoulder secondary to spasticity and decreased functional mobility. This condition is classified by topographic distribution of impairment (hemiplegia, diplegia, quadriplegia) and by clinical findings (spasticity, hypotonia, ataxia, dyskinesia/athetosis). In spastic cerebral palsy, muscles are perceived as stiff, especially during active movement. Velocity-dependent resistance of passive movement produces increased muscle tone; selective control is limited, producing abnormal movement synergies; the active range of motion is limited by coactivation of muscular activity; and the timing of the muscle activation and postural responses is abnormal.[3] Hypotonia is characterized by diminished resting muscle tone, hypermobility, decreased ability to produce voluntary force, and postural instability. Ataxia is a disorder of balance and control and in the timing of coordinated movement. Dyskinesia is associated with uncontrolled or purposeless movements that may present with both hypotonia or hypertonia.

■ Duchenne Muscular Dystrophy

Chief Clinical Characteristics

This presentation typically involves progressive muscular decline with eventual death secondary to respiratory infection or cardiorespiratory insufficiency in those in their late teens or early 20s. There is a high tendency for the development of plantarflexion contractures in this population with a progression to equinovarus deformity. Other muscle groups at risk are the hamstrings, iliotibial band, and hip flexors.[4] Clinically, young boys present with toe walking, excessive lumbar lordosis, and difficulty rising from the floor (positive Gower's sign).

Background Information

This condition is a genetic myopathy that involves a steadily progressive degenerative course. This condition has an X-linked inheritance pattern in which a male baby will inherit the disease from his mother. Symptoms usually begin presenting before the age of 3; however, the symptoms may not be noticed for months or years and may go undiagnosed or misdiagnosed for years.

■ Epidermolysis Bullosa

Chief Clinical Characteristics

This presentation includes blistering over the hands and feet with or without scarring depending on the type. The more severe types involve deeper tissue layers and cause joint deformity.

Background Information

The four types of this condition are all autosomal inherited skin blistering disorders that differ in severity and prognosis. The mildest form is referred to as simplex (epidermolytic) and involves the superficial basal cell layer. This form typically affects the hands and the feet and rarely leaves a scar. The junctional (letalis) form is localized and progressive and typically leaves scarring with pyloric atresia, mucosal lesions, dysplastic teeth, loss of nails, and defects in the basement membrane of the epidermis associated with proteins. The recessive dystrophic and dominant dystrophic types (both dermolytic) affect the deep dermis below the lamina densa. These forms leave severe scarring, including mitten scarring of the hands and feet with marked deformities.[5]

■ Human Immunodeficiency Virus Encephalopathy

Chief Clinical Characteristics

This presentation commonly includes decreased brain growth, developmental delays, weakness with pyramidal tract signs, ataxia, myoclonus, pseudobulbar palsy, and seizures.

Background Information

Infants and children who are congenitally infected with the human immunodeficiency virus often have this form of encephalitis. It usually develops in infancy or may be delayed to as late as 5 years of age. It may have an acute onset with a progressive course or an either static or insidious deterioration.[5] It is the neurological manifestations that lead to the possibility of joint contractures secondary to increased muscular tone, decreased independent mobility, and an increase in time spent in the dependent position of the bed, wheelchair, or seating system.

■ Hydrocephalus

Chief Clinical Characteristics
This presentation involves increased head size with changes in consciousness, muscle tone changes, visual changes, seizure activity, and cardiorespiratory consequences.

Background Information
When suspected, children undergo imaging tests such as magnetic resonance imaging or head ultrasound to determine whether intracranial fluid levels are increased and are with or without ventricular dilation. Children may undergo a ventriculoperitoneal shunt placement or may go untreated under observation if hydrocephalus is showing signs of self-resolving.[6]

■ Immobilization and Prolonged Bedrest

Chief Clinical Characteristics
This presentation typically involves children who are postsurgical or who have a degenerative condition. They may present with some impairment in joint range of motion due to immobilization in a brace or cast, prolonged bedrest, or general disuse.

Background Information
Any joint that is immobilized for treatment purposes or secondary to disuse is at risk for joint contracture. The decreased mobility associated with being bedridden in children with severe illnesses or an inability to move can create complications of decreased joint mobility and therefore limited joint motion as the soft tissues surrounding the joints lose elasticity and available length. These joint contractures can be found in the ankle, knee, hip, shoulder, wrist, and elbow. Gravity-elicited stretch that is achieved during weight-bearing activities is essential for maintaining optimal muscle length in major muscle groups. Prolonged sitting and use of a wheelchair without daily range-of-motion exercises can lead to hip and knee flexion contractures. Children who have experienced a spinal cord injury or any other type of illness or disease process that requires them to be seated in a seating system or wheelchair are at high risk for the development of hip flexion contractures and knee flexion contractures.

■ Infantile Spasms

Chief Clinical Characteristics
This presentation typically involves spasms occurring in clusters of four or five and looks like jack-knifing jolts in which the trunk bends forward at the waist. These spasms occur primarily during periods of drowsiness or when arousing from sleep.

Background Information
This condition begins around 4 to 8 months of age. Neurodevelopmental arrest or regression of skills is common. This condition is commonly treated with an intramuscular injection of adrenocorticotropic hormone.[7]

■ Juvenile Ankylosing Spondylitis

Chief Clinical Characteristics
This presentation typically involves children presenting with back pain or pauciarticular arthritis that can lead to fusion of the spine or classical "bamboo spine" appearance on x-ray.[7]

Background Information
Joints of the legs are usually more involved, with hip joint arthritis at the onset being the earliest and predominant symptom of this condition. There are typically long periods of apparent disease remission; however, systemic symptoms will include low-grade fever and weight loss.[5]

■ Juvenile Dermatomyositis

Chief Clinical Characteristics
This presentation typically involves insidious symptoms of fatigue with low-grade fever, weight loss, and irritability. These symptoms are typically followed by a characteristic rash that appears first over sun-exposed areas. Proximal muscular weakness typically follows within 2 months, as does periorbital and facial erythema. The rash may spread to involve the upper torso, posterior aspect of the arms and legs, medial malleoli, and buttocks. Other complications include partial baldness secondary to chronic scalp inflammation, and hypertrophic and red skin over the metacarpal and proximal interphalangeal joints.

Background Information

Children with the rash only will experience myositis and calcinosis later in the disease course, and more severely affected children will experience nailbed telangiectasia, infarction of oral epithelium and skinfolds, and digital ulceration. As the disease progresses, proximal muscle weakness increases, making even combing hair difficult. Dysphagia and difficulty handling secretions become apparent along with reports of constipation secondary to impaired gastrointestinal smooth muscle function causing abdominal pain or diarrhea. Cardiac myopathy and lymphadenopathy are also common associated diagnoses in the late stages of disease progression. It is the most common of the pediatric inflammatory myopathies.[5] Joint range of motion is primarily affected in children who have the antibody to the polymyositis/scleroderma (Pm/Scl) antigen. These children often present with "bambooing" of the digits with decreased cutaneous elasticity. This leads to "mechanic's hands" with thickened skin and cuticle overgrowth and range-of-motion losses.[5]

■ Juvenile Rheumatoid Arthritis

Chief Clinical Characteristics

This presentation typically involves joint swelling or effusion and the presence of two or more of the following: heat, limitation of range of motion, and tenderness or pain with motion.

Background Information

The three types of this condition are oligoarthritis (pauciarticular), involving four or fewer joints; polyarticular, involving five or more joints; and systemic onset, which is characterized by variable involvement. In addition, nine distinct subtypes have been identified.[5] Children with this condition are at risk for developing anterior uveitis (inflammation of the eye structures), which is typically asymptomatic and should be monitored by an ophthalmologist. Contractures occur in the majority of cases that can lead to functional limitations, growth abnormalities, and secondary postural compensations.[2]

■ Lennox-Gastaut Syndrome

Chief Clinical Characteristics

This presentation consists of an atypical form of absence epilepsy characterized by diffuse slow spike waves often with atonic, tonic, or clonic seizures and mental retardation that persist into adulthood.

Background Information

This condition often affects children with a history of infantile spasm. Onset is between 1 and 8 years of age.[7]

■ Lesch-Nyhan Syndrome

Chief Clinical Characteristics

This presentation can include clinical manifestations of hyperuricemia, mental retardation, dysarthric speech, and compulsive self-biting that usually begins with the eruption of teeth. Orthopedic problems include hip subluxations or dislocations, fractures, and minor scoliosis, and the child is at risk for fractures and infections as well as joint contractures.[8]

Background Information

This condition is a rare X-linked disorder of purine metabolism that ultimately results in hypoxanthine-guanine phosphoribosyltransferase (HPRT) deficiency. HPRT is normally present in every cell of the body, but is highest in concentration in the brain. This condition is often confused with cerebral palsy secondary to its manifestations of early choreoathetosis; however, this eventually progresses to spasticity and dystonia.[5] The increased spasticity and decreased ability to move independently puts these children at risk for joint contractures, especially in the hips, knees, shoulders, and elbows.

■ Leukodystrophies

Chief Clinical Characteristics

This presentation includes pale optic disks, progressive spasticity, and extrapyramidal movements including rigidity, dystonia, and choreoathetosis. Patients may exhibit seizures and gross-motor delay. As the disease progresses, they present with increased spasticity, ataxia, and learning problems with cognitive decline.[9]

Background Information

These disorders are all disorders of the growth and maintenance of the myelin sheath in the central nervous system and are mostly inherited.

■ Myelodysplasia

Chief Clinical Characteristics

This presentation typically involves symptoms that range from mild weakness and limited bowel and bladder control to complete paraplegia associated with hydrocephalus, depending on the level of extrusion.[7] Contractures are present and develop in response to muscle imbalances in the lumbar spine, pelvis, hips, knees, ankles, and feet. Characteristic posturing includes rounded shoulders, kyphosis, scoliosis, excessive lumbar lordosis, anterior pelvic tilt, rotation deformities of the hip or tibia, flexed hips and knees, and pronated feet.[2]

Background Information
This condition involves a cyst containing spinal cord and cerebrospinal fluid outside of the protective spinal column. It is present at birth.

■ Pelizaeus-Merzbacher Disease
Chief Clinical Characteristics
This presentation typically involves progressive psychomotor developmental delays, nystagmus, hypotonia that progresses to hypertonia with spastic quadriplegia, dystonia, and cerebellar ataxia.[10]

Background Information
This is a rare X-linked dysmyelinating disorder in which the myelinating process of the central nervous system is defective. This is secondary to a mutation in the proteolipid protein gene (PLP1).[11]

■ Poliomyelitis
Chief Clinical Characteristics
This presentation typically involves headache, nausea, vomiting, and soreness/stiffness in the posterior muscles of the neck, trunk, and limbs. Other signs and symptoms include muscle atrophy, joint pain, progressive weakness, and progressive skeletal deformity.

Background Information
There are three primary serotypes of the poliovirus that cause direct cellular destruction. These viruses affect the immunologic mechanisms, causing neuronal lesions in the anterior horn cells of the spinal cord, medulla, cerebellum, midbrain, thalamus, hypothalamus, pallidum, and cerebral cortex.[5] Abortive poliomyelitis is usually a brief febrile illness with symptoms including malaise, anorexia, nausea, vomiting, headache, sore throat, constipation, and diffuse abdominal pain. This serotype is short lasting and typically does not result in joint range-of-motion restrictions.

Acute infection from the poliovirus causes a wide range of illness from none at all to severe paralysis and death. It is extremely rare in countries where a vaccination is available. Postpolio syndrome involves diffuse weakness or paralysis of the muscles that were affected in the initial poliovirus attack.

■ Psoriatic Arthritis
Chief Clinical Characteristics
This presentation typically involves an asymmetric pattern of symptoms of the large and small joints such as nail pitting, dactylitis, and onycholysis. There is often a family history. Joint arthritis symptoms are present with symptoms of inflammatory bowel disease.

Background Information
This condition can be present in a polyarthritis that affects large and small joints or as arthritis of the sacroiliac joints that is accompanied by HLA-B12. The severity of this condition is independent of the activity of the gastrointestinal inflammation.[5]

■ Reactive Arthritis
Chief Clinical Characteristics
This presentation commonly involves significant swelling, pain, and erythema present at one or more joints. The inflammatory event typically follows a gastrointestinal or genitourinary infection.

Background Information
This condition usually affects the joints of the lower limbs and may become chronic with duration of several weeks to years.

■ Scleroderma
Chief Clinical Characteristics
This presentation typically includes fibrosis of the dermis and arteries of the lungs, kidneys, and gastrointestinal tract that is chronic in nature with an unknown cause. Raynaud's phenomenon is often the earliest symptom.

Background Information
The destruction of the endothelium results in fibrosis of the dermis, subcutaneous fat, and sometimes the muscles. There is a variation of scleroderma that only affects the skin. There are two types, morphea and linear scleroderma. These cause fibrosis in the dermis and can sometimes extend to the muscle, which can

result in leg-length discrepancies, joint flexion contractions, and/or cosmetic deformities.

■ Seizure Disorders

Chief Clinical Characteristics

This presentation involves abnormal electroencephalographic activity associated with disturbance in development, which causes difficulties with maintaining consciousness and, in cases of muscular involvement, interferes with the child's ability to attain motor skills.

Background Information

There are a number of different seizure disorders, and the reader is referred to a neurology textbook for classification of seizures. This condition may be unexplained or a secondary sign of an organic brain malformation or deficiency. This condition is generally characterized by self-limiting periods of unconsciousness, change in behavior, sensation, or autonomic function due to changes in electrical activity of the brain. This condition is associated with many disabilities with a neurological basis (eg, brain tumor, brain injuries) but can be independent of other conditions.[12] Approximately 25% of children with developmental disabilities have epilepsy.[7]

■ Sjögren-Larsson Syndrome

Chief Clinical Characteristics

This presentation typically involves inflammatory scaling of the skin, typically on the flexures and lower abdomen. Other symptoms include mental retardation, spasticity, degenerative defect of retinal pigment, glistening dots in the foveal area, motor and speech developmental delays, spastic diplegia/tetraplegia, and epilepsy. These symptoms become evident during the first 3 years of life.[5]

Background Information

This syndrome is an inborn error of metabolism that is characterized by increased keratinization of the skin resulting in the noninflammatory scaling of the skin. The increased spasticity and decreased mobility lead to complications including joint contractures.

■ Spinal Muscular Atrophy

Chief Clinical Characteristics

This presentation typically involves muscle wasting and weakness of the proximal musculature.

Sensation remains intact and unchanged during the course of the disorder.[4]

Background Information

The three types of spinal muscular atrophy are inherited as autosomal recessive disorders located on chromosome 5. The pathology of spinal muscular atrophy affects the anterior horn cells containing the motor neurons. Contractures may be present at birth due to decreased fetal movement in the last trimester or may develop over time in response to nonmovement of particular muscle groups.

■ Subacute Sclerosing Panencephalitis

Chief Clinical Characteristics

This presentation can be characterized by initial symptoms that include mild cognitive deterioration with behavioral changes. As the disease progresses, motor function begins to be affected with periodic stereotyped myoclonic jerks, pyramidal and extrapyramidal signs, and possible ataxia, dystonia, and dyskinesia.

Background Information

This condition is a progressive neurological disorder caused by persistent defective measles virus. The virus usually presents itself in early childhood and the affected have a life expectancy of 1 to 3 years with an average of 18 months after onset. In the advanced stages of this condition, individuals become quadriparetic with increased spasticity and eventually comatose, in a persistent vegetative state.[13]

■ Surgical Interventions (eg, Limb Lengthening)

Chief Clinical Characteristics

This presentation includes limited range of motion of the musculature surrounding the bones and/or joints involved in a surgical procedure.[14]

Background Information

Contractures are especially likely to develop if multiple surgeries are required or if wound infections follow the surgery. Open reductions of congenitally dislocated joints are often followed by contractures, and contractures are often a complication following limb-lengthening procedures. Children who have had these procedures are particularly susceptible due to the multiple tissue types involved and the inflammatory sequelae that follow an invasive procedure.[4]

■ Syringomyelia

Chief Clinical Characteristics

This presentation includes loss of sensation, muscle wasting, and absent deep tendon reflexes. The presentation varies with the level and the extent of the lesion. A rapidly progressive scoliosis may be the initial manifestation of syringomyelia. Spastic paraplegia is a common finding.

Background Information

This condition is a cavitation of the spinal cord. In noncommunicating syringomyelia, there is a cystic dilation of the cord and the cerebrospinal fluid pathway is not affected. In communicating syringomyelia, cerebrospinal fluid flow communicates between the central canal of the spinal cord and the cavity. Communicating syringomyelia is often associated with the Arnold-Chiari malformation, which can lead to hydrocephalus, cerebellar ataxia, pyramidal signs, and impaired sensation. Progressive enlargement of the cavity impinges on the anterior horn cells and corticospinal tracts, resulting in the loss of lower level function.

■ Systemic Lupus Erythematosus

Chief Clinical Characteristics

This presentation involves children who most frequently present with fever, fatigue, arthralgia or arthritis, and a rash. Common musculoskeletal findings include arthralgia, arthritis, tendonitis, and myositis.[5]

Background Information

This condition is characterized by autoantibodies directed against self-antigens and results in inflammatory damage to target organs, including the kidneys, blood cells, and central nervous system. Children with this condition may present with a variety of symptoms. If left untreated, or if present for prolonged periods of times, these symptoms may lead to decreased joint mobility and joint contractures.

■ Talipes Equinovarus (Clubfoot)

Chief Clinical Characteristics

This presentation consists of a forefoot curved medially (adducted) with the hindfoot in varus and equinus (plantarflexion) at the ankle.

Background Information

The etiology of congenital clubfoot is unknown. Factors associated with this condition are genetic, male sex, and possibly intrauterine restriction. This condition can also be just one manifestation of other conditions such as myelomeningocele or arthrogryposis.[2] Usually orthopedic intervention is warranted to correct positioning either conservatively (manipulation and serial casting) or surgically.

■ Tethered Cord Syndrome

Chief Clinical Characteristics

This presentation can be characterized by changes in tone, tongue fasciculation, weakness, and bowel/bladder function and the presence of headache.

Background Information

Typically associated with myelodysplasia, this condition occurs when adhesions anchor the spinal cord to the site of the posterior lesion. This usually occurs during fetal development as the spinal cord is supposed to grow into the conus medullaris, but can become a complication as a child grows. This condition results from a persistent filum terminale below the level of L2 that becomes thickened and rope-like.[5] This causes a stretch on the spinal cord that results in metabolic changes and ischemia to the cord itself.[4] The changes in tone or spasticity that result may cause rapid development of contractures.

■ Third-Degree Burns

Chief Clinical Characteristics

This presentation typically involves the history of a severe burn injury, and the child's obvious burn scars determine this diagnosis.

Background Information

Burns are classified into three levels of severity with level 1 being the mildest form and level 3 being the most severe. Third-degree burns often require reconstruction of the area to promote optimal healing. The formation of scar tissue that occurs secondary to the burn and/or the reconstruction may lead to decreased joint mobility.

■ Traumatic Brain Injury

Chief Clinical Characteristics

This presentation typically involves a history of trauma, and the child may present with various states of consciousness and clinical outcomes. Brain injuries that lead to very limited physical function and increased muscle tone in the limbs typically result in joint contractures secondary to spasticity, decreased mobility, and prolonged positioning.

Background Information

Traumatic brain injury is a frequent cause of morbidity and mortality in the pediatric population.[15] This condition can result from a fall, motor vehicle accident, gunshot wound, abuse/assault, etc. The injury may result from an impression injury, in which the head is impacted by a solid object, or an acceleration/deceleration injury such as whiplash. Near-drowning events are also a common cause of this condition in the pediatric population.

References

1. Staheli LT, Hall JG, Jaffe KM, Paholke DO. *Arthrogryposis: A Text Atlas*. Cambridge, UK: Cambridge University Press; 1998.
2. Campbell S, Palisano RJ, Vander Linden DW. *Physical Therapy for Children*. 3rd ed. Philadelphia, PA: W. B. Saunders; 2000.
3. Howie JM. Cerebral palsy. In: Campbell SK, ed. *Decision Making in Pediatric Neurologic Physical Therapy*. New York, NY: Churchill Livingston; 1999.
4. Tecklin JS. *Pediatric Physical Therapy*. 3rd ed. Philadelphia, PA: Lippincott Williams & Wilkins; 1998.
5. Behrman RE, Kliegman RM, Jenson HB. *Nelson Textbook of Pediatrics*. 2nd ed. Philadelphia, PA: W. B. Saunders; 2001.
6. Saukkonen AL, Serlo W, von Wendt L. Epilepsy in hydrocephalic children. *Acta Paediatr Scand*. Feb 1990; 79(2):212–218.
7. Long T, Toscano K. *Handbook of Pediatric Physical Therapy*. 2nd ed. Philadelphia, PA: Lippincott Williams & Wilkins; 2001.
8. Sponseller PD, Ahn NU, Choi JC, Ahn UM. Orthopedic problems in Lesch-Nyhan syndrome. *J Pediatr Orthop*. Sep–Oct 1999;19(5):596–602.
9. Schiffmann R, van der Knaap MS. The latest on leukodystrophies. *Curr Opin Neurol*. Apr 2004;17(2):187–192.
10. Lee ES, Moon HK, Park YH, Garbern J, Hobson GM. A case of complicated spastic paraplegia 2 due to a point mutation in the proteolipid protein 1 gene. *J Neurol Sci*. Sep 15, 2004;224(1–2):83–87.
11. Golomb MR, Walsh LE, Carvalho KS, Christensen CK, DeMyer WE. Clinical findings in Pelizaeus-Merzbacher disease. *J Child Neurol*. May 2004;19(5):328–331.
12. Moshe SL. Seizures early in life. *Neurology*. 2000;55 (5 suppl 1):S15–20; discussion S54–58.
13. Garg RK. Subacute sclerosing panencephalitis. *Postgrad Med J*. Feb 2002;78(916):63–70.
14. Kwan MK, Penafort R, Saw A. Treatment for flexion contracture of the knee during Ilizarov reconstruction of tibia with passive knee extension splint. *Med J Malaysia*. Dec 2004;59(suppl F):39–41.
15. Vogel LC, Hickey KJ, Klaas SJ, Anderson CJ. Unique issues in pediatric spinal cord injury. *Orthop Nurs*. Sep–Oct 2004;23(5):300–308; quiz 309–310.

CHAPTER 57

Torticollis in a Child

Hugh G. Watts, MD ■ *Sharon K. DeMuth, PT, DPT, MS*

Description of the Symptom

Torticollis (also commonly known as "wry neck") is a symptom or physical sign where the neck is turned, and may or may not be tilted. The term is derived from the Latin *tortus* ("twisted") and *collum* ("neck"). This symptom has many causes. This chapter describes possible causes of torticollis in a child.

Special Concerns

- Torticollis of sudden onset (few days)
- Any torticollis where the head is both tilted and rotated to the *same* side
- Any post-traumatic torticollis
- Any neurological signs suggesting an intracranial tumor or space-occupying tumor of the spinal cord

CHAPTER PREVIEW: Conditions That May Lead to Torticollis in a Child

T Trauma

COMMON

Not applicable

UNCOMMON

Muscle strain 1104
Rotary subluxation of C1–C2 1105

RARE

Cervical spine fractures and dislocations 1103
Clavicle fracture with or without brachial plexus injury 1103

I Inflammation

COMMON

Aseptic
Spastic torticollis 1106

Septic
Tonsillitis/adenitis 1107

UNCOMMON

Aseptic
Not applicable

Septic
Pharyngeal abscess 1105

(continued)

Inflammation *(continued)*

RARE

Aseptic
Juvenile rheumatoid arthritis 1104

Septic
Brucellosis 1103
Systemic fungal infection (such as actinomycosis, blastomycosis, coccidioidomycosis, and histoplasmosis) 1106
Tuberculosis of the cervical spine 1107

M Metabolic

COMMON
Not applicable

UNCOMMON
Drug intoxication 1104

RARE
Not applicable

Va Vascular

COMMON
Not applicable

UNCOMMON
Not applicable

RARE
Not applicable

De Degenerative

COMMON
Not applicable

UNCOMMON
Not applicable

RARE
Not applicable

Tu Tumor

COMMON
Malignant Primary, such as:
• Posterior fossa tumor 1105
Malignant Metastatic:
Not applicable
Benign:
Not applicable

Tumor *(continued)*

UNCOMMON

Malignant Primary, such as:
• Posterior fossa tumor 1105
Malignant Metastatic:
Not applicable
Benign:
Not applicable

RARE

Malignant Primary, such as:
• Chordomas 1103
Malignant Metastatic, such as:
• Spinal cord tumors 1106
Benign, such as:
• Syringomyelia 1106
• Thyroglossal duct cyst 1107

Co Congenital

COMMON

Congenital muscular torticollis (infantile torticollis, developmental muscular torticollis) 1103

UNCOMMON

Multiple congenital cervical spine anomalies (Klippel-Feil disorder) 1104
Sprengel's deformity 1106

RARE

Arnold-Chiari malformation (Chiari malformation) 1103

Ne Neurogenic/Psychogenic

COMMON

Not applicable

UNCOMMON

Psychogenic 1105

RARE

Extraocular muscle paresis 1104
Neurological dyskinesias:
• Benign paroxysmal torticollis of infancy 1105
• Dystonia musculorum deformans 1105
• Sandifer's syndrome 1105

Note: These are estimates of relative incidence because few data are available for the less common conditions.

Common Ages at Which Torticollis Presents in a Child

APPROXIMATE AGE	CONDITION
Birth to 3 Years	Benign paroxysmal torticollis of infancy
	Clavicle fracture with or without brachial plexus injury
	Congenital muscular torticollis
	Neurological dyskinesias

(continued)

Common Ages at Which Torticollis Presents in a Child—cont'd

APPROXIMATE AGE	CONDITION
Preschool (3–5 Years)	Chordomas Extraocular muscle paresis Multiple congenital cervical spine anomalies (Klippel-Feil disorder) Pharyngeal abscess Posterior fossa tumor Rotary subluxation of C1–C2 Spinal cord tumors Sprengel's deformity Syringomyelia Tonsillitis/adenitis
Elementary School (6–11 Years)	Juvenile rheumatoid arthritis Muscle strain Neurological dyskinesias: • Dystonia musculorum deformans • Sandifer's syndrome Pharyngeal abscess Psychogenic Rotary subluxation of C1–C2 Tonsillitis/adenitis Tumors: • Chordomas • Posterior fossa tumor • Spinal cord tumors • Syringomyelia
Middle School (12–14 Years)	Juvenile rheumatoid arthritis Muscle strain Pharyngeal abscess Tonsillitis/adenitis Tuberculosis
High School (15–18 Years)	Juvenile rheumatoid arthritis Muscle strain Pharyngeal abscess Tuberculosis

Overview of Torticollis in a Child

"Torticollis" is not a diagnosis, but a symptom or physical sign. Although approximately 80% of children with the problem have congenital (or developmental) muscular torticollis, there are many other causes that, if overlooked, could have serious deleterious consequences for the child.

Torticollis can be long standing or acute. Conditions that cause a torticollis of long standing (many months in an infant or many years in a school-aged child) can lead to cranial deformities, including an asymmetric eye position that aligns the eyes horizontal to the floor while the head remains tilted. In milder form, this is best appreciated by looking at the child's face from an upside-down perspective. (With the child lying supine, stand at the child's head and look at the face.) Acute torticollis is of more immediate concern. In these conditions, the symptom appears over a few days or commonly overnight. Although no specific etiology may be found, and the condition labeled as "spastic torticollis," it is important to rule out the conditions that need more immediate evaluation, such as rotary subluxation of C1 on C2 or posterior fossa tumors of the brain.

Description of Conditions That May Lead to Torticollis in a Child

■ Arnold-Chiari Malformation (Chiari Malformation)

Chief Clinical Characteristics
This presentation typically includes neck and head pain often made worse by coughing or sneezing. There may be blurred vision and complaints of difficulty swallowing or of gagging. Nystagmus may be seen.

Background Information
This congenital malformation is an inferior displacement of the cerebellum and fourth ventricle into the cervical spinal canal. Malformations are classified from I to IV with class I being minimal. Diagnosis is confirmed by magnetic resonance imaging. Treatment, if necessary, may require surgery to enlarge the posterior fossa.[1]

■ Brucellosis

Chief Clinical Characteristics
This presentation involves pain, tenderness, and swelling in the neck and throat. In specific geographic regions of the world, such as the Middle East, infections of the cervical bones may be due to the Brucella organism.

Background Information
The clinical presentation is identical to that of tuberculosis. Differentiation is made by culturing the organisms, when suspected. Treatment is with antibiotics and occasionally surgery.[2]

■ Cervical Spine Fractures and Dislocations

Chief Clinical Characteristics
This presentation can be characterized by a history of severe trauma.

Background Information
Findings resulting from those injuries will alert the examiner to the possibility of this diagnosis. These injuries require major trauma such as a motor vehicle accident or a fall from considerable height.

■ Chordomas

Chief Clinical Characteristics
This presentation can include a child who shows signs of lower motor neuron weakness without cerebellar dysfunction.

Background Information
The specifics will depend on the exact location of the tumor.[3]

■ Clavicle Fracture with or without Brachial Plexus Injury

Chief Clinical Characteristics
This presentation typically involves an infant whose head is noted to be turned to the side (most likely to the fractured side) and who is unwilling to move the ipsilateral arm. A Moro maneuver can be done, at which time the arm on the affected side will not move while the unaffected arm will go through the expected reflex motion. Motion of the affected arm will elicit crying.

Background Information
A particularly difficult delivery may result in this condition, with or without a brachial plexus injury. The newborn baby is unwilling or unable to move the arm when a Moro test is done. Predisposing factors are a child of large birth weight (which can be a feature of maternal diabetes) or malposition of the fetus (eg, shoulder dystocia) resulting in a difficult birth.

■ Congenital Muscular Torticollis (Infantile Torticollis, Developmental Muscular Torticollis)

Chief Clinical Characteristics
This presentation may involve the child's head being turned to one side, while the neck is tilted to the other. It is usually discovered in early infancy. The sternocleidomastoideus muscle on the side toward the tilt and away from the turn is tight. In the early stage of this condition, the tightened sternocleidomastoideus muscle may show a firm small mass. There is a decreased range of motion of the neck.

Background Information
In this condition, the sternocleidomastoid muscle becomes contracted. The condition is a chronic problem noted shortly after birth, and may lead to considerable facial and cranial asymmetry if untreated. Because a baby's neck is relatively short and the child's rooting response keeps the head turned, torticollis may be missed in the first few days unless the neck range of motion is specifically examined. At that time a mass may be palpable in the belly of

the sternocleidomastoid muscle. This mass disappears by 2 or 3 months of age. Initially it was believed that the condition was due to direct trauma, but currently it is hypothesized to be an ischemic event due to a compartment syndrome with subsequent fibrosis (similar to a Volkmann's ischemic contracture of the forearm following a fracture). The head tilted to the affected side but rotated to the opposite side characterizes the child's posture. This is in contradistinction to the posture in a rotary subluxation of C1 on C2 where the head both tilts and rotates to the same direction (Fig. 57-1). Radiographs do not show any anomalies. Treatment is usually exercises. Children who are diagnosed several years after birth may require surgical release of the sternocleidomastoideus muscle.[4]

■ Drug Intoxication

Chief Clinical Characteristics
Rarely, drug toxicity may cause dystonia in childhood. Antipsychotic medications can be a cause, as well as toxicity from serotonin. While such medications are not commonly used in children, accidental overdose is a possibility. Some anti-seizure medications may cause such problems.

Background Information
Whereas in adults, acquired dystonia usually affects one part of the body, such as the neck or hand, in children, the dystonia more often begins in the leg or foot and commonly spreads to involve the entire body. In addition, in

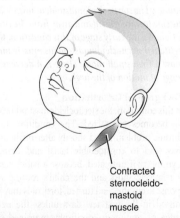

Contracted sternocleido-mastoid muscle

FIGURE 57-1 Head side-bending and rotation in opposite directions.

acquired dystonia the head may tilt forward or backward rather than just to one side. Some symptoms tend to occur after periods of exertion and/or fluctuate over the course of the day.

■ Extraocular Muscle Paresis

Chief Clinical Characteristics
This presentation can be characterized by an inability to move the eyes through a full range of motion.

Background Information
Paresis of the muscles of the eye that results in a rotary malposition of the eyeball may cause a child to tilt the head so that the eyes are orthogonal to the normal horizon. Surgical correction of the eye muscles will usually cause the torticollis to disappear.[5]

■ Juvenile Rheumatoid Arthritis

Chief Clinical Characteristics
This presentation typically involves torticollis in association with the generalized form of this condition (systemic; Still's disease). A forward tilt of the neck is common.

Background Information
Torticollis is not a feature in mono- or pauciarticular juvenile rheumatoid arthritis.[6]

■ Multiple Congenital Cervical Spine Anomalies (Klippel-Feil Disorder)

Chief Clinical Characteristics
This presentation typically includes a child with a short broad neck, low hairline, and torticollis. Restricted neck motion is noted.

Background Information
Neurological problems can develop, albeit very slowly, but do so very late (ie, at 40 or 50 years of age).[7]

■ Muscle Strain

Chief Clinical Characteristics
This presentation may involve a history of the trauma, which is not necessarily severe and which will alert the examiner to the possibility of this diagnosis.

Background Information
Trauma to any of the neck muscles may result in a temporary torticollis. No specific pattern

is noted since the head position will depend on which muscles are strained.

NEUROLOGICAL DYSKINESIAS

■ Benign Paroxysmal Torticollis of Infancy

Chief Clinical Characteristics
This presentation can include torticollis in the presence of a seizure-like disorder.

Background Information
This condition may occur secondary to many neurological causes, including drug intoxication.[8]

■ Dystonia Musculorum Deformans

Chief Clinical Characteristics
This presentation involves torticollis in combination with a number of brain diseases (eg, perinatal brain injury, post-encephalitis, Wilson's and Huntington's diseases).

Background Information
Inheritance may be dominant or recessive, the latter especially in individuals of European descent. The cause is not known, but is thought to be a biochemical aberration of the basal ganglia.[9]

■ Sandifer's Syndrome

Chief Clinical Characteristics
This presentation includes a child who presents with gastroesophageal reflux and sudden posturing of the head in torticollis.

Background Information
There is often an association with a neurological condition such as cerebral palsy.[8]

■ Pharyngeal Abscess

Chief Clinical Characteristics
This presentation involves torticollis due to tonsillitis or adenitis and is more common after a severe inflammation and after several days.

Background Information
The soreness of the mouth and throat with difficulty swallowing make this diagnosis apparent.[9]

■ Posterior Fossa Tumor

Chief Clinical Characteristics
This presentation may involve torticollis in the presence of signs of cerebellar dysfunction.

Strabismus may be seen. Motion sickness and vomiting may be a feature.

Background Information
The mechanism is not understood. This condition is commonly overlooked initially and confused with congenital muscular torticollis.[10,11]

■ Psychogenic

Chief Clinical Characteristics
This presentation involves an atypical cervical spinal condition that may be considered when all other conditions have been excluded.[12]

■ Rotary Subluxation of C1–C2

Chief Clinical Characteristics
This presentation involves a child who is known to be normal and quite suddenly is noted to hold the head tilted.

Background Information
The child will hold the head tilted and rotated to the same direction (Fig. 57-2). This condition is in contrast to congenital muscular torticollis where the head is tilted to one direction and rotated to the opposite (see Fig. 57-1). Rotary displacement alone (type I) is the most common form and is usually benign, resolving in a few days. Occasionally the symptoms may persist, resulting in a fixed deformity. However, a rotary

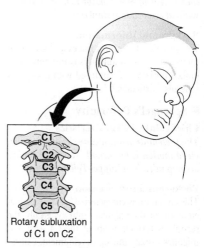

Rotary subluxation of C1 on C2

FIGURE 57-2 Head side-bending and rotation in the same direction.

displacement associated with an anterior shift (type II if the shift is <5 mm; type III if the shift is >5 mm) is particularly dangerous. Vigorous neck motion, manipulation, or an exercise program could lead to paralysis, or even death. The diagnosis is difficult to confirm by plain x-ray and may require computed tomography to be certain.[7]

■ Spastic Torticollis

Chief Clinical Characteristics
This presentation is characterized by an otherwise normal child awakening and finding that the head is turned.

Background Information
A prior upper respiratory infection is frequent, but in the age group where this torticollis is common (approximately 5 to 11 years), a history of an upper respiratory infection is also very common, so the exact relationship is not known. Not infrequently, no specific diagnosis is found. However, the other causes of acute torticollis must be ruled out. Treatment consists mainly of the application of local heat and the use of a cervical collar. Occasionally, gentle cervical collar traction is required, usually on an inpatient basis.[9]

■ Spinal Cord Tumors

Chief Clinical Characteristics
This presentation typically involves a child who shows signs of lower motor neuron weakness without cerebellar dysfunction.

Background Information
The specifics depend on the exact location of the tumor. This condition is commonly overlooked initially and confused with congenital muscular torticollis.[9]

■ Sprengel's Deformity

Chief Clinical Characteristics
This presentation includes an elevated scapula. Head motion is not usually restricted (unless accompanied by a Klippel-Feil disorder).

Background Information
This condition is characterized as a congenital elevation of the scapula. Embryologically, the scapula is formed at about the C4 level and migrates distally during development. Consequently, the condition is now more likely to be described as a congenital undescended scapula.

The scapula is commonly held in the undescended position by a connection between the scapula (*omo* in Greek) and the spine; hence, it is an omovertebral connection that may be fibrous, cartilaginous, or more commonly bone. The condition may be unilateral or bilateral.[7]

■ Syringomyelia

Chief Clinical Characteristics
This presentation may involve loss of sensation, muscle wasting, and absent deep tendon reflexes. The presentation varies with the level and the extent of the lesion.

Background Information
This condition is a cavitation of the spinal cord. In noncommunicating syringomyelia, there is a cystic dilation of the cord and the cerebrospinal fluid pathway is not affected. In communicating syringomyelia, cerebrospinal fluid flow communicates between the central canal of the spinal cord and the cavity. Communicating syringomyelia is often associated with the Arnold-Chiari malformation, which can lead to hydrocephalus, cerebellar ataxia, pyramidal signs, and impaired sensation. Progressive enlargement of the cavity impinges on the anterior horn cells and corticospinal tracts, resulting in the loss of lower level function.[13]

■ Systemic Fungal Infection (Such as Actinomycosis, Blastomycosis, Coccidioidomycosis, and Histoplasmosis)

Chief Clinical Characteristics
This presentation includes pain, tenderness, and swelling in the neck and throat.[14]

Background Information
The particular infecting fungus will depend on the geographic region in which the child lives. *Coccidioidomycosis* is a fungal infection endemic to the southwestern United States and northwestern Mexico. Histoplasmosis is seen characteristically in the northeastern part of the United States in the Great Lakes region. Musculoskeletal involvement is rare; however, lesions of bones and joints result in diffuse soft tissue swelling, bone destruction, and sinus formation. The lesion is readily seen on plain radiographs. Treatment includes long-term antibiotics and irrigation and debridement of the affected area.[14]

■ Thyroglossal Duct Cyst

Chief Clinical Characteristics

This presentation can be characterized by a child who will show a soft mass in the midline of the neck, rather than laterally over the sternocleidomastoideus muscle. The mass is more superficial than the sternocleidomastoideus muscle mass seen in congenital muscular torticollis, and it will move along with tongue movements.[15]

Background Information

Diagnosis is usually based on clinical findings. Treatment often includes surgical excision of the mass, as well as hyoid resection.

■ Tonsillitis/Adenitis

Chief Clinical Characteristics

This presentation involves torticollis several days after a severe inflammation. The soreness of the mouth and throat may lead to difficulty swallowing and breathing.

Background Information

Treatment is usually with antibiotics.[9]

■ Tuberculosis of the Cervical Spine

Chief Clinical Characteristics

This presentation includes torticollis in the presence of pain, tenderness, and swelling in the neck plus in the throat.

Background Information

The likelihood of tuberculosis will depend on the incidence of the disease in the geographic location, and the presence of conditions leading to immuno-incompetence such as other chronic illnesses, human immunodeficiency virus, malnutrition, and use of chemotherapeutic agents or steroids. The disease usually involves the bodies of the cervical vertebrae asymmetrically leading to rotation of the neck together with characteristic kyphosis.

Treatment is usually with antitubercular drugs and sometimes surgery.[2]

References

1. Dure LS, Peraj AK, Cheek WR, et al. Chiari type I malformations in children. *J Pediatr.* 1989;115:573.
2. Watts HG, Lifeso RM. Tuberculosis of bones and joints. *J Bone Joint Surg Am.* 1996;78A(2):288–298.
3. Sibley RK, Day DL, Dehner LP. Metastasizing chordoma in early childhood: a pathological and immunological study with review of the literature. *Pediatr Pathol.* 1987;7:287–301.
4. Cheng JC, Tang SP, Chen TM, et al. The clinical presentation and outcome of treatment of congenital muscular torticollis in infants—a study of 1086 cases. *J Pediat Surg.* 2000;35:1091–1096.
5. Bixenham WW. Diagnosis of superior oblique palsy. *J Clin Neuroophthalmol.* 1981;1:199.
6. Klippel JH, Crofford LJ, Stone JH, Weyand CM. *Primer on the Rheumatic Diseases.* Atlanta, GA: Arthritis Foundation; 2001.
7. Herman MJ, Pizzutillo PD. Cervical spine disorders in children. *Orthop Clin North Am.* 1999;30:457–466.
8. Murphy WJ, Gellis SS. Torticollis with hiatus hernia in infancy: Sandifer's syndrome. *Am J Dis Child.* 1977; 131:564.
9. Loder RT. The cervical spine. In: Morrissy RT, Weinstein SL, eds. *Lovel and Winter's Pediatric Orthopaedics.* Vol II. Philadelphia, PA: Lippincott Williams & Wilkins; 2006:871–919.
10. Gupta AK, Roy DR, Conlon ES, Crawford AH. Torticollis secondary to posterior fossa tumors. *J Pediatr Orthop.* 1996;16:505–507.
11. O'Brien DF, Caird J, Kennedy M, Roberts GA, Marks JC, Allcutt DA. Posterior fossa tumors in children; evaluation, presenting clinical features. *Ir Med J.* 2001;94: 52–53.
12. Snyder CH. Paroxysmal torticollis in infancy. *Am J Dis Child.* 1969;117:458.
13. Oldfield EH, Muraszko K, Shawker TH, Patronas NJ. Pathophysiology of syringomyelia associated with Chiari I malformation of the cerebellar tonsils. Implications for diagnosis and treatment. *J Neurosurg.* 1994;80: 3–15.
14. Kushwaha VP, Shaw BA, Gerardi JA, Oppenheim WL. Musculoskeletal coccidioidomycosis. A review of 25 cases. *Clin Orthop.* Nov 1996;(332):190–199.
15. Brousseau VJ, Solares CA, Xu M, Krakovitz P, Koltai PJ. Thyroglossal duct cysts: presentation and management in children versus adults. *Int J Pediatr Otorhinolaryngol.* 2003;67:1285–1290.

CHAPTER 58

Case Demonstration: Torticollis in a Child

■ *Sharon K. DeMuth, PT, DPT, MS* ■ *Chris A. Sebelski, PT, DPT, OCS, CSCS*

NOTE: This case demonstration was developed using the diagnostic process described in Chapter 4 and demonstrated in Chapter 5. The reader is encouraged to use this diagnostic process in order to ensure thorough clinical reasoning. If additional elaboration is required on the information presented in this chapter, please consult Chapters 4 and 5.

THE DIAGNOSTIC PROCESS

Step 1 Identify the patient's chief concern.
Step 2 Identify *barriers to communication*.
Step 3 Identify *special concerns*.
Step 4 Create a symptom timeline and sketch the anatomy (if needed).
Step 5 Create a diagnostic hypothesis list considering all possible forms of *remote* and *local* pathology that could cause the patient's chief concern.
Step 6 Sort the diagnostic hypothesis list by epidemiology and specific case characteristics.
Step 7 Ask specific questions to rule specific conditions or pathological categories less likely.
Step 8 Re-sort the diagnostic hypothesis list based on the patient's responses to specific questioning.
Step 9 Perform tests to differentiate among the remaining diagnostic hypotheses.
Step 10 Re-sort the diagnostic hypothesis list based on the patient's responses to specific tests.
Step 11 Decide on a diagnostic impression.
Step 12 Determine the appropriate patient disposition.

Case Description

Maria is a 6-month-old girl whose parents noticed at 4 months of age that she held her head turned to the side and that her face seemed somewhat asymmetrical. Maria has two older siblings who are healthy and well.

Their pediatrician referred them to the local general outpatient orthopedic physical therapy practice for exercises for congenital muscular torticollis. Maria's mother states that she has been performing the home exercise program "faithfully every day" for 2 months and there has been no change. The pediatrician has not seen Maria since the appointment 2 months ago. The mother is coming to you, as a Pediatric Certified Specialist, for a second opinion.

Maria's family recently moved here from Mexico. Maria's parents speak some English, but are more comfortable speaking Spanish. You notice as Maria's mother holds her that Maria holds her head turned to the right with her neck tilted to the left.

STEP #1: Identify the patient's chief concern.

- The chief concern of Maria's parents is her asymmetrical head posture and facial features.

STEP #2: Identify *barriers to communication*.

- **Patient's/family's preferred language is different than that of the health care provider.** Maria's parents are most comfortable speaking Spanish; therefore, an interpreter is necessary for the verbal part of the differential diagnosis process. It is important to ensure that the discriminating questions and answers are accurately translated for everyone.

- **Presence of other children in the family.** Because the mother has had two children who are healthy and well, there is a level of experiential wisdom that also needs to be considered when questioning this mother.

STEP #3: Identify *special concerns.*

- **No response to prior physical therapy intervention.** A response would be expected if the child had a typical case of congenital muscular torticollis and the family had been performing the exercises properly.

> **Teaching Comment:** With English as a second language, it is advisable to utilize a translator for this interview to, at the very least, improve rapport with the patient. Additionally, since the differential diagnostic interview is dependent on discriminating questions, it is important to make sure that the discriminating questions and their answers are accurately translated for everyone.

STEP #4: Create a symptom timeline and sketch the anatomy (if needed).

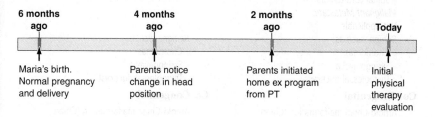

6 months ago	4 months ago	2 months ago	Today
Maria's birth. Normal pregnancy and delivery	Parents notice change in head position	Parents initiated home ex program from PT	Initial physical therapy evaluation

STEP #5: Create a diagnostic hypothesis list considering all possible forms of *remote* and *local* pathology that could cause the patient's chief concern.

T **Trauma**

Cervical spine fractures and dislocations

Clavicle fracture with or without brachial plexus injury
Muscle strain

Rotary subluxation of C1–C2

I **Inflammation**

Aseptic
Juvenile rheumatoid arthritis

Spastic torticollis

Septic
Pharyngeal abscess
Systemic fungal infection
(eg, actinomycosis, blastomycosis, coccidioidomycosis, histoplasmosis)

STEP #6: Sort the diagnostic hypothesis list by epidemiology and specific case characteristics.

T **Trauma** (Don't forget possible child abuse)

~~Cervical spine fractures and dislocations~~ (no trauma associated with onset)
Clavicle fracture with or without brachial plexus injury
~~Muscle strain~~ (no trauma associated with onset, age of patient)
Rotary subluxation of C1–C2

I **Inflammation**

Aseptic
~~Juvenile rheumatoid arthritis~~ (age of patient)
Spastic torticollis

Septic
Pharyngeal abscess
Systemic fungal infection
(eg, actinomycosis, blastomycosis, coccidioidomycosis, histoplasmosis)

Tonsillitis/adenitis
Tuberculosis/brucellosis

M Metabolic

Not applicable

Va Vascular

Not applicable

De Degenerative

Not applicable

Tu Tumor

Malignant Primary, such as:
- Posterior fossa tumors
- Spinal cord tumors

Malignant Metastatic:
Not applicable

Benign, such as:
- Chordomas
- Syringomyelia
- Thyroglossal duct cyst

Co Congenital

Arnold-Chiari malformation (Chiari malformation)

Congenital muscular torticollis (infantile torticollis, developmental muscular torticollis)

Multiple congenital cervical spine anomalies (ie, Klippel-Feil syndrome)

Sprengel's deformity

Ne Neurogenic/Psychogenic

Developmental delay

Extraocular muscle paresis (eg, Brown's syndrome)

Gastroesophageal reflux

Hysterical/psychogenic torticollis

Neurological dyskinesias:
- Benign paroxysmal torticollis of infancy
- Dystonia musculorum deformans

- Sandifer's syndrome

Tonsillitis/adenitis
Tuberculosis/brucellosis

M Metabolic

Not applicable

Va Vascular

Not applicable

De Degenerative

Not applicable

Tu Tumor

Malignant Primary, such as:
- Posterior fossa tumors
- Spinal cord tumors

Malignant Metastatic:
Not applicable

Benign, such as:
- Chordomas
- Syringomyelia
- Thyroglossal duct cyst

Co Congenital

Arnold-Chiari malformation (Chiari malformation)

Congenital muscular torticollis (infantile torticollis, developmental muscular torticollis)

Multiple congenital cervical spine anomalies (ie, Klippel-Feil syndrome)

Sprengel's deformity

Ne Neurogenic/Psychogenic

~~Developmental delay~~ (previous medical history: not first child in family, family good reporters with experience, and child performing age appropriately by parent report)

Extraocular muscle paresis (eg, Brown's syndrome)

Gastroesophageal reflux

~~Hysterical/psychogenic torticollis~~ (age of patient)

Neurological dyskinesias:
- Benign paroxysmal torticollis of infancy
- ~~Dystonia musculorum deformans~~ (age of patient)
- Sandifer's syndrome

STEP #7: Ask specific questions to rule specific conditions or pathological categories less likely.

- **Was the pregnancy and delivery normal?** Yes.

- **Has there been any trauma?** With a normal birth history and no history of trauma, clavicle fracture with or without brachial plexus injury and rotary subluxation of C1–C2 are less likely.

- **Has Maria been running a fever?** No, making pharyngeal abscess, fungal infections, tonsillitis/adenitis, and tuberculosis/brucellosis less likely.

- **Has Maria shown any unusual behaviors such as staring spells, jerking motions or spasms, or potential seizures?** No, which makes less likely spastic torticollis and neurological dyskinesias.

- **Has Maria shown any changes in her eating?** Yes, Maria has been spitting up a lot and she appears to be losing weight. This increases the index of suspicion for gastroesophageal reflux.

STEP #8: Re-sort the diagnostic hypothesis list based on the patient's responses to specific questioning.

T   Trauma (Don't forget possible child abuse)

~~Clavicle fracture with or without brachial plexus injury~~ (normal birth history, no history of trauma)

~~Rotary subluxation of C1–C2~~ (normal birth history, no history of trauma)

I   Inflammation

Aseptic

~~Spastic torticollis~~ (no history of seizures)

Septic

~~Pharyngeal abscess~~ (absence of fever)

~~Systemic fungal infection (eg, actinomycosis, blastomycosis, coccidioidomycosis, histoplasmosis)~~ (absence of fever)

~~Tonsillitis/adenitis~~ (absence of fever)

~~Tuberculosis/brucellosis~~ (absence of fever)

M   Metabolic

Not applicable

Va   Vascular

Not applicable

De   Degenerative

Not applicable

Tu   Tumor

Malignant Primary, such as:
- Posterior fossa tumors
- Spinal cord tumors

Malignant Metastatic:

Not applicable

Benign, such as:
- Chordomas
- Syringomyelia
- Thyroglossal duct cyst

Co   Congenital

Arnold-Chiari malformation (Chiari malformation)

Congenital muscular torticollis (infantile torticollis, developmental muscular torticollis)

Multiple congenital cervical spine anomalies (ie, Klippel-Feil syndrome)

Sprengel's deformity

Ne   Neurogenic/Psychogenic

Extraocular muscle paresis (eg, Brown's syndrome)

Gastroesophageal reflux

~~Neurological dyskinesias:~~
- ~~Benign paroxysmal torticollis of infancy~~ (no history of seizures)
- ~~Sandifer's syndrome~~ (no history of seizures)

STEP #9: Perform tests to differentiate among the remaining diagnostic hypotheses.

Ask parents to undress Maria with the exception of her diaper. The order listed below for the tests is the order the diagnoses are listed in for this sorting. They may not be in the usual or preferred order for doing a physical exam.

- **For concern about possible child abuse, is there any evidence on Maria's skin to suggest multiple bruises from different time periods?** None were found. This finding does not rule out child abuse, but makes it less likely.

- **Does the child have a full range of neck motion, and is there any mass in the sternocleidomastoid muscle on the side to which the head is turned?** Yes, there is a full passive range of motion; no, there is no mass in the muscle. These exclude the diagnosis of congenital muscular torticollis.

- **Examine the neck and back for cervical and scapular abnormalities.** No evidence for an elevated scapula, or webbing of the neck to suggest Klippel-Feil syndrome or Sprengel's.

- **Is there a mass in the neck not associated with the sternocleidomastoid muscle?** No, indicating the child is unlikely to have a thyroglossal duct cyst.

- **Examine the child's eye tracking.** Strabismus found, which raises the index of clinical suspicion for posterior fossa tumors or extraocular paresis.

STEP #10: Re-sort the diagnostic hypothesis list based on the patient's responses to specific tests.

T Trauma (Don't forget possible child abuse)

Not applicable

I Inflammation

Not applicable

M Metabolic

Not applicable

Va Vascular

Not applicable

De Degenerative

Not applicable

Tu Tumor

Malignant Primary, such as:
- Posterior fossa tumors
- Spinal cord tumors

Malignant Metastatic:
Not applicable

Benign, such as:
- Chordomas
- Syringomyelia
- ~~Thyroglossal duct cyst~~ (no sternocleidomastoid mass present)

Co Congenital

Arnold-Chiari malformation (Chiari malformation)

~~Congenital muscular torticollis (infantile torticollis, developmental muscular torticollis)~~ (normal cervical spine passive range of motion)

~~Multiple congenital cervical spine anomalies (ie, Klippel-Feil syndrome)~~ (normal observation findings of the neck)

~~Sprengel's deformity~~ (normal observation findings of the scapula)

Ne Neurogenic/Psychogenic

Extraocular muscle paresis (eg, Brown's syndrome)

Gastroesophageal reflux

STEP #11: Decide on a diagnostic impression.
The differential diagnosis list includes:

- Arnold-Chiari malformation (Chiari malformation)
- Extraocular muscle paresis
- Gastroesophageal reflux
- Posterior fossa tumors
- Spinal cord tumors: chordomas, syringomyelia.

Consultation with other health care practitioners is necessary to further evaluate this patient's condition.

STEP #12: Determine the appropriate patient disposition.

- Refer back to the pediatrician by telephone, providing the results of your evaluation.
- Additionally, fax your report to the pediatrician's office.
- Emphasize to the parents that, although this is not an emergency, following up with the pediatrician is very important.

Case Outcome

The family took Maria to the pediatrician and after further workup Maria was diagnosed with a posterior fossa tumor.

CHAPTER 59

Poor Posture and Scoliosis, Kyphosis, and Lordosis in a Child

■ *Sharon K. DeMuth, PT, DPT, MS* ■ *Stephanie A. Jones, PT, DPT, OCS, NCS*

Description of the Symptom

A parent may state that their child has "poor posture." That may represent the only way in which they can express their concern with their child's spinal shape. While poor posture is a culturally defined concept, scoliosis, kyphosis, and lordosis are significant medical concerns. Spinal curvatures are named for the direction of the convexity or apex and the spinal region (thoracic, lumbar, or cervical). *Scoliosis* is a lateral curvature of the spine and *kyphosis* and *lordosis* are curves in the antero-posterior plane. *Kyphosis* is a curve where the apex is posterior and *lordosis* where the apex is anterior.

The *thoracic* spine is normally kyphotic. However, excessive kyphosis exceeding approximately 40 degrees is abnormal. In the *thoracic spine* kyphosis less than 40 degrees is normal but excessive lordosis, or insufficient kyphosis (less than 20 degrees), is abnormal.[1] In the *lumbar spine* lordosis from approximately 30 to 50 degrees is normal.[1] Greater lordosis is abnormal. In the *lumbar spine* kyphosis is always abnormal. This chapter will discuss poor posture under three separate headings: scoliosis, kyphosis, and lordosis (Figs. 59-1 and 59-2).

This chapter describes possible causes of poor posture and scoliosis, kyphosis, and lordosis in a child.

Special Concerns

- Any acute increase in scoliosis, kyphosis, or lordosis
- Scoliosis, kyphosis, or lordosis associated with pain
- Any curve associated with changes in the foot anatomy (especially cavovarus) suggesting intraspinal anomalies
- Left thoracic scoliosis in adolescents

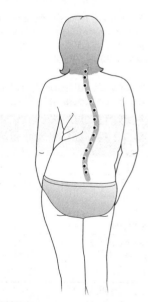

FIGURE 59-1 Adolescent girl with scoliosis.

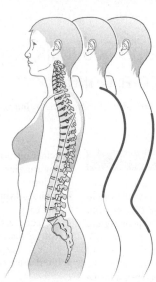

FIGURE 59-2 Lateral curvatures of the spine. In front is an adolescent girl with normal thoracic kyphosis and lumbar lordosis. In the middle is a girl with increased thoracic kyphosis (thoracic hyperkyphosis). At the back is a girl with decreased thoracic kyphosis (thoracic hypokyphosis) and an increase in lumbar lordosis (lumbar hyperlordosis).

CHAPTER PREVIEW: Conditions That May Lead to Poor Posture and Scoliosis, Kyphosis, or Lordosis in a Child

T Trauma		
SCOLIOSIS	**KYPHOSIS**	**LORDOSIS**
COMMON		
Contusion 1130 Muscle spasm 1136	Not applicable	Contusion 1130 Muscle spasm 1136 Spondylolisthesis 1143
UNCOMMON		
Spinal cord injury 1142 Spondylolysis 1143	Spinal cord injury 1142 Vertebral body fracture 1145	Spinal cord injury 1142
RARE		
Lumbar disk herniation 1135 Postradiation sequelae: • Postradiation scoliosis 1139 Rib fracture 1140 Soft tissue scarring 1141 Spondylolisthesis 1143	Postlaminectomy 1138 Postradiation sequelae: • Postradiation kyphosis 1139	Growth arrest from posterior spine fusion 1133 Lumbar disk herniation 1135 Spondylolysis 1143

I Inflammation		
SCOLIOSIS	**KYPHOSIS**	**LORDOSIS**
COMMON		
Not applicable	Not applicable	Not applicable

Inflammation *(continued)*

SCOLIOSIS	KYPHOSIS	LORDOSIS
UNCOMMON		

Aseptic
 Not applicable
 	
 Septic
 Osteomyelitis 1138
   caused by tuberculosis,
   systemic fungal infections
   (eg, coccidiomycosis,
   histoplasmosis, actinomycosis)
 Poliomyelitis 1138
	Aseptic
	 Not applicable
	
	 Septic
	 Tuberculosis 1144
		Aseptic
		 Juvenile ankylosing spondylitis 1134
		 Juvenile rheumatoid arthritis 1135
		
		 Septic
		 Not applicable

RARE		

Not applicable	**Aseptic**
	 Not applicable
	
	 Septic
	 Osteomyelitis 1138
	   caused by tuberculosis,
	   systemic fungal infections
	   (eg, coccidiomycosis,
	   histoplasmosis, actinomycosis)
	 Poliomyelitis 1138
		Aseptic
		 Reactive arthritis (Reiter's
		   syndrome) 1140
		
		 Septic
		 Poliomyelitis 1138

M Metabolic

SCOLIOSIS	KYPHOSIS	LORDOSIS
COMMON		
Not applicable	Not applicable	Not applicable
UNCOMMON		
Osteogenesis imperfecta 1138	Osteogenesis imperfecta 1138	Not applicable
RARE		
Cystic fibrosis 1131 Juvenile osteoporosis 1135 Prader-Willi syndrome 1140	Gaucher's disease 1133 Hyperparathyroidism 1134 Juvenile osteoporosis 1135 Renal osteodystrophy 1140 Rickets 1140	Not applicable

Va Vascular

SCOLIOSIS	KYPHOSIS	LORDOSIS
COMMON		
Not applicable	Not applicable	Not applicable
UNCOMMON		
Not applicable	Not applicable	Not applicable

(continued)

Vascular *(continued)*

SCOLIOSIS	KYPHOSIS	LORDOSIS
RARE		
Not applicable	Not applicable	Not applicable

De Degenerative

SCOLIOSIS	KYPHOSIS	LORDOSIS
COMMON		
Duchenne muscular dystrophy 1132	Scheuermann's disease (vertebral osteochondrosis) 1141	Duchenne muscular dystrophy 1132
UNCOMMON		
Not applicable	Not applicable	Friedreich's ataxia 1133
RARE		
Friedreich's ataxia 1133 Rett syndrome 1140 Spinal muscular atrophies: • Type I (Werdnig-Hoffmann disease) 1142 • Type II (Kugelberg-Welander disease) 1142 • Type III (benign) 1142	Not applicable	Spinal muscular atrophies: • Type I (Werdnig-Hoffmann disease) 1142 • Type II (Kugelberg-Welander disease) 1142 • Type III (benign) 1142

Tu Tumor

SCOLIOSIS	KYPHOSIS	LORDOSIS
COMMON		
Not applicable	Not applicable	Not applicable
UNCOMMON		
Not applicable	*Malignant Primary:* Not applicable *Malignant Metastatic:* Not applicable *Benign, such as:* • Neurofibromatosis (type I, von Recklinghausen's disease) 1145	Not applicable
RARE		
Malignant Primary, such as: • Neuroblastoma 1144 • Neurofibromatosis (type I, von Recklinghausen's disease) 1145 • Spinal cord tumors 1145 • Syringomyelia 1144 *Malignant Metastatic:* Not applicable *Benign, such as:* • Osteoid osteoma 1145	*Malignant Primary, such as:* • Neuroblastoma 1144 • Spinal cord tumors 1145 *Malignant Metastatic:* Not applicable *Benign, such as:* • Osteoid osteoma 1145	Not applicable

Co Congenital

SCOLIOSIS	KYPHOSIS	LORDOSIS
COMMON		
Congenital scoliosis 1130 Myelodysplasia 1137	Myelodysplasia 1137	Compensatory hyperlordosis 1129 Hip flexion contracture 1133 Myelodysplasia 1137
UNCOMMON		

Down syndrome 1132
Sprengel's deformity/
  Klippel-Feil syndrome 1143
	Congenital kyphosis 1130	Developmental dysplasia of
		  the hip with dislocation 1131

RARE		

Amnion rupture sequence 1128
Angelman syndrome 1129
Arthrogryposis 1129
Chondrodysplasia punctata 1129
Cri du chat syndrome (5p-) 1130
Diastrophic dysplasia
  (diastrophic dwarfism) 1131
Dysautonomia (eg,
  Riley-Day syndrome) 1132
Ehlers-Danlos syndrome 1132
Fibrodysplasia ossificans
  progressiva 1132
Fragile X syndrome 1132
Larsen's syndrome 1135
Marfan's syndrome 1135
Metaphyseal chondrodysplasia
  (McKusick type, Pyle
  type) 1136
Metatropic dysplasia
  (kyphoscoliosis) 1136
Mucopolysaccharidoses:
• Type IV (Morquio's
  syndrome) 1136
Noonan syndrome 1138
Pseudoachondroplasia 1140
Rubinstein-Taybi syndrome 1141
Soto's syndrome 1141
Spondyloepiphyseal
  dysplasia congenita 1142
Trisomy 18 (Edwards
  syndrome) 1144
	Achondroplasia 1128
	Diastrophic dysplasia
	  (diastrophic dwarfism) 1131
	Ehlers-Danlos syndrome 1132
	Larsen's syndrome 1135
	Metatropic dysplasia
	  (kyphoscoliosis) 1136
	Mucopolysaccharidoses:
	• Type IH (Hurler
	  syndrome) 1136
	• Type IV (Morquio's
	  syndrome) 1136
	• Type VI (Maroteaux-Lamy
	  type) 1136
	• Type VII (Sly syndrome) 1136
	Pseudoachondroplasia 1140
	Spondyloepiphyseal dysplasia
	  congenita 1142
	Spondyloptosis 1143
		Achondroplasia 1128
		Arthrogryposis 1129
		Congenital lordosis 1130
		Developmental lordosis 1131
		Down syndrome 1132
		Marfan's syndrome 1135
		Mucopolysaccharidoses:
		• Type IV (Morquio's
		  syndrome) 1136
		Pseudoachondroplasia 1140
		Spondyloepiphyseal dysplasia
		  congenita 1142

Ne Neurogenic/Psychogenic

SCOLIOSIS	KYPHOSIS	LORDOSIS
COMMON		
Cerebral palsy 1129 Idiopathic scolioses: • Adolescent 1134	Cerebral palsy 1129 Postural round back 1139	Abdominal muscle weakness 1128 Cerebral palsy 1129

(continued)

Neurogenic/Psychogenic *(continued)*

SCOLIOSIS	KYPHOSIS	LORDOSIS
COMMON		
Nonstructural scolioses: • Leg-length discrepancy 1137 • Postural 1137		
UNCOMMON		
Idiopathic scolioses: • Juvenile 1134	Not applicable	Not applicable
RARE		
Chiari malformation 1129 Congenital myotonic dystrophy 1130 Hydrocephalus 1133 Hysteric scoliosis 1134 Idiopathic scolioses: • Infantile 1134 Myotonic dystrophy 1137	Not applicable	Chiari malformation 1129 Hydrocephalus 1133 Myotonia 1137

Note: These are estimates of relative incidence because few data are available for the less common conditions.

Common Ages at Which Scoliosis, Kyphosis, or Lordosis Presents in a Child

APPROXIMATE AGE	CONDITION
Birth to 3 Years	**Scoliosis** Amnion rupture sequence Arthrogryposis Chiari II malformation Chondrodysplasia punctata Congenital scoliosis Cri du chat Diastrophic dysplasia (diastrophic dwarfism) Down syndrome Ehlers-Danlos syndrome Hydrocephalus Infantile idiopathic scoliosis Larsen's syndrome Metatrophic dysplasia Myelodysplasia Neuroblastoma Spinal cord tumors Spinal muscular atrophy types I and II Sprengel's deformity/Klippel-Feil syndrome Systemic fungal infections Trisomy 18 (Edwards syndrome) **Kyphosis** Achondroplasia Cerebral palsy Congenital kyphosis Diastrophic dysplasia Larsen's syndrome Metatrophic dysplasia

Common Ages at Which Scoliosis, Kyphosis, or Lordosis Presents in a Child—cont'd

APPROXIMATE AGE	CONDITION
	Kyphosis Mucopolysaccharidosis type IH (Hurler syndrome) Myelodysplasia Neuroblastoma Pseudoachondroplasia Spinal cord injury Spinal cord tumors Spondyloptosis Systemic fungal infections
	Lordosis Abdominal muscle weakness Achondroplasia Arthrogryposis Cerebral palsy Chiari malformation Compensatory hyperlordosis Congenital lordosis Developmental dysplasia of the hip with dislocation Developmental lordosis Down syndrome Hip flexion contracture Hydrocephalus Mucopolysaccharidosis type IV (Morquio's syndrome) Myelodysplasia Pseudoachondroplasia Spinal muscular atrophy types I and II Spondyloepiphyseal dysplasia congenita
Preschool (3–5 Years)	**Scoliosis** Cerebral palsy Chondrodysplasia punctata Congenital scoliosis Diastrophic dysplasia Ehlers-Danlos syndrome Hydrocephalus Juvenile idiopathic scoliosis Larsen's syndrome Metaphyseal dysplasia Mucopolysaccharidosis type IV (Morquio's syndrome) Myelodysplasia Neuroblastoma Neurofibromatosis Pseudoachondroplasia Soft tissue scarring Spinal cord injury Spinal cord tumors Spinal muscular atrophy types I and II Sprengel's deformity/Klippel-Feil syndrome Systemic fungal infections
	Kyphosis Achondroplasia Cerebral palsy Congenital kyphosis

(continued)

Common Ages at Which Scoliosis, Kyphosis, or Lordosis Presents in a Child—cont'd

APPROXIMATE AGE	CONDITION
	Kyphosis
	Ehlers-Danlos syndrome
	Gaucher's disease
	Hyperparathyroidism
	Juvenile osteoporosis
	Larsen's syndrome
	Mucopolysaccharidosis type IH (Hurler syndrome)
	Myelodysplasia
	Neurofibromatosis
	Osteogenesis imperfecta
	Osteomyelitis
	Poliomyelitis
	Postlaminectomy
	Postradiation kyphosis
	Postural round back
	Pseudoachondroplasia
	Renal osteodystrophy
	Rickets
	Spina bifida
	Spinal cord injury
	Spinal cord tumors
	Spondyloepiphyseal dysplasia congenita
	Spondyloptosis
	Syringomyelia
	Systemic fungal infections
	Tuberculosis
	Vertebral fracture
	Lordosis
	Abdominal muscle weakness
	Achondroplasia
	Arthrogryposis
	Cerebral palsy
	Chiari malformation
	Compensatory hyperlordosis
	Congenital lordosis
	Developmental dysplasia of the hip with dislocation
	Down syndrome
	Hip flexion contracture
	Hydrocephalus
	Mucopolysaccharidosis type IV (Morquio's syndrome)
	Myelodysplasia
	Poliomyelitis
	Pseudoachondroplasia
	Spinal cord injury
	Spinal muscular atrophy types I and II
	Spondyloepiphyseal dysplasia congenita
Elementary School (6–11 Years)	**Scoliosis**
	Angelman syndrome
	Cerebral palsy
	Chiari I malformation
	Chondrodysplasia punctata
	Congenital scoliosis
	Diastrophic dysplasia

Common Ages at Which Scoliosis, Kyphosis, or Lordosis Presents in a Child—cont'd

APPROXIMATE AGE	CONDITION
Elementary School (6–11 Years)	**Scoliosis** Dysautonomia (eg, Riley-Day syndrome) Ehlers-Danlos syndrome Fibrodysplasia ossificans progressiva Hydrocephalus Juvenile idiopathic scoliosis Larsen's syndrome Metaphyseal dysplasia Myelomeningocele Neurofibromatosis Nonstructural scoliosis Noonan syndrome Osteogenesis imperfecta Osteoid osteoma Osteomyelitis Poliomyelitis Pseudoachondroplasia Rett syndrome Rubinstein-Taybi syndrome Soft tissue scarring Soto's syndrome Spinal cord injury Spinal cord tumors Spinal muscular atrophy types II and III Spondyloepiphyseal dysplasia congenita Sprengel's deformity/Klippel-Feil syndrome Syringomyelia Systemic fungal infections Tuberculosis **Kyphosis** Achondroplasia Cerebral palsy Congenital kyphosis Ehlers-Danlos syndrome Gaucher's disease Hyperparathyroidism Juvenile osteoporosis Mucopolysaccharidosis type IH (Hurler syndrome) Myelodysplasia Neurofibromatosis Osteogenesis imperfecta Osteomyelitis Poliomyelitis Postlaminectomy Postural round back Pseudoachondroplasia Renal osteodystrophy Rickets Scheuermann's disease (vertebral osteochondrosis) Spinal cord injury Spinal cord tumors Spondyloepiphyseal dysplasia congenita Spondyloptosis

(continued)

Common Ages at Which Scoliosis, Kyphosis, or Lordosis Presents in a Child—cont'd

APPROXIMATE AGE	CONDITION
	Kyphosis Systemic fungal infections Tuberculosis Vertebral body fracture
	Lordosis Abdominal muscle weakness Achondroplasia Arthrogryposis Cerebral palsy Chiari malformation Compensatory hyperlordosis Congenital lordosis Developmental dysplasia of the hip with dislocation Down syndrome Duchenne muscular dystrophy Growth arrest from operative procedures Hip flexion contracture Hydrocephalus Juvenile rheumatoid arthritis Mucopolysaccharidosis type IV (Morquio's syndrome) Myelodysplasia Myotonia Poliomyelitis Pseudoachondroplasia Spinal cord injury Spinal muscular atrophy types II and III Spondyloepiphyseal dysplasia congenita Spondylolisthesis Vertebral body fracture
Middle School (12–14 Years)	**Scoliosis** Adolescent idiopathic scoliosis Angelman syndrome Ankylosing spondylitis Arthrogryposis Cerebral palsy Chondrodysplasia punctata Congenital scoliosis Cystic fibrosis Diastrophic dysplasia Duchenne muscular dystrophy Dysautonomia (eg, Riley-Day syndrome) Ehlers-Danlos syndrome Fibrodysplasia ossificans progressiva Fragile X syndrome Friedreich's ataxia Hydrocephalus Hysteric scoliosis Juvenile rheumatoid arthritis Larsen's syndrome Marfan's syndrome Metaphyseal dysplasia Myotonic dystrophy Neurofibromatosis

Common Ages at Which Scoliosis, Kyphosis, or Lordosis Presents in a Child—cont'd

APPROXIMATE AGE	CONDITION
Middle School (12–14 Years)	**Scoliosis** Nonstructural scoliosis Noonan syndrome Osteogenesis imperfecta Osteoid osteoma Osteomyelitis Poliomyelitis Postradiation scoliosis Prader-Willi syndrome Pseudoachondroplasia Rett syndrome Rubinstein-Taybi syndrome Soft tissue scarring Soto's syndrome Spina bifida Spinal cord injury Spinal muscular atrophy types II and III Spondyloepiphyseal dysplasia congenita Spondylolisthesis Spondylolysis Sprengel's deformity/Klippel-Feil syndrome Syringomyelia Systemic fungal infections Tuberculosis
	Kyphosis Achondroplasia Cerebral palsy Congenital kyphosis Ehlers-Danlos syndrome Gaucher's disease Hyperparathyroidism Juvenile osteoporosis Mucopolysaccharidosis type IH (Hurler syndrome) Myelodysplasia Neurofibromatosis Osteogenesis imperfecta Osteomyelitis Poliomyelitis Postlaminectomy Postural round back Pseudoachondroplasia Renal osteodystrophy Rickets Scheuermann's disease (vertebral osteochondrosis) Spinal cord injury Spinal cord tumors Spondyloepiphyseal dysplasia congenita Spondyloptosis Systemic fungal infections Tuberculosis Vertebral body fracture

(continued)

Common Ages at Which Scoliosis, Kyphosis, or Lordosis Presents in a Child—cont'd

APPROXIMATE AGE	CONDITION
	Lordosis Abdominal muscle weakness Achondroplasia Ankylosing spondylitis Arthrogryposis Cerebral palsy Chiari malformation Compensatory hyperlordosis Congenital lordosis Developmental dysplasia of the hip with dislocation Down syndrome Duchenne muscular dystrophy Friedreich's ataxia Growth arrest from operative procedures Hip flexion contracture Hydrocephalus Juvenile rheumatoid arthritis Lumbar disk herniation Marfan's syndrome Myelodysplasia Myotonia Poliomyelitis Pseudoachondroplasia Reactive arthritis (Reiter's syndrome) Spinal cord injury Spinal muscular atrophy types II and III Spondyloepiphyseal dysplasia congenita Spondylolisthesis Spondylolysis Vertebral body fracture
High School (15–18 Years)	**Scoliosis** Adolescent idiopathic scoliosis Angelman syndrome Ankylosing spondylitis Arthrogryposis Cerebral palsy Cystic fibrosis Duchenne muscular dystrophy Dysautonomia (Riley-Day syndrome) Ehlers-Danlos syndrome Fibrodysplasia ossificans progressiva Fragile X syndrome Friedreich's ataxia Hydrocephalus Hysteric scoliosis Juvenile rheumatoid arthritis Lumbar disk herniation Marfan's syndrome Myotonic dystrophy Neurofibromatosis Nonstructural scoliosis Osteogenesis imperfecta Osteoid osteoma

Common Ages at Which Scoliosis, Kyphosis, or Lordosis Presents in a Child—cont'd

APPROXIMATE AGE	CONDITION
High School (15–18 Years)	**Scoliosis** Osteomyelitis Poliomyelitis Postradiation scoliosis (eg, Wilms' tumor) Prader-Willi syndrome Pseudoachondroplasia Rett syndrome Rubinstein-Taybi syndrome Soft tissue scarring Soto's syndrome Spinal cord injury Spinal muscular atrophy types II and III Spondylolisthesis Spondylolysis Syringomyelia Systemic fungal infections Traumatic spinal cord injury Tuberculosis
	Kyphosis Achondroplasia Cerebral palsy Congenital kyphosis Ehlers-Danlos syndrome Gaucher's disease Hyperparathyroidism Juvenile osteoporosis Mucopolysaccharidosis type IH (Hurler syndrome) Myelodysplasia Neurofibromatosis Osteogenesis imperfecta Osteomyelitis Poliomyelitis Postlaminectomy Postural round back Pseudoachondroplasia Renal osteodystrophy Scheuermann's disease (vertebral osteochondrosis) Spinal cord injury Spinal cord tumors Spondyloepiphyseal dysplasia congenita Spondyloptosis Systemic fungal infections Tuberculosis Vertebral body fracture
	Lordosis Abdominal muscle weakness Achondroplasia Ankylosing spondylitis Arthrogryposis Cerebral palsy Chiari malformation Compensatory hyperlordosis

(continued)

Common Ages at Which Scoliosis, Kyphosis, or Lordosis Presents in a Child—cont'd

APPROXIMATE AGE	CONDITION
	Lordosis
	Congenital lordosis
	Developmental dysplasia of the hip with dislocation
	Down syndrome
	Friedreich's ataxia
	Hip flexion contracture
	Hydrocephalus
	Juvenile rheumatoid arthritis
	Lumbar disk herniation
	Marfan's syndrome
	Myelodysplasia
	Myotonia
	Poliomyelitis
	Pseudoachondroplasia
	Reactive arthritis (Reiter's syndrome)
	Spinal cord injury
	Spinal muscular atrophy types II and III
	Spondyloepiphyseal dysplasia congenita
	Spondylolisthesis
	Spondylolysis
	Vertebral body fracture

Overview of Poor Posture and Scoliosis, Kyphosis, and Lordosis in a Child

Poor posture is a physical sign of curvatures of the spine, which can be accentuated or diminished in the sagittal, transverse, and/or frontal planes and are correctable. Almost everyone slumps when fatigued and teenagers frequently slouch in order to aggravate their parents. A child may have poor posture from a variety of causes. A child who wants to imitate the stance common to gymnasts or dancers may stand with an increased lumbar lordosis. Poor self-image may cause a girl who is taller than all her friends to "slouch" or round her back in order to diminish her standing height. Some children slouch in order to see more easily and the problem is visual rather than musculoskeletal. Children who are blind often have difficulty with postural alignment because they are unable to appreciate where their bodies are positioned in space. Once the associated cause of the poor posture has been identified and the child has been referred for glasses, for example, exercises are not usually beneficial. As long as the child has been screened to ensure that the poor posture is just a result of "adolescent" behavior, there is little benefit in attempting to get the child to correct his or her posture with physical therapy.

Scoliosis

Scoliosis may be structural or nonstructural. *Structural scoliosis* includes any scoliosis that does not correct on bending to the opposite side or is associated with rotation (Figs. 59-3A and B). *Nonstructural scoliosis* is reversible and is not associated with rotation of the vertebral bodies. Nonstructural scoliosis is often associated with a leg-length discrepancy that causes the child to posture with a C-shaped curve. A lift under the short leg will make the scoliosis disappear. An injury to the back that causes muscle spasm on one side of the spine may cause the child to hold an asymmetric posture as a result of the pain. Treatment of the muscle spasm will cause the scoliosis to disappear. Structural scoliosis includes any physical alteration in the vertebral bodies, intervertebral disks, muscles, ligaments, or transverse and/or spinous processes that is not reversible and results in a lateral curvature of the spine.

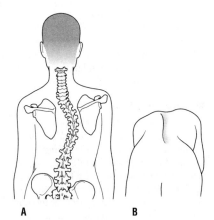

A **B**

FIGURE 59-3 The Adam's test: (A) Standing posteroanterior x-ray of girl with a right thoracic left lumbar scoliosis. Note the marked rotation of the vertebral bodies at the apex of each curve. (B) The same girl in part A seen from behind when she bends forward (the Adam's test), which makes the rotation more obvious. Note the prominence of the ribs on the right in the thoracic region and the prominence of the transverse processes of the lumbar spine on the left.

A child can develop or be born with a musculoskeletal condition (eg, adolescent idiopathic scoliosis) that causes scoliosis as a result of growth. A child may have been injured (eg, a spinal cord injury) or contracted a disease (eg, Duchenne muscular dystrophy) that has caused muscle weakness or paralysis and can develop a scoliosis with growth over time.

It is very important to identify a child with scoliosis early in the course of the disease because treatment options become limited as the curve progresses. If children with idiopathic scoliosis are referred for treatment to a pediatric spine specialist while the curve is less than 40 degrees they may be treated with bracing and avoid surgery. Curves of 50 degrees or more in a growing child usually require treatment with a spine fusion in order to halt progression. It is important to refer any child with scoliosis as soon as you have identified the curve.

Treatment decisions are often predicated on detecting curve progression. Therefore, an accurate baseline radiographic measurement is critical and should be obtained as early as possible. The size of the curve, age of the child, level of physical maturation, and cause of the scoliosis will determine treatment options. Paralytic curves do not respond to bracing but there may be positioning equipment decisions to be made, such as type of wheelchair or support system for children with cerebral palsy or muscular dystrophy.

Structural Kyphosis

Structural kyphosis includes any physical alteration in the vertebral bodies, intervertebral disks, muscles, ligaments, or transverse and/or spinous processes that is not reversible and results in an exaggerated posterior curvature of the spine in the sagittal plane. Surgical procedures for spinal cord tumor resection, traumatic injuries to the vertebrae, and pathological fractures from conditions such as osteoporosis all tend to cause the vertebral body to collapse anteriorly, leading to excessive thoracic kyphosis. The pathological fractures are often painful while many of the other conditions leading to hyperkyphosis are not.

Kyphosis and scoliosis are frequently seen together especially in conditions such as neurofibromatosis where the spinal deformity can be severe. Significant kyphosis is also common in myelodysplasia where the posterior elements of the vertebrae never develop and in syndromes such as Larsen's where congenital malformation of the vertebral bodies leads to life-threatening kyphosis of the cervical spine. Of the spinal deformities, the kyphoses are often the most severe because of the risk of spinal cord impingement and paraplegia. They are also the most difficult surgical challenges and should be handled by experienced practitioners.

Nonstructural kyphosis or postural round back is reversible and the child will be able to completely straighten the forward curve and hyperextend the thoracic spine without difficulty if asked to do so. Slumping forward is a common postural fault and one that distresses parents, but corrective physical therapy exercises are unlikely to help. It just leads to one more issue for the parents and the adolescent to get into conflict over and wastes everyone's time and money.

Lordosis

As with structural scoliosis and kyphosis, *lordosis* also includes any physical alteration in the vertebral bodies, intervertebral disks, muscles, ligaments, or transverse and/or spinous processes that is not reversible and results in a posterior curvature of the spine in the sagittal plane. Lumbar lordosis as a result of abdominal weakness or postural choice is nonstructural and reversible and can be altered with physical therapy intervention. Some cases of congenital lumbar hyperlordosis can be managed successfully with bracing. Lumbar hyperlordosis may be the result of compensation for hip and/or knee flexion contractures as commonly seen in children with the residua of poliomyelitis. These hyperlordoses may be reversible with physical therapy depending on the etiology of the flexion contractures. In children who have contractures caused by a progressive disease such as Duchenne muscular dystrophy, where they ultimately become too weak to shift themselves into any other positions, treatment can only hope to slow the progression of contracture development. For some of these patients with extreme weakness a hyperlordotic lumbar spine position may be their only option for maintaining a sitting position.

Other conditions that are not reversible and again pose a risk for spinal cord compression (eg, a severe spondylolisthesis) may require surgery for stabilization of the deformity. Decreased thoracic kyphosis—or in the extreme, thoracic lordosis—has received increasing attention as a concomitant of idiopathic scoliosis. The specific design of a spinal orthosis for treating a child with idiopathic scoliosis may exacerbate this phenomenon and should be avoided. Pads placed posteriorly to affect the spinal rotation by trying to force the ribs anteriorly may further decrease the thoracic kyphosis and potentially decrease pulmonary capacity.

> ### Description of Conditions That May Lead to Poor Posture and Scoliosis, Kyphosis, and Lordosis in a Child

■ Abdominal Muscle Weakness
Chief Clinical Characteristics
This presentation involves the presence of abdominal weakness and may result in hyperlordosis of the lumbar spine.

Background Information
Such weakness in children might result from a variety of pathologies including Guillain-Barré syndrome, spinal cord injury, and hypotonia. The prognosis for resolution of this condition depends on its underlying etiology.

■ Achondroplasia
Chief Clinical Characteristics
This presentation can include a child with small stature, disproportionate shortening of the proximal limb segment, frontal bossing, macrocephaly, lumbar lordosis, and mild thoracolumbar kyphosis as a result of anterior beaking of the first and/or second lumbar vertebra. Spinal cord compression or root compression can occur as a result of the kyphosis, stenosis of the spinal canal, or injury to the intervertebral disk. A thoracolumbar gibbus occurs frequently. The children are often developmentally delayed and are not able to walk alone until 18 to 24 months of age. Once they start walking, the thoracolumbar gibbus commonly changes into an exaggerated lumbar lordosis. Because the spinal canal is stenotic, they may develop spinal cord compression at the foramen magnum or in the lumbar spine. Stenosis of the foramen magnum often occurs in infants and young children, whereas lumbar stenosis occurs in young adults.[2,3]

Background Information
The incidence of achondroplasia is about 1 in 15,000 to 40,000 live births. This condition is autosomal dominant and about 90% of the cases are a result of a fresh mutation.[3]

■ Amnion Rupture Sequence
Chief Clinical Characteristics
This presentation includes an infant who may present with scoliosis as well as missing digits or partial limb amputations and significant facial deformities.[4]

Background Information
Constrictive tissue bands are caused by a primary amniotic rupture and lead to the formation of fibrotic amniotic strands that become entangled with the fetus and cause various deformities.[5,6] The rupture of the amniotic membrane leads to numerous defects during the course of fetal development and hence the term *sequence* is used. The incidence of

amniotic bands (or constriction bands) is 1 in 10,000 to 45,000.[6]

■ Angelman Syndrome

Chief Clinical Characteristics
This presentation involves severe mental retardation, delay in motor development, and inability to communicate verbally. Many individuals have seizures and paroxysms of inappropriate laughter.

Background Information
Scoliosis may be seen in this population, although not routinely.[7] This disorder is a result of a maternal chromosome interstitial deletion of 15q11q13.[7,8]

■ Arthrogryposis

Chief Clinical Characteristics
This presentation may be characterized by joint contractures of two or more joints and muscle weakness.[9] Scoliosis can result from the muscle imbalances as well from bony spinal involvement.[9] About one-third of the children have C-shaped scoliosis common in neuromuscular diseases.[8] Hyperlordosis may occur in the children born with congenital dislocated hips and fixed hip flexion contractures.

Background Information
One of the main causes of this nonprogressive syndrome may be anterior horn cell degeneration resulting in fetal muscle weakness and joint immobilization *in utero*.[8,9] Other causes may include viral infections, disruption of the vascular supply to the fetus, and myogenic problems.[8,9]

■ Cerebral Palsy

Chief Clinical Characteristics
This presentation involves scoliosis, kyphosis, or hyperlordosis that may develop in these children due to hypotonia, muscle imbalances, spasticity, and positioning in nonambulatory children.[9] Hyperlordosis usually develops as a result of hip flexion contractures.

Background Information
This condition may also be seen as a compensation for a severe thoracic hyperkyphosis. Kyphosis may occur in the lumbar spine as a result of extremely tight hamstring muscles. Scoliosis is more common in children with all types of cerebral palsy, occurring in 50% to 70% of children with spastic quadriplegia. These children often have rapidly progressing curves that require surgical intervention.[10]

■ Chiari Malformation

Chief Clinical Characteristics
This presentation may include suboccipital headache, ocular disturbances, progressive ataxia, spastic weakness, sensory loss, and scoliosis with minimal vertebral body rotation, kyphosis, or lordosis.[11–13] Onset of symptoms may occur after doing an activity that requires prolonged cervical extension.[12] Type II (Arnold-Chiari malformation) presents concomitantly with meningomyelocele and is often symptomatic at birth.[13] Type I may become symptomatic later in childhood or in adulthood and is not associated with meningomyelocele.[13]

Background Information
This is a hindbrain abnormality where the cerebellum or medulla is downwardly herniated through the foramen magnum into the cervical canal, interrupting the flow of cerebrospinal fluid and resulting in hydrocephalus.[13] Syringomyelia or hydromyelia of the cervical spinal cord is often present as well.[11]

■ Chondrodysplasia Punctata

Chief Clinical Characteristics
This presentation may include joint contractures, shortened limbs, and cataracts.[14] The Conradi-Hünermann type presents with atlantoaxial instability, spinal stenosis, kyphosis, and congenital scoliosis.[2]

Background Information
Some of this rare group of disorders can eventually develop into scoliosis from skeletal asymmetries due to the stippled epiphyses.[14]

■ Compensatory Hyperlordosis

Chief Clinical Characteristics
This presentation involves a primary hyperkyphosis and the individual develops a flexible hyperlordosis to compensate for the primary kyphotic deformity. The lordosis can easily be reduced on forward bending.[1]

Background Information
Hyperlordosis may result from diseases that are characterized by neuromuscular weakness

such as myelomeningocele, cerebral palsy, and muscular dystrophy.[9]

■ Congenital Kyphosis

Chief Clinical Characteristics

This presentation is characterized by an increasing degree of kyphosis over time and the individual may develop pain and/or neurological impairments including cord compression. Kyphotic deformity can also be a result of muscle imbalance due to neuromuscular disease.[9,15]

Background Information

A failure of formation of the anterior portion of the vertebrae results in a wedge-shaped bone and the development of kyphosis.

■ Congenital Lordosis

Chief Clinical Characteristics

This presentation involves the failure of formation of the posterior portion of the vertebra, a rare occurrence that results in excessive lordosis.[15]

Background Information

Hyperlordosis may result from diseases that characterized by neuromuscular weakness such as myelomeningocele, cerebral palsy, and muscular dystrophy.[9]

■ Congenital Myotonic Dystrophy

Chief Clinical Characteristics

This presentation involves children who have hypotonia, developmental delay, long, narrow expressionless faces, and mild mental retardation. Around 40% have a severe form, dying as infants, with the other 60% affected later by the disease. Dislocated hips, clubfeet, and scoliosis are common.[16]

Background Information

This disorder has an autosomal dominant transmission.

■ Congenital Scoliosis

Chief Clinical Characteristics

This presentation includes a high incidence of children with other related problems including those affecting the urogenitary, cardiopulmonary, musculoskeletal, and central nervous systems.[15] Scoliosis results from a single- or multiple-level vertebral anomaly due to failure of segmentation or formation or both. Curves are often short and sharp, and present with different patterns than the curve patterns seen in adolescent idiopathic scoliosis.

Background Information

Failure of formation problems include wedge vertebra or fully, partially, and unsegmented hemivertebrae.[15] A wedge vertebra has a height asymmetry with intact pedicles. A hemivertebra is one in which only half of a vertebra is formed and is fused (segmented) to the vertebral bodies above and below (fully segmented), to one vertebral body either above or below (partially), or separated from both by the disk space in the case of the unsegmented hemivertebra. Failures in segmentation include block vertebra, unilateral segmentation (bar) defect, and unilateral bar with a contralateral hemivertebra. The block vertebrae result from bilateral segmentation failures. A unilateral bar results from a unilateral segmentation failure usually on the concave side (Fig. 59-4).[15]

■ Contusion

Chief Clinical Characteristics

This presentation can involve a nonstructural scoliosis; a lateral curve is seen with the concavity on the contused side but there is no vertebral rotation. Pain may be present and lead to muscle spasm in the erector spinae muscles.

Background Information

A contusion is caused by a blow to the back often seen as a consequence of playing a contact sport like American football. There may be swelling and discoloration of the skin but the skin will be intact. Treatment focuses on caring for the contused tissues.[17,18]

■ Cri du Chat Syndrome (5p–)

Chief Clinical Characteristics

This presentation includes mental retardation, hip subluxation or dislocation, clubfeet, hypotonicity, scoliosis, and a high-pitched cat-like cry for which the condition is named.[7,9]

Background Information

This condition is a partial deletion chromosomal disorder on the short arm of chromosome 5. It refers to deletion of a whole host of alleles. The clinical presentation should prompt referral for chromosomal testing, which confirms the diagnosis.

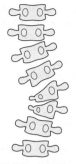
Partial unilateral
failure of formation
(wedge vertebra)

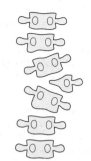
Complete unilateral
failure of formation
(hemi vertebra)

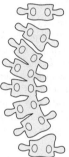
Unilateral failure
of segmentation
(congenital bar)

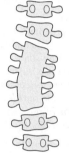
Bilateral failure
of segmentation
(block vertebra)

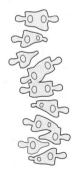
Combined
congenital bars and
wedge vertebrae

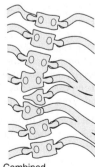
Combined
congenital bars,
wedge vertebrae, and
fused ribs

FIGURE 59-4 Variations of the anomalies of the vertebral spine that can be seen in a child with a congenital scoliosis.

■ Cystic Fibrosis

Chief Clinical Characteristics
This presentation involves a high prevalence of scoliosis in individuals already diagnosed with cystic fibrosis. The curves tend to be single, short mid-thoracic curves, with the apex between T6 and T8 and without a side preference. The curves are usually nonprogressive.[19]

Background Information
Cystic fibrosis is an inherited autosomal recessive disorder affecting multiple systems, but chiefly the lungs and the digestive system. It is most common in white people of Northern and Central European descent, and it is the major cause of severe chronic lung disease in children.[20]

■ Developmental Dysplasia of the Hip with Dislocation

Chief Clinical Characteristics
This presentation consists of limited hip flexion and abduction, pistoning of the femur in the hip joint, femoral shortening, and a positive Barlow or Ortolani sign.[9]

Background Information
Excessive lordosis can be a secondary result from the associated hip flexion contracture. Overall developmental dysplasia is far more common in females, with a ratio of 6:1.[9]

■ Developmental Lordosis

Chief Clinical Characteristics
This presentation is characterized by a flexible, increased lumbar lordosis prior to the onset of puberty.

Background Information
Examination will be completely normal and the condition will resolve with growth.[1]

■ Diastrophic Dysplasia (Diastrophic Dwarfism)

Chief Clinical Characteristics
This presentation involves severe short stature due to short limbs, progressive deformities, contracture development at joints, and hand and foot deformities. All children with this condition will demonstrate increased lumbar lordosis and 80% have progressive scoliosis starting before the age of 2 years. Some children also present with progressive cervical kyphosis. Girls are more frequently affected by scoliosis and congenital

spinal abnormalities than boys with this disorder.

Background Information
Diastrophic dwarfism usually is transmitted by autosomal recession though some are a result of spontaneous mutation. This form of dysplasia is associated with the most severe, numerous, and disparate skeletal abnormalities. It is extremely rare except in Finland.[1,2,7]

■ Down Syndrome

Chief Clinical Characteristics
This presentation includes facial features such as a flattened occiput and a face with up-slanting eyes.[9] Other characteristics of this disease include hypotonia; short, wide feet and hands; joint laxity; and mental retardation.[9] About 50% have congenital heart disease.[7,8] About 50% have an idiopathic type scoliosis, and about 6% spondylolisthesis typically in the lower lumbar spine. Multiple types of cervical defects are common and can lead to cervical instability.[8]

Background Information
Down syndrome occurs due to a chromosomal abnormality called Trisomy 21.[7,9]

■ Duchenne Muscular Dystrophy

Background Information
This presentation includes the onset of scoliosis in association with progressive motor decline and loss of ambulation due to degeneration of muscle fibers.[21] Excessive lumbar lordosis is also common while still ambulatory as a compensation for hip flexion contractures and weakness.[22] Calf hypertrophy is very common.

Background Information
This X-linked disorder it the most common genetic disorder known and the incidence is around 1 in 3,500 live male births. Destruction of myofibrils leads to progressive muscle weakness as a result of loss of muscle contractility. Death occurs during or before the third decade of life.[16]

■ Dysautonomia (eg, Riley-Day Syndrome)

Chief Clinical Characteristics
This presentation can include a lack of overflow tears when the child cries, an absent or weak suck, low tone, decreased deep tendon reflexes, and

labile blood pressure. Children with this condition are often born in a breech presentation. They are delayed in walking and speaking and have poor growth, and 90% will have scoliosis by the age of 13 years. About half develop a significant kyphosis, and fractures and avascular necrosis are frequent in these patients.[8,23]

Background Information
This is an autosomal recessive disorder only seen in families of Ashkenazi Jewish descent with an incidence of 1 in 10,000 to 20,000. It is part of a group of disorders described as hereditary sensory and autonomic neuropathies characterized by widespread sensory and autonomic dysfunction.[23]

■ Ehlers-Danlos Syndrome

Chief Clinical Characteristics
This presentation involves joint hypermobility that can result in spinal deformities including spondylolisthesis, scoliosis, kyphosis, and kyphoscoliosis.[14] Individuals with this condition are prone to dislocate at the hip, knee, shoulder, elbow, and clavicle and typically have cardiac defects. Infants who are hypotonic may have the kyphoscoliotic type of Ehlers-Danlos syndrome.[8]

Background Information
Ten distinct variations of this connective tissue syndrome exist.[7]

■ Fibrodysplasia Ossificans Progressive

Chief Clinical Characteristics
This presentation typically includes ossification that usually begins by 5 years of age, and by 7 years most children will have developed some heterotopic ossification that is restrictive. Common sites for beginning heterotopic ossification are the neck, spine, and shoulder. There is a significant risk of cervical spine fusion and scoliosis.

Background Information
This is an extremely rare autosomal dominant disorder with most cases resulting from spontaneous mutation.[7,24]

■ Fragile X Syndrome

Chief Clinical Characteristics
This presentation is characterized by mild to moderate mental retardation in boys, and about 60% also have autism. Around 50% of girls

with this syndrome have trouble with learning or mental retardation. The children have macrocephaly, large ears, and epicanthal folds. Some children will have kyphoscoliosis, pectus excavatum, flat feet, and cardiac defects.

Background Information
This X-linked disorder is one of the most common causes of mental retardation.[7]

■ Friedreich's Ataxia

Chief Clinical Characteristics
This presentation includes gait ataxia as the initial sign.[12] Children may have difficulty standing as well.[12] Kyphoscoliosis and pes cavus are associated musculoskeletal deformities that may precede the onset of the neurological signs.[12] Severe kyphoscoliosis has been associated with impaired pulmonary function and may contribute to death in these individuals.[12]

Background Information
Individuals with this condition have double major curves or single thoracic or lumbar curves, not the typical C curve seen with other neurological conditions. Children with scoliosis onset prior to age 15 often have more severe and rapidly progressive curves requiring surgery. Individuals with onset of scoliosis after age 15 may show a slower and less severe progression of their scoliosis. Most patients will use a wheelchair for mobility by their early twenties, so increased lumbar lordosis as a result of hip flexion contractures from sitting may also be seen.[16] This inherited, progressive form of spinocerebellar ataxia typically presents before the age of 10.[12] It occurs in about 1 in 50,000 live births.[16]

■ Gaucher's Disease

Chief Clinical Characteristics
This presentation may involve a progressive kyphosis. Many individuals will have osteopenia, pathological fractures, osteonecrosis, and osteomyelitis.

Background Information
The kyphosis usually needs treatment by surgical spine fusion. This is a very rare hereditary glycolipid storage disorder. Gaucher's cells invade the bone marrow and lead to the numerous sequelae.[25]

■ Growth Arrest From Posterior Spine Fusion

Chief Clinical Characteristics
This presentation involves development of hyperlordosis in the spine over the course of several years after a posterior spinal operation.

Background Information
Operations such as isolated posterior spinal fusion, shunt placement for a Baclofen pump, or a selective posterior rhizotomy may disturb the growth of the posterior part of the lumbar vertebrae during the time that the child is still growing, which can lead to the development of a hyperlordosis. Treatment may require anterior spinal fusion.[1]

■ Hip Flexion Contracture

Chief Clinical Characteristics
This presentation can include a limitation of passive and active extension of the hip joint. This can result in excessive lumbar lordosis due to the pelvis being pulled into anterior rotation.

Background Information
A hip flexion contracture can result from a variety of underlying causes including hip dislocation, chondrodysplasia punctata, arthrogryposis, and heterotopic ossification. It might also occur in any child who uses a wheelchair most of the time due to prolonged positioning in hip flexion.[1]

■ Hydrocephalus

Chief Clinical Characteristics
This presentation typically includes altered mental status, papilledema, headache, nausea and vomiting, and change in muscle tone.[26] In infants a bulging anterior fontanel and/or downward deviation of the eyes are other signs.[26]

Background Information
Hydrocephalus or shunt malfunction is also associated with worsening of scoliosis, possibly due to a change in muscle tone, as well as lethargy, headache, vomiting, alterations in personality, and irritability.[9,26] Children with spina bifida often develop this condition as a result of cerebrospinal fluid backup in the ventricles of the brain.[9] Other causes include tumors or masses, intraparenchymal hemorrhage, and congenital malformations.[26] This is usually treated with a ventriculoperitoneal shunt.[26]

■ **Hyperparathyroidism**

Chief Clinical Characteristics

This presentation involves symptoms of hypocalcemia, muscle weakness, anorexia, vomiting, weight loss, and fever in children older than 10 years of age. Bone pain and compression fractures of the vertebrae can occur, leading to severely increased thoracic kyphosis.

Background Information

This condition is rare in children and usually caused by a benign adenoma.[27] Kyphosis is a result of the associated osteoporosis causing vertebral fracture and collapse.[28]

■ **Hysteric Scoliosis**

Chief Clinical Characteristics

This presentation can include a postural or nonstructural scoliosis that is caused by a conversion reaction. The spine will appear normal on x-ray evaluation and no fixed rotation will be seen during the physical exam.

Background Information

Individuals suspected of having this condition require psychological intervention, because the scoliosis is a physical sign of a psychological issue. This is a very rare condition, and it is typically a diagnosis of exclusion.[29]

IDIOPATHIC SCOLIOSES

■ **Adolescent**

Chief Clinical Characteristics

This presentation consists of asymmetrical gluteal folds and shoulder, scapular, or pelvis position.[9] This classification includes children who have a diagnosis of scoliosis from age 10 to skeletal maturity, and scoliosis is more common in females at this stage.[9,30] Prognosis for progression of the curve is greater in this group, especially for those with a larger curve magnitude, females overall, and in particular those with right thoracic or double curves and males with right lumbar curves.[30,31]

Background Information

Approximately 80% of children with scoliosis have the idiopathic type. Scoliosis may be a nonstructural scoliosis type with normal spinal radiographs. Passive or active movement may correct this form of scoliosis.[9] Leg-length inequality, pelvic obliquity, poor posture, and muscle imbalances are some of the causes of this type, also known as a functional curve.[9] It may also be due to idiopathic structural abnormalities in the spine.[9]

■ **Infantile**

Chief Clinical Characteristics

This presentation involves a diagnosis of scoliosis that was confirmed before 3 years of age.[9] It occurs more often in males and usually involves a left thoracolumbar curve. Children with this condition may also demonstrate plagiocephaly, hip dysplasia, congenital heart disease, and mental retardation.[32]

Background Information

These curves usually resolve without any intervention unless they are related to an underlying neuromuscular disease.[9]

■ **Juvenile**

Chief Clinical Characteristics

This presentation is characterized by children whose scoliosis is diagnosed after 3 years of age but before 10 years of age.[30] The incidence is equal for both genders.[9] In children younger than 6 years, both right and left curves are seen equally, but in children older than 6 years, more right curves are seen.[32]

Background Information

Scoliosis is more severe in this group and usually requires intervention.[9] In pre-menses, girls' greater height is associated with a higher incidence of scoliosis.

■ **Juvenile Ankylosing Spondylitis**

Chief Clinical Characteristics

This presentation consists of symmetric lower extremity arthritis.[14] Spinal and sacroiliac pain is common but is usually preceded by pain in other joints and sometimes by several years.[14] The typical child with this condition is a boy of 8 years or older who may have a family history of the disease.[14]

Background Information

Lumbar lordosis, spinal range of motion, and rib cage expansion become progressively diminished over the course of the disease, while thoracic kyphosis increases.[14,33] This is the most common form of the spondyloarthropathies that occur in children.[14]

■ Juvenile Osteoporosis

Chief Clinical Characteristics

This presentation includes an age of onset of between 8 and 14 years for childhood osteoporosis. Note, however, that childhood osteoporosis is sometimes seen in younger children during growth spurts. Children with idiopathic juvenile osteoporosis may present with foot, hip, or lower back pain as well as limping and significantly increased thoracic kyphosis. *Idiopathic juvenile osteoporosis is seen slightly more often in boys than girls.*

Background Information

Osteoporosis is a progressive loss of bone density or inadequate bone formation causing increased vulnerability to fractures. Childhood osteoporosis is often caused by an underlying medical condition such as diabetes or anorexia nervosa but there is a very rare form called idiopathic juvenile osteoporosis. *Idiopathic juvenile osteoporosis* may resolve spontaneously but management of bone loss or reduction of fracture risk through bracing, medication, or physical therapy may be required.[25]

■ Juvenile Rheumatoid Arthritis

Chief Clinical Characteristics

This presentation includes the consistent presence for 6 or more weeks of swelling, or the presence of two or more of the following: limited joint range of motion, palpable tenderness, painful movement, or joint warmth.[14] *There are three subtypes: systemic, polyarticular, and pauciarticular.*[14] *When the spine is involved in the polyarticular form, it becomes flexed throughout, leading to hypolordosis especially in the cervical spine. Severe hip disease may occur in the polyarticular form of this condition and is commonly associated with hyperlordosis in the lumbar spine.*

Background Information

Pauciarticular arthritis affects four or fewer joints.[14] Late-onset pauciarticular arthritis is more common in boys than girls and involves concomitant enthesitis or tendinitis and arthritis that can also involve the spine.[14]

■ Larsen's Syndrome

Chief Clinical Characteristics

This presentation involves congenital joint dislocations of the hips, knees, elbows, and wrists. Spinal segmentation failures result in spinal deformity in this connective tissue disorder.[14] *Scoliosis in the thoracic and lumbar spine occurs along with lordosis and spondylolysis. Hypoplastic cervical vertebrae can cause severe cervical instability leading to quadriplegia and death if not diagnosed and treated.*[2,7]

Background Information

Usually this is an autosomal dominant disorder, but autosomal recessive inheritance has been suggested.

■ Lumbar Disk Herniation

Chief Clinical Characteristics

This presentation commonly includes children who present with their thorax laterally shifted over the pelvis away from the side of the herniation. This is a nonstructural cause of scoliosis since the lateral curve will not show any rotation in the vertebral bodies and the scoliosis will disappear once the pain response to the trauma has disappeared. A child may also show a diminished lumbar lordosis.

Background Information

Herniation of the intervertebral disk due to a disruption in the annulus fibrosis or vertebral end plate is an uncommon phenomenon in adolescents. Diminished lumbar lordosis is seen in individuals with discogenic problems that are thought to predispose them to this type of injury due to increased loading through the disks.[34] Treatment is directed to the disk herniation, after which the scoliosis will resolve.

■ Marfan's Syndrome

Chief Clinical Characteristics

This presentation is characterized by tall stature, hypotonia, and ligamentous laxity. Cardiac defects are often seen with this syndrome.[35] *The spinal abnormalities seen in this condition include abnormal body proportions, chest wall deformities, diminished thoracic kyphosis, and scoliosis.*[14] *Individuals with this condition also have atlantoaxial instability and spondyloloptosis (hypolordosis).*[1]

Background Information

This is an autosomal dominant disorder with a defect in fibrillin, an important component of elastic tissues.[14]

■ Metaphyseal Chondrodysplasia (McKusick Type, Pyle Type)

Chief Clinical Characteristics

This presentation consists of short stature, bowed legs, waddling gait, and vertebral abnormalities associated with increased lumbar lordosis and scoliosis.[7,36]

Background Information

There are several types, and scoliosis is common with the McKusick type and occasionally with the Pyle type. The McKusick type has cupped and ragged metaphyses with mottled calcification at the distal ends of the bones, and the Pyle type is an endochondral defect causing the ends of the long bones to appear splayed. The McKusick type is seen more often in persons of Amish and Finnish descent.[7]

■ Metatropic Dysplasia (Kyphoscoliosis)

Chief Clinical Characteristics

This presentation in newborns includes short limbs and a slender, long trunk.[14] Kyphoscoliosis may develop in late infancy or early childhood and can result in cardiorespiratory complications.[14] Children with this condition have a coccygeal tail that is characteristic of this condition, as well as significant flexion contractures of the limbs.

Background Information

Severe angular kyphosis, which carries the risk of quadriplegia, may also occur.[2] This is a cartilage disorder that results in abnormal bone formation.[14]

MUCOPOLYSACCHARIDOSES

■ Type IH (Hurler Syndrome)

Chief Clinical Characteristics

This presentation may involve impaired growth, contractures, cardiac abnormalities, and kyphotic spinal deformities.[9] A thoracolumbar gibbus (sharply angled kyphosis) may also be present due to anterior vertebral body wedging. Odontoid hypoplasia and C1–C2 subluxation may occur. Most children have hearing loss and cognitive deficits.[7]

Background Information

This is an autosomal recessive condition of lysosomal storage, and prenatal diagnosis is possible.[7,8]

■ Type IV (Morquio's Syndrome)

Chief Clinical Characteristics

This presentation typically involves short stature with severe deformity of the spine and a characteristic prominence of the sternal manubrium, together with long bones with irregular epiphyses, enlarged joints, and flaccid ligaments. There is usually a marked genu valgum, giving a waddling gait.

Background Information

This condition is a genetic disorder of mucopolysaccharide metabolism with excessive urinary keratan sulfate. It is characterized by skeletal abnormalities, joint instability, and the gradual development of cervical myelopathy.[12,37]

■ Type VI (Maroteaux-Lamy Type)

Chief Clinical Characteristics

This presentation includes lumbar kyphosis, genu valgum, mild joint stiffness, and varying degrees of deafness.

Background Information

This autosomal recessive disorder has three clinical subtypes determined by age of onset and rate of progression.[7]

■ Type VII (Sly Syndrome)

Chief Clinical Characteristics

This presentation consists of a child with macrocephaly, a thoracolumbar gibbus, metatarsus adductus, and acetabular dysplasia. Children with this condition have short stature and varying amounts of cognitive deficiency.

Background Information

This autosomal recessive disorder has extensive variation in the clinical presentation.[7]

■ Muscle Spasm

Chief Clinical Characteristics

This presentation usually includes pain with movement and palpation of the lumbar paraspinal muscles, potentially in the presence of change in sagittal spinal curve. The lower extremities are neurologically intact.

Background Information

This condition may be related to a traumatic onset, such as a twist or fall. Muscle guarding may be related to inflammation of underlying articular structures. Typical treatment involves watchful waiting and exercise directed to contributing deficits of body structures and functions. In severe or intractable cases, additional testing may be necessary to exclude fracture, tumor, or congenital condition as a cause of symptoms.

■ **Myelodysplasia**

Chief Clinical Characteristics
This presentation commonly includes scoliosis that may develop as late as age 15 years but usually appears before the age of 9 years.[38] Scoliosis may be more prevalent if the cord lesion or last intact laminar arch is in the thoracic versus lumbar region for children with paraplegia due to myelomeningocele.[38] Lower extremity spasticity and nonambulatory status also may contribute to the development of scoliosis.[38] Hyperlordosis may result from muscle imbalances due to paralysis.[9]

Background Information
This condition includes spina bifida and myelomeningocele, also classified under spinal dysraphism and neural tube defects. Spina bifida is a malformation in which the vertebra does not close completely, resulting in a bifid appearance.[9] This malformation may allow nerve tissue to protrude, which if it is damaged can result in paralysis.[9] The actual structural changes in the vertebrae as well as the effects of muscle paralysis can result in hyperlordosis, kyphosis, or scoliosis in children with this condition.[9]

■ **Myotonia**

Chief Clinical Characteristics
This presentation may be associated with myotonic dystrophy and also with rare syndromes such as myotonic chondrodystrophy (Schwartz-Jampel disease) and myotonia congenita (Thompsen disease). These other conditions tend to have muscular hypertrophy and weakness.

Background Information
Joint abnormalities leading to hip flexion contractures with increased lumbar lordosis may be seen in myotonic chondrodystrophy.[39]

■ **Myotonic Dystrophy**

Chief Clinical Characteristics
This presentation involves muscle weakness that is mild in the first few years of life, with increased weakness developing, especially in the distal muscles such as the hand intrinsics. The accompanying characteristic myotonia is not usually apparent until around 5 years of age.[40] As the disease progresses with age, scoliosis and increased lordosis may be seen in later childhood and adulthood.[7]

Background Information
This is the second most common type of muscular dystrophy in Europe, Australia, and North America with an incidence of 1 in 30,000.[39]

NONSTRUCTURAL SCOLIOSES

■ **Leg-Length Discrepancy**

Chief Clinical Characteristics
This presentation may be characterized by a C-shaped curve that is associated with a lower limb–length discrepancy. Commonly, the curve will demonstrate convexity contralateral to the side of the longer limb and it is correctable with spinal active range of motion and in a seated position.

Background Information
Lower limb–length discrepancies may be caused by a variety of pathologies, including physeal growth arrest, infection, and tumor. However, most minor lower limb–length discrepancies are idiopathic in nature. The diagnosis may be confirmed by measurement of lower limb length on standing anteroposterior x-rays of the lower limbs and pelvic girdle. In severe cases, a shoe lift may be necessary. However, for minor cases of lower limb–length discrepancy (which is the vast majority of cases), primary intervention includes observation for progression and reassurance of the patient, parents, and family.

■ **Postural**

Chief Clinical Characteristics
This presentation includes spinal scoliosis in the presence of limited muscle development or faulty postural habitus.

Background Information
This condition is characterized by normal spinal morphology. In this condition, the appearance of a scoliotic curve is related to functional factors. This condition should

be considered a diagnosis of exclusion. Typical treatment involves correction of underlying deficits in muscle strength, length, and coordination that underlie the clinical presentation.

■ Noonan Syndrome

Chief Clinical Characteristics

This presentation commonly involves short stature, skeletal anomalies, mental retardation, and characteristic facial features including ptosis, low-set ears, and inferiorly slanting palpebral fissures.[41] Severe thoracic scoliosis with or without thoracic lordosis may develop during childhood in this disorder.[41] Other features of this disease include congenital heart disease, sexual immaturity, webbed neck, chest deformities, genu valgum, and cubitus valgus.[41]

Background Information

This is an autosomal dominant condition.[7]

■ Osteogenesis Imperfecta

Chief Clinical Characteristics

The presentation of this disease group includes bowing of the long bones and frequent fractures that may occur as early as birth.[9] Poor collagen synthesis results in brittle bones that develop abnormally, resulting in short stature.[9] Fractures may also result in growth plate disturbance and other bony asymmetries that can result in scoliosis, kyphosis, or kyphoscoliosis.[9] Many children with this condition have bone pain relating to old fractures as well as muscle weakness and ligamentous laxity.

Background Information

Scoliosis in children with osteogenesis imperfecta is usually severe and requires surgical intervention because bracing is not well tolerated in this group of children. Osteogenesis imperfecta is a rare condition with a prevalence of 1 in 15,000 to 20,000.[42]

■ Osteomyelitis

Chief Clinical Characteristics

This presentation commonly involves back pain and in younger children a decreased desire to walk as well as a history of prior trauma. In older children and adolescents, the presentation may include back pain and unusual posture (scoliosis or increased kyphosis). Sometimes abdominal pain and lethargy are also seen.

Background Information

This condition is a localized or widespread infection of bone or bone marrow due to bacteria introduced by trauma or surgery. If present in the spine, it may initially present as discitis, an inflammation of the disk, which can be of infectious or noninfectious origin. The noninfectious variety is often self-limiting and is more common in children than adults. This condition is confirmed if destruction of the vertebral body is observed on x-ray. Discitis does not lead to destruction of bone.[43]

■ Poliomyelitis

Chief Clinical Characteristics

This presentation includes a paralytic form of scoliosis that can develop at any age but is more common from ages 3 to 10. Paralysis of the trunk muscles can result in spinal deformities including scoliosis, hyperlordosis, and excessive kyphosis. Scoliosis in this population tends to be more often severe, concomitant with pelvic obliquity and associated with back pain or respiratory complications, than idiopathic scoliosis. Abnormal thoracic kyphosis with an angle of greater than 40 degrees is also common and may be associated with impaired pulmonary function.[44]

Background Information

Poliomyelitis is a viral infection involving the motor neurons of the central nervous system, especially those in the spinal cord.[12] Although the incidence of poliomyelitis has been reduced dramatically during the past decade, the disease is still an important one in countries such as India, Pakistan, Afghanistan, Niger, and Egypt.[16,45]

■ Postlaminectomy

Chief Clinical Characteristics

This presentation can result from a prior history of spinal surgery and the development of a progressive hyperkyphosis in the thoracic spine over the course of several years.

Background Information

A laminectomy involves removal of some or all of the posterior bone and ligaments of the spine and can involve bilateral removal of facet joints. Removal of these supporting elements may lead to kyphosis in a growing child. More extensive laminectomy procedures may result in more severe kyphosis. This kind of surgical approach is often necessary when resecting spinal cord tumors. Bracing may slow progression, but treatment most likely will require anterior spinal fusion.[25]

POSTRADIATION SEQUELAE

■ Postradiation Kyphosis

Chief Clinical Characteristics
This presentation can include a gradually increasing kyphosis and surgical scarring over the posterior trunk as well as a past history of radiation treatment for a spinal cord tumor such as a neuroblastoma.

Background Information
Radiation damage has a high likelihood of causing a hyperkyphosis.[8,25] About 30% of neuroblastomas occur in the cervical, thoracic, or pelvic ganglia. The neuroblastoma may extend into the spinal foramina and cause compression of the spinal cord and nerve roots. In infants the disease is often localized in the cervical or thoracic region of the spine. Potential damage to the growth plates in the vertebrae is a known risk and if coupled with posterior laminectomy in order to permit tumor resection is a setup for development of a hyperkyphosis with growth after treatment for the tumor. Patients with paraspinal tumors causing cord compression are treated with surgical resection. They will also receive radiation and chemotherapy depending on the disease stage at presentation. Fifty-five percent of children with neuroblastoma survive and since many neuroblastomas present in children under the age of 2 there is a lot of growth left in the spine and the potential for development of a kyphotic deformity.[25,46]

■ Postradiation Scoliosis

Chief Clinical Characteristics
This presentation can be characterized by a gradually developing scoliosis and radiation scarring of the skin over the trunk in the area of the kidney. These children will have a history of treatment for a prior malignancy, commonly nephroblastoma. The scoliosis may develop as late as 10 or more years after radiation treatment for the tumor.

Background Information
In children younger than 15 years of age, nephroblastoma (Wilms' tumor) occurs in 7.8 per million children and is one of the most frequently occurring renal tumors. It is often associated with other congenital anomalies. Three years of age is the median age for occurrence, and the child presents with a mass in the abdomen or flank on one side. Scoliosis develops later as a result of treatment for the tumor. Treatment involves surgical resection of the tumor and chemotherapy and/or radiation depending on the stage of the disease. Radiation damage has a high likelihood of causing a scoliosis.[8,25] Radiation fields have been altered to decrease the incidence of scoliosis, but these children need to be followed carefully until the end of growth. The radiation can damage the growth plates in the vertebral bodies on the side of the lumbar spine exposed to the radiation. This causes asymmetrical growth to occur, leading to scoliosis over time. The scoliosis is likely to increase rapidly during normal growth spurts. There is less risk for asymmetrical growth depending on the age of the child at the time of treatment for the nephroblastoma and depending on the treatment for the tumor (how much radiation the spine receives and where in the spine treatment is directed).[25,47]

■ Postural Round Back

Chief Clinical Characteristics
This presentation includes an increased kyphosis that when evaluated is flexible and corrects completely with active extension of the thoracic spine. No bony changes are seen on x-ray.

Background Information
It is important to make sure there is no pathology such as vertebral osteochondrosis (Scheuermann's disease) or congenital kyphosis. These conditions usually present with a sharply angled kyphosis in comparison to the gentle rounding seen with postural kyphosis.[25]

■ Prader-Willi Syndrome

Chief Clinical Characteristics

This presentation involves hypotonia and difficulty feeding, which characterize infants with this genetic disorder.[9,48] As they mature, scoliosis may develop at any time from age 1 to 15 years; it develops more often in females than males.[49] Children with this condition develop hyperphagia around age 2 to 3 years that often leads to obesity but this is not associated with the onset of scoliosis.[9]

Background Information

Approximately 15% of these children with scoliosis develop severe deformities of the spine.[49] Osteoporosis has been noted to be present in some children with this condition, but it is unclear if there is a relationship between this finding and the scoliosis.[49]

■ Pseudoachondroplasia

Chief Clinical Characteristics

This presentation is characterized by disproportionately short limbs with normal head and face size, joint hypermobility, increased lumbar lordosis, thoracic kyphosis, and scoliosis. Hip flexion contractures may also contribute to an increased lumbar lordosis. The vertebrae have anterior beaking, and odontoid aplasia or hypoplasia. The risks of atlantoaxial instability may be present.[1,7]

Background Information

Children are usually diagnosed with this disorder between 2 and 4 years of age when growth retardation becomes apparent.[2]

■ Reactive Arthritis (Reiter's Syndrome)

Chief Clinical Characteristics

This presentation includes conjunctivitis, arthritis, and urethritis. Sacroiliitis, spondylitis, and painful lower extremity arthritis may occur. The spine tends to flatten in the coronal plane or lose both the normal lordotic and kyphotic curves.

Background Information

This condition has a strong genetic association and the disease is often trigged by sexually transmitted diseases or dysentery.[43,50]

■ Renal Osteodystrophy

Chief Clinical Characteristics

This presentation involves problems that are similar to those seen with rickets. This condition may include growth retardation, bone pain, muscle weakness, skeletal deformity of the spine (increased kyphosis), slipped epiphyses, and varus or valgus of the knees and ankles.[42,51]

Background Information

Renal osteodystrophy is used to describe a variety of bone diseases arising from faulty mineralization because of renal failure.[51]

■ Rett Syndrome

Chief Clinical Characteristics

This presentation includes girls who develop normally until 1 year of age when they begin to lose language and motor skills. The characteristic feature of the disease is repeated hand wringing and loss of purposeful hand use.[52] Scoliosis in these girls is usually progressive and does not respond to bracing or positioning in a wheelchair. About 50% of the girls with the disorder develop scoliosis, usually a long C curve.

Background Information

This X-linked neurodegenerative disorder occurs almost exclusively in girls. Prevalence is around 1 in 15,000 to 22,000.[8,52] Treatment is generally spinal fusion.[1,8]

■ Rib Fracture

Chief Clinical Characteristics

This presentation can be characterized by a nonstructural scoliosis; a lateral curve is seen with the concavity on the side of the fractured rib together with muscle spasm in the region but there is no vertebral rotation.

Background Information

This condition is associated with trauma due to events such as a sports injury, a fall from a height, or a motor vehicle accident. Treatment focuses on caring for the fractured rib.[53,54]

■ Rickets

Chief Clinical Characteristics

This presentation involves children who may have small stature and reduced tension in the ligaments, which can lead to kyphosis and/or scoliosis, as well as other deformities in the extremities.[51,55] Children with severe rickets who present before the age of 2 years may have hypotonia and developmental delay as well as proximal muscle weakness and sweating. Apneic spells, seizures, and cardiomyopathy can also be seen.[42]

Background Information
This condition involves a failure in the mineralization process of growing bone or osteoid tissue. X-rays typically show demineralization at the ends of the long bones. Rickets can be caused by a lack of vitamin D in the diet or a lack of exposure to sunlight such that vitamin D is not absorbed through the skin. Children with darkly pigmented skin are more at risk for this condition, as are children with diseases such as cystic fibrosis or celiac disease. Children taking anticonvulsants also have an increased risk of developing rickets. Two other forms of rickets are vitamin D–resistant rickets (familial hypophosphatemia), an x-linked autosomal dominant disease, and vitamin D–dependent rickets, an autosomal recessive disorder. Both of these forms produce short stature and genu varus.[51,55]

■ Rubinstein-Taybi Syndrome

Chief Clinical Characteristics
This presentation can be characterized by short stature with characteristically short broad thumbs and great toes. Mental retardation, scoliosis, spina bifida occulta, and cervical hyperkyphosis are also seen.

Background Information
Children with this condition are developmentally delayed and often have respiratory infections and feeding difficulties.[7]

■ Scheuermann's Disease (Vertebral Osteochondrosis)

Chief Clinical Characteristics
This presentation commonly includes rigid kyphosis greater than 40 degrees. Excessive lumbar and cervical lordosis are characteristic of the disease when it is present in the thoracic spine.[9,25] If present in the cervical or lumbar spine, it results in a diminished lordosis. Scoliosis may also be present.[9] This condition can occur in any region of the spine, but is most common in the thoracic spine.[9] Onset is usually during the prepubertal growth spurt sometime between 10 and 12 years of age. Children with this condition may present with pain that varies in intensity based on the location of the kyphosis, the stage of the disease, and the severity of the kyphotic deformity.

Background Information
Structural causes include degeneration and growth disturbance of epiphyseal vertebral end plates, leading to wedged vertebrae or narrowed intervertebral disk spaces.[9,25] Vertebral osteochondrosis is seen in 0.4% to 10% of the general population and appears slightly more often in males than females. Curves of 65 to 85 degrees seem to be the most symptomatic.[25]

■ Soft Tissue Scarring

Chief Clinical Characteristics
This presentation includes a history of prior burn scarring or thoracic soft tissue contracture.

Background Information
Children with congenital heart disease who have undergone thoracotomy have a higher incidence of scoliosis associated with the congenital heart defect. Any severe injury to the soft tissues of the trunk such as burns or a severe intrathoracic infection such as an empyema that leads to contracture may cause scoliosis. A child who required multiple surgeries for the treatment of a tracheoesophageal fistula may also present with the same problem. Treatment is difficult and directed to correcting the contractures but may require spinal surgery.[54]

■ Soto's Syndrome

Chief Clinical Characteristics
This presentation consists of delayed motor development, poor coordination, hyperreflexia, hypotonia, and variable cognitive impairment. Children with this condition are large at birth with large hands and feet and increased bone maturation. Most have pes planus and genu valgus, and some have kyphoscoliosis as well as cardiac defects.[7]

■ Spinal Cord Injury

Chief Clinical Characteristics

This presentation includes a history of prior spinal cord injury.

Background Information

Traumatic spinal cord injury in children is rare.[9] Most injuries are due to motor vehicle accidents, but other causes include falls, diving, and sports.[9] The severity and frequency of the scoliosis is greater with a younger age of onset, for paraplegia versus quadriplegia, and for complete versus incomplete spinal cord injuries.[56] Hyperlordosis sometimes associated with hip flexion contractures is often present in children with paraplegia.[56] Thoracic kyphosis is also accentuated more significantly in children with paraplegia compared to those with quadriplegia.[56] Bracing is sometimes used for treatment but lack of skin sensation creates problems. Spinal surgery may be required.

SPINAL MUSCULAR ATROPHIES

■ Type I (Werdnig-Hoffmann Disease)

Chief Clinical Characteristics

This presentation commonly involves decreased fetal movements and often a breech presentation at birth. The infant or child with the disorder has feeding difficulties with a poor suck and swallow and is slow, if at all, to develop head and neck control. Hypotonia and weakness in the legs lead to abduction and external rotation of the hips. Sensation is intact and the child will grimace and cry on exposure to noxious stimuli. Tongue fasciculations are also often present and deep tendon reflexes are absent. Bright, lively facial expressions are common, which is in contrast to infants and children with hypotonia of a more central origin.

Background Information

This autosomal recessive disorder causes a progressive degeneration of the anterior horn cells of the motor neuron. Therapy is supportive and prognosis is poor. Death often occurs with in the first 2 to 3 years due to pneumonia or respiratory failure.[57–62]

■ Type II (Kugelberg-Welander Disease)

Chief Clinical Characteristics

This presentation is characterized by atrophy and weakness of the proximal muscles of the lower extremities and pelvic girdle and then progresses to the distal muscles and muscular fasciculations.[63]

Background Information

This condition is a hereditary juvenile form of spinal muscular atrophy transmitted as an autosomal recessive trait that causes lesions of the anterior horns of the spinal cord. Onset occurs in the first or second decade between the ages of 2 and 17 years; however, it is possible to present in infancy.[60]

■ Type III (Benign)

Chief Clinical Characteristics

This presentation is characterized by atrophy and weakness of the proximal muscles of the lower extremities and pelvic girdle and then progresses to the distal muscles and muscular fasciculations.[63] This variation of spinal muscular atrophy presents with a similar, but milder phenotype as type II and also can present in early infancy.

Background Information

Deoxyribonucleic acid testing is required to distinguish between the various types of spinal muscular atrophy.[60]

■ Spondyloepiphyseal Dysplasia Congenita

Chief Clinical Characteristics

This presentation commonly involves a short neck and trunk as a neonate; the development of thoracolumbar scoliosis and kyphosis occurs in childhood due to this type II collagen disorder.[1,14] Around 40% of children with this condition will show atlantoaxial instability resulting from odontoid deficiencies.[1] They also have hypoplasia of the abdominal muscles, weakness, and easy fatigability as well as decreased motion of the elbows, hips, and knees and delayed ambulation. Severe hip flexion contractures and compensatory lumbar hyperlordosis are seen in patients with more significant disease.[2]

Background Information
This is an autosomal dominant disorder.[7]

■ Spondylolisthesis

Chief Clinical Characteristics
This presentation often involves increased lumbar lordosis, and if the defect is severe enough, the child may also present with a lumbosacral kyphosis in addition to the lumbar hyperlordosis. Scoliosis may be seen concomitantly in 23% to 48% of patients but may be due to muscle spasm.[64] Some children with this condition can have an associated adolescent idiopathic scoliosis where the spondylolisthesis is an unexpected finding in addition to the scoliosis.[65]

Background Information
Spondylolisthesis is defined as the anterior slippage of a superior on inferior vertebrae. In children, the most common types include dysplastic or congenital (type I) and isthmic (type II). Dysplastic spondylolisthesis is most common at the L5–S1 level and is sometimes associated with spina bifida. Isthmic (spondylolytic) spondylolisthesis is associated with a fracture of the pars interarticularis and is also most common at the L5–S1 level.[65] Spondylolisthesis is uncommon in persons of African or African American descent at 1.8%, more common in Caucasian individuals at 3.5% to 5.6%, and there has been a 50% prevalence reported in Inuit people.[65] Treatment depends on the severity of pain and the extent of slipping. Spinal fusion may be required, but bracing occasionally is used for treatment.[64]

■ Spondylolysis

Chief Clinical Characteristics
This presentation may include low back pain, especially with hyperextension and increased lordosis of the lumbar spine and/or hamstring tightness.[66,67] These patients may show a change in their gait and some may have scoliosis. An atypical pattern of scoliosis may be seen as a result of muscle spasm or the child could have adolescent idiopathic scoliosis in addition to the spondylolysis.[65]

Background Information
Spondylolysis is a fracture of the pars interarticularis without slipping of the vertebrae as seen in spondylolisthesis. It is more common in males than females, with an approximately 2:1 ratio.[64] Typically the onset of symptoms is associated with an adolescent growth spurt or a sports-related activity that involves repetitive flexion and extension of the spine such as gymnastics, diving, figure skating, or dancing.[66,67] For nonathletes, Alaskan Native American heritage and a first-degree relative with spondylolysis are significant risk factors.[67,68] Treatment is directed toward pain relief, and bracing may be used if the lesion is thought to be recent and potentially healable.

■ Spondyloptosis

Chief Clinical Characteristics
This presentation involves hypolordosis and flattening.[1] Children with this condition have hamstring tightness, shortening of the waistline, a protuberant abdomen, and a waddling gait. The child may also have back pain.

Background Information
This condition is considered a grade V in the Meyerding classification of spondylolisthesis. The less severe types are classified as grades I through IV based on the degree of slip of L5 on the sacrum.[65]

■ Sprengel's Deformity/Klippel-Feil Syndrome

Chief Clinical Characteristics
This presentation commonly involves a short neck and limited head or neck movement.[69]

Background Information
Sprengel's deformity is a congenitally elevated scapula that is sometimes associated with Klippel-Feil syndrome and scoliosis.[69] Klippel-Feil syndrome results from a failure of segmentation or fusion in the cervical spine and can result in scoliosis.[69] The severity of the scoliosis is greatest in type I of this syndrome, where there is fusion with synostosis of the cervical and upper thoracic vertebrae, followed by type II, which involves the cervical spine in isolation.[69]

■ Syringomyelia

Chief Clinical Characteristics

This presentation can be characterized by asymmetrical numbness, weakness, and lower cranial nerve palsy.[70]

Background Information

Thoracic spine scoliosis is sometimes the first sign of this spinal cord cavitation, especially in children.[70,71] The development of scoliosis may be related to a motor weakness resulting from the cord injury.[70] Syringomyelia is a chronic progressive disease where extended central fluid-filled cavities develop in the spinal cord. It is more commonly seen in males.[8]

■ Systemic Fungal Infections (Such as Actinomycosis, Coccidioidomycosis, and Histoplasmosis)

Chief Clinical Characteristics

This presentation involves scoliosis and/or kyphosis or combined severe kyphoscoliosis related to destruction and collapse of the anterior portion of the vertebral bodies.[25] *Fever, pain, and muscle spasm around the affected joint or joints are commonly seen. Diagnosis is confirmed by tissue culture.*

Background Information

Coccidioidomycosis (also called desert or valley fever)[18] is an infectious fungal disease resulting from inhalation of windborne dust particles carrying *Coccidioides immitis* spores endemic to hot dry areas such as the southwestern United States. Histoplasmosis is an infectious fungal disease resulting from inhalation of *Histoplasma capsulatum* spores from infected soil endemic in the Mississippi and Ohio River Valleys in the United States.[18] Actinomycosis is an infectious fungal disease caused by *Actinomyces israelii*, an organism that normally lives in the human mouth and bowel. The disease occurs worldwide more commonly in people who live in rural areas and who also have another infection that has caused tissue damage. Multiple lumpy abscesses characterize actinomycosis.[18]

■ Trisomy 18 (Edwards Syndrome)

Chief Clinical Characteristics

This presentation consists of mental retardation and hypotonia that may result in scoliosis.[9] *Scoliosis occurs in about 10% of the children with this condition and cardiac defects in 50% or more.*[7] *Long and narrow heads with low-set ears distinguish these children.*[9]

Background Information

This syndrome has a ratio of occurrence of 3:1 females to males.[7,9]

■ Tuberculosis

Chief Clinical Characteristics

This presentation occurs when tuberculosis infection develops in the vertebrae, where it destroys the body anteriorly causing collapse leading to severe scoliosis and kyphosis that can present separately or as combined deformities.[25] *Pain, muscle spasm, and fever may be present and a tissue culture is required to confirm the diagnosis.*

Background Information

This condition is a chronic infection characterized by granulomatous lesions caused by an acid-fast bacillus (an aerobic, gram-positive spore-producing bacteria). The primary target is the lungs, but people develop disseminated tuberculosis involving bone marrow as well as other organs.[18]

TUMORS

■ Neuroblastoma

Chief Clinical Characteristics

This presentation includes large abdominal masses and fever in the child under age 2 years or bone pain and gastrointestinal or respiratory problems in older children.[12] *The onset of scoliosis in children with neuroblastoma is more frequent in children undergoing treatment for a thoracic tumor by laminectomy and/or chemotherapy.*[9,12,72] *Some children with this condition will also receive radiation treatment with the potential for damage to the growth plates in the vertebrae and, when coupled with posterior laminectomy for tumor resection, there is a high likelihood of developing a hyperkyphosis.*

Background Information

This small round cell tumor is the most common solid tumor to present in children.[72]

It occurs in the sympathetic nervous system, most often in the paraspinal ganglions or adrenal glands.[9]

■ Neurofibromatosis (Type I, Von Recklinghausen's Disease)

Chief Clinical Characteristics
This presentation consists of skeletal abnormalities, including scoliosis and kyphosis, which may occur in the thoracic or lumbar spine and can be associated with dystrophic changes of the vertebrae and ribs.[73,74] This autosomal dominant disorder is characterized by diffuse and multiple neurofibromas, hyperpigmentation known as café au lait spots, and Lisch nodules or white spots on the iris.[73,75]

Background Information
The disease affects 1 in 3500 individuals. For most individuals the disease course is benign. Kyphosis, scoliosis and kyphoscoliosis are common, can be severe and rapidly progressive often requiring surgical management.[1,73]

■ Osteoid Osteoma

Chief Clinical Characteristics
This presentation is characterized by night pain typically relieved by aspirin. These benign tumors are most often seen in boys between the ages of 5 and 20 years. They present in the vertebrae, usually in the posterior elements, and may then cause a painful scoliosis or symptoms that imitate neurological concerns.[76,77]

Background Information
An osteoid osteoma in the spine may be difficult to locate by plain radiographs while bone scans are often diagnostic. Elimination of the nidus through surgical excision removes the source of pain and the scoliosis resolves.[1,76]

■ Spinal Cord Tumors

Chief Clinical Characteristics
This presentation commonly includes paraspinal muscle spasm and pain with later development of scoliosis and spastic weakness.[12] Other spinal deformities such as kyphosis in the cervical and thoracic spine may appear after individuals undergo laminectomy to remove the tumor.[78]

Background Information
These types of tumors are relatively rare in children.[12] Tumor types include primary extramedullary tumors (neurofibromas and meningiomas), intramedullary tumors (ependymomas, astrocytomas, oligodendrogliomas), and secondary spinal cord tumors (extradural and intradural metastases).[12]

■ Vertebral Body Fracture

Chief Clinical Characteristics
This presentation involves significant kyphosis with canal compromise without neurological sequelae, or a severe kyphosis with cord compression or fragments displaced into the cord or canal that may cause significant neurological injury. Because of the relatively large size of a child's head in relation to his trunk, cervical and upper thoracic fractures are more common than lower thoracic and lumbar injuries.

Background Information
Vertebral body fractures lead to anterior compression of the vertebral body and kyphosis. Tragically one cause of vertebral body fracture is child abuse. Reports vary from 0% to 3% in large series and the average age for this injury is 22 months. Adolescents are more likely to sustain burst fractures of the thoracic and lumbar spine than children as a result of a fall or a motor vehicle accident. Children less than 13 years of age are more likely to sustain thoracic or lumbar vertebral fractures as a result of compression from the seat belt during a motor vehicle accident since seat belts often do not fit children properly. Treatment will depend on exact location of the fractures, the extent of vertebral fracture, and the presence or absence of neurological loss.[53,79]

References
1. Staheli L. *Practice of Pediatric Orthopedics*. Philadelphia, PA: Lippincott Williams & Wilkins; 2001.
2. Sponseller P, Ain M. The skeletal dysplasias. In: Morrissy R, Weinstein S, eds. *Lovell and Winter's Pediatric Orthopaedics*. Philadelphia, PA: Lippincott, Williams and Wilkins; 2006:205–250.
3. Horton W, Hecht J. Disorders involving transmembrane receptors. In: Behrman R, Kliegman R, Jenson H, eds.

Nelson's Textbook of Pediatrics. 16th ed. Philadelphia, PA: W. B. Saunders; 2000:2120–2123.

4. Waters P. The upper limb. In: Morrissy R, Weinstein S, eds. *Lovell and Winter's Pediatric Orthopaedics.* Vol 2. Philadelphia, PA: Lippincott Williams & Wilkins; 2006:921–985.

5. Jones K. Dysmorphology. In: Behrman R, Kliegman R, Jenson H, eds. *Nelson's Textbook of Pediatrics.* Philadelphia, PA: W. B. Saunders; 2000:535–538.

6. Darmstadt G. Cutaneous defects. In: Behrman R, Kliegman R, Jenson H, eds. *Nelson's Textbook of Pediatrics.* Philadelphia, PA: W. B. Saunders; 2000:1972–1974.

7. Jones K. *Smith's Recognizable Patterns of Human Malformation.* 6th ed. Philadelphia, PA: Elsevier Saunders; 2006.

8. Alman B, Goldberg M. Syndromes of orthopaedic importance. In: Morrissy R, Weinstein S, eds. *Lovell and Winter's Pediatric Orthopaedics.* Philadelphia, PA: Lippincott Williams & Wilkins; 2006:251–313.

9. Ratliffe KT. *Clinical Pediatric Physical Therapy. A Guide for the Physical Therapy Team.* Philadelphia, PA: Mosby; 1998.

10. Renshaw T, Deluca P. Cerebral palsy. In: Morrissy R, Weinstein S, eds. *Lovell and Winter's Pediatric Orthopaedics.* Philadelphia, PA: Lippincott Williams & Wilkins; 2006:551–603.

11. Brockmeyer D, Gollogly S, Smith JT. Scoliosis associated with Chiari I malformations: The effect of suboccipital decompression on scoliosis curve progression: A preliminary study. *Spine.* 2003;28(22):2505–2509.

12. Victor M, Ropper A. *Adam and Victor's Principles of Neurology.* 7th ed. New York, NY: McGraw Hill; 2001.

13. Milhorat TH, Chou MW, Trinidad EM, et al. Chiari I malformation redefined: clinical and radiographic findings for 364 symptomatic patients. *Neurosurgery.* 1999;44(5):1005–1017.

14. Klippel JH, Crofford LJ, Stone JH, Weyand CM. *Primer on the Rheumatic Diseases.* 12th ed. Atlanta, GA: Arthritis Foundation; 2001.

15. Hedequist D, Emans J. Congenital scoliosis. *J Am Acad Orthop Surg.* 2004;12:266–275.

16. Thompson G, Berenson F. Other neuromuscular disorders. In: Morrissy R, Weinstein S, eds. *Lovell and Winter's Pediatric Orthopaedics.* 6th ed. Philadelphia, PA: Lippincott Williams & Wilkins; 2006:649–692.

17. Willis R. Sports medicine in the growing child. In: Morrissy R, Weinstein S, eds. *Lovell and Winter's Pediatric Orthopaedics.* Vol 2. 6th ed. Philadelphia, PA: Lippincott Williams & Wilkins; 2006:1382–1428.

18. Anderson K, Anderson L, Glanze W, eds. *Mosby's Medical, Nursing and Allied Health Dictionary.* 4th ed. St. Louis, MO: Mosby; 1994.

19. Kumar N, Balachandran S, Millner P, Littlewood J, Conway S, Dickson R. Scoliosis in cystic fibrosis: is it idiopathic? *Spine.* 2004;29(18):1990–1995.

20. Boat T. Cystic fibrosis. In: Behrman R, Kliegman R, Jenson H, eds. *Nelson's Textbook of Pediatrics.* 16th ed. Philadelphia, PA: W. B. Saunders; 2000:1315–1327.

21. Alman BA, Raza SN, Biggar WD. Steroid treatment and the development of scoliosis in males with Duchenne muscular dystrophy. *Journal Bone Joint Surg.* 2004; 86-A(3):519–524.

22. Bakker J, de Groot I, Beelen A, Lankhorst G. Predictive factors of cessation of ambulation in patients with Duchenne muscular dystrophy. *Am J Phys Med Rehabil.* 2002;81(12):906–912.

23. Sarnat H. Autonomic neuropathies. In: Behrman R, Kliegman R, Jenson H, eds. *Nelson's Textbook of Pediatrics.* Philadelphia, PA: W. B. Saunders; 2000:1891–1892.

24. Mackenzie W, Gabos P. Localized disorders of bone and soft tissue. In: Morrissy R, Weinstein S, eds. *Lovell and Winter's Pediatric Orthopaedics.* Philadelphia, PA: Lippincott Williams & Wilkins; 2006.

25. Warner Jr W. Kyphosis. In: Morrissy R, Weinstein S, eds. *Lovell and Winter's Pediatric Orthopaedics.* Philadelphia, PA: Lippincott Williams & Wilkins; 2006:797–837.

26. Blumenfeld H. *Neuroanatomy Through Clinical Cases.* Sunderland, MA: Sinauer Associates; 2002.

27. Doyle D, DiGeorge A. Hyperparathyroidism. In: Behrman R, Kliegman R, Jenson H, eds. *Nelson's Textbook of Pediatrics.* 16th ed. Philadelphia, PA: W. B. Saunders; 2000:1719–1721.

28. Brunch R, Schwarten J, Johnson T, Lieberman J. General orthopedics. In: Snider R, ed. *Essentials of Musculoskeletal Care.* Rosemont, IL: American Academy of Orthopedic Surgeons; 1997:51–52.

29. Taft E, Francis R. Evaluation and management of scoliosis. *J Pediatr Health Care.* 2003;17(1):42–44.

30. Jaramillo D, Poussaint TY, Grottkau BE. Scoliosis: evidence-based diagnostic evaluation. *Neuroimaging Clin N Am.* 2003;13:335–341.

31. Soucacos PN, Zacharis K, Soultanis K, Gelalis J, Xenakis T, Beris AE. Risk factors for idiopathic scoliosis: review of a 6-year prospective study. *Orthopedics.* 2000;23 (8):833–838.

32. Newton P, ed. *Adolescent Idiopathic Scoliosis* (Monograph Series No. 28). Rosemont, IL: American Academy of Orthopedic Surgeons; 2004.

33. Wright D. Juvenile idiopathic arthritis. In: Morrissy R, Weinstein S, eds. *Lovell and Winter's Pediatric Orthopaedics.* Vol 1. 6th ed. Philadelphia, PA: Lippincott Williams & Wilkins; 2006:405–437.

34. Lundon K, Bolton K. Structure and function of the lumbar intervertebral disk in health, aging, and pathologic conditions. *J Orthop Sports Phys Ther.* 2001;31(6): 291–306.

35. Robinson L. Marfan syndrome. In: Behrman R, Kliegman R, Jenson H, eds. *Nelson's Textbook of Pediatrics.* 16th ed. Philadelphia, PA: W. B. Saunders; 2000: 2131–2132.

36. Horton W, Hecht J. Disorders involving cartilage matrix proteins. In: Behrman R, Kliegman R, Jenson H, eds. *Nelson's Textbook of Pediatrics.* Philadelphia, PA: W. B. Saunders; 2000:2116–2120.

37. Mikles M, Stanton R. A review of Morquio's syndrome. *Am J Orthop.* 1997;26:533.

38. Trivedi J, Thomson JD, Slakey JB, Banta JV, Jones PW. Clinical and radiographic predictors of scoliosis in patients with myelomeningocele. *J Bone Joint Surg.* 2002;84(8):1389–1394.

39. Sarnat H. Muscular dystrophies. In: Behrman R, Kliegman R, Jenson H, eds. *Nelson's Textbook of Pediatrics.* 16th ed. Philadelphia, PA: W. B. Saunders; 2000:1873–1882.

40. Behrman R, Kliegman R, Jenson H, eds. *Nelson's Textbook of Pediatrics.* 16th ed. Philadelphia, PA: W. B. Saunders; 2000.

41. Lee C-K, Chang B-S, Hong Y-M, Yang SW, Lee C-S, Seo J-B. Spinal deformities in Noonan syndrome. A clinical review of sixty cases. *J Bone Joint Surg.* 2001; 83-A(10):1495–1502.

42. Alman B, Howard A. Metabolic and endocrine abnormalities. In: Morrissy R, Weinstein S, eds. *Lovell and Winter's Pediatric Orthopaedics.* 6th ed. Philadelphia, PA: Lippincott Williams & Wilkins; 2006:167–203.

43. Stans A. Osteomyelitis and septic arthritis. In: Morrissy R, Weinstein S, eds. *Lovell and Winter's Pediatric Orthopaedics.* Vol 1. 6th ed. Philadelphia, PA: Lippincott Williams & Wilkins; 2006:438–491.

44. Lin M-C, Liaw M-Y, Chen W-J, Cheng P-T, Wong AM-K, Chiou W-K. Pulmonary function and spinal characteristics: their relationships in persons with idiopathic and postpoliomyelitic scoliosis. *Arch Phys Med Rehabil.* 2001;82.

45. World Health Organization. Surveillance and immunization 2004–2005. *Polio News.* Autumn;2005:4.

46. McManus M, Gilchrist G. Neuroblastoma. In: Behrman R, Kliegman R, Jenson H, eds. *Nelson's Textbook of Pediatrics.* Philadelphia, PA: W. B. Saunders; 2000:1552–1554.

47. Anderson P. Neoplasms of the kidney. In: Behrman R, Kliegman R, Jenson H, eds. *Nelson's Textbook of Pediatrics.* 16th ed. Philadelphia, PA: W. B. Saunders; 2000:1554–1556.

48. Whitman B, Meyers S, Carrel A, Allen D. The behavioral impact of growth hormone treatment for children and adolescents with Prader-Willi syndrome: a 2-year, controlled study. *Pediatrics.* 2002;109(2):E 35.

49. Butler J, Whittington J, Holland A, Boer H, Clarke D, Webb T. Prevalence of, and risk factors for, physical ill-health in people with Prader-Willi syndrome: a population-based study. *Dev Med Child Neurol.* 2002;44:248–255.

50. Miller M, Petty R. Ankylosing spondylitis and other spondyloarthropathies. In: Behrman R, Kliegman R, Jenson H, eds. *Nelson's Textbook of Pediatrics.* 16th ed. Philadelphia, PA: W. B. Saunders; 2000:710–711.

51. Chesney R. Familial hypophosphatemia and vitamin D–dependent rickets. In: Behrman R, Kliegman R, Jenson H, eds. *Nelson's Textbook of Pediatrics.* 16th ed. Philadelphia, PA: W. B. Saunders; 2000:2136–2137.

52. Haslem R. Miscellaneous disorders. In: Behrman R, Kliegman R, Jenson H, eds. *Nelson's Textbook of Pediatrics.* 16th ed. Philadelphia, PA: W. B. Saunders; 2000:1854.

53. Price C, Flynn J. Management of fractures. In: Morrissy R, Weinstein S, eds. *Lovell and Winter's Pediatric Orthopaedics.* Vol 2. 6th ed. Philadelphia, PA: Lippincott Williams & Wilkins; 2006:1429–1525.

54. Newton P, Wenger D. Idiopathic scoliosis. In: Morrissy R, Weinstein S, eds. *Lovell and Winter's Pediatric Orthopaedics.* Vol 1. 6th ed. Philadelphia, PA: Lippincott Williams & Wilkins; 2006:693–762.

55. Curran J, Barness L. Rickets of vitamin D deficiency. In: Behrman R, Kliegman R, Jenson H, eds. *Nelson's Textbook of Pediatrics.* 16th ed. Philadelphia, PA: W. B. Saunders; 2000:184–187.

56. Bergstrom E, Short D, Frankel H, Henderson N, Jones P. The effect of childhood spinal cord injury on skeletal development: a retrospective study. *Spinal Cord.* 1998;37:838–846.

57. Johnston HM. The floppy weak infant revisited. *Brain Dev.* 2003;25(3):155–158.

58. Jones HR Jr. EMG evaluation of the floppy infant: differential diagnosis and technical aspects. *Muscle Nerve.* 1990;13(4):338–347.

59. Miller VS, Delgado M, Iannaccone ST. Neonatal hypotonia. *Semin Neurol.* 1993;13(1):73–83.

60. Prasad AN, Prasad C. The floppy infant: contribution of genetic and metabolic disorders. *Brain Dev.* 2003;25 (7):457–476.

61. Premasiri MK, Lee YS. The myopathology of floppy and hypotonic infants in Singapore. *Pathology.* 2003;35 (5):409–413.

62. Stiefel L. Hypotonia in infants. *Pediatr Rev.* 1996;17 (3):104–105.

63. Newman Dorland WA. *Dorland's Illustrated Medical Dictionary.* 28th ed. Philadelphia, PA: W. B. Saunders; 1994.

64. Frederickson BE, McHolick WJ, Yuan HA, Lubicky JP. The natural history of spondyloptosis and spondylolisthesis. *J Bone Joint Surg.* 1984;66(5):3–30.

65. Luhmann S, O'Brien M, Lenke L. Spondylolysis and spondylolisthesis. In: Morrissy R, Weinstein S, eds. *Lovell and Winter's Pediatric Orthopaedics.* Philadelphia, PA: Lippincott Williams & Wilkins; 2006: 839–870.

66. Hensinger R. Current concepts review. Spondylolysis and spondylolisthesis in children and adolescents. *J Bone Joint Surg.* 1989;71-A(7):1098–1105.

67. Omey ML, Micheli LJ, Gerbino PG. Idiopathic scoliosis and spondyloptosis in the female athlete: tips for treatment. *Clin Orthop.* 2000;1(372):74–84.

68. Grieve GP. *Common Vertebral Joint Problems.* 2nd ed. New York, NY: Churchill Livingstone; 1988.

69. Thomsen MN, Schneider U, Weber M, Johannisson R, Niethard FU. Scoliosis and congenital anomalies associated with Klippel-Feil syndrome types I–III. *Spine.* 1997;22(4):396–401.

70. Tomlinson RJ, Wolfe MW, Nadall JM, Bennett JT, MacEwen GD. Syringomyelia and developmental scoliosis. *J Pediatr Orthop.* 1994;14:580–585.

71. Özerdemoglzerdemoglu R, Transfeldt E, Denis F. Value of treating primary causes of syrinx in scoliosis associated with syringomyelia. *Spine.* 2003;28(8): 806–814.

72. Katzenstein HM, Kent PM, London WB, Cohn SL. Treatment and outcome of 83 children with intraspinal neuroblastoma: the pediatric oncology experience. *J Clin Oncol.* 2001;19(4):1047–1055.

73. Huson SM, Harper PS, Compston DAS. Von Recklinghausen neurofibromatosis. A clinical and population study in south-east Wales. *Brain.* 1988;111: 1355–1381.

74. Winter R, Moe J, Bradford D, Lonstein J, Pedras C, Weber A. Spine deformity in neurofibromatosis. A review of one hundred and two patients. *J Bone Joint Surg.* 1979;61(5):677–694.

75. Cotran R, Kumar V, Robbins S, Schoen F. *Robbins' Pathologic Basis of Disease.* 5th ed. Philadelphia, PA: W. B. Saunders; 1994.

76. Springfield D, Gebhardt M. Bone and soft tissue tumors. In: Morrissy R, Weinstein S, eds. *Lovell and Winter's Pediatric Orthopaedics.* Philadelphia, PA: Lippincott Williams & Wilkins; 2006:493–549.

77. Shaughnessy W, Arndt C. Benign tumors. In: Behrman R, Kliegman R, Jenson H, eds. *Nelson's Textbook of Pediatrics.* Philadelphia, PA: Nelson's Textbook of Pediatrics; 2000:1567–1569.

78. Yeh J, Sgouros S, Walsh A, Hockley A. Spinal sagittal malalignment following surgery for primary in-tramedullary tumours in children. *Pediatr Neurosurg.* 2001;35(6):318–324.

79. Black B. Spine trauma. In: Richards B, ed. *Orthopedic Knowledge Update Pediatrics.* Rosemont, IL: American Academy of Orthopaedic Surgeons; 1996:273–280.

CHAPTER 60

Bowed Legs and Knock Knees in a Child

■ *Wendi W. McKenna, PT, DPT, PCS*

Description of the Symptom

Bowed legs and *knock knees* describe the position of a child's knees in relation to one another in the frontal plane. The condition may be either unilateral or bilateral.

Bowed legs, or *genu varum*, are defined as excessive space between the femoral condyles (known as the intercondylar distance) when the medial malleoli are in contact, the knees extended, and the tibiofemoral axis is aligned on the frontal plane.[1] *Genu varum* may be associated with excessive medial hip rotation, foot pronation and knee hyperextension.

Knock knees, or *genu valgum*, are defined as excessive space between the medial malleoli (known as the intermalleolar distance) when the medial femoral condyles are in contact, knees extended, and the tibiofemoral axis is aligned on the frontal plane.[1,2] *Genu valgum* may be associated with excessive lateral hip rotation, foot supination, and knee hyperextension. This chapter describes possible causes of bowed legs and knock knees in a child.

Special Concerns

■ Post-traumatic changes in lower extremity alignment or a painful limp
■ Progressive limp leading to refusal to walk with or without pain
■ Grossly asymmetric presentation of lower extremity alignment
■ History of multiple fractures

CHAPTER PREVIEW: Conditions That May Lead to Bowed Legs and Knock Knees in a Child

T Trauma	
BOWED LEGS	**KNOCK KNEES**
COMMON	
Not applicable	Not applicable
UNCOMMON	
Not applicable	Post-traumatic/fracture healing disturbances and abnormal growth 1161
RARE	
Not applicable	Not applicable
I Inflammation	
BOWED LEGS	**KNOCK KNEES**
COMMON	
Not applicable	Not applicable
UNCOMMON	
Not applicable	Not applicable

(continued)

Inflammation (continued)

RARE	
Not applicable	Not applicable

M Metabolic

BOWED LEGS	KNOCK KNEES
COMMON	
Overweight and obesity 1156	Overweight and obesity 1160
UNCOMMON	
Rickets: • Hypophosphatasia 1156	Not applicable
RARE	
Rickets: • Nutritional 1156	Not applicable

Va Vascular

BOWED LEGS	KNOCK KNEES
COMMON	
Not applicable	Not applicable
UNCOMMON	
Not applicable	Hemophilia 1159
RARE	
Not applicable	Not applicable

De Degenerative

BOWED LEGS	KNOCK KNEES
COMMON	
Not applicable	Not applicable
UNCOMMON	
Not applicable	Not applicable
RARE	
Not applicable	Not applicable

Tu Tumor

BOWED LEGS	KNOCK KNEES
COMMON	
Not applicable	Not applicable
UNCOMMON	
Not applicable	Not applicable

Tumor *(continued)*

RARE	
Not applicable	*Malignant Primary:* Not applicable *Malignant Metastatic:* Not applicable *Benign, such as:* • Osteochondromatosis (multiple hereditary exostosis) 1160

Co Congenital

BOWED LEGS	KNOCK KNEES
COMMON	
Idiopathic genu varum 1155 Ligamentous laxity/joint hypermobility 1155	Idiopathic genu valgum 1159 Ligamentous laxity/joint hypermobility 1160
UNCOMMON	
Blount's disease: • Early-onset (infantile and juvenile tibial vara) 1153 • Late-onset (adolescent) 1154 Skeletal dysplasias: • Achondroplasia 1157 • Hypochondroplasias: • Metaphyseal chondrodysplasias 1157 • Multiple epiphyseal dysplasia 1158 • Pseudoachondroplasia 1158 • Spondyloepiphyseal dysplasia 1158	Skeletal dysplasias: • Achondroplasia 1161 • Chondroectodermal dysplasia (Ellis-Van Creveld syndrome) 1162 • Hypochondroplasias: • Metaphyseal chondrodysplasias 1162 • Multiple epiphyseal dysplasia 1162 • Pseudoachondroplasia 1162 • Spondyloepiphyseal dysplasia 1163
RARE	
Focal fibrocartilaginous dysplasia 1155	Focal fibrocartilaginous dysplasia 1159

Ne Neurogenic/Psychogenic

BOWED LEGS	KNOCK KNEES
COMMON	
Not applicable	Cerebral palsy 1158
UNCOMMON	
Not applicable	Not applicable
RARE	
Not applicable	Not applicable

Note: These are estimates of relative incidence because few data are available for the less common conditions.

Common Ages at Which Bowed Legs and Knock Knees Present in a Child

APPROXIMATE AGE	CONDITION
Birth to 3 Years	Blount's disease: early-onset (infantile and juvenile) Cerebral palsy Focal fibrocartilaginous dysplasia

(continued)

Common Ages at Which Bowed Legs and Knock Knees Present in a Child—cont'd

APPROXIMATE AGE	CONDITION
	Idiopathic genu valgum Idiopathic genu varum Ligamentous laxity/joint hypermobility Overweight and obesity Rickets: hypophosphatasia Rickets: nutritional Skeletal dysplasia
Preschool (3–5 Years)	Blount's disease: early-onset (infantile and juvenile) Cerebral palsy Hemophilia Idiopathic genu valgum Idiopathic genu varum Ligamentous laxity/joint hypermobility Osteochondromatosis Overweight and obesity Post-traumatic/fracture healing disturbances and abnormal growth Rickets: hypophosphatasia Rickets: nutritional Skeletal dysplasia
Elementary School (6–11 Years)	Blount's disease (juvenile tibial vara) Cerebral palsy Hemophilia Idiopathic genu valgum Idiopathic genu varum Ligamentous laxity/joint hypermobility Osteochondromatosis Overweight and obesity Post-traumatic/fracture healing disturbances and abnormal growth Rickets: hypophosphatasia Skeletal dysplasia
Middle School (12–14 Years)	Blount's disease: late-onset (adolescent) Cerebral palsy Hemophilia Idiopathic genu valgum Idiopathic genu varum Ligamentous laxity/joint hypermobility Overweight and obesity Post-traumatic/fracture healing disturbances and abnormal growth Rickets: hypophosphatasia Skeletal dysplasia
High School (15–18 Years)	Blount's disease: late-onset (adolescent) Cerebral palsy Hemophilia Idiopathic genu valgum Idiopathic genu varum Ligamentous laxity/joint hypermobility Overweight and obesity Post-traumatic/fracture healing disturbances Rickets: hypophosphatasia Skeletal dysplasia

Overview of Bowed Legs and Knock Knees in a Child

Lower extremity alignment and range of motion change as a child grows, develops, and moves around in his or her environment. Therefore, correctly identifying lower extremity misalignment such as bowed legs and knock knees requires an intimate knowledge of typical lower extremity alignment, bone morphology, and joint range of motion as it relates to a child's age and gross motor skill development. Physical therapists must always assess static and dynamic conditions in order to obtain a complete picture of lower extremity biomechanics, including the effects of one joint on more proximal or distal joints.[3] Only then will more benign, cosmetic issues in normal development be differentiated from structural abnormalities that may contribute to current or future musculoskeletal impairments and functional limitations. Many times concerns regarding knock knees and bowed legs can be sufficiently addressed by educating the parents and grandparents regarding normal development of alignment and biomechanics and scheduling follow-up appointments to monitor progress of alignment.

As mentioned later in the description section, genu varum and valgum can be measured using the intercondylar and intermalleolar distances (Fig. 60-1). The extent of genu varum and valgum can also be documented by measuring the tibiofemoral angle on the frontal plane (Fig. 60-2).[4,5] Values differ significantly depending on the child's age, as illustrated in Figure 60-1. It is, therefore, very important to be familiar with the typical values when determining whether a child presents with physiologically normal alignment that corrects spontaneously or pathological alignment that requires intervention.[6]

Description of Conditions That May Lead to Bowed Legs in a Child

BLOUNT'S DISEASE

■ Early-Onset (Infantile and Juvenile Tibial Vara)

Chief Clinical Characteristics

This presentation includes an infant 0 to 4 years or a juvenile 5 to 10 years with unilateral or bilateral genu varum of idiopathic nature in the absence of other congenital, metabolic, or traumatic etiologies. Other associated clinical presentations may include limb-length discrepancy, gait abnormalities, obesity, extremely high activity levels, recent

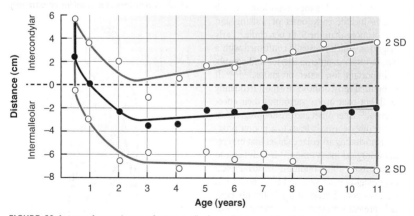

FIGURE 60-1 Age-referenced norms for intermalleolar and intercondylar distance in non-Hispanic white children. (Permission granted by Humana Press to publish from Greene WB. Genu-varum and genu-valgum in children: differential diagnosis and guidelines for evaluation. *Compr Ther.* 1996;22:22–29.)

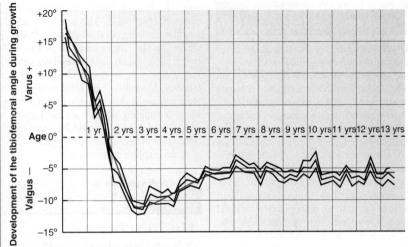

FIGURE 60-2 Typical development of frontal plane knee angulation, ages birth to 14 years. (Reprinted with permission and license from Salenius P, Vankka E. The development of the tibiofemoral angle in children. *J Bone Joint Surg.* 1975;57A:259.)

growth spurt, black or Hispanic heritage, and ligament laxity at the knee.[7–11]

Background Information

This condition is a developmental deformity of the proximal medial physis of the tibia that produces a knee varus deformity (Fig. 60-3).[6,12,13] Etiology is unclear, but risk factors include early onset of walking and weight more than the 95th percentile.[6] Early diagnosis, which is usually confirmed with a patella-forward anteroposterior radiograph, is important for better prognosis.[6,7,13,14] If recognized early, orthoses are most frequently used, but controversy surrounds their effectiveness.[12] Later onset and greater progression of the disease usually leads to a poorer prognosis, including articular changes that may require surgical intervention.[12] It is difficult to differentiate this condition versus typical physiological genu vara and tibial bowing in infants under 2 years of age.[14] Infants typically present with medial tibial torsion, which amplifies the apparent tibial bowing and genu vara.[6] In physiological genu vara there is a smooth angulation that involves both the femur and the tibia. However, in this condition there is a more severe angulation that involves the tibia only and manifests with a visible outward excursion of the knee during the loading response phase of gait.[6]

■ Late-Onset (Adolescent)

Chief Clinical Characteristics

This presentation includes children at least 11 years old with bilateral or unilateral genu vara who have a history of normal lower extremity

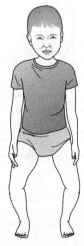

FIGURE 60-3 Genu varum secondary to Blount's disease.

alignment and no history of increased genu vara associated with early-onset Blount's disease. Children may present with obesity and a more complex three-dimensional lower extremity deformity including proximal tibial varus, progressive tibial procurvatum, and possible medial tibial torsion that can contribute to a progressive in-toeing gait pattern. A lateral thrusting of the knee during weight acceptance and knee pain are other signs and symptoms.[8]

Background Information

This condition, like early-onset Blount's, is thought to have a similar pathophysiology where excessive loads produced by body weight inhibit growth of the proximal medial tibial physis.[6,8] Although there have been cases of adolescents of more typical body height and weight presenting with this condition, a majority of patients are at or above the 90th percentile of weight.[8] This condition is diagnosed with radiograph and usually needs to be managed surgically with proximal tibial osteotomies, gradual correction of the varus deformity using an Ilizarov circular external fixator, and/or lateral physeal hemiepiphysiodesis (stapling to selectively close part of the growth plate).[8] Because load-bearing lines are significantly altered in this progressive disease, the distal femur and ankle joint can also be affected. Surgeries may therefore be necessary at multiple sites simultaneously with the goal of restoring proper load-bearing lines and preventing further secondary joint deformity.[6,8,12]

■ Focal Fibrocartilaginous Dysplasia

Chief Clinical Characteristics

This presentation includes young infants and toddlers with a unilateral bowing or angulation deformity of long bones, including the tibia and femur.

Background Information

This condition is a rare benign lesion that is most commonly seen in the proximal tibia (43 of 48 cases) or distal femur (5 of 48 cases).[15] The unilateral cortical defect, identified on radiograph and with histological studies, presents as dense collagenized fibrous tissue with focal areas of fibrocartilaginous changes occurring between the metaphysis and diaphysis.

This defect causes asymmetrical growth and bowing of the long bones, which contributes to angular deformities such as tibial vara or tibial valga.[15–17] Unlike Blount's disease, the lesion does not extend to the physis. Due to the rare nature of this condition, the natural history is largely unknown; however, it has been reported that up to 45% of tibial cases resolved spontaneously, while 86% of femoral lesions progressed and needed surgical intervention to correct.[17] Age of onset ranges from 5 to 28 months with an average of 16.5 months.[17]

■ Idiopathic Genu Varum

Chief Clinical Characteristics

This presentation includes bowed legs two standard deviations or greater from normal, age-matched peers as measured by the tibiofemoral angle or intercondylar distance. Idiopathic genu varum is a diagnosis of exclusion.[6]

Background Information

Excessive genu varum contributes to abnormal loading patterns and ground reaction forces that over time can lead to premature joint deterioration and osteoarthritis.[18,19] Treatment should include referral to an orthopedic surgeon, where imaging studies can be used to exclude other causes for the joint abnormality. Depending on the severity of alignment abnormality, joint instability, and pain that contributes to functional limitations and participation restrictions, conservative bracing or more invasive surgery may be required to correct the alignment.[20]

■ Ligamentous Laxity/Joint Hypermobility

Chief Clinical Characteristics

The presentation includes children, girls more than boys, who score greater than a 4 or 5 on the Beighton score and who may demonstrate increased joint mobility on the nondominant side.[21–24]

Background Information

The Beighton criteria include:

1. Passive extension of the fifth finger at metacarpophalangeal joint to ≥90 degrees
2. Passive apposition of the thumb to the forearm
3. Hyperextension of elbow ≥10 degrees

4. Hyperextension of the knee ≥10 degrees
5. Ability to rest entire palm of hand on floor with forward flexion and extended knees.

The first four maneuvers are assessed bilaterally with a separate score given for right and left sides. Each item receives a score of 0 or 1, with 1 being assigned when the criteria for a maneuver is met. The total score ranges from 0 to 9, with generalized hypermobility diagnosed with a score of ≥4.[24] This condition has been identified in 2.3% to 30% of children screened, depending on the cut-off Beighton score used and the child's age and ethnicity.[25] Many children diagnosed with generalized ligament laxity will not develop significant musculoskeletal issues that will require medical intervention[25] and, in preadolescents, Mikkelsson demonstrated that musculoskeletal pain is not associated with this condition.[26] However, this condition is described as chronic, generalized joint hypermobility that presents with adverse symptoms that contribute to functional limitation. Ligamentous laxity is an associated condition related to Blount's disease,[9] which causes an atypical and excessive genu/tibial varum. Excessive laxity in knee collateral ligaments contributes to poor lateral support of the knee joint, which can lead to asymmetric loading patterns and progressive joint deformity.[27] Nonsurgical care can include bracing to support the knee or correct related malalignment in the foot and ankle. However, severe impairments that cause pain and functional limitation despite conservative care, may need to be surgically corrected.

■ Overweight and Obesity

Chief Clinical Characteristics
This presentation includes a child with a body mass index at or above the 85th percentile and whose genu varum is at least two standard deviations from the normal age-related values as measured by the tibiofemoral angle or intercondylar distance.

Background Information
Though obesity alone has not been identified as a causative factor of bowed legs, it is often associated with infantile/juvenile and late-onset tibial vara or Blount's disease.[8–11] Any child with this condition and his or her family should be educated about the many adverse effects of being overweight and given tools to create a healthier lifestyle. Unfortunately, though physicians appropriately recommend an increase in exercise and the need to improve nutrition and diet, there is no evidence that this advice and awareness is being converted into behavior change.[28] Physical therapists, along with physicians and nutritionists, should play a more active role in identification, education, design of a comprehensive health program, and oversight of implementation to help assist with the lifelong behavior changes that are necessary.

RICKETS

■ Hypophosphatasia

Chief Clinical Characteristics
This presentation includes inadequate bone mineralization and resultant skeletal deformities such as genu valgum or varum.[29] In the childhood form there is a premature loss of deciduous teeth.[30]

Background Information
This condition is a heritable form of rickets that is diagnosed with a biochemical hallmark of subnormal alkaline phosphatase in the serum and impaired activity of the tissue nonspecific alkaline phosphatase.[30,31] This condition presents with a wide range of clinical severity, from death *in utero* to premature loss of adult teeth. At this point, there is no known medical treatment for this rare disease, which has been detected in 70 patients globally.[31] Skeletal abnormalities such as genu varum and valgum should be measured and compared to age-matched peers; if outside the normal range, referral to an orthopedist is appropriate.

■ Nutritional

Chief Clinical Characteristics
This presentation includes children who may be malnourished with a deficiency in vitamin D and/or calcium, have restricted sunlight exposure (limited outdoor play time), or have dark skin pigmentation(eg, African or Asian descent).[32–34] Children may present with unilateral or bilateral genu varum, genu valgum, or windswept deformity.[33]

Background Information
This condition, primarily related to inadequate dietary or environmental vitamin D,

results in a depletion of vitamin D stores and decreased calcium absorption, which decreases the availability of calcium for proper epiphyseal cartilage and skeletal mineralization and development.[32] Any interruption in the development can lead to angular asymmetries, most pronounced at the knee joint. Diagnosis is confirmed with characteristic clinical features, elevated serum alkaline phosphatase activity, reduced serum calcium and circulating vitamin D levels, and radiographic evidence, including impaired mineralization, frayed epiphyses, and/or metaphyseal widening.[32] According to DeLucia, the average age of diagnosis is 20 months with a range from 4 to 38 months. The major clinical signs are patients in the 5th to 10th percentile in height and weight (>50%), leg bowing (76.5%), and ankle and wrist swelling (73.5%). Some children are resistant to lower extremity weight bearing.[32] Treatment includes physician prescription of vitamin D and elemental calcium supplements, which can restore normal serum levels and correct many bony abnormalities.[32] The most severe bony abnormalities may require surgical correction or supportive bracing.

SKELETAL DYSPLASIAS

Chief Clinical Characteristics
This presentation includes children who either at birth or during childhood present with generalized disorders of bone growth and cartilage and bone development. Many persons have disproportionate short stature, which helps to differentiate this presentation from endocrine and metabolic disorders.

Background Information
This group of conditions is a relatively rare group of genetic disorders with 5 affected fetuses in 10,000 pregnancies. However, within that small group 200 different conditions are currently recognized.[35] Historically, skeletal dysplasias were classified according to pattern of bone involvement, but a more recent trend is to categorize them by the causative protein, enzyme, or gene defect that is identified with chromosomal analysis. Management of the various dysplasias includes genetic counseling as well as addressing the various musculoskeletal impairments and

internal medical problems.[35] Some of the most common deformities occur at the knee joint, where varus and valgus angulations can present unilaterally or bilaterally.[35–39] Usually surgery is needed to correct these deformities, but there have been a few cases where the use of distraction with external fixation helped to resolve the joint deformity.[40] In all cases of skeletal dysplasias an orthopedic surgeon should follow the child through development. A few of the more common dysplasias, which can contribute to either or both genu valgus and genu varus abnormalities, are described briefly below.

■ Achondroplasia

Chief Clinical Characteristics
This condition is characterized by short-limbed dwarfism that also involves genu varum, which occurs as the child starts walking.

Background Information
This condition is the most common form of short-limb dwarfism. Achondroplasia is an autosomal dominant condition with two out of three cases resulting from a new, single-point spontaneous mutation in the FGFR3 protein on chromosome 4. Genu varum occurs in 50% of individuals with this condition. No conservative methods of treatment have proved effective, so patients usually must undergo surgery to correct this progressive orthopedic deformity.[35,39] Postoperative rehabilitation is performed by a physical therapist.

HYPOCHONDROPLASIAS

This family of conditions is similar to, but subtler than, achondroplasia. It is characterized by mild short-limb dwarfism, is autosomal dominant, and results in genu varum deformity less than 10% of the time. Significant genu varum may need surgical intervention, but more mild cases can correct spontaneously.[35]

■ Metaphyseal Chondrodysplasias

Chief Clinical Characteristics
This condition is characterized by normal or short stature, but most present with angulation problems at the knee.[35]

Background Information
This condition is a group of disorders that manifests as metaphyseal deformity,

irregularity near the physes, and minimal if any involvement in the epiphysis. The primary defect is in the growth plate. This condition is caused by autosomal dominant or recessive gene patterns of heritability, related to abnormalities involving multiple chromosomes. One type, McKusick metaphyseal chondrodysplasia, must be differentiated from rickets, in which epiphyseal and physeal involvement is severe.[32,35] Usually angulation problems at the knee improve with growth, but if the deformity progresses, proximal tibiofemoral osteotomies are required to correct it. Postoperative rehabilitation is performed by a physical therapist.

Multiple Epiphyseal Dysplasia

Chief Clinical Characteristics
This condition includes limb deformities that manifest in a patient of more typical stature. Children with this condition usually experience functional deficits later in childhood because of gait disturbances, joint pain, and angular problems at the hip and knees.

Background Information
This condition is caused by delayed epiphyseal ossification. Resulting genu valgus deformities usually require surgical intervention to correct, but may recur in children who are still growing. Therefore, surgery is usually performed closer to skeletal maturity.[35,39] One reported case presented with femoral and tibial torsion deformities that led to both significant in-toeing posture and severe genu valgus deformity.[36] Postoperative rehabilitation is performed by a physical therapist.

Pseudoachondroplasia

Chief Clinical Characteristics
This condition is usually characterized by normal head and face morphometry with minor spinal involvement. However, significant varus, valgus, and recurvatum deformities associated with ligament laxity at the knees are common.[35]

Background Information
This condition is one of the most common forms of skeletal dysplasia, with a prevalence of 4 per 1 million. Infants are born with typical proportions and growth retardation is usually identified around the second year of life. Conservative bracing is rarely effective,

and even after multiple osteotomies, the recurrence of knee deformities is common, requiring additional surgery.[35,39] Knee and hip total joint arthroplasty is the most common treatment for premature osteoarthritis when these children reach middle age.[35] Postoperative rehabilitation is performed by a physical therapist.

Spondyloepiphyseal Dysplasia

Chief Clinical Characteristics
This presentation is characterized by significant angular knee deformities.[35]

Background Information
This condition is a category of rare dysplasias with disproportionate short-trunk dwarfism and primary involvement in the spine and epiphyseal centers. The congenital version usually requires osteotomies more often to correct malalignment versus the tarda disorder, which presents with more mild angular deformities at the knees that do not require intervention.

Description of Conditions That May Lead to Knock Knees in a Child

Cerebral Palsy

Chief Clinical Characteristics
This presentation includes excessive genu valgum and gait disturbances accompanied by this neuromuscular disorder.

Background Information
This condition is a movement and posture disorder resulting from nonprogressive damage to the immature central nervous system.[41,42] This damage interferes with the process of development and often manifests with significant gait deviations secondary to osseous deformity, muscle imbalance and weakness, and poor dynamic coordination.[43–45] Gait is often characterized as a "crouch" and includes excessive hip flexion, adduction and medial rotation; genu valgum; and calcaneal eversion with midfoot pronation. Chronic malalignment with posture and movement contributes to many secondary consequences, including permanent muscular and skeletal changes and joint deformity, such as excessive genu valgum.[45] A complete pelvic and lower extremity musculoskeletal

exam, including tibiofemoral angle and inter-malleolar distance, will be necessary at the initial evaluation and over time to identify primary and secondary impairments and to document progression of the joint deformity. Children with this condition should be followed regularly, every 6 to 12 months, by an orthopedic surgeon, who can help assist the family and health care team to make decisions regarding conservative treatment or to identify the need for surgery. Most of the nonsurgical treatment will be performed primarily by a physical therapist, but in the case of severe knee deformities that present with adverse symptoms, surgery (osteotomy) will most often be required.

■ Focal Fibrocartilaginous Dysplasia

Chief Clinical Characteristics
This presentation includes young infants and toddlers with a unilateral bowing or angulation deformity of long bones, including the tibia and femur.

Background Information
This condition is a rare benign lesion that is most commonly seen in the proximal tibia (43 of 48 cases) or distal femur (5 of 48 cases).[15] The unilateral cortical defect, identified on radiograph and with histological studies, presents as dense collagenized fibrous tissue with focal areas of fibrocartilaginous changes occurring between the metaphysis and diaphysis. This defect causes asymmetrical growth and bowing of the long bones, which contributes to angular deformities such as tibial vara or tibial valga.[15–17] Unlike Blount's disease, the lesion does not extend to the physis. Due to the rare nature of this condition the natural history is largely unknown; however, it has been reported that up to 45% of tibial cases resolved spontaneously, while 86% of femoral lesions progressed and needed surgical intervention to correct.[17] Age of onset ranges from 5 to 28 months with an average of 16.5 months.[17]

■ Hemophilia

Chief Clinical Characteristics
This presentation includes knee flexion and valgus deformity caused by asymmetrical growth of the epiphyses. Joint pain usually accompanies these alignment abnormalities.[46]

Background Information
This condition is a hereditary X-linked disease that severely affects 1 out of 10,000 men. Diagnosis and severity of the disease are based on the percentage of serum deficiency of Factor VIII and/or Factor IX, which are necessary for appropriate blood coagulation. These factor deficiencies contribute to early (infantile) and chronic (into adolescence and adulthood) articular complications because minor joint trauma leads to significant hemarthroses causing chronic inflammation, synovitis, and eventually degenerative arthropathy. This disease process results in joint alignment abnormalities and deformities.[47] The knee is the most affected joint, followed by the elbow and ankle.[46] The primary treatment goal is to slow down or stop the progression of joint destruction, which is achieved by comprehensive medical and therapeutic management, emphasizing family education. Acute bleeding episodes are managed by intravenous factor replacement as soon as symptoms such as joint stiffness or discomfort present. However, prophylactic treatment is also available, especially if the child will be engaging in more rigorous activities.[47] Orthopedists will need to be intimately involved throughout the child's development, especially if joint deformities cause significant functional limitations. Surgeries can be helpful to correct severe alignment abnormalities.

■ Idiopathic Genu Valgum

Chief Clinical Characteristics
This presentation includes knock knees two standard deviations or greater from normal, age-matched peers as measured by the tibiofemoral angle or intermalleolar distance. This condition is a diagnosis of exclusion.[6]

Background Information
Excessive genu valgum contributes to abnormal loading patterns and ground reaction forces that over time can lead to premature joint deterioration and osteoarthritis.[18,19] Treatment should include referral to an orthopedic surgeon, where imaging studies can be used to exclude other causes for the joint abnormality. Depending on the severity of alignment abnormality, joint instability, and pain that contributes to functional limitations and participation restrictions, conservative bracing or more invasive surgery may be required to correct the alignment.[20]

■ Ligamentous Laxity/Joint Hypermobility

Chief Clinical Characteristics

This presentation includes children, girls more than boys, who score greater than a 4 or 5 on the Beighton score and who may demonstrate increased joint mobility on the nondominant side.[21–24] This condition can contribute to excessive genu valgum beyond normal values for age-matched peers.

Background Information

Children inherently present with greater range of motion in their joints than adults; this range gradually decreases with age. Hypermobility is often assessed and diagnosed using the Beighton criteria, which depends on the ability to perform the following maneuvers:

1. Passive extension of the fifth finger at metacarpophalangeal joint to ≥90 degrees
2. Passive apposition of the thumb to the forearm
3. Hyperextension of elbow ≥10 degrees
4. Hyperextension of the knee ≥10 degrees
5. Ability to rest entire palm of hand on floor with forward flexion and extended knees.

The first four maneuvers are assessed bilaterally with a separate score given for right and left sides. Each item receives a score of 0 or 1, with 1 being assigned when the criteria for a maneuver is met. The total score ranges from 0 to 9, with generalized hypermobility diagnosed with a score of ≥4.[24] This condition has been identified in 2.3% to 30% of children screened, depending on the cut-off Beighton score used and the child's age and ethnicity.[25] Many children diagnosed with generalized ligament laxity will not develop significant musculoskeletal issues that will require medical intervention[25] and, in preadolescents, Mikkelsson demonstrated that musculoskeletal pain is not associated with this condition.[26] However, this condition is described as chronic, generalized joint hypermobility that presents with adverse symptoms that contribute to functional limitation. This condition has been compared to more serious connective tissue disorders such as Ehlers-Danlos syndrome, osteogenesis imperfecta, and Marfan syndrome.[25] This condition also is associated with arthralgia, abnormal gait, back pain, and joint deformities such as scoliosis and genu valgum; it is most often diagnosed by a pediatric rheumatologist,[25] but even with this confirmed diagnosis, comprehensive clinical assessment of joint alignment and the integrity of surrounding ligaments with appropriate stress tests is essential, especially in the lower extremity and weight-bearing joints. Knee collateral ligament laxity has been associated with genu valgum, which requires referral to an orthopedist for possible surgery to address both the bony abnormality and ligament laxity.[27]

■ Osteochondromatosis (Multiple Hereditary Exostosis)

Chief Clinical Characteristics

This presentation includes children and adolescents with multiple exostoses (osteochondromas) that may cause pain or cosmetic concerns and that can lead to skeletal deformities over time. The most common skeletal deformities include "short stature, limb-length discrepancies, valgus deformity at the knee and ankle, asymmetry of the pectoral and pelvic girdles, bowing of the radius with ulnar deviation of the wrist, and subluxation of the radiocapitellar joint."[48]

Background Information

This condition is an autosomal dominant disorder that affects between 0.9 to 2 persons per 100,000 and diagnosis is confirmed with chromosomal analysis and identification of mutations in the *EXT1* and *EXT2* genes. Osteochondromas, which can be identified clinically and confirmed with radiograph, are benign bone tumors that consist of cartilage-capped exostoses at the metaphyses of rapidly growing ends of long bones.[48,49] Knee valgus deformity is caused by lesions in either the distal femur or proximal tibia.[48,50] Ankle valgus deformity also occurs in up to 50% of patients, which contributes to a flat foot posture. Surgery is often performed to remove exostoses and can also prevent progression or provide correction of secondary orthopedic deformities.[48]

■ Overweight and Obesity

Chief Clinical Characteristics

This presentation includes a child with a body mass index at or above the 85th percentile and whose genu valgum is at least two standard deviations from the normal age-related values as measured by the tibiofemoral angle or intermalleolar distance.

Background Information

The prevalence of obesity is increasing in children of all age ranges,[51] and there is a positive correlation between obesity and increased genu valgum,[52] with a 50% increased incidence of abnormal genu valgum, at least 10 cm of intermalleolar distance, in overweight children when compared to age-matched peers. Genu valgum correction, depending on the child's age, the severity of knee instability, pain and functional limitation, will most likely require orthopedic surgery. If symptoms are significant, referral to an orthopedist for radiograph or computed tomography scan, and possible surgery, is indicated.[6] Physical therapy is indicated in a team approach to treat obesity and for any postsurgical rehabilitation. Physical therapy alone, however, will not alter the bony genu valgum deformity. Any child with obesity and his or her family should be educated about the many adverse effects of being overweight and given tools to create a healthier lifestyle. Unfortunately, though physicians appropriately recommend an increase in exercise and the need to improve nutrition and diet, there is no evidence that this advice and awareness is being converted into behavior change.[28] Physical therapists, along with physicians and nutritionists, should play a more active role in identification, education, design of a comprehensive health program, and oversight of implementation to help assist with the lifelong behavior changes that are necessary.

■ Post-Traumatic/Fracture Healing Disturbances and Abnormal Growth

Chief Clinical Characteristics
This presentation includes tibial valga (knock knee) on the affected side after complete healing of a proximal tibial metaphyseal fracture, known as a Cozen fracture.[53]

Background Information
Tibial metaphyseal fractures are relatively rare fractures that occur in young children an average of 4 years old and are diagnosed by radiograph.[54,55] Despite initial progressive tibial valga angles and leg-length overgrowth discrepancies that occur after fracture healing is complete, follow-up over time usually reveals spontaneous correction in a majority of children.[55,56] Therefore, treatment recommendations include following the growth of children until skeletal maturity with periodic clinical examination and radiographs, but not intervening surgically to correct the malalignment unless secondary complications such as pain and activity restriction are present.[55,56]

SKELETAL DYSPLASIAS

Chief Clinical Characteristics
This presentation includes children who either at birth or during childhood present with generalized disorders of bone growth and cartilage and bone development. Many persons have disproportionate short stature, which helps to differentiate this presentation from endocrine and metabolic disorders.

Background Information
This group of conditions is a relatively rare group of genetic disorders with 5 affected fetuses in 10,000 pregnancies. However, within that small group 200 different conditions are currently recognized.[35] Historically, skeletal dysplasias were classified according to pattern of bone involvement, but a more recent trend is to categorize them by the causative protein, enzyme, or gene defect that is identified with chromosomal analysis. Management of the various dysplasias includes genetic counseling as well as addressing the various musculoskeletal impairments and internal medical problems.[35] Some of the most common deformities occur at the knee joint, where varus and valgus angulations can present unilaterally or bilaterally.[35–39] Usually surgery is needed to correct these deformities, but there have been a few cases where the use of distraction with external fixation helped to resolve the joint deformity.[40] In all cases of skeletal dysplasias an orthopedic surgeon should follow the child through development. A few of the more common dysplasias, which can contribute to either or both genu valgus and genu varus abnormalities, are described briefly below.

■ Achondroplasia

Chief Clinical Characteristics
This condition is characterized by short-limbed dwarfism that also involves genu varum, which occurs as the child starts walking.

Background Information

This condition is the most common form of short-limb dwarfism. Achondroplasia is an autosomal dominant condition with two out of three cases resulting from a new, single-point spontaneous mutation in the FGFR3 protein on chromosome 4. Genu varum occurs in 50% of individuals with this condition. No conservative methods of treatment have proved effective, so patients usually must undergo surgery to correct this progressive orthopedic deformity.[35,39] Postoperative rehabilitation is performed by a physical therapist.

■ Chondroectodermal Dysplasia (Ellis-Van Creveld Syndrome)

Chief Clinical Characteristics

This condition is characterized by short-limb disproportionate dwarfism, polydactyly, hypoplasia of the nails, dental deficiencies, and congenital heart disease. In addition to other orthopedic deformities, a symmetric genu valgus deformity is common.

Background Information

This condition is usually progressive, requiring surgical intervention to correct if greater than 20 degrees.[35] Postoperative rehabilitation is performed by a physical therapist.

HYPOCHONDROPLASIAS

This family of conditions is similar to, but subtler than, achondroplasia. It is characterized by mild short-limb dwarfism, is autosomal dominant, and results in genu varum deformity less than 10% of the time. Significant genu varum may need surgical intervention, but more mild cases can correct spontaneously.[35]

■ Metaphyseal Chondrodysplasias

Chief Clinical Characteristics

This condition is characterized by normal or short stature, but most present with angulation problems at the knee.[35]

Background Information

This condition is a group of disorders that manifests as a metaphyseal deformity, irregularity near the physes, and minimal if any involvement in the epiphysis. The primary defect is in the growth plate. This condition is caused by autosomal dominant or recessive gene patterns of heritability, related to abnormalities involving multiple chromosomes. One type, McKusick metaphyseal chondrodysplasia, must be differentiated from rickets, in which epiphyseal and physeal involvement is severe.[32,35] Usually angulation problems at the knee improve with growth, but if the deformity progresses, proximal tibiofemoral osteotomies are required to correct it. Postoperative rehabilitation is performed by a physical therapist.

■ Multiple Epiphyseal Dysplasia

Chief Clinical Characteristics

This condition includes limb deformities that manifest in a patient of more typical stature. Children with this condition usually experience functional deficits later in childhood because of gait disturbances, joint pain, and angular problems at the hip and knees.

Background Information

This condition is caused by delayed epiphyseal ossification. Resulting genu valgus deformities usually require surgical intervention to correct, but may recur in children who are still growing. Therefore, surgery is usually performed closer to skeletal maturity.[35,39] One reported case presented with femoral and tibial torsion deformities that led to both significant in-toeing posture and severe genu valgus deformity.[36] Postoperative rehabilitation is performed by a physical therapist.

■ Pseudoachondroplasia

Chief Clinical Characteristics

This condition is usually characterized by normal head and face morphometry with minor spinal involvement. However, significant varus, valgus, and recurvatum deformities associated with ligament laxity at the knees are common.[35]

Background Information

This condition is one of the most common forms of skeletal dysplasia, with a prevalence of 4 per 1 million. Infants are born with typical proportions and growth retardation is usually identified around the second year of life. Conservative bracing is rarely effective, and even after multiple osteotomies, the recurrence of knee deformities is common, requiring additional surgery.[35,39] Knee and hip total joint arthroplasty is the most common treatment for premature osteoarthritis when these children reach middle age.[35] Postoperative rehabilitation is performed by a physical therapist.

■ Spondyloepiphyseal Dysplasia

Chief Clinical Characteristics

This presentation is characterized by significant angular knee deformities.[35]

Background Information

This condition is a category of rare dysplasias with disproportionate short-trunk dwarfism and primary involvement in the spine and epiphyseal centers. The congenital version usually requires osteotomies more often to correct malalignment versus the tarda disorder, which presents with more mild angular deformities at the knees that do not require intervention.

References

1. Sass P, Hassan G. Lower extremity abnormalities in children. *Am Fam Physician.* Aug 1, 2003;68(3):461–468.
2. Pretkiewicz-Abacjew E. Knock knee and the gait of six-year-old children. *J Sports Med Phys Fitness.* 2003;43(2):156–164.
3. Lin CJ, Lai KA, Kuan TS, Chou YL. Correlating factors and clinical significance of flexible flatfoot in preschool children. *J Pediatr Orthop.* May–Jun 2001;21(3):378–382.
4. Salenius P, Vankka E. The development of the tibiofemoral angle in children. *J Bone Joint Surg Am.* Mar 1975;57(2):259–261.
5. Long T, Toscano K. *Handbook of Pediatric Physical Therapy.* 2nd ed. Baltimore, MD: Lippincott Williams & Wilkins; 2002.
6. Wallach DM, Davidson RS. Pediatric lower limb disorders. In: Dormans JP, ed. *Pediatric Orthopedics and Sports Medicine.* St. Louis, MO: Mosby; 2004:246–272.
7. Myers TG, Fishman MK, McCarthy JJ, Davidson RS, Gaughan J. Incidence of distal femoral and distal tibial deformities in infantile and adolescent Blount disease. *J Pediatr Orthop.* Mar–Apr 2005;25(2):215–218.
8. Gordon JE, Heidenreich FP, Carpenter CJ, Kelly-Hahn J, Schoenecker PL. Comprehensive treatment of late-onset tibia vara. *J Bone Joint Surg Am.* Jul 2005;87(7):1561–1570.
9. Raney EM, Topoleski TA, Yaghoubian R, Guidera KJ, Marshall JG. Orthotic treatment of infantile tibia vara. *J Pediatr Orthop.* Sep–Oct 1998;18(5):670–674.
10. Thompson GH, Carter JR, Smith CW. Late-onset tibia vara: a comparative analysis. *J Pediatr Orthop.* Mar 1984;4(2):185–194.
11. Wenger DR, Mickelson M, Maynard JA. The evolution and histopathology of adolescent tibia vara. *J Pediatr Orthop.* Jan 1984;4(1):78–88.
12. Schoppee K. Blount disease (idiopathic tibia vara). *Orthop Nurs.* Sep–Oct 1995;14(5):31–34.
13. Cheema JI, Grissom LE, Harcke HT. Radiographic characteristics of lower-extremity bowing in children. *Radiographics.* Jul–Aug 2003;23(4):871–880.
14. McCarthy JJ, Betz RR, Kim A, Davids JR, Davidson RS. Early radiographic differentiation of infantile tibia vara from physiologic bowing using the femoral-tibial ratio. *J Pediatr Orthop.* Jul–Aug 2001;21(4):545–548.
15. Ruchelsman DE, Madan SS, Feldman DS. Genu valgum secondary to focal fibrocartilaginous dysplasia of the distal femur. *J Pediatr Orthop.* Jul–Aug 2004;24(4):408–413.
16. Santos M, Valente E, Almada A, Neves J. Tibia valga due to focal fibrocartilaginous dysplasia: case report. *J Pediatr Orthop B.* Apr 2002;11(2):167–171.
17. Choi HI, Kim CJ, Cho T-J, et al. Focal fibrocartilaginous dysplasia of long bones: report of eight additional cases and literature review. *J Pediatr Orthop.* 2000;20(4):421–427.
18. Wang H, Tan M, Li Z, Yang F, Liang L, Zhang G. [Femoral varus osteotomy combined with interlocking nailing for treatment of genu valgum]. *Zhongguo Xiu Fu Chong Jian Wai Ke Za Zhi.* Mar 15, 2005;19(3):192–194.
19. Brouwer RW, Verhaar JA. [Osteotomy at knee level for young patients with gonarthrosis]. *Ned Tijdschr Geneeskd.* Oct 2, 2004;148(40):1955–1960.
20. Leach J. Orthopedic conditions. In: Campbell SK, ed. *Physical Therapy for Children.* 2nd ed. Philadelphia, PA: W. B. Saunders; 2000:398–428.
21. Jansson A, Saartok T, Werner S, Renstrom P. General joint laxity in 1845 Swedish school children of different ages: age- and gender-specific distributions. *Acta Paediatr.* Sep 2004;93(9):1202–1206.
22. Rikken-Bultman DG, Wellink L, van Dongen PW. Hypermobility in two Dutch school populations. *Eur J Obstet Gynecol Reprod Biol.* Jun 1997;73(2):189–192.
23. van der Giessen LJ, Liekens D, Rutgers KJ, Hartman A, Mulder PG, Oranje AP. Validation of Beighton score and prevalence of connective tissue signs in 773 Dutch children. *J Rheumatol.* Dec 2001;28(12):2726–2730.
24. Gulbahar S, Sahin E, Baydar M, et al. Hypermobility syndrome increases the risk for low bone mass. *Clin Rheumatol.* Nov 26 2005:1–4.
25. Adib N, Davies K, Grahame R, Woo P, Murray KJ. Joint hypermobility syndrome in childhood. A not so benign multisystem disorder? *Rheumatology (Oxford).* Jun 2005;44(6):744–750.
26. Mikkelsson M, Salminen JJ, Kautiainen H. Joint hypermobility is not a contributing factor to musculoskeletal pain in pre-adolescents. *J Rheumatol.* Nov 1996;23(11):1963–1967.
27. Paley D, Bhatnagar J, Herzenberg JE, Bhave A. New procedures for tightening knee collateral ligaments in conjunction with knee realignment osteotomy. *Orthop Clin North Am.* Jul 1994;25(3):533–555.
28. Morrato EH, Hill JO, Wyatt HR, Ghushchyan V, Sullivan PW. Are health care professionals advising patients with diabetes or at risk for developing diabetes to exercise more? *Diabetes Care.* Mar 2006;29(3):543–548.
29. Aronson J, Aronson EA. Rickets and metabolic disorders. In: Staheli LT, ed. *Pediatric Orthopaedic Secrets.* 2nd ed. Philadelphia, PA: Hanley & Belfus; 2003:439–446.
30. Draguet C, Gillerot Y, Mornet E. [Childhood hypophosphatasia: a case report due to a novel mutation]. *Arch Pediatr.* May 2004;11(5):440–443.

31. Mumm S, Jones J, Finnegan P, Henthorn PS, Podgornik MN, Whyte MP. Denaturing gradient gel electrophoresis analysis of the tissue nonspecific alkaline phosphatase isoenzyme gene in hypophosphatasia. *Mol Genet Metab.* Feb 2002;75(2):143–153.

32. DeLucia MC, Mitnick ME, Carpenter TO. Nutritional rickets with normal circulating 25-hydroxyvitamin D: a call for reexamining the role of dietary calcium intake in North American infants. *J Clin Endocrinol Metab.* Aug 2003;88(8):3539–3545.

33. Agaja SB. Factors affecting angular deformities of the knees in Nigerian children—Ilorin experience. *West Afr J Med.* Oct–Dec 2001;20(4):246–250.

34. Allgrove J. Is nutritional rickets returning? *Arch Dis Childhood.* 2004;89(8):699–701.

35. Erol B, Dormans JP, States L, Kaplan F. Skeletal dysplasias and metabolic disorders of bone. In: Dormans JP, ed. *Pediatric Orthopedics and Sports Medicine.* St. Louis, MO: Mosby, Inc.; 2004:111–146.

36. Eddy MC, Steiner RD, McAlister WH, Whyte MP. Bilateral radial ray hypoplasia with multiple epiphyseal dysplasia. *Am J Med Genet.* May 18, 1998;77(3): 182–187.

37. Lindberg EJ, Watts HG. Postosteotomy healing in Pyle's disease (familial metaphyseal dysplasia). A case report. *Clin Orthop Relat Res.* Aug 1997(341):215–217.

38. Patel AC, McAlister WH, Whyte MP. Spondyloepimetaphyseal dysplasia: clinical and radiologic investigation of a large kindred manifesting autosomal dominant inheritance, and a review of the literature. *Medicine (Baltimore).* Sep 1993;72(5):326–342.

39. Kopits SE. Orthopedic complications of dwarfism. *Clin Orthop Relat Res.* Jan–Feb 1976(114):153–179.

40. Givon U, Schindler A, Ganel A. Hemichondrodiastasis for the treatment of genu varum deformity associated with bone dysplasias. *J Pediatr Orthop.* Mar–Apr 2001;21(2):238–241.

41. Spiegel DA. Cerebral palsy. In: Dormans JP, ed. *Pediatric Orthopaedics and Sports Medicine.* St. Louis, MO: Mosby; 2004:373–415.

42. Shapiro BK. Cerebral palsy: A reconceptualization of the spectrum. *J Pediatr.* Aug 2004;145(2 suppl):S3–7.

43. Aktas S, Aiona MD, Orendurff M. Evaluation of rotational gait abnormality in the patients cerebral palsy. *J Pediatr Orthop.* Mar–Apr 2000;20(2):217–220.

44. Waskin MR, Frost JP, Hatalowich GS. Cerebral palsy: a podiatric overview. *J Foot Surg.* Winter 1983;22(4): 362–365.

45. Root L. Varus and valgus foot in cerebral palsy and its management. *Foot Ankle.* Jan–Feb 1984;4(4):174–179.

46. Rodriguez-Merchan EC. Management of the orthopaedic complications of haemophilia. *J Bone Joint Surg Br.* 1998;80B(2):191–196.

47. McGee SM. Hemophilia. In: Campbell SK, cd. *Physical Therapy for Children.* 2nd ed. Philadelphia, PA: W. B. Saunders; 2000:247–259.

48. Stieber JR, Dormans JP. Manifestations of hereditary multiple exostoses. *J Am Acad Orthop Surg.* Mar–Apr 2005;13(2):110–120.

49. Peterson HA. Multiple hereditary osteochondromata. *Clin Orthop Relat Res.* Feb 1989(239):222–230.

50. Nawata K, Teshima R, Minamizaki T, Yamamoto K. Knee deformities in multiple hereditary exostoses. A longitudinal radiographic study. *Clin Orthop Relat Res.* Apr 1995(313):194–199.

51. Ogden C, Flegal K, Carroll MD, Johnson CL. Prevalence and trend in overweight among US children and adolescents, 1999–2000. *JAMA.* 2002;288:1728–1732.

52. Bonet SB, Quintanar RA, Alaves BM, et al. Presence of genu valgum in obese children: cause or effect? *An Pediatr (Barc).* 2003;58(3):232–235.

53. Cozen L. Knock-knee deformity in children. Congenital and acquired. *Clin Orthop Relat Res.* Sep 1990(258): 191–203.

54. Muller I, Muschol M, Mann M, Hassenpflug J. Results of proximal metaphyseal fractures in children. *Arch Orthop Trauma Surg.* Jul 2002;122(6):331–333.

55. Tuten HR, Keeler KA, Gabos PG, Zionts LE, MacKenzie WG. Posttraumatic tibia valga in children. A long-term follow-up note. *J Bone Joint Surg Am.* Jun 1999;81(6): 799–810.

56. Zionts LE, MacEwen GD. Spontaneous improvement of post-traumatic tibia valga. *J Bone Joint Surg Am.* Jun 1986;68(5):680–687.

CHAPTER 61

In-Toeing and Out-Toeing in a Child

■ *Wendi W. McKenna, PT, DPT, PCS*

Description of the Symptom

In-toeing and *out-toeing postures* may be seen during quiet stance or gait.[1-3] These postures are recognized by an excessive bilateral or unilateral angulation of the foot longitudinal axis toward or away from a child's line of forward progression, respectively (Fig. 61-1). This chapter describes possible causes of in-toeing and out-toeing in a child.

Special Concerns

■ Post-traumatic changes in lower extremity alignment or a painful limp
■ Progressive limp leading to refusal to walk with or without pain
■ Grossly asymmetric presentation of lower extremity alignment
■ History of multiple fractures

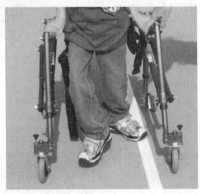

FIGURE 61-1 Out-toeing bilaterally with left foot more affected than right.

CHAPTER PREVIEW: Conditions That May Lead to In-Toeing and Out-Toeing in a Child

T Trauma	
IN-TOEING	**OUT-TOEING**
COMMON	
Not applicable	Slipped capital femoral epiphysis 1175
UNCOMMON	
Not applicable	Not applicable
RARE	
Not applicable	Not applicable

I Inflammation	
IN-TOEING	**OUT-TOEING**
COMMON	
Not applicable	Not applicable

(continued)

Inflammation *(continued)*

UNCOMMON	
Not applicable	Not applicable

RARE	
Not applicable	Not applicable

M Metabolic

IN-TOEING	OUT-TOEING
COMMON	
Not applicable	Overweight and obesity 1175
UNCOMMON	
Not applicable	Not applicable
RARE	
Not applicable	Not applicable

Va Vascular

IN-TOEING	OUT-TOEING
COMMON	
Avascular necrosis of the femoral head (Legg-Calvé-Perthes disease) 1169	Not applicable
UNCOMMON	
Not applicable	Not applicable
RARE	
Not applicable	Not applicable

De Degenerative

IN-TOEING	OUT-TOEING
COMMON	
Not applicable	Not applicable
UNCOMMON	
Not applicable	Not applicable
RARE	
Not applicable	Not applicable

Tu Tumor

IN-TOEING	OUT-TOEING
COMMON	
Not applicable	Not applicable
UNCOMMON	
Not applicable	Not applicable

Tumor *(continued)*

RARE	
Not applicable	Not applicable

Co Congenital

IN-TOEING	OUT-TOEING
COMMON	
Excessive femoral anteversion (torsion) 1171	Femoral retroversion (torsion) 1174
Medial tibial torsion 1171	Lateral tibial torsion 1174
Metatarsus adductus 1171	Muscle imbalance or weakness 1174
Muscle imbalance or weakness 1172	
Talipes equinovarus (clubfoot) 1172	
UNCOMMON	
Not applicable	Not applicable
RARE	
Not applicable	Bladder exstrophy 1173

Ne Neurogenic/Psychogenic

IN-TOEING	OUT-TOEING
COMMON	
Cerebral palsy 1170	Cerebral palsy 1173
UNCOMMON	
Not applicable	Not applicable
RARE	
Tethered cord syndrome 1173	Not applicable

Note: These are estimates of relative incidence because few data are available for the less common conditions.

Common Ages at Which In-Toeing and Out-Toeing Present in a Child

APPROXIMATE AGE	CONDITION
Birth to 3 Years	Abnormal tibial torsion
	Bladder exstrophy
	Cerebral palsy
	Excessive femoral anteversion (torsion)
	Femoral retroversion (torsion)
	Metatarsus adductus
	Muscle imbalance or weakness
	Overweight and obesity
	Talipes equinovarus (clubfoot)
	Tethered cord syndrome
Preschool (3–5 Years)	Abnormal tibial torsion
	Cerebral palsy
	Excessive femoral anteversion (torsion)
	Femoral retroversion (torsion)
	Metatarsus adductus

(continued)

Common Ages at Which In-Toeing and Out-Toeing Present in a Child—cont'd

APPROXIMATE AGE	CONDITION
	Muscle imbalance or weakness
	Overweight and obesity
	Tethered cord syndrome
Elementary School (6–11 Years)	Abnormal tibial torsion
	Avascular necrosis of the femoral head (Legg-Calvé-Perthes disease)
	Cerebral palsy
	Excessive femoral anteversion (torsion)
	Femoral retroversion (torsion)
	Muscle imbalance or weakness
	Overweight and obesity
Middle School (12–14 Years)	Abnormal tibial torsion
	Cerebral palsy
	Excessive femoral anteversion (torsion)
	Femoral retroversion (torsion)
	Muscle imbalance or weakness
	Overweight and obesity
	Slipped capital femoral epiphysis
High School (15–18 Years)	Abnormal tibial torsion
	Cerebral palsy
	Excessive femoral anteversion (torsion)
	Femoral retroversion (torsion)
	Muscle imbalance or weakness
	Overweight and obesity
	Slipped capital femoral epiphysis

Overview of In-Toeing and Out-Toeing in a Child

Lower extremity alignment and range of motion changes as a child grows, develops and moves around his or her environment. Identifying lower extremity misalignment such as in-toeing and out-toeing, therefore, requires an intimate knowledge of typical lower extremity alignment, bone morphology, and joint range of motion as it relates to a child's age and gross motor skill development. Physical therapists must always assess static and dynamic conditions in order to obtain a complete picture of lower extremity biomechanics to differentiate between benign, cosmetic concerns and more functional issues.

Parents and grandparents are often concerned about their child's excessive in-toeing or out-toeing, which may stem from concerns of cosmesis or more functional issues such as increased clumsiness, tripping, and falling. As children, many parents and grandparents received special bracing or orthotic shoes to help "correct" their hip, knee, and foot alignment abnormalities[4] and, therefore, seek similar treatment for their children. However, our current understanding is that many apparent lower extremity alignment abnormalities, including in-toeing and out-toeing, resolve spontaneously over time, cause no long-term functional limitation and participation restriction,[4] and require no treatment.[2] Treatment is usually only indicated and effective if a child presents with:

1. Functional limitations secondary to alignment,
2. Significant developmental history,
3. Abnormal patterns of alignment changes with growth, or
4. Alignment measurements greater than two standard deviations from normal, age-matched values.

Oftentimes, concerns regarding in-toeing and out-toeing can be sufficiently addressed by educating the family regarding normal development of alignment and biomechanics and scheduling follow-up appointments to monitor progress of alignment over time.

After a detailed history is obtained from the child and family, including cosmetic and functional concerns, expectations, and goals, objective measures are necessary to differentially diagnose the origin of the child's stance and gait posture. After observing the child walking and running, in-toeing and out-toeing values are often measured in the clinic setting[1] using the foot progression angle (FPA), the longitudinal axis of the foot during the single leg stance phase of gait as compared to the child's forward direction of movement. The FPA represents a summated rotational profile of the femur, tibia, and foot that can be caused by various combinations of bony and joint configurations or muscle imbalances at the hip, knee, and foot/ankle that ultimately contribute to in-toeing or out-toeing posture. To isolate different joints, however, other tests are necessary, including:

1. Ryder's test to measure femoral anteversion (torsion) values[5];
2. Hip medial and lateral passive range of motion (measured in hip extension) to determine symmetry of range and quality of end feel, which can help to determine whether possible femoral anteversion (torsion) abnormalities exist;
3. Thigh–foot angle to measure tibial torsion; and
4. Non–weight-bearing and weight-bearing relationship between the hindfoot and

forefoot to determine the integrity of the foot and ankle joints.

Refer to Figure 61-2 for typical values of foot progression angle, thigh–foot angle, and medial and lateral hip rotation range of motion in children ages 0 to 15 years. In general, measurements typically are symmetrical on right and left sides; any asymmetry should be more thoroughly investigated with subjective questions relating to developmental and family history and objective tests and measures to determine a cause for the discrepancy.

Description of Conditions That May Lead to In-Toeing in a Child

■ Avascular Necrosis of the Femoral Head (Legg-Calvé-Perthes Disease)

Chief Clinical Characteristics

This presentation includes a gradual onset of limping with or without pain and a reduction of range of motion into hip abduction and medial rotation more limited than lateral rotation.[6] There is controversy as to whether ipsilateral in-toeing due to excessive anteversion or out-toeing due to femoral retroversion is a dominant sign.[7]

Background Information

This condition is a necrosis of the proximal femoral epiphysis due to vascular ischemia. This ischemia injures the cartilage and leads

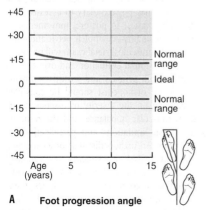

A   **Foot progression angle**

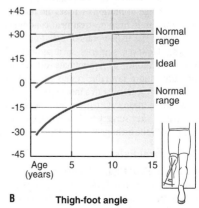

B   **Thigh-foot angle**

FIGURE 61-2 Typical values of (A) foot progression angle, (B) thigh–foot angle,

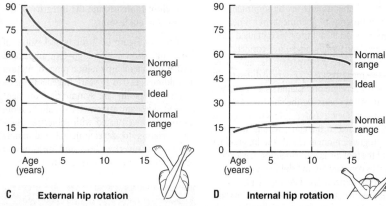

C   **External hip rotation**   **D**   **Internal hip rotation**

FIGURE 61-2 cont'd (C) external, and (D) internal hip rotation range of motion in children ages 0 to 15 years. (Adapted from Rang M, Wenger DR. Toeing in and toeing out: gait disorders. In: Rang M, Wenger DR, eds. The Art and Practice of Children's Orthopaedics. New York, NY: Raven Press; 1993.)

to a cessation of endochondral ossification[8,9] and collapse of the femoral head.[10] This condition is diagnosed with x-ray and the goal for treatment, whether conservative or surgical, is to maximize containment of the femoral head in the acetabulum and to maintain hip joint range of motion.[10,11] This condition affects young children between the ages of 4 and 12 years, presenting in boys four to five times more often than girls.[12] There is also a correlation between this disease and attention deficit hyperactivity disorder, difficulties with school, and poor social interaction skills.[13] The most positive outcomes are with those who contract the disease at a younger age, less than 8 years.[14] Herring and colleagues[14] concluded that bracing and range-of-motion exercises did not differ significantly from no-treatment conditions in children less than 8 years of age at onset of disease. However, surgeries such as femoral varus osteotomy or innominate osteotomy produced more favorable results in children older than 8 years or with a more severe condition classification.[14] Often physical therapy is prescribed after surgery with ongoing consultation with the orthopedic surgeon.

■ Cerebral Palsy

Chief Clinical Characteristics

This presentation includes either an in-toeing or out-toeing gait accompanied by this neuromuscular disorder.

Background Information

This condition is a movement and posture disorder resulting from nonprogressive damage to the immature central nervous system.[15,16] This damage interferes with the process of development and often manifests with significant gait deviations secondary to osseous torsional deformity, muscle imbalance and weakness, and poor dynamic coordination.[17-19] Hip disorders ranging from torsion abnormalities to subluxation and dislocation are common in persons with cerebral palsy.[20] Gait is often characterized by in-toeing. In hemiplegic cerebral palsy the problem is most commonly secondary to posterior tibialis muscle overactivity. In diplegic cerebral palsy, in-toeing may be secondary to excessive medial hip rotation in posture, movement and joint abnormality. A complete pelvic and lower extremity musculoskeletal exam will be necessary at the initial evaluation and over time to identify both primary and secondary impairments. An orthopedist should be consulted depending on the severity of osseous deformity, muscular imbalance, and the resulting functional limitations and participation restrictions. An orthopedist may order imaging and gait analysis assessments that can help guide decisions regarding surgical treatments, including osteotomies and muscle lengthenings or transfers. Assessments can also help guide more conservative treatments, such as stretching, strengthening, positioning, and functional training, carried out primarily by the physical therapist.

■ Excessive Femoral Anteversion (Torsion)

Chief Clinical Characteristics

This presentation includes in-toeing or normal foot progression angle (if compensations exist) as the child walks forward in a straight line. With excessive femoral anteversion, the child usually in-toes and presents with excessive medial hip rotation passive range of motion and reduced lateral hip rotation passive range of motion when compared to age-matched peers.[1,4,21]

Background Information

The twist (or torsion) in the femur at birth orients the femoral neck and head approximately 40 degrees anterior to the transcondylar axis of the knee, thus use of the prefix *ante-* to describe the direction. In typical development, this twist gradually reduces to its mature shape of 15 to 20 degrees of anteversion (torsion) by the time the child is 8 to 10 years old.[4] Excessive femoral anteversion (torsion) is an osseous source of increased hip medial rotation and results in excessive in-toeing. Even though infants and toddlers present with increased femoral anteversion (torsion), they do not in-toe primarily because of the osseous orientation of the pelvis and acetabulum and the soft tissue contracture into lateral hip rotation.[2,4] This condition can be assessed clinically with assessment of passive range-of-motion hip rotation[1] and Ryder's test[5,22]; values outside two standard deviations of typical values are considered abnormal. In these more severe cases, referral to an orthopedic surgeon is indicated, where a more accurate measure of anteversion may be obtained by imaging. After serious pathology is ruled out, nonsurgical treatment should include addressing family concerns, educating the family regarding the natural history of torsion values, and rechecking the child every 6 to 12 months to ensure proper hip development.[23] Nonoperative treatment such as casting, strapping, and shoe wear does not alter the developmental progression of femoral anteversion.[1,24] In more severe cases, or with children who have other pathologies and diagnoses, surgical procedures such as a femoral derotation osteotomy might be necessary, but should be delayed until the child is at least 8 years old.[24,25]

■ Medial Tibial Torsion

Chief Clinical Characteristics

This presentation includes in-toeing, normal foot progression angle, or out-toeing, depending on compensations that may occur in the hip or foot. To diagnose medial tibial torsion, the thigh–foot angle value must indicate a medial orientation. Medial tibial torsion is commonly associated with tibia vara and functional limitations such as clumsy walking, tripping, and falling.[25]

Background Information

This condition is a twist in the tibia from the proximal to the distal end. Medial tibial torsion in an infant can be as much as 30 degrees, but typical ranges with maturity ideally fall around 12 degrees of lateral torsion by the age of 8.[1] Torsion is measured clinically with the thigh–foot angle or transmalleolar axis assessments. This condition is either bilateral or unilateral, affecting the left side more than the right.[22,25] Excessive medial tibial torsion is the most common cause of in-toeing in the toddler ages 1 to 3 years.[25] Because an infant is born with 30 degrees of medial tibial torsion, any delay of the lateral twisting process can contribute to age-matched excessive medial tibial torsion. Other causes that may contribute to this condition are intrauterine positioning, sleeping in the prone position, and sitting on the feet.[1] The resolution of this osseous finding usually occurs by the age of 4,[25] and in 90% of cases by the age of 8,[1] so monitoring over time with parent education about natural history and recommendations to avoid prone sleeping and sitting on the feet are considered the best course of treatment.[1,25] Treatment interventions such as bracing, orthoses, splinting, and exercises have been found to be ineffective, and because long-term complications are minimal, surgery is only recommended in the most severe cases.[1,25]

■ Metatarsus Adductus

Chief Clinical Characteristics

This presentation includes in-toeing with standing and walking. The metatarsals/forefoot deviate medially from the hindfoot to form a "kidney bean–shaped" foot with a deep medial crease and a convex "C-shaped" lateral border.[4] This condition is usually detected in the first year of life, and is the most common cause of in-toeing in infants.[25]

Background Information

Although the etiology is not known, it is believed by some that this condition is secondary to intrauterine position, forces on the foot during development, or an abnormally shaped medial cuneiform.[25] This condition is the most common congenital foot deformity, occurring in as many as 1 out of 1,000 live births[4] and 1 out of 20 live births with siblings or parents with metatarsus adductus.[25] This condition is measured clinically by assessing the position of the forefoot relative to the calcaneus when the hindfoot is placed in subtalar neutral. If the line bisecting the calcaneus extends lateral to the space between the second and third toes, the forefoot is said to be adducted.[4,24] The diagnosis is differentiated from clubfoot deformity because the calcaneus is not in an equino-varus position.[24] Treatment plans and prognosis for this condition are related to the degree of flexibility of the deformity rather than the severity.[25] Flexibility is measured by stabilizing the calcaneus in neutral and abducting the forefoot to end range. A flexible adductus, one that corrects beyond the midline bisector line, usually resolves spontaneously[24,25] and/or with simple stretching exercises performed by the parents.[1] A partly flexible adductus, one that corrects to the midline bisector line, can be treated with serial casting and/or taping or monitored for improvement over time. An in-flexible adductus, one that does not correct to midline, should prompt a referral to an orthopedist. It can then be treated with a course of serial casting for 6 to 8 weeks or manipulation and taping after the age of 6 months.[24] If after the nonsurgical treatment the adductus is not corrected, and if there is pain or functional limitation associated with the deformity, various surgical options may be available for children over the age of 3 or 4.[24,25]

■ Muscle Imbalance or Weakness

Chief Clinical Characteristics

This presentation includes in-toeing gait, often associated with a muscular, neuromuscular, and chromosomal pathology that affects the strength and balance of muscles surrounding the hip, knee, and foot/ankle joints.[17,19,20,26,27]

Background Information

Muscle strength, length, or tone imbalance associated with pathologies such as myelomeningocele or cerebral palsy can be a primary or a secondary/compensatory impairment that affects joint position and alignment in both static and dynamic conditions. Aktas and colleagues concluded that the predicted amount of medial hip rotation (in-toeing) during gait cycle was secondary to dynamic components of muscle use rather than osseous deformities, such as excessive femoral anteversion.[17] Overactive muscles tend to become tight, while underactive muscles become weaker, further contributing to poor alignment and inappropriate muscle coordination. In children without a more definitive diagnosis, muscle imbalance and coordination can also contribute to gait abnormalities. Assessment of any child whose chief complaint is in-toeing should include a lower extremity rotational profile; passive range of motion of hip, knee, and ankle joints; strength testing of opposing muscle groups; and length testing of muscles, especially two/multi-joint muscles such as iliopsoas, hamstrings, and gastrocnemius. Movement analysis gives a picture of dynamic muscle use during functional tasks (eg, walking, climbing stairs, making transitions) and provides additional information on concentric and eccentric muscle strength and coordination. Videotaping and watching movement tasks in slow motion is a feasible method for assessing movement more accurately. Findings that indicate muscle imbalance and weakness can be addressed with exercises for flexibility and strength.[28,29]

■ Talipes Equinovarus (Clubfoot)

Chief Clinical Characteristics

This presentation includes either congenital or acquired hindfoot equinus, midfoot varus, and forefoot adductus,[4] which essentially turns the foot into an in-toe posture with plantarflexion.

Background Information

Acquired clubfoot usually accompanies neuromuscular disorders, such as cerebral palsy, myelomeningocele, and polio. Although no absolute etiology is known, congenital club-foot is most likely a combination of genetics and environment.[4] Increased incidence occurs among families and siblings. Though the foot presents in the same position, each deformity can include different tissues in the lower leg, including osseous deformity or displacement, and dysplasia of muscle, tendon, cartilage, skin, and neurovascular structures.[30] If clubfoot is suspected, an orthopedic surgeon should always be consulted and a systemic assessment should be performed since there is a variable association with other anomalies.[30] This condition can present with various levels of stiffness and will respond to treatment differently. Treatment goals are to (1) provide manipulative correction, (2) restore movement, and (3) maintain correction.[30] Treatment techniques include nonsurgical options such as stretching, serial casting, and orthotics; surgical options exist for those deformities that do not respond to these types of treatment.[4,30]

■ Tethered Cord Syndrome

Chief Clinical Characteristics
This presentation includes progressive gait abnormalities (including increasing in-toeing), recent onset of incontinence, progressive lower extremity muscle weakness or asymmetry, and worsening musculoskeletal deformity. This condition is often associated with other spine or spinal cord malformations such as meningocele, spina bifida occulta, or other spinal dysraphism.[31,32]

Background Information
This condition is a stretch-induced disorder of the spinal cord caused by the anchoring of the caudal end of the spinal cord to the sacrum by inelastic structures formed during infancy and childhood. Although a majority of patients with cord tethering are diagnosed with recognition of cutaneous, musculoskeletal, and vertebral anomalies, some may show slowly progressive or fluctuating signs that are more difficult to detect.[32] Because infants are in the midst of development, this condition can be difficult to differentially diagnose; however, any musculoskeletal deformity such as clubfoot, asymmetric leg length, scoliosis that progresses, or any loss of motor skills

warrants a referral to an orthopedist and neurologist.[32] Imaging can be useful in diagnosing this condition and treatment includes surgery.

Description of Conditions That May Lead to Out-Toeing in a Child

■ Bladder Exstrophy

Chief Clinical Characteristics
This presentation includes out-toeing associated with diastasis of the pubic symphysis, which leads to excessive femoral anteversion and compensatory lateral tibial torsion. Patellar instability can, therefore, be common.[33]

Background Information
This condition is a rare developmental anomaly marked by protrusion and exposure of the posterior bladder through an abdominal defect[34] and is usually accompanied by widely separated ischia. Diagnosed most frequently at birth, infants are immediately referred to a team of medical specialists to begin a series of surgeries for staged reconstruction. The distortion of the pelvis produces an initial lateral rotation deformity in the lower extremities and can contribute to a waddling gait in early childhood; orthopedic complications are less apparent in adolescents.[33] It is hypothesized that an increased femoral anteversion angle compensates for the more retroverted acetabulum such that foot progression angles fall within normal limits by the time children reach a mature gait pattern at age 7.[33] There is no evidence of early onset of osteoarthritis at the hip or tibiofemoral joints; however, there is an increased risk for patellofemoral instability, arthritis and pain, and possible functional limitation and participation restriction.[33]

■ Cerebral Palsy

Chief Clinical Characteristics
This presentation includes either an in-toeing or out-toeing gait accompanied by this neuromuscular disorder.

Background Information
This condition is a movement and posture disorder resulting from nonprogressive damage to the immature central nervous system.[15,16] This damage interferes with the process of

development and often manifests with significant gait deviations secondary to osseous torsional deformity, muscle imbalance and weakness, and poor dynamic coordination.[17–19] Out-toeing gait is often secondary to excessive lateral tibial torsion.[15,17] A complete pelvic and lower extremity musculoskeletal exam is necessary at the initial evaluation and over time to identify both primary and secondary impairments and course of treatment. Orthopedic consultation may be necessary depending on the severity of osseous deformity, muscular imbalance, and the resulting functional limitations and participation restrictions. An orthopedist may order imaging and gait analysis assessments that can help guide decisions regarding surgical treatments, including osteotomies and muscle lengthenings or transfers.

■ Femoral Retroversion (Torsion)

Chief Clinical Characteristics

This presentation includes out-toeing or normal foot progression angle (if compensations exist) as the child walks forward in a straight line. With femoral retroversion, the child usually out-toes and presents with excessive passive range of motion into lateral hip rotation with reduced medial hip rotation, compared to age-matched peers.[1,3,25]

Background Information

The twist (or torsion) in the femur at birth orients the femoral neck and head approximately 40 degrees anterior to the transcondylar axis of the knee, thus use of the prefix *ante-* to describe the direction. In typical development, this twist gradually reduces to its mature shape of 15 to 20 degrees of anteversion (torsion) by the time the child is 8 to 10 years old.[4] Femoral retrotorsion is considered an abnormal finding since the femur is never supposed to present with a posteriorly facing femoral head. Retroversion is an osseous source of increased hip lateral rotation and reduced medial rotation range of motion that results in out-toeing during walking. Other impairments more likely to contribute to out-toeing include lateral hip rotation soft tissue contractures (eg, muscular and capsular restrictions).[25,35] Assess with passive range of motion, noting the end feel, and Ryder's test.[5] If significant out-toeing persists beyond age 3 years, referral to an orthopedist is indicated because this condition can lead to

osteoarthritis, increased risk of stress fracture in the lower extremity, and slipped capital femoral epiphysis.[1] Nonsurgical treatment, including physical therapy, is ineffective.[1]

■ Lateral Tibial Torsion

Chief Clinical Characteristics

This presentation includes out-toeing, normal foot progression angle, or in-toeing, depending on compensations that may occur in the hip or foot. To diagnose lateral tibial torsion, the thigh–foot angle value must indicate a lateral orientation that is two standard deviations greater than that of age-matched peers. Lateral tibial torsion is more commonly seen in children with neuromuscular conditions such as cerebral palsy, spina bifida, and polio.[25]

Background Information

Lateral tibial torsion is a twist in the tibia from the proximal to the distal end. Excessive lateral tibial torsion contributes to out-toeing in children of all ages, but is most often seen in late childhood or early adolescence.[25] It is thought that this condition can contribute to patellofemoral pain and instability.[25] To properly diagnose, educate the family, and plan treatment, it is essential to measure the osseous rotational profile of the entire leg and determine muscle strength balances or imbalances so that deformities and compensations can be detected. Any abnormal findings should lead to referral to an orthopedic surgeon. Nonsurgical treatment to reduce this condition has been found to be ineffective, but surgical intervention is a possibility for children older than 10 years with a greater than 40-degree thigh–foot angle and functional limitation and pain secondary to patellar instability.[1]

■ Muscle Imbalance or Weakness

Chief Clinical Characteristics

This presentation includes out-toeing gait, often associated with a muscular, neuromuscular, and chromosomal pathology that affects the strength and balance of muscles surrounding the hip, knee, and foot/ankle joints.[17,19,20,26,27]

Background Information

Muscle strength, length, or tone imbalance associated with pathologies such as myelomeningocele or cerebral palsy can be a primary or a secondary/compensatory impairment that affects joint position and alignment in both static and dynamic conditions. Overactive muscles tend to become tight, while underactive muscles become weaker, further contributing to poor alignment and inappropriate muscle coordination. In children without a more definitive diagnosis, muscle imbalance and coordination can also contribute to gait abnormalities. Assessment of any child whose chief complaint is out-toeing should include a lower extremity rotational profile; passive range of motion of hip, knee, and ankle joints; strength testing of opposing muscle groups; and length testing of muscles, especially two/multi-joint muscles such as iliopsoas, hamstrings, and gastrocnemius. Movement analysis gives a picture of dynamic muscle use during functional tasks (eg, walking, climbing stairs, making transitions) and provides information on concentric and eccentric muscle strength and coordination. Treatment based on findings should incorporate dynamic stretching techniques, progressive resistance training, and functional task practice to incorporate improved biomechanics and muscle coordination in specific conditions.[28,29]

■ Overweight and Obesity

Chief Clinical Characteristics
This presentation includes a child who seems to carry excess weight for his or her body structure. The child's gait pattern may include slow velocity, reduced cadence, longer stance periods, wider stride, out-toeing, and/or flat feet.[36]

Background Information
Obesity is a pathological increase in fat, which can result from a sedentary lifestyle, excessive intake of high-energy food, and a genetic predisposition to fat storage.[37] Other risk factors in the development of overweight children include overweight parents, low parental concerns about their child's level of thinness, reduced sleep, and child tantrums

over food.[38] The BMI, or body mass index, is used to diagnose children who are overweight or at risk for overweight.[39] In English conversion values, BMI = weight in pounds ÷ height in inches ÷ height in inches × 703, and can easily be measured in the clinic and compared to Centers for Disease Control and Prevention developmental charts (Figs. 61-3 and 61-4).[40,41] Children at or above the 95th percentile are said to be obese and children at or above the 85th percentile are said to be overweight. Children who are overweight and their parents should receive extensive education about the medical and health risks of being overweight. A team of medical-health professionals including but not limited to physicians, nutrition specialists, and physical therapists can help to implement a comprehensive program to reduce overweight and its associated complications.

■ Slipped Capital Femoral Epiphysis

Chief Clinical Characteristics
This presentation includes unilateral out-toeing associated with a limp (decreased weight bearing on affected side) and acute onset of pain in the knee and/or distal thigh or pain in the hip, groin, or proximal thigh region.[42]

Background Information
In this condition, the proximal femoral epiphysis is displaced, usually posteriorly, on the femoral neck. Obesity can be a related factor when suspecting this condition.[43] Because increased pain is associated with hip medial rotation, often the child will position the hip in lateral rotation, which results in an out-toeing posture.[44] If this condition is suspected by the physical therapist, immediate referral to an orthopedist is essential. Diagnosis is confirmed by x-ray and treatment may consist of surgery and postsurgical rehabilitation.

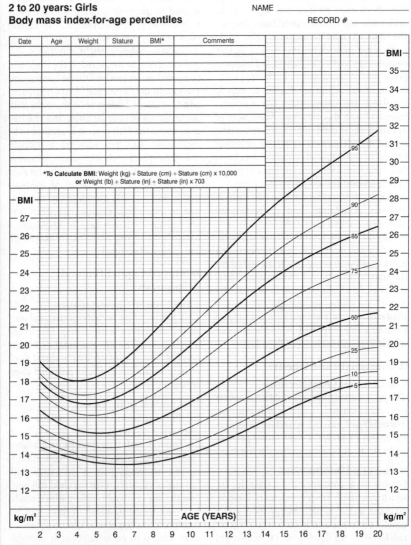

FIGURE 61-3 Developmental chart for body mass index: girls, ages 2 to 20 years.

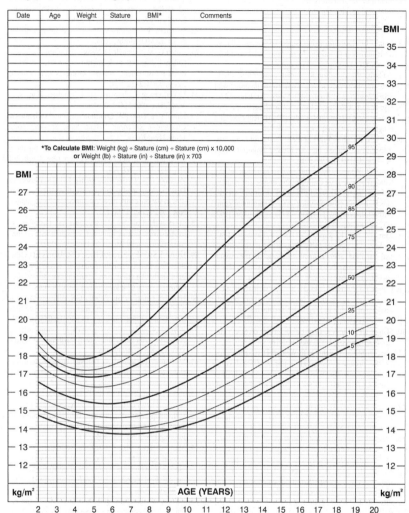

2 to 20 years: Boys
Body mass index-for-age percentiles

NAME _____

RECORD # _____

Published May 30, 2000 (modified 10/16/00).
SOURCE: Developed by the National Center for Health Statistics in collaboration with
the National Center for Chronic Disease Prevention and Health Promotion (2000).
http://www.cdc.gov/growthcharts

FIGURE 61-4 Developmental chart for body mass index: boys, ages 2 to 20 years.

References

1. Sass P, Hassan G. Lower extremity abnormalities in children. *Am Fam Physician.* Aug 1, 2003;68(3):461–468.
2. Staheli LT, Corbett M, Wyss C, King H. Lower-extremity rotational problems in children. Normal values to guide management. *J Bone Joint Surg Am.* Jan 1985;67 (1):39–47.
3. Killam PE. Orthopedic assessment of young children: developmental variations. *Nurse Pract.* Jul 1989;14(7): 27–30, 32–34, 36.
4. Wallach DM, Davidson RS. Pediatric lower limb disorders. In: Dormans JP, ed. *Pediatric Orthopedics and Sports Medicine.* St. Louis, MO: Mosby; 2004:246–272.
5. *Legs & Feet: A Review of Musculoskeletal Assessment Procedures for Children and Adults* [DVD]. Telluride, CO: Progressive GaitWays; 2005.
6. Rao KN, Joseph B. Value of measurement of hip movements in childhood hip disorders. *J Pediatr Orthop.* Jul–Aug 2001;21(4):495–501.
7. Kim HT, Wenger DR. "Functional retroversion" of the femoral head in Legg-Calve-Perthes disease and epiphyseal dysplasia: analysis of head-neck deformity and its effect on limb position using three-dimensional computed tomography. *J Pediatr Orthop.* Mar–Apr 1997; 17(2):240–246.
8. Kim HK, Bian H, Randall T, Garces A, Gerstenfeld LC, Einhorn TA. Increased VEGF expression in the epiphyseal cartilage after ischemic necrosis of the capital femoral epiphysis. *J Bone Miner Res.* Dec 2004; 19(12):2041–2048.
9. Comte F, De Rosa V, Zekri H, et al. Confirmation of the early prognostic value of bone scanning and pinhole imaging of the hip in Legg-Calve-Perthes disease. *J Nucl Med.* 2003;44(11):1761–1766.
10. Skaggs DL, Tolo VT. Legg-Calve-Perthes disease. *J Am Acad Orthop Surg.* Jan 1996;4(1):9–16.
11. Herceg MB, Cutright MT, Weiner DS. Remodeling of the proximal femur after upper femoral varus osteotomy for the treatment of Legg-Calve-Perthes disease. *J Pediatr Orthop.* Nov–Dec 2004;24(6): 654–657.
12. Tamai J, Erol B, Dormans JP. Hip disorders. In: Dormans JP, ed. *Pediatric Orthopedics and Sports Medicine.* St. Louis, MO: Mosby; 2004:175–212.
13. Loder RT, Schwartz EM, Hensinger RN. Behavioral characteristics of children with Legg-Calve-Perthes disease. *J Pediatr Orthop.* Sep–Oct 1993;13(5):598–601.
14. Herring JA, Kim HT, Browne R. Legg-Calve-Perthes disease. Part II: Prospective multicenter study of the effect of treatment on outcome. *J Bone Joint Surg Am.* Oct 2004;86-A(10):2121–2134.
15. Spiegel DA. Cerebral palsy. In: Dormans JP, ed. *Pediatric Orthopaedics and Sports Medicine.* St. Louis, MO: Mosby; 2004:373–415.
16. Shapiro BK. Cerebral palsy: A reconceptualization of the spectrum. *J Pediatr.* Aug 2004;145(2 suppl):S3–7.
17. Aktas S, Aiona MD, Orendurff M. Evaluation of rotational gait abnormality in the patients cerebral palsy. *J Pediatr Orthop.* Mar–Apr 2000;20(2):217–220.
18. Waskin MR, Frost JP, Hatalowich GS. Cerebral palsy: a podiatric overview. *J Foot Surg.* Winter 1983;22(4): 362–365.
19. Root L. Varus and valgus foot in cerebral palsy and its management. *Foot Ankle.* Jan–Feb 1984;4(4):174–179.
20. Flynn JM, Miller F. Management of hip disorders in patients with cerebral palsy. *J Am Acad Orthop Surg.* May–Jun 2002;10(3):198–209.
21. Staheli LT. In-toeing and out-toeing. In: Staheli LT, ed. *Pediatric Orthopedic Secrets.* 2nd ed. Philadelphia, PA: Hanley & Belfus; 2003:213–221.
22. Dormans JP. *Pediatric Orthopedics and Sports Medicine.* St. Louis, MO: Mosby; 2004.
23. Gulan G, Matovinovic D, Nemec B, Rubinic D, Ravlic-Gulan J. Femoral neck anteversion: values, development, measurement, common problems. *Coll Antropol.* Dec 2000;24(2):521–527.
24. Li YH, Leong JC. Intoeing gait in children. *Hong Kong Med J.* Dec 1999;5(4):360–366.
25. Lincoln TL, Suen PW. Common rotational variations in children. *J Am Acad Orthop Surg.* Sep–Oct 2003; 11(5):312–320.
26. Carroll NC. Assessment and management of the lower extremity in myelodysplasia. *Orthop Clin North Am.* Oct 1987;18(4):709–724.
27. Westcott MA, Dynes MC, Remer EM, Donaldson JS, Dias LS. Congenital and acquired orthopedic abnormalities in patients with myelomeningocele. *Radiographics.* Nov 1992;12(6):1155–1173.
28. Morton JF, Brownlee M, McFadyen AK. The effects of progressive resistance training for children with cerebral palsy. *Clin Rehabil.* May 2005;19(3):283–289.
29. Blundell SW, Shepherd RB, Dean CM, Adams RD, Cahill BM. Functional strength training in cerebral palsy: a pilot study of a group circuit training class for children aged 4–8 years. *Clin Rehabil.* Feb 2003;17(1):48–57.
30. Hart ES, Grottkau BE, Rebello GN, Albright MB. The newborn foot: diagnosis and management of common conditions. *Orthop Nurs.* Sep–Oct 2005;24(5):313–321.
31. Roye BD, Davidson RS. Spina bifida. In: Dormans JP, ed. *Pediatric Orthopedics and Sports Medicine.* St. Louis, MO: Mosby; 2004:417–436.
32. Michelson D, Ashwal S. Tethered cord syndrome in childhood: diagnostic features and relationship to congenital anomalies. *Neurol Res.* 2004;26:745–753.
33. Yazici M, Kandemir U, Atilla B, Eryilmaz M. Rotational profile of lower extremities in bladder exstrophy patients with unapproximated pelvis: a clinical and radiologic study in children older than 7 years. *J Pediatr Orthop.* Jul–Aug 1999;19(4):531–535.
34. Martinez-Frias ML, Bermejo E, Rodriguez-Pinilla E, Frias JL. Exstrophy of the cloaca and exstrophy of the bladder: two different expressions of a primary developmental field defect. *Am J Med Genet.* Apr 1, 2001; 99(4):261–269.
35. Pitkow RB. External rotation contracture of the extended hip. A common phenomenon of infancy obscuring femoral neck anteversion and the most frequent cause of out-toeing gait in children. *Clin Orthop Relat Res.* Jul–Aug 1975(110):139–145.
36. Hills AP, Parker AW. Gait characteristics of obese children. *Arch Phys Med Rehabil.* May 1991;72(6):403–407.
37. Piechota G, Malkiewicz J, Karwat ID. [Obesity as a cause and result of disability]. *Przegl Epidemiol.* 2005; 59(1):155–161.
38. Agras WS, Hammer LD, McNicholas F, Kraemer HC. Risk factors for childhood overweight: a prospective study from birth to 9.5 years. *J Pediatr.* Jul 2004; 145(1):20–25.

39. Kuczmarski RJ, Ogden CL, Guo SS, et al. 2000 CDC growth charts for the United States: methods and development. *Vital Health Stat 11.* 2002;246:1–190.

40. BMI chart for girls ages 2–20. National Center for Health Statistics with National Center for Chronic Disease Prevention and Health Promotion; 2000.

41. BMI chart for boys ages 2–20. National Center for Health Statistics with National Center for Chronic Disease Prevention and Health Promotion; 2000.

42. Matava MJ, Patton CM, Luhmann S, Gordon JE, Schoenecker PL. Knee pain as the initial symptom of slipped capital femoral epiphysis: an analysis of initial presentation and treatment. *J Pediatr Orthop.* Jul–Aug 1999;19(4):455–460.

43. Jingushi S, Suenaga E. Slipped capital femoral epiphysis: etiology and treatment. *J Orthop Sci.* 2004;9(2):214–219.

44. Canale ST. Slipped capital femoral epiphysis. In: Staheli LT, ed. *Pediatric Orthopedic Secrets.* 2nd ed. Philadelphia, PA: Hanley & Belfus; 2003:290–293.

CHAPTER 62

Flat Feet in a Child

■ *Wendi W. McKenna, PT, DPT, PCS*

Description of the Symptom

Flat feet, whether rigid or flexible, are defined as having an abnormally low medial longitudinal arch. Flat feet often present symmetric bilaterally, though one side might be slightly more affected than the other. This chapter describes possible causes of flat feet in a child.

Special Concerns

■ Post-traumatic changes in lower extremity alignment or a painful limp
■ Progressive limp leading to refusal to walk with or without pain
■ Grossly asymmetric presentation of lower extremity alignment
■ History of multiple fractures

CHAPTER PREVIEW: Conditions That May Lead to Flat Feet in a Child

T Trauma

COMMON

Ligamentous laxity/joint hypermobility 1184

UNCOMMON

Spring ligament rupture 1186
Tibialis posterior muscle weakness 1187
Tibialis posterior tendon rupture 1187

RARE

Post-traumatic/fracture healing disturbances and abnormal growth 1186

I Inflammation

COMMON

Not applicable

UNCOMMON

Not applicable

RARE

Not applicable

M Metabolic

COMMON

Overweight and obesity 1185

UNCOMMON

Not applicable

RARE

Not applicable

Va Vascular

COMMON

Not applicable

UNCOMMON

Not applicable

RARE

Not applicable

De Degenerative

COMMON

Not applicable

UNCOMMON

Not applicable

RARE

Not applicable

Tu Tumor

COMMON

Not applicable

UNCOMMON

Not applicable

RARE

Malignant Primary:
Not applicable
Malignant Metastatic:
Not applicable
Benign, such as:
• Osteochondromatosis (multiple hereditary exostosis) 1185

Co Congenital

COMMON

Ligamentous laxity/joint hypermobility 1184
Triceps surae muscle contracture 1187

UNCOMMON

Tarsal coalition (peroneal spastic flat foot) 1186

RARE

Congenital vertical talus 1184

FLAT FEET IN A CHILD

Ne Neurogenic/Psychogenic

COMMON

Cerebral palsy 1184
Myelodysplasia 1185

UNCOMMON

Not applicable

RARE

Not applicable

Note: These are estimates of relative incidence because few data are available for the less common conditions.

Common Ages at Which Flat Feet Present in a Child

APPROXIMATE AGE	CONDITION
Birth to 3 Years	Cerebral palsy Congenital vertical talus Ligamentous laxity/joint hypermobility Myelodysplasia Overweight and obesity Tibialis posterior muscle weakness Triceps surae muscle contracture
Preschool (3–5 Years)	Cerebral palsy Congenital vertical talus Ligamentous laxity/joint hypermobility Myelodysplasia Overweight and obesity Tibialis posterior muscle weakness Post-traumatic/fracture healing disturbances and abnormal growth Triceps surae muscle contracture
Elementary School (6–11 Years)	Cerebral palsy Congenital vertical talus Ligamentous laxity/joint hypermobility Myelodysplasia Osteochondromatosis (multiple hereditary exostosis) Overweight and obesity Post-traumatic/fracture healing disturbances and abnormal growth Spring ligament rupture Tarsal coalition Tibialis posterior muscle weakness Tibialis posterior tendon rupture Triceps surae muscle contracture
Middle School (12–14 Years)	Cerebral palsy Ligamentous laxity/joint hypermobility Myelodysplasia Osteochondromatosis (multiple hereditary exostosis) Overweight and obesity Post-traumatic/fracture healing disturbances and abnormal growth Spring ligament rupture Tarsal coalition Tibialis posterior muscle weakness

Common Ages at Which Flat Feet Present in a Child—cont'd

APPROXIMATE AGE	CONDITION
	Tibialis posterior tendon rupture
	Triceps surae muscle contracture
High School (15–18 Years)	Cerebral palsy
	Ligamentous laxity/joint hypermobility
	Myelodysplasia
	Overweight and obesity
	Post-traumatic/fracture healing disturbances and abnormal growth
	Spring ligament rupture
	Tarsal coalition
	Tibialis posterior muscle weakness
	Tibialis posterior tendon rupture
	Triceps surae muscle contracture

Overview of Flat Feet in a Child

Despite the natural progression and spontaneous resolution of flat feet in children, parents and grandparents will often present their children to a physical therapist concerned about their child's seemingly abnormal alignment. Many parents and grandparents, when they themselves were children, received special bracing or orthotic shoes to help "correct" their flat feet[1] and, therefore, often present their children and grandchildren looking for similar treatment. However, our current understanding is that most children typically present with flat feet that resolve spontaneously over time, causing no long-term functional limitations and participation restrictions and requiring no treatment.[2] Treatment is usually only indicated and effective if a child presents with functional limitations and impairments caused by the flat feet such as excessive clumsiness or falling, pain, or alignment values that are two or more standard deviations from normal.

Physical therapists must always assess static and dynamic conditions in order to obtain a complete picture of lower extremity biomechanics, including the effects of one joint on more proximal or distal joints.[3] Only then will more benign, cosmetic issues in normal development be differentiated from functional issues that may contribute to current or future musculoskeletal impairments. Oftentimes, concerns regarding flat feet can be sufficiently addressed by educating the parents and grandparents regarding typical development of alignment and biomechanics and scheduling follow-up appointments to monitor progress of alignment.

The most common structural presentation of flat feet includes excessive calcaneal eversion, excessive subtalar and midtarsal pronation, a dropped navicular, and/or a low medial longitudinal arch.[4] Excessive pronation during the gait cycle can be identified if the foot does not adequately supinate during midstance and terminal stance to provide a rigid lever off of which to progress forward.[5] Flat feet are very common in young children because the medial longitudinal arch does not fully develop until the child is 4 to 5 years old.[5,6] When a concern is raised, the physical therapist must first determine whether the flat foot is flexible or rigid. A flexible flat foot is one in which the medial longitudinal arch is observed in non–weight-bearing positions and collapses down when in a weight-bearing position; a rigid flat foot maintains the low arch position despite the weight-bearing condition.

Flat feet can be either a congenital or an acquired deformity. The foot is a remarkable structure with both passive and dynamic characteristics that allow it to both relax, conforming to surfaces and providing good shock absorption qualities, and to become more rigid, providing a lever for energy conservation and transmission during forward walking. If there is an imbalance in these passive and dynamic forces over time, medial longitudinal arch collapse can result.[7] Some causes of and associations with acquired flat-foot deformities are triceps surae muscle contracture, overweight and obesity, tibialis posterior muscle weakness or dysfunction, and ligamentous laxity.[7]

Neuromuscular dysfunction as seen in cerebral palsy and myelodysplasia can also contribute to flat feet secondary to muscle imbalance and bone growth abnormalities, such as valgus deformity at the distal tibia that can give the appearance of flat feet.[8] Assessing the location and relationship of the medial and lateral malleoli can help to determine whether osseous deformity exists. However, the most common cause of flat feet is ligamentous laxity.[6] When assessing the foot, one must also consider the entire lower extremity, the child's height and weight, and any correlation with the child's balance and functional gross motor skills.[3,5] Although controversy exists as to whether orthotic intervention is appropriate to correct a flexible flat-foot condition,[9] function must always be considered before a decision is made. If a child performs poorly on gross motor and physical tasks or walking velocity is slower than that of her or his peers, possible intervention should be considered.[3]

Description of Conditions That May Lead to Flat Feet in a Child

■ **Cerebral Palsy**

Chief Clinical Characteristics
This presentation includes either a flat-foot gait or equinus gait accompanied by this neuromuscular disorder.

Background Information
This condition is a neurodevelopmental disorder caused by a nonprogressive lesion in the immature brain that occurs *in utero* or during or shortly after birth. Although the initial lesion is unchanging, the associated motor impairments and sensory deficits associated with the lesion can progress as the child grows and develops.[10] Children with cerebral palsy often present with triceps surae muscle contracture combined with foot and ankle muscle weakness and imbalance. These impairments contribute to increased calcaneal valgus deformity, flattened medial longitudinal arch, and secondary forefoot varus deformity.[1,11] Impairments and deformities at the

hip and knee joints also commonly contribute to the overall presentation of static foot alignment and dynamic function, necessitating a comprehensive evaluation. Physical therapists should refer children with cerebral palsy to an orthopedist, who will routinely follow up with these children every 6 to 12 months. Nonsurgical intervention strategies that help align the foot in a more rectus position include dynamic and static stretching, strengthening, bracing, and serial casting. However, if bony changes occur or contractures are significant, surgical intervention may be necessary.[12]

■ **Congenital Vertical Talus**

Chief Clinical Characteristics
This presentation includes a rare rigid flat foot that is present at birth and is caused by a dorsal dislocation of the navicular on the talus and equinus and valgus of the calcaneus.[13–15] The talus head can be palpated as a bump under the plantar surface of the foot. The plantar surface of the foot, therefore, has a convex appearance in weight-bearing and non–weight-bearing conditions and is often referred to as a "congenital rocker-bottom foot."[14]

Background Information
The true congenital vertical talus found at birth has an unknown etiology, but is reported to have familial tendencies; it may also occur in association with myelomeningocele, arthrogryposis, and congenital hip dislocation.[14] Diagnosis, confirmed by radiograph, is followed by required surgical correction,[13–15] with best results occurring in children who have surgery before 2 years of age.[1] Untreated congenital vertical talus will eventually lead to grossly abnormal gait characteristics, callus formation, possible ulceration on the talar head, and secondary changes and impairments in the foot complex.[15] Physical therapists should refer children with congenital vertical talus to a pediatric orthopedic surgeon as early as possible.

■ **Ligamentous Laxity/Joint Hypermobility**

Chief Clinical Characteristics
This presentation includes children with a flexible flat foot and a score greater than a 4 or 5 according to the Beighton criteria.

Background Information

The Beighton criteria include:

1. Passive extension of the fifth finger at metacarpophalangeal joint to ≥90 degrees
2. Passive apposition of the thumb to the forearm
3. Hyperextension of elbow ≥10 degrees
4. Hyperextension of the knee ≥10 degrees
5. Ability to rest entire palm of hand on floor with forward flexion and extended knees.

As previously discussed, the foot and ankle complex relies on a balance of passive constraints and dynamic support to ensure the foot maintains its integrity. Any systemic laxity in foot and ankle ligaments, including the spring ligament and deltoid ligament, can contribute to a flat-foot deformity.[7,16,17] Assessment of the flat foot includes posture analysis, ligament stress tests, observation of the windlass effect (extension of the first metatarsal phalangeal joint in weight-bearing), a manual muscle test of the tibialis posterior, observation of the medial longitudinal arch under weight-bearing and non–weight-bearing conditions and during gait, and assessment of the flexibility of the flat-foot deformity with reconstitution of the arch during a heel rise.[1,18] Often flexible flat foot is a benign condition that does not require treatment; however, if impairments are assessed treatment may include orthoses, strengthening, and neuromuscular re-education aimed at rebalancing the forces causing the malalignment and impairments.[4,7] Rarely is surgery indicated to correct the flat-foot deformity that is secondary to ligament laxity.

■ **Myelodysplasia**

Chief Clinical Characteristics

This presentation includes hindfoot valgus that progresses from a flexible flat foot to a more severe, rigid, and painful deformity as the child grows and develops. Children with this condition typically wear braces from an early age to help align the feet in a more rectus position and provide support for absent or weakened musculature; however, with the long-term influence of gravity, muscle imbalance, ambulation, and insensate feet, children may present with reduced tolerance for brace and shoe wear, increased pain, and incidence of ulceration.[19]

Background Information

This condition, also commonly referred to as spina bifida or myelomeningocele, is defined in *Dorland's Medical Dictionary* as "a defective development of any part (especially the lower segments) of the spinal cord." Hindfoot deformities have been reported in 50% to 75% of children with myelodysplasia; equinovarus foot is commonly seen in newborn infants while progressive valgus hindfoot is seen after the child begins to ambulate and gain weight.[19] Radiographs, especially those taken in weight-bearing positions, can help identify the integrity of talocrural, subtalar, and midtarsal joints, which can often be implicated secondary to bone growth abnormalities. Although treatment usually starts nonsurgically with bracing, if a child experiences pain, difficulty ambulating, increased incidence of skin ulcerations, and intolerance to brace and shoe wear, surgery may be necessary.[19,20]

■ **Osteochondromatosis (Multiple Hereditary Exostosis)**

Chief Clinical Characteristics

This presentation includes children and adolescents with multiple exostoses (osteochondromas) that may cause pain or cosmetic concerns. Ankle valgus deformity, which contributes to a flat-foot posture, can occur in up to 50% of patients with this condition.

Background Information

This condition is an autosomal dominant disorder that affects between 0.9 and 2 people per 100,000; diagnosis is confirmed with chromosomal analysis and identification of mutations in the *EXT1* and *EXT2* genes. Osteochondromas, which can be identified clinically and confirmed with radiograph, are benign bone tumors that consist of cartilage-capped exostoses at the metaphyses of rapidly growing ends of long bones.[21,22] Surgical intervention is necessary to remove exostoses, to prevent progression of exostoses, and to provide correction of secondary orthopedic deformities.[21]

■ **Overweight and Obesity**

Chief Clinical Characteristics

This presentation includes children with a body mass index (BMI) of 85th percentile or higher, indicating overweight and obesity, and flat-foot deformity as defined by a low medial longitudinal arch.[4,7,23]

Background Information

Please refer to the discussion on overweight and obesity in Chapter 61. Bordin and colleagues[23] demonstrated a significant increase in the incidence of flat feet with overweight children ages 8 to 10 years. Diagnosis of the two associated conditions is made by obtaining the BMI to determine overweight and assessing the hindfoot valgus, midfoot pronation, and forefoot abduction to determine level of flat-foot deformity. The flexibility of the flat foot can be diagnosed by observing the reconstitution of the medial longitudinal arch (1) during the windlass effect with extension of the first metatarsal phalangeal joint, (2) during an active heel rise or (3) in non–weight-bearing conditions.[1,14] Diagnosis can be confirmed with standing radiographs of the hindfoot, but this is usually unnecessary unless the foot is symptomatic.[14] Treatment consists of lowering the BMI through a comprehensive weight management program and addressing the abnormal foot alignment with custom or off-the-shelf orthoses, strengthening, and neuromuscular re-education.

■ Post-Traumatic/Fracture Healing Disturbances and Abnormal Growth

Chief Clinical Characteristics

This presentation includes calcaneal valgus or varus deformity following calcaneal fracture, pain, and range-of-motion limitations in the subtalar joint.[24]

Background Information

When the subtalar joint is in a position of valgus, it biomechanically unlocks the midtarsal joints, which lowers the medial longitudinal arch and causes a flat foot. With prolonged flat-foot deformity, ligament, capsule, and muscle supports on the medial aspect of the foot are stretched abnormally and put at risk for secondary dysfunction. As children grow, it is important for muscle/tendon and ground reaction forces to be appropriately aligned because they contribute to the development of bone shape and joint spaces, dictating the joint biomechanics in the lower extremity. Any abnormal forces can cause secondary growth abnormalities and progressive joint deformities that may present with adverse clinical symptoms.[25,26] If a child continues to present with significant pain and deformity following the typical healing time of a calcaneal fracture, referral to an orthopedist is required. In two out of three cases, Jarde and colleagues[24] report that subtalar arthrodesis surgery can yield good results; however, surgery should be avoided if typical subtalar alignment and range of motion can be obtained without pain. Jarde et al.[24] also recommend that talonavicular arthrodesis should be avoided since it must block the movement of a normal joint in order to address a painful joint.

■ Spring Ligament Rupture

Chief Clinical Characteristics

This presentation includes a history of tibialis posterior tendon dysfunction and/or rupture that can lead to progressive tearing, stretching, and finally rupture of the plantar calcaneonavicular (spring) ligament. Pain that progresses from the medial hindfoot to the lateral side near the sinus tarsi while the medial longitudinal arch becomes flatter can accompany this course of events.[27]

Background Information

The spring ligament is a vital stabilizer of the medial longitudinal arch, but as a passive structure, it depends on the dynamic support of surrounding muscles and tendons to maintain its integrity over time. If there is chronic dysfunction of the tibialis posterior muscle and tendon, which is the primary dynamic stabilizer of the hindfoot,[27] then the ligament is required to carry the load of the talus independently, which it can only do for a limited period of time.[17] Usually this rupture occurs later in childhood or adolescence secondary to the time needed to cause the tendon dysfunction, ligament tear and laxity, and complete rupture.[28] Definitive diagnosis requires magnetic resonance imaging and treatment consists of orthopedic surgery to plicate the spring ligament. Often simultaneous surgical repair or reconstruction of the tibialis posterior muscle is also necessary.[17]

■ Tarsal Coalition (Peroneal Spastic Flat Foot)

Chief Clinical Characteristics

This presentation includes rigid flat foot that may be painful and is associated with limited or absent subtalar joint motion. There may be a history of frequent ankle sprains and fractures secondary to poor ability to negotiate uneven terrain.[1] The talocalcaneal coalition (TCC) usually has poorly localized hindfoot pain.[29] The symptoms are more localized to the region of interest in the calcaneonavicular coalition (CNC).[30] Quick inversion of the foot (stretch reflex of the peroneal muscles) causes a spasm or clonus response and immediate, severe pain.[31]

Background Information
Tarsal coalition is an abnormal fusion of two or more tarsal bones, preventing formation of a mobile joint.[1] Coalitions can be formed by fibrous, cartilaginous, or osseous tissue and are commonly diagnosed in childhood and adolescence, when the child is closer to skeletal maturity. Diagnosis is confirmed with use of standing, weight-bearing radiographs.[1,14] There is a greater male-to-female ratio for tarsal coalition[29,30,32] with CNC most commonly diagnosed in children 8 to 12 years old and TCC in children 10 to 14 years old.[29,30,32] Oblique radiographs and computed tomography are the best way to properly identify the union of various joint surfaces.[14] Nonsurgical management to help the symptomatic foot consists of immobilization or casting followed by fabrication of custom orthoses that minimize subtalar motion[1]; however, surgical intervention is usually considered the best option for treatment.[30,32,33]

■ **Tibialis Posterior Muscle Weakness**

Chief Clinical Characteristics
This presentation includes flat foot, including hindfoot valgus and midfoot pronation associated with weakness of the tibialis posterior muscle.

Background Information
Tibialis posterior muscle dysfunction has been implicated as a source of progressive pes planus in adults,[34,35] but weakness in children with flat feet is also a possibility since the position of the foot influences the efficient and consistent recruitment of the tibialis posterior muscle.[34] Diagnosis of this condition can be confirmed clinically with manual muscle test. Treatment is nonsurgical and consists of orthoses and exercise to strengthen the muscle and improve selective recruitment during gait.

■ **Tibialis Posterior Tendon Rupture**

Chief Clinical Characteristics
This presentation includes progressive flat foot of either an insidious onset without discomfort or accompanied by pain, tenderness, and swelling behind the medial malleolus.[36] In children, this tendon injury is commonly associated with the presence of a scar around the medial malleolus secondary to an old laceration injury.[37] It may also be associated with a history of excessive beach walking.

Background Information
This condition in both children and adolescents[28,37,38] can go undiagnosed for a period of time if it presents as an insidious onset of progressive flattening of the foot without pain, even despite nonsurgical treatment such as wearing orthoses or heel cups.[37] Any progressive deformity needs to be identified by assessing dynamic (muscle) and static (ligament, capsule, bone) supports of the medial longitudinal arch. Manual muscle test and palpation of the tendon and muscle belly, comparing both sides, can help to determine the integrity of the tibialis posterior tendon and muscle. In the case of tendon rupture, which on many occasions is definitively diagnosed with surgical exploration, repair or tendon transfer surgery may be necessary.[28,37,39]

■ **Triceps Surae Muscle Contracture**

Chief Clinical Characteristics
This presentation includes contracture of the triceps surae muscle, defined as passive range-of-motion dorsiflexion limited to less than 10 degrees, and resulting flat foot with a low medial longitudinal arch. Older children present with tight triceps surae more often than younger children, and there is a strong correlation between flat feet in adolescence and triceps surae contracture.[11] Lateral tibial torsion combined with shortened triceps surae can also contribute to a flat-foot presentation.[4,40]

Background Information
During typical gait, the ankle must be able to achieve 10 degrees of dorsiflexion during terminal stance as the tibia translates over the talus. However, this condition inhibits this functional range at the talocrural joint. Rather than shortening the step length to accommodate the contracture, the child compensates

with prolonged and excessive subtalar eversion and midfoot pronation when the foot should be supinated into a more rigid lever. Over time, this abnormally prolonged pronation can exacerbate muscle imbalance and weakness and also contribute to ligament laxity and a chronic flat-foot deformity. Reimers and colleagues[11] reported that as children grow older, their feet normally develop a higher medial longitudinal arch, citing a decrease of flat feet from 42% to 6% between the ages of 3 and 17 years. However, Reimers and colleagues[11] also found an increase in the incidence of triceps surae contracture and a 100% correlation with flat-foot deformity. If a child presents with a flat-foot deformity, triceps surae contracture is probably one of the contributing factors. Depending on the severity of the contracture and other adverse symptoms, referral to an orthopedist may be necessary. Treatment may include serial casting with or without botulinum toxin injection to increase range of motion into dorsiflexion, surgical lengthening procedures of the heel cord, and possible bony corrections to reconstitute the medial longitudinal arch.[1]

References

1. Wallach DM, Davidson RS. Pediatric lower limb disorders. In: Dormans JP, ed. *Pediatric Orthopedics and Sports Medicine*. St. Louis, MO: Mosby; 2004:246–272.
2. Staheli LT, Corbett M, Wyss C, King H. Lower-extremity rotational problems in children. Normal values to guide management. *J Bone Joint Surg Am*. Jan 1985;67(1):39–47.
3. Lin CJ, Lai KA, Kuan TS, Chou YL. Correlating factors and clinical significance of flexible flatfoot in preschool children. *J Pediatr Orthop*. May–Jun 2001;21(3):378–382.
4. Napolitano C, Walsh S, Mahoney L, McCrea J. Risk factors that may adversely modify the natural history of the pediatric pronated foot. *Clin Podiatr Med Surg*. Jul 2000;17(3):397–417.
5. Buccieri KM. Use of orthoses and early intervention physical therapy to minimize hyperpronation and promote functional skills in a child with gross motor delays: a case report. *Phys Occup Ther Pediatr*. 2003;23(1):5–20.
6. Sass P, Hassan G. Lower extremity abnormalities in children. *Am Fam Physician*. Aug 1, 2003;68(3):461–468.
7. Van Boerum DH, Sangeorzan BJ. Biomechanics and pathophysiology of flat foot. *Foot Ankle Clin*. Sep 2003; 8(3):419–430.
8. Burkus JK, Moore DW, Raycroft JF. Valgus deformity of the ankle in myelodysplastic patients. Correction by stapling of the medial part of the distal tibial physis. *J Bone Joint Surg Am*. Oct 1983;65(8):1157–1162.
9. Hogan M, Staheli LT. Arch height and lower limb pain: an adult civilian study. *Foot Ankle*. 2002;23(1):43–47.
10. Olney SJ, Wright MJ. Cerebral palsy. In: Campbell SK, Vander Linden DW, Palisano R, eds. *Physical Therapy for Children*. 3rd ed. St. Louis, MO: Saunders Elsevier; 2006:625–664.
11. Reimers J, Pedersen B, Brodersen A. Foot deformity and the length of the triceps surae in Danish children between 3 and 17 years old. *J Pediatr Orthop B*. 1995;4(1):71–73.
12. Root L. Varus and valgus foot in cerebral palsy and its management. *Foot Ankle*. Jan–Feb 1984;4(4):174–179.
13. Badelon O, Rigault P, Pouliquen JC, Padovani JP, Guyonvarch J. [Congenital convex clubfoot: a diagnostic and therapeutic study of 71 cases]. *Int Orthop*. 1984;8(3):211–221.
14. Sullivan JA. Pediatric flatfoot: evaluation and management. *J Am Acad Orthop Surg*. Jan 1999;7(1):44–53.
15. Schwering L. Surgical correction of the true vertical talus deformity. *Orthop Traumatol*. 2005;(2):211–231.
16. Resnick RB, Jahss MH, Choueka J, Kummer F, Hersch JC, Okereke E. Deltoid ligament forces after tibialis posterior tendon rupture: effects of triple arthrodesis and calcaneal displacement osteotomies. *Foot Ankle Int*. Jan 1995;16(1):14–20.
17. Rule J, Yao L, Seeger LL. Spring ligament of the ankle: normal MR anatomy. *Am J Roentgenol*. Dec 1993; 161(6):1241–1244.
18. Rose GK, Welton EA, Marshall T. The diagnosis of flat foot in the child. *J Bone Joint Surg Br*. Jan 1985;67(1): 71–78.
19. Torosian CM, Dias LS. Surgical treatment of severe hindfoot valgus by medial displacement osteotomy of the os calcis in children with myelomeningocele. *J Pediatr Orthop*. Mar–Apr 2000;20(2):226–229.
20. Frawley PA, Broughton NS, Menelaus MB. Incidence and type of hindfoot deformities in patients with low-level spina bifida. *J Pediatr Orthop*. May–Jun 1998;18(3):312–313.
21. Stieber JR, Dormans JP. Manifestations of hereditary multiple exostoses. *J Am Acad Orthop Surg*. Mar–Apr 2005;13(2):110–120.
22. Peterson HA. Multiple hereditary osteochondromata. *Clin Orthop Relat Res*. Feb 1989(239):222–230.
23. Bordin D, De Giorgi G, Mazzocco G, Rigon F. Flat and cavus foot, indexes of obesity and overweight in a population of primary-school children. *Minerva Pediatr*. Feb 2001;53(1):7–13.
24. Jarde O, Trinquier JL, Renaux P, Mauger S, Vives P. [Subtalar arthrodesis for sequelae of calcaneal fractures. Apropos of 57 cases]. *Rev Chir Orthop Reparatrice Appar Mot*. 1994;80(8):728–733.
25. Krivickas LS. Anatomical factors associated with overuse sports injuries. *Sports Med*. Aug 1997;24(2):132–146.
26. Guichet JM, Javed A, Russell J, Saleh M. Effect of the foot on the mechanical alignment of the lower limbs. *Clin Orthop Relat Res*. Oct 2003(415):193–201.
27. Gazdag AR, Cracchiolo A 3rd. Rupture of the posterior tibial tendon. Evaluation of injury of the spring ligament and clinical assessment of tendon transfer and ligament repair. *J Bone Joint Surg Am*. May 1997;79(5):675–681.
28. Brodsky JW, Baum BS, Pollo FE, Shabat S. Surgical reconstruction of posterior tibial tendon tear in adolescents: report of two cases and review of the literature. *Foot Ankle Int*. Mar 2005;26(3):218–223.
29. Drennan JC. Foot pain. In: Staheli LT, ed. *Pediatric Orthopedic Secrets*. 2nd ed. Philadelphia, PA: Hanley & Belfus; 2003.

30. Caselli MA, Sobel E, McHale KA. Pedal manifestations of musculoskeletal disease in children. *Clin Podiatr Med Surg.* 1998;15(3):481–497.

31. Kelo MJ, Riddle DL. Examination and management of a patient with tarsal coalition. *Phys Ther.* May 1998;78(5): 518–525.

32. Kim CW, Shea K, Chambers HG. Heel pain in children. Diagnosis and treatment. *J Am Podiatr Med Assoc.* 1999;89(2):67–74.

33. Wilkens KE. The painful foot in the child. *Instr Course Lect.* 1988;37:77–85.

34. Kulig K, Burnfield JM, Reischl S, Requejo SM, Blanco CE, Thordarson DB. Effect of foot orthoses on tibialis posterior activation in persons with pes planus. *Med Sci Sports Exerc.* Jan 2005;37(1):24–29.

35. Mendicino SS, Quinn M. Tibialis posterior dysfunction: an overview with a surgical case report using a flexor tendon transfer. *J Foot Surg.* Mar–Apr 1989;28(2):154–157.

36. Coady C, Gow N, Stanish W. Foot problems in middle-aged patients: keeping active people up to speed. *Phys Sportsmed.* 1998;26(5):31–36.

37. Masterson E, Jagannathan S, Borton D, Stephens MM. Pes planus in childhood due to tibialis posterior tendon injuries. Treatment by flexor hallucis longus tendon transfer. *J Bone Joint Surg Br.* May 1994;76(3): 444–446.

38. Abosala A, Tumia N, Anderson D. Tibialis posterior tendon rupture in children. *Injury.* Nov 2003;34(11): 866–867.

39. Brodsky JW. Preliminary gait analysis results after posterior tibial tendon reconstruction: a prospective study. *Foot Ankle Int.* Feb 2004;25(2):96–100.

40. Akcali O, Tiner M, Ozaksoy D. Effects of lower extremity rotation on prognosis of flexible flatfoot in children. *Foot Ankle Int.* Sep 2000;21(9):772–774.

FLAT FEET IN A CHILD

CHAPTER **63**

Weakness and Hypotonia in a Child

■ *Elizabeth L. Ege, PT, DPT*

Description of the Symptom

The terms *weakness* and *hypotonia* are often used interchangeably even though they have very different meanings. Weakness is the absence of strength, the inability to exert a force to resist movement, and the absence of power or the inability to exert a force to change position.[1,2] Hypotonia is a state of decreased muscle tone, which is defined clinically as the resistance felt to externally imposed movements in a state of voluntary relaxation.[3] At rest, the muscle is in a state of partial relaxation that requires energy for its full contraction or further muscle relaxation and concurrent contraction of its antagonistic muscle to elongate.[4] It is common for weakness and hypotonia to occur together; however, it is possible to have hypotonia in the absence of weakness and it is dependent on its cause. This chapter describes possible causes of weakness and hypotonia in a child.

Special Concerns

■ Any weakness/hypotonia of sudden onset (few days)
■ Any post-traumatic weakness/hypotonia
■ Any neurological signs suggesting an intracranial tumor or space-occupying tumor of the spinal cord

CHAPTER PREVIEW: Conditions That May Lead to Weakness and Hypotonia in a Child

T Trauma
COMMON
Not applicable
UNCOMMON
Brain and spinal cord injuries:
• Concussion 1197
• Contusion 1197
• Peripheral nerve trauma 1197
• Spinal cord trauma 1197
RARE
Not applicable

I Inflammation
COMMON
Not applicable

Inflammation *(continued)*

UNCOMMON

Aseptic
Acute cerebellar ataxia 1196
Acute demyelinating polyradiculopathy (Guillain-Barré syndrome) 1196
Chronic inflammatory demyelinating polyneuropathy 1197

Septic
Encephalitis 1198
Meningitis 1200
Myelitis 1200

RARE

Aseptic
Polymyositis 1201

Septic
Poliomyelitis 1200

M   Metabolic

COMMON

Not applicable

UNCOMMON

Hyperbilirubinemia 1199
Hypoglycemia 1199
Hypothyroidism 1199
Infantile botulism 1199
Mitochondrial myopathies 1200
Pompe's disease (acid maltase deficiency, glycogen storage disease type 2) 1201
Prader-Willi syndrome 1201

RARE

Not applicable

Va   Vascular

COMMON

Hypoxic/ischemic encephalopathy 1199

UNCOMMON

Hemorrhage 1198

RARE

Not applicable

De   Degenerative

COMMON

Not applicable

(continued)

Degenerative *(continued)*

UNCOMMON

Spinal muscular atrophies:
- Type I (Werdnig-Hoffmann disease) 1201
- Type II (Kugelberg-Welander disease) 1202
- Type III (benign) 1202

RARE

Not applicable

Tu Tumor

COMMON

Not applicable

UNCOMMON

Malignant Primary, such as:
- Posterior fossa tumors/medulloblastomas 1201

Malignant Metastatic:
Not applicable
Benign:
Not applicable

RARE

Not applicable

Co Congenital

COMMON

Not applicable

UNCOMMON

Benign congenital hypotonia 1196
Congenital muscular dystrophy 1198
Congenital myotonic dystrophy (Steinert disease) 1198
Down syndrome (Trisomy 21) 1198
Myasthenia gravis:
- Congenital 1200
- Transient neonatal 1200

RARE

Not applicable

Ne Neurogenic/Psychogenic

COMMON

Not applicable

UNCOMMON

Hereditary spinal motor neuropathies:
- Charcot-Marie-Tooth disease (hereditary sensory motor neuropathy types I and II) 1198
- Dejerine-Sottas disease (hereditary sensory motor neuropathy type III) 1199

Neurogenic/Psychogenic *(continued)*

RARE
Not applicable

Note: These are estimates of relative incidence because few data are available for the less common conditions.

Common Ages at Which Weakness and Hypotonia Present in a Child

APPROXIMATE AGE	CONDITION
Birth to 3 Years	Acute cerebellar ataxia
	Benign congenital hypotonia
	Brain and spinal cord traumas:
	• Concussion
	• Contusion
	• Spinal cord trauma
	Congenital muscular dystrophy
	Congenital myotonic dystrophy
	Down syndrome (Trisomy 21)
	Encephalitis
	Hemorrhage
	Hereditary spinal motor neuropathies
	Hyperbilirubinemia
	Hypoglycemia
	Hypothyroidism
	Hypoxic/ischemic encephalopathy
	Infantile botulism
	Inflammatory demyelinating polyneuropathies:
	• Acute (Guillain-Barré syndrome)
	• Chronic
	Meningitis
	Mitochondrial myopathies
	Myasthenia gravis
	• Congenital
	• Transient neonatal
	Myelitis
	Peripheral nerve trauma
	Poliomyelitis
	Polymyositis
	Pompe's disease (acid maltase deficiency, glycogen storage disease type 2)
	Prader-Willi syndrome
	Spinal muscular atrophy types I, II, and III
Preschool (3–5 Years)	Acute cerebellar ataxia
	Brain and spinal cord trauma
	• Concussion
	• Contusion
	• Spinal cord trauma
	Charcot-Marie-Tooth disease (hereditary spinal motor neuropathy types I and II)
	Encephalitis
	Hemorrhage
	Hypoglycemia
	Hypothyroidism

(continued)

Common Ages at Which Weakness and Hypotonia Present in a Child—cont'd

APPROXIMATE AGE	CONDITION
	Hypoxic/ischemic encephalopathy
	Inflammatory demyelinating polyneuropathies:
	• Acute (Guillain-Barré syndrome)
	• Chronic
	Meningitis
	Myelitis
	Peripheral nerve damage
	Poliomyelitis
	Polymyositis
	Posterior fossa tumors
	Spinal muscular atrophy types I, II, and III
Elementary School (6–11 Years)	Acute cerebellar ataxia
	Brain and spinal cord traumas:
	• Concussion
	• Contusion
	• Spinal cord trauma
	Charcot-Marie-Tooth disease (hereditary spinal motor neuropathy types I and II)
	Encephalitis
	Hemorrhage
	Hypoglycemia
	Hypothyroidism
	Hypoxic/ischemic encephalopathy
	Inflammatory demyelinating polyneuropathies:
	• Acute (Guillain-Barré syndrome)
	• Chronic
	Meningitis
	Myelitis
	Peripheral nerve damage
	Poliomyelitis
	Polymyositis
	Posterior fossa tumors
	Spinal muscular atrophy types I, II, and III
Middle School (12–14 Years)	Acute cerebellar ataxia
	Brain and spinal cord traumas:
	• Concussion
	• Contusion
	• Spinal cord trauma
	Charcot-Marie-Tooth disease (hereditary spinal motor neuropathy types I and II)
	Encephalitis
	Hemorrhage
	Hypoglycemia
	Hypothyroidism
	Hypoxic/ischemic encephalopathy
	Inflammatory demyelinating polyneuropathies:
	• Acute (Guillain-Barré syndrome)
	• Chronic
	Meningitis
	Myelitis
	Peripheral nerve damage
	Poliomyelitis
	Polymyositis
	Spinal muscular atrophy types I, II, and III

Common Ages at Which Weakness and Hypotonia Present in a Child—cont'd

APPROXIMATE AGE	CONDITION
High School (15–18 Years)	Acute cerebellar ataxia Brain and spinal cord traumas: • Concussion • Contusion • Spinal cord trauma Charcot-Marie-Tooth disease (hereditary spinal motor neuropathy types I and II) Encephalitis Hemorrhage Hypoglycemia Hypothyroidism Hypoxic/ischemic encephalopathy Inflammatory demyelinating polyneuropathies: • Acute (Guillain-Barré syndrome) • Chronic Meningitis Myelitis Peripheral nerve damage Poliomyelitis Polymyositis

Overview of Weakness and Hypotonia in a Child

"Floppy infant" syndrome or weakness/hypotonia is a relatively common occurrence in the neonatal period and into childhood. The weak/hypotonic or "floppy" infant presents with a paucity of movement while awake and a "frog leg" posture in the supine position (hips are abducted and externally rotated); in a horizontal suspension with the infant held in prone, the infant's body tends to drape over the examiner's hand.[5] Parents may also report difficulty with feeding, slow or diminished movements, and difficulty breathing.[6,7] This low muscle tone is indicative of an underlying impairment of the central or peripheral neuromuscular system. Differential diagnosis of the disease state producing hypotonia is determined by anatomically localizing the disease state within the neuromuscular system. The first goal is to determine if the source is of a central or peripheral origin. Diseases affecting the brain (specifically the cerebral cortex, basal ganglia, and cerebellum) and spinal cord are considered central and "upper motor neuron disorders" and those affecting the anterior horn cells of the spinal cord, peripheral nerves, and the neuromuscular junction are considered peripheral and "lower motor neuron disorders." The skeletal muscle itself can be a source as well and would be considered a peripheral origin.[4,5,8–10]

To localize the disease producing hypotonia to a central or peripheral origin, the following other characteristic signs in the presence of hypotonia are used to distinguish the location: strength, deep tendon reflexes, infantile reflexes, muscle fasciculations, muscle mass, and sensation. Disorders producing hypotonia that are more central in origin (involving the brain and spinal cord) are likely to present with normal to minimal weakness, normal to hyperactive deep tendon reflexes, persistent infantile reflexes, absent muscle fasciculations, normal muscle mass or some disuse atrophy and normal sensation. In contrast, disorders producing hypotonia that are peripheral in origin tend to present with weakness, decreased to absent deep tendon reflexes, absent infantile reflexes, and normal sensation. Anterior horn cell disorders also would present with prominent muscle fasciculation and muscle atrophy proximally.

Peripheral nerve disorders characteristically have more distal atrophy and may or may not have sensory loss. Neuromuscular junction disorders, unlike other peripheral disorders, would present with normal deep tendon reflexes and muscle mass. Muscle disorders tend to have proximal atrophy with distal pseudohypertrophy.[2,4,5,11,12]

Other diagnostic tests are used to diagnose an infant or child with hypotonia, including the following:

1. A complete history of the pregnancy and birth
2. A family history
3. Laboratory tests including creatine phosphokinase (CPK), lactate dehydrogenase (LDH), transaminases, and deoxyribonucleic acid (DNA) studies
4. Electrophysiological studies including electromyography (EMG) and nerve conduction studies
5. Muscle and nerve biopsy.[2,5,8,10,11,13–17]

Description of Conditions That May Lead to Weakness and Hypotonia in a Child

■ Acute Cerebellar Ataxia

Chief Clinical Characteristics
This presentation typically includes a child who appears healthy and alert with intact sensation and deep tendon reflexes, but may have hypotonia and balance impairments in the absence of measurable weakness. Recovery is commonly rapid and complete.[4]

Background Information
Inflammation is typically due to the varicella virus. There have also been cases of *Haemophilus influenzae* type b meningitis resulting in profound hypotonia and ataxia with a full recovery of normal tone and movement within a year.[18] Treatment initially is focused on medical stabilization. Rehabilitation is individualized and interdisciplinary.

■ Acute Demyelinating Polyradiculopathy (Guillain-Barré Syndrome)

Chief Clinical Characteristics
This presentation involves sensory signs or symptoms that usually present early and are mild. Paralysis usually develops slowly over days and weeks in a relatively symmetrical pattern beginning with the lower extremities and progressing proximally to the abdomen, chest, and upper extremities.

Background Information
Recovery is in the reverse direction and is usually slow, beginning 2 to 4 weeks after halt of progression, but for the majority of the cases recovery is complete. It is the most common acute disease affecting the peripheral nerves and leads to demyelination of both motor and sensory nerves. This disorder is rare in children younger than 2 years of age, but there have been documented cases at term and at 1 month of age.[4,19,20] Treatment initially focuses on medical stabilization. Rehabilitation is individualized and interdisciplinary.

■ Benign Congenital Hypotonia

Chief Clinical Characteristics
This presentation often involves hypotonia that is mild to moderate without significant impairment of cognitive function.

Background Information
This is a diagnosis of exclusion with laboratory studies presenting as normal. It is likely that children with this condition exhibit hypotonia of a central origin due to a variety of central nervous system insults not severe enough to produce permanent motor deficits. The following are the clinical diagnostic criteria:

● Generalized hypotonia with the presence of deep tendon reflexes
● Lack of evidence of neonatal asphyxia
● Lack of developmental delay
● No coexisting systemic diseases
● Normal levels of muscle enzymes
● Progressive improvement in muscle function observed during several months of follow-up.

Testing should be repeated in infants who do not show an improvement in muscle tone. Electromyography should be performed during the neonatal period and at 6 months of age to rule out the presence of motor unit disease. Muscle biopsy should be done at 1 to 2 years of age when the muscles are more mature to prevent misleading results.[4,5,8,10,15,17,21]

BRAIN AND SPINAL CORD INJURIES

■ Concussion

Chief Clinical Characteristics

In its moderate to severe form, this presentation may involve a loss of consciousness and post-traumatic amnesia and may cause transient impairment in function of the brainstem, such as dilation of the pupils, loss of the respiratory reflex, and possibly hypotonia depending on the location and extent of the injury.[22,23]

Background Information

This condition is graded from mild to severe. A mild concussion does not involve a loss of consciousness or post-traumatic amnesia.[24] Treatment initially is focused on medical stabilization. Rehabilitation is individualized and interdisciplinary.

■ Contusion

Chief Clinical Characteristics

This presentation includes a loss of consciousness and oftentimes a skull fracture, which could lead to transient or permanent impairment in function of the brain, resulting in hypotonia again depending on the location and extent of the injury.

Background Information

This condition is a severe concussion with demonstrable cell damage and recovery that is not as rapid or complete.[23,25] Treatment initially is focused on medical stabilization. Rehabilitation is individualized and interdisciplinary.

■ Peripheral Nerve Trauma

Chief Clinical Characteristics

This presentation may include temporary to permanent hypotonia and weakness related to damage to one or more peripheral nerves. The presentation depends on the location of the lesion and the extent of the injury.

Background Information

An example is brachial plexus palsy due to birth trauma with excessive lateral flexion of the cervical spine, away from a fixed shoulder, which leads to stretching and tearing of the neural structures. When the upper trunks of the brachial plexus are involved, the injury is referred to as Erb's palsy. Injury to the lower trunks is referred to as Klumpke's paralysis; however, it is less likely for the lower trunks to be involved.[26] Treatment initially is focused on medical stabilization. Rehabilitation is individualized and interdisciplinary.

■ Spinal Cord Trauma

Chief Clinical Characteristics

This presentation often involves frank trauma to the spinal region with sequelae of hypotonia and hyporeflexia initially, but days to weeks later hyperreflexia and spasticity develop.[17] *It is common for there to be weakness or paralysis of the hands and arms with relative preservation of lower extremity strength with cervical spinal cord trauma due to the neuroanatomy of the corticospinal tract at that level.*[27]

Background Information

Trauma to the cervical spinal cord is commonly a complication of delivery in either a breech or cervical presentation in children under 1 year old. This condition is uncommon in children due to increased translational mobility and enhanced flexion-extension movements within the facet joints. This condition in children ages 2 to 9 usually results from falls or motor vehicle accidents, and for those over 10 years of age, sports injuries begin to be prominent.[28] Treatment initially is focused on medical stabilization. Rehabilitation is individualized and interdisciplinary.

■ Chronic Inflammatory Demyelinating Polyneuropathy

Chief Clinical Characteristics

This presentation involves hypotonia, generalized weakness, and hypoactive reflexes.

Background Information

Cerebrospinal fluid protein is elevated with no family history of neuropathy. Nerve conduction studies reveal a marked slowing consistent with a demyelinating neuropathy. Sural nerve biopsies are also used for diagnosis.[14] Accurate diagnosis is important because children with this disorder are able to show improvement in weakness and hypotonia with steroid treatment. Treatment initially is focused on medical stabilization. Rehabilitation is individualized and interdisciplinary.

Congenital Muscular Dystrophy

Chief Clinical Characteristics

This presentation often varies but presents with hypotonia, weakness, contractures, arthrogryposis, hypoactive reflexes, and hip dislocation.

Background Information

Electromyography reveals small-amplitude polyphasic motor units with a myopathic recruitment pattern and serum muscle enzymes that are only mildly elevated. Muscle biopsy indicates a loss of myofibers, with fatty and connective tissue infiltration. Therapy is individualized and focuses on improving functional mobility.[8,14,15,29]

Congenital Myotonic Dystrophy (Steinert Disease)

Chief Clinical Characteristics

This presentation typically involves an infant with marked temporalis muscle wasting and tenting of the upper lip, severe hypotonia at birth with impaired sucking and swallowing, and severe respiratory distress.

Background Information

This condition is transmitted by an autosomal dominant pattern, most often from the mother. Muscle biopsy does not usually show any specific features and in most cases features consistent with myotonic dystrophy in the mother are used to confirm the diagnosis in the newborn. Overall, the severe weakness, which may require ventilatory support, is transient and gradually improves within days to weeks. However, severe weakness and hypotonia may continue and many infants with myotonic dystrophy also have mental retardation.[14,15,17,30,31]

Down Syndrome (Trisomy 21)

Chief Clinical Characteristics

This presentation includes hypotonia, moderate to severe mental retardation, and dysgenetic features characterized by posteriorly flattened skull, short, flat-bridge nose, epicanthal fold, short phalanges, and widened spaces between the first and second digits of the hands and feet.[17,23,28]

Background Information

This chromosomal disorder characterized by brain dysgenesis has a population frequency of 1 in 600 to 700 live births and is one of the most frequently encountered causes of neonatal hypotonia.[15] Children with Down syndrome tend to have weakness demonstrating significantly lower peak torque values of muscle forces when compared to typically developing children.[32] Therapy is focused on improving functional mobility.

Encephalitis

Chief Clinical Characteristics

This presentation varies and may develop into weakness with spasticity over time.

Background Information

Inflammation of the brain can lead to transient or permanent impairments in tone and strength depending on the location and extent of the damage from the inflammation.[4,12,23,33] Treatment initially is focused on medical stabilization. Rehabilitation is individualized and interdisciplinary.

Hemorrhage

Chief Clinical Characteristics

This presentation may involve a transient or at times permanent hypotonic weakness that may develop.

Background Information

A cerebral hemorrhage is a result of a rupture of one of the intracerebral vessels due to hypertension, vascular anomaly, or other causes.[1] An intracranial hemorrhage may also arise within a malignant primary brain tumor due to its high mitotic activity, the tendency to undergo spontaneous necrosis, and fragile tumor blood vessels.[34] Treatment initially is focused on medical stabilization. Rehabilitation is individualized and interdisciplinary.

HEREDITARY SENSORY MOTOR NEUROPATHIES

Charcot-Marie-Tooth Disease (Hereditary Sensory Motor Neuropathy Types I and II)

Chief Clinical Characteristics

This presentation typically occurs in the late first or early second decade with foot drop, pes cavus, and hammer toes.

Background Information

Types I and II are the demyelinating and axonal forms of the disease. It is dominantly inherited and diagnosis is confirmed by establishing similar electrophysiological abnormalities in one of the child's parents to demonstrate a dominant pattern of inheritance.[10,11,14] Therapy is focused on improving functional mobility.

■ Dejerine-Sottas Disease (Hereditary Sensory Motor Neuropathy Type III)

Chief Clinical Characteristics
This presentation occurs in the first year of life with weakness typically more severe than in other types of this condition with cases of transient respiratory failure. Two-thirds of the cases present with hypotonia and delayed motor development.

Background Information
This condition is autosomally recessive inherited and usually has no family history. Diagnosis is made by demonstrating a severe slowing of nerve conduction velocity and nerve biopsy, revealing prominent onion-bulb formations that indicate repetitive segmental demyelination and remyelination.[10,11,14,16]

■ Hyperbilirubinemia

Chief Clinical Characteristics
This presentation includes signs and symptoms of hypotonia, muscle weakness, and normal to hyperactive reflexes that can be signs that this disorder is progressing.

Background Information
This condition is the result of elevated blood bilirubin levels in infants. It results in jaundice, and if left uncontrolled can be neurotoxic and lead to kernicterus, a condition with severe neural symptoms affecting the basal ganglia and cerebellum.[4,17,23,35]

■ Hypoglycemia

Chief Clinical Characteristics
This presentation involves hypotonia, weakness, and normal to hyperactive reflexes, which can be signs of this metabolic disorder.

Background Information
Abnormally low blood glucose levels can affect the developing brain of infants and children if left unchecked, leading to the above-mentioned symptoms. It is treated medically by balancing glucose and insulin levels.[17,23]

■ Hypothyroidism

Chief Clinical Characteristics
This presentation typically includes few and vague clinical manifestations during the early weeks of life when irreversible brain damage can occur. These clinical manifestations include hypotonia, weakness, feeding difficulties, drowsiness, irritability, and hypothermia.

Background Information
This condition is treated medically with thyroid hormone replacement therapy.[4,17,36]

■ Hypoxic/Ischemic Encephalopathy

Chief Clinical Characteristics
This presentation is characterized by hypotonia, with seizures, craniofacial dysmorphisms, and hypoactive deep tendon reflexes.[10,15,16]

Background Information
Ischemic strokes in neonates are relatively rare, with an incidence of 1.35 per 100,000 live births, and they are predominantly found in the left hemisphere.[37] Causes can include vascular abnormalities, congenital heart malformations, and toxins from analgesics or magnesium given during labor or from recreational drug use, sedatives, or alcohol.[5,37] Diagnosis is on the basis of birth history, neuroimaging evidence, and clinical manifestations. Treatment initially is focused on medical stabilization. Rehabilitation is individualized and interdisciplinary.

■ Infantile Botulism

Chief Clinical Characteristics
This presentation typically involves weakness of the motor cranial nerves, generalized symmetrical muscular paralysis, and autonomic dysfunction.

Background Information
Botulism is common in infancy and is linked to the use of honey or to the ability of the botulism organism to thrive in the immature intestinal tract. The exotoxin is secreted by *Clostridium botulinum* and prevents normal secretion of acetylcholine from the nerve terminal of myoneural junctions. It is diagnosed by finding the botulinum toxin in serum or stool specimens. Antitoxins are available that can be beneficial for treatment.[2,4,5,17]

■ Meningitis

Chief Clinical Characteristics
This presentation may involve hypotonic weakness that may be a resulting symptom of either the bacterial or viral form of meningitis.

Background Information
Recovery from the inflammation can prove the low muscle tone to be transient or permanent or it may become hypertonic.[4,12,23,33] Treatment initially is focused on medical stabilization. Rehabilitation is individualized and interdisciplinary.

■ Mitochondrial Myopathies

Chief Clinical Characteristics
This presentation often includes generalized hypotonia, seizures, and developmental delay.

Background Information
A variety of clinical syndromes can arise in infancy due to abnormal mitochondrial function. The diagnosis is confirmed with observations of elevated serum levels of lactate pyruvate, reflecting abnormal mitochondrial function, electromyographic findings suggestive of myopathy, and sarcolemmal accumulations of mitochondria on muscle biopsy. In some cases, the cause is a delay in the maturation of the enzyme systems and a weak and hypotonic infant may recover with supportive care over a period of months or years as the enzymes become functional.[10,14,31]

MYASTHENIA GRAVIS

■ Congenital

Chief Clinical Characteristics
This presentation typically includes ptosis, ophthalmoplegia, and dysphagia. Hypotonic weakness is common among most patients described with the disorder as well as intermittent episodes of generalized muscular weakness.[9,10,17]

Background Information
In this condition, the mother does not necessarily have myasthenia gravis and the symptoms are intermittent, but persistent. Diagnosis is based on a family history of affected individuals, an abnormal electromyographic response, and a negative test for acetylcholine receptor antibody. There are four discrete disorders of congenital myasthenia gravis, and they are characterized at the ultrastructural level with distinct defects at the level of the presynaptic or postsynaptic region of the neuromuscular junction. Further diagnostic studies are done to determine which disorder and the treatment regimen.[9,15]

■ Transient Neonatal

Chief Clinical Characteristics
This presentation involves floppiness, difficulty feeding, and fatigable bulbar weakness with defective respiration at birth.

Background Information
Transient neonatal myasthenia gravis is a transient condition due to placental transfer of maternal acetylcholine receptor antibodies, which dissipate after several weeks. A diagnosis is made by these clinical signs, examination of the mother, a positive Tensilon test, and an electrophysiological study. Improvement usually occurs over the course of a few weeks as the antibodies clear the infant's system.[9,10,17]

■ Myelitis

Chief Clinical Characteristics
This presentation can involve hypotonic weakness that varies based on the location and extent of damage from the inflammation. It can be transient and develop into spasticity over time.

Background Information
Inflammation of the spinal cord is often part of a more specifically defined disease process such as poliomyelitis, meningomyelitis, or encephalomyelitis.[4,23] Treatment initially is focused on medical stabilization. Rehabilitation is individualized and interdisciplinary.

■ Poliomyelitis

Chief Clinical Characteristics
This presentation involves asymmetrical limb weakness with diminished reflexes and muscle spasms. In some cases there is an associated bulbar palsy and respiratory insufficiency.

Background Information
Although there are widespread immunizations for this disease, it still occurs in areas where children are not well vaccinated. Infected individuals are often left with long-term mobility impairments including

weakness and hypotonia of affected muscles.[4] Recently, there have been reports of an acute flaccid paralysis syndrome associated with acute West Nile virus infection. Reports have referred to the syndrome as West Nile virus poliomyelitis due to the similarity between its presentation and neuropathological and electrophysiological studies pathognomonic with poliomyelitis that suggest anterior horn destruction. Most patients develop acute, asymmetric limb paralysis with generally few sensory findings.[33]

■ **Polymyositis**

Chief Clinical Characteristics
This presentation commonly includes proximal or generalized muscle weakness, hyporeflexia, and hypotonia.

Background Information
In this condition, nerve conduction studies are normal, electromyography suggests myopathic origin, and there is marked elevation of serum creatine phosphokinase. A muscle biopsy can be nonspecifically abnormal or it could be typical of polymyositis with myofiber degeneration and regeneration, perifascicular atrophy, and inflammatory infiltrates. This condition can also be difficult to distinguish from congenital muscular dystrophy, especially if the muscle biopsy is inconclusive. This condition rarely occurs in infants and is potentially treatable.[11,14] Treatment initially is focused on medical stabilization. Rehabilitation is individualized and interdisciplinary.

■ **Pompe's Disease (Acid Maltase Deficiency, Glycogen Storage Disease Type 2)**

Chief Clinical Characteristics
This presentation is characterized by weakness, hypotonia, tongue fasciculations, cardiomyopathy, and hepatosplenomegaly.

Background Information
This autosomal recessive condition causes an acid maltase deficiency leading to glycogen deposits in the liver, brain tissue, and anterior horn cells. Diagnosis is made by a muscle biopsy displaying glycogen vacuoles within myofibers. There is no effective treatment and death is usually due to cardiac or respiratory failure.[10,17,29,38]

■ **Posterior Fossa Tumors/ Medulloblastomas**

Chief Clinical Characteristics
This presentation mainly involves hypotonic weakness that often occurs with ataxia and imbalance of gait, stance, or sitting.

Background Information
These tumors tend to affect the cerebellum and the brainstem adjacent to the roof of the fourth ventricle. They are malignant and tend to occur in children. They are treated with radiation therapy and surgical resection.[4,23,34]

■ **Prader-Willi Syndrome**

Chief Clinical Characteristics
This presentation can be characterized by hypotonia, insatiable appetite with progressive obesity, mental retardation, and dysgenetic features characterized by rounded face, almond-shaped eyes, strabismus, low forehead, and hypogonadism.

Background Information
This genetic disorder occurs in 1 in 10,000 to 16,000 live births and tends to cause both mental and physical abnormalities. Impaired growth hormone secretion is also found and the use of growth hormone replacement therapy coupled with a strictly controlled diet has been found to reduce obesity and increase muscle mass.[16,17,30,39]

SPINAL MUSCULAR ATROPHIES

■ **Type I (Werdnig-Hoffmann Disease)**

Chief Clinical Characteristics
This presentation commonly involves decreased fetal movements and often a breech presentation at birth. The infant or child with the disorder has feeding difficulties with a poor suck and swallow and is slow, if at all, to develop head and neck control. Hypotonia and weakness in the legs lead to abduction and external rotation of the hips. Sensation is intact and the child will grimace and cry on exposure to noxious stimuli. There is often also the presence of tongue fasciculations and absent deep tendon reflexes. Bright, lively facial expressions are common, which is in contrast to infants and children with hypotonia of a more central origin.

Background Information

This autosomal recessive disorder causes a progressive degeneration of the anterior horn cells of the motor neuron. Therapy is supportive and prognosis is poor. Death often occurs within the first 2 to 3 years due to pneumonia or respiratory failure.[5,11,15,17,29,31]

■ Type II (Kugelberg-Welander Disease)

Chief Clinical Characteristics

This presentation is characterized by atrophy and weakness of the proximal muscles of the lower extremities and pelvic girdle and then progresses to the distal muscles and muscular fasciculations.[23]

Background Information

This condition is a hereditary juvenile form of spinal muscular atrophy transmitted as an autosomal recessive trait that causes lesions of the anterior horns of the spinal cord. Onset occurs in the first or second decade between the ages of 2 and 17 years; however, it is possible to present in infancy.[15]

■ Type III (Benign)

Chief Clinical Characteristics

This presentation is characterized by atrophy and weakness of the proximal muscles of the lower extremities and pelvic girdle and then progresses to the distal muscles and muscular fasciculations.[23] *This variation of spinal muscular atrophy presents with a similar, but milder phenotype as type II and also can present in early infancy.*

Background Information

Deoxyribonucleic acid testing is required to distinguish between the various types of spinal muscular atrophy.[15]

References

1. Heaerer A. *DeJong's the Neurologic Examination.* 5th ed. Philadelphia, PA: Lippincott Williams and Wilkins; 1992.
2. Hobdell E. Hypotonia in infants and children. *J Neurosurg Nurs.* Aug 1982;14(4):170–172.
3. Lance JW. The control of muscle tone, reflexes, and movement: Robert Wartenberg lecture. *Neurology.* Dec 1980;30(12):1303–1313.
4. Vannucci RC. Differential diagnosis of diseases producing hypotonia. *Pediatr Ann.* Jul 1989;18(7):404–410.
5. Miller VS, Delgado M, Iannaccone ST. Neonatal hypotonia. *Semin Neurol.* Mar 1993;13(1):73–83.
6. Boheme R. *The Hypotonic Child.* San Antonio, TX: Therapy Skill Builders; 1990.
7. McDonald MS. Parenting a floppy infant. *R I Med J.* Oct 1989;72(10):371–373.
8. Brooke MH, Carroll JE, Ringel SP. Congenital hypotonia revisited. *Muscle Nerve.* Mar–Apr 1979;2(2):84–100.
9. Gay CT, Bodensteiner JB. The floppy infant: recent advances in the understanding of disorders affecting the neuromuscular junction. *Neurol Clin.* Aug 1990;8(3):715–725.
10. Parano E, Lovelace RE. Neonatal peripheral hypotonia: clinical and electromyographic characteristics. *Childs Nerv Syst.* Jun 1993;9(3):166–171.
11. Jones HR Jr. EMG evaluation of the floppy infant: differential diagnosis and technical aspects. *Muscle Nerve.* Apr 1990;13(4):338–347.
12. Zalneraitis EL. The pathophysiology of the floppy infant. *R I Med J.* Oct 1989;72(10):351–354.
13. Aydinli N, Baslo B, Caliskan M, Ertas M, Ozmen M. Muscle ultrasonography and electromyography correlation for evaluation of floppy infants. *Brain Dev.* Jan 2003;25(1):22–24.
14. Maguire HC, Sladky JT. Diagnosis and management of diseases affecting the motor unit in infancy. *R I Med J.* Oct 1989;72(10):361–366.
15. Prasad AN, Prasad C. The floppy infant: contribution of genetic and metabolic disorders. *Brain Dev.* Oct 2003; 25(7):457–476.
16. Richer LP, Shevell MI, Miller SP. Diagnostic profile of neonatal hypotonia: an 11-year study. *Pediatr Neurol.* Jul 2001;25(1):32–37.
17. Stiefel L. Hypotonia in infants. *Pediatr Rev.* Mar 1996;17(3):104–105.
18. King SM, Read SE. Ataxia and hypotonia in *Haemophilus influenzae* type b meningitis. *Pediatr Infect Dis J.* Feb 1988;7(2):140–142.
19. al-Qudah AA, Shahar E, Logan WJ, Murphy EG. Neonatal Guillain-Barre syndrome. *Pediatr Neurol.* Jul–Aug 1988;4(4):255–256.
20. Carroll JE, Jedziniak M, Guggenheim MA. Guillain-Barre syndrome. Another cause of the "floppy infant." *Am J Dis Child.* Jun 1977;131(6):699–700.
21. Carboni P, Pisani F, Crescenzi A, Villani C. Congenital hypotonia with favorable outcome. *Pediatr Neurol.* May 2002;26(5):383–386.
22. Akau CK, Press JM, Gooch JL. Sports medicine. 4. Spine and head injuries. *Arch Phys Med Rehabil.* May 1993;74(5-S):S443–446.
23. Newman Dorland WA. *Dorland's Illustrated Medical Dictionary.* 28th ed. Philadelphia, PA: W. B. Saunders; 1994.
24. Denny-Brown D, Russell WR. Experimental cerebral concussion. *J Physiol.* Dec 20, 1940;99(1):153.
25. Parkinson D. Immediate neurocognitive effects of concussion: graded contusion model of the mouse spinal cord using a pneumatic impact device. *Neurosurgery.* Jun 2003;52(6):1505.
26. de Chalain TM, Clarke HM, Curtis CG. Case report: unilateral combined facial nerve and brachial plexus palsies in a neonate following a midlevel forceps delivery. *Ann Plast Surg.* Feb 1997;38(2):187–190.
27. Levi AD, Tator CH, Bunge RP. Clinical syndromes associated with disproportionate weakness of the upper versus the lower extremities after cervical spinal cord injury. *Neurosurgery.* Jan 1996;38(1):179–183; discussion 183–185.

28. Faillace WJ. Management of childhood neurotrauma. *Surg Clin North Am.* Apr 2002;82(2):349–363, vii.

29. Premasiri MK, Lee YS. The myopathology of floppy and hypotonic infants in Singapore. *Pathology.* Oct 2003;35 (5):409–413.

30. DiMario FJ Jr. Genetic diseases in the etiology of the floppy infant. *R I Med J.* Oct 1989;72(10):357–359.

31. Johnston HM. The floppy weak infant revisited. *Brain Dev.* Apr 2003;25(3):155–158.

32. Mercer VS, Lewis CL. Hip abductor and knee extensor muscle strength of children with and without Down syndrome. *Pediatr Phys Ther.* Spring 2001;13(1):18–26.

33. Sejvar JJ. West Nile virus and "poliomyelitis." *Neurology.* Jul 27 2004;63(2):206–207.

34. Allen JC, Miller DC, Budzilovich GN, Epstein FJ. Brain and spinal cord hemorrhage in long-term survivors of malignant pediatric brain tumors: a possible late effect of therapy. *Neurology.* Jan 1991;41(1):148–150.

35. Scheidt PC, Bryla DA, Nelson KB, Hirtz DG, Hoffman HJ. Phototherapy for neonatal hyperbilirubinemia: six-year follow-up of the National Institute of Child Health and Human Development clinical trial. *Pediatrics.* Apr 1990;85(4):455–463.

36. Virtanen M. Manifestations of congenital hypothyroidism during the 1st week of life. *Eur J Pediatr.* Apr 1988;147(3):270–274.

37. Gunther G, Junker R, Strater R, et al. Symptomatic ischemic stroke in full-term neonates: role of acquired and genetic prothrombotic risk factors. *Stroke.* Oct 2000; 31(10):2437–2441.

38. Verity MA. Infantile Pompe's disease, lipid storage, and partial carnitine deficiency. *Muscle Nerve.* May 1991; 14(5):435–440.

39. Burman P, Ritzen EM, Lindgren AC. Endocrine dysfunction in Prader-Willi syndrome: a review with special reference to GH. *Endocr Rev.* Dec 2001;22(6):787–799.

Index

Note: Page numbers followed by f refer to figures; page numbers followed by t refer to tables.